Te Linde's **Operative Gynecology**

Te Linde's

Operative Gynecology

Sixth Edition

Richard F. Mattingly, M.D.

Professor and Chairman
Department of Gynecology and Obstetrics
The Medical College of Wisconsin
Milwaukee, Wisconsin

John D. Thompson, M.D.

Professor and Chairman
Department of Gynecology and Obstetrics
Emory University School of Medicine
Atlanta, Georgia

 J. B. Lippincott Company *Philadelphia   London   Mexico City   New York   St. Louis   São Paulo   Sydney*

Acquisitions Editor: Lisa A. Biello
Sponsoring Editor: Richard Winters
Manuscript Editor: Patrick O'Kane
Indexer: Barbara S. Littlewood
Art Director: Charles W. Field
Designer: Arlene Putterman
Production Supervisor: J. Corey Gray
Production Coordinator: Charlene Catlett Squibb
Compositor: Tapsco, Inc.
Printer/Binder: Halliday Lithograph

Library of Congress Cataloging in Publication Data

Te Linde, Richard W. (Richard Wesley), 1894-
   Te Linde's Operative gynecology.

   Includes bibliographies and index.
   1. Gynecology, Operative. I. Mattingly, Richard F.
II. Thompson, John D.
III. Title. IV. Title: Operative gynecology.
RG104.T4   1985   618.1'45   84-27859

ISBN 0-397-50526-4

The authors and publisher have exerted every effort to
ensure that drug selection and dosage set forth in this text
are in accord with current recommendations and practice at
the time of publication. However, in view of ongoing
research, changes in government regulations, and the
constant flow of information relating to drug therapy and
drug reactions, the reader is urged to check the package
insert for each drug for any change in indications and
dosage and for added warnings and precautions. This is
particularly important when the recommended agent is a
new or infrequently employed drug.

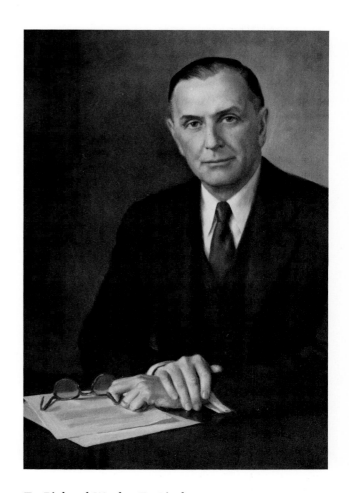

To Richard Wesley Te Linde, M.D.
friend and mentor,
whose intuitive clinical judgment
and masterful surgical skill
have been the inspiration
for the continuation of the philosophy
of pelvic surgery
upon which this book is based

Contributors

LARRY C. CAREY, M.D.
Professor and Chairman
Department of Surgery
Ohio State University Hospital
Columbus, Ohio

PETER J. FABRI, M.D.
Associate Professor of Surgery
Ohio State University Hospital
Columbus, Ohio

MALCOLM G. FREEMAN, M.D.
Professor
Department of Gynecology and Obstetrics
Emory University School of Medicine
Atlanta, Georgia

DAVID A. GRIMES, M.D.
Clinical Research Investigator
Operational Research Branch
Division of Sexually Transmitted Disease
Center for Prevention Service
Centers for Disease Control
Atlanta, Georgia

LEE A. HEBERT, M.D.
Professor of Medicine
Director, Division of Renal Diseases
Ohio State University Hospital
Columbus, Ohio

PAUL KATAYAMA, M.D.
Associate Clinical Professor
Department of Gynecology and Obstetrics
The Medical College of Wisconsin
Milwaukee, Wisconsin

MICHAEL H. KEELAN, JR., M.D.
Professor
Department of Medicine, Cardiology Section
Medical College of Wisconsin
Milwaukee, Wisconsin

JACOB LEMANN, JR., M.D.
Professor
Department of Medicine
Chief, Nephrology Section
The Medical College of Wisconsin
Milwaukee, Wisconsin

RICHARD F. MATTINGLY, M.D.
Professor and Chairman
Department of Gynecology and Obstetrics
The Medical College of Wisconsin
Milwaukee, Wisconsin

GEORGE W. MITCHELL, M.D.
Professor, Department of Obstetrics and Gynecology
The University of Texas
Health Science Center at San Antonio
San Antonio, Texas

DAVID H. NICHOLS, M.D.
Chairman, Section of Obstetrics and Gynecology
Brown University
Obstetrician and Gynecologist in Chief
Women and Infants Hospital of Rhode Island
Providence, Rhode Island

EDWARD J. QUEBBEMAN, M.D., PH.D.
Assistant Professor, Department of Surgery
The Medical College of Wisconsin
Milwaukee, Wisconsin

ELVOY RAINES, J.D.
Associate Executive Director
American Society of Law and Medicine
Boston, Massachusetts

JOHN H. RIDLEY, M.D.
Clinical Professor
Department of Gynecology and Obstetrics
Emory University School of Medicine
Atlanta, Georgia

JOHN A. ROCK, M.D.
Associate Professor
Director, Reproductive Endocrinology
Department of Gynecology and Obstetrics
The Johns Hopkins Hospital
Baltimore, Maryland

FELIX N. RUTLEDGE, M.D.
Head, Department of Gynecology
M.D. Anderson Hospital and Tumor Institute
Houston, Texas

DONALD P. SCHLUETER, M.D.
Professor, Department of Medicine
Chief, Pulmonary Section
The Medical College of Wisconsin
Milwaukee, Wisconsin

ADOLF STAFL, M.D.
Associate Professor
Department of Gynecology and Obstetrics
The Medical College of Wisconsin
Milwaukee, Wisconsin

JOHN D. THOMPSON, M.D.
Professor and Chairman
Department of Gynecology and Obstetrics
Emory University School of Medicine
Atlanta, Georgia

CLIFFORD R. WHEELESS, M.D.
Chief, Obstetrics and Gynecology
The Union Memorial Hospital
Baltimore, Maryland

TIFFANY J. WILLIAMS, M.D.
Professor, Department of Obstetrics and Gynecology
Mayo Medical School
Rochester, Minnesota

J. DONALD WOODRUFF, M.D.
Richard W. Te Linde Professor Emeritus
Gynecologic Pathology
Johns Hopkins University School of Medicine
Baltimore, Maryland

Foreword

The fact that *Operative Gynecology* is in its Sixth Edition is evidence that the need for such a work still exists. As indicated in the preface to the First Edition, operative gynecology is only one part of the general subject of gynecology. If this was true when the First Edition was written, it is doubly true today. Like all branches of medicine, gynecology has broadened. Today it is a multifaceted specialty. In the well-rounded department of gynecology, all aspects of the subject should be represented by some staff member who has special interest and expertise in that subspecialty. For this reason the Sixth Edition has contributions from several authors. Many of these gynecologists have had their operative training at the Johns Hopkins Hospital under myself and, therefore, have the same philosophy regarding pelvic surgery and gynecologic pathology. Hence, the general flavor of the book has not changed.

Since the original author is advancing in years, it is certain that I will not write another Foreword. I wish to thank the present authors, Richard F. Mattingly and John D. Thompson, for carrying on this work so ably. I also wish to thank the gynecologists of this country and abroad for their acceptance of this work. It is my hope that I have made a contribution to operative gynecology and that this text will continue to serve the intellectual and technical needs of all gynecologists who are interested in pelvic surgery.

Richard W. Te Linde, M.D.

ix

Preface

The field of gynecologic surgery is a dynamic specialty. Important changes are occurring continually in our understanding and treatment of pelvic diseases. New advances in biomedical information, diagnostic technology, microbiology, pharmacology, and surgical instrumentation require that a surgical textbook undergo periodic revision and update. Such changes are the basis for the publication of this, the Sixth Edition of *Te Linde's Operative Gynecology*.

During the past decade, the process of subspecialization in gynecology and obstetrics has been accelerated and formalized with the recognition of subspecialties in reproductive endocrinology, maternal–fetal medicine, and gynecologic oncology. The field of pelvic surgery has undergone informal subdivision into surgery for benign gynecologic conditions and surgery for gynecologic malignancies. Despite this proliferation of subspecialties, the goals of this textbook are quite basic: to provide the gynecologist with the essential information about a disease process that will enable him or her to arrive at a proper diagnosis and to select the correct method of treatment.

Having stated our mission, let us examine a related critical issue—the training of the gynecologic surgeon. Many leaders in the discipline believe that improvements in the training of the pelvic surgeon are needed if the skill of the future gynecologist is to equal or surpass that of his predecessor. The pelvic surgeon must be well versed in the general principles of surgery; be experienced in the anatomical dissection of advanced pelvic disease; be capable in the management of complications such as vesicovaginal fistulas and defects involving other adjacent organ systems; have a broad base of operative ex-

perience under the supervision of experienced teachers; and have an understanding of pathology and the basic science aspects of reproductive medicine, and of the clinical manifestations and psychological aspects of pelvic disease. Resident training programs are now required to document the trainee's acquisition of surgical skills more accurately, but in order to accomplish all of these aims, it may be necessary to extend the period of training.

The reader will find many new contributions to the Sixth Edition that update this work and broaden the knowledge of the pelvic surgeon. To help the surgeon be more aware of the broader implications of pelvic surgery for the patient, Malcolm Freeman contributed a chapter on the psychological aspects of pelvic surgery. This important aspect of pelvic surgery is frequently overlooked by the busy surgeon who fails to understand the psychosexual impact of gynecologic surgery on the patient. For example, concerns about loss of libido and impairment of sexual response are very worrisome to a woman who is about to have a hysterectomy and oophorectomy. These and other problems related to the various phases of pelvic surgery are dealt with in great detail in this valuable contribution to the textbook.

The professional liability of the gynecologic surgeon has become a major threat and impediment to the successful performance of pelvic surgery. In a new chapter dealing with these issues, Elvoy Raines, a lawyer knowledgeable in the field of operative gynecology, identifies the various medical-legal conflicts with which the gynecologic surgeon may be faced. More important, this chapter emphasizes procedures that the surgeon can follow to minimize the threat of litigation. The issue of informed consent is dealt with extensively, and the importance of close communication between surgeon and patient is emphasized.

Breast cancer is one of the most frequent and lethal diseases to afflict women. In a new chapter directed to the gynecologist-obstetrician, George W. Mitchell, another author whom we welcome for the first time to this textbook, provides a clear understanding of both benign and malignant diseases of the breast. In this chapter, a new departure in this edition, the current methods of diagnosis and treatment of breast diseases are clearly presented and illustrated and the importance of the gynecologist in the early detection of breast cancer is emphasized.

Chapter 15, Surgery for Anomalies of the Müllerian Ducts, is particularly noteworthy for its careful treatment and illustration of the development of the female reproductive tract from the earliest embryologic features to normal adult female anatomy. A proper understanding of embryology prepares the gynecologist for the management of a variety of anomalies of the female genital tract.

It should be emphasized that the ability to perform gynecologic operations with a low mortality and morbidity rate is not *ipso facto* evidence that gynecologic surgery is being practiced correctly. In addition to a low mortality and morbidity rate, one must be concerned that only patients with proper indications are chosen for surgical treatment. The knowledge that is needed to formulate the proper "indications for surgery" includes, first and foremost, a thorough understanding of the physiology and pathology of the female reproductive organs, as well as of the clinical manifestations of disease process and the normal and abnormal development of psycho-social-sexual behavior. This basic knowledge is the absolute foundation of gynecologic surgery. On the basis of this knowledge, one must decide whether a patient should be offered surgical therapy, remembering that it is only the occasional gynecologic patient who requires surgery for relief of symptoms.

After the right patient has been selected for operation, the right operation must be selected for the patient. For example, it is a mistake to do an abdominal hysterectomy when a vaginal hysterectomy will give better results. The practice of gynecologic surgery includes proper preparation of the patient for operation, proper technical performance of the operation, and proper postoperative care and follow-up. In the practice of gynecologic surgery, mistakes may be made by not performing the operation according to correct technique. Perhaps even more mistakes may be made by not using proper indications for surgery.

It is our hope that the information in this Sixth Edition of *Te Linde's Operative Gynecology* will be beneficial to young men and women who are learning gynecologic surgery as well as to experienced gynecologic surgeons who are interested in bringing their knowledge up to date. Gynecologic surgeons who perform the most common operative procedures will find useful and new information in the text. The pelvic surgeon whose practice is composed of the most complicated, unusual, and difficult problems will also find much useful discussion of specialized operative techniques.

We wish to thank Larry Carey, Peter Fabri, Malcolm Freeman, David Grimes, Lee Hebert, Paul Katayama, Michael Keelan, Jacob Lehmann, George Mitchell, David Nichols, Edward Quebbeman, Elvoy Raines, John Ridley, John Rock, Felix Rutledge, Donald Schlueter, Adolf Stafl, Clifford Wheeless, Tiffany Williams, and Donald Woodruff for their contributions to this edition. We also wish to express our appreciation to Lawrence Wharton, Jr., Howard Jones, and others whose contributions to previous editions provided the continuity that was so important to the evolution of this edition.

John D. Thompson is welcome as a coauthor of the Sixth Edition. Dr. Thompson, like Richard F. Mattingly, is a member of the Hopkins school of pelvic surgery and a former pupil of Richard W. Te Linde's.

It is our wish that the original author, Richard W. Te Linde, should remain a vital part of this ongoing work. It is difficult to believe that in the first three editions of *Operative Gynecology*, the text was written and the illustrations were conceived and supervised in their entirety by this talented author and dedicated surgeon. Richard Te Linde's influence on his pupils, including ourselves, is indelible. There are many schools of pelvic surgery for which the Hopkins philosophy has served as the prototype, and the basic operative procedures described by Te Linde continue to offer the most successful approach for the surgical managment of most gynecologic disorders. Te Linde was an early campaigner for acceptance of carcinoma in situ of the cervix as a distinct clinical disease. One of his many classic contributions to gynecology was his proof of Sampson's theory that retrograde menstruation is a major etiologic factor in the development of endometriosis. Richard W. Te Linde has devoted his entire professional career to the search for new knowledge and to the training of the pelvic surgeon. This text serves as his legacy to the many gynecologists who have known his work but have not had an opportunity to observe the master in his workshop, the operating room. It is a fitting tribute to the work of a lifetime that *Te Linde's Operative Gynecology* has reached the bookshelf of almost every gynecologist in this country and abroad.

Richard F. Mattingly, M.D.
John D. Thompson, M.D.

From the Preface to the First Edition

Gynecology has become a many-sided specialty. No longer is it simply a branch of general surgery. In order to practice this specialty in its broad sense, the gynecologist must be trained in a comprehensive field. He must be a surgeon, expert in his special field; he must be trained in the fundamentals of obstetrics; he must have the technical skill to investigate female urologic conditions; he must have an understanding of endocrinology as it applies to gynecology; he should be well grounded in gynecologic pathology; finally, he must be able to recognize and deal successfully with minor psychiatric problems which arise so commonly among gynecologic patients. With this concept of the specialty in mind this book has been written. It then becomes apparent, when one seeks training in gynecology beyond the simplest fundamentals such as are taught to undergraduates, that special works are necessary for training those who intend to practice it.

The author is a firm believer in the system of long hospital residencies for training young men in the various surgical specialties when their minds are quick to grasp ideas and their fingers are nimble. This volume has been written particularly for this group of men. Unfortunately, there is a paucity of good gynecologic residencies in the United States in the sense that the author has in mind. Many positions bear the name of residency but fail to give the resident sufficient operative work to justify the name. Another excellent method of development of the young gynecologist is an active assistantship to a well-trained, mature gynecologist. If the assistant is permitted to stand at the operating table opposite his chief, day after day, eventually he will acquire skill and judgment which he himself will be able to utilize as an operator. When such a preceptor system is practiced, it is important that the assistant be given some surgery of his own to do while he is still young. If a man is forced to think of himself only as a perennial assistant, this frame of mind will kill his ability to accept responsibility of his own. However, many must learn their operative gynecology under less favorable circumstances than those of the fortunate resident or assistant. This volume should be of value to those who, by self-instruction, must acquire a certain degree of operative skill. Finally, it must be admitted that more gynecology is practiced today by general surgeons in this country than by gynecologists. Although this is not ideal, circumstances make it necessary, and much of this gynecologic surgery is well done. It is hoped that many general surgeons will use this volume as a reference book.

In connection with general surgery, it is only fair to say that much has come to gynecology by way of general surgeons of the old school, who practiced general surgery in the broadest sense. Now that gynecology and/or obstetrics has become a specialty unto itself, it is well in our training of men not to swing too far from general abdominal surgery. In spite of the most careful preoperative investigation, mistakes in diagnosis will be made, and at times the gynecologist will be called upon to take care of general surgical conditions in the region of lower abdomen and the rectum. With this in mind, the author has included in this volume a consideration of a few of the commoner general surgical conditions occasionally encountered incidentally with gynecology or by mistaken diagnosis.

Operative Gynecology is written with the primary purpose of describing the technic of the usual and some of the rarer operative procedures. It also includes indications for and against operations as well as pre- and postoperative care of patients. Although gynecology is divided into several fields, these fields interlock so that it has been found impossible to compose a volume on gynecologic surgery to the exclusion of the other divisions of the specialty. Gynecologic pathology, for instance, is the bedrock upon which good gynecologic surgery is practiced. Without an understanding of it, surgery becomes merely a mechanical job, and errors in surgical judgment are inevitable. Hence, it has become necessary to include in this volume a minimum of gross and microscopic pathology, as it applies directly to the surgical subject under consideration. Also, some consideration is given to psychology and psychiatry in relation to gynecologic surgery. The author believes that getting the young woman on whom a hysterectomy must be done into the proper frame of mind to accept it is as important as possessing the technical skill to perform the operation.

Richard W. Te Linde
Baltimore, Maryland, 1946

Contents

Part One

Aspects of Gynecologic Surgery

Chapter 1

Historical Development of Pelvic Surgery

All specialties in medicine have evolved gradually. Subspecialties continue to emerge as new knowledge is developed within each field. In retrospect, isolated surgical events, especially in the 19th and 20th centuries, served as the foundation of gynecologic surgery as a distinct entity. These historic masterworks highlight the progress in the discipline and, if studied carefully, can have practical value in improving the practice of modern pelvic surgery. A surgeon unlearned in the history of his or her field may repeat the mistakes of the past.

In the early days of medicine in the United States, it was customary for one person to hold a combined chair of anatomy and surgery: obstetrics and gynecology were included with surgery. Philip Syng Physick, often considered the father of American surgery, held the first chair of surgery divorced from anatomy in the United States at the University of Pennsylvania in 1805. John Collins Warren, later to become the founder of the Massachusetts General Hospital, was the first Professor of Anatomy and Surgery at that institution. Gynecology was first recognized in this country as a distinct medical discipline in 1813, when Theodore Woodward was appointed Lecturer in Gynecology at the Medical School of Castleton, Vermont. By the late 19th century, many medical schools had appointed professors of gynecology and obstetrics separate from surgery, although diseases of women and children continued to be taught together as a single course in many schools. Obstetrics was divorced from the chair of surgery during the first part of the 19th century. Gynecology began to be identified as a specialty during this period and its separation from general surgery was more gradual. By the beginning of the 20th century, pediatrics was separated from

gynecology and obstetrics, largely through the efforts of Abraham Jacobi, a pioneer pediatrician of New York. Today, gynecology has been divorced almost completely from general surgery in practice, and in all medical schools in the United States it is combined with obstetrics. The final combination of gynecology and obstetrics as a distinct and major medical specialty in the United States was largely the result of the establishment of the American Board of Obstetrics and Gynecology in 1930, and also the result of the development of residency training programs that combined gynecologic and obstetric education and training. However, attempts continue today to give pelvic surgery the status of a distinct surgical discipline separate from obstetrics.

Important advances in pelvic surgery have been made by many gynecologic surgeons in other countries, in particular Britain and Europe. Therefore, the history of pelvic surgery in the United States must be viewed as a conjoining of surgical concepts and experience from abroad with the rapidly growing technology and science in North America during the 19th and 20th centuries.

Oophorectomy

Pelvic surgery may be said to have begun in the backwoods of Kentucky when Ephraim McDowell (Fig. 1–1) successfully removed a large ovarian tumor from Jane Todd Crawford. He had studied under John Bell of London, who suggested the operation to McDowell. The operation, performed on Christmas morning in 1809, was done without the benefit of anesthesia or asepsis. McDowell considered the operation an experiment, as it truly was, and

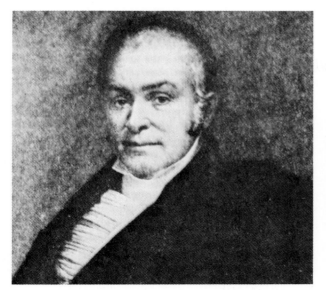

FIG. 1-1 Ephraim McDowell (1771-1830), "father of abdominal surgery."

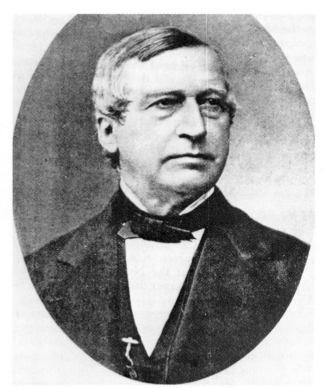

FIG. 1-2 Washington Lee Atlee (1808-1878).

frankly told the patient so. She agreed to accept the risk and demonstrated her faith in her doctor and the Lord by singing hymns during the operation. While McDowell was performing the operation, his house was surrounded by a crowd of the patient's friends, who intended to shoot or hang him if the patient died. Fortunately, she made a rapid recovery and lived for 32 years, to die at the mature age of 78. McDowell's publication of his first three successful cases of ovariotomy (oophorectomy) marks the beginning of abdominal surgery. The operation fell into disrepute shortly thereafter because of misuse. The brothers Atlee of Lancaster, Pennsylvania, were among those who performed the procedure during the middle of the 19th century for a wide range of nonsurgical indications. At the tenth annual meeting of the American Gynecological Society in 1885, Washington Atlee reported that he had performed 255 operations for removal of the ovary.

Myomectomy

Amussat of France performed the first recorded myomectomy in 1840. In the United States, the operation was done shortly thereafter, in 1844, by Washington Atlee (Fig. 1-2). In 1850, Professor Mussey wrote: "Of all the achievements of modern surgery we meet with, none (is) more striking or extraordinary than the operation performed by Professor Atlee for the removal of fibrous tumors." A generation later, J. Marion Sims wrote: "The name of

Atlee stands without a rival in connection with uterine fibroids. His operations were so heroic that no man has as yet dared to imitate him." In more modern times, Victor Bonney in England and Isadore Rubin in this country were the greatest advocates of myomectomy. Their enthusiasm exceeded that of more recent gynecologists, but myomectomy has found a definite place in today's pelvic surgery.

Hysterectomy

It was not until many years after "ovariotomy" was being done rather frequently and with some favorable results that an abdominal hysterectomy was successfully performed. Myomectomy was done before hysterectomy was attempted. In 1843, Charles Clay of Manchester performed abdominal removal of a leiomyomatous uterus, but the patient fell on the floor somewhat violently and died on the morning of the 15th day. The first completely successful removal of a leiomyomatous uterus took place in Massachusetts in 1853. Dr. Walter Burnham of Lowell opened the abdomen to remove what was thought to be an ovarian cyst. Lacking adequate anesthesia, the patient suddenly vomited and extruded the large uterus through the incision. The operator could not replace it and was forced to remove it. The patient survived, and Burnham was encouraged to attempt further hysterectomies. Of his next 15 cases, only 3 survived. Sir James Young Simpson, considered a daring surgeon at the middle of the 19th century, said that the idea of removing uterine leiomyomata should be rejected, "as an utterly unjustifiable operation in surgery." Lawson Tait attempted to solve the problem of leiomyomata by castration, by means of bilateral oophorectomy. At the fifth annual meeting of the American Gynecological Society in 1880, C. D. Palmer reviewed a total of 119 hysterectomies collected from the literature by Pozzi in 1875. Palmer reported a surgical mortality of 64% and estimated that if the unreported cases were included, the mortality rate at that time would have exceeded 75%.

Vaginal hysterectomy was performed in 1813 by Langenbeck in Germany and in 1829 by John Collins Warren in Boston. Both operations were unsuccessful. Fenger described the modern operation of vaginal hysterectomy in 1881. Proponents of the vaginal approach and proponents of the abdominal approach began their arguments in the late 19th century; the argument continues to some extent today. Kelly was an early proponent of vaginal hysterectomy but later changed to a preference for the abdominal approach.

Treatment of Vesicovaginal Fistulas

The history of vesicovaginal fistulas dates from antiquity. That they existed in ancient times is proven by the discovery of a large fistula in the mummy of Queen Henhenit, one of the wives of King Menuhotep, who reigned about 2050 B.C. Avicenna, an Arabo-Persian physician who died in 1037, is said to have been the first to recognize that incontinence of urine in women may be due to a fistula resulting from difficult labor. He considered the condition incurable and advocated contraception in the very young as a preventative. Until the advent of Sims in the mid-19th century, attempts at cure had extremely limited success. Van Roonhuyse of Holland was one of the most ardent experimenters, and deLamelle of France reported some successes; but failures were much more frequent. Mettauer of Virginia also struggled with the problem during this time and was the first to use metallic sutures. In 1838, he performed the first successful closure of a vesicovaginal fistula in this country but did not report it until 1840. In 1847, he reported six such successful cases and in 1855 reported a total of 27 cures.

During these preanesthesia and preasepsis days,

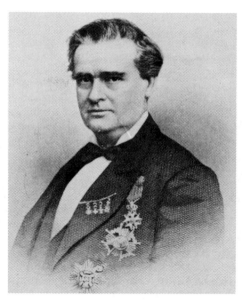

FIG. 1–3 James Marion Sims (1813–1883).

a Southerner, J. Marion Sims, began his experiments on the cure of vesicovaginal fistulas (Fig. 1–3). The term "experiments" is appropriate, since 4 years of experimentation elapsed before his first success. Sims had a successful career in surgery as practiced in those days in Montgomery, Alabama. He had no experience in pelvic surgery; in fact, he disliked it. It was his custom to turn away patients with pelvic disorders, referring them to doctors whom he considered more competent in this field. His slave-holding planter friends owned female slaves who had been delivered by midwives, and some of these slaves suffered from large vesicovaginal fistulas, then considered incurable. With this disturbing condition, the slaves were unacceptable as house servants. One of Sims' planter friends pled with him to attempt to cure the women. At first Sims declined the task, believing it to be hopeless; but finally his compassion for the unfortunate women persuaded him to undertake it. He worked on a group of these black women from 1845 to 1849 before attaining his first cure. During these years he housed and boarded the patients at his own expense in a small building that he constructed for this purpose on his own property. His many failures only stimulated his determination and efforts. The colleagues who at first assisted him at the operations forsook him, and his friends begged him to give up what appeared to be a hopeless effort; so he trained other slave patients to assist him in operation. In his 29th operation on one patient, he was finally successful in closing her vesicovaginal fistula. His ultimate success he attributed to the use of the lateral position (now known as Sims' position), the use of silver-wire sutures, which had initially been described by Mettauer, and the use of special instruments that he devised. The most important and lasting of these instruments was Sims' speculum, which evolved from a pewter spoon he used in earlier cases. However, an almost identical instrument of polished silver had been described by vonMetzler in Prague in 1846. Sims' success in his small private hospital in Montgomery, Alabama soon became known and took him to New York City, where he became one of the founders of the Women's Hospital. From there, his fame spread to the capitals of Europe, where he was received with the greatest esteem, and where he demonstrated his operative technique on several women with fistulas that had been considered incurable. All his operations were done without asepsis and without anesthesia. In the late 1920s, Mahfouz of Egypt reported on his vast experience with the repair of vesicovaginal fistulas utilizing the principles of Sims, with the great advantage of general anesthesia.

Although Sims made one of the important surgical contributions of the 19th century, he overlooked the original canine experiments by Levert (1829) with silver wire and the first successful silver-wire closure of a vesicovaginal fistula by Gosset (1834). To Sims must be accorded the recognition for perfecting and popularizing the technique of vesicovaginal fistula repair from previously developed surgical concepts. Credit for the original pioneering work and initial surgical success with silver wire must go to others.

Anesthesia

Anesthesia and asepsis were the two major developments of the 19th century that advanced the field of gynecologic surgery. Soporifics had been used from time immemorial to lessen the pain of surgery, but none was very successful. The discovery of general anesthesia by chloroform and ether is one of the most fascinating stories in medicine. It introduced a new era in surgery, and progress thereafter was rapid.

There is much discussion as to who first used chloroform (discovered by the great German chemist Justus von Liebig in 1831) as an anesthetic, but it is certain that after a number of personal experiments with it, Simpson administered its beneficent fumes to a woman in the pangs of labor on November 4, 1847. He was the first to apply it in just this way and probably the first to use it for the relief of pain.

The discovery of ether as a general anesthetic was undoubtedly America's greatest contribution to medicine up to that time. A detailed account of the struggle for priority in this great discovery is beyond this short review, but a few salient points may be of interest.

There is little doubt that Crawford Long, a practitioner in a rural community in Georgia, first used ether as an anesthetic in surgery. He was a modest practitioner who did only such surgery and obstetrics as came his way in his general practice; the discovery was somewhat accidental. It was the custom in Long's rural community to hold "ether frolics." The participants would inhale the fumes and become quite intoxicated. During the cavorting about, the merrymakers often fell and bruised themselves. On questioning them, Long was surprised to learn that they had no recollection of falling and suffering no pain at the time of injury. From this experience he conceived the idea that surgery might be made painless by the use of this drug. It was in 1842 that he first used it, though he did not publish his results until 1849.

While Long was using ether as a surgical anesthetic, Horace Wells, a dentist, was experimenting with nitrous oxide and had some of his own teeth extracted under "laughing gas." After an untoward result, however, he abandoned its use. A chemist suggested to William Thomas Green Morton, who was Wells' partner, that he use ether. Morton persuaded John Collins Warren to use it in surgery at the Massachusetts General Hospital—which he did successfully in 1846. A month later, this was reported by an observer of the operation, H. J. Bigelow. Thus, the Massachusetts group was the first to publicize the use of ether anesthesia, although Crawford Long was the first to use it. Long would probably never have received recognition had it not been for J. Marion Sims' bringing it to the attention of the medical public in an article published in 1877. As a result of this, Long's statue now stands in the Hall of Fame in New York and in the Capitol Rotunda in Washington, D.C. In passing, it is of interest to note that the name "anesthesia" was suggested by Oliver Wendell Holmes.

Asepsis, Antisepsis

At the time of the development of gynecologic surgery in the mid- and late 19th century, death from sepsis was the major surgical complication. In the mid-19th century, the development of ether anesthesia extended the surgical treatment of pelvic disease and, at the same time, increased the postoperative mortality from sepsis. Hand washing was sporadic; surgeons operated in their street clothes; ligatures were attached to the outer clothing of the surgical assistant; sea sponges were used, washed, and reused many times without sterilization; and the observers of an operation were frequently invited to examine the operative field with their unwashed fingers. The success of an operative procedure was related principally to the patient's ability to mount sufficient host defenses to prevent the spread of the local tissue infection that invariably occurred.

The discovery of general anesthesia opened the door to rapid progress in pelvic surgery, but other discoveries also stimulated its development. One of these was the proof by Ignaz Semmelweis of the contagiousness of puerperal fever in the Vienna Krankenhaus. His work was published from Budapest, where he became professor in 1845. His insistence on asepsis in the delivery room was responsible for a new era in obstetrics, but his principles were also adopted for surgery. Like many revolutionary discoveries, his ideas were rejected by his colleagues, who ridiculed and persecuted him, eventually forcing him to an insane asylum, where he died at the age of 47—ironically, from septicemia.

Another event that had a profound effect on the development of surgery was the work of Joseph, Baron Lister, who performed the first successful antiseptic treatment of a surgical wound at the Royal Infirmary in Glasgow in 1865, on the day preceding the death of Semmelweis. His method of sterilization included the use of carbolic acid spray, not only to the operative field to prevent the growth of pathologic bacteria, but also to the operating room. His results were published 2 years later, and his ideas were slowly but widely accepted. It is noteworthy that whereas Lister's was the principle of antisepsis, Semmelweis's principle was one of asepsis by thorough scrubbing to sterilize the hands of the operator. So not only did Semmelweis's work precede Lister's by 20 years, but his ideas were more advanced than those of Lister and corresponded more nearly to the customs of modern surgery. Lister also freely acknowledged his contribution to surgical asepsis as an extension of the original bacteriological studies of Louis Pasteur. Pasteur also advanced the principles of surgical asepsis by advocating that a scalpel blade should be passed through a flame before use.

The use of rubber gloves was a great step in aseptic surgery. Although William S. Halsted of Johns Hopkins is generally credited with the introduction of boiled rubber gloves in surgery, the idea was not solely his. Halsted wrote:

The operating in gloves was an evolution rather than an inspiration or happy thought. In the winter of 1889 and 1890, I cannot recall the month, the nurse in charge of my operating room (later Mrs. Halsted) complained that the solutions of mercuric chloride produced a dermatitis of her arms and hands. As she was an unusually efficient woman, I gave the matter my consideration and one day in New York requested the Goodyear Rubber Company to make as an experiment two pair of thin rubber gloves with gauntlets. In the report which I made of the first year's work at the hospital, written in November and December, 1890, and published in March, 1891, I stated that the assistant who passed instruments wore rubber gloves to protect his hands from the solution of phenol—in which the instruments were submerged—rather than to eliminate him as a source of infection. I do not recall having referred again, in my publications, to the employment of rubber gloves. Dr. Hunter Robb in 1894, in his book on aseptic technique, recommended that the operator wear rubber gloves. Dr. Robb was at that time resident gynaecologist of the Johns Hopkins Hospital.

A photograph taken in the Halsted clinic of a breast operation in 1893 shows that gloves were not being worn by him at that time. Halsted states further that it was remarkable that "we could have been so blind as not to have perceived the necessity of wearing them invariably at the operating table." So to Hunter Robb, a gynecologist, belongs the credit of recommending that the operator use rubber gloves.

Horatio Storer of Boston, credited with performing the first successful cesarean hysterectomy in the world in 1869, was actually the first surgeon to wear rubber gloves while operating.

With the adoption of general anesthesia and asepsis, the way was cleared for rapid progress in all fields of surgery. Gynecologic surgery suddenly received renewed life.

Other Advances in Operative Gynecology, 1850–1900

Thomas Addis Emmett, a Virginian who had moved to New York, was an illustrious pupil of Sims' at the Woman's Hospital. He devised operations for the repair of the vagina and cervix. The Emmett vaginal repair has persisted, with some modifications, though the cervical repairs as done by Emmett are seldom used today. Emmett did not follow his mentor, Sims, as chief surgeon at the Woman's Hospital—not from lack of ability but because of personality clashes between him and the governing board of the hospital. Previously, Sims had had clashes with the board over his insistence that women with cervical cancer be admitted to the hospital.

During this era, progress was also being made in England in operative gynecology. Sir Thomas Spencer Wells performed many "ovariotomies" and published his ideas on the subject in his book *Diseases of the Ovaries*. He was one of the first in England to insist on the greatest cleanliness of the operator's hands and instruments. A little later, a Scot, Robert Lawson Tait, transferred to London and Birmingham and made these cities the center of gynecologic surgery in England. He was a violent opponent of antisepsis and antagonistic in his personal relations to the profession, but he made landmark contributions to the surgical management of ectopic pregnancy and pelvic inflammatory disease.

In the United States, leadership in pelvic surgery was transferred from New York to Baltimore. Howard A. Kelly (Fig. 1–4) graduated from the University of Pennsylvania in 1882, the year before Sims died. He spent several years in postgraduate work in Germany when that country led the world in teaching pathology under Virchow and bacteriology under Koch. He was brought to Johns Hopkins as the head of gynecology and obstetrics in 1889, at the age of 31, by Welch and Osler, who had known him in Philadelphia. He was a bold and aggressive surgeon and was given carte blanche to develop his ideas at the new medical school. After several years, realizing that his real interest was in

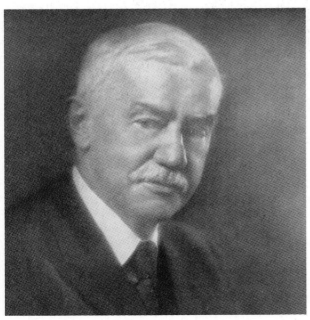

FIG. 1–4 Howard A. Kelly (1858–1943) (Davis AW: Dr. Kelly of Hopkins. Baltimore, Md, The Johns Hopkins Press, 1959)

pelvic surgery, he turned the Department of Obstetrics over to J. Whitridge Williams, whose illustrious career in that specialty justified Kelly's decision. Kelly had great interest in the female urinary system, realizing that the symptomatology of urinary tract disease is often intertwined with that of the reproductive organs. As a means of investigating these symptoms, Kelly invented the air cystoscope and devised ureteral catheters. He was the first to plicate the vesical sphincter for stress incontinence of urine. He also devised many techniques and refinements of pelvic surgery (Fig. 1–5), which were published in his textbook *Operative Gynecology*, a classic on that subject for many years. Kelly's many textbooks were beautifully illustrated by Max Brödel (Fig. 1–6) whom Kelly brought to the United States from Germany as a very young man. Brödel's contribution to operative gynecology was tremendous in his portrayal of operative techniques, pelvic anatomy, and pathologic disease. His contribution was great not only to gynecology, but to all medicine. He set a standard for medical illustrating never before attained and unsurpassed since. His school for medical illustrators supplied medical artists to many medical centers throughout the United States. Brödel's illustrations of Richardson's technique of total abdominal hysterectomy helped turn the tide in favor of total rather than subtotal hysterectomy.

Great as were Kelly's contributions to pelvic surgery, perhaps the most enduring result of his professorship at Johns Hopkins was his establishment of the long-term residency training program, which has been copied generally throughout the United States and to some extent in foreign countries. This plan for training pelvic surgeons, which emphasizes a strong background in and knowledge of gynecologic pathology and female urology, has done more to elevate the quality of gynecologic practice than any other factor.

Treatment of Cervical Cancer

The earliest attempts to cure cervical cancer were made by simple amputation of the cervix. In the early part of the 19th century, Marie Anne Boivin, one of the earliest female surgeons, had amputated a cervix that showed cancerous ulceration. Many others—Osiander, Dupuytren, Recamier, and Lisfranc—had performed the same operation. England was a long way behind France in the diagnosis and treatment of cervical cancer, possibly because of Victorian modesty, which prevented vaginal examinations except in the most desperate cases. Sir James Young Simpson attacked the problem in England and stressed the importance of early diagnosis.

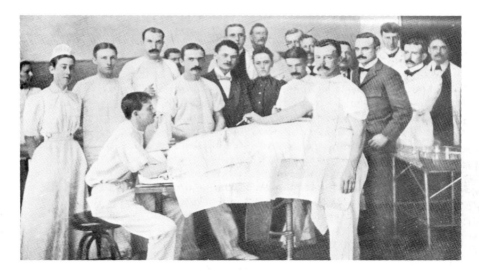

FIG. 1–5 Howard Kelly operates. Grouped about the operating table, left to right, are: Emma Beckwith, head nurse; Jay Durkee (seated); Thomas S. Cullen; Max Brödel; Elisabeth Hurdon; J. E. Stokes; John G. Clark. (Davis AW: Dr. Kelly of Hopkins. Baltimore, Md, The Johns Hopkins Press, 1959)

He observed that cervical amputation "can be employed only in very few cases of cancroid disease of the cervix, seeing that it is only when you can catch the disease, so to speak, before it has reached the line of reflexion between the cervix and the vagina, that you can amputate with any hope or prospect of success."

Following these failures with cervical amputation, simple hysterectomy was done. This, too, was generally unsuccessful, and it became evident that a more radical surgical approach would have to be taken if any measure of success was to be attained. In 1895, Emil Reis of Chicago attacked the problem and developed a radical abdominal operation with pelvic lymph gland dissection, which he performed on dogs and cadavers. In that same year, John Clark, a resident gynecologist at Johns Hopkins Hospital, employed this technique for the treatment of invasive cervical cancer. Three years later, Wertheim of Vienna began doing the same radical abdominal type of hysterectomy with selective pelvic lymphadenectomy and popularized it in Europe and, to a lesser extent, in the United States. His name has been associated with it since, although Clark was the first to perform the operation. Some success was attained with this radical procedure when the disease was limited to the cervix, later defined as Stage I, but when the disease had progressed beyond this stage, the salvage was indeed small. Initially, the operation carried with it a 10% mortality, and ureteral, vesical, and rectal fistulas to the vagina were common. Sampson, who was later to become famous for his work on endometriosis, did special work on the blood supply of the ureter and the pathogenesis of ureteral injury in dogs while he was a resident and young faculty member at the

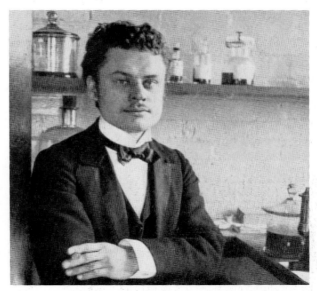

FIG. 1–6   Max Brödel. (Robinson J: Tom Cullen of Baltimore. New York, Oxford University Press, 1949)

Johns Hopkins Hospital. The intention was to preserve ureteral blood supply and thus avoid fistulas from the extensive lymph node dissection. In spite of his work, the percentage of ureteral fistulas remained high with the use of the Wertheim hysterectomy. In recent years, fistulas occur in less than 2% of such cases.

Realizing the shortcomings of operative cure of this disease, Kelly experimented with radium therapy. He and the many gynecologists who followed his early attempts attained greater success in the overall salvage of cervical cancer than had been attained by surgery. Although fistulas and other complications resulted from intravaginal radium therapy, they occurred most often in the advanced cases in which cure was impossible by surgery or irradiation.

In the 1940s, Meigs at the Massachusetts General Hospital revised and extended the Wertheim type of operation. He believed that with modern therapy at his disposal, such as antibiotics, blood replacement, and intravenous control of electrolytes, the operation should be reevaluated. He proved that in expert hands the operation could be done with a mortality rate of not over 1%. He was unable, however, to reduce appreciably the incidence of fistulas.

Another surgical approach to the treatment of cervical cancer was made in 1908 by Schauta, who published a volume on the removal of the uterus and parametrium by the vaginal route, which he had first done in 1901. The greatest proponents of this operation were van Bouwdijk Bastiaanse of Amsterdam and Ernst Navratil of Graz, but it never obtained popularity in the United States. The greatest disadvantage of the procedure was that it did not permit the removal of pelvic lymph nodes, as does the Wertheim procedure. However, the mortality rate in expert hands was only 3% to 4%, in contrast to several times that percentage with the Wertheim procedure.

In 1948, Alexander Brunschwig of New York published his radical surgical method of treating advanced and recurrent cervical cancer. It consisted essentially of exenterating adjacent pelvic organs and the generative organs, with diversion of the urine and feces through the abdominal wall, depending on whether the bladder or rectum or both were removed. Initially, there was a high mortality and morbidity and small salvage. The major usefulness of this procedure was in the en bloc removal of a radioresistant carcinoma of the cervix that had recurred centrally in the cervix and in which extension to the adjacent bladder and rectum could not be disproved. Current improvements in radiation techniques and dosimetry have reduced the frequency of central radiation failure in the treatment of cervical cancer as well as the clinical use of this ultraradical procedure. However, with ample blood replacement, antibiotics, and attention to electrolyte balance, these extensive procedures have found a limited place in the care of cervical cancer in carefully selected cases.

More Milestones

Thomas S. Cullen succeeded Kelly to the chair at Johns Hopkins in 1919 (Fig. 1–7). His contribution to

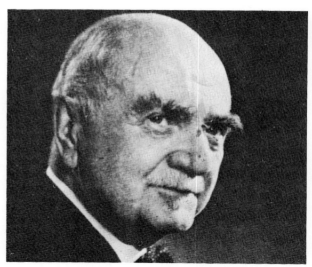

FIG. 1–7 Thomas S. Cullen (1868–1953.) (Robinson J: Tom Cullen of Baltimore. New York, Oxford University Press, 1949)

pelvic surgery was indirect: the establishment of a gynecologic pathologic laboratory. This was somewhat accidental. He went to Baltimore after an internship in Toronto, intending to work with Kelly in pelvic surgery. But there was no position immediately available on Kelly's surgical staff. To mark time, he was sent to the Department of Pathology to work under William Welch. He established a laboratory of gynecologic pathology that remains to this day. Cullen's book *Cancer of the Uterus* (1901) was published from this laboratory and was considered the classic on the subject for many years. Cullen was succeeded in his laboratory by Emil Novak, who published extensively from it, especially in the field of ovarian tumors. Thus, indirectly, with an understanding of the pathology of the pelvic organs, pelvic surgery was placed on a scientific rather than a purely technical level.

Endometriosis, one of the most common conditions requiring pelvic surgery, was first described by Russell in Cullen's laboratory in 1899. The disease was publicized by extensive studies of its histology by Sampson, who had been one of Kelly's early residents. His publications began in the early 1920s and extended to 1940. His theory of retrograde menstruation was the subject of the great controversy during this period. It was greatly strengthened by the experimental work of Scott and TeLinde, who in 1950 created endometriosis artificially in monkeys by permitting them to menstruate into the peritoneal cavity, thus demonstrating the ability of the cast-off endometrium to grow on the serosal surfaces. The effect of hormones on this artificially created endometriosis was studied by Scott and Wharton, and Kistner of Boston proposed the therapeutic use of progesterone to produce a sustained pseudopregnancy. However, surgery, augmented by the use of the carbon dioxide laser, remains the backbone of therapy.

In the realm of vesicovaginal fistulas, the surgical tenets of Sims still hold. Also, Latzko's contribution in 1914 of partial colpocleisis for closure of a high posthysterectomy fistula was a major step in the curability of fistulas of this type. Silver-wire sutures in the vagina have now been superseded by delayed-absorbable suture material.

Rectovaginal fistulas and third-degree perineal tears are today curable in a much higher percentage of cases than before, because of three important advances. The first of these dates from 1882, when Warren described his method of turning down a flap of vaginal mucosa to replace the defect in the terminal end of the anterior wall of the rectum. A better technique was described later by Nobel in 1902. A second advance was the use of sulfasuxidine and neomycin for bowel sterilization. Finally, the cutting of the anal sphincter, as described by Norman Miller in 1939, was considered to be a major step in anal sphincter repair at that time. It made possible the release of pressure from gas and feces, thus preventing the impaction of fecal material in the bowel for several days after the operation. This procedure has been abandoned in modern surgery because it led to weakening of the anal sphincter and persistence of anal incontinence of intestinal gas.

In 1912, Antoine Basset of Paris reported his study of 147 cases of primary carcinoma of the clitoris and described an operation for extensive removal of the malignant tumor and the regional lymph nodes. The Basset operation, which was popularized in the United States by Taussig, was a major contribution to reducing the mortality from cancer of the vulva. This procedure, now individualized for each patient, remains the standardbearer for the treatment of vulvar carcinoma.

Cytology and Carcinoma in Situ

One of the greatest advances in gynecology in the 20th century may be the improvement in the cure rate for cervical cancer that has resulted from the development of cytology and the recognition of carcinoma in situ. In conjunction, these two discoveries have permitted the detection of cervical cancer in the microscopic and, hence, curable stage. Without cytology, very few microscopic carcinomas would be discovered. Without the recognition and proper interpretation of the microscopic picture

known as carcinoma in situ, cytology would be of little value. The first publication of Papanicolaou and Traut appeared in 1941. Subsequent publications by them and others, notably Ruth Graham, demonstrated beyond doubt that cytologic studies could almost infallibly detect cervical cancer. First in 1927 and subsequently in many articles in the 1930s, Walter Schiller of Vienna described a lesion in the surface epithelium of the cervix that we now recognize as carcinoma in situ. The same microscopic picture had been noted by Cullen, Rubin, Schottlander, and Kermauner shortly after the turn of the century, but its relation to invasive cancer was not understood. This relationship was proposed by Galvin and Te Linde in an article published in 1944, and in several subsequent reports. Since then, the relationship has been amply confirmed, and early cervical cancer has become a detectable and a curable disease.

As emphasized in this text, the development of colposcopy in Germany by Hinselmann in 1925 and the introduction of this technique into the United States in the 1960s have provided a new dimension to the assessment of the abnormal cervix as detected by cytology. Colposcopy has also improved the accuracy of diagnosis of early cervical carcinoma. When used by an experienced colposcopist, the stereoscopic magnification provided by colposcopy makes unnecessary blind random cervical biopsies or the routine use of conization for the diagnosis of localized lesions, which can be completely visualized.

Treatment of Uterine Prolapse

The surgical cure of uterine prolapse was first attempted after the advent of anesthesia and asepsis. Up to that time, pessaries of all types had been the vogue. Some of the first surgical attempts were made by ventrofixation, but this proved unsatisfactory, the results often being temporary. Vaginal operations that rarely succeeded included amputation of the elongated cervix; constriction of the vaginal outlet and reconstruction of the perineum; and operations for diminishing the caliber of the vagina, usually by removing a strip or triangle of mucosa and suturing the edges together. The almost complete union of the labia majora was tried in Germany. Then, in 1888, A. Donald of Manchester and his assistant, Fothergill, devised what became known as the Manchester operation. Although infrequently used in the United States today, this operation, with various minor modifications, merits a prominent place in the history of attempts to cure uterine prolapse.

There are still some differences of opinion on the best method of treating uterine prolapse and allied conditions. Vaginal hysterectomy with suitable plastic vaginal repair has gained wide acceptance in the United States. Among the contributors to our present knowledge are Watkins of Chicago (the interposition operation), Spalding of San Francisco and Richardson of Baltimore (the composite operation), Heaney of Chicago (the vaginal hysterectomy), and LeFort of France. Heaney's greatest contribution was the development of a meticulous technique for the vaginal removal of the uterus, applicable in the removal of the benign uterus even when no prolapse exists.

Treatment of Urinary Incontinence

Great progress has been made in the surgical cure of urinary incontinence in the present century. Simple plication of the sphincter with or without cystourethrocele repair, as advocated by Kelly in 1913, and later by Kennedy and others, fails to cure the condition in some cases. In 1910, Rudolf Goebell of Germany first used the pyramidalis muscles to give continence to a child with congenital incontinence (possibly caused by spina bifida occulta). Frangenheim modified the original procedure by using a strip of rectus sheath attached to the pyramidalis muscles. Further modifications were made by Stoeckel in Germany and Aldridge in the United States, and out of this work there has evolved the so-called sling operation in its various modifications. In 1949, Victor Marshall and Andrew Marchetti of New York and Kermit Krantz, now of Kansas City, published their first results on the retropubic technique of vesicourethral suspension, a procedure that has gained considerable popularity in the United States.

During the past three-quarters of a century, more than a hundred abdominal, vaginal, or combined operative procedures have been developed for the control of genuine stress urinary incontinence. These operations are variations of the original Kelly technique of vaginal plication of the urethrovesical sphincter mechanism and the abdominal approach for the retropubic suspension of the urethra as initially described by Marshall, Marchetti, and Krantz.

In recent years, due in part, perhaps, to previous editions of this text, there has been a resurgence of interest in female urology in many gynecologic clinics in this country and abroad. This interest has been heightened by the development of high-technology methods for the advanced study of the urodynamic mechanisms that act as causative factors of urinary incontinence. These sophisticated urodynamic studies, particularly useful for the patient with a previous operative failure, have significantly improved the long-term surgical cure of this socially disabling condition.

Treatment of Congenital Malformations

Significant progress has been made within the last 40 years in reconstructive procedures for congenital malformations of the female generative tract. Many ingenious operations have been devised for forming a vagina when it is congenitally absent. Among the originators of procedures, now only of historical interest, are Baldwin, Frank, Wharton, Graves, and Shirodkar. In 1938, McIndoe devised a simple method of lining the newly formed vaginal cavity with a split-thickness skin graft. The operation has been extremely successful in most hands and has made obsolete other methods, many of which are more complicated and more dangerous.

In 1907, Paul Strassman of Berlin was the first to unify a double uterus. His operation was done through a transverse incision in the uterine fundus and merely bisected, without removing, the septum. More recently, an operation characterized by excision of the septum or the inner aspects of the two horns has been very successfully done. The procedure was described in 1953 by Jones and Jones of Johns Hopkins.

In the 1940s, the epochal work on intersexuality of Lawson Wilkins, a pediatrician, opened the door for surgical work on reconstruction of the genitalia according to the child's physical and emotional instincts. This surgery was initiated chiefly by Howard Jones.

Laparoscopy

The introduction and general acceptance of laparoscopy marks a real milestone in the history of pelvic surgery. The idea of viewing the intra-abdominal organs for diagnosis, however, is not new.

In 1911, Bertram M. Bernheim, an assistant surgeon at the Johns Hopkins Hospital, described two cases in which a proctoscope was passed through a small abdominal incision. He observed the abdominal organs using a reflected light. The next year, Jacobaes in Stockholm reported 115 examinations, 42 abdominal and 27 thoracic. Interest was aroused internationally, and Meirelles of South America, Renon and Rosenthal in France, Roccoi-villa in Italy, and Ordoff in Chicago all described original techniques and ideas of laparoscopy.

In 1929, Kalk, an outstanding German surgeon,

was an avid exponent and promoter of peritoneoscopy. He designed and constructed numerous lens systems and various endoscopes and, with significant detail, described 100 laparoscopy examinations. It is probably through the influence of Kalk that modern laparoscopy acquired credibility. In 1930, Ruddock from the United States became an avid proponent of peritoneoscopy and published reports on over 2500 cases in which local anesthesia and room air was used for the procedure.

In spite of the general use of peritoneoscopy abroad, it was not generally accepted as a diagnostic tool in the United States until Decker published extensively from 1949 to 1967 on visualization of the pelvic organs using the culdoscope. He introduced the culdoscope into the cul-de-sac after puncturing it through the posterior fornix. The patients were placed in the knee-chest position, allowing air to rush in by suction. Culdoscopy has been almost completely replaced by laparoscopy in most clinics.

The rebirth and modernization of laparoscopy can be traced to the early work of Palmer in Paris in 1940. His careful experiments on creation of a pneumoperitoneum and the control of intra-abdominal pressure were valuable contributions to the science of laparoscopy. He used the term "gynecological celioscopy" rather than "laparoscopy" and preferred this procedure to culdoscopy because it reduced the risk of pelvic infection. He believed that surgical techniques could be better applied through the laparoscope than the culdoscope. In recent years, many operative procedures formerly requiring a major pelvic operation have been successfully performed through the laparoscope. Among these are tubal sterilization, lysis of pelvic adhesions, an evaluation of chronic pelvic pain and infertility, evaluation of treated pelvic malignancies, and, more recently, the use of the carbon dioxide laser for vaporization of endometriosis implants throughout the pelvis.

Bibliography

Bernheim BM: Organoscopy. Ann Surg 53:764, 1911

Bonney V: Technique and results of myomectomy. Lancet 220:171, 1931

Brunschwig A: Whither gynecology? Am J Obstet Gynecol 100:122, 1968

Castiglioni A: A History of Medicine. New York, AA Knopf, 1941

Clark JG: A more radical method of performing hysterectomy for cancer of the uterus. Bull Johns Hopkins Hosp 6:120, 1895

Davis AW: Dr. Kelly of Hopkins. The Johns Hopkins Press, Baltimore, 1959

Decker A: Culdoscopy: Its diagnostic value in pelvic disease. JAMA 140:378, 1949

————: Culdoscopy. Am J Obstet Gynecol 63:654, 1952

————: Culdoscopy. Philadelphia, FA Davis Co, 1967

deLamelle J: Traite des Fistulas Vesicouterines et Vesicouterine-Vaginales, Paris, 1892

Eskew PN, Watt GW: Postgraduate medical education in obstetrics and gynecology. Obstet Gynecol 58:642, 1981

Galvin GA, Te Linde RW: The minimal histological changes in biopsies to justify a diagnosis of cervical cancer. Am J Obstet Gynecol 48:774, 1944

Gosset M: Calculus in the bladder: Incontinence of urine—Vesico-vaginal fistula. Advantages of gilt-wire suture. Lancet 1:345, 1834

Graham H: Eternal Eve: The History of Gynecology and Obstetrics. Garden City, NJ, Doubleday and Co, 1951

Halsted WS: An Account of the Introduction of Gloves etc. Menasha, Wisc, George Banta Publishing Co, 1939

Harris S: Woman's Surgeon. New York, Macmillan, 1950

Kelly HA: Operative Gynecology. New York, Appleton and Co, 1898

Latzko W: Behandlung hochsitzender Blasen und Mastdarm Scheiden Fistlen Noch Uterus exterpetion Mit hohen Scheidenverschluss. Zbl Gynaek 38:906, 1914

Levert HS: Experiments on the use of metallic sutures, as applied to arteries. Am J Med Sci 4:17, 1829

Mahfouz Bey NJ: Urinary and recto-vaginal fistulae in woman. J Obstet Gynaec Brit Empire 36:581, 1929

Mettauer JT: Vesico-vaginal fistula. Boston Med Surg J 22:154, 1840

Richardson EH: A simplified technique for abdominal panhysterectomy. Surg Gynecol Obstet 48:248, 1929

Robinson J: Tom Cullen of Baltimore. Oxford University Press, New York, 1949

Robb H: Aseptic Surgical Technique. Philadelphia, JB Lippincott, 1904

Rubin IC: Progress in myomectomy. Am J Obstet Gynecol 44:197, 1942

Ruddock JC: Peritoneoscopy. West J Surg 42:392, 1934

————: Application and evaluation of peritoneoscopy. Calif Med 71:110, 1949

————: Peritoneoscopy: A critical clinical review. Surg Clin N Am 37:1249, 1957

Schiller W: Untersuchen zur Entstehung der Geschulste. Collumearzinom des Uterus. Virchow Arch Path Anat 263:279, 1927

Schottlander J, Kermauner F: Zur Kenntnis des Uterus Karzinoms. Berlin, Karger, 1912

Sims M: The Story of My Life. New York, D Appleton & Co, 1884

————: On the treatment of vesico-vaginal fistulas. Am J Med Sci 23:59, 1852

Speert H: Obstetrics and Gynecology in America, a History. Baltimore, Waverly Press, 1980

————: Obstetrics and Gynecologic Milestones, Essays in Eponymy. New York, The Macmillan Co, 1958

Te Linde RW, Scott RB: Experimental endometriosis. Am J Obstet Gynecol 60:1147, 1950

Wertheim E: Zur Frage der Radical Operation beim Uterus Krebs. Arch Gynak 61:627, 1900

Wilkins L: The Diagnosis and Treatment of Endocrine Disorders in Childhood and Adolescence. Springfield, Ill., Charles C Thomas, 1950

Chapter 2

Psychological Aspects of Pelvic Surgery

Malcolm G. Freeman, M.D.

Gynecologists are so familiar with the science and technology of gynecologic surgery, and we deal with it so regularly, that there is a considerable risk of losing perspective about the impact of surgery on the life of the individual woman who is subjected to this stress. Indeed, what is for us an ordinary and daily event of usually simple dimensions may be for the patient a unique ordeal that challenges the central core of her identity. It behooves us to remind ourselves from time to time of the psychological stresses that are routinely and extraordinarily precipitated by the extirpation of a body part that is emotionally synonymous with a woman's feminine nature. What follows will largely be familiar material to any gynecologic surgeon. If there is a virtue associated with the presentation, it will not consist of new and astounding insights into a process that has become familiar to many of us. Instead, what is intended is to create some organization and system within which fragmented knowledge can be seen in a clear and recognizable pattern; a pattern that can be remembered and utilized to facilitate the patient care process and ease the anxiety and emotional stress of the surgical subject.

The patient who experiences ablative genital or breast surgery is influenced by many emotional factors. These vary in degree from subject to subject but are usually additive in nature. The patient, as she passes through the presurgical, surgical, and postsurgical experience, often feels beset on every hand and may, in fact, be inundated beyond her capacity to compensate. If help is not available to facilitate emotional healing and rehabilitation as well as physical healing and rehabilitation, then permanent emotional damage may be the result.

Most of us have seen the postsurgical cripple:

The woman who complains of continuing pelvic pain

The woman whose vagina is dry and whose sexual excitement has vanished

The woman who feels desexed and damaged

The woman who has lost her ability to trust and lives in rage and bitterness

The woman who no longer has desire

The woman who feels old before her time

The woman who is abandoned by her lover or drives her lover away

The woman who terminates her sexual identity and begins to draw in the edges of her life

These women have been stressed beyond their ability to compensate and heal.

Most women, of course, do heal and take up their lives, raise their children, work their jobs, and relate to their husbands or lovers. For some the healing is quick and the stress is modest. For others the healing is harder and the struggle to be well and whole leaves tender scars that slowly fade as life goes on. It is of all of these women that we will speak.

Emotional Response to Surgery

Massler and Devanesan have said there is an emotional response to any physical assault on the body. The magnitude of the response is expected to be proportional to the degree of emotional investment one has in the part of the body being assaulted. Among women, the parts of the body that are most vulnerable to this emotional reaction to assault are the face, hair, breasts, genitalia, and perhaps intestine (colostomy, ileostomy). Barnes and Tinkham have said that on the whole patients tend to react to current stress in much the same way as they have reacted to past crises and personal losses. Well-established patterns of behavior repeat themselves at such critical moments. This gives an opportunity to predict some of the patient's reactions by taking a history of her reactions to stress in the past.

Roeske has defined 13 factors related to poor prognosis for mental health after hysterectomy (see below). These factors begin to define the patient whose emotional stability in response to genital surgical stress is apt to be less certain. I would add to Roeske's list the woman who has a hysteric personality, since patients of this kind often require additional emotional support to handle life stresses.

FACTORS RELATED TO POOR PROGNOSIS FOR MENTAL HEALTH AFTER HYSTERECTOMY (3 MONTHS TO 3 YEARS POST-OP)

Gender identity (the intimate sense of herself as a woman)—the hyperfeminine cope less well

Previous adverse reactions to stress

Previous depressive episodes

Depression or other mental illness in her family of origin

A history of multiple physical complaints (especially low back pain)

Numerous hospitalizations and surgeries

Age less than 35 years at time of hysterectomy

A wish for a child or more children

Anticipation that the surgery will produce a loss of interest in and satisfaction from coitus

Husband's or other significant person's negative attitude toward hysterectomy

Marital dissatisfaction and instability

Disapproving cultural and religious attitudes

Lack of vocational or avocational involvement

Common emotional responses to surgery in general are listed below. For the most part, they are self-explanatory. Dependency and regression are particularly severe when recovery is prolonged and the patient has come to define herself in a "sick role." When the surgical illness involves a part of the patient's body that she feels is an essential element of her feminine identity, the emotional response is apt to be proportionately increased. Even when the physical and emotional stresses of the surgical procedure and physical healing have passed, there may be a prolonged period of grief.

COMMON EMOTIONAL RESPONSES TO SURGERY

Insecurity and vulnerability
  Surrender of control
  Sense of being manipulated
  Depersonalization (hospital)
  Helplessness
  Feelings of being attacked
Anxiety
  Fear of dying (may be expressed as anesthesia fear)
  Fear of pain
  Fear of loss of identity (role, independence, attractiveness, etc.)
  Fear of unknown
Emotional lability, sadness, tearfulness, irritability
Regression and dependency
A feeling of illness—a state of nonhealth ("sick" role)
Grief

Medical staff often do not appreciate the important role of grief when considering a patient's reaction to her illness. Grief is a normal and natural emotional response to loss of any kind and can be considered essential to emotional healing. The stages of grief are well enough defined to make behavior that otherwise seems incomprehensible understandable. The first and most primitive emotional response to loss is denial. Denial takes many forms. The patient may demonstrate denial, for instance, by not going to see the physician if she has a breast mass or by simply pretending that it isn't there. Not remembering things she has been told by the physician may be denial. The patient, on returning home, may say, "Well, I don't really remember what he said." She may forget the important things or deny the seriousness of the problem. Denial is a very primitive response but one that allows people to function and survive emotional stresses that they may not be able to handle otherwise.

The second stage of grief is bargaining with God. The patient has the opportunity to bargain with God only when anticipating a loss. The surgical patient commonly does this: "I promise to be a good person if only I don't have to die." "I will be kind to my children and I will not complain to my husband and I will go to church regularly."

The next stage of grief is guilt. Guilt occurs whether the grief reaction is before the loss or after the loss. Many of us feel that whatever bad happens is likely to be a punishment from God. Therefore, if something bad happens, we feel guilt as if we had done wrong. This gives rise to a series of "if onlys." "If only I had had my annual Pap smear. If only I had gone to the doctor regularly." When a mother has died: "If only I had gone to see my mother more often or taken her out to dinner or if only I had paid her rent instead of letting her do it on her social security." The guilt feelings come from a belief in magical or supernatural cause and effect. Guilt may sometimes be devastating and incapacitating but is usually transitory.

Following guilt, people who go through grief usually go into a stage of depression. Depression is characterized by feelings of helplessness, hopelessness, and worthlessness. To get a history of depression we ask the patient if she feels helpless, if she feels hopeless, and if she feels worthless. Depressed patients will quickly agree with you that those feelings characterize their day-to-day responses. Post-surgical depression is very common. When prolonged, it indicates that the patient has not been able to work through the grief process and find resolution. Depression is often rage turned inward (that is, suppressed rage), and when the patient is able to identify her rage and begin to express it, then the depression usually begins to lift and the patient begins to feel much better. When the patient begins to take charge of her life again and make decisions, even small ones, she begins to feel better and feelings of helplessness, hopelessness, and worthlessness abate. The stage during which the patient ventilates anger can be difficult for those providing care, but it should be accepted as healthy. The patient who is becoming angry is, in fact, beginning to deal with her grief and moving along toward final resolution of it. During the stage of anger, the patient may write letters to the newspaper or sue us. She may complain bitterly about the nursing staff, or the doctors, or the size of the bill, or read all of the literature that has to do with unnecessary surgery. All of these are a form of protest at the stress that has been dealt to her body and to her mind. When this behavior is seen, it means, in the great majority of instances, that the depression is beginning to lift and the patient is beginning to move toward the end of her grief.

Finally, there is resolution and integration. The stressful experience of loss eventually becomes an accepted part of one's life, the memory of which causes sadness and regret but no longer causes the devastating immobilization that is found in the earlier stages of grief. The integration of this experience does not mean that it is forgotten, only that it has less affect tied to it.

When a person is dealing with grief, she may have worked through the majority of the process and still, for a period of several years, have flashes of grief. There will be a word, an image, something that happens on television, that brings all of the acute grief feelings back in a very severe form for a few moments and then passes. It is important to note about grief that the stages of grief do not always follow in the orderly sequence described above. For many people, they are mixed up. The patient may feel fragments of anger, fragments of depression, or fragments of guilt at the same time that she is going through other phases. Grief is a common experience, and whenever the behavior of a patient seems excessive, bizarre, or out of the realm of what would usually be anticipated, it is a useful idea to look for the role that grief may be playing.

Some of the diseases with which we deal, cancer in particular, have special stresses. Schain has described fairly universal concerns among cancer patients, no matter where in the body the cancer may be located. The fear of death is, of course, common. There is fear of the morbidity associated with cancer treatments. Patients sometimes may fear that the treatment will be as severe as the disease. In the case of irradiation for carcinoma of the cervix, the vagina may sometimes be totally destroyed as a sexual organ. There may be fear of cancer recurrence. Even if the patient has been told that she has reason to expect a cure, she may feel as though she is carrying a time bomb around in her abdomen. We speak of five-year cure rates, which say that we are never quite sure that malignancy is gone forever. There is fear of abandonment. The patient often feels that having cancer is like having leprosy; she becomes untouchable and unclean in some way. There is a small but real risk (and a major anxiety) that the partner of the woman who has cancer might abandon her. The loss of functional ability, of social value, and of self-esteem are major concerns.

Patients fear the loss of economic competence. A woman who has worked hard every day of her life fears that she will be partially or totally disabled so that she is no longer able to work. The loss of familiar role behavior is important. All of us define part of our identities by the way that we carry out our expected tasks or responsibilities. If the patient is unable to do these tasks, she may lose her sense of identity because she has lost her usual role.

Finally there are site-specific function problems. The man who has had a leg amputated because of disease has a different function problem than the woman who has had a pelvic exenteration. Breast and gynecologic diseases are, in a sense, unique in that they attack sexual identity directly, as well as body image and self-esteem. Genital organs are one of the important ways in which we define our sexual identity.

There are specific emotional issues related to hysterectomy. Physicians tend to deal directly with the anatomical, physiologic, and pathologic situations that justify uterine removal. We spend little time considering the magical or symbolic value of the uterus. To the patient, the symbolic or magical value of the uterus is often of great importance and must be dealt with in some manner by the patient before uterine removal can be reconciled. Roeske points out that most premenopausal women express some form of ambivalence about giving up this valued part of self. When hysterectomy offers relief from fear of pregnancy, relief from pain, relief from continuous or excessive bleeding, relief from disability, relief from incontinence, or relief from cancer, it is apt to be viewed as a positive and appropriate procedure. This is particularly true for women over 35 years of age in whom childbearing expectations have been met.

Even when hysterectomy offers relief from distress, however, the loss of the uterus often stirs up ambivalent feelings related to its symbolic value. The first symbolic significance of the uterus is related to menstruation. The onset of menstruation is a rite of passage into feminine adulthood. When a girl has her first period, she often feels that she has become a woman. There are many women for whom menstruation is not just a bother; in fact it is a sign of their femininity, and its presence confirms that femininity. There are women who feel that menstruation offers them a cyclic cleansing; they feel that during the month poisons build up in the body and cause premenstrual tension, grumpiness, or change in emotional status. With the beginning of menstrual flow, these unpleasant emotional feelings and physical feelings fade away, and, in their minds, this means that the menstruation itself is a way to cleanse accumulated poisons from the body. Some women feel the rhythmicity of the menstrual cycle as a sort of timing and ordering of their life. Like the phases of the moon, it gives them a sense of routine, of regularity, of predictability in their lives that has emotional significance. The loss of that rhythmicity leaves them feeling empty.

For many women, the uterus has symbolic significance as a sexual organ, and they feel that it is essential to sexual response. If the patient feels that a uterus is essential to sexual response, then, in fact, it often is. Such women may become sexually dysfunctional when the uterus is removed. Women may also feel that their uterus is closely tied to feelings of attractiveness and sexual desirability. Removal of it constitutes a de-sexing, a destroying of their identity and function as women. Many women who have all of the children they want and who do not want to get pregnant again are still disturbed that sterilization or hysterectomy removes the possibility of pregnancy. The possibility of pregnancy in their lives has a symbolic feminine meaning that they regret losing. The uterine presence means completeness and wholeness and its removal means that there is a hole left in them, a vacancy, a cavity.

For some women, the uterus is regarded as a source of youth, of strength, of energy, of well-being, the regulator of general body health. Such a woman may feel that she has lost her youth because she has lost her uterus.

Many women feel that a partner will be able to tell that she has no uterus and that because of its absence her partner will experience sex differently and see her as less feminine, less of a woman, as old or defective. There is the fear that the partner will despise her or will abandon her for a woman who is complete; either complete in the sense of being able to offer him a child or complete in the sense of not having been de-sexed, or damaged, or made worthless. All of these terms are commonly used by women in describing their reaction to loss of their uterus.

Lamont, who studied rehabilitation among exenterative surgery patients, says that sexual happiness is not a question of anatomy or endocrinology, especially in the female who previously has been sexually well-adjusted. Loss of sexual function is more likely to be related to a patient's feeling of unattractiveness. Lamont's view may be extreme. There are certainly surgical procedures that damage a woman's ability to be sexually responsive and happy. The woman who has an irradiated vagina, for instance, may lose that ability. Most women who have learned to be sexually responsive, however, can continue to be sexually responsive even with the loss of breasts, vulva, vagina, uterus, tubes, ovaries, or rectum so long as their brain is intact and so long as they feel like sexually attractive people.

Derogatis has said that "sexual dysfunction is attendant upon gynecologic surgery even . . . when it does not involve dramatic procedures or a malignancy. In cases where threat to life and external disfiguration are added, the incidence of dysfunction is considerably higher." The incidence of sexual dysfunction among postoperative hysterectomy patients has been the subject of several studies. Table 2-1 is from Derogatis's paper describing hysterectomy patients who report postoperative sexual dysfunction. The percentage of women reporting dysfunction increases as these studies become more recent. In 1950, with Huffman's study, the frequency was believed to be about 10%. In the last two studies, from 1974 and 1977, the frequency was up to 38% and 37%. We are beginning to get a more sophisticated concept of what sexual dysfunction is, and perhaps we ask better questions. Certainly, this is a high percentage of dysfunction.

There are direct and indirect sexual disorders in gynecologic patients (and sometimes in their partners) that result from surgery or disease. The direct physiologic effects cause dyspareunia and have to

TABLE 2-1 *Proportion of Hysterectomy Patients Reporting Postoperative Sexual Dysfunction*

STUDY, YEAR	SEXUAL DYSFUNCTION, %
Huffman, 1950	10
Dodds, et al., 1961	15
Patterson and Craig, 1963	18
Munday and Cox, 1967	28
Richards, 1974	38
Dennerstein, et al., 1977	37

Derogatis LR: Breast and gynecologic cancers: Their unique impact on body image and sexual identity in women. In Vaeth JM, Blomberg RC, Adler L (eds): Body Image, Self-Esteem and Sexuality in Cancer Patients, p 8. New York, S Karger, 1980

do with estrogen loss (with subsequent vaginal atrophy, pain, or scarring), with loss of lubrication secondary to atrophy or to autonomic nerve fiber disruption, and with vaginal shortening (when it is extreme). There may be loss of vulva, clitoris, or vagina depending on the type of surgery, and there may also be loss of strength and health. The indirect effects result from the loss of self-esteem, the change in body image, and the loss or change in the patient's sense of sexual identity. These changes may cause loss of desire, loss of excitement (which includes lubrication and dyspareunia), and loss of orgasm (anorgasmia). Sexual dysfunctions may lead to the loss of the partner or to deterioration of a relationship as an indirect effect.

Direct effects on the male partner sometimes have to do with the loss of the female partner's physical attractiveness. A response of this type seems to be much less common than most women suppose. A woman's physical attractiveness to her partner is usually less important than she fears it might be. In most instances in which one partner complains of the other's physical appearance, the complaint is a mask for deeper interpersonal issues. Among most men, the requirement of "prettiness" in a beloved partner rapidly declines as they reach their mid-thirties, and other factors of compatibility and mutual caring tend to become more important. Even though men continue to appreciate physical attractiveness in other women, it seldom is a crucial factor in a valued relationship. Women tend to be very critical of their own appearance and quite realistic about their own physical faults and about those of their husbands. Concerning their wives' appearance, men tend to have a fantasy that changes relatively little as the years pass.

There is also a "fantasy" identity. People relate to their own perception of their partner's identity rather than to the person himself or herself. This perception may be quite different from the partner's own self-perception. When a woman has had a surgical procedure and extirpation of reproductive organs, it is quite possible for her partner to begin to perceive her in a different way, and this change may change the relationship for better or worse.

There is sometimes a fear of contagion. One of the reasons that male partners sometimes leave women who have had gynecologic cancer is a subtle feeling that the cancer may be contagious. Even though this seems unrealistic, it is a common fear.

A loss or change in the female partner's sexual availability may have an impact on her male partner. The fear of causing pain or injury has a major inhibiting effect on many men, and feelings of isolation and loss of nurturing result from the disability of the patient.

There may also be indirect effects on the male partner as a result of such things as a change in the patient's assertive role. The woman's usual assertive sexual role may be temporarily or permanently lost as a result of the surgical experience. Her usual sexual response may change. Her dependency and insecurity, particularly during the healing phases, may lead to a major change in the male partner. All of these changes may result in loss of desire, excitement, or orgasm in the male partner.

The Surgeon's Influence on Emotional Response to Surgery

How does the surgeon help or hinder the patient's emotional response to surgery? Barnes and Tinkham have said:

> Surgeons tend to be activists rather than empathetic listeners and many of them need to distance themselves from the patient's feelings and fears as a kind of protective insulation against the things they see every day. Some do not hear the patient and instead relate to a uterus or a breast or an appendix, and not a human being in distress. At times one observes a kind of cut and run syndrome in some surgeon-patient relationships. There are also doctors with a tendency to react to their patient's problems in terms of their own personal and moral value systems.

In other words, not all of us are as supportive or empathetic as we might be. Even though we see ourselves as pragmatic problem-solvers who do all that is reasonable and logical to contribute to our patient's health, our patients sometimes see us in quite another and less flattering way.

To be satisfied, the patient needs two assurances from her surgeon, besides technical competence and professional efficiency. The patient needs to feel that she has the surgeon's complete attention during the patient-physician interaction, and she needs to feel that the surgeon is willing and able to accept and help her to cope with her feelings as well as her physical dysfunction. Actually, neither of these requirements is difficult. It is not hard to give the patient the impression that she has our full attention if, in fact, she does. When the surgeon pushes other things out of mind, looks directly at the patient continuously, and listens carefully, the patient is apt to think she has her listener's attention. When the surgeon responds appropriately to what she is saying, she is sure of it. Dealing with the patient's feelings is usually not difficult if the surgeon accepts the viewpoint that the patient's feelings are a part of the gynecologic disorder. Most of the feelings surgical patients have are predictable and familiar to the surgeon but not to the patient. The application of common sense on the part of the surgeon will be enormously helpful to the patient.

The surgeon should begin by finding out what the patient's expectations may be about what will be done to her body and what the consequences of surgery will be on her life. As she tells the surgeon these things, her knowledge, fears, and biases fairly quickly emerge. The surgeon is then able to cope with these by supplementing her knowledge with appropriate explanations of anatomy and physiology and by describing in detail the usual preoperative, operative, and postoperative routines and experiences. The patient should be told in detail exactly what is likely to happen, and what she and her family can expect. Physical feelings, bandages, incisions, catheters, tubing, medications, and so on should all be described. The anticipated amount of discomfort and techniques to handle discomfort should be outlined. The patient's own role in convalescence and recovery should be defined. The nature of common complications should be mentioned, although a true "informed consent" may be a nearly impossible task. A timetable for discomfort, medication, ambulation, bowel movements, and discharge from the hospital should be given. The patient's questions and fears should be heard and answered.

This interaction should never be assigned to anyone other than the surgeon. A physician's assistant, resident, or nurse is not a satisfactory substitute, although each may reinforce this training process. When preparation for surgery is properly carried out, the patient's anxiety is greatly allayed, her postoperative care is simplified, and her need for pain medication is apt to be greatly reduced. Instead of feeling like a powerless victim, she is likely to feel like an important partner in a cooperative enterprise—which she is.

It is important to remember that whatever the patient's feelings may be, they must be accepted. However, information, reassurance, and support will usually quickly modify many dysfunctional feelings and lead toward a more healthy attitude and understanding of the surgical process. The surgeon also needs to remember that not all of the patient's feelings must be changed. It is enormously helpful for most patients to be able to talk about fears and ventilate their anxiety even if nothing definitive can be done about them at that moment.

The surgeon also needs to remember that a patient's family is an important part of her support system and can be a potent ally or a bitter enemy to the health care team. The family's need for information, reassurance, support, and attention cannot be neglected.

It is important that the surgeon be available to patients. Too often, receptionists or secretaries seem to feel that their role is to shield the physician from patients rather than to facilitate that contact. Often the physician is unaware of this behavior or covertly may encourage it. Few dissatisfactions make patients more angry than not being able to reach their physician within a reasonable length of time.

The art of touching—the therapeutic laying on of hands—is important. Human beings need to be and enjoy being touched, providing the toucher is a person they trust and accept. The touch itself is soothing, supportive, reassuring, and accepting, particularly to the sick or emotionally vulnerable patient. Physicians should be taught not to *paw* the patient but to *touch* the patient when they have some reason to. Being lonely, frightened, and sick is a reason for the patient to be touched by her physician. To hold the patient's hand while talking to her, or to touch her shoulder is therapeutic. In the old days before fetal monitoring, we evaluated the quality of labor by sitting at the patient's bedside with our hand on her abdomen feeling uterine contractions. It was interesting to see how often the presence of the physician and a warm hand on her abdomen made the patient relax, rest, and become more comfortable even during active labor. It is important to recognize how powerful and positive touching is when it is done in a therapeutic way, that is, for the patient's benefit rather than the surgeon's. Often a gentle touch can say things that words do not express.

Psychosexual Rehabilitation

Psychosexual rehabilitation after gynecologic or breast surgery has as its goal the restoration of sexual identity, body image, and self-esteem. Most of this rehabilitation is a gradual process that the patient does for herself, but it can be facilitated by the health care team at several places.

As healing takes place, there is a gradual loss of dependency with resumption of strength and usual roles. The resumption of her usual roles helps the patient feel more like her old self. She gradually begins to lose the sick role, and see herself again as a well person.

Every patient who undergoes surgery will go through the grief process to some extent. Though grief is inevitable and normal, it is also uncomfortable. The grief process can be speeded by encouraging the patient to ventilate, to talk about her feelings rather than repressing them or brooding unnecessarily. Everybody needs support systems, particularly when under stress. Support systems are people who are able to supply emotional support when stress is heavy and the need for ventilation and encouragement is great. The physician and other health care workers can and do function as part of a patient's support system, but most of the support is given by spouse, family, and friends. A good friendship offers mutual but often not simultaneous support. Rarely is a spouse alone sufficient support; usually others are necessary to share the load. Sometimes, to the patient her spouse may seem part of the problem rather than part of the solution.

Part of rehabilitation comes from validation of the patient's sexual identity from herself, from others, and from her roles. As she begins to see herself as a sexual person, and as her sexual partner, family, and friends indicate their continuing acceptance of her as an important, powerful, sexual person, that mantle rests more and more comfortably on her shoulders. The woman who has had a mastectomy, for example, needs the affirmation of knowing that her partner sees her as attractive and sexually desires her, and without that affirmation she may have trouble seeing herself as a sexual person.

Cosmetics, dress, and grooming are an important part of rehabilitation. We live in a culture that places great emphasis on women's physical appearance. When a postoperative patient combs her hair, puts on lipstick, and demands her own nightgown instead of a hospital gown, she has begun to heal. When the patient feels that surgery has been disfiguring in some way, she needs to find a way to compensate with dress or grooming in order to feel whole and complete again. This need cannot be neglected.

THE FOUR PLEASURES

When sexual functional loss has occurred, real compensation is needed. The patient's surgical treatment cannot be said to be complete until she has been returned to a level of sexual functioning that she judges to be gratifying and satisfactory. Patients who talk about their sexual lives regularly describe four different pleasures associated with sexuality. They describe these same four pleasures so regularly that we can assume they are universal in our culture. Understanding the four pleasures offers the key to sexual rehabilitation of men or women who have lost some portion of their usual sexual function.

THE PLEASURE OF TOUCHING. This pleasure—the pleasure of being held, caressed, cuddled, stroked, kissed, hugged, of feeling warm—is not necessarily sexual; it is actually a basic human need. In our society it is difficult for adults to have their touching needs met in any way outside of sexual interaction. For many women who have never experienced an orgasm, sexual interaction is nevertheless profoundly enjoyable because of the touching and concentrated attention they perceive during the experience. Women who have orgasm easily and regularly often complain about their sexual interactions if insufficient time is devoted to "foreplay" and "afterplay"—in other words, when insufficient touching has taken place to gratify their needs. Often, when something has happened to interfere with genital sexual expression in a couple, all physical contact abruptly stops so that touching and affection needs are no longer met. The couple's relationship actually may suffer more from loss of touching and simple affection than from loss of intercourse. When touching has ceased and needs for simple affection and nurturing are no longer met, the partners begin to feel alienated and needy. Encouraging the couple to resume and emphasize touching usually brings them closer together and decreases tension, and good feelings increase. Simple touching can be carried out even when a patient is in early convalescence. Touching also helps affirm feelings of being accepted, wanted, needed, and of being sexually desirable.

THE PLEASURE OF GENITAL CARESSING. Genitalia (including breasts and nipples in both sexes) are extremely sensitive to touch. Genital and breast play is a regular part of courtship and intensely gratifying to most people, whether it is followed by orgasm or not. Orgasm itself is a brief sensation, whereas genital caressing can and sometimes does continue for hours with a relatively low expenditure of energy. During premarital courtship, whole body touching and genital caressing is a major focus, and both male and female partners go to great lengths to make sure it can take place without outside interruption.

When a patient is recovering from surgery or has

had surgical loss of sexual function, genital caressing as a giver or receiver is often possible and intensely gratifying. Although excessive sexual excitement in women who are in their first few weeks after pelvic surgery is not advisable, the pleasure of breast caressing may be comforting to the patient.

Women who have lost the ability to have vaginal intercourse because of vaginal loss may substitute interfemoral or anal intercourse if either is acceptable to them. Women who have lost their vulva from surgery or disease may still be able to have vaginal intercourse or may receive intense sexual pleasure from abdominal, inguinal, perianal, or inner thigh caressing. A sexual gratification substitute can usually be found for any genital loss unless the inhibitions or ethical code of the couple prohibit alternatives or experimentation. When a woman has already learned to be orgasmic with genitalia intact, she can often learn to be orgasmic again in spite of major genital loss, including loss of the clitoris.

THE PLEASURE OF ORGASM. An orgasmic response tends to be pleasurable and relieves sexual tension. An orgasm may be painful, but that is a rare occurrence. In general, men and women enjoy orgasms whether produced by dreams, fantasy, caressing, masturbation, vaginal intercourse, anal intercourse, or any other means. Most people tend to value one means of producing orgasms more than another, but this is a matter of personal preference. Although all orgasms may be physiologically identical, there are major differences in the way orgasm is perceived as well as valued by different people.

When the ability to have orgasm by one favorite means is temporarily or permanently impossible following pelvic surgery, the patient can be encouraged to try alternative ways to achieve orgasmic relief, so long as the alternatives do not violate her value system. Sometimes the patient will need help reconsidering her value system, where it came from, and what it means to her.

THE PLEASURE OF GIVING PLEASURE TO A PARTNER. Most people value their ability to be a source of pleasure for a beloved partner. To give pleasure and have a role in creating excitement and gratification gives a person a sense of identity and a feeling of being needed and valued. Men often carry this feeling to an extreme so that they may feel responsible for their partner's pleasure. This attitude can become a performance trap and should be avoided.

Women who lose their ability to engage in vaginal intercourse may still feel they fulfill their feminine role if they can be a source of pleasure for a sexual partner. When a patient has functional loss, her ability to compensate may be evaluated by reviewing the "four pleasures" and defining alternative ways of feminine response.

OFFERING HELP

Whenever a patient's psychosexual rehabilitation after surgery seems to have become impaired and she fails to make steady progress toward resumption of her usual role with appropriate self-esteem, energy, identity, and ability to handle life stresses, she should be offered help. Help should be offered early (after a period measured in days to weeks or, at most, a few months) rather than late (months to years), since intervention, if early, is often easy and brief rather than the long-term psychotherapy that can be required if confirmed patterns of emotional dysfunction must be dealt with. Help should be given first by the surgeon and then, if more help is needed, by a psychotherapist who is interested in and familiar with these problems.

Some gynecologists suggest that the time to do a hysterectomy on a patient is when she begs for it. It is not necessary for a patient to beg for surgery before the surgeon decides to do it, but when a patient feels the procedure will be of enormous benefit, wants it done, and chooses it without any coercion, she is very likely to be pleased by the procedure and gratified by having had it done. She is also apt to recover from it quite well and to resume her life after a reasonable period of convalescence. When she goes into the procedure with reluctance and anxiety and a feeling that she will come out as a different and damaged person, her recovery may well be delayed and stormy.

The pelvic surgeon's responsibility transcends the performance of the surgical procedure, no matter how technically skillful that may be. The appropriate decisions about whether to operate, when to operate, and what procedure to do and the considerate management of the patient's return to health are the hallmarks of an accomplished surgeon. They distinguish the specialist from the surgical technician. The informed gynecologic surgeon possesses the knowledge and ability to do a better job of helping the patient return to health.

Bibliography

Barnes AB, Tinkham CB: Surgical gynecology. In Notman MT, Nadelson CC (ed): The Woman Patient: Medical and Psychological Interfaces. New York, Plenum Press, 1978

Cutler WB, García CR: The Medical Management of Menopause and Premenopause. Philadelphia, JB Lippincott, 1984

Derogatis LR: Breast and gynecologic cancers: Their unique impact on body image and sexual identity in women. In Vaeth JM, Blomberg RC, Adler L (eds): Body Image, Self-Esteem, and Sexuality in Cancer Patients. New York, S Karger, 1980

Lamont JA, DePetrillo AD, Sargeant EJ: Psychosexual rehabilitative and exenterative surgery. Gynecol Oncol 6:236, 1978

Massler DJ, Devanesan MM: Sexual consequences of gynecologic operations. In Comfort A (ed): Sexual Conse-quences of Disability. Philadelphia, George F. Stickley, 1978

Roeske NCA: Hysterectomy and other gynecological surgeries: A psychological view. In Notman MT, Nadelson CC (eds): The Woman Patient: Medical and Psychological Inter-faces. New York, Plenum Press, 1978

Schain WS: Sexual functioning, self-esteem, and cancer care. In Vaeth JM, Blomberg RC, Adler L (eds): Body Image, Self-Esteem, and Sexuality in Cancer Patients. New York, S Karger, 1980

Chapter 3

Professional Liability of the Gynecologic Surgeon

Elvoy Raines, J.D.

The gynecologic surgeon shares the company of a small number of other medical and surgical specialists who have experienced in recent years an astonishing expansion of their risk of lawsuit related to the practice of their profession. This growth in the significance of their professional liability is reflected in the sizable insurance premiums they must pay (as much as ten times that paid by other physicians), in the protocols and restrictions or limitations on privileges imposed by hospitals, and, unfortunately, in an evolution in the physician/patient relationship and a collateral adjustment in the manner of surgical practice not necessarily dictated by medical or scientific considerations.

There are important practical and professional considerations that should be understood by the gynecologic surgeon, both to prevent unjustified exposure to a legal claim and also to preserve the scientific integrity of the decision-making process. The final outcome of these protective actions should be one in which the physician may practice without the specter of a lawsuit clouding his or her judgment. This chapter is *not* a legal treatise or a substitute for appropriate legal counsel, nor is it an exhaustive explanation of tort (personal injury) law. Physicians interested in full treatment of the subjects and legal theories raised herein are referred to the bibliography for further reading.

The Physician/Patient Relationship

ESTABLISHMENT OF THE RELATIONSHIP

There are circumstances when the liability of the physician is nonexistent or limited (as in emergencies), but this discussion will focus upon the common physician/patient relationship where a duty of some sort is owed by the physician to the patient: a duty to perform as agreed between the parties and a duty not to injure the patient.

In general, the physician/patient relationship is contractual: one party is paid for services provided another. But there is also a personal, physical aspect since the physician (and especially the surgeon) actually touches the patient, either topically or invasively. Legal consequences attach in either instance, and lawsuits against physicians may be based upon contract or tort law. For this reason, the relationship of the parties may determine, first, whether a basis for a claim ever arises and then how the claim is resolved.

The manner in which the physician/patient relationship is established and maintained may be as important as the quality of the care actually provided as a determinant of whether the patient files a claim. The physician must be diligent in the early stages of the relationship to make certain that he or she is the appropriate provider for that particular patient, that his or her training and skills are adequate, and that the patient clearly understands the respective roles of the physician and patient in the pursuit of a mutually satisfactory outcome.

The patient should be involved—actually encouraged to participate—in her care, even in the mundane and simple activities of compliance with a therapeutic plan and monitoring of symptoms. Involvement of the patient improves the likelihood that communication will be free and effective, that potential misunderstandings will be avoided, and that any actual incidents will be managed in a more efficient and timely manner.

INFORMED CONSENT

A developing body of law (and much confusion and concern in some parts of the medical community) surrounds the concept of informed consent—that process by which the patient acquires an understanding of the contemplated surgical procedure and gives the physician permission to act. If the physician acts without permission, or beyond the limits or scope of permission, he or she may violate the agreement (contract) that is the basis of the physician/patient relationship or may be liable, under tort law, for personal injury, however slight.

It should be emphasized—and integrated into a physician's practice habits—that informed consent is a *process*. While its manifestation is generally a form signed by the patient that asserts that she understands the contemplated procedure, risks, alternatives, and so on, the form is only incidental to the process: it simply serves to show in writing that the process did indeed occur. The process is the key, essential to appropriate professional practice, and not at all mysterious or complicated.

The patient is the final decision-maker. Of course there are exceptions due to age, intelligence, mental or legal capacity, and so on, but in general dealings with patients, the surgeon must acknowledge that there are shared responsibilities and respective responsibilities between physician and patient, and the decision to accept a physician's recommendation of surgery is ultimately the patient's alone.

If permission is given, and if the act is to be legally defensible, it must be based upon all elements *material* to the patient. Generally, courts will expect the patient to act on the value system of the fictional "reasonable man," that creation of the law which approximates the average person in terms of education and intellectual capacity. Material elements will almost always include a description of the procedure and why it is recommended; the risk of complication, side effect, or injury associated with the procedure; alternatives to the procedure, including taking no action; the projected outcome and relative chances of success for the procedure; and information about costs for both the procedure and aftercare. Those risks that are known to exist and occur with some frequency should be explained, even if slight in terms of impact; rare but severe complications (those that cause permanent impairment or death) should also be explained.

COMMUNICATION BETWEEN PHYSICIAN AND PATIENT

The patient and the physician both have obvious reasons for striving to maximize the quality of their communications. It might be argued that the physician has the added incentive of knowing that if a failure of communication leads to a lawsuit, he or she is the one who will suffer most, legally, for that failure.

The most effective means of reducing exposure to professional liability is effective communication: it prevents mistakes, misunderstandings, and inaccurate expectations; it also prevents lawsuits. The surgeon may improve the quality of communication by attending to details that may require extra time initially but that ultimately save time and energy for the physician, and consequences and costs for the patient: allow time for uninterrupted discussions with the patient, encourage the patient to ask questions, see that the patient follows directions and is a participant in her care, and reference and record all conversations (including telephone conversations) in the patient's file.

SPECIAL DUTIES OF THE SPECIALIST

The existence of a duty owed the patient by the physician is necessary for liability. Also necessary is a breach of that duty, and an injury that is caused by that breach of duty. The gynecologic surgeon, like other specialists, will be held to a higher standard of care in a court's analysis of the duty and the breach than would a generalist, perhaps even one performing the same procedure. In the past, a "locality rule" was in effect, even for specialists, which set the standard as that which a similarly trained physician in that locality would be expected to meet; today, except in a very few jurisdictions, specialists are held to a nationally applied standard of care, rigidly enforced by courts and easily established by a plethora of expert witnesses.

LIABILITY FOR THE ACTS OF OTHERS

The surgeon is responsible for his own actions, but he may also bear the legal responsibility for acts of those providing care and services to the patient under his direction. Courts explain this transference of liability in terms of "vicarious liability" or "respondeat superior." Simply stated, the primary physician may be liable for the acts of another person, even another physician, where the second person causes injury to the patient during the course and scope of his or her employment and there is some relationship between the providers that would give the primary physician control or right of control over the second person's actions.

A second, and less easily applied, rule of liability for the actions of others, is established under the legal theory of *res ipsa loquitur*. It is a concept that means roughly "the thing speaks for itself" and is a form of strict liability, wherein by circumstantial proof negligence may be inferred from the fact that an injury occurred that does not normally occur in the absence of negligence. This inference shifts the burden of proof to the defendant physician. Requisite elements, in addition to the presumption of negligence, are that the injury is caused by an instrumentality within the exclusive control of the physician and that there is no contributing action by the patient.

The surgeon must be aware that the theory of *respondeat superior* may apply in the operating room as well as in the office: employees may place him or her in positions of liability, but members of the health care team providing surgical assistance, laboratory and record interpretation, and follow-up care also may cause injury for which he or she is liable. For that reason, adequate, effective communication between the surgeon and colleagues, other providers, and staff is essential to meaningful risk management.

TERMINATION OF THE PHYSICIAN/ PATIENT RELATIONSHIP

Just as the physician/patient relationship is a product of agreement between the parties, so, too, should be the termination of the relationship. Unless treatment is no longer required or the patient terminates the relationship, the physician wishing to terminate his or her obligation to provide professional services should give adequate and timely notice to the patient, refer the case if necessary and advisable, and provide all records and information necessary to a proper response by the replacing physician. Failure to adequately ensure continuous coverage may result in a lawsuit for abandonment and negligence. If the physician wishes to limit the relationship from the outset, that should be made clear in the initial formation of the relationship; the surgeon, for instance, may wish to explain that his or her services will be provided with the understanding that the patient will return to her referring physician, who provides her routine gynecologic care.

Practice Management

RECORDKEEPING

After effective communication, the single most important aspect of liability risk management is the maintenance of good records. As a determinant of the defensibility of a case, it may be the most important element. There is no substitute for an articulate, fully informative record as a mechanism for communication among members of the health care team, and as a permanent written record of treatment decisions and effects. In the absence of a record or elements of a record, only the memories of the parties are available, and that places the allegations of the plaintiff on a par with the defenses of the defendant.

Gynecologic surgeons must devote considerable attention to recordkeeping, since their exposure to a lawsuit is so high. For 1980, statistics indicate that six of the eight most frequently performed operative procedures were among those commonly performed by gynecologists. [The eight most frequently performed procedures, in order of frequency, are: biopsy, diagnostic dilatation and curettage; excision of lesion of skin or tissue; hysterectomy; ligation and division of fallopian tubes; cesarean section; repair of inguinal hernia; and oophorectomy.] In simple numbers, gynecologic surgeons have a greater degree of exposure to lawsuit because they have a greater number of patient/surgical encounters. Therefore, prompt, accurate recording of information is essential.

Completeness, accuracy, and adequacy are critical elements in recordkeeping. For completeness, the physician should pay special attention to the medical history, and the record should include progress notes (as well as information regarding a patient's failure to comply with therapeutic plans), consent forms, lab reports, consultant reports, correspondence, and notes of conversations, both in person and on the telephone. Questions asked should have answers in the record; lab tests ordered should be followed by a reading and interpretation in writing. Flat, unqualified predictions ("_____ is not a threat to her general health") should not appear in the record, and self-deprecating humor or other irrelevant asides should not appear. In order to ensure an up-to-date record, timely writing or dictation of the operative record is essential; dictated records should be reviewed for typographical errors or other mistakes. Written remarks must be legible. The chart is a clinical record of care rendered, and remarks should be precise, professional, complete, and accurate. And finally, completeness includes making sure that the record is internally consistent; inconsistencies in the physician's comments or in those added by others should be explained in the record.

Any blank spaces or alterations in the record can be especially damaging to the defensibility of a physician's actions. Unanswered questions or absence of comments suggests that important matters went unattended, and alterations suggest inconclusiveness or an attempt at subterfuge. Something should be written at *every* patient visit, and the surgeon should never delay in completing essential information. There should be no obliteration of already recorded information, and if a mistake is made or a change is necessary for any reason, the incorrect statement should be lined through once (so the original may be still legible) and the correction made, dated, and initialed with an explanation for the change. When sharing records, surgeons should provide copies, retaining the originals in their files at all times.

CONSULTATION, SECOND OPINION, OR REFERRAL

The surgeon should resort readily to consultation, or referral if necessary, rather than relying upon "hopes" or "odds" for achieving a positive outcome; no surgeon should expect that his or her knowledge is complete and superior in all instances, for a court will quickly demonstrate that theirs is the final judgment of appropriate medical practice. Information should be explained to the patient in a correct, timely, and responsible manner, with bad news conveyed in a serious and professional manner rather than jokingly or casually.

Too frequently, physicians will decide that they can perform a given procedure as well as anyone, or that they do not wish to risk losing a patient to a competing physician; such short-sightedness leads only to lawsuits. Timely consultation suggests prudence on the part of the physician, and recorded opinions of two physicians make the defensibility of the primary physician much greater.

AWARENESS OF CURRENT LITERATURE AND PROCEDURAL SPECIFICATIONS

The surgeon is expected to be current to the date of the procedure on readings related to all relevant professional practice considerations. Any lapse reflects badly on the competence of the physician and reduces the defensibility of his or her actions. State-of-the-art opinions and guidelines should be followed closely, and technical information and standards must be a functional part of the surgeon's knowledge. Expert witnesses need only display the professional literature to establish a failure in professional performance.

OFFICE STAFF APPRECIATION OF LIABILITY ISSUES

As explained in relation to vicarious liability, the actions of others may cause the physician to acquire an unnecessary liability risk. This is true also of behavioral considerations for the physician's staff. Inappropriate behavior or antagonistic remarks by nurses, clerks, and secretaries can sour the best physician/patient relationship. Therefore, all staff members should be involved in risk management. Among the basic considerations: retain copies of all telephone messages and conversations with patients; record all missed appointments or variances in compliance with therapy; note inconsistencies in patient statements about history or progress; and keep all financial and billing records separate from medical and surgical records.

COMMUNICATION WITH THE INSURANCE CARRIER

Surgeons who do not communicate freely and regularly with their insurance carrier may find it difficult to understand the true role of an insurer. It is important to understand that the risk of the physician is the risk of the insurer, at least to a degree, and that the physician has no greater ally in risk management efforts. A basic yet thorough understanding of the policy is essential. In addition, the names and locations of claims managers and the criteria for reporting incidents to the insurer are essential items to know.

Early reporting of incidents is critical to maintaining a defensible practice. For the surgeon, this is an even more important habit, and one that will be fairly commonly practiced, since surgery naturally involves a core percentage of unanticipated outcomes or incidents. It is impossible to perform as a surgeon for any considerable period without committing an act or being identified with an outcome that could become the basis for a lawsuit. Therefore, perception of the occurrence of incidents, and a prompt reporting to the insurer, allows time and perspective for insurer and insured to anticipate and prepare a defense against claims of potential plaintiffs. If no case arises, the exercise of incident management (described in more detail below) will permit the physician to examine critically his or her own performance.

COMMUNICATION WITH OTHER PHYSICIANS, NURSES, AND STAFF

"Physicians get physicians sued" is a statement that the surgeon will hear repeatedly. And it is true. And nurses get physicians sued, and residents, and other hospital staff members. The failure of these providers to confine their observations to clinical facts and objective analysis of patient care is the primary cause of lawsuits generated from the medical community. The solution is not a conspiracy of silence but a more professional pattern of behavior within the confines of the hospital and in the physician's office. A basic rule is never to write or say anything that you would be reluctant to repeat on a witness stand.

The quality of communication is critical as well. Studies have shown a significant variance in the understanding of terminology, especially quantifying terms such as "sometimes" and "always," with variations from region to region and between professions. Specificity, opportunities for questions, and periodic review of the effectiveness of communication aid the surgeon in ensuring that correct understandings occur.

Zones of Risk

The gynecologic surgeon will find the majority of his or her practice related to diseases of the female genital tract. However, aspects of other specialties find application in good gynecologic practice: endocrinology, internal medicine, and obstetrics, for example. Therefore, the gynecologic surgeon must have a thorough knowledge of female reproductive physiology and of the concurrent mental and emotional factors that are so integral to reproductive ability and sexual function. Furthermore, the interaction and interdependence of the gynecologic surgeon with other specialists mandates an ability to coordinate efforts and cooperate toward a positive outcome.

Common gynecologic conditions may not necessarily require surgery, and the surgeon should exercise prudence in selecting and recommending treatment modalities.

The initial examination of the patient, and all preoperative evaluations, should be comprehensive and detailed. This early and preliminary investigation is critical to correct management of care thereafter.

Accurate diagnosis is essential prior to any elective operative procedure. Especially important is the identification of pregnancy, and any suggestion of pregnancy should forestall elective procedures until all factors are known.

Gynecologic surgery generally involves fewer complications than some other surgical encounters, and therefore potential liability is somewhat reduced; however, there is no special immunity from error or injury in gynecologic surgery, and the surgeon must direct special attention to a variety of zones of risk inherent in such surgical encounters.

DIAGNOSIS AND TREATMENT

Diagnostic issues account for about 15% of claims. Treatment issues are the basis for legal claims in about 40% of cases. For the surgeon, these factors present a formidable risk that must be translated into a manner of practice that will minimize the risk of delay in diagnosis, misdiagnosis, or failure to diagnose.

For gynecologists, special areas of risk involve breast disease, surgical injury, infection, and problems related to contraception and sterilization.

Adequate training in the techniques and procedures for breast examination, diagnosis, and follow-up is essential. Moreover, the appropriate referral of patients, or consultation, is basic to a defensible practice.

Surgical injury, particularly bowel and urinary tract injuries, are also common enough to merit special consideration and anticipation; postoperative infection is the most common complication. When such an injury occurs (nicked ureters, perforations of the uterus, and so on) the appropriate steps in incident management must be taken.

Problems related to contraception and sterilization account for many of the claims against gynecologists. Incomplete abortion, failure to diagnose or mismanagement of ectopic pregnancy, and failed sterilization procedures are common areas of risk.

INJURIES FROM MEDICATION OR EQUIPMENT AND FACILITIES

Medication issues account for about 7% of claims, and equipment or facilities-related injuries account for about 3%—both percentages are small, but nevertheless, both areas contribute to the liability exposure of the surgeon. The administration of drugs and the care and maintenance of office and hospital equipment are matters that require the surgeon's awareness and understanding. No drug or item or equipment should ever be used without a full knowledge of its function and of possible complications.

SPECIAL AREAS OF RISK FOR THE GYNECOLOGIC SURGEON

In addition to the issues raised above, the gynecologic surgeon has a unique level of liability exposure in the performance of laparoscopy, laparotomy, cancer screening, hysterectomy, oophorectomy, abortion, and conception control. Professional services related to these special areas of risk should incorporate the highest degree and quality of communication, informed consent, and attention to detail in recordkeeping and case follow-up. The surgeon who knows the areas of legal risk is forearmed and able to anticipate the occasional poor outcome or small error and deal more effectively with it.

Fistulas

Pelvic surgery—particularly total abdominal hysterectomy or vaginal hysterectomy and repair—may lead to the development of vesicovaginal or ureteral fistulas. Rectovaginal fistulas are likely to occur with vaginal repair, abdominal hysterectomy, incision and drainage of a Bartholin abscess, sigmoid resection, and hemorrhoidectomy.

When injury is recognized while an operation is in progress, it should be repaired at once. However, some fistulas will be recognized in the first days after a surgical procedure; in such instances, the surgeon may wish to delay repair until inflammation, local swelling, and identified infection have diminished.

Hysterectomy

Total hysterectomy is the fourth most frequently performed surgical procedure in the United States. Today, many hysterectomies are performed for conditions that are potentially dangerous, partially disabling, or simply uncomfortable. Therefore, because of the relatively elective nature of the procedure in some instances, and because of the risk of infection or injury to the urinary tract and other organs, special attention to medical-legal concerns such as informed consent is appropriate.

Dilatation and Curettage

Dilatation and curettage ranks second in frequency among surgical procedures. Although most physicians consider it to be a minor operative procedure, there is a risk of complication, such as perforation of the uterus, and the surgeon should be fully prepared to deal with any complications arising during or after the procedure.

Abortion

Another procedure considered relatively routine, abortion is a zone of risk for the gynecologist who is less than experienced or who is providing services to women at high risk, in the later stages of pregnancy, or in inadequately equipped facilities. Complications and injuries that often lead to lawsuits include uterine perforation, cervical laceration, hemorrhage, incomplete removal of the fetus and placenta, and anesthetic problems.

Sterilization and Contraception

Two emerging zones of risk for the gynecologist in terms of professional liability are contraception and sterilization procedures. Inappropriately prescribing or inserting of contraceptive methods or devices, ignoring or failing to identify contraindications, and failing to adequately manage complications all expose the physician to lawsuits.

Surgical laparoscopy for sterilization may lead to electrosurgical injuries or hemorrhage, but more commonly the gynecologist is sued on the basis of failures of informed consent or of negligence in the performance of the procedure: the patient expects to be sterile and then becomes pregnant. Such cases lead to claims of "wrongful birth" or "wrongful conception." There may be recovery even if the fetus is aborted. Therefore, it is imperative that the gynecologist explain in detail and to the patient's full understanding the possibility of a sterilization procedure's being unsuccessful and the consequent risk, however remote, of a pregnancy. Since most states now recognize the right of action of wrongful birth, this is one area of professional liability risk that must be effectively managed. It can be, with a careful discussion of the procedure with the patient.

Incident Management

Every physician encounters unexpected problems, unanticipated complications, and actual errors of skill or judgment. The management of these events is critical to whether a lawsuit results. The techniques of incident management have been mentioned in previous sections of this chapter, but a full treatment follows.

The occurrence of an incident involving injury to the patient, however insignificant to the physician, should be treated professionally and diligently. At the first opportunity, a full report of the incident should be shared with the insurer; in a hospital, the incident should be reported to the risk management team or the legal counsel, as well as the chief of service or department head. But first, attention must be paid the patient and her problem resolved.

The first and most important step is to avoid concealment, subterfuge, lying, or minimization of the injury in communicating with the patient and her family. Honesty is the best protection from a legal viewpoint and the most effective medical course to follow. A calm, uninterrupted conversation should be conducted with the patient, explaining precisely what occurred and what will be necessary to mitigate the damage. A full disclosure of what occurred is absolutely essential, but the surgeon should avoid embellishing the facts with details that will create anxiety or apprehension beyond the scope of the actual problem. Certain terms should be avoided in conversation: the surgeon should not mention "negligence" or "malpractice"; similarly he or she should not confess to "fault" but rather explain that complications occur and, referring back to the properly conducted process of informed consent, remind the patient that such an event was discussed as a possibility.

For the repair of injuries caused in the course of surgery, a second process of informed consent may be necessary, unless the error is corrected during the course of the original procedure. In either case, the explanation of the repair procedure must be quite detailed, and the risk and complications that relate to that procedure must be fully explained. The scope of permission granted in the process of informed consent will weigh heavily in a court's

consideration of whether the additional surgery was necessary, and whether the patient was appropriately prepared with information and explanations.

Informed Consent: Surgery by Residents and Substitutes

Hospitals affiliated with institutions for health care education and training are faced with the special problem of consent to surgery extending to physicians other than the attending physician who is known to the patient. Although the hospital and medical staff may understand the rather routine

---

[NAME OF HOSPITAL]
CONSENT TO HOSPITAL ADMISSION AND
MEDICAL TREATMENT

Name of Patient: _____

Name of Attending Physician(s): _____

Date of Admission: _____ Time: _____ (AM) (PM)

1. I, (or [NAME OF AUTHORIZED REPRESENTATIVE] acting on behalf of) [NAME OF PATIENT], suffering from a condition requiring hospital care, hereby consent to the rendering of such care, which may include routine diagnostic procedures and such medical treatment as the named attending physician(s) or others of the hospital's medical staff consider to be necessary.

2. I understand that the practice of medicine and surgery is not an exact science and that diagnosis and treatment may involve risks of injury, or even death. I acknowledge that no guarantees have been made to me as to the result of examination or treatment in this hospital.

3. I understand that:
   (A) It is customary, absent emergency or extraordinary circumstances, that no substantial procedures are performed upon a patient unless and until he or she has had an opportunity to discuss them with the physician or other health professional to the patient's satisfaction;
   (B) Each patient has the right to consent, or to refuse consent, to any proposed procedure or therapeutic course; and
   (C) No patient will be involved in any research or experimental procedure without his or her full knowledge and consent.

4. I understand that many of the physicians on the staff of this hospital, including the attending physician(s) named above, are not employees or agents of the hospital but, rather, are independent contractors who have been granted the privilege of using its facilities for the care and treatment of their patients. Further, I realize that among those who attend patients at this hospital are medical, nursing, and other health care personnel in training who, unless requested otherwise, may be present during patient care, as a part of their education. Still or motion pictures and closed circuit television monitoring of patient care also may be used for education purposes, unless a patient expressly requests otherwise.

5. This form has been fully explained to me, and I am satisfied that I understand its content and significance.

Date of Execution: _____

_____   _____
[SIGNATURE OF PATIENT]   [SIGNATURE OF WITNESS]

(If patient is unable to consent or is a minor, complete the following:) Patient [is a minor _____ years of age] (is unable to consent because]:

_____

_____   _____
[SIGNATURE OF LEGAL GUARDIAN OR CLOSEST AVAILABLE RELATIVE]   [SIGNATURE OF WITNESS]

FIG. 3–1 Consent form.

and necessary involvement of surgeons-in-training and the performance of surgery by physicians other than those to whom the patient has specifically granted consent, it is unwise to presume that the patient gives "implied consent" by entering a teaching hospital.

Consent forms for the teaching hospital should include a reference to the fact that residents and substitute physicians may either perform the surgery in its entirety, or assist in the surgery to which the patient has been asked to consent (Fig. 3–1). Additionally, the attending physician should explain to the patient that such participation or substitution may occur. If the patient objects, such objection should be noted in the record and every effort made to prevent violation of the objection. If the institution cannot ensure compliance, then, except in an emergency, the patient should be encouraged to utilize a different institution.

Emergencies provide the only defensible exception to consent to substitutes, and they should be thoroughly documented as such.

Conclusion

Gynecologic surgeons have several opportunities to manage and control their legal risk, and several corresponding periods of special exposure. Diligence in practice, both in the office and the hospital, and attention to those occasions and the procedures which carry heightened risk for the physician, will permit the most effective risk and incident management and the diminution of liability problems. Surgeons should create and maintain a strong, complete presurgical record; they should personally perform the functions involved in the process of obtaining informed consent; they should respond to complications in a timely and responsible manner, involving the patient when possible; and they should give equal attention to the postoperative relationship with the patient.

The law offers protection and privilege for the gynecologic surgeon, and careful practitioners will familiarize themselves with local rules and regulations, as well as general concepts such as those explained here. In this way, they may not only function as surgeons but also be comfortable with the liability that is a basic element of their position of trust and their professional relationship with patients.

Bibliography

Alton W: Malpractice: A Trial Lawyer's Advice for Physicians. Boston, Little, Brown, 1977

Fiscina SF: Medical Law for the Attending Physician: A Case Oriented Analysis. Carbondale, Ill, Southern Illinois University Press, 1982

Holder AR: Medical Malpractice Law, 2 ed. New York, Wiley, 1978

King JH, Jr: The Law of Medical Malpractice in a Nutshell. St. Paul, Minn, West Publishing Company, 1977

Kramer C: Medical Malpractice. New York, Practising Law Institute, 1976

Levine M: Surgical Malpractice. LaMesa, California, Trans-Media, 1970

Pegalis S, Wachsman H: American Law of Medical Malpractice. 3 vols. Rochester, New York Lawyers Co-operative Publishing Company, 1980

Pollack R: Clinical Aspects of Malpractice. Oradel, New Jersey, Medical Economics Books, 1980

Prosser WL: Handbook of the Law of Torts. St. Paul, Minn, West Publishing Company, 1971

Richards EP III, Rathbun KC: Medical Risk Management: Preventive Legal Strategies for Health Care Providers. Rockville, Maryland, Aspen Publications, 1983

Rosoff J: Informed Consent. Rockville, Maryland, Aspen Publications, 1981

National Center for Health Statistics: Utilization of Short-Stay Hospitals, Annual Summaries and Surgical Operations in Short-Stay Hospitals, U.S., selected years 1973–1980. U.S. Dept. of Health and Human Services, Government Printing Office; Socio-Economic Factbook for Surgery, 1982 Edition. Chicago, American College of Surgeons

Chapter 4

Anatomy of the Female Pelvis

For the pelvic surgeon, a knowledge of the precise anatomical relationships of the parietal and visceral structures of the female pelvis is as essential as are the diagnostic and technical skills. The foundation stones of successful gynecologic surgery are laid by visualizing the anatomical components of the abdomen and pelvis with such a keen understanding of the various surgical planes and spaces that an operative procedure could be performed as though the tissue layers were transparent. Without this knowledge of pelvic anatomy, surgery ceases to be a science and an art and becomes merely a technical procedure that may be both hazardous to the patient and a constant threat to the surgeon. Although a discussion of the anatomy of the female pelvis in its entirety is beyond the scope of this presentation, certain anatomical details should be a part of the fundamental knowledge of every gynecologic surgeon. The student who wishes to pursue the intricacies of pelvic anatomy in greater detail is directed to a standard anatomy text.

The anatomy of the female pelvis has a different perspective for the pelvic surgeon than for the basic scientist. The gynecologic surgeon has some difficulty in integrating basic anatomy into surgical practice until extensive practical experience in operative gynecology has been acquired. For this reason, errors in surgical judgement confront the surgeon more frequently during earlier surgical experiences than at a later period of practice.

The key anatomical landmarks that are important to the pelvic surgeon in performing a gynecologic operation include the planes and spaces in the pelvis; the close relationships between the urinary, reproductive, and gastrointestinal tracts; the vascular, lymphatic, and collateral circulation of the female pelvis; and the neuromuscular innervation and support of the pelvic viscera. Many of these subjects, particularly the lymphatic drainage of the pelvis, are discussed as they pertain to a specific operative procedure and so will not be discussed here.

The Pelvic Viscera

The female reproductive tract occupies a unique yet precarious position in the pelvis. It is developmentally interposed between the bladder anteriorly and the rectum posteriorly. The embryologic anlagen of these three visceral structures are so intimately entwined that it is impossible to envision a disease process occurring in one organ that does not have the potential to involve the others. Removal of the uterus from its location between the adjacent bladder and rectum requires not only surgical skill but an understanding of the fascial planes, ligaments, and vessels that involve the uterus and adjacent viscera.

When the female pelvis is viewed from the anterior and superior aspects (Fig. 4–1), the close approximation of the sigmoid colon, the uterus, and the bladder can be seen. The broad ligament, which is adjacent to the uterus, is a filmy structure that is composed of a double layer of peritoneum between which the important blood vessels, nerves, and lymphatics course to the uterus and adjacent structures. It passes from the lateral margins of the uterus to the lateral pelvic wall. Its upper margins contain three diverging structures. The most anterior of these is the round ligament, which passes laterally and ventrally to reach the abdominal inguinal ring.

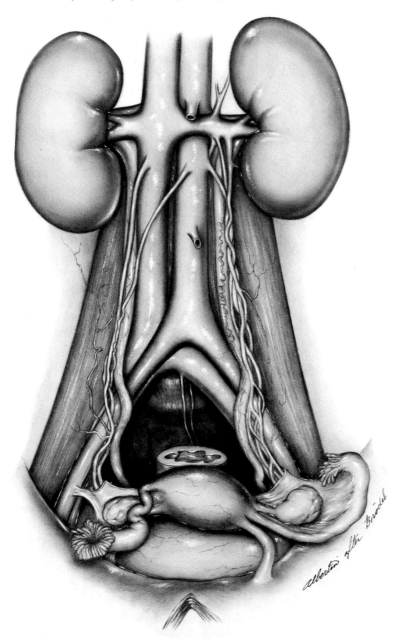

FIG. 4-1 Abdominal and pelvic anatomy of the female reproductive tract.

The most posterior structure is the ovarian ligament, which is attached to the posterior leaf of the broad ligament and extends from the uterine pole of the ovary to the side of the uterus just below the origin of the fallopian tube. Adjacent to the mesovarium is the suspensory ligament of the ovary, the infundibulopelvic ligament, which extends laterally between the two layers of the broad ligament from the tubal extremity of the ovary to the lateral pelvic wall. This ligament forms the lateral portion of the free boundary of both broad ligaments. The central and most superior of the three structures running in the upper border of the broad ligament is the fallopian (uterine) tube. The fallopian tube has four parts, the first of which is the infundibulum, a funnellike dilatation that opens into the abdominal cavity by way of the external ostium, which is surrounded by numerous diverging processes, the fimbriae. One of these is much longer than the rest and extends along the free border of the mesosalpinx to the tubal extremity of the ovary. This structure, the fimbria ovarica, has recently been shown to contain smooth muscle fibers, which contract at the time of ovulation. It is important in drawing the fimbriae of the tube to the ovary. The second part of the fallopian tube is the ampulla, which progressively narrows, terminating at the third portion of the tube, the narrow isthmus. The ampullary-isthmic junction is an important anatomical landmark that is involved in gamete migration through the oviduct. The lumen of the isthmus is relatively straight but is indented by longitudinal folds that have an important physiologic role in the transport mechanism of the fertilized ovum to the uterine ostia. The fourth part of the fallopian tube is the intramural or interstitial portion, which passes through the uterine wall, opening into the uterine cavity at both cornua. Although this is one of the narrowest portions of the tube, surprisingly it has the lowest incidence of tubal pregnancy because if it becomes infected, it is more likely to become totally obstructed than partly so.

The *bladder* is a retroperitoneal viscus that is located behind the symphysis pubis and rests on the anterior portion of the urogenital diaphragm, vaginal fornix, and lower uterine segment (Fig. 4–2). The base of the bladder is closely related to the lower uterine segment and the anterior fornix of the vagina. The trigone of the bladder is contiguous with the upper one-third of the vagina and anterior fornix, while the remainder of the bladder base rests intimately on the cervix and inferior portion of the lower uterine segment. Therefore, when the bladder is being dissected free from the uterus and cervix during the course of a total hysterectomy, the most vulnerable portion of the bladder wall is the portion that is above the trigone. These anatomical relationships are the principal reason that injury to the bladder base during a total hysterectomy rarely causes any damage to the trigone or ureterovesical junction. Should injury to the bladder occur during hysterectomy, it usually occurs approximately 3 cm to 4 cm or more above the trigone and is easily repaired at the time of surgery. Should the injury fail to be recognized at surgery, a vesicovaginal fistula may result. Fortunately, this defect may be repaired through the vagina without concern for injury to the trigone or ureter, which are rarely involved. The peritoneum over the superior and posterior wall of the bladder is reflected onto the lower uterine segment and becomes densely fused to the uterus as its serosal surface. This vesicouterine plica forms the anterior cul-de-sac of the pelvis, although it is only of limited clinical importance. In rare cases, when the uterus has been removed and a subsequent hernia occurs in this region

of the pelvic floor, the small bowel may herniate through the anterior segment of the urogenital diaphragm. Such rare cases of pelvic enterocele formation are more difficult to correct anatomically. The exact location of an enterocele should be carefully evaluated before any reparative attempt is undertaken.

The bladder has been opened for a view of the interior in Figure 4–3. The three openings in the base of the bladder are the orifices of the two ureters and the urethra. The interureteric ridge is a slightly curved, transverse fold of the mucosa that extends between the two ureteral orifices and forms the superior boundary of the vesical trigone. The three angles of the trigone are represented by the orifices of the urethra and the two ureters. This area is redder in color and is free from the folds that characterize the remainder of the bladder mucosa. Should the bladder become chronically infected for a prolonged period of time, the bladder mucosa becomes thicker and marked by deep, irregular trabeculations that are the result of the thickened and fibrosed submucosa that develops in response to the inflammatory process. Such changes are characteristic of chronic cystitis and produce not only thickening of the wall but also a reduction in the bladder capacity, which causes the symptoms of urinary frequency and urgency. The ureteral orifices are separated by 3 mm to 5 mm, depending on the contraction or distention of the bladder wall. The terminal ureters pass through the vesical wall (5 mm–7 mm) and into the bladder at the lateral and superior angles of the trigone. During their medial diversion into the trigone, the terminal 3 cm to 4 cm of ureter passes along the anterior fornix from a position immediately adjacent to the lateral vaginal wall. Although the precise position of the trigone may vary slightly, depending on the length of the anterior vaginal wall, it can be identified easily, since the female urethra is approximately 4 cm in length and opens into the bladder at the base of the trigone. The trigone itself is approximately 2.5 cm to 3.0 cm in length from the internal urethral orifice to the interureteric ridge. Since the length of the anterior vaginal wall is 8 cm or slightly more in the adult female, the superior margin of the trigone of the bladder is 1 cm or more inferior to the apex of the vaginal fornix. Anatomically, it is important to understand that the trigone rests on the upper one-third of the vagina and anterior fornix.

The relationships of the abdominal and pelvic ureter are important. In general, the ureter measures approximately 25 cm to 30 cm in total length in the adult. The abdominal ureter is approximately 13 cm to 15 cm in length and courses retroperitoneally along the anteromedial aspect of the psoas

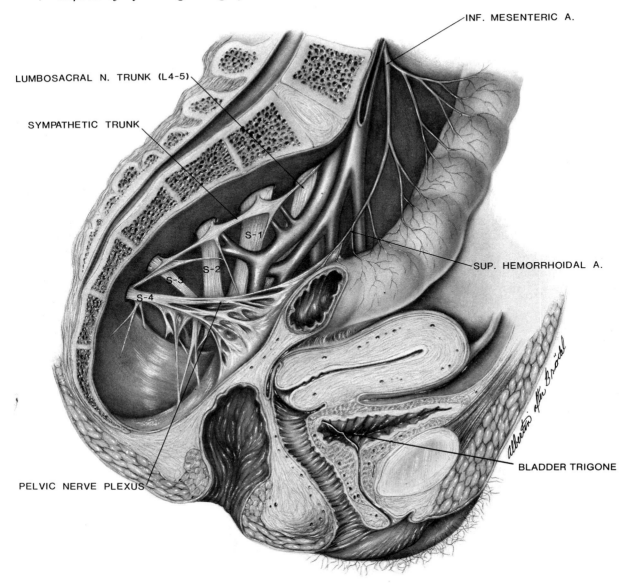

LUMBOSACRAL N. TRUNK (L4-5)

SYMPATHETIC TRUNK

INF. MESENTERIC A.

S-1

S-2

S-3

S-4

SUP. HEMORRHOIDAL A.

BLADDER TRIGONE

PELVIC NERVE PLEXUS

FIG. 4–2 Sagittal view of female pelvis, including relationships of pelvic viscera, vasculature, and nerve plexuses. S2, S3, and S4 include both somatic nerves to the pelvic diaphragm and parasympathetic nerves to the bladder detrusor. These fibers join with the sympathetic fibers from T11, T12, S1, and S2 (hypogastric nerve) to form the pelvic plexus.

muscle throughout its abdominal route to the pelvis as shown in Figure 4–1. The medial border of the right ureter lies in close approximation to the lateral margin of the vena cava. This has created some anatomical difficulty in dissecting the paracaval lymph nodes from the inferior vena cava and necessitates the careful lateral retraction of the ureter, should a lymph node dissection be performed in this region. The right ureter crosses the common iliac artery at or just beyond its bifurcation. The pelvic ureter, which is approximately equal in length to the abdominal segment (13 cm–15 cm), passes along the posterolateral aspect of the pelvis and anterior to the hypogastric artery. Here it courses along the obturator muscle to the region in the greater sciatic notch to the level of the ischial spine. In this part of its course, the ureter lies between the obturator nerve and the anterior division

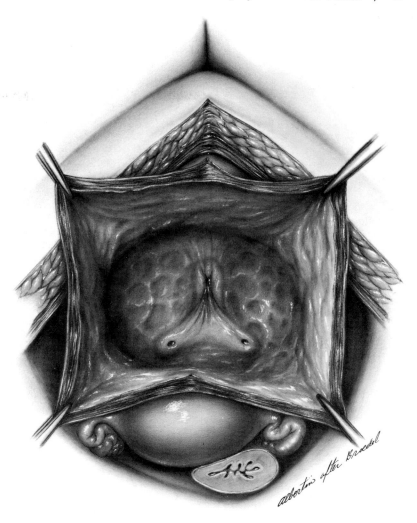

FIG. 4–3 Opened view of bladder showing relationship of trigone and bladder base to adjacent uterus and vagina.

of the hypogastric artery on its lateral side and the peritoneum of the cul-de-sac of Douglas on its medial side. At this point, the ureter turns forward and medially, passing lateral to the uterosacral ligament, through the cardinal ligament and beneath the uterine artery and vein, approximately 1.5 cm to 2 cm lateral to the internal cervical os. It continues slightly medially for approximately 2 cm to 3 cm where it comes in close approximation to the anterior vaginal fornix and passes medially to enter the base of the bladder at the trigone. Its intramural (3 mm) and submucosal (7 mm) portions give a combined length to the bladder segment of the ureter of 1 cm or more. The ureter opens obliquely into the ureterovesical junction. The critical anatomical points where ureteral injury can occur include the juxtaposition of the ureter beneath the uterine artery, its medial course along the lower portion of

the cardinal ligament and anterior vaginal fornix before it enters the base of the bladder, its course along the base of the broad ligament just lateral to the uterosacral ligament, and its position along the medial aspect of the infundibulopelvic ligament where it crosses the pelvic brim.

The lower portion of the sigmoid colon passes medially into the midline of the pelvis, where it becomes closely related to the uterus and vagina and is continuous with the rectum below the peritoneal reflection of the cul-de-sac of Douglas (see Fig. 4–2). The rectum is closely situated against the posterior fornix and vaginal wall, from which it is separated by a thin layer of loose areolar tissue. Fortunately, the rectum is rarely in direct line of surgical injury at the time of hysterectomy because it passes retroperitoneally beneath the cul-de-sac of Douglas and is not normally attached to the uterus or the cervix proper. However, the rectum and terminal sigmoid can become densely adherent to the cervix as a result of scarring and fixation of the cul-de-sac, as is frequently seen in cases of pelvic endometriosis and pelvic inflammatory disease. The rectum passes through the posterior aspect of the pelvic floor, directly behind the urogenital diaphragm, where it is supported by the puborectalis portion of the levator ani muscles (Fig. 4–4). It terminates in the anal canal and anus and serves principally as a reservoir for the fecal content of the lower colon prior to the voluntary fecal expulsion through the anal canal during the process of defecation. The anal canal is approximately 3 cm to 4 cm in length and serves as a flattened, empty conduit of the lower colon that terminates in the anus. Unless there has been relaxation of the pelvic diaphragm, caused by age or multiple childbearing, the anal canal usually remains empty except during the process of defecation. This portion of the colon is bounded superiorly by the levator ani muscles and inferiorly by the anus (see Fig. 4–4). Its principal function is in producing fecal continence. The physiology of defecation and the extrinsic and intrinsic sphincter mechanisms are discussed further in Chapter 28. There is little opportunity to traumatize the anterior wall of the rectum during a hysterectomy if the proper tissue plane has been entered by reflecting the cul-de-sac peritoneum from the posterior aspect of the cervix. This space is usually quite avascular unless the dissection extends into the lateral margins of the rectum where it receives its blood supply from the inferior hemorrhoidal vessels. Because of these favorable anatom-

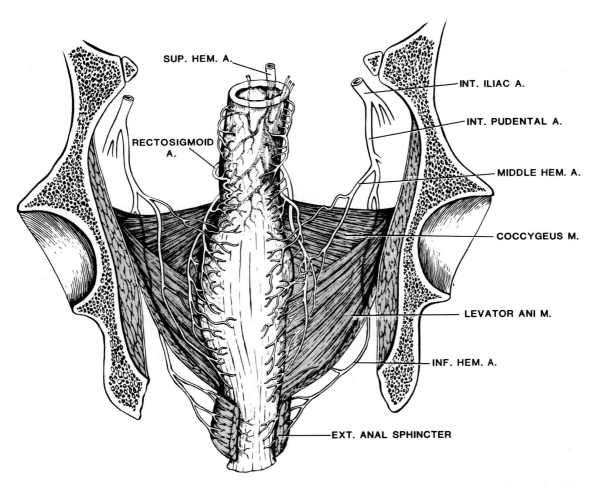

FIG. 4–4 Rectosigmoid colon and anal canal, showing collateral arterial circulation from superior hemorrhoidal (inferior mesenteric), middle hemorrhoidal (hypogastric or internal iliac), and inferior hemorrhoidal (internal pudendal) arteries.

ical relationships, the rectum is injured infrequently during pelvic surgery in a ratio of approximately 1 to 4, as compared to the bladder.

Musculofascial Support of the Pelvis

The uterus is principally supported by the reflection of the endopelvic fascia into two principal ligaments, the cardinal and uterosacral ligaments. The cardinal ligaments are a component of the pubovesicocervical fascia, which surrounds the cervix and the base of the bladder and urethra, passes forward to join the paravesical fascia, and continues laterally to attach to each pelvic wall. Each ligament is located at the base of the broad ligament. These ligaments are extensive and strong and provide the major support to the uterus above the pelvic diaphragm.

The posterior reflection of this endopelvic fascia continues as the uterosacral ligaments, which pass around the lateral margins of the rectum. These ligaments form the lateral boundaries of the cul-de-sac of Douglas before inserting onto the periosteum of the fourth sacral vertebra (Fig. 4–5). The uterosacral ligaments serve to pull the cervix and

lower uterine segment backward at the point where they are attached to the posterior aspect of the cervix. The ligaments assist in maintaining the uterus in an anteflexed position and provide some anatomical support to prevent descensus of the uterus through the urogenital diaphragm. In addition to the fascial component, the uterosacral ligaments contain important nerve fibers from the hypogastric and sacral plexuses, with both pre- and postganglionic fibers of the parasympathetic and sympathetic nerves. The sympathetic nerves include pain fibers to the uterus and cervix.

The third and most prominent ligament is the round ligament, which arises from the anterior surface of the uterus near the origin of the fallopian tube. It courses beneath the anterior leaf of the broad ligament and passes laterally to enter the abdominal (internal) inguinal ring. This ligament is a homologue of the gubernaculum testis that becomes attached to the Müllerian ducts during embryologic development. It passes through the inguinal canal, accompanied by the ilioinguinal nerve and the vulvar branch of the genitofemoral nerve, and inserts into the labium majus. During its development, this ligament brings segments of peritoneum into the

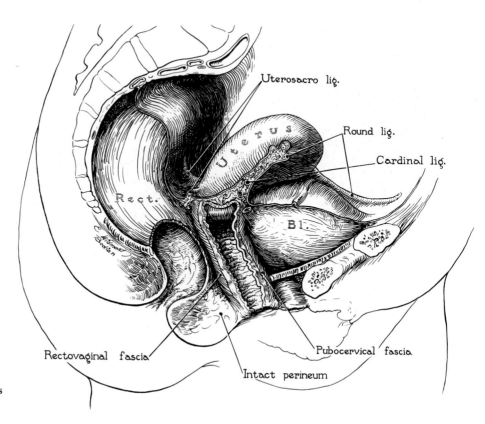

FIG. 4–5 Ligamentous supports of the uterus.

inguinal canal, which may become cystic during adult life; a condition known as a cyst of the canal of Nuck. Endometriosis has also been found in this segment of the inguinal canal. The round ligament is accompanied by a small arterial branch from the ovarian artery and vein (Sampson's artery) and by a small branch from the inferior epigastric artery, which it crosses in its course through the internal inguinal ring, as shown in Figure 4–6. Therefore, the round ligament receives its blood supply from two sources: proximally, from the ovarian artery (Sampson's artery) and more distally, in the region of the inguinal canal, from the inferior epigastric artery. In this region of the anatomy, the boundaries of Hesselbach's triangle are clearly evident (see Fig.

4–6), including the inferior epigastric artery as the lateral boundary, the edge of the rectus muscle as the medial boundary, and the medial portion of the inguinal ligament as the inferior boundary. It is easy to visualize the sites of inguinal hernias from this view, noting the easy access of small bowel or omentum through a dilated internal inguinal ring (indirect hernia) should the attenuated fibers of the transversalis muscle surrounding the entrance to the inguinal ring become weakened. A direct, congenital hernia on the medial side of the inferior epigastric vessels passes through the center of Hesselbach's triangle. An inguinal hernia is uncommon in the female. A femoral hernia is more common, occurring through the larger aperture beneath the

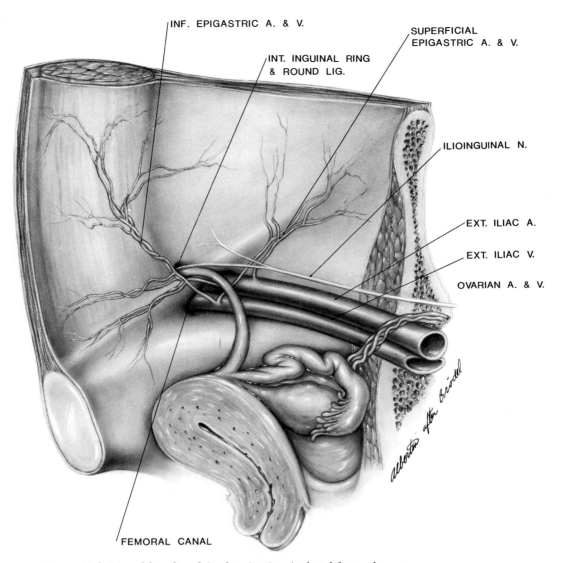

INF. EPIGASTRIC A. & V.

INT. INGUINAL RING & ROUND LIG.

SUPERFICIAL EPIGASTRIC A. & V.

ILIOINGUINAL N.

EXT. ILIAC A.

EXT. ILIAC V.

OVARIAN A. & V.

FEMORAL CANAL

FIG. 4–6 Sagittal view of female pelvis, showing inguinal and femoral anatomy.

inguinal ligament where the external iliac vessels pass through the femoral canal. With age, the femoral ring may dilate because of weakening of the ligament and of the lacunar fascia that attaches the inguinal ligament to the underlying pectineus muscle on the anterior pubic ramus. Hernias in this region are usually present on the medial side of the femoral vessels, adjacent to the lacunar ligament, where the canal contains mostly adipose tissue (see Fig. 4–6).

Posteriorly, the cul-de-sac of Douglas is bounded by the uterosacral ligaments that pass from the posterior aspect of the cervix along the lateral margins of the rectum, to insert into the anterior surface of the fourth sacral body. At the deepest part of the cul-de-sac of Douglas, the peritoneum reverses its direction and passes from the posterior surface of the cervix to the anterior wall of the rectum. This peritoneal space is an important anatomical land-

mark because it identifies the position of the lower colon where this becomes attached to the posterior vagina and vaginal fornix. A recent study by Kuhn and Hollyock of the anatomy of the cul-de-sac of Douglas demonstrates that it extends from the attachment of the uterosacral ligaments to a depth of approximately 5.0 cm to 5.5 cm adjacent to the rectovaginal septum, in both nulliparous and multiparous women. Therefore, it is quite evident that when this peritoneal space is placed on a stretch, it can extend nearly halfway along the posterior vaginal wall. In the Kuhn and Hollyock study, there appears to be no relationship between the depth of the cul-de-sac and the presence of an enterocele, a correlation that was previously considered to be anatomically important.

The pelvic floor is principally composed of the levator ani and coccygeus muscles. As shown in Figure 4–7, the coccygeus muscle forms the posterior

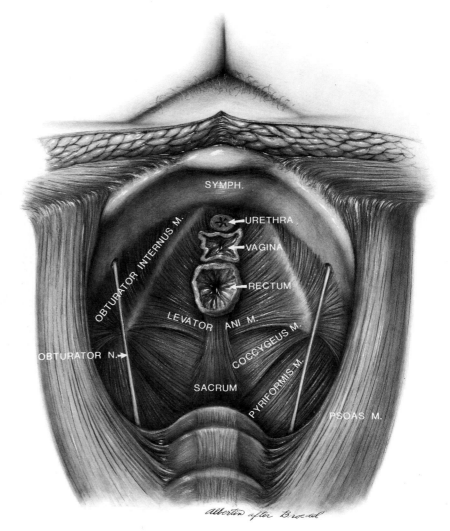

FIG. 4–7 Anatomy of the pelvic floor.

part of the pelvic floor, arising from the ischial tuberosity and inserting into the lateral margins of the lower sacral and upper coccygeal vertebrae. The levator ani muscle is composed of three parts: the ileococcygeus muscle, which lies most posteriorly and attaches to the coccyx; the pubococcygeus, which lies in an intermediate position and attaches posteriorly to the anococcygeal raphe; and the puborectalis muscle, which lies most medially, encircles the anus and vagina, and passes superior to the urogenital diaphragm. This third portion serves as a skeletal muscular support for the anus, vagina, and upper urethra. As shown in the lateral view (Fig. 4–8), the most anterior portion of the levator ani muscle is seen to arise from the inferior ramus of the pelvic bone. The remainder of the

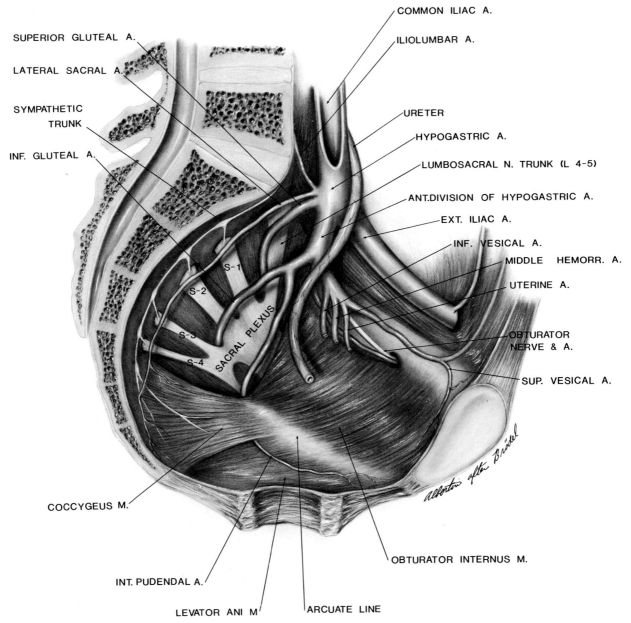

FIG. 4–8 Anatomy of the pelvic floor, showing relationships of pelvic musculature, divisions of hypogastric artery, the pelvic ureter, and lumbosacral and sacral nerve plexus.

muscle arises from the arcuate line or tendinous arch of the obturator internus muscle along the lateral wall of the pelvis. The fascia overlying the obturator internus muscle is thickened to form this tendinous arch, from which most of the levator ani muscle arises. Only the most medial part of the levator muscle arises from pubic bone. The three portions of the levator ani compose the principal part of the pelvic floor, which is the primary support of the pelvic viscera. This muscular diaphragm is pierced in the midline by the urethra, vagina, and rectum, each of which is supported by fibers from the medial portion of this striated muscle (see Fig. 4–7). The uterus may herniate through the pelvic diaphragm to produce descensus uteri, should the muscles become weakened and stretched by age or childbirth. When the pelvic floor weakens, the cardinal and uterosacral ligaments weaken as well, with subsequent descent of the uterus. This is followed by elongation of the round ligaments, which permits retrocession and retroversion of the uterus to occur (Fig. 4–9). Further weakening of the pelvic floor and urogenital diaphragm with elongation of the pelvic ligaments permits uterine de-

scensus, which may finally reach the degree of total procidentia.

The obturator internus muscle arises from the inner surface of the anterior or lateral wall of the pelvis, where it surrounds the obturator foramen, being attached to the inferior ramus of the pubis and ischium. Its lower part is covered by a portion of the levator ani muscle. Its posterior margins arise from the inner surface of the iliac bone near the hip. It also arises from the pelvic surface of the obturator membrane. It converges to insert on the surface of the ischium between its spine and tuberosity. The ischiorectal fossa is bounded laterally by the obturator internus and medially by the external surface of the levator ani muscle. The internal pudendal nerve and vessels pass through this space, called Alcock's canal, to reach the perineum and vulva.

Nerve Supply to the Abdomen and Pelvis

The nerve supply to the abdominal wall, including sensory and motor fibers to the skin and abdominal

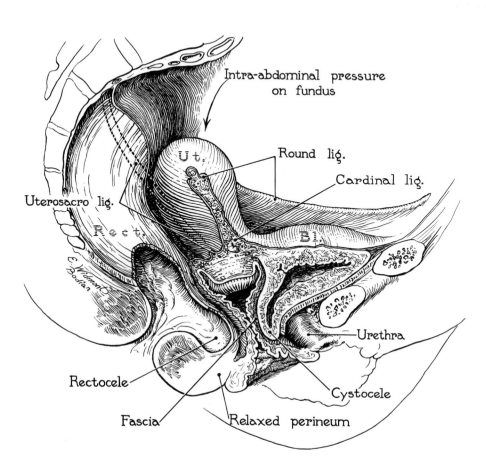

FIG. 4–9 Failure of normal supports permits descent of uterus, as well as cystocele and rectocele formation.

muscles, arises from the thoracic nerves T6 to T12 (Fig. 4–10). The thoracic nerves continue from their intercostal branches along the lower rib cage and enter the abdominal wall, where they pass forward between the internal oblique and transversalis muscles. After entering the rectus sheath and rectus muscles, the terminal branches of the nerves pass through the anterior rectus fascia and supply the skin as cutaneous nerves. The 12th thoracic nerve is joined by L1 and forms the iliohypogastric nerve that supplies motor fibers to the internal and external oblique and transversalis muscle along with sensory fibers to the skin of the upper and lateral aspect of the thigh. It passes medially, where it communicates with the ilioinguinal nerve and car-

ries sensory fibers to the subcutaneous tissue and skin of the external inguinal ring and the skin over the symphysis pubis. The umbilicus, an important gynecologic landmark, is innervated by the T10 dermatome. It is a reference point for the fourth lumbar vertebra and the bifurcation of the aorta.

As shown in Figure 4–2, the pelvic organs are innervated by both sympathetic and parasympathetic nerves. The abdominal sympathetic nerves pass to the pelvis through four pathways: (1) some fibers follow the abdominal sympathetic chain into the pelvis; (2) other fibers traverse the sympathetic plexus with the ovarian and (3) superior hemorrhoidal vessels; while (4) most of the sympathetic fibers enter the para-aortic plexus and leave the

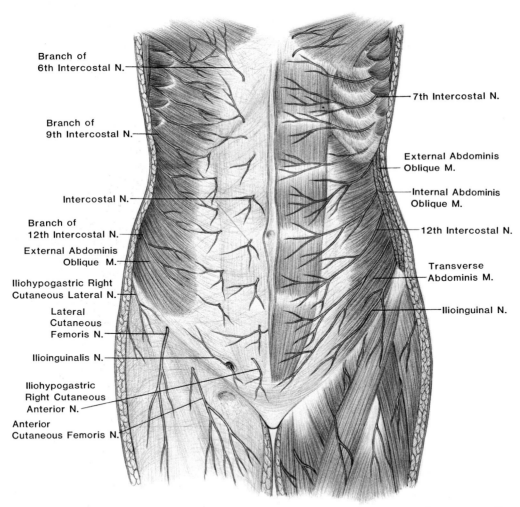

FIG. 4–10 Nerve supply to the abdomen. (*Right*) Deep innervation of T6–T12 to the transversalis, internal oblique, and rectus muscles. (*Left*) Superficial distribution, including cutaneous nerves, after penetration and innervation of the external oblique muscle and fascia. Innervation of the groin and thigh is also shown.

abdomen as the hypogastric (presacral) plexus, principally from spinal cord levels L1 through L4. The presacral plexus crosses the pelvic brim and divides into right and left parts to enter two pelvic nerve bundles. These presacral nerves pass deep into the pelvis to become a part of the pelvic plexus (Fig. 4–11). The deep pelvic plexus is further divided into an anterior subdivision, which provides a vesical plexus where it innervates the base of the bladder and urethra, and a posterior division, which sends fibers to the uterine fundus, cervix, vagina, rectosigmoid colon, and anal canal. The parasympathetic nerves enter the pelvis through the second, third, and fourth sacral nerves (S2, S3, S4) and their preganglionic fibers are distributed to the pelvic organs through the pelvic nerve plexus. This plexus also receives sympathetic postganglionic fibers that originate in spinal cord levels L1 through L4 and reach the pelvis by the described pathways. These sympathetic fibers pass through the pelvis through the hypogastric plexus, and both the sympathetic and parasympathetic nerves enter the uterus from within the broad ligaments, as well as along the uterosacral ligaments. The major sensory nerves from the pelvic viscera are carried along the sympathetic nerve plexus to reach their origin in the spinal cord, principally along L2 to L4. For this reason, uterine discomfort is usually registered in the lower abdomen or hypogastrium, which is the regional area innervated by the lumbar nerves. This neurologic phenomenon is understandable in view of the fact that the uterus arose, embryologically, from the mesothelium of the abdominal cavity, along the developing lumbar vertebrae. Pain stimuli originating from the cervix are usually registered through the sacral sympathetic chain and conducted through the uterosacral ligaments to the sacral sympathetic plexus from S2, S3, and S4. Therefore, pain from the cervix is frequently referred to the lumbosacral region.

The obturator nerve is the only motor nerve that arises from the lumbar plexus and passes through the pelvis without innervating any of the pelvic structures. It arises from the anterior divisions of

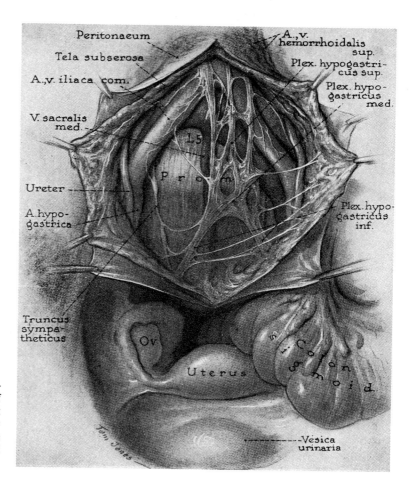

FIG. 4–11 Presacral nerve plexus, showing passage of sympathetic trunk over bifurcation of aorta. Note division of trunk into left and right presacral nerves. (Curtis AH, Anson BJ, Ashley FL, et al: The anatomy of the pelvic autonomic nerves in relation to gynecology. Surg Gynecol Obstet 75:743, 1942.)

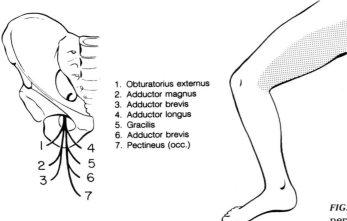

1. Obturatorius externus
2. Adductor magnus
3. Adductor brevis
4. Adductor longus
5. Gracilis
6. Adductor brevis
7. Pectineus (occ.)

FIG. 4–12 Obturator nerve (L2–L4) motor and sensory innervation.

L2, L3, and L4, emerges from the medial border of the psoas muscle near the brim of the pelvis beneath the common iliac vessels and passes lateral to the hypogastric vessels and ureter, where it runs along the lateral wall of the pelvis to enter the obturator foramen with the obturator vessels. It is a motor nerve to the adductor muscles of the thigh (adductor magnus, longus, and brevis, and the gracilis). Injury to this nerve may occur during radical pelvic surgery when the obturator fossa is dissected and will produce not only motor adductor dysfunction but sensory loss over the medial aspect of the thigh (Fig. 4–12). In general, this loss of adductor function can be compensated for by other adductor muscles of the lower extremity.

The lumbosacral nerve trunk contains the major fibers that innervate the striated muscles of the pelvic floor and the lower extremities. As shown in Figure 4–8, this large nerve trunk rests on the piriformis muscle against the posterolateral aspect of the pelvis. It is also directly adjacent to the deep branches of the hypogastric artery and vein and can be damaged inadvertently during pelvic surgery when there is troublesome bleeding in the sacroiliac fossa. The lumbosacral trunk contains fibers that originate from a part of the L4 and L5 nerves. After descending into the pelvis, they are joined with the anterior divisions of S1, S2, and S3, forming with them the large sacral plexus. The *tibial nerve* is composed of fibers from the anterior divisions of L4, L5, S1, S2, and S3. It is joined by the common peroneal nerve, which is composed of fibers from the posterior divisions of L4, L5, S1, and S2; together they compose the all-important *sciatic nerve* trunk. This nerve trunk passes through the greater sciatic foramen to innervate the muscles of the lower extremity (Figs. 4–13, 4–14). Injury to the main nerve trunk causes weakness of the hamstring muscles

and compromises flexion of the leg. The peroneal nerve innervates the extensor muscles of the ankle and the abductor muscles of the foot. Injury to the peroneal nerve may cause footdrop and an inversion of the foot and produce difficulty in walking. The tibial nerve innervates the calf muscles. Injury to this section of the nerve trunk causes difficulty flexing the foot and also interferes with walking. The lateral popliteal (peroneal) division of the sciatic nerve is generally more likely to suffer injury than the medial (tibial) division. The medial division descends in a more vertical direction from the sciatic notch than does the popliteal division and continues to the leg and into the muscles that it innervates

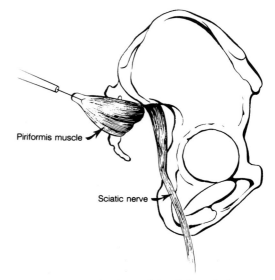

Piriformis muscle

Sciatic nerve

FIG. 4–13 Anatomical relationship of the sciatic nerve (L4–L5, S1–S3), passing through greater sciatic foramen to innervate the muscles of the lower extremity.

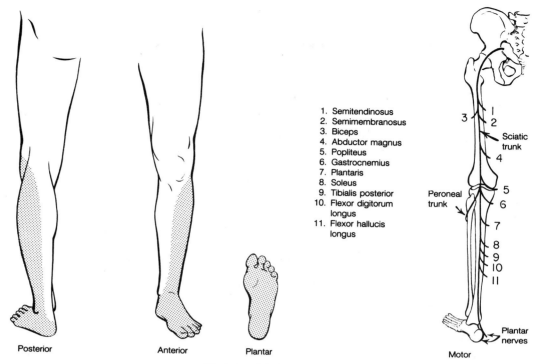

1. Semitendinosus
2. Semimembranosus
3. Biceps
4. Abductor magnus
5. Popliteus
6. Gastrocnemius
7. Plantaris
8. Soleus
9. Tibialis posterior
10. Flexor digitorum longus
11. Flexor hallucis longus

FIG. 4-14 Sciatic nerve distribution of motor and sensory fibers.

with little fixation by its branches. The lateral (peroneal) popliteal division is more angulated and is relatively fixed at both the sciatic notch and the neck of the fibula. Lateral displacement of the thigh subjects the nerve to stretch between two fixed points, although the sciatic nerve may stretch normally for 2 cm to 3 cm when the hip is flexed and the leg is extended. With flexion of the leg and the hip as occurs in the dorsal lithotomy position, the peroneal nerve can be inadvertently injured. Overstretching of the nerve can produce serious injury. More commonly, the peroneal nerve is injured by overstretching along the sacrospinous ligament as it passes through the greater sciatic foramen. This stretching is caused by exaggerated positions of the lower extremity during pelvic surgery, such as when the patient is in the "jack-knife" position, in which the lower extremity is bent at the knee and the knee is unsupported and adducted laterally. This position is used by many surgeons in performing the Marshall–Marchetti–Krantz procedure. It is also commonly used for observing the pelvis during laparoscopy. Although nerve damage of this kind is usually temporary and will respond to conservative physiotherapy, it is a complication of pelvic surgery that can be prevented by supporting the knees in leg stirrups, by avoiding undue lateral rotation of

the legs while leg stirrups are being used, and by refraining from hyperflexion of the thigh on the hip joint. Most of these problems arise from exaggerated modifications of the dorsal lithotomy position that may produce tension on the sciatic nerve trunk as it passes through the greater sciatic foramen. Undue traction on the lower extremity, sufficient to elevate the buttocks off the operating table, will also produce this type of complication. Wide lateral displacement of the knee by an assistant during vaginal surgery can produce damage to the lateral (peroneal) component of the sciatic nerve.

The femoral nerve is one of the largest nerves of the lumbar plexus and arises from L2, L3, and L4. It pierces the substance of the psoas muscle and emerges lateral to the psoas muscle where it passes beneath the inguinal ligament, assuming a medial position, and then divides into a number of branches to supply motor function to the pectineal, sartorius, and quadriceps muscles. It also provides sensory nerves to the anterior and medial surface of the thigh and leg. Injury to the femoral nerve produces early symptoms of paresthesia and a gradual numbing sensation along the anterior and medial surface of the thigh from the cutaneous branches of the nerve. This paresthesia extends to the medial side of the lower leg and the foot. If the more terminal branch of the nerve (saphenous nerve) is involved, depending on the degree of femoral nerve palsy, motor dysfunction can impair the extension of the leg, limiting the ability to walk and climb stairs. This limitation is caused by palsy of the quadriceps muscles that extend the leg at the knee. If the sartorius and pectineus muscles are involved, there will be limitation of flexion of the thigh on the abdomen. These nerve injuries can occur from femoral nerve entrapment by the use of self-retaining retractors with compression or impingement of the nerve against the lateral pelvic wall in the region of the psoas muscle. In particular, a retractor with a very deep blade may cause pressure on the femoral nerve in its intra-abdominal position adjacent to the psoas muscle. One of the common sites of retractor compression is approximately 4 cm proximal to the inguinal ligament. Whether pressure is applied directly against the nerve or whether the psoas muscle is diverted firmly against the lateral pelvic wall, the femoral nerve can undergo undue pressure and damage. Transverse incisions, either muscle-cutting or modified Pfannenstiel, permit lateral placement of the retractor blade and increase the chance of femoral nerve injury. The O'Connor–O'Sullivan self-retaining retractor may cause lateral femoral nerve entrapment, since it may encroach deeper along the lateral pelvic wall and compress the psoas muscle. In the placement of the lateral retractor it is important to make certain that the retractor blade is superficial to the psoas muscle. The muscle and nerve can be further protected by a well-positioned laparotomy pad beneath the inferior margin of the blade. The duration of surgery is also an important factor in nerve damage, with more frequent nerve palsy associated with operations that exceed 2 hours. These precautions should be carefully considered when operating on a thin patient and when a Pfannenstiel or transverse incision is used. Although most patients with femoral nerve injury show complete recovery, many have gait disturbances and muscular dysfunction of the thigh for many months following surgery.

One potential complication should be particularly considered when operating on a very thin patient who has limited subcutaneous fat in the abdominal wall. This pertains to the patient who is placed in an exaggerated dorsal lithotomy position in which the thighs are hyperflexed and the femoral nerve may be compressed against the fixed, fibrous inguinal ligament. There have been many reported cases of femoral nerve palsy in which the nerve has become impinged or stretched against the inguinal ligament for prolonged vaginal operations in this hyperflexed position.

The pudendal plexus is formed by parts of the anterior divisions of S2, S3, and S4. The sacral plexus is formed from part of S4 and all of S5, along with the coccygeal nerves. The visceral branches of the pudendal plexus, both sympathetic and parasympathetic, enter the pelvic plexus as described above. Its motor branches include the perineal branch to the levator ani muscle, arising from S3 and S4, as well as branches to the coccygeus muscle. The terminal and largest branch, the internal pudendal nerve, arises from S2 and S3, enters the greater sciatic foramen medial to the inferior gluteal vessels, returns to the pelvis through the lesser sciatic foramen, passes through the ischiorectal fossa (Alcock's canal), and courses toward its distribution to the muscles of the perineum and vulva.

The external genitalia are innervated by four groups of nerves: (1) the iliohypogastric nerve (T12 and L1); (2) the ilioinguinal nerve (L1); (3) the genitofemoral nerve (L1 and L2); and (4) branches of the pudendal nerve (S2, S3, and S4). The iliohypogastric nerve, arising from T12 and L1, passes between the internal oblique and transversalis muscles to the lateral aspect of the iliac crest, where it divides into an anterior and posterior branch (see Fig. 4–10). The anterior branch innervates the skin over the symphysis pubis, the superior aspect of the labia majora and the mons pubis. The posterior (iliac) branch passes over the iliac crest to the gluteal region. The ilioinguinal nerve (L1) passes in a similar course but slightly inferior to the iliohypogastric nerve, traverses the inguinal canal, and innervates the medial aspect of the labium majus. The genitofemoral nerve (L1 and L2), however, emerges from the anterior surface of the psoas muscle and sends a deep branch into the substance of the labium majus to supply the dartos muscle. It also gives off a lumboinguinal branch that continues on to the upper part of the medial aspect of the thigh. Finally, the pudendal nerve (S2, S3, and S4) reaches the perineum through Alcock's canal and gives sensory branches to the medial and lateral aspects of the labium majus (Fig. 4–15). Nerve entrapment from lower abdominal surgery can involve the ilioinguinal and iliohypogastric nerves. Such injuries can follow appendectomy, inguinal herniorrhaphy and various gynecologic procedures performed through the true transverse and Pfannenstiel incisions. The nerves may be injured either directly by suture or indirectly by pressure against the nerve producing nerve root pain from the superior aspect of the labia and the mons pubis. Treatment frequently requires secondary surgical exploration with excision of the involved segment of the nerve to relieve the symptoms.

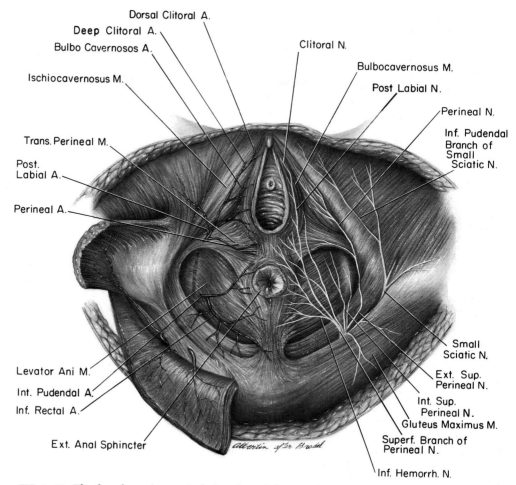

Dorsal Clitoral A.
Deep Clitoral A.
Bulbo Cavernosos A.
Clitoral N.
Bulbocavernosus M.
Ischiocavernosus M.
Post. Labial N.
Perineal N.
Inf. Pudendal Branch of Small Sciatic N.
Trans. Perineal M.
Post. Labial A.
Perineal A.
Levator Ani M.
Int. Pudendal A.
Inf. Rectal A.
Small Sciatic N.
Ext. Sup. Perineal N.
Int. Sup. Perineal N.
Gluteus Maximus M.
Ext. Anal Sphincter
Superf. Branch of Perineal N.
Inf. Hemorrh. N.

FIG. 4–15 The female perineum. Inferior view of the muscles of pelvic floor in relation to rectal, vaginal, and urethral openings. On left, distribution of terminal branches of pudendal nerves. On right, distribution of branch of internal pudendal artery.

One additional nerve from the sacral plexus, the posterior femoral cutaneous nerve arising from the posterior division of S1 and S2 and the anterior divisions of S2 and S3, innervates the medial aspect of the thigh as well as the lateral aspects of the labium majus.

Blood Supply to the Pelvis

ABDOMINAL AORTA AND INFERIOR VENA CAVA

Although the pelvic surgeon is rarely called upon to dissect the aorta and vena cava, an awareness of the relationships of these great vessels as they enter the pelvis is particularly important for the proper understanding of the major blood supply to the pel-

vis. Recently, the field of gynecologic oncology has incorporated the para-aortic lymph nodes as a part of the complete assessment of a pelvic tumor. Therefore, the lower portions of the aorta and vena cava have become a familiar anatomical sight for many pelvic surgeons.

The abdominal aorta begins at the aortic hiatus of the diaphragm in front of the lower border of the body of the last thoracic vertebra. It descends along the front of the vertebral column, where it bifurcates at the fourth lumbar vertebra and divides into the left and right common iliac arteries (see Fig. 4–1). The level on the abdominal wall of the aortic bifurcation at L4 is at or near the umbilicus. An incision to permit the surgical approach to the lower portion of the aorta must be extended somewhat above the umbilicus. Infrequently, the aortic bifurcation may occur as high as the third lumbar vertebra. Prior to its bifurcation, the abdominal aorta gives off two major branches that supply arterial blood to the pelvic viscera: the ovarian artery and the inferior mesenteric artery. The right ovarian artery is seen to cross the anterior surface of the vena cava and the lower portion of the abdominal ureter, where it courses on the lateral side of the ureter to enter the pelvis through the infundibulopelvic ligament. In contrast, the left ovarian artery crosses the ureter immediately after arising from the anterolateral aspect of the abdominal aorta approximately 1 cm below the site of the origin of the renal artery and vein. The left ovarian artery courses along the lateral side of the ureter to cross the bifurcation of the common iliac artery at the pelvic brim. It enters the infundibulopelvic ligament to supply the ovary and to communicate with an arcade that fuses with the uterine artery in the broad ligament. The course of the two ovarian veins is different. The left ovarian vein passes along the surface of the psoas muscle to drain into the left renal vein before the latter enters the vena cava. In contrast, the right ovarian vein passes along the infundibulopelvic ligament, crosses the pelvic brim, where it passes over the lower portion of the abdominal ureter with the ovarian artery, and ascends along the vena cava to enter the vena cava approximately 1 cm below the right renal vein. Enlargement and distention of the right ovarian vein during pregnancy have been associated with dilatation of the abdominal ureter above the pelvic brim and have been questioned as factors causing right hydronephrosis during pregnancy.

The inferior mesenteric artery arises approximately 3 cm to 4 cm above the bifurcation of the aorta and passes into the root of the mesentery of the sigmoid colon, where it supplies the rectosigmoid colon through the superior hemorrhoidal artery, which communicates freely with the middle and inferior hemorrhoidal arteries. The inferior mesenteric artery is an important landmark in para-aortic lymph node dissection because it can be easily traumatized and bleeds vigorously. Fortunately, accidental transection of the inferior mesenteric artery produces no serious compromise to the blood supply of the lower colon, since the collateral circulation from the middle and inferior hemorrhoidal arteries provides an adequate arterial blood supply to the rectum and lower portion of the sigmoid colon.

At the aortic bifurcation, the right common iliac artery crosses over the proximal portion of the left common iliac vein before the left and right iliac veins give rise to the vena cava. It has been suggested that this vascular overcrossing may impair venous return and increase the incidence of venous thrombosis of the left leg. Recent vascular studies, however, have documented that venous thrombosis occurs with equal frequency in both lower extremities. The right common iliac artery continues along the medial border of the psoas muscle to the pelvic brim, where it divides into the external iliac and hypogastric arteries. It continues obliquely and laterally along the medial border of the psoas muscle to pass below the medial portion of the inguinal ligament, where it continues as the femoral artery. It is important to note that the right common iliac artery courses on the medial side of the common iliac vein near its proximal portion, but deviates to the lateral side of the external iliac vein as it approaches the femoral canal. These anatomical relationships are important during the dissection of the lymphatics of the external and common iliac vessels because the thin walls of the iliac veins may be traumatized easily if their precise boundaries are not fully appreciated. The left common and external iliac artery, however, remain on the lateral side of the corresponding iliac vein at all times throughout their course along the pelvic brim before the external iliac artery and vein enter the femoral canal. Therefore, the lateral aspect of the left common and external iliac artery can be dissected without danger of trauma to the vein, which always courses along the medial side of the artery. The right common iliac artery is usually slightly longer than the left and courses more obliquely across the body of the last lumbar vertebra. Immediately lateral to its origin is the right common iliac vein. The left common iliac artery continues along the medial border of the psoas muscle on the lateral side of the left common iliac vein before dividing into the external iliac and hypogastric arteries near the lumbosacral joint. The external iliac artery provides no arterial blood directly to the pelvis except for the infrequent anomalous obturator artery that may arise from its distal end. When this anomaly occurs, there is an important source of collateral circulation with the hypogastric artery.

The middle sacral artery arises from the postero-inferior aspect of the aorta at its bifurcation (see Fig. 4–1) and courses under the left common iliac vein to pass over L5 before emerging over the pelvic brim and along the anterior surface of the sacrum together with the presacral nerve. The middle sacral vein(s) courses over the sacral vertebrae and enters the inferior vena cava at its origin from the common iliac veins.

The hypogastric artery provides the blood supply to the pelvic viscera and musculature. It continues through the ischiorectal fossa as the internal pudendal artery to the perineum and vulva, where it extends within the labia to reach the urogenital diaphragm and the clitoris. For descriptive purposes, the hypogastric artery may be divided into an anterior and a posterior trunk. The posterior division gives off parietal branches only, while the anterior division gives off mainly visceral branches but also some parietal branches.

BRANCHES OF THE HYPOGASTRIC ARTERY

Anterior Division	Posterior Division
Visceral Branches	*Parietal Branches*
Uterine	Iliolumbar
Superior vesical	Lateral Sacral
Middle vesical	Superior Gluteal
Inferior vesical	
Middle hemorrhoidal	
Inferior hemorrhoidal	
Vaginal	
Parietal Branches	
Obturator	
Inferior Gluteal	
Internal Pudendal	

As shown in Figure 4–8, the anterior division gives off its most medial visceral branch, the uterine artery, prior to continuing along the medial aspect of the paravesical space to supply the superior and inferior vesical branches to the bladder. The bladder obtains its superior vesical branch from the segment of the anterior division that continues as the obliterated umbilical artery and passes along the inferior surface of the rectus muscle to insert in the umbilicus along with the urachus from the bladder. The branches of the anterior division supply the uterus, the uterine tube, the vagina, and the bladder. The uterine artery passes through the base of the broad ligament, where it deviates sharply medially along with the uterine vein to course over the ureter and to send collateral branches to the fundus, where it forms a collateral anchor with the ovarian artery (Fig. 4–16). The uterine artery also gives off descending branches to the cervix and vagina. The inferior vesical artery usually arises from the anterior division of the hypogastric artery, either separately or as a branch from the cervical or vaginal artery. It anastomoses freely with the middle and superior vesical arteries. In addition to the visceral branches, the anterior division gives origin to three parietal branches: the obturator, the internal pudendal, and the inferior gluteal arteries. The obturator artery is the most proximal parietal branch of the anterior division and runs forward and posteriorly into the base of the obturator space, where it courses along with the obturator nerve above it and the obturator vein below, to leave the pelvis through the obturator foramen. The terminal portion of the anterior division of the hypogastric artery continues as the internal pudendal artery. This artery continues

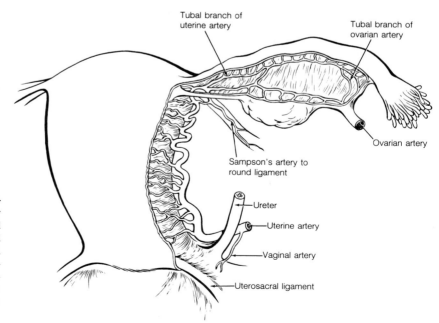

FIG. 4–16 Collateral circulation of uterine and ovarian arteries. Uterine artery crosses over the ureter in the cardinal ligament, gives off cervical and vaginal branches before ascending in the wall and serosal surface of uterus and anastomosing with medial end of ovarian artery. Note the small branch of the uterine or ovarian artery that nourishes the round ligament (Sampson's artery).

along the piriformis muscle and passes down to the lower border of the greater sciatic foramen, where it turns inferiorly to pass through the ischiorectal fossa, giving branches to the perineum, labia, and clitoris (see Fig. 4–15). In its course, the internal pudendal artery gives off the inferior hemorrhoidal artery, which passes along the pelvic floor to reach the rectum and anal canal, where it anastomoses freely with the other hemorrhoidal vessels. The inferior gluteal artery arises from the anterior division of the hypogastric artery and passes out of the pelvis between the piriformis and coccygeus muscles to supply the muscles of the thigh and to anastomose with the superior gluteal and other vessels that surround the hip.

The bladder is supplied by the superior, the middle, and the inferior vesical arteries. The superior vesical artery arises from the umbilical artery, which is obliterated distal to the point of branching;

it supplies the superior surface of the bladder and anastomoses with the other vesical arteries. The middle vesical artery may arise from either the umbilical artery or from one of the branches of the superior vesical. The inferior vesical artery usually arises from the anterior trunk of the hypogastric or as a branch from the cervical or vaginal artery and is distributed to the base of the bladder.

The rectosigmoid colon is supplied by three arteries (see Fig. 4–4): the superior hemorrhoidal, which continues from the inferior mesenteric artery; the middle hemorrhoidal from the anterior trunk of the hypogastric; and the inferior hemorrhoidal, which arises from the internal pudendal artery. These hemorrhoidal vessels anastomose freely. Any compromise of the blood supply to the rectum from one of these vessels is easily compensated for by the rich collateral circulation from the other vessels.

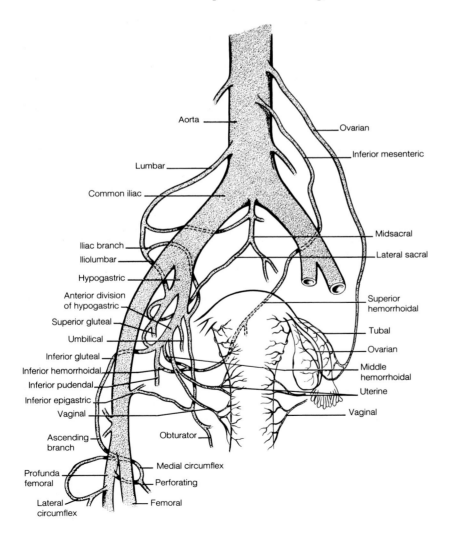

FIG. 4–17 Collateral circulation of pelvis.

All branches of the posterior division of the hypogastric artery are parietal. They include the iliolumbar, the lateral sacral, and the superior gluteal arteries. As seen in Figure 4–8, the iliolumbar artery originates most proximally from the posterior division of the hypogastric artery and immediately divides into lumbar and iliac branches. The lateral sacral artery may be paired or may arise as a single trunk, giving branches to the first, second, third, and fourth anterior sacral foramina. Some of the branches of the lateral sacral artery communicate directly with branches from the middle sacral artery. The superior gluteal artery, which is the third and largest branch of the posterior division of the hypogastric, passes posteriorly, usually between the first sacral nerve and the lumbosacral trunk and continues posteriorly, where it leaves the pelvis through the greater sciatic foramen above the piriformis muscle.

Collateral Arterial Circulation of the Female Pelvis

The collateral circulation of the female pelvis is extensive and provides a variety of intercommunicating sources of arterial blood from various sites along the arterial tree (Fig. 4–17). These collateral vessels anastomose with the hypogastric artery and the blood supply to the uterus through a number of circuitous arterial pathways in the pelvis. During a difficult hysterectomy, the collateral circulation may create problems in achieving adequate hemostasis. Therefore, it is important to have a clear understanding of the various extrapelvic arteries that communicate with the pelvic circulation.

The collateral circulation of the pelvis may be divided into three main arterial groups: those vessels that communicate with branches from the aorta; those that communicate with branches from the external iliac artery; and those that communicate with branches from the femoral artery.

The Female Perineum

When the female pelvis is viewed from below, the center of the pelvic floor is seen to project down like the center of a funnel. The anal canal passes through the center of the pelvic floor, which is made up of the levator ani and coccygeus muscles. Between the projecting floor and side of the bony pelvis is a space, the ischiorectal fossa. In front of the anal canal, the pelvic floor is penetrated by the

---

COLLATERAL CIRCULATION

Branches from the Aorta

Ovarian artery—anastomoses freely with uterine artery (Fig. 4-18)
Inferior mesenteric artery—continues as superior hemorrhoidal artery to anastomose with middle and inferior hemorrhoidal arteries from hypogastric and internal pudendal (Fig. 4-19)
Lumbar and vertebral arteries—anastomose with iliolumbar artery of hypogastric (Fig. 4-20)
Middle sacral artery—anastomoses with lateral sacral artery of hypogastric (Fig. 4-21)

Branches from External Iliac Artery

Deep iliac circumflex artery—anastomoses with iliolumbar and superior gluteal of hypogastric (Fig. 4-22)
Inferior epigastric artery—gives origin to obturator artery in 25% of cases, providing additional anastomoses of external iliac with medial femoral circumflex and communicating pelvic branches (Fig. 4-23)

Branches from Femoral Artery

Medial femoral circumflex artery, superficial and deep—anastomoses with obturator and inferior gluteal arteries from hypogastric (Fig. 4-24)
Lateral femoral circumflex artery—anastomoses with superior gluteal and iliolumbar arteries from hypogastric (Fig. 4-22)

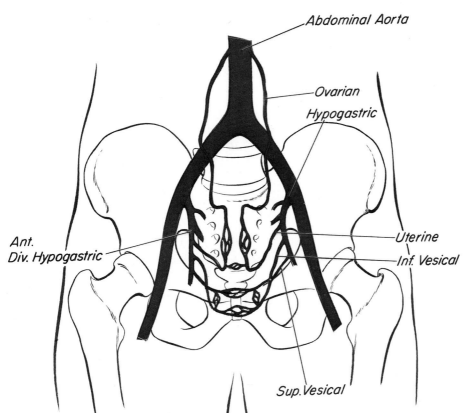

Abdominal Aorta

Ovarian

Hypogastric

Ant.
Div. Hypogastric

Uterine

Inf. Vesical

Sup. Vesical

FIG. 4-18 Arterial arcade and anastomosis between ovarian and uterine arteries.

vagina and urethra and is consequently weakened. This area is reinforced by the urogenital diaphragm, which is also called the *triangular membrane* or *triangular ligament* because it fills a triangular space between the inferior pubic rami (see Fig. 4–15). In the erect position, the pelvic contents are supported jointly by the medial part of the pelvic floor and by the urogenital diaphragm.

The urogenital diaphragm contains a superficial and a deep compartment. The deep compartment consists of a layer of fascia that separates the deep transverse perineal muscle from the underlying levator ani. This fascia attaches to the inferior borders of the pelvic rami and fuses in the midline to fill the gap between the medial borders of the levator ani, where it binds together the borders of the pubococcygeus muscles. The deep compartment of the urogenital diaphragm is supported by a group of muscles in the superficial compartment, including the superficial transverse perineus, the bulbocavernosus, and the ischiocavernosus muscles. The superficial transverse perineus muscles arise from the inferior ramus and tuberosity of the ischium, extend transversely to the midline, and insert into the central tendon of the perineum, with some of the fibers crossing to the opposite side. The bulbocavernosus muscle arises from fibrous tissue dorsal to the clitoris and from the superficial fascial layer of the urogenital diaphragm between the crura of the clitoris. The muscle inserts mainly into the central tendon of the perineum. The ischiocavernosus muscles arise from the interior ramus of the ischium and from behind and on each side of the attachment of the crus of the clitoris. It inserts into the medial and inferior surface of the crus near the pubic symphysis. The innervation of these muscles is supplied by the perineal branch of the internal pudendal nerve. The blood supply is furnished by the perineal artery and vein.

The greater vestibular glands of Bartholin lie in the interval between the ischiocavernosus and bulbocavernosus and are partly covered by the latter muscle. These glands discharge their secretion into the vestibule of the vagina through an orifice along the posterolateral aspect of the introitus, just external to the hymenal ring. Just superior to the Bar-

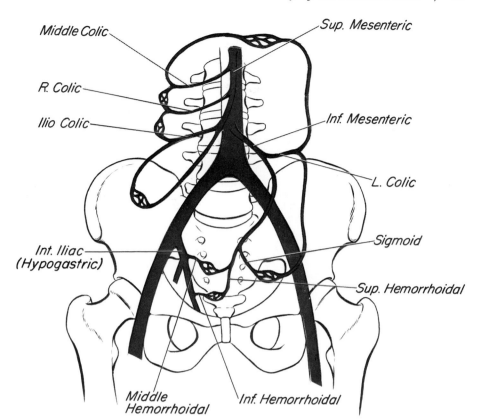

Middle Colic

Sup. Mesenteric

R. Colic

Ilio Colic

Inf. Mesenteric

L. Colic

Sigmoid

Int. Iliac
(Hypogastric)

Sup. Hemorrhoidal

Middle
Hemorrhoidal

Inf. Hemorrhoidal

FIG. 4-19 Collateral circulation of inferior mesenteric artery to branches of hypogastric artery, from superior hemorrhoidal to middle and inferior hemorrhoidal arteries.

tholin gland is the vestibular bulb, which is composed of venous sinusoids and erectile tissue that are drained by the internal pudendal veins. These vascular structures are easily traumatized during attempts to remove the underlying Bartholin gland and may produce a postoperative hematoma that can extend from the anterior perineal compartment into a more superficial space beneath the superficial (Colles') fascia. Colles' fascia extends over the mons pubis to fuse eventually with the fascia of the external oblique muscles of the abdominal wall. A hematoma developing in this region of the urogenital diaphragm clearly delineates the attachments of the superficial compartment. Colles' fascia is a continuation of the superficial fascia of the anterior abdominal wall (Scarpa's fascia). It fuses laterally with the inferior rami of the ischium, which prevents the spread of the vulvar hematoma into the thigh, and inferiorly with the deep fascia over the transverse perineal muscle. These fascial attachments provide a potential space for a hematoma to extend over the urogenital diaphragm and symphysis pubis and to dissect beneath Scarpa's fascia of the lower abdominal wall. The vestibular bulbs

extend forward to form the pars intermedia, which provide erectile tissue to the base of the clitoris. The crura of the clitoris attach to the inferior border of the pubic rami, pass forward and medially and then sharply upward, converging to form the corpora cavernosa of the clitoris.

The structures deep within the deep perineal compartment include the dorsal nerve to the clitoris, the internal pudendal artery and its terminal branches, the vein to the clitoris, and the deep transverse perineal muscle. The dorsal nerve of the clitoris runs in the lateral part of the compartment adjacent to the inferior pubic rami. It is accompanied by the internal pudendal artery, which gives off the artery to the vestibular bulb and the dorsal artery of the clitoris. The deep transverse perineal muscle occupies most of the deep compartment. This thin layer of muscle, with its counterpart on the opposite side, forms a weak sphincter around the urethra and vagina.

In summary, the construction of the urogenital diaphragm or triangular ligament is as follows: The deepest component includes the deep perineal compartment with the deep and superior fascia

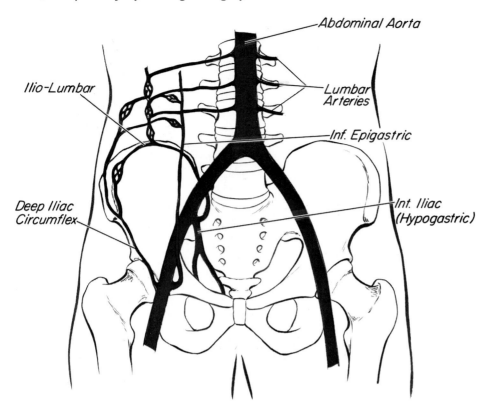

FIG. 4-20 Collateral circulation of aorta and hypogastric arteries through lumbar and iliolumbar anastomoses.

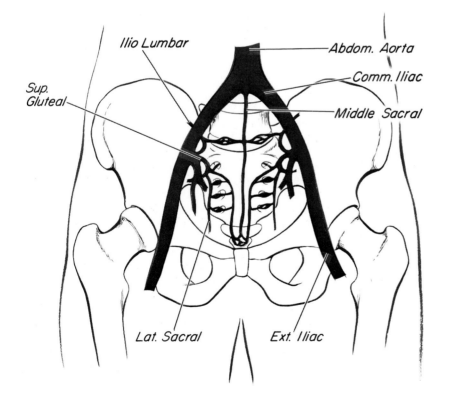

FIG. 4-21 Anastomosis of middle sacral artery from aorta with hypogastric branches, including lateral sacral and iliolumbar arteries.

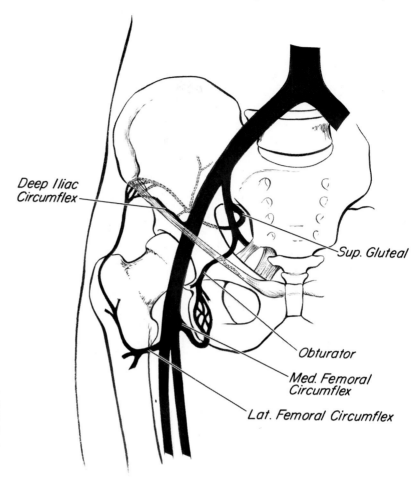

Deep Iliac Circumflex

Sup. Gluteal

Obturator

Med. Femoral Circumflex

Lat. Femoral Circumflex

FIG. 4-22 Collateral arterial circulation between external iliac and hypogastric arteries through anastomoses with iliolumbar and superior gluteal arteries. Note anastomoses from medial and lateral femoral circumflex vessels with obturator and superior gluteal branches of hypogastric artery.

laying on either side of the muscle. The superficial compartment includes the crus of the clitoris, the ischiocavernosus muscle overlying it, the vestibular (Bartholin) gland and the vestibular bulb, the bulbocavernosus muscle covering them, and the superficial transverse perineus muscle. The perineal branch of the internal pudendal nerve innervates the muscles in this compartment, and the perineal artery and vein furnish their blood supply. The external perineal fascia is the most superficial layer of the fascia that invests the muscles and structures of the superficial compartment and fuses with the underlying superficial fascia. A potential space exists between the anterior compartment and the overlying fascia of the subcutaneous fat (Colles' fascia) that is limited by the boundaries of the urogenital diaphragm but is contiguous over the suprapubic region with Scarpa's fascia of the anterior abdominal wall.

The nerves in this region arise from S2, S3, and S4, which fuse to form the pudendal nerve. The pudendal nerve leaves the pelvis through the greater sciatic foramen and passes lateral to the sacrospinous ligament, reentering the pelvis through the lesser sciatic foramen, and then passes along the lateral wall of the ischiorectal fossa in a fascial space called Alcock's canal. As it enters the canal, the pudendal nerve divides into three main branches (see Fig. 4–15). The first of these is the inferior hemorrhoidal nerve in the anal region; the second is the perineal nerve, which itself divides into the posterior labial nerves and the deep perineal nerve to the pelvic floor and urogenital diaphragm. The third branch is the dorsal nerve of the clitoris. There is an overlapping of the sensory innervation of the mons pubis and the superior portion of the labia from the ilioinguinal nerve of the lumbar plexus, which reaches the perineum

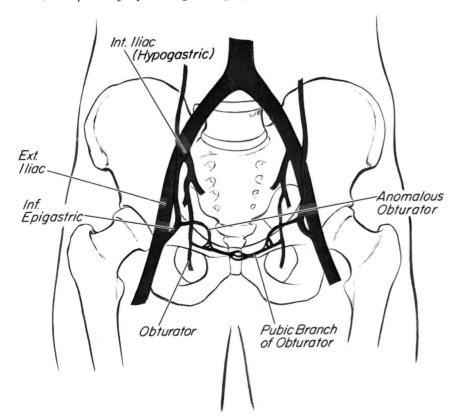

Int. Iliac
(Hypogastric)

Ext.
Iliac

Inf.
Epigastric

Anomalous
Obturator

Obturator

Pubic Branch
of Obturator

FIG. 4-23 Anastomosis of external iliac and hypogastric arteries through obturator originating anomalously from inferior epigastric artery.

through the inguinal canal. The pattern of the nerve supply resembles that of the vascular supply (see Fig. 4–15). The main artery in this region is the internal pudendal artery, which continues to the perineum from the anterior division of the hypogastric artery. It passes out of the pelvis through the greater sciatic notch, then through the lesser sciatic foramen to enter Alcock's canal, where it gives off the first of three main branches, the inferior hemorrhoidal branch. Toward the end of Alcock's canal, the internal pudendal artery gives off the second main branch, the perineal artery. This branch in turn gives off the transverse perineal artery, which supplies the perineal musculature, and usually the posterior labial artery, which continues on to supply the labia. As the internal pudendal artery runs through the deep perineal compartment of the urogenital diaphragm, it gives off a branch to the bulb and crus of the clitoris. Finally, the artery terminates as the dorsal artery to the clitoris.

The external genitalia of the female perineum include the labia majora and minora, the vaginal introitus, or vestibule of the vagina, and the clitoris. The labia majora are the homologues of the male

scrotum and extend along the lateral side of the labia minora from the perineal body to the inferior aspect of the mons pubis. The labia minora surround the vaginal introitus, continue forward, and spread into medial and lateral folds which insert into the clitoris. The component parts of the clitoris include two corpora cavernosa and the glans clitoris. Each of the corpora consists of two parts, a crus and a body. Extending downward from the glans is the pars intermedia, which receives the anterior end of the right and left vestibular bulb. The two folds from the superior aspect of the labia minora extend forward into the clitoris. The medial folds unite, passing to the inferior aspect of the gland of the clitoris. The lateral folds unite, forming the prepuce of the clitoris at the base of the glans. The vestibule is the area between the labia minora. The opening of the urethra is located in the anterior part of the vestibule and the paraurethral glands of Skene are located laterally along the caudal margin of the external urethral orifice. The opening of the vagina is located in the posterior part of the vestibule. The Bartholin ducts open into the vestibule on either side of the vagina just external to the hymenal ring.

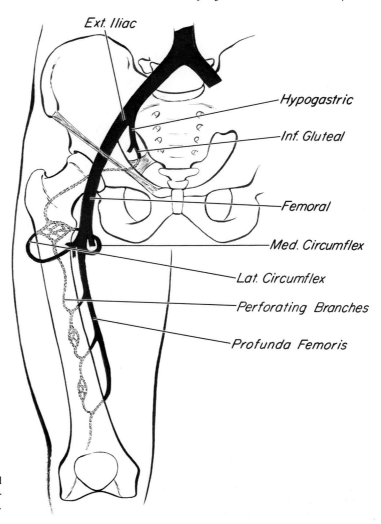

Ext. Iliac

Hypogastric

Inf. Gluteal

Femoral

Med. Circumflex

Lat. Circumflex

Perforating Branches

Profunda Femoris

FIG. 4-24 Anastomoses of deep medial and lateral femoral circumflex arteries around hip joint to posterior division (inferior gluteal) of hypogastric artery.

The lower abdomen and groin contain the external inguinal ring. The superior crus of the external oblique fascia forms the superior and medial margins of the ring, while the inferior crus of the external oblique fascia forms the lateral and inferior boundaries. Four structures pass through the external inguinal ring: the ilioinguinal nerve from the lumbar plexus, which supplies the mons pubis as well as the superior part of the labia majora and the medial part of the thigh; the arteries and the veins of the round ligament from the ovarian (Sampson's) artery and the inferior epigastric vessels; and the round ligament of the uterus, which continues lateral to the pubic tubercle to insert into the labium majus. Inguinal hernias are uncommon in the female and, when they do occur, they are of the indirect, congenital type that arise from the area

of the abdominal wall that is outlined by Hesselbach's triangle.

Bibliography

Bossy J: Atlas of Neuroanatomy and Special Sense Organs. Philadelphia, WB Saunders, 1970

Burchell RC: Physiology of internal iliac artery ligation. J Obstet Gynaecol Br Commw 75:642, 1968

Clemente DC: Anatomy: A Regional Atlas of the Human Body. Philadelphia, Lea and Febiger, 1975

Curtis AH, Anson BJ, Ashley FL, et al: The anatomy of the pelvic autonomic nerves in relation to gynecology. Surg Obstet Gynecol 75:743, 1942

Figge FHJ (ed): Sabotta's Atlas of Human Anatomy, 8th ed, Vols 1–3. New York, Hafner, 1962

Georgy FM: Femoral neuropathy following abdominal hysterectomy. Am J Obstet Gynecol 123:819, 1975

Goss CM (ed): Gray's Anatomy of the Human Body, 29th ed. Philadelphia, Lea and Febiger, 1973

Hopper CL, Baker JB: Bilateral femoral neuropathy complicating vaginal hysterectomy. Obstet Gynecol 32:543, 1968

Hudson AR, Hunter GA, Waddell JP: Iatrogenic femoral nerve injuries. Can J Surg 22(1):62, 1979

Kelly HA: Gynecology. New York, D Appleton and Co, 1928

Kopell HP, Thompson WAL: Sciatic notch. In Kopell HP, Thompson WAL (eds): Peripheral Entrapment Neuropathies. Baltimore, Williams and Wilkins, 1963

Krantz KE: Anatomy of the female reproductive system. In Benson RC (ed): Current Obstetrics and Gynecologic Diagnosis and Treatment. 2nd ed. Los Altos, Calif., Lange Medical Publications, 1978

Kuhn RJP, Hollyock VE: Observations on the anatomy of the rectovaginal pouch and septum. Obstet Gynecol 59:445, 1982

Leff RG, Shapiro SR: Lower extremity complications of the lithotomy position: prevention and management. J Urol 122:138, 1979

Loffer FD, Pent D, Goodkin R: Sciatic nerve injury in a patient undergoing laparoscopy. J Reprod Med 21:371, 1978

McQuarrie HG, Harris JW, Ellsworth HS et al: Sciatic neuropathy complicating vaginal hysterectomy. Am J Obstet Gynecol 112:223, 1972

Meldrum DR: Femoral nerve compression injury in tubal microsurgery. Fertil Steril 32:345, 1979

Pernkopf E: Atlas of Topographical and Applied Human Anatomy. WB Saunders, Philadelphia and London, 1964

Stulz P, Pfeiffer KM: Peripheral nerve injuries resulting from common surgical procedures in the lower portion of the abdomen. Arch Surg 117:324, 1982

Vosburg LF, Finn WF: Femoral nerve impairment subsequent to hysterectomy. Am J Obstet Gynecol 882:931, 1961

Part Two

Preoperative and Postoperative Management

Chapter 5

Preoperative Care

The hallmark of a competent surgeon is embodied in the type of patient that he or she selects for a specific operative procedure. A succinct but inclusive history and physical examination should clarify the severity of the patient's symptoms, identify the disease process or anatomical defect, and verify the need for the recommended surgery. At a moment in medical history when such judgments are commonly being challenged by second surgical opinions and medical-legal scrutiny, the gynecologic surgeon is well advised to give the highest priority to this patient selection process. Reports of second surgical opinions may exaggerate in suggesting that over 50% of the gynecologic symptoms used as indications for major pelvic surgery could be alleviated by more conservative nonoperative treatment (McCarthy, Finkel, 1980). Nevertheless, there is a growing consumer concern that the indications for pelvic surgery may have become too lax in recent years for the patient's welfare. For example, is it in the patient's best interest when a 45-year-old female has a hysterectomy for no other symptoms or clinical findings than a history of menometrorrhea when neither a dilatation and curettage nor medical management has been utilized? We disagree with a popular tendency to consider the uterus to be a superfluous organ at the completion of childbearing that preferably should be removed. The view that the retained uterus is merely a potential site for cancer is at odds with a rational understanding of the true risk of cervical and endometrial malignancy with modern medical care in comparison to the risks of major surgery, including the potential psychological sequelae.

No longer is a surgeon judged solely on technical skill; to the patient, the proper clinical judgement and the indications for surgery are of equal importance. Although it is a delight to observe an operation by a technically adept surgeon, if the operation is done on poor indications, the patient may suffer a loss, rather than a gain. Too often, a patient is subjected to an unnecessary major operation when a minor procedure would have sufficed. Not infrequently, the surgeon operates without knowledge of the basic pathologic lesion and without having conducted a proper diagnostic investigation.

Surgery may be indicated on solid grounds, or it may be done without defensible indications. It may be adequate or inadequate. It may be excessive and only add to the patient's misery. Before performing surgery, the surgeon would do well to consider one of three basic indications. As students, we frequently heard them and they are, we believe, worthy of repetition: the indications for surgery are (1) to save life, (2) to relieve suffering, and (3) to correct deformity. If a contemplated surgery cannot be justified on the basis of one or more of these indications, the surgeon should take another long look at the problem.

History Taking

The preoperative care of the patient begins in the office or outpatient department with the careful taking of a complete history. Good history taking, careful preoperative examination, and the preparation of the patient, physically and mentally, are essential to good surgical results. No matter how busy the gynecologist may be, it is essential that he or she take the history personally. When the patient comes for gynecologic advice, the personal talk with the physician may result in great benefit to her.

Personal contact is also of the greatest value to the physician since the evaluation of the case can be guided by an overall clinical impression of the patient's symptoms rather than by a complete reliance on findings on the pelvic examination. The maxim that "the patient will tell you what is wrong with her, if you will only give her time" is disregarded too often by the busy surgeon. Good history taking requires time and patience, and neither of these is found easily by the gynecologist, and in particular by a gynecologist-obstetrician who has a large obstetrical practice in addition to a heavy surgical schedule. However, the reward for following such a course is the avoidance of unnecessary surgery. Unindicated operations, particularly when performed upon those mentally troubled by some difficult problem of life, may not only prove to be unsuccessful in relieving the patient's symptoms but may concentrate her attention on the pelvic organs and aggravate invalidism. It is our practice not to make a rapid decision regarding the recommendation for major pelvic surgery on the first consultation if the condition is not urgent. Preferably, the patient should be counseled on the need for surgery after all aspects of her physical and emotional makeup are thoroughly evaluated. The surgeon who is quick with the knife and short on words of explanation is usually the one who has the poorest doctor–patient relationship and the greatest malpractice experience.

The history should be concise, but accuracy should not be sacrificed for the sake of brevity. For several years it has been our custom to use a form in obtaining the history. There are objections to any form, for no one has ever devised a perfect form for every case. However, if one uses records for clinical research, important omissions are far more infrequent when information is compiled on a form. There should be no restriction in recording the present illness, and the greatest freedom is permitted the physician in documenting the details of the patient's present condition. Often, there are events in the patient's history that do not fit into any medical form but that may have an important bearing on the present illness; these, too, should be recorded properly and completely in the present illness.

There are a few points which should be stressed in taking a gynecologic history. The menstrual history must be accurate and detailed, since the clue to a correct diagnosis of the gynecologic condition for which surgery is being considered often appears in the pattern of the menstrual irregularity. This holds true whether the menstrual disturbance is caused by an organic lesion or has a dysfunctional cause. In fact, differentiation between dysfunctional

and early organic disease is one of the most common and difficult clinical distinctions that must be made. Of major importance are the accurate dates of the last and the previous menstrual period. When there is great discrepancy between menstrual dates and pelvic findings in a patient with a suspected pregnancy, the sensitive radioimmunoassay tests for hCG are invaluable for the diagnosis. In women under the age of 30, a history of maternal use of intrauterine diethylstilbestrol (DES) during the first trimester of pregnancy is important in alerting the gynecologist to the potential presence of various anatomical abnormalities, such as vaginal adenosis, an anatomical (cockscomb) alteration of the cervix, or a T-shaped deformity of the uterus. A documented history of Herpes (Type 2) viral infection of the lower genital tract has longterm implications for future recurrences and symptomatology.

The reproductive history is of great importance to the gynecologist, particularly the history of previous pregnancies and their complications—such as, for example, dystocia, postpartum infection, abortions, urinary-tract infections, excessive-size infants, vaginal tears, or pulmonary embolism, to list but a few. A well-taken marital history may reveal dyspareunia and unsatisfactory sexual relations, which may, in turn, explain symptoms that resemble organic pelvic disease.

The symptomatology of urinary-tract disease is so closely related to that of disease of the reproductive tract that it is important to obtain a complete urological history and, on occasion, an investigation of the urinary tract before making a final diagnosis and a decision about treatment. All too commonly, women have a vaginal repair with plication of the bladder neck for symptoms of urinary frequency, urgency, and dysuria, while the real problem lies undiagnosed as a chronic infection or a neurogenic dysfunction of the bladder. It is well to remember that a disorder of the lower urinary tract may produce symptoms suggestive of reproductive tract disease, and vice versa. For this reason, we have advocated basic urologic training for every gynecologist. The gynecologist who is adept at using the cystoscope is better prepared to evaluate the case than one who must depend completely on the urologist's report.

Gynecologic Examination

It is incumbent upon the gynecologist to make a complete assessment of the patient's general medical health as well as to perform a gynecologic examination. As the primary physician for women, the gynecologist-obstetrician frequently is the only physician who has seen the patient, particularly if her initial physician consultation concerns a problem involving the reproductive tract. It is important, therefore, to perform a complete physical examination, which must include a blood pressure assessment, weight measurement, examination of the thyroid, auscultation of the heart and lungs, and examination of the breasts, abdomen, and pelvis. Particular attention must be placed on any evidence of abnormal sexual development, including ambiguity of the external and internal female genitalia and abnormal hair growth on the extremities, chest, abdomen, and pubic regions. A critical evaluation of cardiac and pulmonary function before any proposed surgical procedure is carried out must be the responsibility of the gynecologist. Whether additional medical consultation is required must be determined before a general anesthetic is administered. A meticulously collected, midstream, clean catch or catheterized urine specimen should be examined and a urine culture obtained in all cases in which the symptoms even remotely suggest the possibility of urinary tract disease. Although there is a reported 2% to 3% incidence of urinary tract infection or significant bacteriuria (Kass) following a single catheterization, recent evidence suggests that such complications occur more frequently among patients in whom urinary tract infection or abnormal bladder function existed prior to the catheterization. Hence, we still believe that transurethral catheterization, if properly performed, is not a hazard to the normal bladder and may provide valuable information in the total assessment of the patient's gynecologic symptoms.

BREASTS

The breasts are first inspected for symmetry, size, the condition of the nipples, and the presence of a gross lesion. Normal breast tissue, which feels rather shotty to the fingertips, is often erroneously considered to be tumor by the patient and even by physicians who are unfamiliar with the proper method of breast palpation. The breasts should be examined with the patient in both the upright and the supine positions for symmetry, contour, and a palpable mass. In the supine position, the patient's shoulder should be raised slightly with a towel to bring the lateral aspect of the breast tissue level with the remaining portion of the breast. The arm should be raised above the head to flatten the breast against the thoracic cage, which will permit easy examination of the full thickness of the breast tissue. The examination should be done with the flat surface of the physician's fingers and palm; a significant lesion will almost always be detected in this manner. Any suspicious lesion should be evaluated by mammography (xeroradiography), needle aspiration, or biopsy to confirm or discount the existence of a significant breast lesion (see chapter 10). The nipples and adjacent areolar tissue are then gently compressed, and the presence and character of any secretions are noted. Cytologic (Papanicolaou) examination of breast secretions has been reported by Masukawa and others to diagnose very early cases of breast carcinoma prior to the clinical discovery of a gross lesion. The finding of secretions often gives valuable information when pregnancy is suspected, but minimal galactorrhea is not uncommon in parous women many years after the last child and occasionally is found in women who have never been pregnant.

ABDOMEN

Examination of the abdomen includes both inspection and palpation; percussion and auscultation are also useful. Bulging of the flanks suggests free abdominal fluid, but thin-walled ovarian cysts and irregularly shaped uterine leiomyomata may give a similar clinical picture. Although large ovarian cysts and leiomyomata most commonly cause protrusion of the anterior abdominal wall, there are many confusing exceptions. Palpation for a fluid wave through the lateral quadrants of the abdomen is also a useful procedure. Percussion for areas of flatness or tympany and for shifting dullness may aid in determining whether the distention is due to intraperitoneal fluid or to intestinal gas. Auscultation is especially useful in differentiating among a large tumor, a distended bowel, or an advanced pregnancy as the cause of abdominal enlargement.

PELVIS AND RECTUM

An accurate evaluation of the female reproductive tract is essential in establishing the underlying cause of the patient's gynecologic symptoms. Although a detailed description of a pelvic examination is not given here, it is important to stress some of the steps in evaluating the female pelvis. The bladder should be emptied by voiding prior to an adequate pelvic examination. If the patient has urinary tract symptoms, a clean-catch or catheterized urine specimen should be obtained for complete urinalysis and for culture and antibiotic sensitivity studies. Should the patient complain of urinary incontinence, she should be examined with a full bladder in the lithotomy and erect positions to demonstrate stress incontinence of the urethral sphincter (Bonney test). On inspecting the vulva for gross lesions, the Bartholin and Skene glands should be examined for evidence of cyst formation and for purulent exudate as sources of gynecologic infection. Particular attention should be given to the mons pubis and the labia majora and minora for subtle changes in skin pigment, for vesicle formation, or for small raised lesions that may represent evidence of viral infection or early neoplasia. The outlet should be closely inspected for relaxation of the anterior and posterior vaginal walls, and the vaginal mucosa should be observed for infection and estrogen effect. The patient should be encouraged to bear down and to cough in order to demonstrate the degree of relaxation of the anterior and posterior vaginal walls and the extent of uterine descensus, without the use of a tenaculum. The urethra should be compressed along its entire length to test for a possible suburethral diverticulum, often manifested by the expression of purulent material from the urethral meatus or by a tender suburethral mass. The cervix should be evaluated for abnormal gross pathology, particularly ulceration, neoplastic growths, and abnormal discharge. A Papanicolaou smear should be taken, combining a sample of posterior vaginal pool material with cells scraped from the entire circumference of the external os and adjacent endocervical canal. This type of combined cytologic smear is extremely valuable in detecting cervical and endometrial lesions and should always be included in a complete gynecologic examination. A remote history of a negative Papanicolaou smear does not exclude the possibility of a cervical or endometrial neoplasm, because of the frequency (10%–20%) of false-negative cervical-vaginal smears. A patient

should not undergo pelvic surgery without having had a recent cytologic study of the cervix performed by the gynecologist. In view of the fact that 80% to 90% of all preclinical malignancies of the cervix demonstrate no significant gross lesion, it is impossible to be certain of the condition of the cervix without a Papanicolaou smear or a colposcopically directed cervical biopsy (see chapter 31). The uterus is examined bimanually by the abdominal-vaginal route for position, size, mobility, irregularity, and tenderness to motion. Both adnexal regions are evaluated vaginally and by rectovaginal examination.

Rectal examination should never be neglected in the routine pelvic examination. In addition to giving information about the competence of the anal sphincter and about lesions in the anal canal and lower rectum, it is an effective method of detecting pelvic pathology and especially in evaluating the broad and uterosacral ligaments, the cul-de-sac of Douglas, the uterus, and the adnexa. In this procedure, the index finger is inserted into the vagina and the middle finger into the rectum (Fig. 5–1). This technique permits examination of the rectum to a higher level than does examination with the index finger, as well as an opportunity to evaluate the ovaries, the cul-de-sac, and the posterior aspect of the broad ligament. When the pelvic findings are doubtful or inconclusive, a more adequate examination should be done under general anesthesia before a final decision for or against surgery is made. In fact, pelvic examination under anesthesia

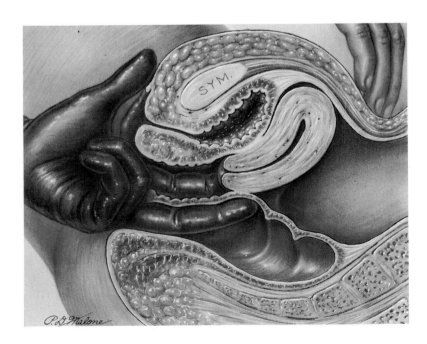

FIG. 5–1 Rectovaginal-abdominal examination.

should always precede any gynecologic procedure, whether major or minor. Frequently, suspected pelvic pathology is completely ruled out by thorough preoperative pelvic examination and a needless laparotomy is avoided. The most common area of clinical confusion is in establishing the presence of an ovarian cyst, which may be confused with bowel, bladder, or a uterine leiomyoma. If a normal ovary can be palpated and a cyst is not identified under anesthesia, the patient has been spared a needless operative procedure. All patients having a dilatation and curettage should have a pelvic examination under anesthesia and the pelvic organs should be described in detail for future reference.

Laboratory Examinations

A determination of hemoglobin level, a hematocrit, a white blood count and differential count, and a complete urinalysis should be a part of every preoperative work-up of a gynecologic patient. Symptoms suggestive of hepatic, renal, or metabolic disease should be thoroughly investigated by specifically related laboratory studies, such as liver function studies, assessments of fasting or 2-hour postprandial blood glucose levels, enzyme determinations, assessments of total protein with albumin/globulin ratio and of thymol turbidity, cephalin flocculation, prothrombin time, and total bilirubin levels. A history of renal disease requires evaluation with an intravenous pyelogram, and blood urea nitrogen, serum creatinine, and possibly creatinine clearance studies, along with complete urinalysis and urine culture. When masculinizing or feminizing ovarian tumors are suspected, determinations of plasma androgen and estrogen levels are frequently helpful. For all patients having extensive pelvic surgery, a baseline electrolyte panel is important as a basis for postoperative fluid and electrolyte replacement therapy. An intravenous pyelogram should be obtained in the differential diagnosis of a pelvic mass. Chest x-ray examination with anteroposterior and lateral views are routine hospital admission procedures. Patients over 40 years of age should have an electrocardiogram prior to major pelvic surgery. Ultrasonography may be a useful diagnostic tool in separating uterine from adnexal disease, in diagnosing an intrauterine from an extrauterine pregnancy, and in measuring the growth of uterine myomata. However, it should never be considered as exceeding the diagnostic accuracy of a thorough pelvic examination; to do so may subject the patient to unnecessary diagnostic studies and the risk of unnecessary surgery.

Preoperative Evaluation

The outcome of pelvic surgery is related to four major factors: (1) the severity and reversibility of the organic disease, (2) the presence of a surgically resectable disease process, (3) the skill and judgement of the pelvic surgeon, and (4) the surgeon's knowledge of the disease process. Diminished cardiac, pulmonary, or renal reserve produces an unstable physiologic background for extensive or emergency surgery. Arteriosclerosis, with its ischemic and compromising effects on the heart, produces myocardial changes detectable by electrocardiogram (ECG) in more than 75% of such patients. Full cardiac stabilization and digitalization should be afforded all patients in whom there is a significant dysfunction as evidenced by diminished cardiac reserve.

Dehydration and hypovolemia are serious and frequently critical factors in the development of postoperative complications. Without adequate interstitial fluid and vascular volume replacement prior to surgery, the patient's cardiac reserve may fail to maintain a normal circulation, and vasomotor collapse or acute renal tubular necrosis may result. In an effort to maintain an ideal urinary output of approximately 50 ml/hr to 60 ml/hr, dehydration must be avoided for any prolonged period of time preoperatively, during surgery, and postoperatively. Proper hydration is assured if approximately 250 ml/hr to 300 ml/hr of intravenous fluids is given during surgery. This rate, which is approximately twice the average fluid replacement rate given in the postoperative state, compensates for the insensible fluid loss from the exposed peritoneal surfaces. Because the cardiovascular tree in elderly patients lacks resilience, adequate blood and fluid replacement during surgery is essential in order to avoid the devitalizing effects of hypovolemia, shock, and hypoxia.

Chronic pulmonary disease is a frequent respiratory complication, although less so in women than in men. Such obstructive changes in the bronchial tree and alveoli, including bronchiectasis and emphysema, produce an excellent environment for respiratory infection, impair oxygen exchange, and result in respiratory acidosis. Atelectasis, pneumonia, and the Adult Respiratory Distress Syndrome (ARDS) are difficult to control in such a setting, to the degree that ARDS is one of the major postoperative complications that may terminate in a postoperative death.

Particular attention must be given to the elderly patient, whose cardiac, pulmonary, or renal reserve requires meticulous evaluation and preoperative correction of any physiologic and functional abnormality. In a survey at the Milwaukee County

Medical complex of 500 male and female surgical patients 80 years of age or older, Carey noted the following preoperative complications: (1) nearly one-third were malnourished (below 100 pounds); (2) anemia was present in 15% of the patients, and among these, 1 in 4 required preoperative blood transfusions; (3) hypertension, cardiomegaly, or arteriosclerotic heart disease was present in more than 50% of the patients, and the ECG was abnormal in 80%; and (4) acute or chronic lung disease was present in over 25%. Of paramount importance was the fact that the mortality rate among such patients was 4 to 5 times higher than the expected rate when emergency surgery prevented their proper evaluation and preparation.

Age as a Factor in Pelvic Surgery

Having defined the potential medical complications and operative risks that pertain to elderly women, it is important to state that chronologic age, by itself, is no longer an accurate indicator of organ function. Atheromatous changes in the cardiovascular system are uncommon in women until well past the climacteric. This biologic phenomenon is but one of the many factors that promote increasing female longevity. The average female lifespan has increased to 78 years during the past half century. As a consequence, more women are entering the period of their life where gynecologic disease is more prevalent and surgery is necessary.

The predictable life expectancy at various ages in the elderly has likewise changed. According to actuarial life tables, an 80-year-old woman has an additional life expectancy of 6.5 years; at 85 there is a 5-year life expectancy, and at 90 years, a 3.5-year expectancy. It is an acknowledged fact that such changes in longevity have influenced the need for surgery in the aging female. Many clinics show the current incidence of major surgery to be highest in the 60- to 69-year-old age group. However, when surgery is combined with meticulous medical control of concurrent disease, physiologic and pharmacologic competence in the field of anesthesiology, and excellent surgical skill, there is only a minimal increase in surgical risks for the elderly female (*i.e.,* over the age of 65) above those for the premenopausal patient.

Pulmonary Evaluation*

Despite continuing advances in anesthesia, surgical techniques, pharmacology, and our understanding

* The section on pulmonary evaluation was contributed by Donald P. Schlueter, M.D.

of the physiologic events during the postoperative period, pulmonary complications associated with abdominal surgery remain a major problem. Preexisting pulmonary disease, especially chronic obstructive lung disease, is one of the most significant factors predisposing to operative and postoperative respiratory complications. Overall, pulmonary complications have been reported in 5% to 56% of patients having lower abdominal surgery. Stein and associates have shown that 70% of patients with chronic bronchitis and emphysema develop atelectasis and pneumonia postoperatively whereas only 3% of patients with normal preoperative lung function encounter similar difficulties. Gold and Helvich reported a 24% incidence of operative and postoperative complications in an asthmatic population as compared with 14% in the control group. Although respiratory complications occur most frequently with obstructive lung disease, factors that alter lung elasticity—such as fibrosis—or thoracic mechanics—particularly obesity—will also lead to an increased incidence of postoperative problems. The importance of age as a factor in all types of postoperative complications, especially those involving the respiratory system, increases sharply after age 50. With aging there are changes in air flow rates, lung volumes, lung elasticity, physiologic dead space, arterial oxygen tension (P_aO_2), and alveolar-arterial oxygen gradient: all of which result in less efficient respiratory function. Tissue hypoxia is more likely to occur in this group, since circulatory responses to hypoxia are diminished.

Few data are available dealing specifically with the effects of smoking on the incidence of postoperative complications. However, there is ample evidence implicating smoking as a significant factor in the production of respiratory symptoms and in the etiology of obstructive lung disease. Physiologic alterations, including increased airway resistance, decreased flow rates, impaired ventilation distribution, increased carboxyhemoglobin levels, and decreased P_aO_2 levels have been reported in smokers. Even smoking a single cigarette has been shown to result in a significant increase in airway resistance. Tobacco smoke can lead to a decrease in surfactant activity and thus promote alveolar instability and microatelectasis. Defense against infection is altered due to depression of mucociliary function and alveolar macrophage activity. All of these factors combined place the smoker at a higher risk for anesthesia and surgery. Shapiro has estimated that patients who smoke quadruple their risk of pulmonary complications; age over 65 triples the risk; and body weight more than 20% greater than ideal doubles the normal rate of complications.

An often-neglected factor in pulmonary evaluations is chronic alcoholism. Alcoholics have more respiratory symptoms and an increased incidence of pulmonary infections because of altered host defenses. Physiologic changes resulting in a decreased diffusing capacity, increased shunting, and decreased surfactant production are frequently found.

The operative site and type of procedure will have a significant effect on the incidence of postoperative respiratory complications following abdominal surgery. The incidence following lower abdominal surgery is somewhat lower than that for upper abdominal procedures. With these procedures, pain as well as associated abdominal distention are frequent causes of respiratory complications because of their limiting effects on ventilatory capacity.

PREOPERATIVE PULMONARY EVALUATION

The question of who should have a preoperative pulmonary evaluation beyond the usual routine history and physical exam is frequently raised. Certain observations that can be made by the physician to alert him to potential respiratory complications are summarized below. These high-risk patients should undergo a more extensive pulmonary evaluation. However, any patient in whom a history of respiratory symptoms has been elicited is a candidate. She should be questioned specifically about the frequency, volume of sputum, and productivity of a cough. An attempt should be made to quantitate the degree of dyspnea; is it present at rest or is it worse in certain positions; what level of exercise causes symptoms; and what particular activity is most aggravating. The presence or absence of wheezing and precipitating factors should also be noted. A careful smoking history is extremely important. The past medical history should elicit any prior illnesses involving the lungs or thorax, and it is helpful to determine from surgical history whether the patient had experienced any postoperative respiratory complications.

The preoperative assessment of the patient with pulmonary impairment actually begins with the physician's first impression, that is, with the patient's general appearance. The robust, energetic individual with a trim figure and good musculature certainly is more likely to handle satisfactorily the stress of the postoperative period than is the sedentary person with poor posture, flabby musculature, and obesity. Inspection of the thorax for deformities, mobility limitations, and muscle weakness and atrophy is vitally important, since any one of these abnormalities may interfere with adequate ventilation. Such simple tests as having the patient blow out a match at arm's length will demonstrate the presence of obstruction. This can be further substantiated by timing her forced expiration, which should be complete in 3 seconds, and listening with a stethoscope for the presence of wheezes. Respiratory excursions can be determined by percussion in the full inspiratory position (normally 4–6 cm). Thorough auscultation of the chest should be carried out, both with quiet breathing and with forced expiration, to detect rales, rhonchi, or wheezes that may be indicative of the presence of secretions or airway obstruction. Differences in the intensity of breath sounds should be noted, since they may indicate the presence of pleural disease or of decreased ventilation. The abnormalities can then be verified by percussion. Obviously, a chest roentgenogram should be routine in all candidates for surgical procedures. Pulmonary function studies provide an objective measurement of the degree of respiratory impairment. A wide variety of test procedures are available and, carefully selected, they can provide information about a specific physiologic abnormality without unnecessary stress to the patient.

PHYSIOLOGIC EVALUATION

In general, pulmonary function tests should be performed in all patients in whom respiratory symp-

---

**BEDSIDE INDICATORS OF
POTENTIAL POSTOPERATIVE RESPIRATORY COMPLICATIONS**

Historical	*Physical*
Age > 50 years	Tachypnea
Smoking history	Wheezing
Chronic alcoholism	Cyanosis
Respiratory symptoms	Prolonged expiration
Known lung disease	Generalized weakness
Body weight > 20% over ideal	Poor mental status
Abdominal surgery	Thoracic musculoskeletal abnormality

---

toms are elicited or in whom significant abnormalities have been demonstrated on chest examination, as well as in heavy smokers and those at increased risk of postoperative respiratory complications, as previously described.

The basic screening test of pulmonary function is spirometry. This test requires a maximum forced expiration by the patient from full inspiration while the change in volume with time is traced on a recording spirometer. From this tracing, measurements of forced vital capacity (FVC), one-second forced expired volume ($FEV_{1.0}$/FVC) ratio, forced expiratory flow from 200 ml to 1200 ml ($FEF_{200-1200}$) and forced expiratory flow from 25% to 75% of the forced vital capacity (FEF_{25-75}) are obtained. In many laboratories a flow–volume curve is generated simultaneously during the forced expiration. This test can detect obstruction in the upper airway and trachea as well as obstruction in the small airways. The latter finding is important, since obstruction in the small airways is not usually detected on auscultation of the chest but can lead to significant disturbances in ventilation–perfusion relationships and to hypoxemia.

Since these tests are effort-dependent, adequate cooperation from the patient is necessary for meaningful results. It is obvious that in a patient who is seriously ill or incapable of understanding instructions, the results are not reliable in quantitating the impairment. The two major kinds of defects that will be demonstrated by spirometry are restrictive defects and obstructive ones. *Restrictive pulmonary disease* includes those conditions in which there is actual reduction in the volume of air-containing tissue, and it affects primarily the volume of air that can be inspired. In these conditions, the FVC and the $FEV_{1.0}$ are reduced, while the $FEV_{1.0}$/FVC ratio and expiratory flow rates are normal. *Obstructive disease* includes those conditions in which there is reduction and prolongation of air flow during expiration. This results in a normal or low FVC and a reduction in $FEV_{1.0}$, $FEV_{1.0}$/FVC ratio, and expiratory flow rates. In order to quantitate the changes in lung volume and to determine if the reduction in FVC is secondary to airway obstruction or restriction, a determination of lung volume is necessary. This can be accomplished by gas dilution technique using helium. With this method, the functional residual capacity (FRC) is measured and the total lung capacity (TLC) and residual volume (RV) are derived. In restrictive disease all lung volumes are decreased, and in obstructive disease they are elevated. The degree of air trapping can be estimated from the RV/TLC ratio (Fig. 5–2). In addition, the time required for equilibration of the marker gas will give some indication of the distribution of inspired gas, being prolonged when distribution is abnormal. Problems in oxygen transfer due either to disturbance in ventilation–perfusion relationships or to alveolar capillary membrane abnormalities can be evaluated by measuring the carbon monoxide diffusing capacity. Regional ventilation–per-

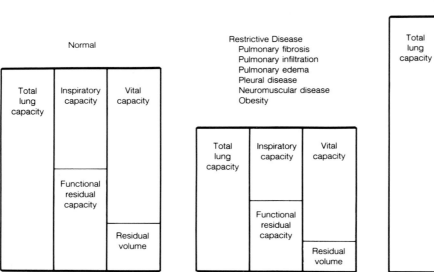

FIG. 5–2 Normal lung compartments and changes that are found in obstructive and restrictive lung disease.

fusion disturbances can be visually demonstrated by radioactive scanning techniques using xenon.

Arterial blood gas studies should be performed preoperatively in all patients with evidence of pulmonary disease. An elevated P_aCO_2 is indicative of inadequate ventilation, while a low P_aO_2 is most frequently associated with ventilation–perfusion mismatching, diffusion defect, or anatomical shunting. Shunting can be verified by the inability to raise the P_aO_2 above 550 mm Hg after breathing 100% oxygen for 30 minutes. Hemoglobin concentration should also be measured since this determines the oxygen-carrying capacity of the blood. The laboratory indicators of potential postoperative respiratory complications are summarized below.

LABORATORY INDICATORS OF POTENTIAL POSTOPERATIVE RESPIRATORY COMPLICATIONS

COPD on chest x-ray
Severe thoracic deformity on chest x-ray
FVC less than 50% of predicted
$FEV_{1.0}$ less than 2 liters or less than 50% of predicted
MVV less than 50% of predicted
FEF_{25-75} less than 1.0 liter/sec
P_aO_2 less than 65 mm Hg
P_aCO_2 greater than 45 mm Hg

FVC = forced vital capacity; $FEV_{1.0}$ = one-second forced expired volume; MVV = maximum voluntary ventilation; FEF_{25-75} = forced expiratory flow from 25% to 75% of FVC; COPD = chronic obstructive pulmonary disease

PROBLEMS ASSOCIATED WITH OBSTRUCTIVE LUNG DISEASE

The three most common obstructive pulmonary diseases are chronic bronchitis, emphysema, and asthma. Although bronchitis and emphysema fre-

quently occur together and the discussion is facilitated by considering them in one section, there are significant differences that alter the approach to therapy and the expected response. The following definitions have been proposed by the World Health Organization and are generally accepted. Chronic bronchitis is a clinical disorder characterized by excessive mucous secretion in the bronchial tree. Chronic cough is present on most days for a minimum of 3 months in the year and for not less than 2 successive years. Emphysema is an anatomical alteration of the lung characterized by an abnormal enlargement of the air spaces distal to the terminal nonrespiratory bronchiole, accompanied by destructive changes of the alveolar walls. Table 5–1 lists some of the distinguishing clinical and laboratory features of these two diseases. Obviously, with combined disease these differences become less distinct. It is important to consider the mechanisms of obstruction in these two diseases, since they will provide some idea of what to expect from the various therapeutic modalities employed. Bronchitis is essentially intrinsic airway disease, with the obstruction resulting from bronchoconstriction, mucosal edema, and the accumulation of secretions. The bronchoconstriction can be reversed with a variety of bronchodilators, the mucosal edema can be reduced with decongestants, and the secretions can be mobilized with humidification, expectorants, and mucolytic agents. In emphysema, although the above mechanisms may play a role, the major cause of obstruction is the loss of the normal tractional support of the airways provided by the connective tissue structure of the lung. It is a destructive process in the lung and is therefore irreversible. For this reason, response to therapy is usually not dramatic. With these facts in mind, the preoperative preparation of the patient will be considered.

Patients with obstructive lung disease should be

TABLE 5–1 *Differential Characteristics in Chronic Obstructive Lung Disease*

CHARACTERISTIC	BRONCHITIC TYPE	EMPHYSEMATOUS TYPE
Body build	Stocky, obese	Thin, wasted
Age	40–60 years	Usually > 50 years
Dyspnea	Sustained, progressive	Variable
Cough	Major symptom	Minor problem
Sputum	Often profuse	Scanty
Wheezing	Episodic	Uncommon
Cyanosis	Common	Uncommon
P_aO_2	Frequently low	Normal or slightly low
P_aCO_2	Frequently elevated	Usually normal
Heart failure	Common	None
Respiratory failure	Frequent	Infrequent
Response to therapy	Good	Poor

admitted to the hospital several days prior to surgery. The first step in preparation is the cessation of exposure to inhaled irritants; namely, the patient must stop smoking. This will probably do more to prevent postoperative complication than any other measure. An air-conditioned room will be helpful when the weather is hot and humid. In addition, fellow patients and visitors will not be allowed to smoke in the room.

Bronchial infection may be present, particularly if the cough is very productive or symptoms severe. Therefore, a sputum smear and culture should be obtained. If the sputum is purulent, even if a specific pathogen is not isolated, the patient should receive a course of antibiotics. Ampicillin or tetracycline in a dosage of 2.0 g/day are preferred, since they are effective against the most common pathogens involved, *Streptococcus pneumoniae* and *Haemophilus influenza*. With isolation of a specific organism, other antibiotics may be indicated. In some cases it may be advisable to postpone surgery to a later date.

Bronchodilators should be used on a round-the-clock basis when bronchospasm is present. An adrenergic agent such as terbutaline, metaproterenol, or albuterol is indicated. Theophylline should form the basis of bronchodilator therapy. Many slow-release preparations are available that can be given orally at 12-hr intervals. With this dosage schedule, relatively uniform theophylline blood levels can be obtained in the therapeutic range of 10 mg/ml to 20 mg/ml. Determination of the serum concentration of theophylline, which can be done in most hospitals, facilitates maintaining therapeutic levels and avoiding toxicity. For patients unable to take medications orally, a continuous intravenous infusion of aminophylline at a rate of 0.5 to 0.7 mg/kg/min will usually provide therapeutic levels. Aerosolized bronchodilators such as isoproterenol (Isuprel), isoetharine (Bronkosol) or metaproterenol (Alupent) with saline given by nebulizer or intermittent positive pressure breathing (IPPB) every 4 to 6 hours is often very effective in reversing bronchospasm and stimulating cough and clearing of secretion. Metaproterenol may have some advantages because of its longer duration of action. The nebulizer usually provides better distribution of aerosol, although some patients are able to coordinate their inspiration better with the IPPB treatment. Controlled studies have failed to show any statistically significant differences between these two methods of administration in the incidence of postoperative respiratory complications. If IPPB is to be used postoperatively in these patients, they should be introduced to its use preoperatively at a time when they are alert and free of pain and are able to cooperate completely. Since this type of therapy is most frequently employed in the immediate postoperative period in patients with airway obstruction, the patient is already experienced and consequently therapy is more effective. When the patient has recovered enough to use a nebulizer effectively for delivering the bronchodilator, IPPB can be discontinued. The use of a metered dose inhaler is discouraged because of difficulties with coordination during this period and potential overuse.

Bronchial secretions should be reduced by the foregoing medical measures. Removal of remaining secretions can be accomplished by reducing their viscosity with mist therapy. Mist therapy can be provided by a heated aerosol, a pressure nebulizer, or an ultrasonic generator and administered with a face mask. It may be somewhat more effective if given after the IPPB treatment. Thick mucous secretions may be thinned by nebulizing N-acetylcysteine (Mucomyst). A bronchodilator should be added to this agent, since the mucolytic agent may cause bronchospasm. Expectorants have been in use for many years, but there is little evidence that they are more effective than water. Adequate hydration is extremely important, and patients should be encouraged to drink at least eight glasses of water daily.

Physical therapy is very helpful in teaching the patient with obstructive lung disease to breathe more efficiently, and instruction in postural drainage and effective coughing will improve her ability to mobilize secretions.

Bronchial asthma, in general, involves a younger age group. It is an episodic disease with symptoms occurring during certain seasons of the year, allowing some selectivity for surgical procedures; and the physiologic disturbances are usually almost completely reversible. Asthma is defined as a disease characterized by an increased responsiveness of the trachea and bronchi to various stimuli and is manifested by a general narrowing of the airways that changes in severity either spontaneously or as the result of therapy. The preoperative preparation of the asthmatic patient is much the same as that for the patient with chronic bronchitis or emphysema. She should be removed from all irritants, not only cigarette smoke but pollens, dusts, fumes, and any other materials known to trigger an acute attack in the patient. Emotional stress is an important precipitating factor in this disease, and the period of preoperative preparation can be used to lessen tension and anxiety through reassurance and sympathetic discussion of the problem. The use of a mild tranquilizer may be helpful. The therapeutic program should include regular oral and aerosolized bronchodilators, humidification, hydration, and antibiotics if the sputum is purulent. If the sputum is very viscid and difficult to raise, N-acetylcysteine (Mucomyst) can be helpful but must be used with caution and not without a bronchodilator, since it may cause severe bronchospasm. It is extremely important to question the patient thoroughly regarding medications to determine if she is receiving corticosteroids or has taken them within the previous 6 months. They should be continued orally until surgery and then given parenterally. If steroids have been used during the previous 12 months, adrenal response to the stress of surgery may be diminished. Acute adrenal insufficiency can be prevented by administration of hydrocortisone preoperatively in a dose of 100 mg IM the night before surgery and 100 mg IM the morning of surgery. If the surgery is particularly prolonged or complicated, it may be necessary to give additional hydrocortisone during and after surgery.

Preanesthetic agents must be used cautiously in all patients with obstructive lung disease because of their ventilatory depressant potential. Morphine and meperidine are particularly prone to reduce the ventilatory response to hypercapnea, and this effect may be potentiated by promethazine. Atropine and scopolamine tend to decrease liquid secretions, which may result in the formation of mucous plugs and contribute to postoperative atelectasis and pneumonia.

Inhalation anesthesia by way of an endotracheal tube is preferred when moderate to severe obstructive lung disease is present, since it provides complete control of ventilation during surgery and the postoperative period. It also provides a ready access to the bronchial tree for removal of secretions during the period when the cough mechanism is depressed. Halothane has proved to be a very satisfactory agent because it relaxes bronchial smooth muscle, is nonirritating to the airways, does not stimulate tracheobronchial secretions, and is associated with rapid induction of and recovery from anesthesia.

Much discussion has focused on the preoperative preparation of the patient with obstructive lung disease; however, this is important because a program such as that outlined, if assiduously applied, can significantly reduce respiratory complication and hence the postoperative recovery period.

PROBLEMS ASSOCIATED WITH RESTRICTIVE LUNG DISEASE

The incidence of postoperative respiratory complications tends to be lower in patients with restrictive lung disease, particularly those limited to the lung, than in those with obstructive disease.

This is probably because patients with restrictive lung disease are usually able to compensate for the increased work of breathing and maintain adequate ventilation. In addition, hypercapnea is infrequent in these patients, and oxygen can be administered without fear of depressing ventilation. Because of the increased retractive force of the respiratory system, the cough mechanism remains effective in removing secretions. The major exceptions to these statements involve markedly obese patients and patients with neuromuscular disease involving the thorax. Figure 5–2 lists the predominantly restrictive diseases that result in a reduction in the volume of air-containing tissue. Physiologically, this reduction results in a decrease in vital capacity and lung volumes without airway obstruction except when the disease is very severe. Oxygen transfer is usually impaired, as shown by a low diffusion lung carbon monoxide (low D_LCO) level, and hypoxemia without hypercapnea is the rule.

Hypoxemia can be corrected in most cases of restrictive pulmonary disease by increasing the inspired oxygen concentration. However, in some patients with primarily thoracic cage disease or with extreme obesity, hypercapnea may accompany the hypoxemia, and suppression of ventilation may occur with high inspired oxygen concentration.

The patient with restrictive disease limited to the lungs requires only brief preoperative preparation, including instruction in the use of IPPB, deep breathing, and coughing. More recently, incentive spirometers and similar devices have been used to achieve a maximum sustained inspiration that appears effective in preventing and reexpanding the atelectatic lung. However, a recent study by Jung and associates (1980) of patients undergoing abdominal surgery failed to show any advantage of one method over the other in reducing postoperative respiratory complications.

Since patients with restrictive disease may be taking corticosteroids or may have taken them in the recent past, they should be questioned specifically about this, and therapy should be instituted as previously described. Special attention should be given to patients with evidence of impaired ventilation as indicated by the presence of hypercapnea. IPPB or incentive spirometry and measures directed at liquefying secretions should be instituted several days prior to surgery along with chest physiotherapy and instruction in coughing. Oxygen should be administered carefully, particularly to obese patients with hypercapnea, since correction of the hypoxemia may significantly depress ventilation. Measurement of the ventilatory response to carbon dioxide preoperatively is helpful in determining which individuals are likely to experience depression of ventilation with oxygen. Weight reduction will usually decrease or eliminate this type of response. Retention of fluid and congestive heart failure occur relatively frequently in patients with restrictive disease, so diuresis and cautious digitalization, if indicated, should be accomplished prior to surgery. Olgivie cautions that preoperative evaluation by an experienced chest physician may be indicated in patients with severely impaired respiratory function.

Cardiovascular Evaluation*

Advances in medical and surgical therapy have been responsible for prolongation of productive life in a significant number of patients with cardiovascular disease. Antibiotics and surgical procedure have altered the natural history of congenital and rheumatic heart diseases. Coronary artery disease continues to be the major cause of death in this country, but mortality has declined in recent years. Aggressive management of this disease now includes transluminal angioplasty and direct intracoronary thrombolysis in addition to surgical revascularization. Recognition and treatment of hypertension have resulted in a decreased incidence of malignant progression of this disease. In summary, the likelihood of facing problems of unrelated medical and surgical illnesses in the cardiac patient continues to increase.

Patients with severe preoperative cardiac disease including ECG evidence of severe ischemia, heart block, or congestive heart failure are most likely to experience postoperative cardiac problems. The evaluation and management of these patients presents a challenge to surgeon, anesthesiologist, and cardiologist alike. Cadanelli and associates reported a 13.5% incidence of heart disease in 1664 patients presenting for gynecologic surgery. Twelve percent of the cardiac patients demonstrated clinical or ECG deterioration, and overall mortality among these was less than 1%. The anticipation of potential problems depends on the preoperative recognition and understanding of the fundamental cardiac disease process.

The clinical history will readily identify the patient with overt cardiorespiratory symptoms. Interpretation of atypical symptoms tests the skill of the most experienced clinician. This is particularly evident in the evaluation of chest pain syndromes. The classic description of ischemic chest pain is well known and easily recognized. Angina pectoris should also be suspected, if discomfort of any qual-

itative description is localized between the waist and the jaw and is predictably evoked by effort or emotion. Coronary risk factors must be carefully weighed in any patient whose history suggests possible angina pectoris. Anginal pain that occurs at rest, particularly in the early morning, suggests the diagnosis of vasospastic disease. The association of other vasoregulatory disorders, such as migraine or Raynaud's phenomenon, enhances the probability of coronary artery spasm as a diagnosis. A prominent heart murmur, pulmonary rales, or peripheral edema direct immediate attention to the cardiovascular system. Vascular bruits, gallop sounds, or abnormal venous pulsations are more subtle findings but are equally important signs of cardiac or vascular disease.

Routine laboratory studies in the preoperative patient often fail to reveal the extent of underlying cardiac pathology. The resting ECG is helpful if it is abnormal, but a normal tracing is no reassurance in a patient with classic symptoms of progressive angina pectoris. Furthermore, the ECG reverts to normal in approximately 25% of patients with proven myocardial infarction. The exercise ECG is frequently used to assess patients with suspected angina pectoris. The test is not sufficiently sensitive to be helpful if the patient has a typical history of ischemic pain. The history alone is 90% predictive of coronary disease whereas the stress test has only 75% to 80% sensitivity. In recent years, nuclear scanning has assumed a prominent role in the diagnosis of coronary artery disease by noninvasive testing. Stress tests are performed using either Thallium-201 or Technetium-99M. Thallium-201 is an analog of potassium and it is distributed to and taken up by the myocardium in proportion to blood flow. It is injected intravenously at peak exercise, and scanning is performed in at least three projections within 15 minutes of the completion of exercise. The scan is repeated 3 to 4 hours later using similar projections. Failure of uptake in a region of myocardium suggests stenosis or occlusion of the artery to the corresponding region. If the delayed scan shows reperfusion of the previously underperfused area, the test is considered positive for ischemia. Failure to reperfuse identifies severe ischemia or old infarction. The ^{201}Tl perfusion scan enhances the sensitivity of stress testing in both males and females, but it is worth noting that false-positive scans are more frequent in females. The ^{99m}Tc blood pool scan is combined with a computerized program that permits analysis of left or right ventricular wall motion. Radioisotope angiocardiography can be performed before and during graded exercise. This study yields valuable information concerning cardiac reserve. It is a less reliable predictor of coronary

---

* The section on Cardiovascular Evaluation was contributed by Michael H. Keelan, Jr., M.D.

disease than is the ^{201}Tl perfusion scan because of the low specificity of the test.

The standard chest x-ray provides adequate evaluation of the cardiac silhouette and lung fields in most patients. Accurate determination of individual chamber size and thickness is best provided by ultrasonic (echo) cardiography. The sector scan (2D) echo is a useful technique for evaluation of ventricular wall motion, valve orifice size, and intracardiac masses such as thrombus or myxoma.

Preoperative attention to electrolyte concentrations and renal function help to avoid "surprise" arrhythmias during the perioperative period. All medications must be reviewed, since many patients will be taking one or more cardiac drugs. Serum drug level determinations are available for digitalis and a variety of antiarrhythmic agents. Routine assessment of serum digoxin level is not recommended. The test should be obtained if there is a question of drug intoxication or a lack of patient compliance with the prescribed regimen. Blood volume measurements may be useful in elderly patients or in those with extensive malignancies, whose total volumes are often contracted.

CORONARY ARTERY DISEASE

Coronary artery disease rarely afflicts premenopausal women without major risk factors such as hyperlipidemia, hypertension, diabetes mellitus, or smoking. Use of an anovulatory drug appears to increase the risk of coronary disease in patients over 40 years of age. Realistically, ischemic heart disease is a disease of men and postmenopausal women. The diagnosis is made by history (angina pectoris or prior documented myocardial infarction) or by ECG evidence of infarction. Various electrocardiographic changes, including left bundle branch block and ST–T changes, suggest the diagnosis of ischemic disease, but they are not definitive. Even significant Q waves, the hallmark of transmural myocardial infarction, are not always diagnostic. Hypertrophic cardiomyopathy and mitral valve prolapse are noncoronary diseases in which the cardiogram may demonstrate a pseudoinfarction pattern. A preoperative diagnosis of coronary artery disease increases the surgical risk for complications, but multiple factors influence the overall prognosis. Unstable coronary disease is a major risk factor. Patients with recent onset of angina, progressive angina, or rest angina should be fully evaluated by a cardiac consultant prior to elective surgery. Surgery should be deferred until the patient has stabilized with appropriate pharmacologic or surgical therapy. Myocardial infarction within the previous 6 months should also be considered a potentially unstable

condition. Surgery performed within this interval is accompanied by an unacceptably high incidence of both reinfarction and fatality. Emergency surgery is occasionally necessary in patients with unstable coronary syndromes. Most patients will have been treated with combinations of vasodilators, including nitrates, calcium channel blockers, or β-adrenergic blocking agents. Whenever possible, these drugs should be continued through the perioperative course or tapered off gradually if they must be discontinued. The availability of direct invasive monitoring of left ventricular filling pressure using the balloon-tipped floating pulmonary artery catheter has made it possible to monitor hemodynamic parameters throughout the critical perioperative period. Filling pressures and systemic arterial pressure is optimized, thereby avoiding inadvertent fluid overload and unnecessary increase in myocardial oxygen demand. Of course, ECG monitoring is also used. In patients with exceptionally unstable disease, the preoperative insertion of the intra-aortic counterpulsation balloon catheter has provided stabilization during the operative procedure. This device augments the central aortic diastolic pressure, thereby increasing coronary perfusion. The balloon deflates rapidly, producing a dramatic fall in end-diastolic aortic pressure. The impedence to ejection is reduced and systolic cardiac emptying is enhanced.

Congestive heart failure, overt or covert, is the single most important predictor of cardiac complications in the surgical patient. Because of its overall frequency, coronary disease is the likely cause for heart failure in most patients presenting for surgery. Elective surgery should not be done in patients whose signs and symptoms are overt. Patients with gross cardiomegaly or gallop rhythm should be carefully assessed with either echocardiography or nuclear ventriculography. Invasive hemodynamic monitoring is indicated for patients with a severe reduction in resting left ventricular function who may urgently require surgery. Similar monitoring should be considered for any patient with a recent history of heart failure regardless of the current findings. Cardiac rhythm disturbances, particularly ventricular premature beats, are also associated with increased surgical risk. This risk is most prominent, however, when the ectopic beats are associated with a decrease in left ventricular function. In the absence of defined cardiovascular disease, premature ventricular beats are not harbingers of sudden death or symptomatic ventricular tachycardia and need not be treated at all. Commonly used antiarrhythmics such as quinidine, procainamide, and, particularly, disopyramide are cardiac depressants, and routine use of these drugs preoperatively is not recommended. Patients with known coronary artery disease and frequent ventricular ectopic beats, especially couplets or salvos, should be treated instead with intravenous lidocaine. Infusion is begun prior to induction. An initial bolus injection of 1 mg/kg to 1.5 mg/kg is followed 15 to 20 minutes later by a similar dose. After the first bolus an infusion of 1 mg/min to 4 mg/min is begun. The doses should be reduced by half in elderly patients or those with liver disease. Atrial ectopic beats are often predictors of more complex atrial arrhythmias, such as atrial flutter or fibrillation. They may be the first sign of impending cardiac failure. Digitalis is recommended for this reason. Routine preoperative administration of digitalis is *not* recommended for all patients with coronary disease. This drug may be detrimental to some patients with reduced coronary reserve because of the increased oxygen demand associated with the augmented contractile state. Its use should be restricted to: (1) patients with clinical congestive heart failure; (2) patients with objective evidence of poor left ventricular function without decompensation; or (3) patients with atrial arrhythmias. Rapid "eleventh-hour digitalization" should be avoided to reduce the incidence of toxicity.

Contrary to popular belief, the greatest risk for myocardial infarction is not necessarily within the immediate intraoperative period. High rates of perioperative myocardial infarction are noted on the third and the fourth postoperative days. Surveillance with daily ECGs during this time is recommended. When indicated, creatine phosphokinase (CPK) enzymes should be obtained with myocardial brain fraction analysis. The enzymes are not obtained routinely unless there is a change in the cardiogram or the patient's clinical status suggests a cardiac event.

In summary, elective surgery should be deferred in patients with unstable syndromes. Following myocardial infarction, a 6-month delay is advised. Patients with unstable angina should be stabilized by appropriate pharmacologic and/or surgical therapy. Optimal perioperative assessment should include hemodynamic as well as electrocardiographic monitoring for unstable patients in need of urgent surgery.

VALVULAR HEART DISEASE

The incidence of rheumatic fever has declined dramatically in recent years. Mitral valve prolapse is now widely recognized as perhaps the most common of all valvular abnormalities. Its predilection for the female is also well known. The etiology is diverse, but in most patients it is not well known. The disease may be familiar, and it is often accompanied by a variety of poorly explained symptoms including chest pain and fatigue. Multiple arrhythmias have been described. These include ventricular ectopic beats, atrial tachyarrhythmias, bradycardiac rhythms, and, rarely, sudden death. Autonomic dysfunction has also been identified in many patients involving abnormalities of both sympathetic and parasympathetic tone. This syndrome has often been described as being a nuisance rather than a threat.

Innovative advances in valvular repair may defer or delay valve replacement in some patients, but in most patients with advanced valvular disease, defective valves still require replacement with a prosthetic device. Bioprostheses are available and are used primarily in elderly patients or others in whom the risk of long-term anticoagulation is excessive. Because of the relatively poor durability of these valves, they have not displaced the synthetic prosthesis as the valve of choice for most young or middle-aged patients. Improved long-term results following valve replacement mean that more patients with prosthetic valves survive to endure the trials of other medical and surgical disorders.

Patients with valvular disease generally exhibit more predictable courses than do patients with coronary disease. Those in functional classes III–IV (NHHA classification) have symptoms that limit their daily activities either moderately or severely. The surgical risk is greatest for these patients. Most of these patients will be taking digitalis, a diuretic, and, perhaps, a vasodilator. Surgery should be deferred until overt heart failure has improved and the patient is clinically stable. Invasive monitoring is also recommended during the operative procedure. All patients with valvular disease should be treated with antibiotic prophylaxis against endocarditis. Patients with severe aortic stenosis have an increased risk for surgery and this group is not always symptomatic. Echocardiographic evaluation is recommended for all patients with harsh ejection murmurs.

The anticoagulated patient poses a special challenge. It had been recommended that Coumadin be stopped several days before surgery, allowing the prothrombin time to decline to approximately 15 seconds, at which time surgery would be done. Postoperatively, the Coumadin was resumed as soon as it was deemed safe to do so. This protocol has been successful in a number of patients, but both clotting and hemorrhagic complications have been reported. The risk for thromboembolism is greater in patients with mitral prostheses. For this group we prefer to administer fresh frozen plasma (NOT vitamin K) immediately before surgery, and begin IV heparin as soon as possible postoperatively. The regular Coumadin dose is reinstituted at the same time. This regimen has proven to be both effective and safe.

Patients with valvular disease are at risk according to their functional status. Those with critical aortic stenosis are exceptions, and ultrasonic cardiac examination is helpful in the evaluation of these patients. Special attention to endocarditis prophylaxis is necessary in all patients with valvular disease. Anticoagulation poses a minimal problem in the performance of routine surgical procedure if proper protocol is employed.

CONGENITAL HEART DISEASE

The natural history of most forms of serious congenital heart disease dictates that surgical correction be performed early in life. If surgery is not possible, mortality is high and the patients do not survive to adulthood. Exceptions to this rule include patients with cyanotic heart disease such as Eisenmenger's complex and tetralogy of Fallot, who may live well into the adult years without cardiac surgical intervention. Patients with acyanotic disorders such as congenital aortic stenosis, artial septal defect, and small ventricular septal defects often survive into adulthood without major complications. Functional classification may be misleading, particularly in patients with cyanotic disease, who may seem to be surprisingly free of symptoms despite marked erythrocytosis, hypoxemia, and cyanosis. Low-level stress tests combined with arterial oximetry give a better assessment of the true cardiac reserve in these patients. Increased blood viscosity may lead to problems of thrombosis, and decreased platelets frequently are associated with a bleeding tendency. In general, patients with congenital heart disease should be treated prophylactically for endocarditis, although those with atrial septal defect need not be.

HYPERTENSION

In the absence of cardiac or renal complications, hypertension of itself adds little risk to surgical procedures. Since a variety of antihypertensive medications are currently available, it is imperative to carefully review drugs well in advance of anticipated surgery. Agents commonly used in the management of mild to moderate hypertension include diuretics, rauwolfia, and beta blockers. Other currently available drugs capable of inducing significant cardiovascular affects include monoamine-oxidase inhibitors, guanethedine, hydralazine, prazosin, and captopril. In patients with mild hypertension, medications can generally be discontinued completely during the preoperative period without ill effect. If severe diastolic hypertension exists (diastolic pressures in excess of 115 mm Hg), it is best to continue antihypertensives to the time of surgery and reinitiate them in the early postoperative period. Rarely, it may be necessary to continue antihypertensives by the intravenous route. Nitroprusside and hydralazine are suitable drugs. With evidence of cardiomegaly or past congestive heart failure it is advised that the patient receive digitalis in anticipation of surgery.

The approach to the surgical patient with cardiac disease should include a cooperative effort on the part of the gynecologist, anesthesiologist, and the internist-cardiologist. Although the risk of mortality and morbidity understandably is greater in this patient, the risks, as summarized in Table 5–2, can be minimized by careful preoperative, intraoperative, and postoperative management.

Preparation of the Patient for the Operation

A povidone-iodine (Betadine) douche and a vaginal suppository of nitrofurazone (Furacin), inserted high in the vagina, each night for 2 or 3 nights preceding surgery, has been useful in decreasing the frequency of cuff cellulitis postoperatively. Many gynecologists routinely prepare the atrophic vagina of the postmenopausal patient with estrogen vaginal suppositories or cream for 4 to 6 weeks preoperatively. This has been particularly useful for patients undergoing vaginal surgery, since thickening the vaginal mucosa makes the tissues easier to dissect. There is no clinical evidence, however, that the vaginal flora are significantly altered or reduced by an increase of intracellular glycogen in the vaginal epithelium or by a drop in the vaginal pH—changes which are produced by estrogen preparations and the lactobacillus organisms.

The evening meal on the day before an operation should be light and easily digestible. Overloading the alimentary tract shortly before the operation is particularly hazardous, not only as an anesthetic risk but also because it increases postoperative discomfort from nausea and gas formation. It is important that the patient have an adequate night's rest prior to the operation. Since the hospital environment usually causes apprehension, a mild sedative is advisable to ensure a good night's sleep. We commonly use pentobarbital sodium, 100 mg orally, or its equivalent.

The patient should be in the fasting state overnight, with nothing by mouth from midnight, unless the operation is scheduled for late in the day. In such cases, a light breakfast of a liquid diet is per-

TABLE 5–2 *Risks in Surgical Patients with Cardiovascular Disorders*

DISORDER	RISK FACTORS	PRECAUTIONS
Atherosclerotic heart disease	Unstable angina Recent myocardial infarction Arrhythmias* Congestive heart failure*	Delay elective surgery 6 months ECG and hemodynamic monitoring Nuclear or ECHO evaluation of left ventricular function
Valvular heart disease	Endocarditis Congestive heart failure Critical aortic stenosis Anticoagulants†	Antibiotic prophylaxis ECHO Hemodynamic monitoring
Congenital heart disease	Endocarditis (endarteritis) Thrombosis, hemorrhage	Antibiotic prophylaxis Evaluation of clotting factors
Hypertension	Drug interactions	Maintenance of therapy for severe hypertension only
Cardiomyopathy	Arrhythmias Congestive heart failure Anticoagulants	As for arteriosclerotic heart disease and valvular heart disease

* Arrhythmias and reduced functional capacity are potentially serious risk factors to patients regardless of etiology of heart disease. They require careful consideration of renal status, electrolyte balance, and drug therapy during the preoperative period. Monitoring central venous pressure and daily weights will help to maintain optimal fluid balance.
† See text

missible, not later than 6 hours preoperatively. The lower colon should be cleansed by a preoperative enema on the evening prior to surgery and again before the operation is scheduled. Adequate time should be scheduled to permit complete evaluation of the enema. If necessary, repeat enemas should be given until the colon is completely empty of fecal material. A patient should not be awakened at dawn by an attendant to be given an enema when the operation is posted at noon. Not only is such a procedure a discourtesy to the patient, but the lower bowel may become refilled with fecal material because of increased intestinal peristalsis from the anxiety of awaiting the operative procedure. Preoperative sedation is usually requested by the anesthesiologist when he or she examines the patient on the night before surgery.

The use of prophylactic broad-spectrum antibiotics has become commonplace in recent years for certain patients undergoing vaginal and abdominal surgery. Although this practice has as many opponents as it has advocates, there are certain types of pelvic surgery that have shown specific benefit. Patients undergoing vaginal hysterectomy, for example, have a high incidence of cuff cellulitis, particularly patients who are premenopausal and have a highly vascular reproductive tract. In these cases, postoperative collections of serum and blood from venous sinusoids in the vaginal cuff provide an excellent nutrient in which vaginal flora can grow

and multiply. Postoperative cuff cellulitis occurs in as many as 30% to 50% of these cases. Here, a broad-spectrum, single antibiotic agent has proven useful in producing a significant reduction in the incidence of febrile morbidity to no more than 5% to 10%. When given as intraoperative treatment (2 hours before surgery and every 6 hours, for a total of 3 doses), one of the new generation cephalosporins, semisynthetic penicillins, or semisynthetic broad-spectrum β-lactamase antibiotics are highly effective agents.

The infections that occur following surgery on the female reproductive tract arise from the introduction of the normal vaginal flora into the surgical field. Pelvic surgery provides ideal conditions for the development of both aerobic and anaerobic infections, principally those that are polymicrobial rather than monomicrobial in origin. When surgery is performed on the reproductive tract through a bacteriologically contaminated field, such as the vagina, bacteria are seeded into the pedicles and surgical margins of pelvic tissues. This provides an excellent nidus for infection in the devitalized tissue bed. The destruction of tissue by clamps and sutures lowers the tissue oxidation-reduction potential, frequently referred to as the redox potential. This process of lowering tissue oxygen levels enhances the growth of facultative anaerobes that normally inhabit the vagina. As the tissue hypoxia progresses, strict anaerobes are the primary bacteria that survive and proliferate. Therefore, the usual postoperative infection in the vaginal vault, although initially polymicrobial, can be prevented if an adequate tissue level of a broad-spectrum antibiotic is present at the time of the operative contamination. The short-term (24-hour), intraoperative use of a broad-spectrum antibiotic has proven to be as effective as long-term (5–7 days) use in preventing postoperative infectious morbidity. Therefore, a preoperative, intraoperative, and postoperative dose of a broad spectrum antibiotic that has particular sensitivity to gram-negative organisms, given at 6-hour intervals, will inhibit the growth of aerobic organisms. The reduced utilization of oxygen, by inhibiting the growth of aerobic organisms, will interrupt the oxidative-reductive cycle and prevent lowering of the redox potential. The secondary benefit of maintaining a high tissue oxygen level is the suppression of the growth of anaerobic bacteria. This simple technique of controlling the microbiologic environment of bacteria has proven effective in controlling the growth of both aerobic and anaerobic bacteria in a potentially contaminated operative field such as the vaginal vault.

In 1973, Ledger, Sweet, and Headington were among the first to demonstrate the effectiveness of short-term prophylactic antibiotic therapy. Since that time, innumerable studies have demonstrated that the various aminoglycoside or cephalosporin antibiotics each have predictable effects in suppressing the growth of gram-negative aerobic bacteria, which are the most common type of bacterial infective agents in the operative site following vaginal or abdominal hysterectomy. Because the most common complication associated with vaginal hysterectomy is infection, the available data clearly indicate that with the intraoperative use of short-term antibiotics, the incidence of postoperative pelvic infection can be reduced dramatically. Although originally this benefit from prophylactic antibiotics was considered to be effective principally for the premenopausal patient, a decrease in infectious morbidity has also been demonstrated in the postmenopausal patient, particularly when a vaginal repair has been undertaken in conjunction with a vaginal hysterectomy. Recent reviews of this subject by Duff and Park, and by Polk and associates, provide clear evidence of the clinical benefit of this technique of controlling pelvic infection as a result of gynecologic surgery.

By reducing infection, postoperative short-term antibiotic prophylaxis results in a shortened hospital stay and a decrease in medical expense for the majority of patients. A prophylactic antibiotic should be a drug that is *not* used as a treatment of choice for overt pelvic infection. Further, the antibiotic should have a low incidence of toxic side effects and should be capable of achieving an effective tissue concentration at the operative site within a short period following administration. Several agents have been shown to be effective in reducing pelvic infection following vaginal and abdominal hysterectomy, including ampicillin, cephaloradine (Loridine), cephalothin (Keflin), cephradine (Anspor), cefazolin (Ancef), and doxycycline (Vibramycin), to list but a few.

Prophylactic antibiotics may be effective in reducing the incidence of postoperative infectious morbidity, but they should never be used as a substitute for time-honored principles of adequate hemostasis and gentle handling of tissues. Although Wangensteen has made the uncomplimentary statement that "antibiotics will turn a third-class surgeon into a second-class surgeon, but will never turn a second-class surgeon into a first-class surgeon," there is a changing attitude regarding the effectiveness of the short-term, intraoperative use of broad-spectrum antibiotics in modern pelvic surgery.

Preoperative Procedures in the Operating Suite

The patient is brought to the operating room area and is transferred to the operating table in the anesthesia room adjoining the surgical suite. A Kelly pad is placed on the foot of the operating table so that liquids used for the vaginal cleanup will drain into a floor basin. A nurse shaves the patient's lower abdomen or vulva or both in the anesthesia room prior to surgery. Since several minutes are required to attain a surgical plane of anesthesia, no time is lost as a result of shaving while the patient is unconscious.

After shaving and catheterization, the patient is usually sufficiently anesthetized for a careful bimanual pelvic examination. The operator may obtain, in this examination, very valuable information that may not be obtainable when the patient is awake. Following the pelvic examination, the perineum and the vagina are cleansed before all pelvic surgery. There is always the possibility that the findings at operation may make a total abdominal hysterectomy advisable, even when the preoperative plan in the operator's mind did not include such an extensive procedure. It is extremely disconcerting to find that a total hysterectomy must be performed at the time of a laparotomy if the vagina is not properly prepared. To prevent this circumstance, we have made the preoperative vaginal cleanup a routine procedure. To clean the perineum and the vagina, the nurse or surgical assistant first scrubs the vulva and the perineum with a sponge that is soaked with surgical soap or povidine iodine solution and held in the gloved hand. Then the vagina is scrubbed with a soapy sponge held in the fingers. Following the vaginal scrub, the fingers are spread, the outlet is enlarged, and the perineum is depressed to permit the soapy water or iodine solution to run out of the vagina. The solution is flushed away with sterile water that is poured into the vagina by the nurse. From this point on, the cleanup is done with a sterile sponge on a sponge forceps. This is used several times to clean the vagina with the appropriate antiseptic solution. After the vaginal cleansing, the vagina and the perineum are rinsed with a 70% alcohol solution.

Next, an unfolded sterile sponge is inserted into the vagina. The end of the vaginal sponge is left protruding from the outlet and the sponge forceps is left attached to facilitate its removal during the operation. The sponge absorbs any secretions that may come from the cervical canal as the result of operative manipulation and removes any residual alcohol from the vagina. At operation, the sponge is removed by a nurse who pulls on the sponge forceps just before the vagina is opened at the time of total hysterectomy. If a hysterectomy is not done, the vaginal sponge is removed at the completion of the laparotomy.

After the vaginal cleanup, the abdomen is washed with ether. Particular attention is paid to cleansing the umbilicus with a Q-tip sponge. The abdomen is prepared by the nurse or surgical assistant with a 5-minute scrub using a povidone-iodine (Betadine) or similar antiseptic solution. The surgically prepared area should extend from the abdominal wall midway between the umbilicus and the rib cage, superiorly, to the lower aspect of the mons pubis, inferiorly. The lateral margins of the skin preparation should extend to the anterior iliac crest and anterior axillary line. In recent years, many clinics have used Viodrape placed over the skin to protect the incision from contamination by skin bacteria.

Bibliography

Alexander S: Surgery in the cardiac patient. Surg Clin North Am 50:567, 1970

American Heart Association Committee Report. Prevention of Bacterial Endocarditis. Circulation 56(1):139A, 1977

Anderson DO, Ferris BC: Role of tobacco smoking in the causation of chronic respiratory disease. N Engl J Med 267:787, 1962

Antman EM, Stone PH, Muller JE, et al: Calcium channel blocking agents in the treatment of cardiovascular disorders. Part I: Basic and clinical electrophysiologic effects. Ann Intern Med 93:875, 1980

Appel GB, Neu HC: The nephrotoxicity of antimicrobial agents. N Engl J Med 296:663, 1977. First of three parts
————: The nephrotoxicity of antimicrobial agents. N Engl J Med 296:722, 1977. Second of three parts
————: The nephrotoxicity of antimicrobial agents. N Engl J Med 296:784, 1977. Third of three parts

Arkins R, Smessaert AA, Hicks RG: Mortality and morbidity in surgical patients with coronary artery disease. JAMA 190:485, 1964

Behrendt DM, Morrow AG: General operative procedures after cardiac valve replacement—results and methods of management of 33 patients. Arch Surg 96:824, 1968

Berger SA, Nagar H, Gordon M: Antimicrobial prophylaxis in obstetric and gynecologic surgery: A critical review. J Reprod Med 24:185, 1980

Beta-Blocker Heart Attack Study Group: The beta-blocker heart attack trial. JAMA 246:2073, 1981

Bomalski JS, Phair JG: Alcohol, immunosuppression, and the lung. Arch Int Med 142:2073, 1982

Cadanelli GP, Cavatorta E, Verrilli D: Chirurgia gynecologia e cardiopatie. Quad Clin Obstet Gynec 22:911, 1967

Cohn JN, Franciosa JA: Vasodilator Therapy in Cardiac Failure. N Engl J Med 297:27, 1977

Criteria Committee of the New York Heart Association: Diseases of the Heart and Blood Vessels: Nomenclature and Criteria for Diagnosis, 6th ed. Boston, Little, Brown & Co., 1964

Cunningham FG, Hamsell DL, DePalma RT, et al: Moxalactam for obstetric and gynecologic infections: In vitro and dose-finding studies. Am J Obstet Gynecol 139:915, 1981

Dana JB, Ohler RL: Influence of heart disease on surgical risk. JAMA 162:878, 1956

Devereaux RB, et al: Mitral valve prolapse. Circulation 54:3, 1976

Dodek A: The serum digoxin test: A clinical perspective. Cardiology Digest 14:19, 1979

Dreifus LS, Rabbino MD, Watanabe Y, Tabesh E: Arrhythmias in the Postoperative Period. Am J Card 12:431, 1963

Duff P, Park RC: Antibiotic prophylaxis in vaginal hysterectomy: A review. Obstet Gynecol (suppl) 55:193, 1980

Eidenmiller LR, Awe C, Hodam RP, et al: General surgical procedures in valve replacement patients. Am Surg 35:559, 1969

Gazes PC: Non-cardiac surgery in cardiac patients—preoperative and operative management. Postgrad Med 49:171, 1971

German PM, Stackpole DA, Levenson DK, et al: Second opinion for elective surgery. N Engl J Med 302:1169, 1980

Gold MJ, Helvich M: A study of the complications related to anesthesia in asthmatic patients. Anesth Analg (Cleve) 42:283, 1963

Goldman L, Caldera DL, Southwick FS, et al: Cardiac Risk Factors and Complications in Noncardiac Surgery. Medicine (Baltimore) 57:357, 1978

Greene HG: Cephalosporin therapy of soft tissue infections: An overview. J Int Med Res (suppl 1) 8:53, 1980

Hoeprich PD: Current principles of antibiotic therapy. Obstet Gynecol (suppl) 55:121, 1980

Horan LG, Flowers NC, Johnson JC: Significance of the diagnostic Q wave of myocardial infarction. Circulation 43:428, 1971

Jarkuberm JS, Braunwald E: Present status of digitalis treatment of acute myocardial infarction. Circulation 45:891, 1972

Jung R, et al: Comparison of three methods of respiratory care following upper abdominal surgery. Chest 78:31, 1980

Kannel WB, Feinlieb M: The natural history of angina pectoris in the Framingham Study—prognosis and survival. Am J Cardiol 29:154, 1972

Kass EH: The Role of Asymptomatic Bacteriuria in the Pathogenesis of Pyelonephritis. In Quinn EL, Kass EH (eds): Biology of Pyelonephritis, p 399. Boston: Little Brown & Company, 1960

Katholi RE, Nolan SP, McGuire B: Living with prosthetic heart valves, subsequent noncardiac operations and the risk of thromboembolism or hemorrhage. Am Heart J 92:162, 1976

Keelan MH, Jr: Evaluation of the gynecological patient with heart disease. Clin Obstet Gynecol 16:80, 1973

Ledger WJ: Prevention, diagnosis and treatment of postoperative infections. Obstet Gynecol (suppl) 55:203, 1980

Ledger WJ, Sweet RL, Headington JT: Prophylactic cephaloridine in the prevention of postoperative pelvic infections in premenopausal women undergoing vaginal surgery. Am J Obstet Gynecol 115:766, 1973

Masukawa T, Levinson EF, Forst JK: The cytologic examination of breast secretions. Acta Cytol (Baltimore) 10:261, 1966

Mattingly RF: Surgery in the aging female. Clin Obstet Gynecol 7:573, 1964

Mattingly RF: The prophylactic use of antibiotics in pelvic surgery: A discussion. Obstet Gynecol (suppl) 55:267, 1980

Mattingly TW: Patients with coronary disease as a surgical risk. Am J Cardiol 12:279, 1963

McCarthy EG, Finkel ML: Second consultant opinion for elective gynecologic surgery. Obstet Gynecol 56:403, 1980

Mills P, Rose J, Hollingsworth J, et al. Long term prognosis of mitral valve prolapse. N Engl J Med 297:13, 1977

Norwegian Multicenter Study Group: Timolol-induced reduction in mortality and reinfarction in patients surviving acute myocardial infarction. N Engl J Med 304:801, 1981

Okada RD, Boucher CA, Strauss HW, et al: Exercise radionuclide imaging approaches to coronary artery disease. Am J Cardiol 46:1188, 1980

Olgivie C: Physician among surgeons: Thoughts on preoperative assessment. Thorax 35:881, 1980

Polk BF, Shapiro M, Goldstein P, et al: Randomised clinical trial of perioperative Cefazolin in preventing infection after hysterectomy. Lancet 8166:437, 1980

Schlueter DP: Pulmonary risks. Clin Obstet Gynecol 16:91, 1973

Selzer A, Cohn KE: Some thoughts concerning prophylactic use of digitalis. Am J Cardiol 26:214, 1970

Shapiro B: Evaluation of respiratory function in the perioperative period. ASA Refresher Courses 221:1, 1979

Skinner JF, Pearce ML: Surgical risk in the cardiac patient. J Chronic Dis 17:57, 1964

Stahlgren LH: An analysis of factors which influence mortality following extensive abdominal operations upon geriatric patients. Surg Gynecol Obstet 113:283, 1961

Stein M, Koota GM, Simon M, et al: Pulmonary evaluation of surgical patients. JAMA 181:765, 1962

Stone PH, Antman EM, Muller JE, et al: Calcium channel blocking agents in the treatment of cardiovascular disorders. Part II: Hemodynamic effects and clinical applications. Ann Int Med 93:886, 1980

Swartz MH, Teichholz LE, Donoso F: Mitral valve prolapse—a review of associated arrhythmias. Am J Med 62:377, 1977

Swartz WH: Prophylaxis of minor febrile and major infections morbidity following hysterectomy. Obstet Gynecol 54:285, 1979

Tarhan S, Moffitt EA, Taylor WF, et al: Myocardial infarction after general anesthesia. JAMA 220:1451, 1972

Tinker JH, Tarhan S: Discontinuing anticoagulant therapy in surgical patients with cardiac valve prostheses: Observations in 180 operations. JAMA 239:738, 1978

U.S. Department of Health and Human Services, National Center for Health Statistics. Monthly Vital Statistics Report, vol 29, No 13, September 17, 1981 (published and unpublished data).

Wann LS, Dillon JC: Echocardiography of the Aortic Valve. In DeVlieger M (ed): Handbook of Clinical Ultrasound, p 453. New York, John Wiley and Sons, 1978

Wightman JA: A prospective survey of the incidence of postoperative pulmonary complications. Br J Surg 55:85, 1968

Chapter 6

Postoperative Care

Immediate Postoperative Care

The most critical period of a patient's postoperative course falls within the first 72 hours following surgery. During this period, the patient's physiologic reserve must be accurately assessed. Precise monitoring of the cardiovascular, renal, and respiratory systems provides the most valuable information about the patient's postoperative condition. Proper function of these three vital organ systems assures the surgeon of accurate control of the patient's physiologic response to pelvic surgery.

Cardiovascular Changes

Although blood pressure is one of the most valid indicators of cardiovascular reserve, postoperatively there may be wide variations in blood pressure recordings. Changes in peripheral vasodilatation or constriction as related to shifts in plasma volume in the intravascular compartment, as well as lability of the autonomic nervous system, result in blood pressure fluctuations in the immediate postoperative period. Compensatory tachycardia and peripheral vasoconstriction may temporarily mask major blood loss during or immediately following surgery. It is not until at least 25% to 30% of the normal blood volume has been lost that blood pressure will drop significantly and remain persistently low. For a 60-kg female, this would indicate a blood loss of approximately 1400 ml (*i.e.,* blood volume = 70 ml/kg). Although the pulse rate is quite sensitive to pressure changes in the great vessels, an increase in pulse rate, in itself, is not pathognomonic of impending cardiac decompensation. It is true that pressure receptors in the aortic arch and the carotid sinuses stimulate cardioaccelerator response, but acceleration of the heart is frequently seen in many conditions other than a fall of pressure in the aorta or great vessels. Among such causes are excitement, fear, and anxiety, and, in particular, the stress of surgery. In addition, changes in pulse rate in elderly people are frequently delayed and fail to predict impending cardiac failure accurately. Nonetheless, persistent tachycardia, combined with other clinical signs of cardiac decompensation, such as peripheral vasoconstriction with cold, clammy extremities, skin pallor, oliguria, and hypotension, is classic evidence of hypovolemia and cardiovascular decompensation.

Central Venous Pressure Monitoring

Central venous pressure (CVP) monitoring provides a sensitive clinical method of evaluating four measurable independent forces: (1) the volume and flow of blood in the central veins; (2) distensibility and contractility of the right chambers of the heart during filling; (3) vasomotor activity in central veins; and (4) intrathoracic pressure. Although all four factors may vary with profound blood loss, one of the primary clinical purposes of CVP monitoring is to monitor the central venous compartment while intravascular volume is being augmented. A high CVP (*i.e.,* more than 12–15 cm of water) may indicate a full intravascular compartment and an adequate circulating blood volume, but it may also indicate impending cardiac decompensation with right-sided heart failure. Consequently, blood volume studies, combined with continuous CVP recordings, provide useful information about both intravascular and cardiac reserve. In more difficult cases of cardio-pulmonary decompensation that require precise monitoring and resuscitation, the Swan–Ganz, multichannel pulmonary catheter has been of invaluable assistance in defining specific cardiac and pulmonary reserve, separate from vascular volume deficits. In the usual uncomplicated case, such as an abdominal or vaginal hysterectomy with the patient making a normal postoperative recovery, CVP monitoring is not necessary.

ANATOMY OF INFRACLAVICULAR SUBCLAVIAN VEIN

In 1952, Aubaniac, a French physician, was among the first to advocate the use of the subclavian vein for intravenous infusions. J. N. Wilson cannulated the superior vena cava through a percutaneous puncture of the subclavian vein. He reported a high percentage of successful cannulations and a low incidence of complications. There are five percutaneous sites for CVP monitoring: the groin, the antecubital fossa, the shoulder, the jugular vein, and the subclavian vein. Infraclavicular catheterization of the subclavian vein has had wide clinical use and has many advantages. Because of the obscured position of this vessel, an understanding of the anatomy of this region is important in mastering the technique of subclavian venipuncture.

As Figure 6–1 shows, the subclavian vein is located within the costoclavicular-scalene triangle, which is bounded anteriorly by the medial end of the clavicle, posteriorly by the upper surface of the first rib, and laterally by the anterior scalene muscle. The anterior scalene muscle separates the subclavian vein from the subclavian artery, which lies beneath and along the lateral aspect of the muscle. The subclavian vein is covered by 5 cm of the clavicle medially and joins the internal jugular vein near the medial border of the anterior scalene muscle to form the innominate vein. The innominate vein descends behind the sternum and joins with the opposite innominate vein to form the superior vena cava. The subclavian vein, which is approximately 3 cm or 4 cm long, continues as the axillary vein below the clavicle, en route to the axilla. Several other significant structures occupy this region. The phrenic nerve courses across the anterior surface of the anterior scalene muscle near its attachment to the first rib and courses medially to lie posterior to the subclavian vein. It can be injured if the posterior wall of the vessel is penetrated. The internal thoracic nerve and the apical pleura are in contact with the posterior surface of the subclavian vein at its junction with the internal jugular vein. The roots of the brachial plexus formed by the 5th, 6th, 7th,

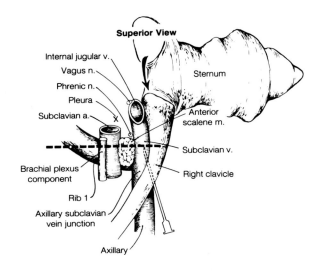

FIG. 6–1 Anatomical relationships of subclavian vein. Dotted line represents the location of transverse section for lateral view. (Adapted from Moosman DA: The anatomy of infraclavicular vein catheterization and its complaints. Surg Gynecol Obstet 136:71, 1973.)

and 8th cervical and the 1st thoracic nerves lie lateral to the anterior scalene muscle on the lateral side of the subclavian artery. If a cannulating needle is directed too far laterally, the brachial nerve plexus could be injured or the subclavian artery could be punctured. The thoracic duct on the left side and the lymphatic duct on the right, cross the anterior scalene muscle on either side of the thorax to enter the superior aspect of each subclavian vein near its junction with the internal jugular vein. These lymphatic vessels are rarely encroached upon during subclavian catheterization.

CENTRAL VENOUS PRESSURE MONITORING BY SUBCLAVIAN CATHETER

As illustrated in Figure 6–2A, the subclavian catheter is inserted with the patient in the supine position,

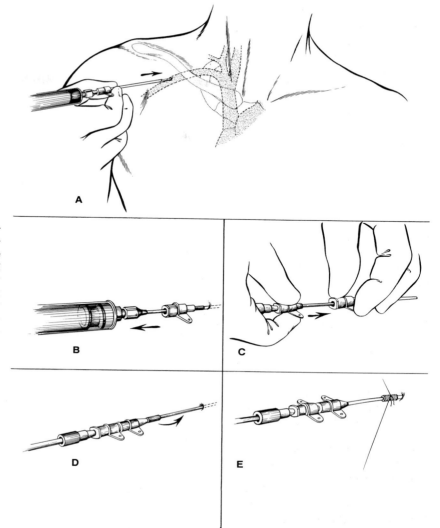

FIG. 6–2 Insertion of subclavian catheter for monitoring central venous pressure. (*A*) After locally anesthetizing the puncture site, the needle with overlying introducer catheter is directed medially between the first rib and the clavicle at the junction of the middle and inner third of the clavicle. Needle is held parallel to the anterior chest wall and advanced along the undersurface of the clavicle. Entry into the vein is evident with aspiration of blood in attached syringe. (*B*) The needle and syringe are removed from the Teflon sheath and a finger is held over end of open catheter to prevent entry of air. (*C*) The silicone infusion catheter is now inserted through introducer catheter until the two connectors meet and lock firmly. (*D*) The intravenous fluid line is connected to the silicone infusion catheter. (*E*) The suture sleeve is advanced to the skin surface where the catheter is sutured firmly to the skin.

with the foot of the bed elevated 6 to 12 inches to increase the pressure in the subclavian vein and produce venous distention. After meticulous aseptic preparation of the skin with povidone-iodine (Betadine), the skin and subcutaneous tissues are infiltrated with a 1% solution of lidocaine (Xylocaine) if the patient is awake. The point of needle insertion is approximately 1 cm below the junction of the inner and middle third of the clavicle. Most central venous catheter units include an external introducer catheter (Teflon) and an internal (silicone) infusion catheter. The outer, Teflon sheath accommodates a No. 12 gauge needle, which fits snugly into and protrudes beyond the end of the Teflon catheter. The needle and sheath are introduced into the skin with the shaft of the needle held almost parallel with

the anterior chest wall (Fig. 6–2A). The needle is directed medially and advanced along the undersurface of the clavicle. It is not necessary to scrape the posterior surface of the clavicle to ensure that the pleura are protected from puncture. By applying suction constantly, the needle passes beneath the skin and immediately aspirates dark red blood, which confirms entry into the vein. If the vein is not entered, the needle is withdrawn and readvanced in a similar manner but in a slightly more cranial or caudal direction. As soon as a free flow of blood is obtained, the introduced Teflon sheath is advanced far enough to be certain that it is securely placed within the vein. The sheath is held in place by the connector, the finger is placed over the end of the needle to prevent air embolism, and the internal needle is replaced (Fig. 6–2B) by the silicone infusion catheter that accompanies the CVP kit (Fig. 6–2C). A thin wire stylet inside the infusion catheter allows the catheter to be advanced easily; occasionally, the stylet must be withdrawn slightly in order to advance the catheter as far as possible into the innominate vein and superior vena cava. The silicone infusion catheter is advanced until the attached connector can be securely wedged into the connector of the Teflon sheath (Fig. 6–2C). After the infusion catheter is connected to an intravenous fluid line, the Teflon sheath is carefully withdrawn from the vein, remaining partially in the subcutaneous tissue while leaving an ample length of the infusion catheter in the vena cava (Fig. 6–2D). A suture sleeve on the introducer sheath is slid down to the puncture site and sutured to the skin (Fig. 6–2E). The tip of the catheter is preferably positioned in the superior vena cava and should not be advanced into the right atrium or ventricle, where it could cause accidental trauma to the heart wall or cardiac arrhythmias. To ensure its continued sterility and proper function, the subclavian vein catheter should not be used for fluid replacement or for the withdrawal of blood for laboratory studies, if it is at all possible to avoid these uses. A central venous line for hyperalimentation is an exception to this rule. The dressing should be changed daily and the catheterization site cleaned with povidone-iodine or similar antimicrobial solution.

The zero reference point on the CVP manometer is adjusted to a point approximately 5 cm posterior to the 4th costochondral junction. Others choose a point 10 cm anterior to the skin of the back in the plane of the 4th costochondral junction, and some select a point equidistant between the anterior and the posterior chest wall. Although the specific external reference point for the right atrium is not critical, it is important to continue to use the same manometer site in subsequent recordings. Normal CVP is considered to be within the range of 5 cm to 12 cm of water. Since pressure readings depend on the integrated effects of blood volume, pulmonary circulation, cardiac output, and vascular tone, there is wide variation in the normal CVP level.

Factors that tend to elevate CVP include cardiac failure, increased venous return (as in hypervolemia, increased venous tone, or reduced venous-capillary resistance of the peripheral microcirculation), and vasoconstriction of the pulmonary microcirculation.

Factors that tend to lower CVP include improved cardiac output and diminished venous return (as in hypovolemic shock, increased peripheral resistance, or venous pooling).

Perhaps the most precise method of monitoring the effect of fluid replacement including blood, plasma, water, and electrolytes, is by repeated monitoring of CVP levels. This method permits adequate fluid replacement with relative assurance that cardiac overloading will be avoided. As the CVP rises to a level of 12 cm of water, fluid replacement is restricted until the CVP level is gradually reduced.

CVP monitoring cannot be assumed to be infallible, but must be used in conjunction with critical evaluation of other clinical methods of cardiovascular monitoring. By itself, CVP does not indicate blood volume or the adequacy of fluid replacement. It indicates the ability of the heart to pump effectively the volume of fluid returned to it. It may also indicate a deficiency of venous return. When more specific information is required to differentiate cardiopulmonary function from excessive intravascular volume replacement, the insertion of a Swan-Ganz catheter into the pulmonary artery may be critical for the proper management of a postoperative patient. In general, we prefer not to leave a catheter in the subclavian vein for more than 3 to 5 days, although we have, on specific occasions, left it in place for as long as 2 to 3 weeks. The longer the catheter is maintained in the vena cava or great veins, the greater is the risk of seeding the bloodstream with bacteria from the skin.

The complication rate of catheterization of the superior vena cava and major central veins varies in frequency from 1% to 10% of reported cases. Most of the serious complications of the subclavian puncture, such as pneumothorax, hemothorax, hydrothorax, brachial nerve injury, and subclavian artery puncture, result from introducing the needle with too great a posterior or lateral angulation. These problems can be prevented by keeping the needle in a medial direction, almost parallel to the anterior chest wall as it is introduced, and by directing it between the first rib and the clavicle, close to, but not against, the posterior surface of the clavicle. Additional complications include air embolization during insertion, cellulitis and sepsis, thrombosis, and catheter embolization into the right atrium. The most common complications of catheter insertion are pneumothorax and hemothorax.

The risk of bacteremia is one of the major disadvantages of an indwelling central intravenous catheter. A culture of the catheter tip, upon removal, reportedly has been positive in between 5% and 45% of the cases studied. However, a catheter-induced bacteremia has been reported in less than 0.5% of cases. *Staphylococcus* is the most common organism cultured, and the infection rate increases with the length of time that the catheter is in place. Meticulous attention must be given to daily maintenance of a central venous catheter, which requires that the catheter be redressed and the skin scrubbed with isopropyl alcohol and povidone-iodine every 24 hours. The catheter should be removed whenever there is clinical suspicion of a systemic infection if the cause cannot be otherwise identified.

SWAN–GANZ CATHETER

In the absence of serious cardiopulmonary dysfunction, CVP monitoring is usually sufficient to evaluate both right and left heart hemodynamics. However, in a critically ill patient, such as the patient in the state of advanced hemorrhagic shock, it is essential to distinguish cardiac and pulmonary dysfunction from hypovolemia. The appropriate fluid management in such cases depends on the accurate hemodynamic assessment of cardiac output, pulmonary arterial pressure, pulmonary capillary wedge pressure, and the ultimate ability to differentiate cardiogenic from noncardiogenic pulmonary edema. The CVP method of continuous cardiopulmonary monitoring is essential with patients who develop adult respiratory distress syndrome. In particular, there is good evidence to show that pulmonary artery pressure and pulmonary capillary wedge pressure are much more reliable indicators of the variations of left ventricular filling pressure than is CVP.

The Swan–Ganz flow-directed catheter was introduced in 1970 for the purpose of measuring right ventricular and pulmonary artery pressures. Since that time, various multiple-lumen, radiopaque, balloon-tipped catheters have been developed to permit easy insertion and the advancement of the catheter by direct blood flow into the pulmonary artery (Fig. 6–3). The catheter is inserted by a cutaneous approach, usually through the right or left internal jugular vein, although the subclavian vein has also been utilized. After a No. 16-gauge Teflon catheter is placed into the vein, a No. 8 French, radiopaque, triple-balloon catheter is inserted and the balloon is inflated. The catheter is carried by the force of the bloodstream and is allowed to pass directly through the right atrium and the right ventricle and into the pulmonary artery. Its progress can be monitored by the characteristic pressure tracings on a bedside oscilloscope. Once the catheter has advanced until it lodges in a wedged position in the pulmonary vasculature, a characteristic pulmonary capillary wedge pressure tracing is observed on the oscilloscope. At this point the balloon is deflated and a pulmonary artery tracing can be obtained con-

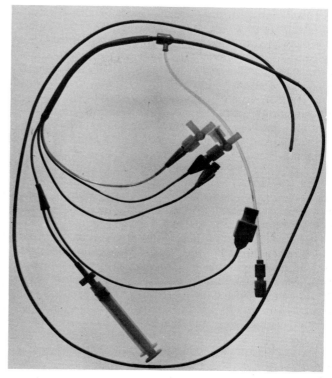

FIG. 6–3 Swan–Ganz multilumen, triple-balloon catheter.

tinuously. The pulmonary wedge pressure can be determined intermittently by reinflating the balloon. The pulmonary wedge pressure is closely related to the left atrial pressure, which in turn reflects the left ventricular end-diastolic pressure if there is no significant mitral valvular disease. A normal pulmonary wedge pressure is less than 12 mm Hg; pressures above this level indicate pulmonary vascular congestion or pulmonary edema. Regardless of the cause, an elevated pulmonary wedge pressure reflects an increase in intravascular volume, and the patient should be treated accordingly. In contrast, CVP values may provide misleading information about cardiac ventricular activity and can misguide the physician in the accurate replacement of intravascular fluid volume.

The indwelling Swan-Ganz catheter allows continuous monitoring of pulmonary artery pressure, pulmonary capillary wedge pressure, CVP, arterial blood pressure, and cardiac output. In addition, arterial gas pressures, including the percent of oxygen saturation, can be obtained. These are the essential data for computation of all cardiac indices and for calculation of the extent of right-to-left pulmonary vascular shunting. When pulmonary wedge pressure rises above 12 mm Hg to 15 mm Hg, suggesting impairment of left cardiac output or an increase in intravascular volume, the infusion fluid volume should be restricted to avoid progressive cardiopulmonary failure. For the critically ill patient with severe cardiopulmonary compromise due to hypovolemia, hypoxemia, and progressive acidosis, the Swan-Ganz catheter is an invaluable aid to the proper replacement of intravascular volume.

Shock

Shock may be defined in various ways, but in practical terms it is a state of inadequate tissue perfusion, characterized by cardiac output inadequate to provide normal circulation in the major organs. Whether the basic underlying factor is myocardial failure, obstruction of the arterial pathways (pulmonary embolus or coronary occlusion), increased peripheral capillary resistance, widespread peripheral vascular pooling, or direct blood loss, the end result is the same: insufficient circulating blood volume to ensure adequate tissue perfusion. Historically, Blalock at the Johns Hopkins Hospital was one of the earlier investigators to propose a classification for shock according to various causative mechanisms, and the general categories in use today are similar to those proposed by him. They include: (1) hemorrhagic shock, (2) septic shock, (3) neurogenic shock, (4) cardiogenic shock, and (5) various combinations of these.

Although each type of shock is related to a particular pathophysiologic pattern, in practice a combination of interrelated factors is usually involved in the more serious forms of circulatory collapse. Sepsis, with its adverse effect on cellular metabolism, is a frequent complication in patients with acute blood loss. Irrespective of whether shock initiated by a single factor or a combination of factors, the end stage of shock is the same—a decreased cardiac output, diminished circulatory blood volume with progressive hemoconcentration, alterations in cell metabolism, hypoxia and acidosis, peripheral capillary dilatation, and, finally, failure of return of blood to the heart, resulting in cardiac standstill.

PATHOPHYSIOLOGY OF HEMORRHAGIC SHOCK

Shock, regardless of its precipitating cause, is a molecular disorder. The basic pathophysiologic problem in all types of shock is hypoxia, which produces metabolic disarrangements that revolve about anaerobic glucose metabolism. This anaerobic process produces increased blood levels of lactic acid, amino acids, fatty acids, and phosphoric acids, which lower the blood pH and produce systemic acidosis. Metabolic acidosis causes disruption of the lysosome membrane within the cell with an outpouring of lytic enzymes, principally acid phosphatase and hydrolases, which destroy the cell. This anaerobic metabolism also decreases the production of ATP, which governs the exchange of extracellular sodium and intracellular potassium and limits the synthesis of proteins and enzymes. A decrease in ATP synthesis causes a loss of the sodium-pump mechanism and permits an influx of sodium and water into the cell and an escape of potassium from the cell. The net metabolic effect of these changes is an increased serum level of blood pyruvate and lactate, an increase in serum potassium (hyperkalemia), an intracellular shift of sodium and water, a depletion of serum sodium, and a gradual process of hemoconcentration—all changes that are characteristic of metabolic acidosis. Intracellular release of lysosomal enzymes causes both lysis of the cell membrane and degradation of proteins, carbohydrate, and fat.

In order to prevent the effects of shock from becoming irreversible, it is essential that the patient be maintained in appropriate hemodynamic balance. This balance depends on three interrelated factors: (1) an adequate cardiac output—an effective pump; (2) a reasonably normal blood volume—an effective circulatory fluid; and (3) a normal vascular tone—an open conducting system. Alterations in any one of these basic hemodynamic prerequisites will produce compensatory changes in the remaining two. Consequently, the early compensatory changes that accompany acute blood loss, which include an increase in cardiac rate and an increase in peripheral vascular resistance, will result in an adequate circulation without significant change in blood pressure. These autonomic changes will temporarily mask the symptoms and clinical signs of an altered circulating blood volume. When blood volume loss reaches 30% or more, these adaptive changes fail to support a normal cardiac output and an adequate peripheral circulation and systemic blood pressure falls. As the hypovolemia progresses, the cell becomes more anoxic, sodium and water enter the cell, and potassium and lactate are forced into the serum. The clinical effect of this metabolic shift is the accumulation of an increasing amount of blood lactate in the serum, which is reflected by progressive acidosis, and the development of dehydration and hemoconcentration.

The barometer of hemorrhagic shock is at the capillary level, where increased peripheral vascular constriction, caused by the release of sympathomimetic amines, produces arteriovenous shunting and accelerates the process of cellular anoxia, anaerobic metabolism, and lactic acidosis. As the lysosomes rupture and destroy the cell, the anoxic process becomes irreversible. The process is complicated by the fact that the arterial precapillary sphincter mechanism is apparently more sensitive to low pH than is the distal venous sphincter. As acidosis advances and the precapillary sphincter decompensates, the venous sphincter maintains its tone, and an increase in capillary stagnation or pooling is produced. Consequently, blood is trapped or pooled in the peripheral capillary bed, which is estimated to be capable of accommodating a blood volume 500 times greater than normal.

Clinically, hemorrhagic shock may be divided into three phases; early, intermediate, and late or irreversible. A dramatic example of *early hemorrhagic shock* is seen in the gradual intraperitoneal accumulation of blood from a ruptured ectopic pregnancy. Such cases clearly demonstrate the early stage of shock by a temporary decrease in cardiac output and arterial blood pressure. This is followed by compensatory changes of the sympathetic nervous system and decreased vagal nerve activity. In effect, these adaptive measures tend to increase the heart rate and restore cardiac output and arterial pressure temporarily. These changes are augmented by an increase in peripheral arterial resistance and an inotropic effect on the cardiac muscle, producing more forceful myocardial contractions. At this stage, the patient with an ectopic pregnancy will experience increasing symptoms of abdominal and pelvic pain, but the magnitude of the intraperitoneal blood loss may be masked by these adaptive hemodynamic responses. If the patient is seen at this time, the compensatory mechanisms of early shock will maintain a relatively normal blood pressure while she is in the supine position. This process can be unmasked by having the patient sit or stand erect, which will demonstrate orthostatic hypotension. The pulse rate will be rapid and the patient will be hypovolemic from intraperitoneal hemorrhage. This form of early, "warm" shock is reversible and is not associated with prolonged cellular acidosis. However, if not treated promptly, the hemodynamic compensatory changes may fail. When patients are delayed in obtaining prompt medical care, the blood loss may progress to a more critical, and frequently irreversible phase.

Plasma refill is an important compensatory mechanism in hemorrhagic shock. It was previously thought that the fastest rate at which humans could refill plasma volume by the intravascular absorption of interstitial water was 90 ml/hr. More recent studies have demonstrated that interstitial fluid can reenter the vascular space to compensate for severe hypovolemia at about ten times this rate, or approximately 900 ml/hr. Hemorrhagic shock, then, is a phenomenon that is related to intravascular volume, the rate of blood loss, and the rate of plasma refill. Over a long period, one can slowly lose an enormous amount of blood without clinical evidence of hypotension or shock. However, a very rapid loss of a small amount of blood can result in clinical shock. One of the major differences between these two hemodynamic conditions is related to plasma refill. The continuous refill of the intravascular compartment by interstitial fluid will prevent shock in cases of insidious and slow blood loss. However, this physiologic mechanism is insufficient to compensate for rapid blood loss, even though the loss is of a smaller total volume. It is evident that the individual is shielded from the state of hemorrhagic shock by a number of physiologic mechanisms and adaptations that will temporarily avert vascular collapse. When the limits of these physiologic adaptations have been exceeded, the patient will enter a phase of hypovolemia, impairment of venous return, and cardiac output inadequate to sustain normal tissue perfusion.

The *intermediate stage* of shock is the pivotal stage of this disease in terms of reversibility (Fig. 6–4), since compensatory mechanisms alone are no longer effective in producing an adequate circulation. During the intermediate phase, cardiac output may be decreased more than can be counterbalanced by the reflex inotropic mechanisms and, as a consequence, many vital organs will have an inadequate circulation. There is a preferential distribution of blood to the heart and brain from less vital organs. Prolonged impairment of oxygen supply to the kidneys will produce progressive renal shutdown and will accelerate the metabolic acidosis by changes in cellular function of the distal renal tubules. Peripheral ischemia, associated with sympathetic stimulation of the sweat glands, produces cold clammy extremities and the early signs of advanced, or "cold" shock.

If the intermediate phase of shock goes untreated, it will progress to the terminal phase. Diminished cardiac output and impaired cerebral perfusion is manifested by progressive mental confusion and, later, by coma. The decrease in blood flow to the gastrointestinal tract may produce a secondary bacteremia from breakdown of the mucosal–endothelial barrier. A decrease in renal blood flow is immediately sensed by the juxtaglomerular apparatus of the afferent renal arterioles, leading to the release of renin into the plasma and the subsequent conversion of renin to an inactive polypeptide, angiotensin I, which is metabolized to the vasoactive form, angiotensin II, in the liver. This potent arteriolar constrictor induces the secretion of cate-

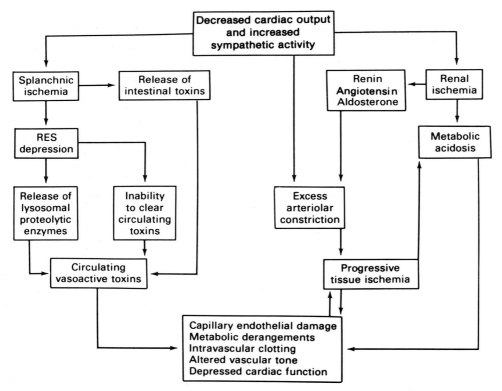

FIG. 6–4 Pathophysiologic changes in intermediate shock.

cholamine from the adrenal medulla and aldosterone from the adrenal cortex. The action of aldosterone in conserving salt and water to improve the depleted circulating blood volume is only temporarily beneficial. Renal ischemia also produces a decrease in the glomerular filtration rate, with progressive oliguria or anuria. Bicarbonate solutions and other alkaline buffers are of limited value in controlling progressive acidosis. Unless the circulation is restored to normal, changing the blood pH will have no effect on this metabolic process and the lactic acidosis will persist.

The final, *irreversible phase* of hemorrhagic shock produces the clinical picture of progressive cerebral and cardiovascular ischemia (Fig. 6–5) due to intense peripheral vasoconstriction. The patient becomes unresponsive to external stimuli, is ashen-gray in color, and is anuric. Cardiac arrhythmia develops, and the patient finally expires in cardiac arrest. Heroic attempts to reverse this stage of the metabolic process are usually unsuccessful because the myocardium and central nervous system have undergone cellular death and are unable to respond to any kind of stimulation or aggressive therapy.

TREATMENT OF SHOCK

Each patient must have accurate hemodynamic evaluation before beginning any type of treatment. However, the basic goals of all types of treatment are similar: (1) to improve the effective circulating blood volume, and (2) to improve cellular perfusion and oxygenation. The major effect of this therapy is to increase the effective blood flow to organs and tissues, regardless of the causative factors. In recognition of the unified concept of shock as a decreased perfusion of vital organs, the essential steps of treatment are to ventilate and to infuse. Pharmacologic drugs and surgery are essential components in the treatment of hemorrhagic shock. The general objectives in the treatment of shock that are included in this discussion are outlined in Table 6–1.

Fluid Replacement

Although the most essential requirement in the management of hemorrhagic shock is the immediate control of the source of bleeding, before surgery can be performed, it is first necessary to replace

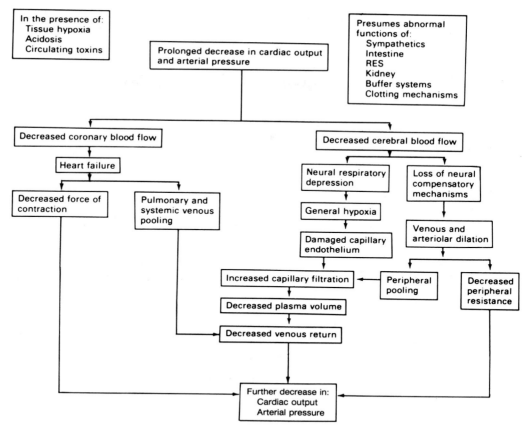

FIG. 6–5 Pathophysiologic changes in irreversible shock.

the patient's blood volume. The establishment of adequate vascular volume is more important than the specific type of fluid administered, although whole blood has no equal in the treatment of hemorrhagic shock. Delay in blood replacement may require the immediate use of noncolloidal solutions, principally the sodium-containing crystalloids, such as sodium chloride or the so-called balanced salt solution, Ringer's lactate. These crystalloid solutions, including 5% glucose and water, have molecules that are quite small and rapidly filter through the vessel wall into the interstitial space. Although this interstitial transfer may be beneficial, since it will offset the previous intracellular transfer of water and sodium from the interstitial compartment, care must be taken to avoid interstitial overload and the production of harmful edema. As a rule of thumb, at least three times as much crystalloid solution as whole blood is required to replace a specific amount of vascular volume.

Instead of crystalloids, some prefer intravascular colloid replacement, including the use of plasma, albumin, and such hypertonic solutions as high or low molecular weight dextran and polyethyl starches. These molecules are large enough to stay within the vascular tree and do not permeate the capillary wall easily. However, the risk of serum

TABLE 6–1 *General Objectives in Treating Shock*

INDICATION	OBJECTIVE
Systolic blood pressure	$\geqslant$90 mm Hg
Urine output	>40 ml/hr
Central venous pressure	12–15 cm H_2O
Pulmonary capillary wedge	
pressure	12–15 mm Hg
Skin	Warm, no cyanosis
Sensorium	Oriented
Blood gases	
P_aO_2	80–100 mm Hg
P_aCO_2	30–35 mm Hg
pH	7.35–7.50
Hemoglobin	12–14 g%

hepatitis is always present with the use of large volumes of plasma, and therefore most clinics prefer to use salt-poor albumin rather than plasma. Hauser, Shoemaker, and associates have shown, in controlled hemorrhagic shock studies, that 200 ml of 25% albumin produced improvement in plasma volume, cardiac output, stroke volume, and oxygen consumption equivalent to that produced by 1 liter of Ringer's lactate solution. Therefore, salt-poor albumin is an excellent plasma expander. It is used as one of the major components of fluid replacement therapy to combat hypovolemia. High (mol wt 70,000) or low (mol wt 40,000) molecular weight dextran has been used cautiously as a plasma expander during the past decade for several reasons. Initially, its osmotic activity as a colloid pulls extracellular fluid very rapidly into the vascular compartment and keeps the tissues dehydrated. Although dextran does have a beneficial effect on preventing the aggregation of red blood cells and platelets, which decreases the frequency of venous thrombosis, it also has thromboplastinlike properties and may cause further bleeding from disseminated intravascular coagulation. This intracapillary coagulation is more active with the use of high molecular weight dextran than with the low molecular weight solution; nonetheless, it is present in both dextran solutions and caution should be used to avoid the replacement of more than 20% of the total blood volume with these colloids.

An important laboratory method of monitoring colloid and crystalloid fluid replacement is through the use of serum osmolality (normal = 290 mOsm/liter). Regardless of the type of fluids given—whole blood, albumin, crystalloids, or other colloids—adequate intravascular volume replacement therapy may require several times the normal blood volume in fluid replacement before there is evidence of clinical improvement, since the amount of peripheral pooling is unpredictable. With such large amounts of intravenous fluids, it is essential that the fluid volume be monitored carefully with frequent assessment of CVP or pulmonary wedge pressure recordings to avoid the complication of cardiac overload and pulmonary edema. Nonetheless, until the low CVP or pulmonary wedge pressure levels return to normal, aggressive replacement of intravascular volume is the key to improvement in tissue perfusion and in the patient's clinical response. Fluid replacement should also be monitored by accurate recording of urinary output. In general, urinary output is an excellent clinical indicator of tissue perfusion. If the kidneys produce at least 30 ml/hr to 40 ml/hr of urine, it is probable that all other organs are being adequately perfused. Urine specific gravity is also an excellent index of the extent of hydration (normal sp gr = 1.010–1.015).

Meticulous control of fluid and electrolyte balance is essential in altering peripheral cellular metabolism. Correction of tissue oxygenation is important in the prevention or treatment of potentially fatal hyperkalemia due to shock. The extracellular release of potassium into the serum is a frequent complication of shock that may develop with alarming rapidity. The clinical signs of hyperkalemia include decreased deep tendon reflexes, muscle weakness, acroparesthesias, and cardiac arrhythmias. The use of the following agents is beneficial in the management of hyperkalemia: calcium gluconate (10 ml of 10% solution given slowly, intravenously); sodium bicarbonate (1 ampule [45 mEq] given slowly, intravenously); or insulin and glucose (30 units of crystalline insulin in 500 ml of 20% dextrose over 30 to 60 minutes, intravenously). These agents either counteract the physiologic effect of extracellular potassium or produce a temporary shift of potassium into the cell and rapidly lower the serum level. This effect may also be achieved by cation exchange,

TABLE 6–2 *Adrenergic Receptors, Agents, and Response in the Treatment of Shock*

RECEPTOR	AGENT	RESPONSE
α	Norepinephrine* Dopamine†	Vasoconstriction (postcapillary > precapillary)
β_1	Isoproterenol‡	Positive inotropic (contractility) and chronotropic (rate) stimulation of heart
	Dopamine	(inotropic > chronotropic)
	Dobutamine§	(inotropic ≫ chronotropic)
β_2	Isoproterenol	Vasodilatation
	Dopamine	"Dopaminergic" (specifically, renal and splanchnic vasodilatation)

* Levophed   † Intropin   ‡ Isuprel   § Dobutrex

TABLE 6–3   *Adrenergic Receptors and Organ Response*

ORGAN	RECEPTOR	RESPONSE	BLOCKING AGENTS
Heart	β_1	↑Heart rate, ↑contractility, ↑AV conduction rate	Propranolol (Inderal) Metoprolol (Lopressor)
Blood vessels	β_2 α	Dilatation Constriction	Propranolol Phentolamine (Regitine) Phenoxybenzamine (Dibenzyline) Chlorpromazine (Thorazine)
Bronchioles	β_2	Dilatation	Propranolol

whereby 1 g of polystyrene sulfonate (Kayexalate) removes 1 mEq of serum potassium by exchanging 3 mEq of sodium. This may be given rectally (50 g of Kayexalate and 50 g of sorbitol in 200 ml of water) as an enema, which should be retained for 30 to 60 minutes; it may be repeated every 6 to 12 hours as needed or given orally (15 g of Kayexalate in 15 ml of 70% sorbitol solution in water every 4 to 12 hours as needed).

Vasoactive Drugs

The pharmacologic effects of most agents used in the treatment of shock are mediated through adrenergic receptors in various organs and blood vessels. These receptors are designated as α and β; the latter having been divided into β_1 and β_2 components (Table 6–2). The α and β receptors have specific adrenergic responses in various organs (Table 6–3). It is important to emphasize that there is a variable and graded response of various organs to sympathetic stimulation as outlined in Figure 6–6. Further, for any given α-adrenergic stimulation (vasoconstriction), the precapillary sphincters are less responsive than the postcapillary sphincters. As a result, venous return and cardiac output are diminished due to peripheral vascular pooling and loss of fluid into the extravascular space. An increase in intravascular colloid and osmotic pressure will counteract this increase of interstitial fluid accumulation and will improve the circulating blood volume. Several adrenergic agents have an important role in providing hemodynamic support to patients in shock: only one or two, however, are of major clinical value.

Potent vasopressor substances such as norepinephrine (Levophed) are not appropriate agents for the treatment of hemorrhagic shock. Since the hemodynamic changes following shock have produced a marked increase in peripheral vascular constriction, the use of potent pressor-amines may cause further impairment of peripheral tissue perfusion. The net effect of this treatment would be to produce further tissue anoxia and to perpetuate and compound the metabolic acidosis. If there is clinical evidence of vasoconstriction with cold, clammy extremities, the use of a potent vasoconstricting agent is unwarranted.

In early shock with mild peripheral vasoconstriction (warm shock), the use of α-blocking agents such as chlorpromazine (Thorazine) or phenoxybenzamine (Dibenzyline) has been quite successful. When used in intravenous doses of 10 mg to 25 mg every 4 to 6 hours, chlorpromazine has proven to be an effective α-blocker with rapid improvement in renal blood flow and urinary output. The beneficial effect of this drug lies in the fact that it can be used in small doses with relative safety and immediate vasomotor response. In most cases, dopamine or dobutamine is the agent of choice for more advanced stages of shock. As shown in Table 6–2, dopamine stimulates both α and β_1 receptors, thereby producing controlled vasoconstriction and improved inotropic cardiac contractility at doses

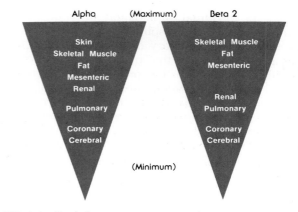

FIG. 6–6   Graded receptor response of various organs to α and β-2 adrenergic stimulation.

between 8 mcg/kg/min and 15 mcg/kg/min. Dopamine also has a specific pharmacologic effect on producing renal and splanchnic vasodilatation which is beneficial in improving renal blood flow. At doses of greater than 15 mcg/kg/min to 20 mcg/kg/min, the drug acts as a vasoconstrictor and the effects are comparable to those of norepinephrine; such doses should be avoided. The following pharmacologic effects of dopamine make it a preferable drug for hemorrhagic shock: (1) it stimulates the β_1 receptors in the heart, producing a positive inotropic (contractive force) and a lesser chronotropic (rate) effect on the myocardium; (2) it produces vasodilatation of the renal and splanchnic vascular beds; (3) it has a controlled α-adrenergic, vasoconstrictive effect on other vascular beds at therapeutic levels. The most sensitive clinical indication of the pharmacologic level of this drug is a urinary output of 30 ml to 40 ml per hour. When this clinical response has been achieved, one should make no further demands on the patient's adaptive vascular mechanisms, and no additional increase in this agent should be used. An ideal urinary ouput of 50 ml to 60 ml per hour may not be immediately achievable during the acute recovery phase of shock.

Pulmonary Ventilation in Hemorrhagic Shock

The adult respiratory distress syndrome (ARDS) may result as a latent sequela to the hemodynamic changes of shock. The patient may show signs of tachypnea and develop rales throughout the lungs within a period of 24 hours following the restoration of the blood pressure to normal values. The clinical picture of respiratory distress is associated with a reduction of P_aO_2 (as low as 40–60 mm Hg) along with an elevated P_aCO_2. Administration of 100% oxygen may not improve the situation and may give clinical evidence of pulmonary shunting from areas of the lung that are partially perfused but not ventilated. The use of controlled mechanical ventilation should be instituted immediately in an attempt to compensate for the respiratory acidosis that may develop. The respiratory distress appears to be a result of changes in the integrity of the alveolar capillary membrane that produce diffuse pulmonary interstitial edema without cardiomegaly. As a result, severe hypoxemia is difficult to correct, despite use of 100% oxygen and mechanical ventilation. The apparent loss of alveolar surfactant leads to atelectasis and exaggeration of the right-to-left pulmonary shunt of unoxygenated blood. The physiologic mechanism that is responsible for this pulmonary insult appears to be the initial damage to the alveoli and pulmonary capillaries from the transient or prolonged state of shock and hypoxemia.

The treatment of shock lung is frequently more difficult than cardiac and hemodynamic resuscitation. Although the overzealous and aggressive use of intravascular volume replacement can produce pulmonary edema, it is questionable whether this physiologic derangement is the mechanism responsible for the development of the shock lung. However, it is essential that meticulous fluid and electrolyte balance be maintained to avoid further insult to the damaged lung. The use of oxygen is obligatory for the hypoxemic state. Oxygen must be used with endotracheal intubation and with a volume-cycled mechanical ventilator. If there is no improvement in P_aO_2 after 12 hours of increasing concentrations of oxygen from 60% to 100%, it is important to institute positive end-expiratory pressure (PEEP) to improve the inflation of the pulmonary alveoli and to enhance oxygen exchange. The etiology and treatment of ARDS are discussed in more detail in the section on Pulmonary Complications, below in this chapter.

Treatment of Acidosis

The effect of progressive metabolic acidosis due to hypoxia and anaerobic glycolysis is cytotoxic, with the release of lysosomal lytic enzymes and cell death. Acidosis also increases the tone of both afferent arteriolar and efferent venous sphincters, the efferent more than the afferent vessels, with progression of peripheral pooling and cellular anoxia. The biologic effect of alkali in counteracting the metabolic acidosis is its potential benefit on the arteriolar sphincter and on improving lysosomal membrane integrity. Sodium bicarbonate and tris(hydroxymethyl)aminomethane (TRIS buffer or THAM) are used occasionally in the treatment of metabolic acidosis. It must be understood, however, that the acidosis will not improve until the anaerobic cellular metabolism is corrected. If it is to be clinically effective, alkali therapy should be initiated early in the treatment of shock. The usual dosage of bicarbonate is 45 mEq to 60 mEq per liter of parenteral fluid. However, the only effective treatment of metabolic acidosis is the reestablishment of an adequate vascular volume that is sufficient to produce tissue perfusion and arrest the process of anaerobic cellular metabolism.

Corticosteroids

Pharmacologic doses of hydrocortisone have shown more favorable clinical response when used in the treatment of gram-negative septic shock than in hemorrhagic shock. The principal effects of hydrocortisone in the management of shock are related to its inotropic effect, its theoretical enhancement of the microcirculation by the reduction of peripheral vascular resistance, and its effect on lysosomal membrane stabilization. When used, corticosteroid agents should be given in dosages equivalent to 2 g/24 hr to 6 g/24 hr of hydrocortisone. Dexamethasone (Decadron) is used in large dosages of 6 mg/kg/24 hr. Methylprednisolone (Solu-Medrol), 30 mg/kg every 8 to 12 hours, may also be used. If the agent is used for 48 hours without clinical response, its efficacy is doubtful. It can be discontinued abruptly without evidence of adrenal insufficiency or other untoward effects. Corticosteroids are more beneficial in the early stage of hemorrhagic shock than in the later phase of this metabolic dysfunction when the syndrome has become very advanced or irreversible.

The Surgical Control of Pelvic Hemorrhage

The most important step in the treatment of hemorrhagic shock is the control of hemorrhage. The pelvic bleeding must be controlled as soon as the patient's vital signs and blood volume have been stabilized. Life-threatening pelvic hemorrhage is more frequently a complication of obstetrics, where it is frequently associated with a ruptured gravid uterus, than of gynecology. Uncontrollable gynecologic hemorrhage is seen most commonly with extensive or radical pelvic surgery and postoperatively as a result of retraction of either an ovarian or a uterine vessel from its ligature with a consequent retroperitoneal hemorrhage.

Identifying the specific bleeding vessel in intraoperative and postoperative hemorrhage from the pelvis may be technically difficult or, occasionally, impossible. The anatomy is altered as a result of surgery, and the vessels are retracted beneath the pelvic peritoneum. However, the blood should be rapidly suctioned away and a search should be made for the bleeding source. If the vessel is not found promptly, one should not lose valuable time by continuing the search while the patient's condition deteriorates. Instead, ligation of the anterior division of the hypogastric artery should be performed. This procedure more often becomes necessary following a difficult operative dissection from advanced pelvic disease, both benign and malignant, than after more conservative pelvic surgery.

HYPOGASTRIC ARTERY LIGATION. One of the most effective and rapid methods of controlling severe pelvic hemorrhage is by ligation of both hypogastric arteries. Because of the major collateral circulation with the aorta and femoral artery (see chapter 4), including the lumbar, iliolumbar, middle sacral, lateral sacral, superior and middle hemorrhoidal, and gluteal arteries, it is important to ligate the anterior division of the hypogastric artery *distal* to the posterior parietal branch(es), as demonstrated in Figure

6–7. In ligating the hypogastric artery, the peritoneum is opened on the lateral side of the common iliac artery near its bifurcation, with the ureter left attached to the medial peritoneal reflection to avoid disturbing its blood supply. The posterior branch of the hypogastric artery must be clearly identified prior to the selection of the point of dissection and double ligation of the anterior division. After the artery is dissected and mobilized free from the adjacent vein, nonabsorbable suture (No. 0 silk) is free-tied and passed around the artery with an Adson or right-angle clamp. A second free-tie is placed distal to the initial ligature to avoid recanalization. Transfixion of the vessel is not essential or desirable in this procedure. The major advantages of ligating the anterior division of the hypogastric artery are in isolating the collateral arterial circulation from the pelvis and in reducing the pulse pressure on the bleeding artery, as has been demonstrated by Burchell. This reduction in pulse pressure will permit thrombosis of the bleeding vessel to occur. Since the uterine artery is the first visceral branch of the hypogastric artery, it is occasionally feasible to identify this artery and ligate it separately, should this vessel be the origin of the pelvic bleeding. However, this is a much more difficult procedure than ligating the entire anterior division of the hypogastric artery and should not be attempted in the face of massive pelvic bleeding, distorted pelvic anatomy, and shock.

In the presence of massive bleeding when the uterus has not been removed, (as may occur in certain obstetric operations,) it is important to separately identify and ligate each ovarian artery after each hypogastric artery has been ligated because

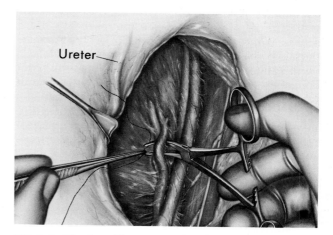

FIG. 6–7 Ligation of hypogastric artery, showing peritoneal reflection with attached ureter from bifurcation of iliac artery, and silk ligature placed around anterior division of hypogastric artery.

Ureter

of the important collateral communication of the aorta with the ovarian and uterine arteries. This procedure is easily accomplished by extending the peritoneal incision above the pelvic brim and the bifurcation of the common iliac artery, being careful to remain lateral to the ureter and to avoid traumatizing the ovarian vessels. If there is difficulty in distinguishing the artery from the ovarian vein, ligation of both the ovarian artery and vein within the infundibulopelvic ligament is acceptable. Even though ligating both the arterial and venous circulation to the ovary leads to a high incidence of postoperative cystic enlargement of the ovary, this complication is preferable to the risk of recurrent pelvic bleeding when the ovarian arteries are not ligated. Each ovarian artery should be dissected free from its retroperitoneal position at or above the pelvic brim and free-tied with No. 0 silk suture. Only one ligature is necessary for each. The artery should not be cut, to avoid the need for multiple ligatures and the risk of retraction and retroperitoneal bleeding of the vessel. A single hemoclip can also be placed on each ovarian artery as a quicker and easier method of occlusion. Care must be taken to avoid injury to the ovarian vein when the artery is being freed for ligation. If injury occurs, control of bleeding may be troublesome. The left vein can be particularly troublesome because, should it retract beneath the peritoneum, its drainage into the left renal vein makes it difficult to trace.

INTRA-ARTERIAL EMBOLIZATION. Although hypogastric artery ligation is an effective and direct method of controlling postoperative hemorrhage in the female pelvis, many patients are poor surgical risks for additional major surgery while in the hypotensive state. In particular, patients with cardiopulmonary compromise or debilitating disease or who are of an advanced age may develop more serious complications should major surgery be undertaken when they are in a precarious hemodynamic state. Recently, transcatheter arterial embolization by angiography has been added to the various methods of controlling pelvic hemorrhage. In 1969 Nusbaum and coworkers described using this method to control bleeding from esophageal varices by selectively cannulating the superior mesenteric artery and infusing small doses of vasopressin into terminal vessels. The subsequent use of particulate matter to achieve hemostasis within bleeding viscera developed rapidly. Numerous embolic materials have been used, one of the more effective being Gelfoam sliced into 2-ml to 3-ml fragments and mixed with a small amount of saline to facilitate injection through an arterial catheter. Although many other compounds are used for transcatheter embolization, including autologous clot, subcutaneous tissue, small Silastic spheres, and metal coils, Gelfoam is one of the most practical and easily injected materials. It is sterile, nonantigenic, remains in the vessels for 20 to 50 days and forms a fibrin mesh framework upon which blood clot may develop. Its immediate effect is to obstruct the distal artery or arteriole and reduce the pulse pressure in the bleeding vessel, thereby permitting clot formation and cessation of bleeding. Although initially developed for use in the gastrointestinal tract, this method has wide application for the control of bleeding in many areas of the body, including the central nervous system, kidney, head, and neck, as well as the control of hemorrhage from genitourinary organs. One of its earliest uses in the field of gynecology was for the control of massive vaginal hemorrhage in patients with advanced carcinoma of the cervix.

The method of intravascular injection is quite simple, although it requires the expertise of a person skilled in angiography. Percutaneous catheterization of the femoral artery under local anesthesia provides direct access in a retrograde manner to the hypogastric artery. If prior hypogastric artery ligation has obstructed this pathway, an arteriogram of the pelvic vasculature through one of the collateral arteries will usually localize the specific bleeding vessel. When the site of bleeding is identified by angiography, either the hypogastric artery or the specific collateral vessel is cannulated and small pieces of Gelfoam, small metal coils, or other hemostatic materials are injected into the peripheral vessel under direct angiographic observation. When it becomes evident by repeat angiography that the vessel has been occluded, the catheter is removed and the patient is monitored carefully for evidence of further bleeding. This technique is quick, safe, and effective and may remove the need for additional surgery. However, no procedure is without risk of complication and this angiographic procedure is no exception. Pelvic pain and fever can occur as a result of localized ischemia and secondary cellulitis, but these symptoms and signs are usually transient. Cases of bladder ischemia and vesicovaginal fistula have been reported after vascular embolization, usually following occlusion of the hypogastric artery in patients who have also received prior megavoltage pelvic irradiation.

Other Methods of Control of Hemorrhage

Despite the major emphasis that has been given to hypogastric artery ligation and intra-arterial embolization, the immediate procedure that should be undertaken in a patient with postoperative vaginal hemorrhage is an examination of the vaginal cuff. In general, this examination is more effective if done under general anesthesia, which permits an accurate determination of whether there is an associated retroperitoneal pelvic hematoma in the operative site. If a hematoma has developed, it is important that proper drainage be established and that Penrose drains be inserted to avoid further loculation and secluded bleeding. If the bleeding is found to arise from the angles of the vagina in the area of the descending vaginal artery or vein, figure-of-eight transfixion sutures are placed, using No. 1 delayed-absorbable suture material. The hemostatic suture should include the vaginal mucosa and a deep bite into the underlying paravaginal tissues. Care must be taken to avoid the inadvertent placement of a ligature into the musculature of the bladder wall or underlying rectum. If bleeding has not been completely controlled by this technique, it is unwise to continue to add suture upon suture in a frantic effort to control the vaginal bleeding. In such cases, it is probable that the bleeding vessels have retracted well above the vaginal margins and cannot be reached by this approach. It is advisable at this time to insert a vaginal pack firmly against the vaginal vault to compress the vascular pedicles against the pelvic diaphragm. If the bleeding subsides, the pack may be advanced in 24 hours and, if no further bleeding occurs, it may be removed in 48 hours. The patient should be ambulated slowly to avoid undue pelvic pressure, which might reactivate the bleeding source.

Some surgeons have found the Logothetopulos vaginal pack to be of assistance in compressing the retracted, bleeding vessels in the pelvis. This technique includes the formation of a large pack of loose gauze within an outstretched, opened piece of gauze. This can be used in an umbrella fashion within the pelvic cavity by bringing the four corners of the opened gauze together and placing traction on the free margins of the pack when it is pulled through the vaginal vault. This approach attempts to compress the bleeding vessels against the pelvic floor by the traction and pressure exerted with the umbrella pack. It may be used at the time of either abdominal or vaginal surgery for compression of bleeding vessels that cannot be controlled by other means. The pack can be left in place with perineal traction for 24 to 48 hours until the bleeding has ceased.

The use of microfibrillar collagen for the local control of intraoperative bleeding was mentioned previously. This bovine collagen material can be applied directly and compressed against an area of a small bleeding vessel. It acts as a fibrin nidus to accelerate thrombus formation on the surface of the vessel. Caution must be exercised in the use of this material because it has been found to produce

secondary fibrosis in the pelvis. There have been recent reports of retroperitoneal fibrosis and ureteral obstruction secondary to the use of this material. These sequelae have cautioned the pelvic surgeon against applying this agent near the ureter. When used in other sites, we have found no adverse reactions. If a localized hemostatic agent is considered necessary, the use of Gelfoam or topical thrombin may prove to be more efficacious with less fibrosis. More important, the surgeon should not rely on any agent for control of a significant amount of arterial or venous bleeding. Instead, every effort should be made to identify the bleeding vessel and to occlude it with either a hemoclip or a ligature.

External counterpressure by means of antishock trousers has been used for the temporary control of acute, profuse intra-abdominal hemorrhage while the patient is being prepared for surgery. In some cases, the bleeding can be controlled and surgery can be avoided. This technique has been used in more than 175 cases of surgically uncontrollable hemorrhage, as reported in the literature, with temporary or complete control of the hemorrhage. The counterpressure technique was borrowed from the experience of the military services: the anti-G suit was used to prevent pooling of blood in the extremities during certain flight maneuvers. The suit is made of polyvinyl and wraps around the patient and secures with Velcro fasteners. It contains an abdominal pneumatic bladder that extends from the xyphoid to the pubis and has two separate leg bladders. It is inflated to a pressure between 25 mm Hg and 40 mm Hg (some clinics have used pressures of 100 mm Hg or higher). When applied for periods of from 2 to 48 hours, results have been excellent in increasing intra-abdominal pressure to a level that controls the source of arterial or venous bleeding. We have found this technique to be most effective in cases where all previous surgical attempts to identify and control the source of intra-abdominal bleeding following pelvic surgery were found to be unsuccessful. We have also used it for the patient in profound shock from intra-abdominal hemorrhage, such as that caused by a ruptured tubal pregnancy, while the blood volume is being rapidly replaced prior to surgery.

Pulmonary Complications[*]

HYPOVENTILATION

One of the most frequent and dangerous complications in the immediate postoperative period, even

* The section on Pulmonary Complications was contributed by Donald P. Schlueter, M.D.

in patients with normal lungs, is hypoventilation. To assess ventilation, the expired gas can be collected and the volume expired per minute (minute volume = V_E) can be determined. However, a portion of this gas ventilates non–gas-exchanging areas of the lung, namely, conducting airways referred to as dead space. This ventilation is wasted, since it does not participate in gas exchange. The normal dead space volume is approximately equal in pulmonary milliliters to the person's ideal weight in pounds (*i.e.*, a 150-pound female has a dead space volume of 150 ml). To calculate the effective or alveolar ventilation, the dead space must be subtracted from the tidal volume and the difference multiplied by the respiratory rate. Gross errors in the estimation of ventilation can be made if only V_E is considered. If tidal volume decreases from 500 ml to 250 ml, but respiratory rate doubles from 14 rpm (respirations per minute) to 28 rpm, minute volume remains at 7.0 liters. However, assuming a dead space of 150 ml, the alveolar ventilation under these conditions decreases from 4.9 liters to 2.8 liters, resulting in significant alteration in blood gases. This type of respiratory pattern is common in the patient with abdominal surgery, who tends to decrease tidal volume to avoid pain. Hypoventilation is defined as a level of alveolar ventilation that is insufficient to prevent accumulation of carbon dioxide. The causes include depression of central respiratory control from obesity, neuromuscular disease, pain, restrictive dressings, immobility, hypomobility, and increased carbon dioxide production. Obviously, patients with obstructive and restrictive respiratory impairment are much more likely to develop hypoventilation during this critical early postoperative period.

Inadequate ventilation may not be clinically obvious unless an estimate of alveolar ventilation is made. Ultimately, arterial blood gas studies are the most accurate measure of alveolar ventilation. Table 6–4 shows the effect of decreasing alveolar ventilation on the arterial blood gases. From this data, it can be seen that although the P_aCO_2 rises almost linearly as alveolar ventilation decreases, changes

in oxygenation (S_aO_2 = arterial oxygen saturation) are modest until respiratory acidosis is severe. Thus, the best indicator of adequate ventilation is the P_aCO_2. A normal P_aO_2 in the presence of a severe respiratory acidosis (elevated P_aCO_2) would implicate the administration of oxygen as a causative factor in the hypoventilation.

ACUTE VENTILATORY FAILURE

The treatment of acute ventilatory failure manifested by hypoventilation and a P_aCO_2 greater than 50 mm Hg is mechanical ventilatory support until the causative factors can be alleviated. This may require several hours to several days. It is important, therefore, to leave the endotracheal tube in place following surgery until adequate spontaneous ventilation and arterial blood gas levels have been demonstrated. The adequacy of respiratory mechanics can be determined by measuring tidal volume and inspiratory effort. The tidal volume should exceed 10 ml/kg and inspiratory pressure should be greater than −20 cm H_2O. The tidal volume alone is not a reliable indicator of respiratory adequacy in a patient with abnormal lungs because of changes in physiologic dead space. Under these circumstances, P_aCO_2 is used as a guide, since an elevated or rising P_aCO_2 is the best clinical indicator of inadequate alveolar ventilation and progressive respiratory acidosis. Weaning is accomplished either by taking the patient off the ventilator with supplemental oxygen and periodic monitoring of arterial blood gas levels or by intermittent mandatory ventilation. The latter technique allows the gradual reduction of ventilator support with the advantage of providing a known minimum minute ventilation and the security of the monitoring systems of the ventilator. This method is particularly helpful in patients who have poor ventilatory reserve, or who have been intubated for prolonged periods. After extubation, treatment can be continued with supplemental oxygen and IPPB until the patient's respiratory status is stabilized.

ACUTE RESPIRATORY FAILURE (ARDS)

Acute respiratory failure can be defined as a disturbance in respiratory function that results in a P_aO_2 of less than 50 mm Hg with or without carbon dioxide retention. Although a number of conditions can result in this finding, notably, a large pulmonary embolus, this discussion will be limited to ARDS. In 1967, Ashbaugh described sudden respiratory failure in 12 adult patients who had dyspnea, hypoxemia, reduced respiratory compliance, and diffuse alveolar infiltrates that resembled pulmonary

TABLE 6–4 *Effect of Decreasing Alveolar Ventilation on Arterial Blood Gases*

ALVEOLAR VENTILATION (Liter/min)	P_aO_2 (mm Hg)	S_aO_2 (%)	P_aCO_2 (mm Hg)	pH
5.0	100	96	40	7.40
4.0	82	94	50	7.32
3.0	68	87	75	7.20
2.0	30	40	105	7.05

edema without evidence of prior lung disease or congestive failure. This syndrome is a form of non-hydrostatic pulmonary edema that represents the final pathway of the response of the lungs to acute diffuse alveolar injury from a variety of causes. A broad spectrum of disorders has been associated with ARDS. These disorders are listed in Disorders Associated with Adult Respiratory Distress Syndrome. ARDS has been found to be relatively com-

tional oxygen therapy. Suggested criteria are listed in Criteria for the Diagnosis of Adult Respiratory Distress Syndrome. Initially, it may be difficult to distinguish ARDS from cardiac failure and pulmonary edema. The use of the Swan-Ganz catheter to monitor pulmonary capillary wedge pressure has been extremely helpful in making this distinction. It also provides a method of determining cardiac output and tissue oxygen delivery.

DISORDERS ASSOCIATED WITH ADULT RESPIRATORY DISTRESS SYNDROME

Shock of any etiology
Infections and sepsis
Trauma
Liquid aspiration
Fat and amniotic fluid embolism
Drug overdose
Inhaled toxins, including oxygen
Intravascular coagulation
Pancreatitis
Eclampsia

CRITERIA FOR THE DIAGNOSIS OF ADULT RESPIRATORY DISTRESS SYNDROME

1. Clinical history of predisposing condition
2. Clinical respiratory distress
   a. tachypnea greater than 20 breaths per minute
   b. labored breathing
3. Chest x-ray showing diffuse pulmonary infiltrates
4. P_aO_2 less than 50 mm Hg or F_iO_2* greater than 0.6
5. Increased shunt fraction
6. Increased dead space ventilation
7. Decreased total respiratory compliance

---

* F_iO_2 = Forced inspiratory oxygen concentration
Adapted from Petty TL, Fowler AH, 1982

mon, affecting about 150,000 persons per year, with a mortality rate approaching 50% despite current supportive measures. The hallmark of ARDS is progressive hypoxemia that is refractory to conven-

The pathogenesis of ARDS is complex; a summary of potential mechanisms is shown in Figure 6–8. A recent review by Divertie found that damage to the alveolar capillary membrane resulting in the in-

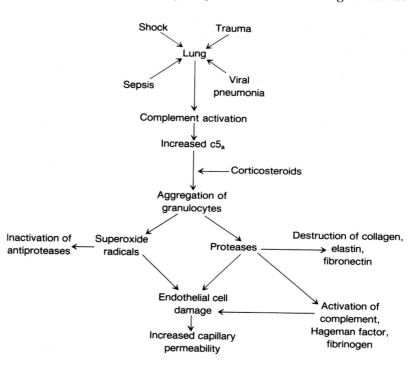

FIG. 6–8 Summary of the mechanisms involved in the pathogenesis of ARDS.

creased capillary permeability is precipitated by complement activation, subsequent aggregation of granulocytes, and liberation of proteases and superoxide radicals. Obviously, therapy must be directed at reversing the primary physiologic abnormality, which is, basically, progressive hypoxemia. The cornerstone of therapy is ventilatory support with positive end-expiratory pressure (PEEP) until repair of the capillary damage can occur. PEEP improves ventilation–perfusion relationships, and consequently oxygenation, by increasing functional residual capacity and stabilizing the alveoli at low levels of inflation. Particularly at high levels, PEEP may have an adverse effect on tissue oxygen delivery (cardiac output $\times$ P_aO_2); therefore, careful monitoring of this product is necessary as the PEEP level is increased. The use of corticosteroids in ARDS has been controversial, but recent studies suggest potential therapeutic benefit. Steroids have been shown to inhibit complement-induced granulocyte aggregation, to cause disaggregation of neutrophils, and to block the increase in sheep-lung vascular permeability after endotoxemia. Sibbald and coworkers demonstrated decreased passage of radiolabeled albumin from serum into pulmonary edema fluid in patients with ARDS after methylprednisolone had been administered. Steroids may be beneficial if given early in the emergency of ARDS in a dosage of 1 g to 2 g per day (methylprednisolone sodium-succinate, Solu-Medrol) but should be discontinued after 48 hours to avoid the possible complications of sepsis.

Judicious management of fluid intake is essential in maintaining adequate perfusion of vital organs and avoiding further complications. Since one of the major determinants of fluid flux in the lung is the hydrostatic pressure in the pulmonary capillaries, this pressure assumes greater than normal importance in the presence of increased capillary permeability. Measurement of pulmonary capillary wedge pressure is the only reliable method of monitoring fluid administration. If adequate perfusion cannot be maintained when the pulmonary wedge pressure is within the upper limits of the normal range (10–12 mm Hg) the use of pressor agents should be considered. Colloid should be administered only if the serum protein level is low because rapid equilibration of protein concentrations between the capillary and interstitial spaces occurs.

With an increasing understanding of the mechanisms of ARDS, early recognition, and aggressive intervention, the prognosis in ARDS has improved. The long-term outlook has been variable, but, in general, most patients who survive are left with surprisingly few pulmonary sequelae.

ATELECTASIS

That airway obstruction can lead to atelectasis is a well-known fact that is readily recognized clinically and roentgenographically. The cause may be mucous plugs or inappropriate endotracheal tube placement. A more common and less obvious postoperative problem is so called microatelectasis, which results from failure to inspire deeply or from constant volume ventilation of the lung. It appears that occasional large inflations are necessary to replenish surfactant and prevent alveolar collapse. Secretions accumulating during anesthesia may result in obstruction of small airways and also contribute to the problem. Specifically, during inhalation of a high concentration of oxygen, atelectasis may develop rapidly in areas of the lung where small airways have become obstructed.

Microatelectasis is difficult to detect clinically and roentgenographically. The earliest indication of its occurrence is a fall in P_aO_2 and oxygen saturation in the presence of a normal to low P_aCO_2.

In the early stages of development, the P_aO_2 can usually be returned to normal by increasing the inspired oxygen concentration. Chest physiotherapy, deep breathing, coughing, incentive spirometry, and IPPB will be helpful in resolving the problem. As atelectasis becomes more widespread, the application of positive pressure ventilation and hyperinflation may be necessary to reverse the process. For extensive atelectasis, bronchoscopy to remove mucous plugs may be necessary.

PNEUMONIA

Postoperative pneumonia has become less frequent with the introduction of early ambulation and intensive respiratory therapy in the immediate postoperative period. Since pneumonia is frequently associated with atelectasis and hypoventilation, prevention or prompt reversal of these conditions is the best prophylactic measure. Animal studies have shown that even with instillation of infected material directly into the lower respiratory tract, pneumonia could not be produced without addition of such other factors as atelectasis and hypoventilation. A decrease in the activity of cilia caused by drugs or altered humidity may interfere significantly with bacterial clearing. This is particularly true in patients with obstructive lung disease. In patients with an endotracheal tube in place, the normal protective mechanisms of the upper respiratory system are abolished. Infection is much more likely to develop in this group and is directly related to the duration of intubation. Gram-negative organisms, usually *Proteus* or *Pseudomonas,* are most frequently encountered under these circumstances. Deep tracheal secretions should be aspirated into a sterile sputum trap for culture and antibiotic susceptibility studies. Pathogenic organisms are invariably isolated, but it must be emphasized that a positive sputum culture cannot be equated with pulmonary infection requiring antibiotic therapy. Treatment must be based on such other criteria as fever, persistence of purulent sputum, leukocytosis, positive blood culture, and physical and roentgenographic signs of pneumonia. Prophylactic antibiotic therapy rarely has a place in the treatment of patients on assisted ventilation except in emergency situations, such as acute aspiration or fulminating infection, in which the gram-stained sputum smear should be used as a guide for initial therapy. Meticulous aseptic technique must be used in suctioning to prevent the introduction of infection. Adequate humidification is essential to facilitate the removal of secretions.

Care of the Gastrointestinal Tract

Every surgeon of experience has developed confidence in a particular routine for feeding the postoperative patient and for stimulation of the gastrointestinal tract. The early and progressive use of soft and solid foods postoperatively has been beneficial in encouraging return of normal bowel function following pelvic surgery. A full liquid diet is started on the second or third postoperative day, but should coincide with the appearance of active bowel sounds or the passage of gas per rectum. Rapid progression to a full soft diet on the following day and a full diet as desired thereafter has stimulated early bowel function without significant complications. Seriously ill patients, however, must remain on parenteral fluids until bowel activity is well established, regardless of the length of time that this might require.

PARALYTIC ILEUS AND DISTENTION

Postoperative ileus and distention associated with peritonitis, bowel surgery, or prolonged packing of the bowel during pelvic surgery frequently require gastric suction and gentle intestinal stimulation in the immediate postoperative period. Prevention of intestinal distention should be the aim of every surgeon. In cases such as ruptured tubo-ovarian abscess or prolonged surgery, where distention is anticipated, a nasogastric tube should be inserted at the time of surgery and the placement of the tube should be checked by the operating surgeon.

At the first indication of tympanites, treatment should be prompt and vigorous, for paralytic ileus is much more easily conquered early than when fully developed. A course of pantothenic acid has frequently proven to be helpful in the uncomplicated case. Our usual order is for 1 ml pantothenic acid, given hypodermically every hour for 3 doses, unless there is reason to suspect organic obstruction of inflammatory bowel lesions; bowel anastomosis or repair also contraindicate such stimulation. After this initial short, vigorous course, the drug is given every 4 hours for 2 or 3 days as necessary. A rectal tube is inserted and left in place long enough to permit the gas forced along by the peristaltic stimulants to be expelled. Enemas are given not oftener than twice a day.

Within the first 48 hours to 72 hours after operation, we use an enema composed of 130 ml of Fleet's phosphosoda in disposable containers. Later, enemas of larger volume, such as a 500-ml soapsuds enema, may be more effective. An enema of 240 ml milk and 240 ml molasses is a particularly effective old-time remedy for the production of gas and the stimulation of peristalsis.

A nasogastric tube should be passed and attached to suction if gastric dilatation is prominent or if nausea and vomiting are associated with distention of the small bowel. Fluid and electrolyte balance should be maintained while the bowel is placed at rest under alternating suction. The tube is clamped initially and removed when bowel sounds have returned to normal and the patient can tolerate oral fluids. Premature removal of the nasogastric tube requires reinsertion should the patient's bowel continue to be hypoactive. We have found the insertion of 30 ml to 60 ml of mineral oil into the stomach before removal of the nasogastric tube to be helpful in augmenting peristalsis of the bowel.

In the presence of a normally functioning bowel, mild laxatives of the surgeon's choice, such as milk of magnesia or senna granules (Senokot), may be administered on the third postoperative day. When mechanical obstruction is seriously suspected, cathartics are contraindicated. Likewise, when the wall of the large bowel has been weakened by operative injury or inflammation, laxatives and enemas should be used with great caution. Often, a rectal tube inserted to a low level, just beyond the anal sphincter, will permit the patient to expel gas, and usually a small volume of Fleet's enema may be given safely. When chronic distention without obstruction persists for several days, we occasionally give oral Fleet's phosphosoda (30 ml). Although the latter stimulant may be somewhat harsh, the distention is usually relieved once the gas and liquid bowel contents have passed through the intestinal tract.

It is important to differentiate between postoperative ileus and postoperative obstruction if proper therapy is to be initiated promptly with beneficial results (Table 6–5). The distinction may be difficult. This is because partial bowel obstruction is frequently accompanied by a secondary ileus as part of the clinical picture. Only by close clinical observation of the bowel sounds, serial abdominal x-ray studies, and frequent white blood-cell counts can one clearly separate these two postoperative complications. Obviously, adynamic ileus is the more frequent clinical entity, a fact that may mislead the surgeon into a false sense of security unless he remains acutely aware of the distinguishing features of intestinal obstruction. Serial monitoring of the white blood-cell count and differential count is an important method for differentiating bowel obstruction from paralytic ileus. A key feature of advancing bowel obstruction is necrosis of the bowel wall, which will cause a progressive leukocytosis, along with distention and peritonitis. The most common gynecologic disease process associated with both ileus and intestinal obstruction is severe pelvic inflammatory disease. Notoriously, acute exacerbation of pelvic inflammatory disease or rupture of a pelvic abscess is associated with prolonged ileus. Occasionally, fibrous adhesions form and secondary bowel obstruction will occur. Postoperative pelvic peritonitis from any cause, including cellulitis resulting from hematoma formation and secondary infection of the vaginal cuff, is frequently associated with ileus, whereas intestinal obstruction only rarely results from such a complication.

In contrast to pelvic surgery for benign disease, any cancer surgery, including pelvic exenteration for cervical carcinoma, is frequently complicated either by postoperative adynamic ileus or by intestinal obstruction. When radical surgery is preceded by preoperative irradiation, the small bowel is frequently compromised by a protracted ileus.

Care of the Urinary Bladder

The most common postoperative problem of the female bladder is atony caused by overdistention and the reluctance of the patient to initiate the voluntary phase of voiding. Following abdominal surgery, the patient is frequently unwilling to contract the abdominal muscles to produce sufficient intra-abdominal pressure against the dome of the bladder to initiate the voiding reflex. Following vaginal surgery, spasm, edema, and tenderness of the pubococcygeus muscles following anterior colporrhaphy may obstruct the process of voiding. The operative trauma from plication of the pubovesicocervical fascia causes edema of the urethral wall and submucosa, especially at the urethrovesical junction, thus contributing to the urinary obstruction.

For spontaneous voiding to occur, the parasym-

TABLE 6–5 *Differential Diagnosis Between Postoperative Ileus and Postoperative Obstruction*

CLINICAL FEATURES	POSTOPERATIVE ILEUS	POSTOPERATIVE OBSTRUCTION
Abdominal pain	Discomfort from distention but not cramping pains	Cramping, progressively severe
Relationship to previous surgery	Usually within 48–72 hours of surgery	Usually delayed; may be 5–7 days for remote onset
Nausea and vomiting	Present	Present
Distention	Present	Present
Bowel sounds	Absent or hypoactive	Borborygmi with peristaltic rushes and high-pitched tinkles
Fever	Only if related to associated peritonitis	Rarely present unless bowel becomes gangrenous
Abdominal x-rays	Distended loops of small and large bowels; gas usually present in colon	Single or multiple loops of distended bowel, usually small bowel with air fluid levels
Treatment	Conservative with nasogastric suction; enemas; cholinergic stimulation	Partial: conservative with nasogastric decompression; or Complete: surgical

pathetic function of the bladder detrusor must be coordinated with the voluntary motor function of the abdominal wall and the levator muscles. In the past, it has been customary to insert an indwelling urethral catheter for 5 or more days following vaginal plastic surgery. Although this technique is still used in many clinics, the use of a suprapubic catheter has proven to be very effective in urinary drainage. The suprapubic technique was developed and introduced to the gynecologic literature from this clinic in 1964. When inserted at the time of surgery, the suprapubic Silastic tube eliminates the necessity for repeated bladder catheterization until spontaneous voiding occurs. Although used preferentially following anterior vaginal colporrhaphy, suprapubic bladder catheterization is also useful when the need for prolonged bladder drainage is anticipated, such as after radical Wertheim hyster-

ectomy. We also insert a suprapubic catheter when performing a Marshall–Marchetti–Krantz urethral suspension.

The procedure for suprapubic bladder drainage is easy to perform either before or after the operative procedure. It includes the insertion of a No. 12 French gauge Silastic (silicone) catheter into the bladder through a needle trocar (Fig. 6–9). A No. 12 French gauge pigtail (Bonano) Teflon catheter and other modifications have also been used by many clinics. The bladder is filled with 300 ml of sterile water and the needle trocar is inserted through the surgically cleaned anterior abdominal wall, approximately 2 cm above the symphysis pubis. When the stylet is removed from the trocar, clear fluid should pass from the bladder under pressure. Approximately 10 cm of the suprapubic catheter is threaded through the trocar, following which the

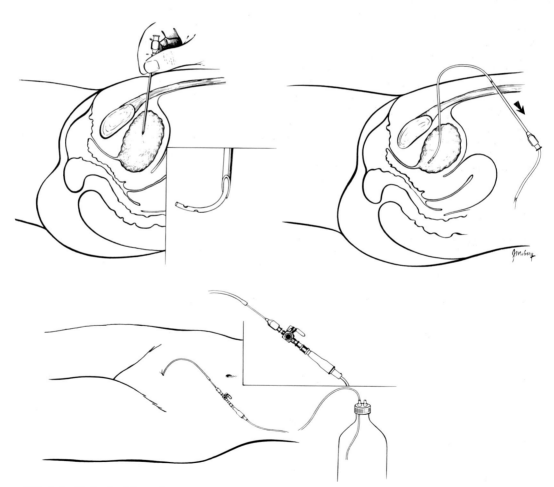

FIG. 6–9 Method of inserting suprapubic tube through needle and drainage into bottle. Suprapubic catheterization avoids the trauma to the urethra caused by repeated catheterization or an indwelling catheter.

trocar is removed by sliding it over the indwelling tube. The opposite end of the Silastic catheter is connected to a sterile, 1-liter drainage bottle or to a sterile closed drainage urinometer bag. The tubing should be filled with fluid at all times and should be anchored to the skin with silicone paste or sutured to the skin to avoid accidental removal. A two-way stopcock is inserted between the catheter and drainage tubing for easy opening and closing of the system. The system is not irrigated unless there is plugging of the bladder catheter and failure of drainage. In approximately 5% of our cases, particularly among obese patients, the catheter fails to drain adequately and requires either replacement or removal.

Aside from a decrease in the chances of developing urinary tract infection, the major advantage of suprapubic drainage is clearly an increase in patient comfort. As is evident to the nursing staff, 85% to 90% of our patients do not require a single catheterization following vaginal hysterectomy and repair. This fact alone, plus the comfort of the suprapubic catheter to the patient, has encouraged us to continue using this method of bladder drainage. The patient who has had a radical hysterectomy is an ideal candidate for suprapubic catheter drainage while the bladder is left at rest until return of normal bladder function occurs. In these cases, the patient may be discharged from the hospital with the suprapubic catheter attached to a leg drainage bag and with instructions on how irrigation should be done if the catheter becomes occluded. If a normal voiding pattern is delayed following an anterior colporrhaphy with plication of the vesical neck, the patient may continue the voiding exercises at home when an indwelling suprapubic catheter is used. The catheter is removed when there is less than 100 ml of residual urine after spontaneous voiding.

It is our opinion, as well as that of others, that prophylactic antibiotics, when given with the use of an indwelling bladder catheter, are ineffective in preventing urinary tract infection. Although urinary tract symptoms may be delayed with the use of prophylactic antibiotics, it is our experience that the incidence of infection is unchanged but that a subsequent urinary tract infection may result from resistant organisms that are more difficult to treat at a later time. For these reasons, we prefer to treat only patients who have significant bacteriuria and pyuria, which includes approximately 10% to 15% of the patients with suprapubic drainage. This incidence of bladder infection is a significant improvement from the common rate of 70% to 90% (Kass and Sossen) when a urethral catheter is retained for more than 72 hours.

Vascular Complications

VENOUS THROMBOSIS

The sudden occurrence in a postoperative patient of respiratory distress that is followed promptly by irreversible hypotension, chest pain, coma and finally death is a complication that converts a successful operative procedure into a postoperative mortality. Fortunately, the incidence rate for fatal postoperative pulmonary emboli is low, varying between 0.1% and 1% of patients undergoing major gynecologic surgery. This complication is also dependent on the type of operative procedure and the patient-risk factors involved. However, venous thrombosis of the deep veins in the lower extremities is a common complication of major gynecologic surgery, occurring, on average, in 15% of cases. The rate of occurrence ranges from 5% to 45%, depending on the type of surgery performed. In recent years, diagnostic studies have provided more accurate information on the frequency of this vascular complication and have identified those patients with deep thrombosis who are candidates for embolization. The opportunity for earlier, prophylactic use of anticoagulation therapy for these high-risk patients has reduced the incidence of pulmonary embolus significantly.

With the recent use of ^{125}I labeled fibrinogen scanning of the lower extremities and other diagnostic techniques, including Doppler ultrasound, impedence plethysmography, thermography, and venography, silent venous thrombosis of the lower extremities has been identified as occurring far more frequently than had been previously recognized. Regrettably, the classic clinical symptoms and signs of leg pain, calf tenderness, unilateral leg swelling, and a positive Homans' sign occur with equal frequency in patients who have proven venous thrombosis and in those who do not. A positive Löwenberg sign—leg pain produced by blood pressure cuff compression with a systolic reading of less than 160 mm Hg—that suggests an underlying deep vein obstruction has proven to be a more sensitive clinical test. It is evident, therefore, that these time-honored clinical findings of deep thrombosis occur late in the genesis of this disease and are not useful in the early detection of thrombosis and prevention of embolization. Unfortunately, 50% of patients who die from a pulmonary embolus have no preceding clinical symptoms or signs. Yet, at autopsy, over 90% of such cases have leg vein thrombosis. Prevention of death in these patients requires effective prophylactic measures prior to surgery or the early detection and effective treatment of subclinical cases of venous thrombosis in the postoperative period, before embolization occurs.

Essentially all of the major factors contributing to postoperative venous thrombosis were described by Virchow more than 125 years ago. These factors include (a) an increase in blood coagulability; (b) venous stasis; and (c) trauma to the vessel wall. Tissue injury activates blood coagulation by the extrinsic and intrinsic pathways (Fig. 6–10), either by exposing the blood to increased levels of tissue thromboplastin (extrinsic) or to subendothelial collagen in the vessel wall, which activates Factor XII (intrinsic). Venous damage is particularly prevalent in patients undergoing radical surgery where skeletonization of the pelvic vasculature is performed. When postoperative infection and pelvic cellulitis occur, there is an acceleration of the clotting mechanism due to the release of tissue thromboplastin (extrinsic) and the activation of Factor VII (intrinsic) by collagen. The activation of both extrinsic and intrinsic pathways results in the conversion of Factor X to an active form that, in turn, interacts with Factor V, calcium, and phospholipid from platelet Factor III to convert prothrombin to thrombin (Fig. 6–11). Thrombin is the rate-regulating proteolytic enzyme that controls the conversion of fibrinogen to fibrin, the basic component of a venous thrombus. Other coagulation factors that are known to be increased following surgery are, principally, Factors XI, IX, and VIII, which increase as a result of activating the intrinsic pathway, and Factor XII, which is ac-

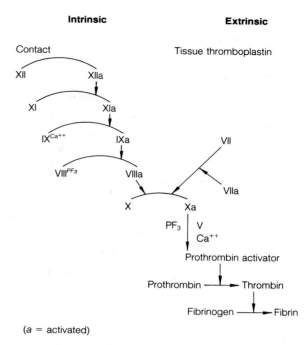

(a = activated)

FIG. 6–11 Schematic representation of the cascade clotting mechanism, illustrating the role of extrinsic and intrinsic factors. Increases in tissue thromboplastin–like substance and collagen-activated factor XII initiate the formation of fibrin through the extrinsic and intrinsic pathways, principally by the activation of factor X.

tivated by tissue collagen. There is also an increase in circulating platelets, platelet adhesiveness and aggregation within 72 hours to 96 hours following surgery. In addition, there is an increase in fibrinogen and in circulating fibrinolysin inhibitors. Normally, the fibrinolytic system, which is principally plasmin formed from its inactive precursor, plasminogen, balances the clotting mechanism by digesting fibrin and fibrinogen and inactivating Factors V and VIII. An acceleration of the clotting mechanism leads to a thrombus in either the venous or the arterial system. An excess of fibrinolytic activity causes blood to fail to clot and can produce serious hemorrhage. A proper balance of both is required for normal circulation.

Venous stasis is known to be the cornerstone of postoperative thrombus formation. Venous stasis in the lower extremities and pelvis results in platelet aggregation and the adhesion of platelets to the vein wall with the release of a thromboplastinlike substance that forms a platelet-fibrin-red cell network with resultant thrombus formation. These physiologic changes in venous hemodynamics occur in the preoperative, operative, and postoperative periods. Many investigators have found it advisable

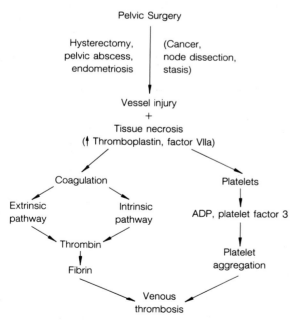

FIG. 6–10 Formation of venous thrombus following various surgical procedures with the activation of clotting factors and aggregation of platelets.

to perform the preoperative studies on high-risk patients on an ambulatory basis or, if the patient has been hospitalized for a significant period of time, to discharge her home for several weeks in order to increase her physical activity prior to elective surgery. Doran and others have shown that venous return from the lower extremities is decreased to one-half its normal rate during the operative procedure. The decrease results from the loss of muscle tone that is caused by muscle relaxation from anesthetic agents. [125]I labeled fibrinogen scanning studies have demonstrated that venous clot is initiated during the operative procedure in 50% of the patients who develop thrombosis in the postoperative period. Blood flow from the lower extremity has been shown to undergo further reduction to approximately 75% the normal drainage flow immediately following surgery. This reduced flow rate persists for 10 to 14 days, due to the loss of pump action of the leg muscles. The major site of clot formation is in the soleal venous sinuses of the calf, a portion of the venous arcade that joins the posterior tibial and peroneal veins that drain the soleal muscle. Thrombi from these sinuses occur frequently behind the valves that are located at the point at which the sinuses drain into the collecting veins. Thrombi form frequently in these large sinuses or valve cusps in bedridden patients.

Another factor conducing to venous stasis is prolonged surgery with tight packing of the intestines in the upper abdomen and obstruction of the underlying vena cava. The type and length of operation is directly related to the incidence of postoperative venous thrombosis, as outlined in Table 6–6.

Diagnosis of Venous Thrombosis

The traditional clinical methods used to diagnose venous thrombosis of the lower extremity are of limited value. Such methods may be in error in 50% of the cases and provide both false-positive and false-negative information. This diagnostic problem is due to the silent and insidious nature of the venous thrombus formation process, which takes place principally in the deep soleal veins in the lower extremity. Because the clinical diagnosis of this vascular complication is so inaccurate, more objective methods of diagnosis were required. In recent years, venography, ^{125}I labeled fibrinogen scanning, Doppler ultrasound, and impedance plethysmography have been used along with a variety of other imaging techniques. Venography is regarded as the most definitive method for the diagnosis of venous thrombosis and has been used as the reference source against which other techniques are measured.

VENOGRAPHY. The venogram has had the widest clinical use of all available techniques in the study of venous thrombosis with the most extensive clinical correlation in the large veins of the lower extremities. Venography is generally reserved for cases where there is clinical suspicion of venous

TABLE 6–6 *Risk Categories of Thromboembolism in Gynecologic Surgery*

RISK CATEGORY	LOW RISK	MEDIUM RISK	HIGH RISK
Age	40 years	40 years	50 years
Contributing factors			
Surgery	Uncomplicated or minor	Major abdominal or pelvic	Major, extensive malignant disease
Weight		Moderately obese—75 to 90 kg or >20% above ideal weight	Morbidly obese—>115 kg or >30% above ideal weight Previous venous thrombosis Varicose veins Cardiac disease Diabetes (insulin dependent)
Calf vein thrombosis	2%	10–35%	30–60%
Iliofemoral vein thrombosis	0.4%	2–8%	5–10%
Fatal pulmonary emboli	0.2%	0.1–0.5%	1%
Recommended prophylaxis	Early ambulation	Low-dose heparin or intermittent pneumatic compression	Low-dose heparin and/or intermittent pneumatic compression

thrombosis or pulmonary embolus. Because it is an invasive technique, venography has limited usefulness as a screening procedure.

125I LABELED FIBRINOGEN SCANNING. Recent studies have used scintillation counter scanning of the lower extremities following the administration of 125I labeled fibrinogen. The incorporation of iodinated fibrinogen into a developing thrombus was first tested by Hobbs and Davies in 1960. The large, collaborative English study of Kakkar and coworkers (1975) was one of the first to give clear evidence of the clinical accuracy of this technique in a collaborative, random study of more than 4000 patients. This study demonstrated a 93% correlation of the fibrinogen scanning technique with venography in the identification of a developing venous thrombus in the lower extremity. Preoperative monitoring is initiated 24 hours after the intravenous injection of 100 microcuries of 125I labeled fibrinogen; subsequently, monitoring is performed in the immediate postoperative period and daily thereafter. An iodine preparation is administered to prevent 125I uptake by the thyroid. Scintillation readings along the lower leg at 2-inch intervals that monitor the venous flow in the deep veins of the calf are compared with precordial readings, and a percentage of the heart count is plotted graphically for each leg. Venous thrombosis is suspected when the level of radioactivity at any point in the leg is 20% greater than either the reading taken 24 hours earlier at the same point or the reading taken at the same point in the other leg. A diagnosis of venous thrombosis can be made if the scan remains abnormal for more than 24 hours. However, the test has specific limitations. It is unreliable in the upper thigh because of the close proximity of the bladder, where the iodine is excreted in the urine, and because of the large veins and arteries in the pelvis, which increase the background noise. It is relatively insensitive in the diagnosis of established venous thrombosis, being positive in only 70% of the cases. Further, as long as 72 hours may be required before enough iodinated fibrinogen is deposited in the formed thrombus to give a positive result. Its major use, therefore, is in the prophylactic screening of high-risk patients to detect the earliest stage of deep vein thrombus formation.

DOPPLER ULTRASOUND. The use of Doppler ultrasound, a noninvasive technique, has become more prevalent during the past decade for the diagnosis of venous thrombosis. In its major physiologic use, in the measurement of the velocity of blood flow in large vessels, a reflected signal is converted to the audible range and directed through a loudspeaker. In the case of venous thrombosis, the absence of the signal signifies an obstructed vein.

When used in the upper thigh, the technique is highly sensitive to venous thrombosis in the lower iliac, femoral or popliteal vessels. However, sensitivity decreases rapidly in smaller vessels, particularly in the solear sinuses of the calf, where the accuracy rate, in most series, is less than 60%. The technique is of limited value as a routine screening test for high-risk patients.

IMPEDANCE PLETHYSMOGRAPHY. Impedance plethysmography is based on the measurement of the electrical resistance in a specific area of the body, such as the lower extremities. When blood flow has been reduced by venous outflow obstruction, such as with venous thrombosis, there is a marked reduction in the electrical resistance over the involved vessel. This technique is most specific in venous occlusion in the larger veins of the thigh—namely, the lower iliac, femoral and popliteal—having an overall accuracy of 95% in comparison to venography. It is much less useful for the detection of small calf vein thrombi, due to the caliber of the small soleus sinuses and the subtle changes in blood flow through these vessels. The ability of the technique to detect asymptomatic venous thrombi in the calf veins has been found to be less than 50% that of venography.

In summary, the early diagnosis of deep vein thrombosis of the lower extremity following pelvic surgery is difficult to establish. Since clinical signs and symptoms are absent in more than 50% of cases, the early diagnosis must be established by a routine screening procedure if early treatment is to be established. Of the reliable methods available, 125I labeled fibrinogen is perhaps the most accurate method of detecting small thrombi in the calf veins. However, it would not be cost effective to screen all patients who undergo gynecologic surgery. If very high-risk patients were screened for deep vein thrombosis in the calf veins by 125I fibrinogen scanning, along with impedance plethysmography or Doppler ultrasound of the thigh, a highly accurate surveillance system would be achieved. However, since few proximal thrombi occur in the upper thigh in the absence of deep vein thrombosis in the calf vessels, fibrinogen scan of the lower extremity appears to be adequate. Since all of these techniques are both costly and time consuming, the practical approach to this problem is to screen only patients who are known to be at high risk for the development of this complication.

RISK FACTORS FOR VASCULAR COMPLICATIONS

Several factors have been observed that present a clinical profile of the patient who is prone to venous thrombosis and pulmonary embolism (Table 6–7).

TABLE 6-7   *Profile of Patient at High Risk*
           for Venous Thrombosis

FACTOR	CONDITION
Age	>age 45 years
Obesity	
Moderate	75 to 90 kg or >20% above ideal weight
Morbid	>115 kg or >30% above ideal weight with reduced fibrinolysin and immobility
Immobility	
Preoperative	Prolonged hospitalization; venous stasis
Intraoperative	Prolonged operative time; loss of pump action of calf muscles; compression of vena cava
Postoperative	Prolonged bed confinement; venous stasis
Trauma	Damage of wall of pelvic veins Radical pelvic surgery
Malignancy	Release of tissue thromboplastin Activation of Factor X; reduced fibrinolysin
Medical diseases	Diabetes mellitus Cardiac disease, heart failure Large varicose veins Previous venous thrombosis with or without embolization Chronic pulmonary disease

Among the many clinical factors that predispose to venous thrombosis in women, the following are the most prevalent: age greater than 45, obesity greater than 20% above ideal weight, prolonged surgery, and immobility in the preoperative, operative, and postoperative periods. Pelvic malignancy, previous thromboembolism, severe diabetes, heart failure, and chronic pulmonary disease also increase the risk of vascular thrombi.

Age

In autopsy studies by Sevitt and Gallagher, the incidence of deep vein thrombosis was greatest in patients over 60 years of age. Many additional studies have demonstrated a linear increase in fatal pulmonary emboli as patient age increases. The major correlation in such patients relates to degenerative changes in the vascular tree. The incidence of pulmonary embolism following major surgery increases sharply in women over 45 years of age.

Obesity

The risk of thromboembolism is decidedly increased in the obese patient. Breneman recognized obesity as one of the most significant factors in thromboembolic disease in the operative patient. His study of patients with thromboembolic disease demonstrated that they were 21.6% above their ideal weight. The major way that obesity influences thrombus formation is by venous stasis, which is aggravated by postoperative immobility.

Immobility

Prolonged inactivity in the preoperative patient causes an impairment in the venous circulation of the lower extremities. Preoperative immobilization, such as that required for prolonged diagnostic evaluation, produces a decrease in muscle tone of the lower extremity with diminished venous flow. These hemodynamic changes result in sludging of the platelets and red cells and set the stage for venous thrombosis during the operative period. Flanc and associates and Kemble have clearly demonstrated this fact, using ^{125}I labeled fibrinogen scanning before and immediately after surgery. They observed that in 50% of patients who ultimately developed postoperative thrombosis, the onset of the clot formation was during the operative procedure. Similarly, the patient who has undergone prolonged anesthesia with generalized muscle relaxation will have an increased incidence of venous stagnation of the lower extremities and a higher incidence of thromboembolism postoperatively. It is important to reemphasize the fact that the nidus for venous thrombosis is frequently initiated either before or, more commonly, during the time of the operative procedure. Consequently, prophylactic treatment for the high-risk patient should be initiated *prior* to surgery and should be continued until the patient is fully ambulatory.

Postoperative immobilization provides an added physiologic insult to preexisting venous stasis. As many as 66% of patients who develop postoperative venous thrombosis will have evidence of thrombosis within 48 hours following surgery as detected by ^{125}I labeled fibrinogen scanning. Such anatomical positions as sitting with the legs crossed, dangling from bed, and exaggerated Fowler's position produce impairment in venous return from the lower extremities. The high-risk patient, in particular, should be ambulated vigorously and when confined to bed, should have the legs and trunk elevated approximately 15 degrees above the horizontal. Sharnoff has demonstrated that immobilization in bed is perhaps more hazardous than the physiologic impact of advancing age.

Other Factors

Other factors that lead to increased risk of thrombosis and pulmonary embolism include varicose veins, previous thromboembolism, severe diabetes, cardiac failure, and chronic pulmonary disease—all of which produce impairment of circulation with resultant stasis and an increased frequency of venous thrombosis. Malignancy is also a recognized factor in venous thrombosis, although the exact mechanism is not fully understood. Many tumors undergoing tissue breakdown are known to elaborate a thromboplastinlike substance that may predispose to increased thrombosis.

It is evident that a clinical profile can be developed for the high-risk patient. The paradigmatic high-risk patient is a woman who is more than 45 years of age, is morbidly obese (greater than twice her ideal weight), is diabetic, has varicose veins and/or heart disease, has been in the hospital for a prolonged period for medical evaluation or treatment, and has a malignant tumor. Regardless of the nature of the pelvic disease, the greater the number of risk factors, the longer the operation, and the more difficult the surgical procedure, the more frequent is the occurrence of venous thrombosis and pulmonary embolus. Patients who embody one or more of these surgical risks should have intensive monitoring and prophylactic treatment for venous thrombosis.

TREATMENT OF VENOUS THROMBOSIS

Prophylaxis

The most effective treatment of venous thrombosis is prevention. In view of the evidence that between 5% and 45% of patients undergoing major gynecologic surgery develop venous thrombosis of the lower extremity, a prophylactic method of preventing this complication should be considered prior to surgery. In about 20% of cases, venous thrombi in the calf veins extend to the popliteal or femoral vessels, and in an estimated 40% of these, the patient will develop pulmonary emboli. These facts are sufficient to warrant the prophylactic treatment of the high-risk patient in an effort to avoid this life-threatening sequence of events.

LOW-DOSE HEPARIN. Many randomized prospective studies document the reduction of deep vein thrombosis from an incidence of 35% to 45% in untreated high-risk patients to approximately 7% in similar patients treated prophylactically with low-dose heparin. These studies have been conducted during the past two decades and have been verified recently by Kakkar and coworkers (1975) in a multicenter study of more than 4000 surgical patients over 40 years of age (Table 6–8). This study evaluated the effectiveness of low-dose heparin given prophylactically at doses of 5000 USP units of calcium heparin, subcutaneously, 2 hours before surgery

TABLE 6–8 *Pulmonary Embolism and Deep Vein Thrombosis in Patients on Low-Dose Heparin and in Controls*

	LOW-DOSE HEPARIN	CONTROL
Number of patients	2045	2076
Number of deaths from all cases	80	100
Deaths caused by pulmonary embolism (verified at autopsy)	2	16
Deep vein thrombosis	8%	25%

(Adapted from Kakkar VV, et al: Prevention of postoperative pulmonary embolism by low dose heparin. Lancet 2:45, 1975).

and every 8 hours after for the subsequent 7 postoperative days. The study demonstrated the benefit of low-dose heparin by reducing the incidence of thrombi from 24% in the untreated control group to 8% in the low-dose heparin-treated group. The most significant observation from this study was that 16 patients in the control, untreated group and only 2 patients in the heparin-treated group died of acute massive pulmonary embolism as revealed on autopsy. Of interest is the fact that in the prophylactic use of low-dose heparin, there is no significant alteration of clotting time and, as a consequence, there is no increase in operative or postoperative bleeding. This phenomenon is attributed to the mechanism of action of heparin, which binds to antithrombin III and exerts its major anticoagulant effect in combination with this naturally occurring inhibitor. Together they inhibit the activated coagulation Factors XIIa, XIa, Xa, and thrombin. Low doses of heparin interfere with the early stages of coagulation before thrombin is formed, thereby preventing thrombus formation without significantly altering the clotting factors in the plasma. These results as well as other studies recorded in Table 6–9 indicate that this method of prophylactic heparin therapy has been eminently successful in reducing the incidence of deep vein thrombosis in the surgical patient.

OTHER METHODS. It has been demonstrated by ^{125}I scanning techniques, both preoperatively and postoperatively, that more than 50% of cases of deep vein thrombosis in the soleal veins of the calf occur during the operative procedure as a result of venous stasis. Many methods have been devised to improve venous return from the legs. In particular, various mechanical devices have been used for intermittent calf compression during surgery and in the immediate postoperative period. An external pneu-

TABLE 6-9   *Results of Prophylactic Treatment of Venous Thrombosis Following Gynecologic Surgery**

STUDY	DATE	TYPE OF SURGERY	NUMBER OF PATIENTS	VENOUS THROMBOSIS (%)			
				Control	Heparin	Dextran	Oral AC+
Bonnar, et al	1973	Simple hysterectomy	260	15.0	—	0.1	—
		Radical malignant	62	33.0	—	5.0	—
Ballard, et al	1973	Major gynecol age 40	110	29.0	3.6	—	—
McCarthy, et al	1974	Major gynecol	130	—	10.9	16.2	—
Baetschi, et al	1975	Major gynecol	458	—	2.3	—	4.7
Gjonnaess and Abildgaard	1976	Major gynecol age 50	95	8.0	2.0	—	—
Adolf, et al	1978	Major gynecol	454	29.3	7.0	—	—
Taberner, et al	1978	Major gynecol	146	23.0	6.0	—	6.0

* Detected by ^{125}I labeled fibrinogen scan
+ AC = anticoagulants
(Adapted from Genton E, Turpie AGG, 1980)

matic compression device or boot appears quite promising. Eight randomized prospective clinical studies reported by Joist and Sherman (1979) have demonstrated a definite benefit to pneumatic calf compression in high-risk patients. These studies have documented a reduction in the incidence of postoperative deep vein thrombosis from 25% in control patients to 6% in patients who wore the pneumatic compression device. This technique has been studied recently by Clarke-Pearson and Creasman for patients undergoing gynecologic cancer surgery. The benefit for these high-risk patients appears to be similar to that for general surgical patients. It is important, however, that the compression device be worn by the patient in the early postoperative period until she is fully ambulatory. Since the results of these early studies resemble those for low dose heparin in the prophylaxis against deep vein thrombosis, the technique shows promise for increased use in gynecologic surgery.

Venous drainage during surgery can also be enhanced by simple elevation of the legs to 15 degrees above the horizontal or, when the patient is in Trendelenburg's position, by keeping the legs straight rather than bent at the knees. Cushioning the heels on the operating table will also prevent compression of the deep leg veins by the soleus muscle and will enhance venous return. These physical methods provide only limited improvement of venous drainage from the lower extremity and must be augmented in the early postoperative period with early ambulation and avoidance of dangling of the legs from the bedside or prolonged sitting following surgery. For patients who need prolonged bed confinement following radical surgery, physical therapy should be instituted immediately following surgery with encouragement of flexion and extension of the foot to stimulate calf muscle contraction and improvement in venous return.

Anticoagulant Therapy

There is general agreement that deep vein thrombosis should be treated initially with intravenous heparin, using 5,000 to 10,000 units as an intravenous bolus. This will produce therapeutic levels for anticoagulation in most patients. Since the major effect of an intravenous bolus of heparin will be cleared from the plasma within 4 hours, maintenance doses of heparin should be either by intermittent intravenous injections at 4 to 6 hour intervals or, preferably, by continuous intravenous infusion at a rate of 1,000 to 1,200 units per hour. We prefer to use a constant-infusion intravenous pump that is reliable in delivering small continuous doses of heparin because when heparin is administered by intermittent intravenous bolus, 15% to 25% of patients will receive either an inadequate or an excessive dosage. Continuous heparinization by the intravenous route prevents the rise and fall of the heparin level and avoids recurrent thrombosis during the period of inadequate anticoagulation and potential bleeding complications during the period when heparin levels are increased. The level of anticoagulation should be carefully monitored 30 minutes prior to each scheduled intermittent bolus. In patients receiving continuous intravenous infusion, the level of anticoagulation may be assessed at any time. An anticoagulation level equivalent to a Lee–White clotting time that is two to three times the control level is considered adequate. Alternatively, an activated partial thromboplastin time of 1.5 to 2 times the control levels indicates adequate anticoagulation. Obviously, the monitoring method should be in accordance with the local preference of the clinical laboratory being used. Once optimal levels are established, clotting studies may be done at 24-hour intervals to determine proper maintenance doses of heparin. The duration of intravenous treatment is difficult to specify, but treatment should be continued for at least 5 to 7 days until there has been resolution of the thrombus in the leg veins or until thrombi have become firmly organized and attached to the vessel wall. If clinical signs of improvement are not clearly demonstrated, more than 7 days of treatment may be required. The symptomatic patient with acute thrombophlebitis should also be maintained at bedrest until the symptoms of pain and fever have subsided. The patient's leg should be maintained in an elevated position until the edema has completely subsided, at which time progressive ambulation is permitted. It is our policy to restrict ambulation until the leg edema has subsided. After a period of 5 to 7 days of heparin therapy, oral anticoagulation is initiated. The combined medication of oral Coumadin medication and tapered doses of heparin is used for approximately 48 hours to 72 hours, after which Coumadin therapy is continued alone. Proper Coumadin therapy is aimed at maintaining a prothrombin time approximately 2.5 times the normal control. The Coumadin therapy is usually continued for a period of 4 to 6 weeks and then discontinued.

The rationale for the treatment of asymptomatic deep vein thrombosis of the lower extremity has been questioned by many surgeons. In brief, there are those who simply ignore this subclinical diagnosis and consider this vascular phenomenon to be an innocuous sequela of pelvic surgery. However, if patients with established venous thrombosis are not treated, the risk of serious morbidity or possibly mortality must be considered. The major risk is the extension of the venous thrombus into the popliteal and proximal veins of the thigh, which reportedly occurs in approximately 20% of cases. The use of a Doppler scan, plethysmography, or venogram is required to identify the occurrence of proximal thrombosis. It is estimated that 40% of these patients, or 8% of the group with thrombosis of the calf veins, will have pulmonary emboli and, more important, recurrent embolization. On the conservative side, one might question the advisability of treating the 80% of patients who do not have proximal migration of the venous clot into the thigh to protect the 20% who do. If the 8% risk of pulmonary embolization is not sufficient reason for treatment, one should consider that once extension of the thrombosis into the proximal vessels has occurred, nearly two-thirds of the patients will have residual disease in the venous system of the leg with loss of valve function and impairment of venous return. This complication will lead frequently to the postphlebitic syndrome of chronic pain and lymphedema of the lower extremity. Because of these unhappy consequences, the prudent surgeon should consider the brief treatment of documented deep venous thrombosis to be a relatively cost-efficient method of managing this vascular complication of pelvic surgery.

Acute iliofemoral thrombosis is one of the most serious and hazardous complications of venous thrombosis of the lower extremity. An estimated 40% of such patients develop pulmonary emboli. This condition is difficult to misdiagnose because in the acute stage, commonly called *phlegmasia cerulea dolens*, the leg becomes exquisitely tender, edematous, and cyanotic. The acute stage is high morbidity from gangrene as well as high mortality from pulmonary embolism. This condition also results in a high incidence of chronic postphlebitic venous obstruction with chronic pain and peripheral edema. Effective therapy requires immediate anticoagulation as outlined. If complete occlusion occurs, surgical treatment is usually required. Unless the clot is removed from the iliofemoral vessels, propagation into the vena cava and pulmonary embolization may occur in as many as 50% of cases, according to Mavor.

Venography is useful in confirming the diagnosis of iliofemoral thrombosis and is essential in evaluating the extent of involvement of the contiguous deep veins. When a pulmonary embolus has occurred, venography is also helpful in determining the presence of nonocclusive contralateral thrombosis from the opposite leg, which may be the site of origin of the embolus.

Most cases of iliofemoral thrombosis are insidious in origin and can be treated medically with heparin therapy if diagnosed early, thereby avoiding complete vascular occlusion and gangrene formation. When gangrene occurs, the vascular occlusion leads to massive swelling of the leg with pooling of blood, which may produce hypovolemia in some cases. Although the risk of mobilization of an embolus is always present, when gangrene has set in it is urgent that immediate thrombectomy be performed with clearance of the iliofemoral segments. With the use of intravenous heparin therapy and early thrombectomy, the incidence of pulmonary emboli has been extremely low. In these acutely ill patients, intravenous heparin must be maintained continuously until there is complete resolution of the leg edema, inflammation, and pain in the calf and thigh. Only then can the patient be ambulated and the process of oral anticoagulation be initiated. These patients require not only early and aggressive management, both medical and surgical, but continuation of the anticoagulation therapy for a period of 6 to 9 months for complete vascular canalization and prevention of recurrent thrombosis.

Routine Orders

When the patient has fully recovered from the anesthetic and is suitable for return to the nursing floor and routine postoperative care, we have found the following basic postoperative orders to be useful. This list should be expanded to include the special needs of each postoperative patient.

1. Vital signs:
   - _____ q 15 min × 4
   - _____ q ½ hr until stable
   - _____ q 2 hr × 24 hr, then b.i.d.
2. Position:
   - _____ Low Trendelenburg
   - _____ Semi-Fowler
   - _____ Flat
   - _____ Other
3. Turn, cough, hyperventilate:
   - _____ q 2 hr × 24 hr
   - _____ q 4 hr until ambulatory
4. Suction trachea and aspirate pharynx p.r.n.
5. Fluid intake and output chart
6. Sedation:
   - _____ Morphine sulphate
   - _____ Codeine sulphate
   - _____ Demerol
   - _____ Other
7. Diet
8. Ambulation
9. Fluid orders
10. Catheterize q 6 hr if patient is unable to void or if urethral catheter is used, connect to straight drainage.

Estrogen Replacement Therapy

During the past decade, few subjects in medicine have engendered greater controversy than has the use of estrogen by postmenopausal women. In the postoperative patient who has undergone bilateral oophorectomy at the time of pelvic surgery, important metabolic changes occur as a result of estrogen deficiency. The most significant effects include vasomotor symptoms, genitourinary atrophy, and osteoporosis. In counselling the patient about the advisability or the necessity of oophorectomy and surgical castration at the time of surgery, it is important that the surgeon take the time to explain all the benefits and risks of postoophorectomy estrogen replacement.

In most cases, the uterus will be removed with any gynecologic disease that requires bilateral oophorectomy. This prophylactic measure of oophorectomy is reasonable if the patient is approaching the menopause since ovarian cancer is the major cause of death from gynecologic malignancy and its cure rate has remained unchanged for the past three decades. These facts have encouraged many gynecologists to remove the ovaries from hysterectomy patients who are 45 years of age or older and approaching the menopause. The ease of oral estrogen replacement has made this surgical approach quite acceptable.

Among the most important sequelae of the castration or postmenopause is bone demineralization or osteoporosis. With the sudden decrease in plasma estrogen following oophorectomy, there is bone reabsorption without change in the chemical composition of the bone. This reabsorption involves the entire skeleton, although the soft cancellous bone undergoes the demineralization process before the hard cortical bone. For this reason the earliest effects of advancing osteoporosis are seen in spontaneous fracture of the distal radius, the weight-bearing vertebral bodies, and the neck of the femur.

In 1979, more than 125,000 women in the United States suffered a fracture of the proximal femur, and 12% died as a direct result. Of white women over 60 years of age, 25% have radiographic or clinical evidence of vertebral crush injuries. Although bone loss is a normal aging process for both men and women, the most significant physiologic event associated with skeletal fractures in women is the loss of ovarian function, whether due to oophorectomy or to spontaneous menopause. While there are apparently no estrogen receptors in bone, estrogen plays an important role in calcium metabolism. Osteoporosis is perhaps the most significant abnormality resulting from estrogen deficiency and is a major cause of morbidity and mortality.

Several theories have been proposed to explain the mechanism of action of estrogen in retarding bone reabsorption. Estrogen is known to suppress the action of parathyroid hormone at the osteoclastic cellular level and thereby suppress the effect of parathormone on bone reabsorption. A diminished plasma level of estrogen results in an increased sensitivity in these cells to parathyroid hormone stimulation, which in turn results in an acceleration of bone reabsorption. As a result of the estrogen deficiency, bone demineralization increases serum calcium. This, in turn, suppresses parathyroid hormone secretion. Consequently, the beneficial effect of parathyroid hormone on renal tubular reabsorption of calcium and the formation of the active, dihydroxy form of vitamin D is diminished. The low level of 25-dihydroxyvitamin D results in an increased renal excretion of calcium and a diminished calcium absorption from the gastrointestinal tract. If low-dose estrogen is provided on a continued basis, the action of the parathyroid hormone on bone reabsorption is decreased. This, in turn, lowers the serum calcium level. The lowered serum calcium level enhances parathyroid hormone release, which has a positive effect on calcium metabolism by increasing renal tubular reabsorption of calcium. Calcium absorption from the gastrointestinal tract is also increased because activated vitamin D levels are higher.

Although the foregoing may be a plausible explanation of the role of estrogen in bone reabsorption, the exact mechanism is by no means fully understood. Many investigators believe that estrogen does not affect osteoclast activity directly, since estrogen receptors have not been shown to be present in bone. There is some evidence that the effect of estrogen on bone metabolism is mediated by its control of calcitonin secretion. Calcitonin, a peptide hormone synthesized by the C-cells of the thyroid gland, is decreased in the postmenopausal patient; calcitonin is known to reduce both the number of osteoclasts and their physiologic activity. The administration of estrogen not only prevents bone loss but also raises the plasma level of calcitonin to premenopausal levels. Therefore, another possible explanation of the pathogenesis of postmenopausal osteoporosis is the accelerated decline in calcitonin secretion that is associated with loss of ovarian function.

Photon absorbitometry studies have made it eminently clear that premature castration and the cessation of ovarian function at the menopause are both associated with a dramatic and continued decline in bone density. Lindsay and associates demonstrated that when oophorectomized, perimenopausal patients were treated with estrogen for periods of up to 8 years, significant bone loss did not occur. When estrogen was withdrawn, bone mineral content fell at a normal postmenopausal rate, demonstrating the long-term prevention of bone loss by estrogen. This group also demonstrated a significant reduction in height loss among post-oophorectomized women who were treated prophylactically with small doses of mestranol (mean dosage was 20 mcg/day). It seems evident, therefore, that bone demineralization can be delayed with estrogen replacement therapy. Although no therapy now available can restore bone mass in a patient with osteoporosis, women who have premature ovarian failure or bilateral oophorectomy before 50 years of age would be benefited if treated prophylactically with estrogen. At particular risk of osteoporosis are slender white women who smoke and are physically inactive.

There are many orally active estrogen compounds. Conjugated equine estrogen in the dosage of 0.625 mg/day for 3 weeks of each month is one of the more common agents used. Ethinyl estradiol in a dosage of 0.02 mg/day or Mestranol in a dose of 25 to 30 mcg/day will produce similar biologic effects. In the prematurely castrated patient, estrogen should be given at least until she reaches 50 years of age, the normal age of menopause, and may safely be continued for the next 5 or 10 years if the major estrogen target organ, the uterus, has been removed. However, the prophylactic use of estrogen must be decided on an individual basis.

The remaining major physiologic changes associated with loss of estrogen—namely, vasomotor symptoms and genitourinary atrophy—may or may not be clinically symptomatic. Although the hot flush appears to occur in synchrony with a pulsatile surge of luteinizing hormone (LH), the change in hormone level is not the major causative factor. The major defect is in the heat regulatory mechanism in the intact hypothalamus. It has been postulated that gonadotropin releasing hormone (GnRH) and the heat regulatory center are affected concomitantly by α-adrenergic stimulation. This stimulation produces a secondary autonomic response that causes a hot flush. Although the precise stimulatory mechanism is as yet incompletely explained, estrogen replacement has a dampening effect on both the pulsatile gonadotropin release mechanism and the thermogenic center. The treatment for vasomotor symptoms and genitourinary atrophy, however, may be given on a very temporary basis until the patient has adjusted to the change in circulating estrogen level. Genitourinary symptoms are less frequent and have a delayed onset. A troublesome clinical problem of estrogen deprivation is the urethral syndrome. This is a recurrent abacterial urethritis, that causes dysuria, nocturia, and urinary frequency and urgency. The syndrome is usually well controlled with estrogen replacement therapy, with the most immediate response being produced by local vaginal estrogen.

The atrophic changes of the vagina are late sequelae of the diminished plasma estrogen level and do not occur for many months or years following the removal of the ovaries. Such changes as vaginal dryness, dyspareunia, irritation, and, occasionally, postcoital bleeding are associated with atrophy of the vaginal epithelium. Although vasomotor and genitourinary symptoms are troublesome, they produce no serious long-term health hazards to the patient. The major advantage of estrogen replacement following oophorectomy is in preventing the more serious problem of bone demineralization with resultant osteoporosis.

Bibliography

Adolf J, Buttermann G, Weidenbach A, et al: Optimization of postoperative prophylaxis of thrombosis in gynecology. Geburtsh Frauenheilk 38:98, 1978

Alexander S: Surgery in the cardiac patient. Surg Clin North Am 50:567, 1970

American Heart Association–National Research Council: Standards on cardiopulmonary resuscitation and emergency cardiac care. JAMA (Suppl) 227:833, 1974

Ashbaugh DG, Bigelow DB, Petty TL, et al: Acute respiratory distress in adults. Lancet 2:319, 1967

Athanasoulis CA: Therapeutic applications of angiography Part 1. N Engl J Med 302:1117, 1980

Aubaniac R: L'injection intraveineuse sousclaviculaire: advantages et technique. Presse Med 60:1456, 1952

Baertschi U, Schaer A, Bader P, et al: A comparison of low dose heparin and oral anticoagulants in the prevention of thrombo-phlebitis following gynaecological operations. Geburtsh Frauenheilk 35:754, 1975

Ballard RM, Bradley–Watson PJ, Johnstone FD, et al: Low doses of subcutaneous heparin in the prevention of deep vein thrombosis after gynaecological surgery. J Obstet Gynaecol Br Commonw 80:469, 1973

Bates GW: On the nature of hot flash. Clin Obstet Gynecol 24:231, 1981

Baxter CR: Shock and metabolism. Surg Gynecol Obstet 142:216, 1976

Bernstein K, Ulmsten U, Astedt B, et al: Incidence of thrombosis after gynecologic surgery evaluated by an improved ^{125}I-fibrinogen uptake test. Angiology 3(9):606, 1980

Blalock A: Consideration of present status of shock problem: Problems of shock. Surg 14:487, 1943

Bonnar JJ, Walsh J: Prevention of thrombosis after pelvic surgery by British Dextran 70. Lancet 1:614, 1972

Bonnar J, Walsh JJ, Haddon M, et al: Coagulation system changes induced by pelvic surgery and the effect of dextran 70. Bibl Anat 12:351, 1973

Breneman JC: Postoperative thromboembolic disease: Computer analysis leading to statistical prediction. JAMA 193:576, 1965

Buchanan EC: Blood and blood substitutes for treating hemorrhagic shock. Am J Hosp Pharm 34:631, 1977

Buchanan EC, Murray WJ: Hemorrhagic shock. Am J Hosp Pharm 34:636, 1977

Burchell RC: The umbrella pack to control pelvic hemorrhage. Conn Med 32:734, 1968

Burchell RC: Physiology of internal iliac artery ligation. J Obstet Gynaecol Brit Comm 75:642, 1968

Chung AF, Menon J, Dillon TF: Acute postoperative retroperitoneal fibrosis and ureteral obstruction secondary to the use of avitene. Am J Obstet Gynecol 132:908, 1978

Clarke–Pearson DL, Creasman WT: Diagnosis of deep venous thrombosis in ob-gyn by impedance phlebography. Obstet Gynecol 58:52, 1981

Clarke–Pearson DL, Jelovsek FR, Creasman WT: Thromboembolism complicating surgery for cervical and uterine malignancy: Incidence, risk factors, and prophylaxis. Obstet Gynecol 61:87, 1983

Clayton JK, Anderson JA, McNicol GP: Effect of cigarette smoking on subsequent postoperative thromboembolic disease in gynecological patients. Br Med J 2:402, 1978

Collins CG: Suppurative pelvic thrombophlebitis. Am J Obstet Gynecol 108:681, 1970

Cranley JJ, Canos AJ, Sull WJ: The diagnosis of deep vein thrombosis. Arch Surg 111:34, 1976

Criteria Committee of the New York Heart Association, Inc.: Diseases of the Heart and Blood Vessels: Nomenclature and Criteria for Diagnosis. ed. 6. Boston, Little, Brown & Co, 1964

Czer LSC, Appel P, Shoemaker WC: Pathogenesis of respiratory failure (ARDS) after hemorrhage and trauma: II. Cardiorespiratory patterns after development of ARDS. Crit Care Med 8:513, 1980

Czer LSC, Shoemaker WC: Optimal hematocrit value in critically ill postoperative patients. Surg Gynecol Obstet 147:363, 1978

Dalen N, Lamke B, Wallgren A: Bone-mineral losses in oophorectomized women. J Bone Joint Surg 56:1235, 1974

Divertie MB: Adult respiratory distress syndrome. Mayo Clin Proc 57:371, 1982

Doran FSA: Prevention of deep vein thrombosis. Br J Hosp Med 6:773, 1971

Endl VJ, Auinger W: Early detection of postoperative deep-vein thrombosis in gynaecological patients by the ^{125}I-fibrinogen test. Wien Klin Wochenschr 89:304, 1977

Everett HS, Ridley JH: Female Urology. New York, Harper-Horber, 1968

Flanc C, Kakkar VW, Clarke MB: The detection of venous thrombosis of the legs using ^{125}I-labeled fibrinogen. Br J Surg 55:742, 1958

Furman RH: Coronary heart disease and the menopause. In Ryan KJ, Gibson DC (eds): Menopause and Aging. DHEW Publication No. (NIH) 73-319, 1971

Gallagher JC, Nordin BEC: Estrogens and calcium metabolism. In van Keep PA, Lauritzen C (eds): Frontiers of Hormone Research, Vol. 2, Ageing and Estrogens. Basel, S Karger, 1973

———: Calcium metabolism and the menopause. In Curry AS (ed): Biochemistry of Women. Cleveland, CRC Press, 1974

Gazes PC: Non-cardiac surgery in cardiac patients: Preoperative and operative management. Postgrad Med 49:171, 1971

Genton E: Pulmonary embolism and infarction. In Chung ED, (ed): Cardiac Emergency Care. Philadelphia, Lea & Febiger, 1979

Genton E, Turpie AGG: Venous thromboembolism associated with gynecologic surgery. Clin Obstet Gynecol 23:209, 1980

Gjonnaess H, Abildgaard U: Bleeding in gynecological surgery: Influence of low dose heparin. Int J Gynaecol Obstet 14:9, 1976

Gordon GS: Postmenopausal osteoporosis: Cause, prevention and treatment. Clin Obstet Gynecol 4:169, 1977

Gray LA, Christopherson WM, Hoover RN: Estrogens and endometrial carcinoma. Obstet Gynecol 49:385, 1977

Hammond CB, Ory SJ: Endocrine problems in the menopause. Clin Obstet Gynecol 25:19, 1982

Hardaway RM, III: Monitoring of the patient in a state of shock. Surg Gynecol Obstet 148:339, 1979

———: Treatment of shock. Comp Ther 53:14, 1979

Hauser CJ, Shoemaker WC, Turpin I, et al: Oxygen transport responses to colloids and crystalloids in critically ill surgical patients. Surg Gynecol Obstet 150:811, 1980

Helgason S: Estrogen replacement therapy after the menopause. Acta Obstet Gynecol Scand (Suppl) 107:1, 1982

Hirsh J, Genton E, Hull R: Venous Thromboembolism. New York, Grune & Stratton, 1981

Hobbs JT, Davies JW: Detection of venous thrombosis with ^{131}I-labeled fibrinogen in the rabbit. Lancet 2:134, 1960

Hodgkinson CP, Hodari AA: Trocar suprapubic cystostomy for postoperative bladder drainage in the female. Am J Obstet Gynecol 96:773, 1966

Holcroft JW: Impairment of venous return in hemorrhagic shock. Surg Clin North Am 62:17, 1982

Horan LG, Flowers NC, Johnson JC: Significance of the diagnostic Q wave of myocardial infarction. Circulation 43:428, 1971

Jeffcoate TNA, Tindall VR: Venous thrombosis and embolism in obstetrics and gynecology. Aust NZ J Obstet Gynaecol 5:119, 1965

Joist JH, Sherman LA (eds): Venous and Arterial Thrombosis: Pathogenesis, Diagnosis, Prevention and Therapy. New York, Grune & Stratton, 1979

Judd HL, Cleary RE, Creasman WT, et al: Estrogen replacement therapy. Obstet Gynecol 58:267, 1981

Kakkar VV, Corrigan TP, Fossard DP: Prevention of postoperative pulmonary embolism by low dose heparin. Lancet 2:45, 1975

Kannel WB, Feinlieb M: The natural history of angina pectoris in the Framingham study: Prognosis and survival. Am J Cardiol 29:154, 1972

Karliner JS, Braunwald E: Present status of digitalis treatment of acute myocardial infarction. Circulation 45:891, 1972

Kass EH, Sossen HS: Prevention of infection of urinary tract in presence of indwelling catheters. JAMA 169:1181, 1959

Keelan MH, Jr: Evaluation of the gynecological patient with heart disease. Clin Obstet Gynecol 16:80, 1973

Kemble JVH: Incidence of deep vein thrombosis. Br J Hosp Med 6:721, 1971

King CR, Daly JW: The prevention of postoperative pulmonary emboli with low-molecular-weight dextran. Am J Obstet Gynecol 123:46, 1975

Kotz KL, Geelhoed GW: Lethal thromboembolism and its prevention in pelvic surgery: A review. Gyn Oncol 12:271, 1981

Ledingham I McA, Routh GS: The pathophysiology of shock. Brit J Hosp Med 22:472, 1979

Lillehei RC, Motsay GJ, Dietzman RH: The use of corticosteroids in the treatment of shock. Int J Clin Pharmacol 5:423, 1972

Lindquist O: Relationship between menstrual status and development of osteoporosis. Acta Obstet Gynecol Scand (Suppl) 110:22, 1982

Lindsay R, Aitken JM, Anderson JB, et al: Long-term prevention of postmenopausal osteoporosis by oestrogen. Lancet 1:1038, 1976

Lindsay R, Hart DM, MacLean A, et al: Bone response to termination of estrogen treatment. Lancet 1:1325, 1978

Lindsay R, Hart DM, Forrest C, et al: Prevention of spinal osteoporosis in oophorectomised women. Lancet 2:1151, 1980

Logothetopulos L: Eine Absolut Sichere Bultstill-Ungsmethode bieVaginalen Und Zentralbl. Gynakologe 50:3202, 1926

Longerbeam JK, Vannix R, Wagner W, et al: Central venous pressure monitoring. Am J Surg 110:220, 1965

McCarthy TG, McQueen J, Johnstone FD, et al: A comparison of low dose subcutaneous heparin and intravenous dextran 70 in the prophylaxis of deep venous thrombosis after gynaecological surgery. J Obstet Gynaecol Br Commonw 81:486, 1974

McDevitt E: Thromboembolic complications following gynecologic operations: Role of prophylactic anticoagulant therapy. In Sherry S, Brinkhous KM, Genton E, et al (eds): Thrombosis. Washington, D.C., National Academy of Sciences, 1969

Mammar EF (ed): Venous thromboembolism. Semin Thromb Hemost 2:4, April 1976

Marshall DH, Horsman A, Nordin BEC: The prevention and management of post-menopausal osteoporosis. Acta Obstet Gynecol Scand (Suppl) 65:49, 1977

Mattingly RF, Moore DE, Clark DO: Bacteriologic study of suprapubic bladder drainage. Am J Obstet Gynecol 114:732, 1972

Mattingly TW: Patients with coronary disease as a surgical risk. Am J Cardiol 12:279, 1963

Mavor GE: Surgery of deep vein thrombosis. Br J Hosp Med 6:755, 1971

Meema HE, Bunker ML, Meema S: Loss of compact bone due to menopause. Obstet Gynecol 26:333, 1965

Mobin-Uddin K, Callard GM, Bolooki H, et al: Transcaval interruption with umbrella filter. N Engl J Med 286:55, 1972

Moosman DA: The anatomy of infraclavicular subclavian vein catheterization and its complications. Surg Gynecol Obstet 136:71, 1973

Moser KM, LeMoine JR: Is embolic risk conditioned by location of deep venous thrombosis? Ann Int Med 94:439, 1981

Moss GS, Lowe RJ, Jilek J, et al: Colloid or crystalloid in the resuscitation of hemorrhagic shock: A controlled clinical trial. Surgery 89:434, 1981

Nusbaum M, Baum S, Blakemore WS: Clinical experience with the diagnosis and management of gastrointestinal hemorrhage by selective mesenteric catheterization. Ann Surg 170:506, 1969

Oliver JA, Jr, Lance JS: Selective embolization to control massive hemorrhage following pelvic surgery. Am J Obstet Gynecol 135:431, 1979

Petty TL, Fowler AA: Another look at ARDS. Chest 82:98, 1982

Poole GV, Meredith JW, Pennell T, et al: Comparison of colloids and crystalloids in resuscitation from hemorrhagic shock. Surg Gynecol Obstet 154:577, 1982

Proudfit CM: Estrogens and menopause. JAMA 236:939, 1976

Prout WB: Relative value of central venous pressure monitoring and blood volume measurement in the management of shock. Lancet 1:1108, 1968

Quigley MM, Hammon CB: Estrogen replacement therapy: Help or hazard? N Engl J Med 301:646, 1979

Rinaldo JE, Rogers RM: Adult Respiratory Distress Syndrome. N Engl J Med 306:900, 1982

Safar P (ed): Advances in Cardiopulmonary Resuscitation. New York, Springer-Verlag, 1977

Safar P: Cardiopulmonary–cerebral resuscitation. Including emergency airway control. In Schwartz G (ed): Principles and Practice of Emergency Medicine. Philadelphia, WB Saunders, 1977

Schlueter DP: High-risk gynecology: Pulmonary risks. Clin Obstet Gynecol 16:91, 1973

Schumer W, Nyhus LM: Corticosteroids in the treatment of shock. Chicago, University of Illinois Press, 1970

Selzer A, Cohn KE: Some thoughts concerning prophylactic use of digitalis. Am J Cardiol 26:214, 1970

Sevitt S, Gallagher NG: Venous thrombosis and pulmonary embolism: a clinical pathological study in injured and burned patients. Br J Surg 48:475, 1961

Shoemaker WC, Appel P, Czer LSC, et al: Pathogenesis of respiratory failure (ARDS) after hemorrhage and trauma: I. Cardiorespiratory patterns preceding the development of ARDS. Crit Care Med 8:504, 1980

Sibbald WJ, Anderson RR, Reid B, et al: Alveolo-capillary permeability in human septic ARDS: Effect of high dose corticosteroid. Ther Chest 79:133, 1981

Smith DC, Prentice R, Thompson DJ, et al: Association of exogenous estrogen and endometrial carcinoma. N Engl J Med 293:1164, 1975

Smith DC, Wyatt JF: Embolization of the hypogastric arteries in the control of massive vaginal hemorrhage. Obstet Gynecol 49:317, 1977

Stephenson HE (ed): Cardiac Arrest and Resuscitation. St Louis, CV Mosby, 1974

Sturdee DW, Wilson KA, Pipili E, et al: Physiological aspects of menopausal hot flush. Brit Med J 2:79, 1978

Swan HJC, Ganz W, Forrester J, et al: Catheterization of the heart in man with use of a flow-directed balloon-tipped catheter. N Engl J Med 283:447, 1970

Taberner DA, Poller L, Burslem RW, et al: Oral anticoagulants controlled by the British comparative thromboplastin versus low-dose heparin in prophylaxis of deep vein thrombosis. Br Med J 1:272, 1978

Taussig FJ: Bladder function after confinement and after gynecological operations. Trans Am Gynecol Soc 40:351, 1915

Thomas D (ed): Thrombosis. Br Med Bull 2:34, May 1978

Tice DA: Low dosage of heparin. Surg Gynecol Obstet 143:970, 1976

Twombly GH: Hemorrhage in gynecologic surgery. Clin Obstet Gynecol 16:135, 1973

Utian WH: Menopause In Modern Perspective. New York, Appleton-Century Crofts, 1980

Virchow R: Handbuch der speciellen Pathologie and Therapie. Vol II. Erlangen and Stuttgart, F Enke, 1854

Walsh JJ, Bonnar J, Wright FW: A study of pulmonary embolism and deep leg vein thrombosis after major gynaecological surgery using labelled fibrogen-phlebography and lung scanning. J Obstet Gynaecol Br Commonw 81:311, 1974

Weinstein MC: Estrogen use in post-menopausal women: Costs, risks, and benefits. N Engl J Med 303:308, 1980

Weiss NS, Szekely DR, Austin DF: Increasing incidence of endometrial cancer in the United States. N Engl J Med 294:1259, 1976

Williams TJ, Julian CG: Tidal drainage in the postoperative bladder. Am J Obstet Gynecol 83:1313, 1962

Wilson JE: Diagnostic methods for deep venous thrombosis (editorial). Arch Int Med 140:893, 1980

Wilson JN, Grow JB, Demony CV, et al: Central venous pressure in optimal blood volume maintenance. Arch Surg 85:563, 1962

Ziel HK, Finkle WD: Increased risk of endometrial carcinoma among users of conjugated estrogens. N Engl J Med 293:1167, 1975

Chapter 7

Total Parenteral Nutrition

Edward J. Quebbeman, M.D.

Malnutrition can now be eliminated from the list of stresses that patients must endure during illness, surgery, or trauma. Many patients can tolerate no food intake by mouth for 1 to 2 weeks whereas others can be given a specialized diet or tube feeding mixture. A few will require total parenteral nutrition (TPN) for prolonged periods. For these patients, all the nutrients and compounds required for preserving or increasing their body cell mass must be supplied intravenously, without causing metabolic stress.

Indication for Total Parenteral Nutrition

Patients who require TPN have been hospitalized for disease processes such as gastrointestinal tract obstruction, prolonged ileus, short bowel syndrome, radiation enteritis, intra-abdominal abscess, pancreatitis, regional enteritis, or enterocutaneous fistula. A patient with any condition that will prevent oral intake of adequate amounts of food for more than 7 to 10 days will probably require TPN. Since it is much easier to maintain an adequate nutritional state than to improve a poor one, the decision to use TPN should not be delayed.

If a patient is already suffering from malnutrition, TPN should be started immediately, unless oral intake is possible and likely to remain so. The degree of malnutrition can be assessed by taking measurements of several physical and chemical indicators, such as serum albumin levels, total lymphocyte count, actual and ideal body weight ratio, creatinine/height index, and triceps skin fold thickness in conjunction with a clinical assessment of the patient. A detailed history of weight loss, nu-

trient intake, nausea and vomiting, diarrhea, and associated chronic illnesses should be part of the assessment. The physical examination should evaluate subcutaneous fat, muscle strength and wasting, edema, and skin condition.

Physical and chemical measurements of malnutrition are subject to many influences during illness, so although helpful as guides, they should not be used alone. For example, albumin values less than 3.2 g/dl are frequently used to indicate malnutrition, but Starker and coworkers found that in hospitalized patients, albumin and body weight measurements in conjunction provided a better indication of sodium balance and extracellular fluid volume. Bistrian and coworkers found that according to the five physical and chemical measurements, 40% to 50% of hospitalized patients were malnourished. Buzby's research group developed an equation using the same five measurements to correlate nutritional status to morbidity and mortality. Immunologic skin testing for recall antigens has been correlated to both nutritional status and morbidity and mortality but is not useful in the assessment of nutritional status.

Starvation and Stress

The starvation seen in severely ill, hospitalized patients is essentially different from simple starvation in the way it affects the metabolic benefits of infused nutrients. Most patients can tolerate a weight loss of 5% to 10%. But a 40% loss of body weight is uniformly fatal, because, in addition to the fat supplies and skeletal muscle, vital body proteins are depleted, affecting the liver, spleen, and pancreas.

Even though the 70-kg human stores approximately 100,000/kcal as fat for energy, the enzymes needed to convert this fat to glucose are not intrinsic, so, instead, the body makes glucose from protein. This protein degradation is used for gluconeogenesis because several vital organs, including the central nervous system, and red cells and white cells require glucose as their principal energy source.

If the body is to withstand starvation, an adaptive process to conserve vital body proteins must take over. After 3 weeks of starvation, nitrogen output in the urine will fall to 3 g/day from the normal level of 10 g/day to 15 g/day, indicating a lesser rate of protein breakdown and conservation of body cell mass. Physical activity will decrease, and the basal metabolic rate will fall by approximately 12% to 20%.

The body's adaptation to starvation involves many parts of the metabolic process. The central nervous system converts to using ketones and ketoacid substrates for energy, which allows the breakdown rate of protein to drop by about 70%. Another adaptive process decreases the use of glucose by muscle tissue; when insulin levels fall, muscle uses an energy substrate of fatty acids, and, therefore, less glucose. Later in the process of starvation, the elevated levels of ketoacids and ketones directly depress further gluconeogenesis.

Most of the endocrine systems are involved in the response to starvation. The insulin level falls rapidly, but levels of glucagon, growth hormone, and catecholamines increase, generating more glucose from protein substrate, which depletes the body cell mass rapidly. Later in the starvation process, glucagon returns to normal, growth hormone levels remain elevated, catecholamines decrease, and gluconeogenesis is slowed.

The kinds of changes that allow for conservation of body cell mass during simple starvation do not operate after injury, trauma, or infection. Afferent information, such as pain and other nerve responses to injury, along with hypovolemia and hypotension, is integrated in the central nervous system and hypothalamus, causing efferent responses, which adjust the body to the stress condition. Levels of catecholamines and glucocorticoids become elevated, accentuating gluconeogenesis and preventing decreases in basal metabolic rates. Antidiuretic hormone levels are increased and the renin-angiotensin system is activated, allowing fluid retention, which prevents early detection of the degree of weight loss.

During stress, urinary nitrogen levels may increase to 20 g or more per 24 hours, corresponding to a loss of 600 g of hydrated body protein. Body weight decreases, since proteins, carbohydrates, and fats are all being degraded for energy, but the adaptive responses seen in simple starvation do not operate in the different hormonal milieu created by the stress condition.

Provision of nutrients can offset some of this nitrogen loss and even produce positive nitrogen balance. During starvation, the provision of 150 g glucose (the amount in 3 liters of 5% dextrose IV solution) will reduce nitrogen loss even further than the maximum physiologic adaptive mechanisms because glucose prevents much of the obligatory gluconeogenesis, creating a protein sparing effect. As Moore explained in his concise review, if high levels of glucose are supplied (up to 750 g/24 hr), protein sparing can be optimized and nitrogen output decreased to 1.8 g/m^2/day.

During periods of injury and stress, patients must receive energy intake at least equal to energy expenditure; and to attain positive nitrogen balance, they must receive amino acid nitrogen in excess of urinary losses. Although fat alone cannot provide this energy intake, a combination of glucose and fat is effective.

Initiating Total Parenteral Nutrition

Safe venous access is required for initiating TPN. A reliable intravenous catheter should be placed into a large central vein with the catheter tip located so that blood flow will dilute the highly concentrated nutritional fluids. The insertion site should also allow easy fixation of the catheter at the entrance site, minimum catheter movement during body movements, and easy dressing changes. A subclavian vein approach satisfies the requirements for safe catheter placement, but neither internal jugular vein nor antecubital fossa placements provide safe access.

Catheter placement should be performed by experienced personnel under sterile conditions, and never as an emergency procedure. The procedure should be performed in an operating room, an intensive care unit, or an area designated for catheter placement, but not in the usual patient bed space. Adequate lighting and a table that can tilt into the Trendelenburg position are essential, as are space and equipment to recognize and treat any complications that occur.

The patient's shoulder and neck should be scrubbed as for any surgical procedure. All personnel should wear caps and masks, and the surgeon should wear a sterile gown and gloves. The patient should be flat on the table with arms at the sides and in the Trendelenburg position to promote distention of the subclavian vein. The needle is inserted one fingerbreadth below the clavicle at the bend in the medial one-third of the clavicle. The needle is then directed in a horizontal position toward a spot one fingerbreadth above the sternal notch (Fig. 7–1). Entry into the vein is confirmed when dark blood flows freely into the syringe. Subsequent manipulation depends on the type of catheter used.

Catheters of polyvinyl chloride, Teflon, or polyethylene can be used for subclavian vascular access. The most appropriate material, Silastic, is less thrombogenic, causes fewer reactions with body tissue, has a very low potential for surface adherence of bacteria, and is very soft and pliable, reducing the chance of damage to the veins. If TPN is to be used for several weeks or months, safety considerations become more important.

Following insertion, the catheter should be secured to the skin with a suture (*e.g.,* No. 3-0 silk) and a transparent dressing applied (*e.g.,* Tegaderm or OP-Site). This type of dressing prevents catheter movement and ingress of bacteria while allowing evaporation of moisture. Additional tape should be used to secure the catheter.

Before starting the first fluid, the position of the catheter must be identified using an upright chest x-ray. The catheter tip should be in the superior vena cava or right atrium. If it is in the internal jugular vein, the catheter should be repositioned before TPN is begun. Occasionally, Silastic catheters that have been inadvertently placed in the jugular vein will follow the flow of blood and move into the vena cava spontaneously. The x-ray should also be examined to exclude the occurrence of a pneu-

mothorax or hemothorax or the accidental placement of the catheter into the chest cavity or arterial circulation.

Several other complications of attempted subclavian catheterization have occurred. These include hematoma from damage to the subclavian artery, nerve damage from hitting the brachial plexus, and tracheal puncture. Air embolism has occurred when the needle or catheter were left open to air while the central venous pressure was low, and has also occurred when the IV tubing became disconnected. Catheter embolism can be minimized or eliminated by properly understanding how to use the catheter selected and by using catheters that do not require introduction through a large sharp-edged needle.

Late complications of central venous catheterization also occur, most commonly technical problems caused when the catheter is inadvertently removed or disconnected, resulting in contamination or clotting. Such problems are usually overcome by educating both the patient and the nursing staff about proper methods of catheter care.

The more serious problem of subclavian vein thrombosis should be suspected if the patient complains of a stiff or sore neck, swelling and discomfort in the supraclavicular area, increase in diameter of the ipsilateral arm, or venous prominence over the arm or shoulder. Complete occlusion of the subclavian vein that can be diagnosed clinically occurs in 5% of patients with nonsilicone catheters. When venography is used, the rate increases to 30% to 42%, because most problems are asymptomatic.

If thrombosis is suspected, a venogram should be

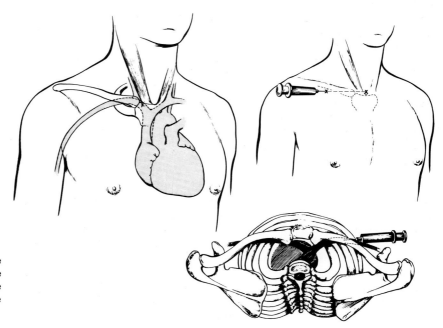

FIG. 7–1 Anatomical relationships of the subclavian vein, demonstrating that the needle must be advanced parallel to the patient's back and toward a point one fingerbreadth above the sternal notch.

obtained, and, if necessary, the catheter should be removed. If the catheter cannot be easily replaced in another site, or if the catheter is one of the more permanent Hickman-type Silastic catheters, streptokinase or urokinase can be used to dissolve the clot. Anticoagulation therapy used prophylactically for pulmonary embolus or to prevent progression of a clot is not generally necessary, but should be used if the patient is severely symptomatic or if the catheter is not removed.

Catheter-related sepsis is difficult to differentiate from other causes of sepsis. More common causes of febrile episodes in hospitalized patients receiving TPN are pneumonia, urinary tract infection, wound infection, and intra-abdominal abscess. If TPN catheters were routinely removed during any febrile episode, as many as 90% would be removed unnecessarily. Even when bacteremia is documented, only 25% of the infections are caused by the patient's TPN catheter.

The sudden occurrence of septic shock or erythema with purulent exudate at the catheter insertion site is an indication for immediate catheter removal. If a sudden febrile episode occurs in a previously afebrile patient receiving TPN, the procedure listed below should be followed:

1. Culture the TPN fluid and change the bag and tubing.
2. Obtain blood cultures from peripheral veins and through the catheter. Include fungal cultures.
3. Search for other sources of fever, such as pneumonia, wound infection, and so on.
4. Withhold antibiotics unless overwhelming sepsis is suspected.
5. If no other source of sepsis is found and blood cultures are positive, remove the catheter and culture the tip.

Primary catheter sepsis is confirmed if the tip is positive, if the blood cultures are positive for the same organism, if fever disappears within 24 hours of removal, and if no other source of infection is present. Infected Silastic catheters that are required for long-term care may be successfully treated using parenteral antibiotics. *Staphylococcus epidermidis*, *Staphylococcus aureus*, *Candida albicans*, and, less often, the gram-negative bacteria are the most common infecting organisms, emphasizing the need for sterile technique during catheter insertion and dressing changes.

Prevention of catheter-related problems is an important treatment goal. The catheter should only be used for TPN and not for other medications or blood products. Only personnel who are knowledgeable and trained in the techniques should care for the catheter and intravenous system. Dressings should be changed under sterile conditions. The new dressing should be occlusive, dry, and placed to prevent catheter movement. Routine follow-up consultation should be sought from the nutritional support team.

Prescribing Fluids in Total Parenteral Nutrition

TPN mixtures are composed of a calorie source (glucose or fats), a protein source (usually crystalline amino acids), and an assortment of electrolytes, vitamins, and trace elements sufficient to prevent a multitude of deficiency states. The solution chosen should meet the patient's energy needs. Resting energy expenditure (REE) can be calculated using the following equation, which includes body surface area (BSA) and specific constants:

$$\text{Male} \quad \text{REE} = 789 \times \text{BSA} + 137$$

$$\text{Female} \quad \text{REE} = 544 \times \text{BSA} + 414$$

To allow for individual variation, and to be certain that sufficient energy is available for protein synthesis and physical activity, provide 20% more than the calculated energy need. The equation need not be changed for accompanying conditions. For example, patients under stress, with sepsis, or with trauma do not need more energy, and malnourished patients do not need less, although excessively obese patients should receive less energy than calculated.

Solutions consist of a nonprotein energy substrate, generally a combination of glucose and fat in the form of triglycerides derived from a soybean extract. Using glucose as the only energy substrate for prolonged periods can cause hyperglycemia, a high respiratory quotient, fat deposition in the liver, and essential fatty acid deficiency syndrome. A desirable proportion of fat calories is between 10% and 50% of the total energy intake. This proportion is usually well tolerated.

The protein component for the solution is provided by a mixture of crystalline amino acids. The recommended daily requirement for protein is 0.7 g/kg/24 hr, but patients under stress will require a greater amount. The initial value chosen for TPN is usually between 1 g/kg/24 hr and 1.5 g/kg/24 hr, but the amount is substantially influenced by the level of energy intake. As energy intake increases up to the resting energy expenditure, the amount of protein needed to allow net protein synthesis decreases. After TPN has begun, the final adjustments to the protein intake can occur based on the results of a 24-hour urine collection to determine nitrogen output. While well-nourished, stable subjects are in a net zero nitrogen balance, malnourished patients requiring TPN are generally retaining 20 mg/kg/24 hr to 60 mg/kg/24 hr more than they lose. Attempting to achieve greater nitrogen retention may cause elevation of the BUN and degradation of the expensive amino acids that were meant to be incorporated into protein.

Electrolytes are provided to replace ongoing loss and to allow protein synthesis to occur. If insufficient potassium, phosphate, or zinc are given, positive nitrogen balance cannot be obtained. The addition of such trace elements, as zinc, copper, manganese, and chromium is necessary to prevent clinically significant deficiency syndromes during prolonged TPN. Recommended compounds and daily intakes are listed in Suggested Daily Additives to TPN Fluids.

SUGGESTED DAILY ADDITIVES TO TPN FLUIDS

Electrolytes

Sodium chloride	70 mEq
Potassium phosphate	60 mEq
Magnesium sulfate	10 mEq
Calcium gluconate	10 mEq

Vitamins (MVI-12)*

A	3,300.0 IU
D	200.0 IU
E	10.0 IU
C	100.0 mg
Thiamine (B_1)	3.0 mg
Riboflavin (B_2)	3.6 mg
Niacin	40 mg
Pyridoxine (B_6)	4.0 mg
Pantothenic acid	15 mg
Biotin	60 mcg
B_{12}	5 mcg
Folic acid	400 mcg

Trace Elements

Zinc	4.0 mg
Copper	1.0 mg
Manganese	0.5 mg
Chromium	10.0 mcg

---

* MVI-12 = multivitamin-12
These values are approximate and exact requirements are not known. Electrolyte concentrations may need to be altered substantially.

Vitamin supplementation is required during TPN, but the exact doses are uncertain and estimates vary widely. While the water-soluble vitamins, B and C, can be given in large doses without harm, the fat-soluble vitamins A, D, and E have been associated

with toxicity, and should be limited. A typical solution contains 1 ampule of a multivitamin-12 (MVI-12) per day, supplemented with 10 mg of vitamin K intramuscularly once every week.

The last value to be calculated is the IV rate, which is based on the quantity of protein, glucose, and fat necessary per day and on the total fluid requirements of the patient. Fluid requirements for patients needing TPN are calculated as for any other patient, with consideration for basal requirements and ongoing losses. The nutritional fluid administered should be substituted for other IV fluids to avoid the problem of excess fluid accumulation.

The solutions prescribed should not only be chosen with appropriate consideration for the requirements of the patient, but should also be as easy as possible for the pharmacist to mix. Failure to understand this last requirement will increase pharmacy time and cost, allow possible inaccuracies in mixing, and increase the likelihood of solution contamination. Some of the commonly available solutions for mixing TPN are listed in Table 7–1. These are generally packaged in 500 ml quantities and are easy to use in 250 ml quantities.

Monitoring

While patients are receiving TPN, they require close observation to prevent metabolic complications and to measure progress (Table 7–2).

One of the most important values to measure is the nitrogen balance. This simple measurement is indicative of protein synthesis, since there are no other nitrogen stores in the body, excluding that measured by the BUN. This measurement requires an *accurate* collection of *all* urine during a 24-hour period. Ideally, the total nitrogen should be measured, but often urea nitrogen is the only measurement available from the clinical laboratory. If only urea nitrogen is available, a 2 g factor is frequently added to account for nonurea urine nitrogen losses. Loss of nitrogen from feces, skin, hair, and other secretions must also be added, approximately 20 mg/kg/24 hr. The total of all these losses is then subtracted from the total amount of nitrogen being infused to determine the balance. A negative balance requires a reevaluation of the level of energy and protein intake, and, probably, an increase in the protein component of the solution to achieve a positive balance.

Stopping Total Parenteral Nutrition

The use of TPN is expensive and puts the patients at some risk of developing technical or metabolic

TABLE 7–1   *Values for Parenteral Solutions (per liter)*

SUBSTRATE	CONCENTRATION (%)	CALORIES (kcal)	OSMOLALITY (mosm/liter)	NITROGEN (g)
Glucose	10.0	340	505	—
	50.0	1700	2520	—
	70.0	2380	3530	—
Lipid	10.0	1100	270	—
	20.0	2000	340	—
Protein	5.5	—	550	9.27
	7.0	—	700	11.80
	8.5	—	850	14.33
	10.0	—	1000	16.86

complications, so it should not be continued for prolonged periods unless absolutely necessary. Before TPN is stopped, the patient should be able to ingest adequate nutrition either orally or by tube feeding in order to maintain weight, and improve clinically. Often, TPN support is stopped prematurely because adequate intake is anticipated rather than actually achieved. On the other hand, TPN is occasionally continued indefinitely in the hopes that the patient will improve more quickly than on oral intake, but there is no justification for this practice.

When TPN is to be stopped, a short period (2–4 hours) of reduced infusion rate is usually begun before the infusion is stopped. Prolonged weaning to prevent reactive hypoglycemia is not necessary since solutions no longer contain excessively high infusion rates of concentrated glucose mixtures.

The Team Approach to Total Parenteral Nutrition

TPN can now be safely administered to patients in many hospitals because of the existence of a team of individuals from different disciplines. Although the composition and exact function of the team

TABLE 7–2   *Values Monitored Routinely During TPN*

VALUE MEASURED	PURPOSE
Sodium	Avoid excess free water or hypernatremia
Potassium	May decrease with glucose administration or protein synthesis
Chloride	Avoid hyperchloremia from high chloride content of some amino acid solutions
Phosphate	May decrease during protein anabolism even with renal failure
Osmolality	Avoids hyperosmotic nonketotic dehydration and coma
BUN	May increase with excessive amino acid intake or improper protein/calorie ratio
Glucose	Early increase with sepsis, diabetes, excessive intake
Urine S/A	Indicates need for insulin if glucosuria occurs
Weight	Decrease may indicate inadequate nutrition, rapid increase is overhydration
Intake/output	Avoid fluid overload
SGOT, alkaline phosphatase, Bilirubin	Alteration may suggest changing total energy intake or proportion of fat and glucose
HCT, HGB	To detect the frequently progressive anemia
Albumin iron-binding capacity	May be indicative of nutritional status and severity of disease

CALCULATION AND SOLUTION ADMIXTURES IN TPN

Patient = male, Weight = 70 Kg, Height = 170 cm
Body surface area = 1.81 m² Resting energy expenditure = 1565 kcal
Estimated requirements = 1878 kcal/day, 14 g/day nitrogen

Solution	Mostly Glucose	50% Fats	Fluid Restricted
Glucose	50% 500 ml	50% 250 ml	70% 250 ml
Amino acids	8.5% 500 ml	8.5% 500 ml	10% 500 ml
Rate (ml/hour)	80	60	50
Fats	10% 500 ml qod	10% 1000 ml/day	20% 500 ml/day
Total volume (ml/day)	2170	2440	1700
Total nitrogen (g/day)	13.7	13.7	13.5
Total calories (kcal/day)	1882	1916	1952

These examples illustrate some of the many possible solution admixtures that can easily be performed by the pharmacist.

members vary between hospitals, most teams consist of a physician, a nurse, a pharmacist, and a dietician. Although usually the TPN team act as consultants for the primary physician caring for the patient, at some institutions the team is primarily responsible for the patient, and some hospitals have a designated area for TPN care.

The team approach by either method is highly beneficial, providing a high concentration of personnel with knowledge, expertise, and interdisciplinary communication at the patient's bedside. Team members can provide continuing education on nutritional therapy, they can continuously audit and collect quality control data, and they can investigate ways to improve the safety and efficacy of TPN as a treatment modality. Most teams operate with a standardized protocol that covers patient assessment, catheter insertion techniques, solutions used, and monitoring functions performed.

Special Problems

Although most patients requiring TPN can tolerate a standard solution mixture as illustrated in Calculation and Solution Admixtures in TPN, there are several reasons that a solution may need to be altered for various patients with certain disease processes.

CARDIAC AND RESPIRATORY INSUFFICIENCY

Patients with congestive heart failure require decreased sodium and decreased total fluid volume.

The best solution can be prepared from the most concentrated solutions of glucose, amino acid, and fat available (see Calculation and Solution Admixtures in TPN). Fluid-restricted solutions may also be beneficial for patients with respiratory failure, who should receive less total glucose in favor of more fat, since the respiratory quotient (CO_2/O_2) of glucose (1.00) is greater than fat (0.70), and excess glucose will increase the load of CO_2 the lungs must excrete. Excessive total caloric intake resulting in fat synthesis from glucose substrate may severely compromise respiratory function, since large amounts of CO_2 are released (respiratory quotient > 8.0).

RENAL FAILURE

Patients with renal failure develop high body fluid volumes, BUN and potassium among other abnormalities. These patients need to receive a concentrated solution of glucose and fat to avoid high fluid volumes, and they also need a low protein intake of 0.7 g/kg/24 hr or less. When hemodialysis or peritoneal dialysis is readily accessible, there is no need to prevent the patient from receiving adequate nutrition.

A controversy exists over the type of amino acid infusion to use for patients with renal failure. The rationale for using a standard solution is to be certain that all amino acids are readily available for protein synthesis, but some nutritionists advocate a solution of only the eight essential amino acids (e.g., Nephramine) because the other amino acids may possibly be synthesized by transamination. At this time, there is no definitive proof that solutions of essential amino acids are more beneficial than a mixture including nonessential amino acids.

LIVER FAILURE

Nutritional support during hepatic failure is especially demanding because of the wide variety of metabolic functions performed by the liver. The metabolic derangements associated with liver failure are numerous; among them are decreased insulin/glucagon ratio with consequent gluconeogenesis, causing net catabolism of body protein. Ureagenesis is also impaired, and toxic nitrogenous compounds, including ammonia, may accumulate. So although the need for protein is increased, the patient is also intolerant of protein.

Fisher demonstrated that intravenous protein is actually better tolerated than oral protein and can be given to 50% to 60% of patients without causing encephalopathy. The remaining 40% to 50% of patients require a mixture of amino acids high in branch chain amino acids (leucine, isoleucine, valine) and low in the aromatic amino acids (phenylalanine, tyrosine, tryptophan), which cross the blood-brain barrier and cause encephalopathy. Branch chain amino acid mixtures are commercially available now; their exact function in liver failure or in trauma and sepsis is unclear, although it is being studied.

Peripheral Vein Nutrition

There is a choice between giving full nutrional support by the complex, central vein technique or giving less complete nutritional support by the simpler, peripheral vein method. Peripheral solutions generally include amino acids, with 5% glucose to provide about 600 kcal in 3 liters of total volume. Peripheral solutions provide some degree of protein sparing, and limited amounts of electrolytes and fats can be added. The factor preventing adequate nutritional support through peripheral veins is the osmolality of the solution (see Suggested Daily Additives to TPN Fluids, above). Peripheral veins are at risk for phlebitis if osmolality exceeds 600 mOsm, which is almost equal to a 10% glucose solution.

Several other problems exist when using the peripheral route: patients who most need therapy rarely have adequate peripheral veins remaining after receiving other intravenous therapies. The volume of the infusion has to be higher to reduce the osmolality of the solution. The caloric support is suboptimal unless very high (85%) amounts of fat are used. Too frequently, patients could have tolerated a short period of starvation without peripheral vein nutrition, or they should actually have received TPN, but their physician was procrastinating.

Conclusion

Parenteral nutrition is a valuable adjunctive therapy to prevent complications of malnutrition and starvation in patients unable to absorb nutrients from the gastrointestinal tract. Ongoing research is attempting to identify the appropriate place for this expensive therapy in the care of patients. A patient's morbidity and mortality risk are still predominantly determined by the underlying disease process; TPN should be used to prevent additional metabolic stress. TPN is a safe procedure when performed by knowledgeable personnel, and the treatment should be available in all hospitals caring for severely ill patients.

Bibliography

AMA Department of Foods and Nutrition. Guidelines for essential trace element preparation for parenteral use. JAMA 241:2051, 1979

Askanazi J, Carpentier YA, Elwyn DH, et al: Influence of total parenteral nutrition on fuel utilization in injury and sepsis. Ann Surg 191:40, 1980

Askanazi J, Elwyn DH, Silverberg PA, et al: Respiratory distress secondary to a high carbohydrate load. Surgery 87:596, 1980

Ausman RK, Quebbeman EJ, Altmann CL: Liver malfunction associated with parenteral nutrition. In Johnston IDA (ed): Advances in Clinical Nutrition. Boston, MTP Press 1983

Baker JP, Detsky AS, Wesson DE, et al: Nutritional assessment: A comparison of clinical judgement and objective measurements. N Engl J Med 306:969, 1982

Bistrian BR, Blackburn GL, Hallowell E, et al: Protein status of general surgical patients. JAMA 230:858, 1974

Bjornson HS, Colley R, Bower RH, et al: Association between microorganism growth at the catheter site and colonization of the catheter in patients receiving total parenteral nutrition. Surgery 92:720, 1982

Blackburn GL, Bistrian BR, Maini BS, et al: Nutritional and metabolic assessment of the hospitalized patient. Journal of Parenteral and Enteral Nutrition 1:11, 1977

Blackburn GL, Etter G, Mackenzie T: Criteria for choosing amino acid therapy in acute renal failure. Am J Clin Nutr 31:1841, 1978

Brismar B, Hardstedt C, Jacobson S: Diagnosis of thrombosis by catheter phlebography after prolonged central venous catheterization. Ann Surg 194:779, 1981

Brown R, Bancewicz J, Hamid J, et al: Delayed hypersensitivity skin testing does not influence the management of surgical patients. Ann Surg 196:672, 1982

Buzby GP, Mullen JL, Mathews DC, et al: Prognostic nutritional index in gastrointestinal surgery. Am J Surg 139:160, 1980

Colley R, Wilson J, Kapusta E, et al: Fever and catheter-related sepsis in total parenteral nutrition. Journal of Parenteral and Enteral Nutrition 3:32, 1979

Dillon JD, Schaffner W, Van Way CW, et al: Septicemia and total parenteral nutrition: Distinguishing catheter-related from other septic episodes. JAMA 223:1341, 1973

Elwyn DH: Nutritional requirements of adult surgical patients. Crit Care Med 8:9, 1980

Fischer JE: Surgical Nutrition. Boston, Little Brown & Co, 1983

Hoshal VL: Total intravenous nutrition with peripherally inserted silicone elastomer central venous catheters. Arch Surg 110:644, 1975

Maki DG, Weise CE, Sarafin HW: A semiquantitative culture method for identifying intravenous-catheter-related infection. N Engl J Med 296:1305, 1977

Mirtallo JM, Schneider PT, Mauko K, et al: A comparison of essential and general amino acid infusions in the nutritional support of patients with compromised renal function. Journal of Parenteral and Enteral Nutrition 6:109, 1982

Moore FD: Energy and the maintenance of the body cell mass. Journal of Parenteral and Enteral Nutrition 4:228, 1980

Moosman DA: The anatomy of infraclavicular subclavian vein catheterization and its complications. Surg Gynecol Obstet 136:71, 1973

Mullin TJ, Kirkpatrick JR: The effect of nutritional support on immune competency in patients suffering from trauma, sepsis, and malignant disease. Surgery 90:610, 1981

Nordenstrom J, Carpentier YA, Askanazi J, et al: Metabolic utilization of intravenous fat emulsion during total parenteral nutrition. Ann Surg 196:221, 1982

Padberg FT, Ruggiero J, Blackburn GL, et al: Central venous catheterization for parenteral nutrition. Ann Surg 193:264, 1973

Quebbeman EJ: Estimating energy requirements in patients receiving parenteral nutrition. Arch Surg 117:1281, 1982

Quebbeman EJ: A re-evaluation of energy expenditure during parenteral nutrition. Ann Surg 195:282, 1982

Sanders RA, Sheldon GF: Septic complications of total parenteral nutrition: A five year experience. Am J Surg 132:214, 1976

Sitges-Serra A, Puig P, Jaurrieta E, et al: Catheter sepsis due to *Staphylococcus epidermidis* during parenteral nutrition. Surg Gynecol Obstet 151:481, 1980

Starker PM, Gump FE, Askanazi J, et al: Serum albumin levels as an index of nutritional support. Surgery 91:194, 1982

Stewart RD, Sanislow CA: Silastic intravenous catheter. N Engl J Med 265:1283, 1961

Valerio D, Hussey JK, Smith FW: Central vein thrombosis associated with intravenous feeding: A prospective study. Journal of Parenteral and Enteral Nutrition 5:240, 1981

Welch GW, McKeel DW, Silverstein P, et al: The role of the catheter composition in the development of thrombophlebitis. Surg Gynecol Obstet 138:421, 1974

Chapter 8

Water, Electrolyte, and Acid–Base Metabolism

Lee A. Hebert, M.D., and
Jacob Lemann, M.D.

In the normal adult, about 50% to 70% of body weight is water. Fatty tissue contains very little water; therefore, with increasing degrees of obesity, the percentage of body weight that is water approaches 50%. With increasing degrees of leanness, the percentage of body weight that is water approaches 70%. The approximate distribution of body water in health is shown in Table 8–1. Osmotic and oncotic forces are important determinants of water distribution; thus we must begin with a review of these concepts.

Osmotic Forces (Osmolality, Osmotic Pressure)

If a solute is added to pure water, the presence of the second molecular species interferes with the normal "activity" of water molecules. As a result, water diffuses more slowly through the solution, and the solution must be raised to a higher temperature before boiling will occur and lowered to a cooler temperature before freezing will occur. These effects of solute on the colligative properties of water are related principally to the number of molecules present per unit volume rather than to the specific kind of molecule or to the total weight of solute present. The determination of osmolality is a measure of the number of molecules in the solution that are effective in reducing the concentration and, therefore, the chemical properties of water. The slower rate of diffusion of water caused by the solute accounts for the fact that water diffuses from zones of low osmolality (high water concentration) to zones of high osmolality (low water concentration). The hydrostatic pressure that must be applied to the zone of high osmolality to oppose exactly osmotic pressure is equal to the osmotic pressure between the zones of high and low osmolality. The effect of solute concentration on the freezing point vapor pressure of water is the basis for the clinical measurement of osmolality in body fluids.

The osmolality of normal extracellular fluid (ECF) is determined almost entirely by sodium and its accompanying anions. However, under certain conditions such other substances as glucose, mannitol, alcohol, and urea can accumulate and contribute importantly to plasma osmolality. The contribution of each of these solutes to plasma osmolality can be determined directly in the clinical laboratory, by measuring freezing-point depression, or by calculation. Calculation of plasma osmolality (P_{osm}) from the known concentration of solutes is as follows:

$$P_{osm} = 2 \times [Na] \text{ mEq/liter} + \text{glucose mM/liter}$$
$$+ \text{ urea mM/liter}$$
$$+ \text{ osmolar concentration of other solutes.}$$

For normal plasma,

$$P_{osm} = 2 \times 140 \text{ mEq/liter} + (900 \text{ mg glucose/liter})/$$
$$(180 \text{ mg glucose/mOsm})$$
$$+ (140 \text{ mg urea nitrogen/liter})/$$
$$(28 \text{ mg urea nitrogen/mOsm})$$
$$+ \text{ other solutes (negligible in}$$
$$\text{normal plasma)}$$
$$= 290 \text{ mOsm/liter.}$$

(mM = millimoles; mOsm = milliosmoles.)

TABLE 8–1 *The Body Water Compartments in Health*

PARAMETER	TOTAL BODY WATER	INTRACELLULAR WATER	EXTRACELLULAR WATER*
Percentage of total body water	100%	67%	33%
Percentage of body weight	60%	40%	20%
Actual volume (liters) in a 60-kg person	36	24	12
Osmolality (mOsm/kg of water)	290	290	290

* The intravascular water space is about one-fourth of the extracellular water space. However, the intravascular volume is substantially larger than the intravascular water space because of the additional space occupied by blood cell and plasma proteins. The intravascular volume (blood volume) is about 7% of body weight or slightly more than 4 liters in a 60 kg person.

The osmolalities of intracellular fluid (ICF) and (ECF) are equal because cell walls (except for the collecting duct of the kidney) are always freely permeable to water. Potassium is the major intracellular cation and is found in concentrations of approximately 150 mEq/liter of cell water. Thus, potassium plus its accompanying anions, principally phosphate and protein, account for almost all of the osmolality of intracellular fluid. In health, Na^+ is excluded from cells by active pumps located in cell walls, and K^+ is maintained in cells, probably because of the active and selective exclusion of Na^+.

Oncotic Forces (Oncotic Pressure, Colloid Osmotic Pressure)

Just as crystalloids in solution, such as Na^+, Cl^-, and urea, reduce the concentration of water, so also do colloids such as albumin and globulins. However, in biological solutions the contribution of proteins in lowering the effective concentration of water is far less than that of crystalloids, since there are far fewer protein molecules than crystalloid molecules. One gram of albumin (mol wt 68,000) theoretically yields 0.015 mOsm [(1,000 mg/68,000 mg/mM) × 1 mOsm/mM], whereas one gram of sodium chloride theoretically yields 34.3 mOsm [(1,000 mg/58.5 mg/mM) × 2 mOsm/mM]. Thus, gram for gram, sodium chloride is theoretically 2300 times more effective in increasing the osmolality of a solution than albumin. The oncotic pressure of solutions is expressed in mm Hg for the same reason that osmotic forces are expressed in units of hydrostatic pressure.

Even though oncotic forces are small relative to osmotic forces, they are very important in biologic systems because plasma proteins are selectively retained in the intravascular space. Thus, the effective concentration of water and electrolytes is selectively reduced in the intravascular compared to the interstitial space. All other things being equal, this will result in diffusion of water and electrolytes from the interstitial to the intravascular space. However, at the capillary level, where these oncotic forces are at work, the capillary blood hydrostatic pressure opposes the inward diffusion of water and electrolytes. At the arterial end of the capillary, the effect of capillary blood hydrostatic pressure (about 35 mm Hg) pushing fluid outward is greater than the effect of capillary blood oncotic pressure (equivalent to 25 mm Hg) causing inward diffusion of fluid. Therefore, net outward movement of water and electrolytes occurs. However, at the venous end of the capillary, the capillary blood oncotic pressure (equivalent to about 25 mm Hg) exceeds capillary blood hydrostatic pressure (now about 15 mm Hg) and, therefore, net inward movement of water and electrolytes occurs. In health, the rate of fluid outflow from the arterial end of the capillary equals the rate of uptake at the venous end of the capillary.

Regulation of Water and Electrolyte Distribution Between Intracellular and Extracellular Compartments

Osmotic forces regulate the distribution of water between ECF and ICF, and under all steady-state conditions, ECF osmolality equals ICF osmolality. The implications of these principles when water or solute is added to body fluids are as follows.

EFFECT OF ADDITION OF WATER ON ECF AND ICF VOLUME AND OSMOLALITY

The ingestion of water or the intravenous infusion of water, as 5% solution of glucose in water (which is the same as water when the glucose is metabolized to $H_2O + CO_2$) results in expansion of all body fluid compartments. Since the osmolality of all body compartments is the same, the water is distributed in the body water compartments in proportion to their size. For example, 1000 ml of a 5% solution of dextrose in water is infused into a normal 60-kg individual with plasma osmolality $(P_{osm}) = 290$ mOsm/liter and serum sodium = 140 mEq/liter. Assuming that there is no excretion of the water and complete metabolism of the glucose to CO_2 and water, the change in volume of the body water compartments (see Table 8–1) when complete mixing has occurred is as follows: The ICF is increased by about 666 ml and the ECF is increased by about 333 ml. The intravascular water, which is one-fourth of the ECF, is increased by only about 83 ml. Plasma osmolality decreases by about 2%. This is sufficient to completely suppress antidiuretic hormone (ADH) release and cause a maximum water diuresis in a normal person.

EFFECT OF ADDITION OF SOLUTE ON ECF AND ICF VOLUME AND OSMOLALITY

If solutes are ingested or infused that penetrate cells slowly (*e.g.*, glucose) or are actively excluded from cells (*e.g.*, Na^+), water is obligated to remain with these solutes in the ECF so that conditions of osmotic equilibrium between ICF and ECF are met. If these solutes are given in isotonic solutions (*i.e.*, if the osmolality of the solution equals that of body fluids), conditions of osmotic equilibrium are met without shifts of water between ICF and ECF. Thus, the ECF is selectively expanded. On the other hand, if these solutes are ingested without water or given as hypertonic solutions, ECF osmolality will rise as these solutes move into the ECF, and water will diffuse from ICF to ECF until osmolality in the two compartments is equal. Thus, the ECF is expanded as the ICF is contracted.

Although certain other solutes, such as urea and ethyl alcohol, increase plasma osmolality, they do not affect the steady-state distribution of water between ECF and ICF because these solutes readily penetrate cells and eventually distribute throughout the body water space. Nevertheless, in non–steady states, such as rapid removal of urea by hemodialysis, or rapid addition by intravenous infusion, transient redistribution of water between ECF and ICF does occur. Such shifts of fluid in brain tissue can lead to significant changes in brain function.

Regulation of Water and Electrolyte Distribution Between the Intravascular and Interstitial Compartments

As discussed above, the regulation of fluid and electrolyte transfer at the capillary level is determined by the balance among oncotic forces, hydrostatic forces, and capillary permeability to plasma proteins. These forces can be perturbed in the following ways.

Hypoalbuminemia results in a fall in plasma oncotic pressure, a rise in the effective concentration of water and electrolytes in the intravascular space, and, all other things being equal, net movement of water and electrolytes into the interstitial space. As a consequence, intravascular volume decreases and the kidney responds by retaining sodium and water in an attempt to restore intravascular volume to normal. If the hypoalbuminemia is sufficiently pronounced (usually less than 2.5 g/100 ml), and the expected renal retention of sodium and water occurs, edema will develop before a new equilibrium between outflux and influx of fluid at the capillary level is achieved.

The sequence of events that leads to edema formation is depicted in Figure 8–1. Note that the stimulus to renal sodium and water retention in hypoalbuminemia is a decrease in intravascular volume. In many hypoalbuminemic patients, the retention of sodium and water does not completely restore intravascular volume to normal. In fact, in some patients with marked hypoalbuminemia, massive edema (expansion of the interstitial volume) may be present, yet the intravascular volume may be dangerously low, even to the point of shock.

Acute major venous thrombosis or a diffuse increase in capillary permeability (as can occur in acute ischemic injury to a limb) can also cause a serious perturbation of the distribution of fluid between the intravascular and interstitial space. These

Decrease in plasma albumin
↓
Decrease in plasma oncotic pressure
↓
Capillary outflux exceeds influx
↓
Intravascular volume decreases, interstitial volume increases
↓
Renal sodium and water retention develops
↓
Intravascular volume is restored toward normal; however, interstitial volume is expanded further and interstitial fluid pressure rises
↓
The rise in interstitial fluid pressure diminishes excessive capillary outflux
↓
Edema develops when a large interstitial fluid volume is needed to raise interstitial pressure enough to prevent the excessive capillary outflux caused by the hypoalbuminemia

FIG. 8-1 Sequence of events leading to edema formation in hypoalbuminemia.

conditions lead to edema formation by exactly the same mechanism as depicted in Figure 8–1. Thus, the patient who acutely develops marked edema below a venous obstruction, or who sustains an extensive ischemic injury to a limb, can also exhibit a contracted intravascular volume in the presence of marked peripheral edema.

Marked edema can also develop in the presence of extensive lymphatic obstruction—for example, following extensive surgical destruction of the lymphatic vessels to a limb. However, in these situations the edema rarely, if ever, accumulates at such a rate that a serious decrease in intravascular volume becomes clinically evident.

Furthermore, once the edema in such patients is established, the intravascular volume and the renal, endocrine, and hemodynamic factors regulating the intravascular volume will return to normal. Thus, if diuretic therapy is used to reduce the lymphedema, it can do so but intravascular volume will be decreased below normal, possibly adversely affecting hemodynamics.

Regulation of Water and Sodium Exchanges with the External Environment

The following discussion focuses on the normal response of the kidney to perturbations of sodium or water balance because an examination of the state of renal sodium and water excretion is often the key to the understanding of the pathogenesis of a disorder of fluid and electrolyte balance and usually provides the basis for planning appropriate fluid and electrolyte therapy.

WATER BALANCE

Water balance equals water intake minus water output. It is sometimes assumed that the measurement of fluid intake and output, as it is performed clinically, is a measure of water balance. However, the difficulty in assessing the state of water balance from the measurement of intake and output is indicated in Table 8–2, which lists all the sources of intake and output of water from the body. It is evident from this table that only a few of the important components of water balance are included in the measurement of intake and output. For this reason, some serious disturbances of water balance may not be reflected in the intake and output record. Fortunately, the accurate measurement of water balance does not require that special techniques be used to measure the various sources of intake and output of water from the body. Instead, in most

clinical situations, changes in water balance can be assessed simply by following changes in body weight.

In the great majority of clinical situations, changes in water balance occur secondarily to changes in sodium balance. For example, in the pathogenesis of fluid retention in congestive heart failure, the primary event is positive sodium balance because of a decreased renal capacity to excrete sodium. The ingested water that is retained is retained as a secondary event to maintain plasma osmolality at some level set by the thirst mechanism. If sodium had not been retained, water would not have been retained. For this reason, the key to preventing fluid retention in such patients is the regulation of sodium intake and output, not water intake.

Less commonly, a change in water balance is the primary event, and changes in sodium balance are secondary to the change in water balance. In order to recognize such situations, it is necessary to understand the normal renal response to primary changes in water balance. Since the capacity of the kidneys to concentrate and dilute the urine is commonly evaluated by measurement of urine specific gravity, it is first necessary to consider the relationship between urine osmolality (U_{osm}) and specific gravity (sp gr).

$$\text{sp gr} = W_s / W_{H_2O}$$

where

W_s = weight of the solution

W_{H_2O} = weight of an equal volume of water.

In normal urine there is, on the average, a linear relationship between urine osmolality and specific gravity, as shown in Figure 8–2. This relationship is disturbed when molecules that have molecular weights much higher than the predominant normal urinary solutes are excreted in large amounts. Thus, in the presence of large numbers of molecules with high molecular weight, specific gravity is no longer a reliable index of osmolality. The normal, predominant urinary solutes are sodium, potassium, and chloride ions, and urea, which have molecular weights of 23, 39, 35, and 60, respectively. The commonly encountered urinary solutes that cause large increases in specific gravity but small increase in urine osmolality are glucose (mol wt 180), mannitol (mol wt 181), dextran (mol wt 20,000–40,000), iodine-containing radiographic contrast materials such as those used for angiography or intravenous pyelography (mol wt 600–800), and protein (but only with heavy proteinuria). If these substances are absent, urine specific gravity can be relied upon to reflect

TABLE 8–2   The Components of Water Balance*

SOURCES	MEASURED CLINICALLY	COMMENTS
	WATER INTAKE	
Oral intake of liquids, intravenous fluids.	Yes	
Water in solid food	Rarely	Water content of solid food in diet of normal adult averages 800–1000 ml/day
Metabolic water	No	The average adult forms about 200–300 ml of water daily by oxidation of carbohydrate and fat to water and CO_2
Water absorbed by way of respiratory tract during use of gases hydrated by ultrasonic nebulizer.	No	Up to 350 ml of water can be absorbed daily at respiratory volumes of 10 liter/min
	WATER OUTPUT	
Sensible losses Urine	Yes	Output variable in health, depends on water intake. Usual range is 600–2500 ml/day. With renal insufficiency and loss of renal concentrating capacity, urine flow rate depends principally on rate of solute excretion.
Sweat	No	In hot environments, several liters of water can be lost daily
Stool	Rarely	A normally formed stool contains 80–100 ml of water. Diarrheal stools are principally water.
Other sensible losses Gastric drainage, transudation from skin, etc.	Variable	
Insensible losses Evaporation from skin	No	Normally 450 ml lost daily. In the average-size adult, with fever, losses increase about 10% per degree F.
Evaporation from lung surfaces	No	Normally 450 ml lost daily. Losses increase by 50% with doubling of ventilatory rate.

* Water balance = Water intake − water output

urine osmolality. If these substances are present, urine osmolality must be measured directly to determine the true extent to which the kidneys have concentrated or diluted the urine.

Normal Renal Response to Water Deprivation

The permeability of the collecting duct to water is markedly increased when ADH is released. Thus, as the tubular fluid enters the collecting duct, water diffuses from the collecting duct into the hypertonic medullary interstitium until osmotic equilibrium is achieved between tubular fluid and medullary interstitium. This results in a marked reduction in urine volume and a marked increase in urine osmolality. In health, the osmolality of the medullary interstitium is 900 mOsm/liter to 1200 mOsm/liter.

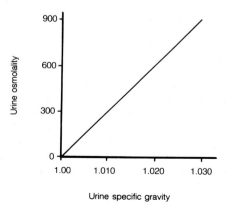

FIG. 8–2   Approximate relationship between specific gravity and osmolality in normal urine.

Thus, in states of maximum water conservation, the urine osmolality approaches 900 mOsm/liter to 1200 mOsm/liter. In such circumstances, urine flow rates approximate 0.5% or less of the normal glomerular filtration rate, resulting in urine flow rates of about 0.3 ml/min, 20 ml/hr, or 500 ml/day.

Normal Renal Response to Water Loading

The administration of water or hypotonic solutions results in a reduction in the osmolality of body fluids. A 2% reduction in plasma osmolality (e.g., P_{osm} 290 → 284 mOsm/liter, serum sodium 140 → 137 mEq/liter) is sufficient to result in a complete suppression of ADH secretion. In an average, healthy adult, the ingestion of 1000 ml of water is more than enough to elicit such a response and the formation of a maximally dilute urine. When ADH secretion is inhibited and renal function is normal, urine osmolality will usually be less than 100 mOsm/liter, urine specific gravity will be less than 1.005 and urine flow rates will approach 15% to 20% of the glomer-

ular filtration rate (i.e., 10–15 ml/min, 600–900 ml/hr).

SODIUM BALANCE

Sodium balance equals sodium intake minus sodium output. The components of sodium balance are shown in Table 8–3. From this table it is evident that the kidneys play the central role in the regulation of sodium balance by adjusting sodium excretion to match sodium intake. Unless there are abnormal losses of sodium through the skin or gut, sodium balance can thus be assessed simply by determining dietary sodium intake and measuring the urinary excretion of sodium. However, these measurements are not usually necessary because if the patient has free access to water and an intact thirst mechanism, water will be ingested and retained in proportion to the level of sodium retention. Thus, changes in sodium balance will be reflected by changes in body weight. Occasionally, the mea-

TABLE 8–3   The Components of Sodium Balance*

SOURCES	COMMENTS
	SODIUM INTAKE
Dietary	Normal adult intake of salt is about 10 g NaCl daily (~170 mEq Na^+ and Cl^- or 4.0 g Na^+). Restricted dietary salt intake usually is 2 g sodium (87 mEq NaCl) daily.
Parenteral	1000 ml normal saline (0.9% saline) = 9 g NaCl = 155 mEq Na^+ + 155 mEq Cl^-
	SODIUM OUTPUT
Urine	Variable. In health, reflects intake since virtually all ingested NaCl is excreted in urine.
Skin	Negligible except with sweating. Sweat contains 50–60 mEq Na^+/liter and several liters of sweat may be lost each day in hot environments.
Gastrointestinal secretion Normally formed stool	$Na^+ \sim 1$ mEq/24 hr
Diarrheal stool Secretory (infectious) Fermentative (malabsorption)	$Na^+ \sim 130$ mEq/liter $Na^+ \sim 50$ mEq/liter
Vomitus or gastric aspirate Normally acid gastric juice Achlorhydria	$Na^+ \sim 40$ mEq/liter $Na^+ \sim 130$ mEq/liter
All other GI secretions (bile, pancreatic juice, small bowel secretions)	$Na^+ \sim 130$ mEq/liter

* Sodium balance = Sodium intake − sodium output

surement of urine sodium excretion may be useful. For example, when body weight and serum sodium concentration are stable and there are no abnormal extrarenal sodium losses, the measurement of the 24-hour urinary excretion of sodium will accurately reflect sodium intake.

Normal Renal Response to Sodium Restriction and Sodium Loading

When sodium intake is abruptly reduced from a normal (*e.g.*, 170 mEq/24 hr) to a very low level (*e.g.*, 10 mEq/24 hr), approximately 3 to 4 days are required until maximum renal sodium conservation occurs. During this period of adjustment, renal sodium output exceeds intake, and water is lost with sodium in isosmotic proportion from the ECF. Usually, 1 to 2 liters of ECF are lost in the change from a normal to a very low sodium intake. Thus, normal individuals come into balance on a low sodium intake, but the ECF volume may then be regulated at a suboptimal level. The potential danger to such a patient lies in the fact that the person is then more vulnerable to the potential hypotensive effects of anesthesia or additional volume losses that may occur during surgery.

The normal renal response to salt loading is analogous to that of salt restriction in that it takes several days for the renal excretion of sodium to increase in response to the higher level of sodium intake. Thus, when balance is finally achieved, ECF volume is being regulated at an expanded level. This can be undesirable. For example, the patient with underlying heart disease who comes into sodium balance on a high sodium chloride intake will be more vulnerable to the development of congestive heart failure if additional fluids are administered.

Clinical Assessment of Disorders of Water and Electrolyte Metabolism

Disorders of ECF electrolyte composition may be detected by measurement of the serum electrolyte concentrations. However, identification of the process (or processes) behind the disturbance of electrolyte composition and the planning of subsequent therapy are critically dependent upon one's being able to assess accurately whether the disturbance in ECF electrolyte composition is associated with volume expansion, volume contraction, or a normal volume.

In the evaluation of a patient's ECF volume status, it must be kept clearly in mind that the critical volume is that portion of the intravascular volume that is effective in determining the filling pressure of the ventricles and, hence, the cardiac output.

Hereafter, this theoretical volume will be referred to as the effective intravascular volume (EIVV).

In light of the above definition, an optimum EIVV is that intravascular volume that maintains an optimum cardiac output and thus optimizes tissue perfusion. Although in many clinical situations the actual intravascular volume and the EIVV are the same and can be expected to change in direct proportion, in a number of important clinical states the actual intravascular volume is different from the EIVV. For example, in acute metabolic acidosis, increased venoconstriction can develop, resulting in an abnormal increase in central venous pressure (CVP) and cardiac output. Under this circumstance, the actual intravascular volume could be less than normal while the EIVV is greater than normal. That is, because of the increase in venous tone, a lower than normal intravascular volume can maintain a normal EIVV.

Acute changes in venous tone induced by drugs (*e.g.*, morphine, furosemide, norepinephrine), changes in acid–base status, or the presence of bacterial endotoxin can also disrupt the normal relationship between the actual intravascular volume and the EIVV.

Currently, the most reliable clinical means for assessing the status of the EIVV is the measurement of the pulmonary capillary wedge pressure. This measurement is an estimate of the pulmonary capillary pressure, which, in turn, is a measure of the filling pressure of the left ventricle. Factors that increase pulmonary capillary wedge pressure tend to increase cardiac output by increasing capillary outflux. When EIVV is considered within these constraints, it becomes clear that, under virtually any physiologic or pathophysiologic circumstance, an optimum EIVV is that intravascular volume which results in a pulmonary capillary wedge pressure that is high enough to promote optimal cardiac output and yet low enough to prevent pulmonary edema.

Fortunately, in the great majority of clinical situations, it is not necessary to resort to measuring pulmonary wedge pressure in order to assess whether a disturbance of ECF composition is associated with an EIVV that is abnormally high, abnormally low, or normal. Instead, an accurate assessment of the EIVV can usually be made by a careful clinical assessment using the criteria listed in Table 8–4. This table lists the bedside and laboratory means to assess volume status according to whether the findings are consistent with an EIVV that is less than normal, or an EIVV that is nearly normal or expanded.

Also shown in Table 8–4 are the conditions under which the given means for evaluating the intra-

TABLE 8-4 *Assessment of Effective Intravascular Volume (EIVV)*

SUGGESTIVE EVIDENCE	QUALIFYING CONDITIONS*
SIGNIFICANTLY DECREASED EIVV	
History of fluid and electrolyte deprivation or loss (*e.g.,* vomiting, diarrhea)	Difficulty in establishing by history whether the magnitude of loss or deprivation is sufficient to result in negative balance of water and electrolytes
Decrease in body weight below normal not explained by inadequate calorie intake.	None
Blood pressure less than usual for patient or orthostatic hypotension	(*a*) Patients receiving methyldopa (Aldomet), guanethidine (Ismelin), or other drugs that interfere with vascular α-receptors; (*b*) peripheral neuropathy as in diabetics, (*c*) prolonged bedrest
Elevated serum creatinine associated with concentrated urine ($U_{osm}/P_{osm} > 1.5$), and Na^+ conservation: ($U_{Na} < 20$ mEq/liter) or $\%E/F_{Na} < 1\%$†	Decreased renal perfusion due to: (*a*) severe hepatic failure (hepatorenal syndrome); (*b*) severe cardiac failure. Acute, high-grade urinary tract obstruction. (See text)
Low central venous pressure (CVP) or pulmonary capillary wedge pressure.	(See text)
Decreased tissue turgor	(See text)
Hematocrit above normal	Presence of conditions that may cause erythrocytosis
Decreased intravascular volume measured by indicator dilution method	(See text)
NEARLY NORMAL OR EXPANDED EIVV (*I.E.,* ABSENCE OF SIGNIFICANT INTRAVASCULAR VOLUME DEPLETION)	
Hypertension with patient in sitting or standing position and no orthostatic fall in blood pressure.	None
Presence of cardiac failure: Left ventricular failure: audible third heart sound (S_3), or pulmonary edema	None
Right ventricular failure: peripheral edema with increased venous pressure (neck vein distention, increased CVP)	Right ventricular failure but normal left ventricular function (See text)
Increase in weight above normal not explained by increased caloric intake	(*a*) Significant hypoalbuminemia; (*b*) development of "third spaces" (*e.g.,* ascites, bowel obstruction)
Increased CVP	(See text)
Increased pulmonary capillary wedge pressure	(See text)

TABLE 8–4 *(Continued)*

SUGGESTIVE EVIDENCE	QUALIFYING CONDITIONS*
Edema, ascites, or pleural effusion	(See text)
Hematocrit less than normal	Presence of conditions that may cause loss, destruction, or decreased production of red blood cells
Normal to increased intravascular volume as assessed by indicator dilution methods	(See text)

* Qualifying conditions are circumstances that may render the meaning of the finding indeterminant with respect to the evaluation of the EIVV.
† %E/F$_{Na}$ = percent excretion of filtered sodium. (See text)

vascular volume must be qualified (*i.e.*, the conditions that may render the meaning of the finding indeterminant with respect to the evaluation of intravascular volume). For example, the relationship between an increase in weight and change in intravascular volume is rendered indeterminant if at the same time the patient has developed a third space, as in bowel obstruction. In this instance, the entire weight gain could be caused by the accumulation of fluid outside the intravascular volume. Thus, the finding of weight gain in this setting cannot be used as evidence of an increase in EIVV.

We suggest that the evaluation of EIVV, using the criteria in Table 8–4, be approached in the following manner: First, whenever a finding can be significantly qualified, it should not be used in arriving at a final decision. Second, as many independent means as practical should be used to assess the EIVV in order to minimize the effect of possible error on the final decision. Obviously, the greater the number of independent, unqualified findings that can be marshalled in favor of a given clinical decision, the more likely it is that the decision is correct. If such a systemic approach to clinical decision-making is used, it should be possible to arrive at an accurate evaluation of volume status in most circumstances.

Data Base for Assessment of the Effective Intravascular Volume (EIVV)

BODY WEIGHT

All patients should be weighed on admission to the hospital and then periodically during their hospital stay. In patients undergoing surgery, or in whom problems in fluid and electrolyte balance are anticipated, weight must be measured daily.

Alterations in body weight are the result of changes in body water content plus solid tissue content (fat, protein, bone). Gains or losses of solid tissue are almost always related to changes in caloric intake and rarely exceed 0.25 kg/24 hr. For example, a patient who takes no calories for 24 hours is forced to consume her endogenous stores of fat and protein to meet the energy requirements for continued life. The complete oxidation of fat yields 9 calories per gram, and protein yields 4 calories per gram. It can be readily calculated that the complete oxidation of 0.25 kg solid tissue (in starvation, a mixture of about 87% fat, 13% protein) will yield enough calories to meet basal daily energy needs. Thus, changes in weight exceeding 0.25 kg/24 hr are almost always attributable to changes in water balance. Although the relationship between body weight and EIVV can be variable, usually the relationship between changes in body weight and intravascular volume can be correctly assessed by the application of the following guidelines: (1) A decrease in body weight below normal (for the patient), and not explainable on the basis of inadequate caloric intake, can be assumed to be accompanied by a decrease in intravascular volume. (2) An increase in body weight above normal not explainable by increased nutrition can be assumed to be accompanied by an increase in intravascular volume except when the weight gain develops in association with the following conditions: (a) Significant hypoalbuminemia: serum albumin less than 2.5 g/100 ml; (b) Venous obstruction; or (c) Development of third spaces (*e.g.*, obstructed or ischemic bowel). Under these three general conditions, an increase in body weight may not reflect an increase in the EIVV.

RENAL FUNCTION

Creatinine is a byproduct of muscle energy metabolism and is produced at a constant rate that is related to muscle mass. Normal males produce 20 mg/kg to 25 mg/kg (ideal body weight) per 24 hours, while females produce 15 mg/kg to 20 mg/kg (ideal body weight) per 24 hours. Nearly all of the creatinine produced is excreted by glomerular filtration. Therefore, changes in the concentration of serum creatinine reflect changes in the glomerular filtration rate (GFR), and the clearance of creatinine (C_{cr}) is an index of the GFR:

$$C_{cr} = U_{cr} V/S_{cr} \sim GFR$$

where

U_{cr} = urinary creatinine concentration;

V = urine volume per unit time; and

S_{cr} = serum creatinine.

Thus, by rearranging the above equation:

$$S_{cr} \sim U_{cr}V/GFR.$$

Normally, as muscle mass (which is proportional to $U_{cr}V$) increases, the glomerular filtration rate increases proportionately less. Therefore, on the average, children have lower serum creatinine values than adults, and large adults have higher serum creatinine levels than small adults. Because of these considerations, a single range of serum creatinine values cannot be applied to everyone. The suggested normal ranges of serum creatinine for adults according to ideal body weight are shown in Table 8–5. Azotemia is arbitrarily defined here as a serum creatinine greater than the upper limit of normal for body size, as shown in Table 8–5. The BUN is influenced by dietary protein intake, tissue metabolism, and urine flow rate, in addition to the glomerular filtration rate, and generally should not be relied upon to assess changes in the glomerular filtration rate.

The following guidelines are suggested for the evaluation of the intravascular volume in light of the state of renal function. The azotemia can be assumed to be due to decreased renal perfusion if the serum creatinine is elevated, and the urine is concentrated ($U_{osm}/P_{osm} > 1.5$; sp gr > 1.015), and

TABLE 8–5 *The Normal Relationship Between Body Size and Serum Creatinine*

IDEAL BODY WEIGHT	EXPECTED RANGE OF SERUM CREATININE*
<55 kg (120 lb)	0.6–1.0 mg/100 ml
55–80 kg (120–175 lb)	0.8–1.2 mg/100 ml
>80 kg (175 lb)	1.0–1.4 mg/100 ml

* Autoanalyzer picric acid method

renal sodium conservation is present ($U_{Na} < 20$ mEq/liter or % $E/F_{Na} < 1.0\%$, where

% E/F_{Na} = percent fractional excretion

of filtered sodium

= (Excreted sodium)

$\times$ 100/(Filtered sodium)

= ($U_{Na} \times S_{cr}$) $\times$ 100/($S_{Na} \times U_{cr}$)

where

U_{Na} = urinary sodium concentration;

S_{cr} = serum creatinine concentration,

S_{Na} = serum sodium concentration;

U_{cr} = urine creatinine concentration.

If severe cardiac failure and severe liver failure (hepatorenal syndrome) can be excluded, the decreased renal perfusion can be assumed to be due to a decreased EIVV.

EDEMA, ASCITES, PLEURAL EFFUSION

Guidelines for interpreting the status of intravascular volume in the presence of edema, ascites, or pleural effusions are as follows: (1) EIVV is increased when edema, pleural effusion, or ascites occur in the setting of congestive heart failure. (2) Increased EIVV cannot be assumed in the presence of edema, ascites, or pleural effusion if there is significant hypoalbuminemia or venous obstruction, or if the accumulation of fluid is in a relatively small area of capillary injury (*e.g.*, pleural effusion due to pulmonary infarction).

TISSUE TURGOR

Tissue turgor is a function of the elasticity of the solid components of tissue and the degree of distention of the tissues by interstitial fluid. If tissue becomes depleted of interstitial fluid, it is less elastic (*i.e.*, it less readily returns to its original shape after being deformed). Skin turgor is best assessed on the forehead and anterior chest. In patients under 50 years of age, the turgor of the dorsum of the hand can also be used. In older patients, the elasticity of the solid components of tissue is decreased, and the turgor of the skin becomes unreliable in interpreting changes in interstitial volume.

CENTRAL VENOUS PRESSURE

The measurement of CVP is a relatively simple but useful means for monitoring cardiac function and the interaction of cardiac function with factors affecting the cardiovascular status, such as intravenous fluid therapy. For the valid measurement of the CVP, the catheter must be placed in the large intrathoracic veins near the right atrium (as assessed by chest x-ray), and the catheter must be patent (as assessed by the cyclic variation of CVP with ventilatory movements: decreased CVP during inspiration, increased CVP during expiration). In the normal adult, CVP is about 5 to 12 cm of water.

A CVP of less than 3 cm of water is commonly seen in children and young adults who have no evidence of a decreased EIVV. However, in older adults and the elderly, a CVP of less than 3 cm of water can be assumed to reflect a significant decrease in EIVV.

The CVP is an index of the filling pressure of the right atrium, which in turn is an index of the filling pressure of the right ventricle. In uncomplicated circumstances, expansion of the intravascular volume results in an increased CVP, while contraction of the intravascular volume results in a decreased CVP. It must be emphasized, however, that the CVP cannot be used to assess the adequacy of left ventricular function in patients in whom left ventricular function may be impaired relative to right ventricular function. In such patients, left ventricular function can be monitored by observing the patient for the signs and symptoms of left ventricular failure (dyspnea, development of an audible third heart sound [S_3], or pulmonary edema), or by direct measurement of pulmonary capillary wedge pressure.

PULMONARY CAPILLARY WEDGE PRESSURE

Technical refinements of the Swan–Ganz catheter make it possible to measure pulmonary wedge pressure and cardiac output with the same catheter. This permits a definitive assessment of the volume status of the patient, since it can be determined whether the cardiac output is appropriate for a given pulmonary wedge pressure. Specific guidelines for the interpretation of the relationship between pulmonary wedge pressure and cardiac output are as follows:

The patient with normal volume status: Pulmonary wedge pressure can be expected to be between 8 and 12 mm Hg in patients with a normal cardiopulmonary system and a normal EIVV volume. Cardiac output will be normal. Occasionally, pulmonary wedge pressure can be less than 8 mm Hg without indicating volume contraction. However, in that circumstance, the cardiac output will be normal despite the unusually low pulmonary wedge pressure.

The patient who is volume contracted: Patients who have a normal cardiopulmonary system but who are significantly volume depleted will usually have a pulmonary wedge pressure of less than 8 mm Hg, and cardiac output will be less than normal. In patients with chronic pulmonary hypertension—for example, those with chronic left ventricular failure, a higher than normal pulmonary wedge pressure is needed to drive in a satisfactory cardiac output. Thus, in such patients, pulmonary wedge pressure can be above the normal range but be inappropriately low for the patient. This situation can be identified by showing that: (1) cardiac output is less than normal, despite the elevated pulmonary wedge pressure; (2) volume infusion causes an increase in cardiac output toward a more favorable range; and (3) despite further increase in pulmonary wedge pressure with volume expansion, pulmonary function does not deteriorate (P_aO_2 does not decrease, P_aCO_2 does not increase, pulmonary compliance does not worsen) indicating that the lungs are adapted to functioning at a higher than normal pulmonary wedge pressure.

The patient who is volume expanded: In patients with a normal cardiopulmonary system, pulmonary wedge pressure is usually above 18 mm Hg when volume expansion is substantial. Cardiac output is above normal. If cardiac function is impaired, cardiac output will be inappropriately low for the level of pulmonary wedge pressure.

When a given pulmonary wedge pressure is being interpreted, the serum albumin level should also be taken into consideration, since it is the serum albumin level that opposes the effect of capillary hydrostatic pressure to cause migration of fluid from the capillary lumen to the interstitial space. Thus, at any given elevated pulmonary wedge pressure, pulmonary edema will develop more rapidly in the patient who is hypoalbuminemic compared to a patient who has a normal serum albumin concentration.

In some patients, it is not possible to obtain a reliable pulmonary wedge pressure. In most of these patients, the pulmonary artery diastolic pressure is a good estimate of the pulmonary wedge pressure. However, if pulmonary hypertension is present, pulmonary vascular resistance is increased; thus, pulmonary artery diastolic pressure may not be a good index of the pulmonary wedge pressure. In such patients, it is important to be able to obtain a wedge pressure. Finally, in patients being ventilated with high levels of positive end-expiratory pressure (PEEP), pulmonary wedge pressure may become an unreliable index of left atrial filling pressure because the high intrapulmonary pressures may cause obstruction of the catheter orifice.

BLOOD PRESSURE

The following guidelines are suggested for the evaluation of the EIVV from measurement of blood pressure: (1) A nearly normal or expanded EIVV can be assumed in patients with hypertension that is demonstrated in the sitting or standing position; (2) EIVV may be decreased in patients who previously were hypertensive, but who now have become normotensive; and (3) EIVV may be decreased in patients who develop orthostatic hypotension (a drop in systolic pressure greater than 10 mm Hg in changing from the supine to sitting or standing position). However, orthostatic hypotension can also be present, in the absence of volume contraction, as a result of prolonged bedrest, during the use of such antihypertensive agents as methyldopa (Aldomet) or guanethidine (Ismelin), or in certain autonomic neuropathies such as those associated with diabetes mellitus.

INDICATOR DILUTION TECHNIQUES

Indicator dilution techniques directly measure intravascular volume, and serial measurements can be made to monitor changes in intravascular volume. Nevertheless, as discussed above, the measurement of the actual intravascular volume does not necessarily solve the problem of the status of the EIVV. For this reason, the measurement of the actual intravascular volume is not generally used in the assessment of volume status.

Clinical Assessment of Disorders of Extracellular Fluid Composition (Sodium and Water)

The schema for the evaluation of the hyponatremic patient has as its point of departure the assessment of volume status. That is, a determination must first be made of whether the patient's hyponatremia is associated with a decreased, a normal, or an increased EIVV. Once this initial separation is made, based on the assessment of intravascular volume, a further separation, based only on the state of renal sodium and water excretion, is made. Each of the final categories contains relatively few diagnostic possibilities and, in most instances, the presence or absence of each of these conditions in a given patient can be readily determined. The schema for the evaluation of the hypernatremic patient is analogous except that it has as its point of departure the assessment of the state of renal water excretion.

CLINICAL ASSESSMENT OF HYPONATREMIA

In the discussion that follows, only patients with "true" hyponatremia will be considered (i.e., hyponatremia in which serum osmolality is decreased in proportion to the reduction in serum sodium concentration, after appropriate correction for any elevation in the plasma urea nitrogen). By making this distinction, hyponatremia due to the abnormal accumulation of extracellular fluid (ECF) solutes such as glucose or mannitol can be excluded. In this type of hyponatremia, the decreased concentration of ECF sodium is the result of the shift of water from cells to the ECF in response to the osmotic gradient caused by the accumulation of the solute. As a consequence, the hyponatremia is associated with an increased plasma osmolality. These patients can also be readily identified by the presence of hyperglycemia sufficient to explain the decrease in serum sodium concentration, or by a history of administration of large amounts of mannitol—for example, in adults, more than 100 g—usually in the presence of a decreased capacity to excrete mannitol (decreased glomerular filtration rate).

We also exclude spurious hyponatremia resulting from the abnormal accumulation of plasma lipids or proteins. In such circumstances, the concentration of sodium in plasma water is normal; however, the concentration of sodium expressed per liter of whole plasma is reduced because an abnormally large volume of whole plasma is occupied by the lipids or proteins, which do not contain plasma water and electrolytes. Thus, when aliquots of hyperlipemic or hyperproteinemic plasma are analyzed, a lesser amount of sodium is determined to be present in a given volume of whole plasma. Plasma osmolality, however, is normal because lipids and proteins do not contribute importantly to plasma osmolality (see Osmotic Forces above). These patients can also be readily identified by the presence of markedly elevated total serum protein levels (e.g., multiple myeloma), or by the presence of grossly lipemic serum.

Hyponatremia and Volume Depletion Associated with Renal Sodium Wasting

The normal renal response to volume depletion and hyponatremia is the virtual elimination of sodium from the urine (see Sodium Balance, above, and Fig. 8–3). Thus, the presence of excessive amounts of urinary sodium under these conditions indicates that renal sodium loss is the cause or a major contributing factor to the state of sodium depletion. A spot urine sodium concentration greater than 40 mEq/liter, a $\%E/F_{Na}$ greater than 1%, or a urinary

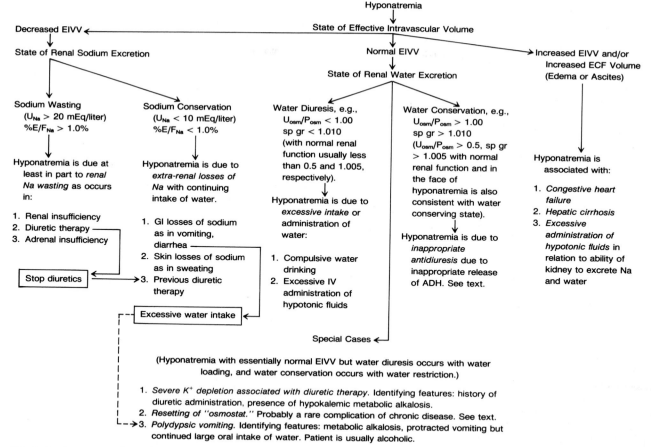

FIG. 8–3 An approach to the assessment of the hyponatremic patient. This approach considers only patients with true hyponatremia (*i.e.*, in nonazotemic patients, serum osmolality is reduced in proportion to the decrease in serum sodium). Thus, patients are excluded who have lowered concentrations of serum sodium because of hyperlipidemia, hyperproteinemia, or the abnormal accumulation of solutes in the ECF, such as glucose or mannitol. %E/F$_{Na}$ = Fractional intake of sodium. See text.

sodium excretion rate greater than intake indicates such renal sodium wasting. The following conditions are associated with hyponatremia, intravascular volume depletion, and renal sodium wasting:

CHRONIC RENAL DISEASE. All types of renal disease can be associated with renal salt wasting. In adults with such a disorder, the serum creatinine is virtually always greater than 2.0 mg, and usually much higher before a significant salt leak develops. These azotemic patients usually require 85 mEq to 170 mEq of sodium daily (5–10 g sodium chloride) to maintain salt balance at a normal EIVV. Thus, if sodium intake is decreased in azotemic patients by anorexia or vomiting, or if additional sodium losses occur (*e.g.*, diarrhea or diuretic therapy), the inability of the diseased kidney to conserve sodium

and water normally may rapidly lead to the development of significant sodium and water deficits. Usually, water intake continues and, thus, sodium balance is more adversely affected than water balance. As a consequence, the patient becomes volume-contracted with hyponatremia. With the onset of congestive heart failure or the nephrotic syndrome, the salt leak of chronic renal failure usually disappears, and salt intake must be restricted.

DIURETIC THERAPY (THIAZIDES, FUROSEMIDE, OR ETHACRYNIC ACID). Diuretics induce a renal salt-wasting state, and, if the urinary output of sodium exceeds intake, sodium depletion ensues. Diuretics may rarely cause hyponatremia without evidence of volume depletion if severe potassium depletion has been a result of their use (see Fig. 8-3).

ADRENAL INSUFFICIENCY (ADDISON'S DISEASE). Destruction of the adrenal gland or sudden withdrawal of chronic, daily glucocorticoid therapy results in inadequate adrenal function. The lack of mineralocorticoid causes renal salt wasting but renal potassium retention and leads to sodium depletion. The lack of glucocorticoid results in a decreased capacity to excrete a water load and leads to hyponatremia, but not to volume depletion or hyperkalemia.

Hyponatremia and Volume Depletion Associated with Renal Sodium Conservation

A spot urine sodium concentration of less than 20 mEq/liter or $\%E/F_{Na}$ less than 1% in a hyponatremic, volume-contracted patient is evidence of normal renal sodium conservation and indicates that the cause of the sodium depletion is nonrenal in origin or that it occurred during prior diuretic therapy. The fact that the serum sodium concentration is lower than normal indicates that water balance is less negative than sodium balance. The following conditions may result in volume depletion and hyponatremia as a result of extrarenal losses of sodium.

GASTROINTESTINAL LOSSES (e.g., vomiting, diarrhea, gastric aspiration). If losses of fluid from the upper gastrointestinal tract cause the hyponatremia and if the gastric juice is normally acid, metabolic alkalosis will be present. If diarrheal losses cause the hyponatremia, metabolic acidosis may be present. In patients with gastric achlorhydria, upper gastrointestinal losses can also lead to metabolic acidosis.

LOSSES OF SODIUM FROM THE SKIN. Sweat contains about 50 mEq/liter of sodium and is a hypotonic fluid. Thus, the effect of sweat losses that are not replaced is the development of hypernatremia. However, in most situations the water losses from the skin are replaced more adequately than the sodium losses. Thus, most patients who develop significant sodium losses from sweating become hyponatremic. Skin losses of fluid and electrolytes can also occur following burns or other skin injuries. These are isotonic losses of sodium and will also lead to hyponatremia if the water losses are more adequately replaced than the sodium losses.

LOSSES OF SODIUM BECAUSE OF PRIOR DIURETIC THERAPY. The natriuretic action of most diuretics is less than 24 hours.

Hyponatremia and Normal Volume Status Associated with Water Diuresis

In a patient with normal renal function who has become hyponatremic from the administration or ingestion of excessive amounts of water, intravascular and ECF volume are normal to slightly expanded, and one can expect to find high rates of urine flow in association with maximally, or nearly maximally, dilute urine (see Water Balance, above). In patients with preexisting renal functional impairment, water loading also results in increases in urine flow rate and dilution of the urine; however, maximally dilute urine cannot be formed. Hyponatremia secondary to water loading may be seen in compulsive water drinkers, who are usually severely neurotic or psychotic, or after excessive intravenous administration of hypotonic fluids.

Hyponatremia and Normal Volume Status Associated with Water Conservation

As discussed above, in a patient with normal renal function who is hyponatremic and has evidence of normal or nearly normal intravascular volume, it is appropriate to observe a brisk water diuresis. When high flow rates of hypotonic urine are not observed, the patient is exhibiting an inappropriate antidiuresis. This may be due to the inappropriate release of antidiuretic hormone, although other mechanisms can also be involved (e.g., decreased renal blood flow, certain drugs). Additional characteristics of such patients are that administered sodium is promptly excreted in the urine because volume contraction is not associated with the hyponatremia. On the other hand, when sodium intake is curtailed, renal sodium conservation is observed. These patients also exhibit normal adrenal and renal function, and are not edematous. The syndrome of inappropriate antidiuresis has been associated with a variety of clinical states, including malignant tumors (e.g., in the lung or pancreas), central nervous system disorders (e.g., head trauma, meningitis), infections (e.g., tuberculosis, bacterial pneumonias), the postoperative state, hypopituitarism, and myxedema, and with such drugs as chlorpropamide. Infusion of oxytocin to induce uterine contraction can also cause hyponatremia because of the antidiuretic effects of oxytocin.

Under the category of hyponatremia associated with normal intravascular volume are three special categories. The feature that sets these apart is that patients in these categories may exhibit evidence of water conservation when water is withdrawn, or an appropriate or nearly appropriate water diuresis when water is administered. That is, it appears that osmoregulation has been reset to "defend" a lowered plasma osmolality. The first special case is an unusual response to diuretic therapy characterized by hyponatremia, severe potassium depletion, and metabolic alkalosis. Despite the hyponatremia and normal intravascular volume, exchangeable sodium is near normal, suggesting intracellular movement of sodium. The second special case is an unusual manifestation of chronic illness, such as pulmonary tuberculosis. The third special case involves patients with sodium depletion from gastrointestinal sodium loss in whom the decrease in EIVV is minimized by excessive water intake and water retention. This effect of excessive water intake can occur in any of the causes of sodium depletion.

Hyponatremia Associated with Increased EIVV or Increased ECF Volume (Edema or Ascites)

CONGESTIVE HEART FAILURE. When hyponatremia develops spontaneously in the course of chronic congestive heart failure (*i.e.*, is not the result of excessive water administration or diuretic therapy), it is usually indicative of severe cardiac insufficiency and a poor prognosis. The cause of the hyponatremia in such patients has been ascribed to a decreased capacity to increase renal free water clearance, perhaps because of increased fractional reabsorption of glomerular filtrate proximal to the renal diluting sites of the distal nephron.

CIRRHOSIS OF THE LIVER. Patients with cirrhosis and ascites have a decreased capacity to excrete a water load, possibly because of the same mechanisms operative in patients with congestive heart failure.

EXCESSIVE ADMINISTRATION OF HYPOTONIC FLUIDS. This is usually an iatrogenic situation and readily recognized.

CLINICAL ASSESSMENT OF HYPERNATREMIA

All patients with hypernatremia (Fig. 8–4) are volume-contracted, except those in whom hypernatremia develops as a result of excessive adminis-

tration of hypertonic saline or in those rare examples of essential hypernatremia. The following discussion considers only the first group of patients; however, the section on treatment (see below) considers both forms of hypernatremia.

Hypernatremia Associated with Formation of Concentrated Urine

The normal renal response to decreased intake of water or increased extrarenal losses of water is the formation of a maximally concentrated urine (see Water Balance, above). In most clinical situations in which hypernatremia is the result of water depletion, the expected renal response is $U_{osm}/P_{osm} > 1.5$, and sp gr > 1.015. Thus, the finding of hypernatremia with evidence of renal conservation of water indicates that the hypernatremia is due to excessive nonrenal losses of water or to solute diuresis.

EXCESSIVE NONRENAL WATER LOSS. Hypernatremia typically develops in patients with accelerated rates of nonrenal water loss because of a hot environment, fever, or hyperventilation in whom water losses are not replaced because the patient cannot perceive or communicate thirst. Despite the hypernatremia, sodium deficits are also usually present because initially, as water deficits develop, renal sodium excretion increases in order to maintain normal plasma osmolality and serum sodium concentration. However, when more than about 15% of ECF volume is lost, renal conservation of sodium occurs and, if the water losses continue, hypernatremia necessarily develops. The presence of volume deficits is indicated by the signs of intravascular

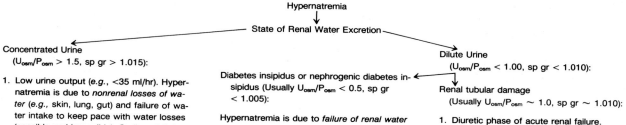

Hypernatremia
↓
State of Renal Water Excretion

Concentrated Urine
($U_{osm}/P_{osm} > 1.5$, sp gr > 1.015):

1. Low urine output (*e.g.*, <35 ml/hr). Hypernatremia is due to *nonrenal losses of water* (*e.g.*, skin, lung, gut) and failure of water intake to keep pace with water losses (sensible and insensible). Sodium deficits are also usually present.

2. Normal urine output (*e.g.*, >35 ml/hr). Hypernatremia is due to *solute diuresis in face of inadequate water intake* (*i.e.*, solute intake requiring renal excretion is high), thereby necessitating a high urine output relative to intake (*e.g.*, high-protein tube feeding mixtures given with inadequate amounts of "free water"). Sodium deficits are also usually present.

Diabetes insipidus or nephrogenic diabetes insipidus (Usually $U_{osm}/P_{osm} < 0.5$, sp gr < 1.005):

Hypernatremia is due to *failure of renal water conservation* because of lack of ADH (diabetes insipidus) or inability of the renal tubule to respond to ADH (nephrogenic diabetes insipidus), and failure of water intake to keep pace with water losses (sensible and insensible).

Dilute Urine
($U_{osm}/P_{osm} < 1.00$, sp gr < 1.010):

Renal tubular damage
(Usually $U_{osm}/P_{osm} \sim 1.0$, sp gr ~ 1.010):

1. Diuretic phase of acute renal failure.
2. Postobstructive diuresis.
3. Severe potassium depletion.
4. Severe hypercalcemia.
5. Chronic renal disease.

Hypernatremia is due at least in part to *failure of normal renal water conservation* and failure of water intake to keep pace with water losses (sensible and insensible). Sodium deficits are also usually present.

FIG. 8–4 An approach to the assessment of the hypernatremic patient. This approach does not consider patients with hypernatremia secondary to excessive administration of hypertonic saline.

volume depletion as previously described. Urine flow rate is usually less than 35 ml/hr.

SOLUTE DIURESIS. The amount of water that must accompany the excretion of a given amount of solute in the urine is determined by the osmolality of the renal medullary interstitial fluid (with which the collection duct fluid must equilibrate), and the plasma level of ADH activity (which determines the permeability of the collecting duct to water and, therefore, the rate at which water will move from the collecting duct to medullary interstitial fluid to achieve osmotic equilibrium). Hypernatremia will result if water intake does not keep pace with renal water losses, because, although renal sodium excretion is also increased in solute diuresis, renal sodium reabsorption is affected proportionately less than water reabsorption. Large amounts of mannitol infused intravenously or high-protein mixtures fed by nasogastric tube (each gram of protein yields 8 mOsm, as urea, phosphate, and potassium) can cause a solute diuresis sufficient to cause hypernatremia if water intake is inadequate. In solute diuresis, urine volume is usually greater than 35 ml/hr.

Hypernatremia Associated with Formation of Dilute Urine

The finding of an isotonic or hypotonic urine in the face of hypernatremia indicates that, at least in part, the hypernatremia is due to failure of normal renal conservation of water. Failure to concentrate the urine under these conditions may be due to lack of ADH (hypothalamic-pituitary diabetes insipidus), inability of ADH to increase collecting duct permeability to water (nephrogenic diabetes insipidus), or impaired renal tubular function that interferes with the development of a hypertonic medullary interstitium (renal tubular damage).

Diabetes insipidus or nephrogenic diabetes insipidus should be suspected immediately in a patient with hypernatremia when the urine is very dilute (*i.e.*, $U_{osm}/P_{osm} < 0.5$, or sp gr < 1.005).

In patients with renal tubular damage, the ability to concentrate and dilute the urine is decreased. As a result, under all conditions, the urine is isotonic or nearly isotonic with plasma. Hypernatremia can supervene when water losses exceed sodium losses and water intake does not keep pace with water losses. Despite the hypernatremia, significant sodium deficits are usually present because renal sodium wasting is also usually a feature of these disorders. The following are examples of clinical situations in which renal tubular damage can be associated with hypernatremia.

THE DIURETIC PHASE OF ACUTE RENAL FAILURE. Occasionally, in a patient recovering from acute renal injury, tubular function is more severely affected than glomerular function. Thus, an inordinately large fraction of the glomerular filtrate escapes reabsorption, resulting in high urine flow rates. The period of inappropriate diuresis can persist for a period lasting from a few days to several weeks.

POSTOBSTRUCTIVE DIURESIS. The sudden release of chronic urinary tract obstruction is often followed by a period of several days or several weeks in which urine flow rates are abnormally high.

Management of Water and Electrolyte Balance

The approach to the management of water and electrolyte balance has two parts. First, a plan must be formulated to correct the patient's existing deficits or excesses of sodium or water. This plan must take into consideration the magnitude of the imbalances, the rate at which correction should be attempted, and the criterion that must be applied to assess the adequacy of correction. Second, a plan must be formulated to provide replacement of normal and abnormal ongoing losses of water and electrolyte. General guidelines are presented in Tables 8–6 and 8–7 and are discussed below.

CORRECTION OF VOLUME DEFICITS

Estimating the Magnitude of Sodium or Water Deficits

If the patient has been weighed daily, the magnitude of the water deficit due to external losses of water can be closely estimated from the decrease in body weight. The coexisting sodium deficits can be estimated by examining the weight deficits in light of the serum sodium concentration. For example, if the patient has acutely lost 3 kg in weight and the serum sodium concentration is within ±10% of normal serum sodium concentration (*i.e.*, 126–154 mEq/liter), little error is incurred by assuming that the patient has lost 3 liters of extracellular fluid (*i.e.*, isotonic saline) and, therefore, replacement therapy should be about 3 liters of 0.9% saline (155 mEq/liter). There is no advantage in using an equivalent amount of Ringer's lactate, since the kidneys will adjust electrolyte excretion to make up for small differences between the composition of the extracellular fluid and the isotonic saline.

In patients in whom sodium and water deficits cannot be documented by changes in body weight, or in whom the losses are from the intravascular volume into internal "third spaces," approximate but very useful guidelines are available to estimate the magnitude of the intravascular volume deficit. These guidelines are as follows. A loss equivalent

TABLE 8-6   *General Guidelines for Planning Fluid and Electrolyte Therapy in Complicated Cases*

VOLUME-CONTRACTED PATIENTS (FROM WATER AND ELECTROLYTE LOSS)

Replace deficits:

Moderate volume contraction (e.g., decreased EIVV causing azotemia but no hypotension). Plan to replace deficits in about 24 hours (e.g., 0.9% saline at 200–250 ml/hr). If patient is hypernatremic, 0.9% and 0.45% saline may be alternated.

Severe volume contraction (e.g., decreased EIVV causing hypotension). Give 0.9% saline as rapidly as practicable until the hypotension is corrected.

Estimate maintenance needs and add this amount to the fluids used to correct the preexisting water and electrolyte deficits.

For patients with normal renal function and no abnormal losses:

MAINTENANCE	EQUIVALENT INTRAVENOUS FLUID ORDERS
Water: 2500–3000 ml/24 hr	Alternate: 5% dextrose in 0.45% saline with
Sodium: 150 mEq/24 hr	5% dextrose in 0.25% saline Each day add:
Potassium: 40 mEq/24 hr	Multivitamins to 1st liter Potassium chloride 20 mEq to 1st and 2nd liter Infuse at 100–125 ml/hr
Nutrition (Short-Term):	At least 400 carbohydrate calories/24 hr

For patients with acute renal failure with no urine output and no abnormal losses:

MAINTENANCE	EQUIVALENT INTRAVENOUS FLUID ORDERS
Water: 600 ml/24 hr	600 ml 20% glucose in water and multivitamins per 24 hrs
Sodium: 0 Potassium: 0 Nutrition:	At least 400 carbohydrate calories/24 hr

See Table 8-7 if patients have abnormal losses of water and electrolytes.

Monitor patient frequently:

Weigh daily.

Measure serum creatinine and electrolytes daily or more frequently if necessary.

Measure CVP or pulmonary wedge pressure in complicated cases. If patient has normal cardipulmonary function, CVP is sufficient. If cardiac disease or pulmonary hypertension is suspected, pulmonary wedge pressure measurement is preferred.

Evaluate water and electrolyte needs daily or more frequently in patients with high rates of abnormal losses.

VOLUME-EXPANDED PATIENTS (INCREASED EIVV)

Correct volume excess:

Mild (e.g., simple edema): Decrease NaCl intake.

Moderate (e.g., mild pulmonary vascular congestion). Induce diuresis with diuretic and allow the sodium and water losses to go unreplaced.

Severe volume excess (e.g., severe pulmonary edema). Steps 1 and 2 and phlebotomy or plasmaphoresis (if the patient is anemic) and digitalis if heart disease is present.

Estimate ongoing losses (as above) and begin replacing when volume excesses have been corrected.

Monitor patient frequently.

TABLE 8-7 *Major Sources, Loss Rates, and Replacement Fluids in Abnormal Water and Electrolyte Loss*

SOURCES	RATE OF LOSS	REPLACEMENT FLUID
Fever	Insensible water losses (normally 450 ml/24 hr from skin and 450 ml/24 hr from lung) increase by about 10% per degree F or 20% per degree C for each degree of temperature above normal	Replace with 5% dextrose in water
Hyperventilation	Doubling alveolar ventilation (*i.e.*, 50% reduction in P_aCO_2) increases insensible water losses from lung by 50%. Thus, the increase in alveolar ventilation required to reduce P_aCO_2 from 40 to 20 mm Hg increases insensible loss from lung from 450 to 675 ml/24 hours.	Replace with 5% dextrose in water
Gastric fluid	Rates of loss from nasogastric suction are usually 1 to 2 liters/24 hr but can be much greater. Normal composition of gastric juice is approximately H^+ 100 mEq/liter; sodium 40 mEq/liter; potassium 10 mEq/liter; and chloride 150 mEq/liter.	Replace with 0.45 normal saline and potassium chloride (usually 20 to 40 mEq/liter) as needed*
Diarrheal fluid	Losses can vary from trivial to several liters daily. In adults, diarrheal fluid usually resembles ECF except that the bicarbonate concentration is higher (about 30–50 mEq/liter) and chloride concentration is lower (about 80 mEq/liter). Potassium concentration is variable (10 to 40 mEq/liter)	Replace with 0.45 normal saline and 50 mEq of sodium bicarbonate/liter and potassium chloride (usually 20 mEq/liter), as needed*
Urine in acute renal failure	Because of tubular injury, urine sodium concentration generally is between 40 and 80 mEq/liter and is largely independent of urine flow rate.	Replace with 0.45 normal saline and potassium chloride, as needed*

* The rate of potassium replacement is usually determined by the serum potassium concentration rather than the rates of potassium loss. For example, even though a patient in acute renal failure may be losing 30 mEq/24 hr potassium in the urine, it may not be necessary to replace this amount since potassium may be entering the ECF at an even faster rate because of catabolism of cellular proteins. On the other hand, the potassium losses in gastric fluid may amount to only 10 to 20 mEq/24 hr, yet far greater amounts of potassium may have to be administered to maintain a normal serum potassium level since gastric aspiration may lead to metabolic alkalosis, causing renal potassium wasting and extensive diffusion of potassium into ICF.

to 15% of ECF volume (about 2–3 liters in the average adult) results in a decrease in tissue turgor, but blood pressure and renal function as judged by serum creatinine are usually normal. Losses of sodium and water in excess of 15% of ECF volume are usually accompanied by decreased tissue turgor, orthostatic or frank hypotension, and significant elevation of serum creatinine.

Correction Rates for Volume Deficits and Criteria for Assessment

Sodium and water losses great enough to result in hypotension represent a medical emergency, and rapid intravenous administration of isotonic saline is indicated until the hypotension is reversed. Thereafter, the rate of intravenous therapy is guided by the adequacy of the intravascular volume as assessed by other criteria, particularly the measurement of blood pressure and pulse in the supine and sitting positions, urine flow rate, and CVP or pulmonary wedge pressure. In patients with less severe degrees of volume depletion, salt and water deficits can often be corrected by increasing oral intake. Salt can be added to food (the salt packets commonly present on hospital trays provide slightly more than 1 g sodium chloride), or plain sodium chloride tablets can be given, with water ad libitum, letting the patient's thirst mechanism dictate water intake. As a guide to the amount of sodium chloride that should be added to the diet to restore the deficits, it should be recalled that 1 liter of ECF contains 140 mEq sodium or about 9 g sodium chloride. The adequacy of replacement therapy can be assessed over the ensuing days by measurement of change in body weight and blood pressure and by the decrease in serum creatinine.

CORRECTION OF VOLUME EXCESS

Expansion of EIVV sufficient to precipitate pulmonary edema is a medical emergency and requires the usual treatment of pulmonary edema, including placing the patient in the sitting position or elevating the head of the bed, as well as the administration of oxygen, digitalis, and diuretics, as needed. If the pulmonary edema does not improve, phlebotomy may be needed to relieve the vascular congestion. If the volume excess is less severe (*e.g.*, simple edema) the problem can usually be controlled by decreasing salt intake or adding a diuretic drug, or both. The effectiveness of treatment can be guided by the decrease in body weight and periodic measurement of serum electrolytes and creatinine.

CORRECTION OF HYPONATREMIA

The approach to the correction of hyponatremia depends upon whether the patient has significant central nervous system symptoms as a result of the hyponatremia (coma or seizures), and the cause of the hyponatremia. If the patient has coma or seizures as a result of hyponatremia, the serum sodium is usually less than 125 mEq/liter, and, usually, the reduction has occurred rapidly, over a few hours to days. In these situations, regardless of the cause of the hyponatremia, serum sodium should be rapidly raised toward normal by the intravenous administration of hypertonic (3%–5%) saline. Sufficient sodium chloride should be given to raise serum sodium by about 10 mEq/liter to 15 mEq/liter. The infusion of hypertonic saline results in diffusion of water from ICF to ECF until isosmotic conditions are restored. This results in reduction of cell volume and an increase of ICF osmolality toward normal, but also in an expansion of ECF volume (see Effect of Addition of Solute on ECF and ICF Volume and Osmolality, above). The expansion of the ECF by the hypertonic saline may precipitate congestive heart failure, particularly if there is underlying heart disease. Therefore, patients receiving hypertonic saline should be carefully observed for signs of volume expansion.

In order to raise serum sodium by 10 mEq/liter, 10 mEq sodium must be given for each liter of body water. Example: It is desired to raise serum sodium from 100 mEq/liter to 110 mEq/liter in a patient weighing 60 kg who is obtunded from hyponatremia. Body water makes up about 50% of body weight. Therefore, body water = 0.5 × 60 kg = 30 liters. Serum sodium is to be raised by 10 mEq/liter, or 10 mEq/liter × 30 liters = 300 mEq. Thus, approximately 600 ml of 3% saline (855 mEq/liter) will be required. Generally this amount of solute can be given safely over 2 to 4 hours. In patients with coma or seizures from hyponatremia who cannot tolerate the infusion of this amount of solute because of underlying heart disease, hyponatremia can be rapidly corrected by inducing a brisk diuresis (5 ml/min–10 ml/min) with an intravenous diuretic, such as furosemide. The urinary losses of sodium, chloride, and potassium are simultaneously replaced with intravenous hypertonic solutions whereas the urinary water losses are not replaced.

Hyponatremia Associated with Volume Depletion

The administration of isotonic saline in amounts sufficient to replace existing sodium deficits will usually result in complete correction of the hyponatremia, as discussed in connection with the treatment of volume depletion, since restoration of EIVV toward normal allows a water diuresis. If specific disease states, such as adrenal insufficiency or diarrhea, are associated with the development of the hyponatremia and volume depletion, these, of course, also require treatment.

Hyponatremia Associated with Normal Intravascular Volume

If the hyponatremia is associated with excessive intake of water, restricting water intake to normal will correct the hyponatremia. If the hyponatremia is due to an inappropriate antidiuresis, water intake must be restricted below normal: for example, to about 800 ml of measured liquid intake daily in an average size adult (see Table 8–2). This will usually result in negative water balance, a fall in body weight, and a rise in serum sodium concentration toward normal. If a specific cause for the inappropriate antidiuresis can be identified, such as oxytocin infusions or chlorpropamide therapy, it should, of course, be eliminated.

Hyponatremia Associated with Expanded Intravascular Volume and Extracellular Fluid

The spontaneous development of hyponatremia in the course of severe congestive heart failure or liver failure is an ominous sign. The hyponatremia does not usually cause any clinical symptoms, and although it can be successfully treated by water restriction, clinical improvement usually does not follow. Furthermore, during such treatment, patients complain bitterly of thirst. Thus, water restriction sufficient to raise serum sodium to normal is not indicated. It does seem prudent, however, to restrict water to prevent the serum sodium from decreasing to less than 120 mEq/liter in an effort to prevent possible central nervous system symptoms of hyponatremia.

CORRECTION OF HYPERNATREMIA

Hypernatremia Secondary to Water Depletion

The amount of water needed to correct the serum sodium toward normal is given in the following example: A patient weighing 60 kg has a serum sodium level of 172 mEq/liter and osmolality of 360 mOsm/kg. Assuming body water to be $0.5 \times$ body weight, and desiring to reduce serum sodium to 155 mEq/liter; the body water of 30 liters (0.5×60 kg) must be increased to 30 liters $\times$ 172/155 = 33.2 liters. Thus, the water deficit is (33.2 − 30) liters = 3.2 liters. Generally, this deficit would be corrected with hypotonic saline given over a period of 24 to 48 hours along with the water and electrolyte needed to maintain day-to-day water and electrolyte balance (see below).

If remediable causes of hypernatremia are present, these, of course, must also be treated.

Hypernatremia Secondary to Excessive Administration of Hypertonic Saline

In this circumstance, which does rarely occur when intra-amniotic infusion of hypertonic saline is used to induce abortion, hypernatremia is due solely to positive sodium chloride balance. Therefore, treatment consists simply in inducing a state of negative sodium chloride balance while maintaining a slightly positive water balance. If the hypernatremia is associated with impairment of central nervous system function (usually Na > 160 mEq/liter), 2 to 3 liters 5% solution of glucose in water should rapidly be given intravenously, together with sufficient furosemide to induce a urine flow rate of about 10 ml/min to 20 ml/min. About 100 mg furosemide intravenously is an appropriate initial dose. This will result in the excretion of urine containing about 140 mEq/liter sodium and chloride and 10 mEq/liter potassium. If, at the same time, only the water and potassium are replaced (e.g., replacement of each 1000 ml urine with 1000 ml 5% solution of glucose in water + 10 mEq to 20 mEq potassium chloride, given intravenously) the patient will be selectively depleted of sodium chloride, and within several hours plasma electrolytes can be restored to normal. During this period of correction, serum and urinary electrolytes must be frequently monitored to assess the adequacy of intravenous replacement therapy, particularly the rate of potassium administration.

Potassium Metabolism

Disorders of potassium metabolism frequently coexist with disorders of sodium and water balance. When, for example, there are gastrointestinal losses of water and electrolytes, sodium and potassium losses often go hand-in-hand. The recognition and management of potassium depletion under these circumstances is discussed above in connection with the management of disorders of sodium and water balance. It is also important, however, to recognize those disorders in which disturbances of potassium balance are the primary abnormality or the major feature of the electrolyte disturbances.

HYPERKALEMIA

Hyperkalemia is defined as a serum potassium greater than 5.0 mEq/liter. Generally, serum potassium levels between 5 and 6 mEq/liter cause little or no functional abnormality, but such levels indicate that an abnormality of potassium regulation is present. This sign should be heeded and its cause investigated, since further small elevations in serum potassium concentration can seriously impair cardiac and skeletal muscle function. At a serum potassium level of 6 or 7 mEq/liter, the ECG begins to show tall, peaked T-waves, and skeletal muscle weakness may be present. At a serum potassium level greater than 7 mEq/liter, severe ECG abnormalities may be present, including complete suppression of atrial activity and an idioventricular rhythm that can then lead to ventricular tachycardia and fibrillation. Profound skeletal muscle weakness leading to respiratory arrest can also develop. If serious hyperkalemia is suspected, an ECG should be obtained immediately along with a blood specimen for potassium measurement. The ECG findings will establish whether life-threatening hyperkalemia is present. Table 8–8 lists the principal clinical conditions associated with hyperkalemia.

Pseudohyperkalemia can result from hemolysis of red cells as a result of the mechanical trauma of venipuncture. Such pseudohyperkalemia can be readily recognized, since both potassium and hemoglobin are released by the damaged cells. If the serum potassium level has been significantly raised by *in vitro* hemolysis, the serum will be visibly pink owing to the presence of free hemoglobin. Patients with extraordinarily high white blood cell counts or platelet counts can also exhibit pseudohyperkalemia from excessive traumatic *in vitro* lysis of these cells.

Pseudohyperkalemia can be avoided by drawing venous blood samples under low pressure into a heparinized syringe.

TABLE 8–8 *Causes of Hyperkalemia*

CAUSE	EFFECT
Excessive intake of potassium	
Transfusion of blood stored for prolonged periods	Shortened life span of stored RBCs after transfusion leads to excessive release of RBC potassium to ECF. Plasma potassium of stored blood is also increased (30 mEq/liter) after 14 days of storage.
Excessive oral or intravenous intake of potassium	Acute ingestion of 500 mEq potassium chloride can cause fatal hyperkalemia with normal renal function. If renal function is impaired, even normal potassium intake can cause severe hyperkalemia.
Excessive release of intracellular stores of potassium	
Chemotherapy of malignancies	The potential for any of these conditions to cause serious hyperkalemia is greatly increased when they coexist with impaired renal function.
Catabolism of hematomas	
Rhabdomyolysis	
Succinyl choline action on muscle	
Sepsis with excessive catabolism of muscle protein	
Acute digitalis poisoning	
Familial hyperkalemic periodic paralysis	
Intravenous hypertonic glucose or mannitol	
Intravenous arginine	
Metabolic acidosis	H^+ displaces K^+ from intracellular sites causing increased diffusion of K^+ into ECF.
Impaired renal capacity to excrete potassium	
Grossly reduced glomerular filtration rate	Almost all of filtered potassium is reabsorbed. Excreted potassium represents almost exclusively potassium secreted by the tubules. Nevertheless, grossly reduced glomerular filtration rate is associated with grossly reduced tubular function and hence the tendency to hyperkalemia.
Impaired tubular function	Occasionally, patients with nearly normal glomerular filtration rate can have substantial impairment of potassium secretion (*e.g.*, the diuretic phase of acute tubular necrosis).
Decreased aldosterone secretion	
Addison's disease	Aldosterone is necessary for normal potassium and H^+ secretion and normal Na^+ absorption in the distal renal tubule
Primary hypoaldosteronism	
Impaired renin production by kidneys causing impaired aldosterone secretion	
Drugs that suppress angiotensin formation (β-blocking agents, *e.g.*, propanolol; prostaglandin synthetase inhibitors, *e.g.*, indomethacin; angiotensin converting enzyme inhibition, *e.g.*, Captopril	Angiotensin II causes aldosterone secretion; β-blockers and nonsteroidal anti-inflammatory agents directly suppress angiotensin formation by suppressing renin production. Captopril prevents angiotensin II formation by blocking conversion of angiotensin I.
Drugs that interfere with renal potassium secretion.	Spironolactone competitively inhibits the action of aldosterone. Triamterene and amiloride block potassium secretion even in the absence of aldosterone.
Ureteral implantation into jejunal loop	Increased reabsorption of potassium from jejunum causes predisposition to hyperkalemia.

Treatment of Hyperkalemia

LIFE-THREATENING HYPERKALEMIA. (ECG shows sine waves or loss of atrial activity and a broad QRS complex. Serum potassium is usually greater than 7.0 mEq/liter).

1. Infuse intravenously one ampule (5 mEq/liter) of calcium chloride or calcium gluconate over 15 minutes with ECG monitoring to observe for reversal of ECG changes toward normal. The infusion can be repeated once. Calcium ion directly antagonizes the effect of potassium on myocardial metabolism.
2. At the same time, begin an intravenous infusion of glucose, insulin, and sodium bicarbonate (e.g., 500 ml 10% dextrose in water plus 15 units of regular insulin plus three ampules [150 mEq] of sodium bicarbonate). Infuse over 1 to 2 hours. This maneuver causes potassium to move intracellularly.
3. As soon as practical, give cation exchange resin (Kayexalate) by mouth, by nasogastric tube, or by retention enema (e.g., 20 g–50 g of Kayexalate). An equal number of grams of sorbitol should be given if the Kayexalate is given into the upper gastrointestinal tract. Sorbitol, a sugar that is poorly absorbed from the intestine, causes an osmotic diarrhea and prevents concretions of Kayexalate from forming within the gut. Kayexalate is an ion-exchange resin in the sodium cycle. It removes potassium from the body by binding potassium and releasing sodium into body fluids.

MODERATE HYPERKALEMIA. (ECG shows only peaked T-waves; potassium is usually less than 7.0 mEq/liter).

1. Reduce potassium intake (normal potassium intake is 60–100 mEq/24 hr). Reducing dietary potassium to 50 mEq/24 hr to 60 mEq/24 hr is usually sufficient to correct mild hyperkalemia.
2. Kayexalate may be needed periodically to control serum potassium.
3. Correct metabolic acidosis if present.

HYPOKALEMIA

Hypokalemia (Table 8–9) is defined as a serum potassium level less than 3.5 mEq/liter. Usually significant symptoms do not result from hypokalemia unless the serum potassium level is less than 3.0 mEq/liter. An important exception is the patient receiving digitalis preparations. In such patients, hypokalemia, or even low normal serum potassium, can increase myocardial irritability and lead to serious arrhythmias. In addition to causing increased myocardial irritability, hypokalemia can also cause profound muscle weakness and ileus. Chronic severe hypokalemia can also cause metabolic alkalosis and decreased capacity to concentrate the urine. The ECG in hypokalemia often shows U-waves, although this finding is not diagnostic of hypokalemia.

Treatment of Hypokalemia

Mild asymptomatic hypokalemia can usually be corrected simply by eliminating the cause of the potassium wasting or by increasing potassium intake. If the hypokalemia is due to diuretic therapy, potassium depletion generally can be avoided by adding spironolactone or triamterene. Potassium supplementation can also be used, but if the patient is on a low sodium chloride intake, the potassium supplement must be given as potassium chloride. The use of the other, more palatable, potassium salts, such as gluconate, citrate, or acetate, and all forms of potassium in food, are much less effective in correcting hypokalemia and are used primarily in patients on a low chloride intake.

Severe or symptomatic hypokalemia usually requires intravenous administration of potassium chloride. In general, the use of intravenous solutions containing greater than 40 mEq/liter potassium should be avoided, since infusing high concentrations of potassium could cause hyperkalemia. In correcting even severe potassium deficits, it is seldom necessary to infuse more than 120 mEq/24 hr to 160 mEq/24 hr potassium chloride. When higher rates are used, it is advisable to monitor the patient's ECG and serum potassium frequently.

Disorders of Acid–Base Metabolism

The major acid–base buffer system of the extracellular fluid is the carbonic acid/bicarbonate system. Thus, it has been traditional to define acid–base disturbances in terms of alterations of this buffer system:

$$[1] \qquad H^+ + CO_3 - \underset{R_2}{\overset{R_1}{\rightleftarrows}} H_2CO_3 \underset{R_4}{\overset{R_3}{\rightleftarrows}} CO_2 + H_2O$$

In the steady state, according to the law of mass action, the H^+ concentration of body fluids is determined by the following relationships:

$$[2] \qquad H^+ = \frac{K \cdot H_2CO_3}{HCO_3^-}$$

H_2CO_3 is not measured clinically. However, $H_2CO_3 = pCO_2$, and pCO_2 can be measured clinically

TABLE 8–9   *Causes of Hypokalemia*

CAUSE	COMMENTS ON PATHOGENESIS
Decreased potassium intake	With 0 mEq potassium intake, stool potassium is about 10 mEq/24 hr, urinary potassium is < 30 mEq/24 hr or is < 20 mEq/liter
Excessive renal losses of potassium	Urinary potassium usually greater than 30 mEq/24 hr or 20 mEq/liter
Diuretic therapy	All diuretics except for spironolactone, triamterene, and amiloride cause renal potassium wasting. Mechanism: Diuretics cause increased sodium delivery to distal tubular sites where sodium is reabsorbed in exchange for potassium or hydrogen ion.
Diuretic phase of acute tubular necrosis and other causes of osmotic diuresis.	Mechanism: Same as above
Metabolic alkalosis	Mechanism: Large amounts of bicarbonate are filtered. Because of the decreased permeability of bicarbonate relative to sodium ion, sodium reabsorption proceeds slightly faster than bicarbonate reabsorption causing the tubular lumen to develop increased electronegativity. In the distal tubule, this favors increased inward migration of potassium and hence, increased renal potassium excretion.
High-dose intravenous carbenicillin therapy	Carbenicillin is a poorly reabsorbed anion. The filtration of large amounts of poorly reabsorbed anion leads to renal potassium wasting for the same reason that increased renal bicarbonate excretion leads to increased renal potassium wasting.
Gentamicin or amphotericin B nephrotoxicity	Renal tubular damage presumably causes increased back flux of potassium into renal tubules.

Increased renal mineralocorticoid effects
  Mineralocorticoid therapy (DOCA, 9 α fluorocortisone)
  Primary aldosteronism
  Secondary aldosteronism (*e.g.*, cirrhosis of the liver, renal artery stenosis, malignant hypertension)
  Cushing's syndrome
  Excessive licorice ingestion
	Increased activity of distal tubular site which reabsorbs sodium in exchange for potassium or H^+

Renal tubular acidosis (RTA)	Mechanism:
	  Distal RTA: Increased renal potassium secretion in exchange for sodium at the distal tubular site because of decreased availability of H^+ for secretion
	  Proximal RTA: Increased bicarbonate excretion leads to increased renal potassium excretion.

Excessive gastrointestinal losses of potassium Vomiting, gastric drainage, diarrhea	Renal potassium excretion also increased (see metabolic alkalosis)
Villous adenoma of rectum	Loss of potassium-rich mucus per rectum
Shift of potassium from the extracellular to the intracellular fluid Correction of metabolic acidosis	H^+ leave cells, K^+ enter cells during correction of metabolic acidosis.
Correction of hyperglycemia	K^+ enter cells with glucose to provide cation to balance anion that forms during metabolism of glucose.
Hypokalemia periodic paralysis	Unexplained familial disorder

TABLE 8-10 *Primary Disorders of Acid-Base Regulation*

ACID-BASE DISTURBANCE	PRIMARY (INITIATING) EVENT	SECONDARY (COMPENSATORY) EVENT	RESULTANT CHANGE IN BLOOD H^+ AND pH
Metabolic acidosis	↓HCO_3^-	↓pCO_2	H^+↑, pH↓
Metabolic alkalosis	↑HCO_3^-	↑pCO_2 (Minimal and only with severe increase in HCO_3^-)	H^+↓, pH↑
Respiratory acidosis			
Acute (24 hours)	↑P_aCO_2	Negligible ↑HCO_3^-	H^+↑, pH↓
Chronic (3–7 days or longer)	↑P_aCO_2	Important ↑HCO_3^-	
Respiratory alkalosis	↓P_aCO_2	↓HCO_3^-	H^+↓, pH↑

(a is the solubility coefficient of carbon dioxide). Thus, Equation 2 can be rewritten as

$$[3] \quad H^+ = \frac{K \cdot a \cdot pCO_2}{HCO_3^-} = \frac{K'pCO_2}{HCO_3^-}$$

This is the Henderson equation. It states that, in the steady state, the H^+ concentration in body fluids is determined by the ratio of the P_aCO_2 (the respiratory component of acid–base regulation) to HCO_3^- (the metabolic component of acid–base regulation). From these considerations, the basic nomenclature of acid–base disorders follows. The Henderson–Hassabalch equation is the logarithmic form of the Henderson equation. In the logarithmic form, the equation is more difficult to analyze. Thus, for the purposes of the present discussion, we prefer to analyze acid–base disturbances in terms of the Henderson equation. Table 8–10 shows the directional changes in acid–base parameters for the primary acid–base disorders. Figure 8–5 shows the expected range of arterial blood pH, P_aCO_2, and bicarbonate concentrations for the primary acid–base disturbances.

THE PRIMARY ACID–BASE DISORDERS

Metabolic Acidosis

Metabolic acidosis begins as a reduction in plasma HCO_3^- and a rise in H^+. In response to these changes, alveolar ventilation is increased, resulting in a decrease in pCO_2 and restoration of H^+ toward normal (see Figure 8–5 for appropriate decrease in pCO_2 for given HCO_3^- reduction in metabolic acidosis). The decrease in plasma HCO_3^- can be the result of the following.

1. An excessive rate of production of nonvolatile acids requiring buffering by HCO_3^- (e.g., diabetic ketoacidosis, lactic acidosis, methanol ingestion).
2. A normal rate of production of nonvolatile acids, but a decreased ability of the kidney to regenerate the HCO_3^- consumed in the buffering reaction (e.g., chronic azotemic renal disease, distal renal tubular acidosis).
3. Excessive losses of HCO_3^- (e.g., gastrointestinal losses from diarrhea, renal losses in proximal renal tubular acidosis).
4. Combinations of the above.

CAUSES OF METABOLIC ACIDOSIS.

Increase in Unmeasured Anions

Mechanism: Increased nonvolatile acid production
    Diabetic ketoacidosis
    Lactic acidosis
    Salicylate poisoning
    Ethylene glycol poisoning
    Paraldehyde poisoning

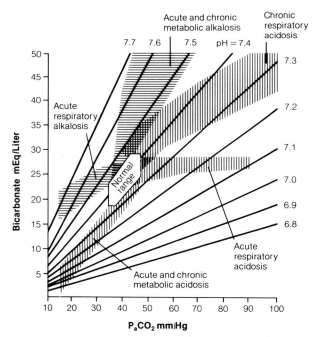

FIG. 8-5 Range of arterial blood pH, P_aO_2, and bicarbonate concentrations in the primary acid–base disturbances. The width of the bands indicates the 95% confidence limits of the range of the variables. (Adapted from Arbus, 1973.)

Mechanism: No increase in nonvolatile acid production
  Renal failure

No Increase in Unmeasured Anions
(Hyperchloremic Metabolic Acidosis)

Mechanism: Excessive HCO_3^- loss
  Diarrhea
  Drainage of pancreatic juice
  Ureterosigmoidostomy
  Proximal renal tubular acidosis
  Carbonic anhydrase inhibiting diuretics
Mechanism: Excessive HCl production
  Ammonium chloride, arginine HCl or lysine HCl
  administration
  Intravenous hyperalimentation solution con-
  taining cationic amino acids
Mechanism: Decreased renal HCO_3^- production
  Distal renal tubular acidosis

Although classification based on rates of acid production and excretion is useful for teaching acid–
base pathophysiology, it is not satisfactory as a diagnostic approach to the individual patient with
metabolic acidosis because there are no readily
available means to measure acid production or excretion. Instead, the diagnostic approach should be
to determine whether the decrease in plasma HCO_3^-
is associated with a normal or an increased concentration of unmeasured anion in the plasma,
which is calculated as follows:

Unmeasured anion

$$= Na\ mEq/liter - (Cl + HCO_3)\ mEq/liter.$$

Normal unmeasured anion concentration is from 8
mEq/liter to 12 mEq/liter. In health, the unmeasured anions are mostly protein anions along with
small quantities of sulfate, phosphate, and organic
acids. In metabolic acidosis associated with increased
unmeasured anions, the increase in unmeasured
anions can be due to accumulation of sulfate and
phosphate (as in renal failure) or nonvolatile organic
acids (such as ketoacids, as in diabetic ketoacidosis).

In patients with metabolic acidosis, increased unmeasured anions, and increased acid production,
the fall in serum bicarbonate is a result of the rise
in unmeasured anion. For example, in lactic acidosis,
each lactic acid anion produced reacts with body
buffers as follows:

$$H\ lactate + NaHCO_3 \rightarrow Na\ lactate + H_2CO_3$$
$$\downarrow$$
$$H_2O + CO_2\uparrow$$

Thus, the rise in blood lactate level is accompanied
by a fall in blood bicarbonate level.

In metabolic acidosis with increased unmeasured
anion and no increase in acid production (renal failure), the fall in bicarbonate is due to inadequate
renal acid excretion (renal bicarbonate production).
The rise in unmeasured anion in renal failure is
due principally to retention of sulfate and phosphate anions because of the reduced renal capacity
to excrete these ions by glomerular filtration.

In hyperchloremic metabolic acidosis, the decrease in serum bicarbonate is accompanied by an
equivalent increase in serum chloride above normal.
In these disorders, the sodium bicarbonate stores
are low and sodium chloride is retained in excessive
amounts in order to preserve the volume status of
the patient. Thus, the body opts to preserve volume
status by retaining sodium as the chloride salt, rather
than excrete the sodium chloride, contract around
the reduced bicarbonate stores, and raise plasma
bicarbonate concentration. Thus, the retention of
sodium chloride in these disorders is another example of the primacy of the maintenance of normal
volume over the maintenance of normal composition of body fluids.

TREATMENT OF METABOLIC ACIDOSIS. Moderate degrees of metabolic acidosis (plasma bicarbonate
greater than 15 mEq/liter to 18 mEq/liter) are usually well tolerated for short periods. However, if
metabolic acidosis is acute and moderately severe
to severe (plasma bicarbonate less than 10 mEq/
liter), dyspnea, depressed cardiac function, and ob-
tundation can result. In such a setting, it is often
necessary to infuse sodium bicarbonate intravenously to correct the acidosis. The effective space
of distribution of bicarbonate is approximately equal
to body water (about 50% of body weight). Thus, for
a 60-kg woman with severe metabolic acidosis in
whom it is desired to acutely raise plasma bicarbonate from 6 mEq to 10 mEq, approximately 120
mEq sodium bicarbonate are required (4 mEq/liter
× 30 liter = 120 mEq). Normally this would be infused over 1 to 2 hours. Bicarbonate could then be
given at a slower rate until the acidosis was corrected. In general, serum bicarbonate should not
be acutely raised to levels greater than 15 mEq/
liter to 18 mEq/liter. Too-rapid correction requires
infusion of large amounts of sodium bicarbonate,
and this may cause overexpansion of the ECF and
congestive heart failure. Finally, rapidly restoring
the plasma bicarbonate to normal may produce alkalosis because of persistence of a low pCO_2. That
is, if plasma bicarbonate is rapidly restored to normal or above in the treatment of metabolic acidosis,
alveolar ventilation will frequently persist at elevated levels for an additional 24 to 48 hours. Thus,

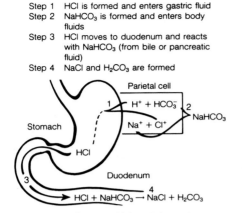

Step 1   HCl is formed and enters gastric fluid
Step 2   NaHCO₃ is formed and enters body
          fluids
Step 3   HCl moves to duodenum and reacts
          with NaHCO₃ (from bile or pancreatic
          fluid)
Step 4   NaCl and H₂CO₃ are formed

Summation: No net effect on acid–base balance since:
One H⁺ and one HCO₃⁻ are formed in Steps 1 and 2.
One H⁺ and one HCO₃⁻ are destroyed in Step 4.

FIG. 8–6 Normal disposal of hydrochloric acid and sodium bicarbonate formed by gastric mucosa.

the low pCO_2 with normal plasma bicarbonate can result in severe alkalosis, which, in turn, can cause cardiac arrhythmias, tetany, and seizures.

Metabolic Alkalosis

CAUSES OF METABOLIC ALKALOSIS.

Mechanism: Chloride depletion (responds to sodium chloride and potassium chloride repletion).
  Vomiting
  Gastric drainage
  Certain diuretics
  Abrupt relief of hypercapnia
  Congenital chloride diarrhea
  Cystic fibrosis
Mechanism: Potassium depletion (responds to potassium chloride and sodium chloride repletion).
  Hyperaldosteronism
  Bartter's syndrome
  Cushing's syndrome
  Licorice ingestion
  Chronic diarrhea
Mechanism: Increased renal acid excretion (responds to removal of offending mechanism).
  "Milk alkali" syndrome
  Hypercalcemia
  High dose carbenecillin or other anionic penicillins
Mechanism: Massive alkali administration
  Massive blood or plasma transfusions
  Massive NaHCO₃ ingestion

A detailed discussion of metabolic alkalosis is beyond the scope of this review. Instead, attention will be focused on the metabolic alkalosis that can follow gastric drainage (gastric alkalosis) because it is, perhaps, the form of metabolic alkalosis most commonly encountered in surgical patients.

Figure 8–6 depicts the normal handling of HCl and NaHCO₃ produced by the gastric mucosa. Note that the initial reactants (NaCl + H₂CO₃, step no. 1) are the same as the final products (NaCl + H₂CO₃, step no. 4). Thus, normally, gastric acid secretion has no net effect on acid–base regulation. However, if the gastric HCl is lost from the body and the chloride loss is not replaced, metabolic alkalosis will ensue as depicted in Figure 8–7.

Severe potassium depletion alone can also cause metabolic alkalosis. Although the mechanism is not clearly established, apparently severe potassium depletion causes intracellular acidosis, which, at the renal tubular cell level, results in increased renal acid excretion (renal bicarbonate production) and an increased renal threshold for bicarbonate so that the high filtered loads of bicarbonate can be retained by the kidney. Hypercalcemia is also said to cause metabolic alkalosis by causing increased renal acid excretion.

TREATMENT OF METABOLIC ALKALOSIS.   Metabolic alkalosis can have serious consequences, such as tetany, major motor seizures, production of hypokalemia and cardiac arrhythmias (particularly in patients receiving digitalis), suppression of alveolar ventilation, and decrease in cerebral blood flow. Furthermore, the presence of metabolic alkalosis is often a sign that the patient is significantly volume-contracted. For these reasons, it is important to treat metabolic alkalosis and its underlying causes. Effective treatment consists in making good sodium, potassium, and chloride deficits as they occur, as discussed above. Rarely is it necessary to treat metabolic alkalosis with intravenous infusion of hydrochloride acid, ammonium chloride, or arginine hydrochloride. This form of treatment is necessary in a patient who cannot undergo the sodium bicarbonate diuresis necessary to correct the metabolic alkalosis. Usually, this inability is the result of severely impaired renal or cardiac function.

Respiratory Acidosis

Respiratory acidosis results from decreased alveolar ventilation. This causes decreased CO_2 excretion by the lungs and an increase in blood P_aCO_2. With acute rises in P_aCO_2, H⁺ rises linearly with increasing P_aCO_2, because there is little change in plasma HCO_3^- concentration. However, after 24 hours of hypercapnia there is a significant increase in renal acid

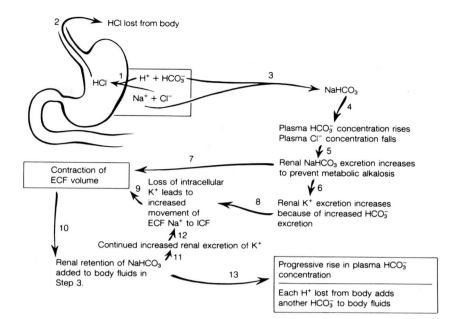

FIG. 8–7 Pathogenesis of metabolic alkalosis from loss of gastric hydrochloric acid.

excretion (bicarbonate production), which results in a rise in plasma HCO_3^- concentration and a fall in plasma H^+. These plasma concentrations usually reach a steady state by 3 to 7 days. (See Figure 8–5 for HCO_3^- elevation appropriate for acute and chronic P_aCO_2 elevations).

CAUSES OF RESPIRATORY ACIDOSIS.

Mechanism: Any condition that decreases alveolar ventilation
 "Bellows" failure (*e.g.*, respiratory muscle paralysis, fractured ribs)
 Obstructive pulmonary disease (*e.g.*, asthma, pulmonary emphysema, foreign body in the trachea)
 Decrease in respiratory center drive (*e.g.*, sedative drugs, particularly narcotics. O_2 therapy in chronic hypercapnia, Pickwickian syndrome)

TREATMENT OF RESPIRATORY ACIDOSIS. The only treatment for respiratory acidosis is to increase alveolar ventilation (by such means as endotracheal tube, mechanical ventilators, or bronchodilators). Within minutes, severe respiratory acidosis can be reversed with adequate ventilation. In patients with chronic respiratory acidosis, posthypercapneic alkalosis will develop if P_aCO_2 is rapidly restored to normal and the patient is unable to initiate and sustain a bicarbonate diuresis. This inability is usually because of sodium chloride or potassium chloride deficits. If sodium chloride or potassium chloride is provided to correct volume contraction and intracellular potassium deficits, a bicarbonate diuresis will ensue and correction of metabolic alkalosis will be achieved.

Respiratory Alkalosis

Respiratory alkalosis results from an increase in alveolar ventilation. This causes an increase in CO_2 excretion along with a fall in blood P_aCO_2. Concomitantly, plasma HCO_3 is reduced primarily as a result of the action of intracellular buffers (see Fig. 8–5 for HCO_3^- concentrations appropriate for acute P_aCO_2 reductions).

CAUSES OF RESPIRATORY ALKALOSIS.

Mechanism: Any condition that increases alveolar ventilation:
 Hyperventilation syndrome—a manifestation of an anxiety reaction
 Hepatic failure
 Fever
 Aspirin intoxication
 Central nervous system disorders (*e.g.*, tumors, cerebrovascular accident, infection, trauma)
 Hypoxemia (heart failure, pulmonary emboli, restrictive lung disease, altitude, severe anemia)
 Iatrogenic (excessive ventilator therapy)

TREATMENT OF RESPIRATORY ALKALOSIS. The symptoms of acute respiratory alkalosis (*e.g.*, paresthesias, light-headedness, tetany) can be rapidly controlled by raising P_aCO_2 to normal (*e.g.*, by rebreathing into a paper bag). Definite treatment consists in removing the cause of hyperventilation. Respiratory alkalosis can also cause tetany and seizures and predispose to cardiac arrhythmias (by causing an intracellular shift of K^+), particularly in patients receiving digitalis.

Bibliography

Arbus GS: An in vivo acid-base nomogram for clinical use. Can Med Assoc J 109:291, 1973

Cohen JJ, Kassirer JP: Acid Base. Little, Brown and Company, 1982

Crexells C, Chatterjee K, Forrester JS, et al: Optimal level of filling pressure in the left side of the heart in acute myocardial infarction. N Engl J Med 289:1263, 1973

Dick DAT: Cell Water. London, Butterworth, 1966

Dudrick SJ, Rhoads JE: Metabolism in surgical patients: Protein, carbohydrate and fat utilization by oral and parenteral routes. In Davis L (ed): Textbook of Surgery, 10th ed. Philadelphia, WB Saunders, 1972

Fleming CR, McGill DB, Hoffman HN III, et al: Subject Review total parenteral nutrition. Mayo Clin Proc 51:187, 1976

Forrester J, Diamond G, McHugh T, Swan HJC: Filling pressures in the right and left sides of the heart in acute myocardial infarction. N Engl J Med 285:190, 1971

Hebert LA, Lemann J, Jr: Operative risks: The clinical evaluation and management of disorders of water and electrolyte balance. Clin Obstet Gynecol 16:195, 1973

Kassirer JP, Berkman PM, Laurenz DR, et al: The critical role of chloride in the correction of hypokalemic alkalosis in man. Am J Med 38:172, 1965

Lennon EJ, Lemann J, Jr: Fluid and Electrolyte Balance. In TeLinde RW, Mattingly RF (eds): Operative Gynecology, 4th ed. Philadelphia, JB Lippincott, 1970

Maxwell MH, Kleeman CR: Clinical Disorders of Fluid and Electrolyte Metabolism, 3rd ed. New York, McGraw-Hill, 1980

Pitts RF: Physiology of the Kidney and Body Fluids, 3rd ed. Chicago, Year Book Medical Publishers, 1974

Schrier RW (ed): Renal and Electrolyte Disorders, 2nd ed. Boston, Little, Brown and Company, 1980

Part Three

Operations for Non-neoplastic Conditions

Chapter 9

Opening and Closing the Abdomen

Opening the Abdomen

In selecting the location and type of an abdominal incision, the pelvic surgeon must consider many important requirements: (1) adequate operative exposure; (2) strength of the healing scar; (3) postoperative comfort of the patient; and (4) simplicity and speed of the procedure. Although many other factors enter into the choice of an abdominal incision, such as cosmetic considerations, abdominal contour, previous scars, and the pelvic pathology, the requirement for adequate exposure of the underlying pelvic organs far exceeds all others in importance. The surgeon must be completely familiar with the anatomy of the anterior abdominal wall before an intelligent decision can be made on a particular type of incision. As Figure 9–1 illustrates, the anatomy of the abdominal wall includes two striated muscles coursing obliquely between the lower margin of the rib cage and the brim of the pelvis. These are the external and internal oblique muscles. Beneath these is the transversalis muscle, which lies directly above the peritoneum. These three muscles fuse in the midline at the linea alba by means of their fascial aponeuroses. The central portion of the abdominal wall receives its major support from the paired rectus abdominis muscles, which extend on either side of the linea alba from the costal margins of the 5th, 6th, 7th, and 8th ribs and insert into the superior pubic rami. A cross-section of the lower abdominal wall shows that the fascia of the abdominal muscles envelop the anterior and posterior surface of the rectus muscles and anchor the external oblique, the internal oblique, and the transversalis muscles with the vertical (rectus) mus-

cles (Fig. 9–2). There is excellent fascial support anteriorly and posteriorly to the rectus muscles above the arcuate (semicircular) line. Here the fascial aponeurosis of the external oblique and the split fascial aponeurosis of the internal oblique fuse together anterior to the rectus muscle and insert in the midline (linea alba). Above the arcuate line, the posterior lamella of the internal oblique aponeurosis fuses with the aponeurosis of the transversalis muscle, passes posterior to the rectus muscle, and inserts in the midline. The lower one-half of the lower abdominal wall is weakened below the arcuate line, at a level approximately horizontal to the anterior superior iliac spine, where the posterior division of the rectus sheath disappears. Here, the divided lamella of the internal oblique muscle combines and passes anterior to the rectus muscle. From this lower portion of the lower abdominal wall to the pubic rami, only the attenuated transversalis fascia and the peritoneum lie adjacent to the posterior surface of the muscle. It is in this weakened section of the lower abdomen that most of the incisional hernias occur following pelvic surgery (see Fig. 9–1). The distribution and course of the nerves and blood vessels of the abdominal wall bear directly on the postoperative healing and function of the abdominal wall. The quality of the tissues, including the abdominal fascia and muscles, the lines of elasticity, and the direction of muscular contractility are factors that influence healing and affect the strength of the resultant scar.

The anterior abdominal wall has an excellent blood supply except at the linea alba. The limited vascularity of this central line of fascial fusion accounts for the higher incidence of impaired healing

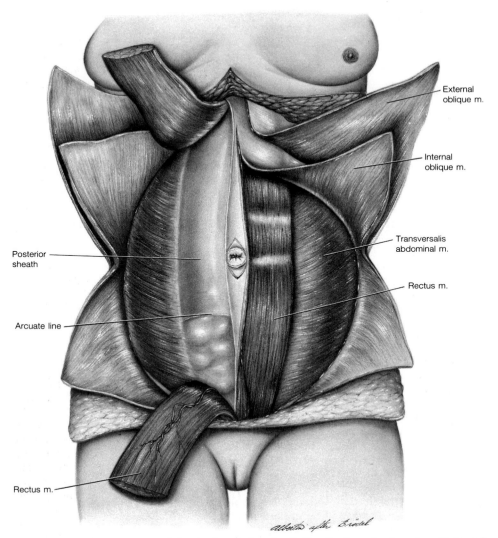

FIG. 9–1 Musculature of the abdominal wall showing (*left*) reflection of external and internal oblique muscles along with anterior division of rectus sheath, which exposes the transversalis and rectus muscles. Note tendinous inscriptions in rectus sheath above the umbilicus. The rectus muscle has been reflected (*right*) to demonstrate the posterior rectus sheath and the abrupt cessation of the posterior lamella of the internal oblique at the linea semicircularis (*arcuate line*). Below the arcuate line the intestines are separated from the abdominal wall by the peritoneum and the attenuated fascia of the transversalis muscle.

from midline incisions and the more frequent occurrence of incisional hernias and evisceration, as compared to transverse abdominal incisions.

The rectus muscles are supplied by two vascular systems: from above, by the superior epigastric artery and vein, which are terminal branches of the internal mammary vessels; from below, by the inferior epigastric artery and vein, which arise from the external iliac vessels beneath Poupart's ligament (Fig. 9–3). This freely anastomosing vascular system provides one continuous arterial and venous channel on either side of the anterior abdominal wall, extending from the subclavian artery and vein, above, to the external iliac vessels, below. The intercostal vessels (T8–12 and L1) also send branches to the external and internal oblique and the transversalis muscles and join the circulation of the rectus muscles to complete the blood supply to the abdominal wall. Bleeding into the rectus abdominis muscle can produce confusing acute abdominal symptoms, as discussed by Cullen and Brödel in a classic description of the anatomy of the rectus muscle and more recently, by Fletcher and Joseph. This entity usually results from trauma to the unprotected portion of the inferior epigastric artery below the arcuate line (linea semicircularis), where the protection of the vessels is limited to the attenuated fascia of the transversalis muscle.

There are three major incisions through which practically all pelvic surgery is done: (1) the midline, (2) the transverse incision, and (3) the gridiron (muscle-splitting) incision.

MIDLINE INCISION

Most abdominal operations on the female reproductive tract are performed through a low midline incision. The incision can be made rapidly and easily and can be extended above the umbilicus when necessary. Consequently, it has the greatest advantage of operative exposure with the least time requirement. The length of the incision is important in the healing process, even though it is frequently stated that "the incision heals from side to side." As measured by Sloan, tension on a midline incision is roughly proportional to the square of the length of the incision; that is, a 30-lb force is necessary to approximate the edges of a 3-inch incision, whereas an 80-lb force is necessary to approximate a 5-inch incision. The skin incision is continued through the fat to the linea alba, using a clean knife other than the one used on the skin (Fig. 9–4A). Bleeders are occluded with Halsted clamps and tied with No. 3-0 plain catgut.

The aponeurosis is incised at the linea alba for the full length of the incision (Fig. 9–4B). The adherent fat is separated from the fascial margins only to the extent necessary to permit adequate exposure of the edges. In parous women there is usually no difficulty in finding the midline because the underlying rectus muscles are usually separated because of previous stretching of the abdominal wall (diastasis recti). In nulliparous women, the midline may not be immediately evident. In such cases, the pyramidalis muscles, which arise from the symphysis pubis, are the most useful landmarks in directing the surgeon to the midline. The medial border of each muscle passes upward and inward and inserts into the lower one-third of the linea alba. Near the umbilicus, the rectus muscles are usually separated and can be divided further by using the handle of the scalpel. At this point, the skin edges of the incision are covered with towels before the peritoneal cavity is entered.

The peritoneal fat is incised, and the peritoneum becomes visible beneath. The urachus, the embry-

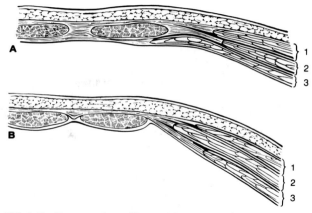

FIG. 9–2 Cross-section of lower abdominal wall. (*A*) The anterior fascial sheath of the rectus muscle from external oblique (*1*) and split aponeurosis of internal oblique muscles (*2*). The posterior sheath is formed by aponeurosis of transversalis muscle (*3*) and split aponeurosis of internal oblique. (*B*) Lower portion of abdominal wall below arcuate line (*linea semicircularis*) with absence of a posterior fascial sheath of the rectus muscle and all of the fascial aponeuroses (*1, 2, 3*) forming the anterior rectus sheath.

ologic remnant of the allantois, is frequently seen as it courses from the dome of the bladder to the umbilicus; it identifies the midline of the lower abdomen. The peritoneum is picked up with mouse-tooth forceps by the operator and the assistant and is carefully incised to avoid accidental laceration of the underlying bowel, which may be adherent beneath the peritoneum (Fig. 9–4C). Pushing the fat away with the knife handle before incising the peritoneum allows good visualization of the underlying bowel and is an excellent surgical precaution. The cut edges of the peritoneum are grasped with Kelly clamps, and the peritoneal incision is enlarged with the knife and scissors while the assistant and the operator elevate the abdominal wall (Fig. 9–4D). Enlargement of the peritoneal incision downward is done under direct vision, with care being exercised to avoid injury to the dome of the bladder.

Special care must be taken in entering the peritoneal cavity, particularly when there has been a previous laparotomy; when the bladder is distended or possibly displaced upward by a tumor; when there is a large tumor such as a uterine leiomyoma or an ovarian tumor pressing tightly against the parietal peritoneum; and when the history and clinical findings suggest the presence of extensive pelvic inflammatory disease. In entering the abdomen through a previous scar, it is advisable to incise the peritoneum at a higher level to avoid

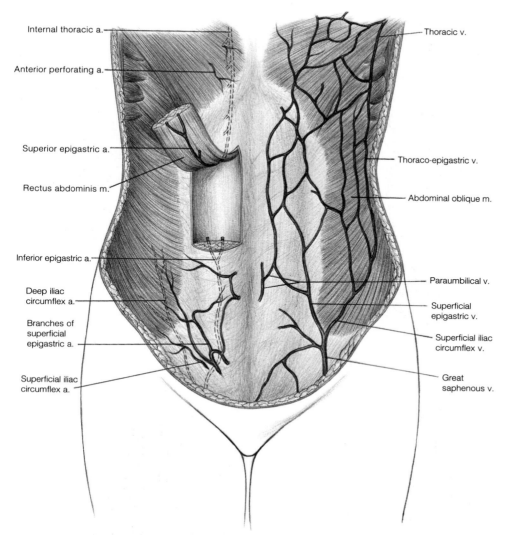

FIG. 9–3 Collateral arterial and venous circulation of abdominal wall. The superior and inferior epigastric arteries provide a rich arcade for the rectus muscles, arising superiorly from the internal thoracic artery and inferiorly from the external iliac artery. The venous system has a similar origin, with the exception that the superficial inferior epigastric vein communicates with the saphenous vein of the leg.

possible injury to an adherent bladder. When a large tumor presses against the parietal peritoneum, it is best to attempt entrance above the tumor by nicking the peritoneum slightly and listening for the rush of air into the peritoneal cavity. Injury to the bladder occurs more frequently at the time of entry into the peritoneal cavity, in the experience of Everett and Mattingly, than at any other time during pelvic surgery. It is therefore important for the gynecologist to observe the thickness of tissues that he is incising. If they appear muscular or vascular, it is well to abandon entrance at that point and attempt an opening at a higher level. Adherent bowel from previous surgery or pelvic inflammatory disease must be identified by gently opening the thin layer of peritoneum if there is no other available site of entry, and removing the adherent bowel from the peritoneum with careful scissor or digital dissection under direct vision.

After the peritoneal cavity has been entered, the abdominal walls are retracted with either self-retaining or wide-bladed retractors. It is advisable to

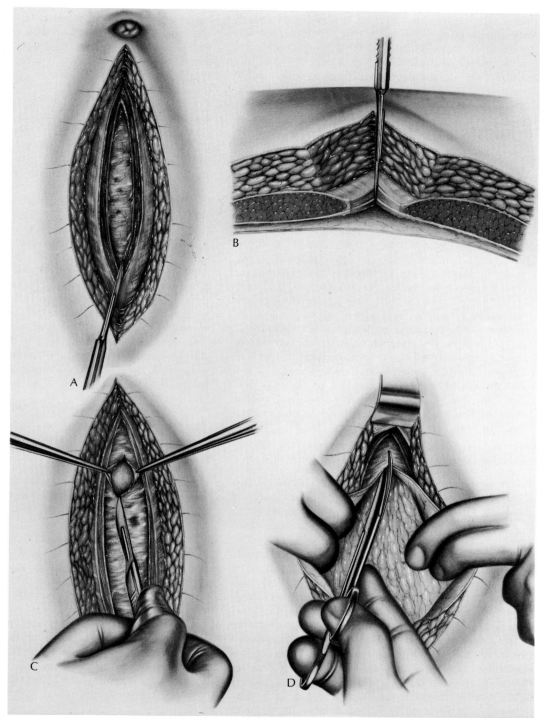

FIG. 9–4 *(A)* Cutting of linea alba in low midline incision with scalpel. *(B)* Cross-section of abdominal wall showing skin, subcutaneous fat, anterior and posterior rectus sheaths, and underlying peritoneum. *(C)* Opening of peritoneum with knife and demonstration of small bowel protruding into peritoneal opening. *(D)* Enlargement of peritoneal opening to the region of the umbilicus with Mayo scissors.

protect the abdominal muscles with moist laparotomy packs placed beneath the retractor blades, particularly in cases in which prolonged surgery is anticipated. Although the Trendelenburg position is helpful in displacing the intestines in the upper abdomen, a steep position is neither necessary nor desirable with the use of modern methods of anesthesia and muscle relaxants. In particular, any patient with limited cardiac reserve should not be subjected to steep Trendelenburg's position, as this may compromise the adequacy of pulmonary ventilation during surgery. The intestines may be gently held in the upper abdomen with two or three moist laparotomy packs; multiple packs may place undue pressure on the bowel. If the bowel does not remain out of the operative field with two laparotomy packs placed carefully over the small intestines and anchored well in the lateral corners of the abdomen, it is probable that the anesthesia is inadequate and that the bowel needs further relaxation. It is well to remember, also, that the average moist laparotomy pack, when formed into a sphere, occupies approximately 240 cc of available intra-abdominal space; consequently, excessive packs will crowd the upper abdomen and restrict movement of the diaphragm. In addition, excessive compression of the small bowel between laparotomy packs will produce temporary damage to the terminal motor nerve endings and may result in postoperative adynamic ileus.

TRANSVERSE INCISION

Three principle types of transverse incisions are used in the lower abdomen for pelvic surgery: (1) the true transverse or muscle-cutting incision; (2) the modified Pfannenstiel; and (3) the true Pfannenstiel incision.

Pfannenstiel is reported to have first recommended a transverse low abdominal incision in 1900, but this surgical approach was initially advocated in 1823 by Baudelocque, a French obstetrician. Although this incision has been championed by a number of surgeons, it has been less popular in the United States than the low midline incision. The critics of this incision emphasize the longer time required for opening and closing the abdomen as well as the increased amount of bleeding caused by dissecting the fat from the rectus fascia, in particular, with the modified Pfannenstiel procedure. In addition, exposure is somewhat less than with a midline incision, with no opportunity for enlargement of the incision should the disease process be found to extend above the pelvic brim. In the event that bowel surgery is contemplated, the transverse

incision may limit access to the upper abdomen and interfere with the location of the colostomy site in the lower abdomen. Consequently, the transverse technique is not advised for large pelvic tumors or when any surgical procedure is contemplated in the upper abdomen.

The advantages cited for the transverse incision include the well-known fact that incisional hernias are infrequent with this method, whereas they are more common following vertical incisions. This is undoubtedly one of the strongest points in favor of the transverse incision, but the incision also has a cosmetic advantage, since the scar is located in the lower abdomen or hidden near the margin of the pubic hairline. The incision is also reported to entail less postoperative discomfort.

As discussed in the chapter on pelvic anatomy, the transverse type of incision is associated with a higher frequency of femoral nerve injury, as emphasized by Hudson and colleagues. This complication occurs more commonly in thin patients in whom the lateral margins of the incision extend close to the lateral abdominal wall and in whom a self-retaining retractor is used. The ilioinguinal and iliohypogastric nerves that innervate the mons pubis and labia may also be damaged by retractor entrapment or excision.

Transverse Muscle-Cutting Incision

The limitation of operative exposure encountered with the Pfannenstiel incision can be improved by using the transverse muscle-cutting incision as advocated by Maylard. By cutting the rectus and abdominal muscles transversely, excellent exposure is obtained for any type of pelvic procedure. The incision, illustrated in Figure 9–5A and B, requires identification and ligation of the inferior epigastric vessels to avoid retraction and hematoma formation in the lateral margins of the incision. Anatomically, this incision produces a strong scar, since the nerves and blood vessels enter the abdominal wall muscles in the same direction as the incision. Consequently, the incision does not cut across nerve endings excessively or devitalize segments of the abdominal wall, unlike the midline or lateral rectus incisions. The peritoneum and attenuated transversalis fascia are incised transversely, as shown in Figure 9–5C. In closing the transverse incision, it is preferable to include the fascia with each muscle stitch since the sutures may pull through muscle tissue alone. No. 1 polyglactin (Vicryl) suture is used for this closure. Major disadvantages of this incision include the time required for incising and reapproximating the abdominal muscles and the potential injury to the ilioinguinal, iliohypogastric, and femoral nerves.

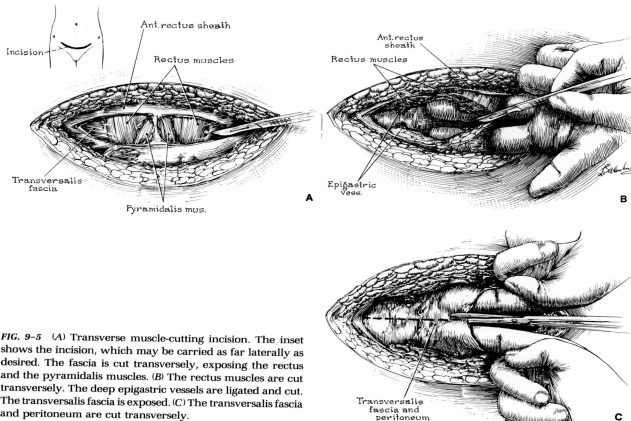

FIG. 9–5 (*A*) Transverse muscle-cutting incision. The inset shows the incision, which may be carried as far laterally as desired. The fascia is cut transversely, exposing the rectus and the pyramidalis muscles. (*B*) The rectus muscles are cut transversely. The deep epigastric vessels are ligated and cut. The transversalis fascia is exposed. (*C*) The transversalis fascia and peritoneum are cut transversely.

Pfannenstiel Incision

The original, true Pfannenstiel incision is described as a transverse incision that is slightly curved (concavity upward) and may be made at any level suitable to the surgeon. It is usually 10 cm to 15 cm in length and extends through the skin and subcutaneous fat to the level of the rectus sheath. The rectus sheath is incised transversely on either side of the linea alba, which is cut separately, joining the two lateral incisions. The rectus sheath is separated from the underlying muscle by inserting the fingers on either side of the cut edge of the sheath and pulling the fascia in opposite directions, with one hand toward the head and the other hand toward the feet. This maneuver will free the sheath from the anterior surface of the rectus muscle as far as desired. The rectus muscles are then separated in the midline and the peritoneum is opened vertically. This procedure avoids the necessity of dissecting the subcutaneous fat away from the anterior rectus sheath, as is done in the modified Pfannenstiel incision. However, it separates the perforating nerves

and small blood vessels that enter the fascia from the underlying muscles and nourish the sheath, which may weaken the incision somewhat.

Modified Pfannenstiel Incision

The modified Pfannenstiel incision is shown in Figure 9–6A, B. The slightly curved transverse incision begins at the level of the anterior superior iliac spine and extends just below the pubic hairline, through subcutaneous fat, down to the aponeurosis of the external oblique muscle and the anterior sheath of the recti. The superficial branches of the inferior epigastric artery and vein may be encountered at the lateral margin of the incision. When encountered, they are ligated. The fascia is cleaned superiorly and inferiorly until a sufficient area is exposed from the region of the umbilicus to the symphysis to permit a vertical incision in the linea alba (Fig. 9–6B). Excessive separation of the fat from the fascia in the lateral margins of the incision is unnecessary and may provide sites for a small postoperative hematoma. Separation of the rectus muscles and entrance into the peritoneum are as in the ordinary

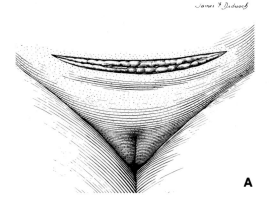

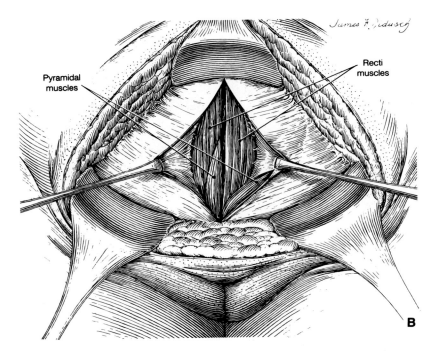

FIG. 9–6 Modified Pfannenstiel incision. (*A*) Skin incision just below hairline. (*B*) Midline incision through fascia, exposing rectus and pyramidalis muscles.

midline incision. Because of the importance of obtaining adequate hemostasis in the subcutaneous fat of the skin flaps, the modified procedure is definitely more time-consuming than the low midline incision or the true Pfannenstiel incision.

GRIDIRON (MUSCLE-SPLITTING) INCISION

The gridiron incision is our choice for an uncomplicated appendectomy and may be used for the extraperitoneal drainage of an abscess from pelvic inflammatory disease. In pelvic inflammatory disease, when drainage becomes necessary for an indolent broad ligament abscess that does not point into the cul-de-sac, drainage through a gridiron in-

cision is most effective. The incision is made as for an appendectomy except that it is made a little lower, and the peritoneal cavity is not entered. Similarly, should drainage of the pelvis be required during a pelvic laparotomy, we prefer to avoid draining the abscess through a midline incision and use a small gridiron (stab wound) incision by placing drains in the pelvis. In treating a large tubo-ovarian abscess that extends out of the pelvis and does not respond to antibiotic therapy, drainage may be required. Abdominal drainage through a muscle-splitting incision is made directly over the abscess. This permits entrance into the center of the site of infection without soiling the peritoneal cavity.

The gridiron incision is made obliquely downward and inward over McBurney's point (Fig. 9–7A). The location may be varied when the incision is done for appendectomy during pregnancy or when it is used for abscess drainage, as mentioned. The incision is carried through the skin and subcutaneous fat to the external oblique muscle. The fibers of the muscle are separated in the direction in which they run (Fig. 9–7B). The internal oblique and the transversus abdominis are separated in the

line of their fibers (Fig. 9–7C). At this point, the internal oblique and the transversus abdominis course in the same direction and are closely fused. Retractors are placed to widen the divided muscle fibers, and the preperitoneal fat is exposed. This is incised and the peritoneal cavity is entered. The cecum lies very close to the peritoneum at this point, and care must be taken to avoid injury to the bowel.

On specific occasions, other lower abdominal in-

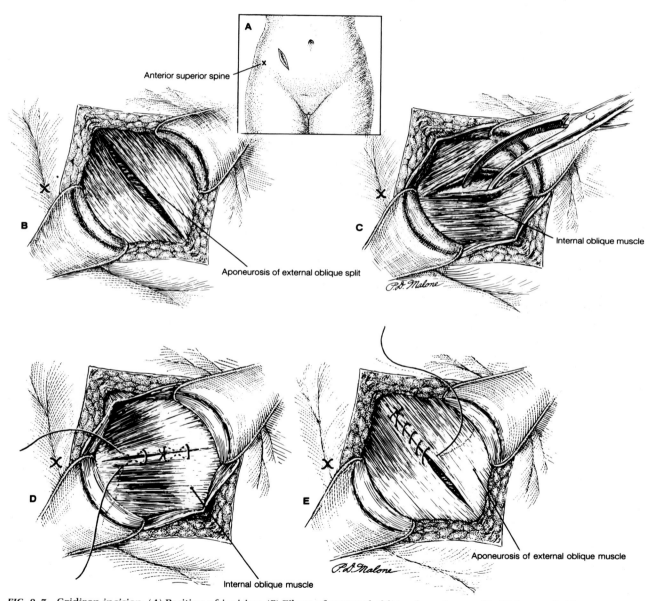

FIG. 9–7 Gridiron incision. (*A*) Position of incision. (*B*) Fibers of external oblique have been split. (*C*) Internal oblique muscle being split with Kelly clamp. (*D*) Gridiron incision closing: internal oblique fibers approximated with figure-of-eight of No. 0 delayed-absorbable sutures. (*E*) Aponeurosis of external oblique is closed with continuous or interrupted No. 0 delayed-absorbable polyglactin sutures.

cisions are used, including the paramedian, the transverse paraumbilical, and the Cherney incisions. Historically, only the Cherney transverse suprapubic incision has been used with any frequency in gynecologic surgery. Although it is one of the strongest of all transverse incisions, excising and replacing the inferior aspect of the rectus muscles from the superior rami of the pubis is time-consuming. Further, the inferior epigastric artery and vein are frequently injured and must be ligated and excised to permit upward reflexion and mobility of the rectus muscles for adequate exposure of the pelvis.

Closing the Abdomen

After completion of the pelvic operation, the sigmoid is placed over the operative field to prevent adhesions of the small intestines. The omentum is drawn down over the viscera, and the peritoneum is closed.

MIDLINE INCISION

In closing the midline incision, the margins of the peritoneum are approximated, beginning at the up-

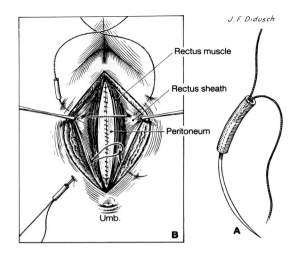

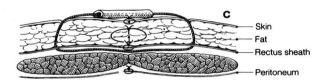

FIG. 9–9 Method of placing tension sutures. (*A*) Long cutting needle threaded with No. 2 nylon or braided silk and shod with rubber tubing. (*B*) Method of placing sutures through skin, fat, and fascia. (*C*) Layer-for-layer closure of the abdomen and position of tension suture through skin and subcutaneous fat, and beneath anterior rectus fascia.

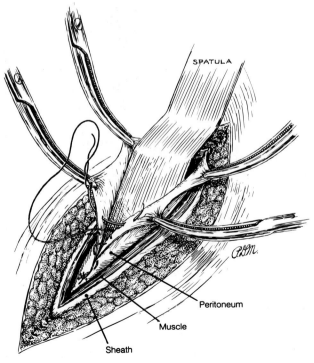

FIG. 9–8 Method of closure of the peritoneum that results in everted peritoneal three-point edges.

per end; both the peritoneum and the posterior rectus sheath are sutured together with a continuous suture of No. 2-0 plain catgut. Nonchromatized catgut is used on the peritoneum because it is more pliable, there is less tissue reaction, and possibly there is less adhesion formation. A three-point stitch is used to evert the cut peritoneal edges and to make the intraperitoneal suture line as smooth as possible (Fig. 9–8). To improve the exposure of the peritoneal edge, the peritoneum is grasped with Kelly clamps that exteriorize the margins for the operator to suture. If the intestines should interfere with the closure, they may be retracted with a malleable spatula or, if great difficulty is experienced, a Mikulicz pad may be inserted over the intestines and withdrawn just before completion of the closure. In high-risk patients, two or three tension sutures of braided silk or No. 2 nylon are placed in the abdominal wall (Fig. 9–9A). These sutures pass through the skin, fat, and anterior rectus sheath; but to prevent bleeding, pain and partial muscle necrosis from a distended abdomen, they avoid the muscles (Fig. 9–9B). In cases where additional support to the abdominal incision is required, such as with secondary closure following evisceration, the rectus muscle is encircled, making certain that the sutures remain outside the peritoneal cavity. Small pieces of fine rubber tubing are placed on each suture to ensure that, when tied, the sutures do not cause pressure necrosis of the skin over the incision (Fig. 9–9C).

It is important to qualify our routine use of tension sutures: we ordinarily tie them loosely enough across the incision to permit two fingers to pass between the suture and the skin. They are used primarily to hold the incision together in the event of abdominal distention. Constricting tension sutures can impair circulation to the incision and produce local ischemia, which may result in poor healing.

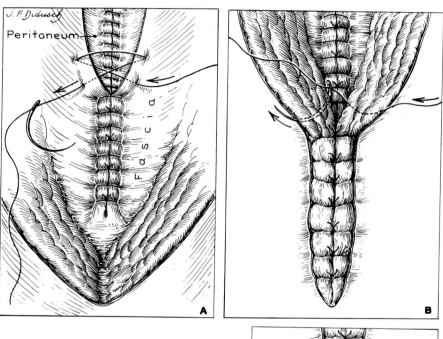

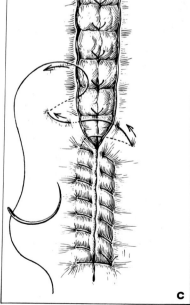

FIG. 9–10 Layer-for-layer closure of abdomen. (*A*) The peritoneum has been closed with a continuous No. 2-0 plain catgut suture. The fascia is being closed with figure-of-eight sutures. (*B*) Fat is approximated with interrupted suture of No. 3-0 catgut. (*C*) Skin is approximated with a continuous on-end mattress suture of No. 3-0 silk.

Healing of the incision is more effective when the skin edges fall together without tension and without undue pressure from deep sutures.

To avoid the problem of skin necrosis beneath the retention suture, some surgeons employ an alternate method of using a retention suture bridge. In this method, a plastic bridge is positioned over the incision, overlapping the place where the retention sutures emerge from the skin on either side of the incision. The ends of the sutures are passed through the appropriate holes and the suture is tied loosely over the bridge. The tied suture is then slipped into the groove in the raised center cap of the bridge; rotation of the cap permits the surgeon to increase or decrease tension on the stay suture in the abdominal wall, following which the cap is depressed and locked into position. Postoperatively, the center cap and retention suture may be loosened or tightened to accommodate the abdominal distention without producing undue pressure on the incision.

The rectus muscles are not sutured together in the midline incision unless there is sufficient diastasis to cause symptoms. In that case, a special closure resembling a ventral hernia repair is used. In the routine closure, the fascial edges are approximated with single, figure-of-eight sutures of No. 1 polyglactin (Vicryl) suture or similar delayed-absorbable suture material. These stitches are shown in Fig. 9–10A. A stronger fascial closure is the Smead–Jones technique, in which a far-near, near-far modification of the horizontal mattress stitch is used. This technique offers the advantage of a wider fascial anchor of the suture and avoids the problem of suture pull-through along the fascial edge (Fig. 9–11).

Experiments on wound healing (Jenkins 1976) demonstrate clear superiority of the placement of musculofascial sutures in the abdominal wall at 1 cm to 2 cm intervals, allowing a generous 2 cm margin of fascia, including the medial border of the underlying muscle, in patients who are high-risk for poor wound healing. The musculofascial margins should not be approximated snugly, as formerly taught, but should be tied loosely enough to permit 2 cm to 3 cm distention of the abdominal wall postoperatively. The analogy is to the technique for bowel closure, in which tight, necrosing sutures in the mucosal margins of a bowel anastomosis are avoided to prevent ischemia and suture pull-through or knot failure. In many cases of incisional hernia or evisceration, the surgeon frequently finds free loops of the tied suture that have cut through the fascia.

After closure of the fascia, the subcutaneous fat is approximated with interrupted sutures of No. 3-0 plain catgut (Fig. 9–10B), and the skin is closed with silk by the preferred stitch of the operator. Figure 9–10C and Figure 9–12A demonstrate skin closure with a continuous on-end mattress suture. This skin suture requires a little more time than the simple continuous suture, but it makes an excellent closure and is particularly useful when one is dealing with the lax skin of a parous woman, since it prevents inversion of skin margins. Figure 9–12B shows a horizontal mattress stitch. We prefer a lock stitch (Fig. 9–12C) when hemostasis is desired and the skin bleeders are too superficial to ligate; these are usually controlled by pressure on the skin margins. Figure 9–12D demonstrates a continuous suture, which is quite satisfactory when the texture of the skin is firm. Figure 9–12E demonstrates a simple interrupted stitch. Interrupted stitches, particularly the vertical mattress, are placed with a straight Keith needle instead of the usual curved skin needle. This interrupted technique makes an ideal skin closure, although it is more time-consuming than the continuous suture. Recently, we have found the use of disposable skin staples to be a more rapid method of skin closure that has less foreign body reaction

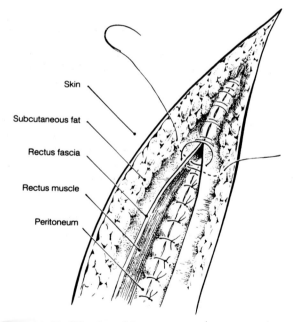

Skin

Subcutaneous fat

Rectus fascia

Rectus muscle

Peritoneum

FIG. 9–11 Modification of far-near, near-far suture (Smead–Jones). Suture passes deeply through lateral side of anterior rectus fascia and adjacent fat, crosses the midline of the incision to pick up the medial edge of the rectus fascia, then catches the near side of the opposite rectus sheath, and finally returns to the far margin of the opposite rectus sheath and subcutaneous fat. (Adapted from Baggish MS, Lee WK: Abdominal wound disruption. Obstet Gynecol 46:533, 1975.)

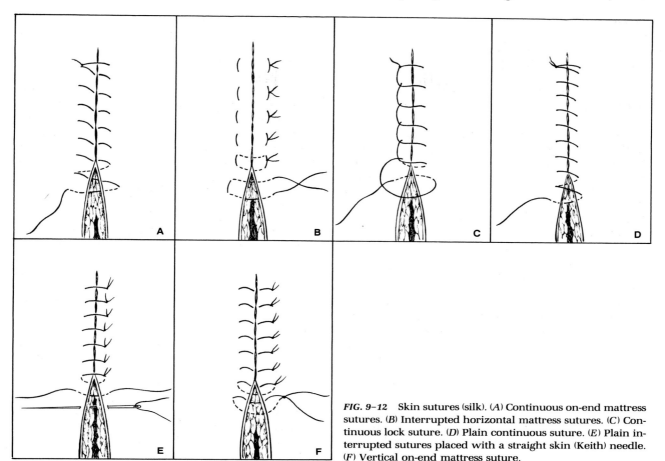

FIG. 9–12 Skin sutures (silk). (*A*) Continuous on-end mattress sutures. (*B*) Interrupted horizontal mattress sutures. (*C*) Continuous lock suture. (*D*) Plain continuous suture. (*E*) Plain interrupted sutures placed with a straight skin (Keith) needle. (*F*) Vertical on-end mattress suture.

and stitch abscess from skin bacteria than various other suture techniques.

TRANSVERSE INCISION

When the true Pfannenstiel incision is being closed, the peritoneum and rectus fascia are closed separately, as in the midline incision, but tension sutures are not used. When the modified Pfannenstiel incision is being closed, special attention must be directed to obliterating the dead space by anchoring the subcutaneous fat to the underlying fascia with sutures of No. 3-0 plain catgut. Additional sutures are used to approximate the opposing margins of subcutaneous fat. The skin margins may be closed with a subcuticular suture of No. 3-0 plain catgut or a removable No. 2-0 monofilament nylon suture.

The transverse muscle-cutting incision is closed by suturing the peritoneum transversely and approximating the abdominal wall muscles with horizontal figure-of-eight sutures that incorporate both fascia and muscle in the stitch. A separate layer of fascia stitches may be placed for reinforcement of the muscle closure even though the incision is anatomically stronger than a midline incision. Contraction of the oblique muscles of the abdomen or strain on the incision tends to draw the muscles and edges of aponeurosis tighter together and strengthen the closure. The edges of the subcutaneous fat are approximated with No. 3-0 catgut, and the skin is closed according to the preference of the surgeon.

GRIDIRON INCISION

The gridiron incision is closed with similar sutures to those used for the midline incision, although there is less strain on the suture line. As is true for the transverse incision, tension on the gridiron incision from contraction of the abdominal muscles draws the edges of the muscle and fascia closer together. The peritoneum is closed with a continuous suture of No. 2-0 plain catgut. The internal oblique and the transversus abdominis are closed as a single layer with figure-of-eight sutures of No. 0 delayed-absorbable suture (see Fig. 9–7D). The margins of the external oblique are closed with interrupted or figure-of-eight sutures (see Fig. 9–7E). The fat and skin are closed as described. We close the skin of this incision with interrupted sutures of fine silk, by which a firm approximation can be obtained.

Complications

The important complications of abdominal wall incisions are characterized by their time of occurrence following surgery. Wound infection and dehiscence or evisceration occur early in the postoperative period. Incisional hernias are late manifestations of impairment of primary wound healing.

WOUND INFECTION

The frequency of postoperative wound infections varies from one clinic to another and is related to many factors, including the experience of the surgeon, the type of procedure performed, the clinic population operated upon, and the surgical condition of the patient. The usual rate of significant wound infections is 5% or less for all major abdominal operations. The incidence is somewhat higher in patients with pelvic inflammatory disease.

One of the most frequent causes of wound infection is the direct implantation of bacteria at the operating table. An inoculum of bacteria may reach the incision from either the skin of the patient or the skin of the operator. A study at Duke University by Moylan and Kennedy demonstrated the importance of gown and drape barriers in the prevention of wound infection. In 2253 consecutive general surgical operations, the use of a disposable gown and drape system in place of a reusable cotton cloth material reduced the incidence of postoperative infection from 6.4% to 2.3%. Earlier work by Beck and Collett demonstrated conclusively that cotton materials, when wet, actually wick bacteria through the fabric and cause contamination of the wound. Of interest in the Duke study was the fact that the disposable gown and drape system resulted in a lowered infection rate in clean as well as in clean-contaminated operations. Further, their study showed that there was no difference in the infection rate between clean and clean-contaminated procedures when prophylactic antibiotics were given preoperatively, intraoperatively, and postoperatively. Operative procedures that exceeded 90 minutes in length had a much higher infection rate than did the less lengthy operations. It is a well-known fact that elderly patients, especially those older than 60 years of age, are more prone to wound infection complications than younger patients. This may be the result of poor nutrition, decreased immune response, or other aging factors. It was also shown in the Duke study and in other investigations that women have a statistically higher wound infection rate than do men. This phenomenon may be related to wound seeding from subclinical infections in the vaginal tract. Cole and Bernard determined that 20% to 40% of all surgical gloves are punctured during the course of an average operation and that such puncture sites could contaminate the wound with 4,000 to 18,000 staphylococci within 20 minutes.

Newer antiseptic scrub techniques have been developed, including povidone-iodine (Betadine), 4% chlorhexidine gluconate (Hibiclens) and the standard 3% hexaclorophene (pHisoHex). A study by Peterson and coworkers evaluating these compounds as surgical scrub preparations showed that of the three, chlorhexidine gluconate in detergent solution produced the best immediate and persistent reduction in normal hand flora. Preoperative baths and scrubbing the patient's abdomen the night before surgery with an antiseptic solution, such as povidone-iodine, has reduced the frequency of postoperative wound infection in many clinics operating primarily on patients from low socioeconomic groups. However, the patient's abdomen should not be shaved until immediately prior to surgery to avoid superficial skin lacerations that would permit bacterial invasion. During most operations, the patient's skin is inadequately isolated from the incision with skin towels or adherent plastic drapes, although the latter are considered to be more effective than loose skin towels. Recent studies suggest that the use of disposable drapes and towels, and adherent skin drapes may contribute to a reduction in wound infections.

Whenever a bacteria-containing organ is opened —mainly the bowel, gallbladder, or urinary tract— there is a marked increase in the infection rate of the abdominal incision. Frequently, small areas of infection occur in low midline incisions, particularly at the lower end of the incision, where the hair follicles may harbor bacteria that are not sterilized by the surgical scrub. As mentioned, these cases are benefited by scrubbing the abdomen for 20 minutes the evening before surgery. The number of wound infections also correlates with the obesity of the patient. An incision through a large panniculus is a favorite place for anaerobic and aerobic bacteria to multiply. The fact that folds in the skin, moistened by perspiration, harbor more bacteria than dry skin is the rationale upon which many surgeons leave the incision exposed postoperatively in a very obese patient. The incision should be thoroughly irrigated with saline prior to closure of the subcutaneous tissues to make certain that a hematoma is not overlooked in the operative site, particularly when the patient is obese. Prophylactic antibiotics and subcutaneous drains are useful in controlling wound infections when infection has been encountered in the pelvis, particularly when a stab wound is required for drainage. However, for the antibiotic to prove effective in reducing incisional infections, that is, for it to result in a therapeutic tissue level at the time of surgery, it must be given at least 2 hours preoperatively.

Coliform bacilli, particularly *Escherichia coli* and *Aerobacter aerogenes*, are the most frequent contaminants of the incision in postoperative patients, along with *Staphylococcus aureus*. In most cases, the wound infection develops to the stage of clinical recognition within 5 to 6 days postoperatively. Usually the temperature remains slightly elevated and the patient may frequently complain of tenderness in the incisional area, although this symptom is not consistently present. In most instances, the wound infection is discovered in a routine search for the cause of a temperature elevation and is noted by the presence of reddening of the skin with fluctuation or induration of the subcutaneous tissues.

The wound should be cultured and bacterial sensitivity studies should be obtained in order to treat the patient with appropriate antibiotics. The wound is cleaned daily with hydrogen peroxide and povidone-iodine solution. Hot compresses are used if there is considerable induration of the adjacent tissue, as moist heat is superior to dry heat in aiding drainage of the infected tissue. The area of the incisional infection should be stimulated to granulate from the base upward by the use of an iodoform wick, urea crystals, and the like. After healing has been initiated, the skin edges may be debrided and drawn together by narrow strips of sterile adhesive tape (Steri-strips) or, if necessary, by secondary closure.

Although a rare complication of gynecologic surgery, the fulminating course of necrotizing fascitis due to hemolytic *Streptococcus* and *Staphylococcus*, as well as a variety of virulent gram-negative bacteria, deserves early diagnosis and vigorous antibiotic treatment. The wound harboring this necrotizing process is excruciatingly painful, initially, and demonstrates dark vesicles, dusky discoloration, and widespread ecchymosis. There is rapid progression of subcutaneous and fascial necrosis, septicemia, and death occurs in 20% to 30% of the pa-

tients. This condition, which has been reviewed recently by Borkowf, must be differentiated from gas gangrene (*Clostridium*) and progressive synergistic bacterial gangrene for proper management.

WOUND DEHISCENCE AND EVISCERATION

In the broadest sense, the term *dehiscence* includes the separation of any of the suture layers of the abdominal wall, although it is usually used synonymously with the terms evisceration, wound disruption, and burst abdomen. In the latter definitions, the disruption includes all layers of the abdominal wall and protrusion of the intestines through the incision.

Reports of the frequency of actual dehiscence and evisceration vary considerably in the surgical literature, between 0.3% and 3% of all cases of pelvic surgery. Pratt reports the occurrence of eight dehiscences in approximately 2500 gynecologic laparotomies (0.3%) at the Mayo Clinic and all eight cases had vertical incisions and extensive operations. Baggish and Lee report a reduction in the incidence of wound disruption from 0.4% to 0.1% as a result of utilizing polyglycolic acid suture material and the far-near, near-far (Smead-Jones) fascial closure. Keill and coworkers reported an incidence of wound dehiscence of 0.68% in cases with transverse incisions compared to 2% in cases with vertical incisions. Mowat and Bonnar observed a decrease in the incidence of wound dehiscence from 2.9% to 0.3% when the transverse incision was used for cesarean section. As noted by Rollins, approximately 50% of patients with a serious wound complication have had prior abdominal or pelvic surgery. Complete disruption and evisceration is one of the most serious of all wound complications. A 10-year study by Helmcamp at the New York Hospital found a mortality rate of 2.9%, or 2 deaths among 70 cases.

Etiologic Factors

The various reported factors associated with wound dehiscence may be summarized in four general categories: (1) the type and location of the incision, (2) the specific type of suture, (3) the inherent strength of the tissues, and (4) mechanical factors.

The importance of the type of incision has been previously discussed. It is well recognized that low midline incisions have a higher rate of wound dehiscence than transverse or gridiron incisions. In addition, the strength of the incision is inversely proportional to its length.

The choice of a permanent or absorbable suture in the closure of an incision has been long debated as a factor in wound healing. Previous reports failed to document a difference between the frequency of wound disruption in cases in which the fascial closure was accomplished by nonabsorbable suture and those in which absorbable catgut was used. However, recent evidence has established that a difference does exist. In a study of more than 1000 major abdominal procedures, Baggish and Lee demonstrated a reduction in the incidence of wound disruption from 0.4% to 0.1% when polyglycolic, delayed-absorbable suture material and the Smead–Jones fascial closure were used. In a similar comparative study, Wallace and colleagues showed a definite benefit to the use of delayed-absorbable suture (polyglactin) in conjunction with the Smead–Jones fascial closure: the incidence of wound separation and disruption was none among 747 cases, compared to 5 among 708 cases when abdominal closure with absorbable suture material was used. In an important study on wound healing, Jenkins showed that when a tightly sewn laparotomy wound becomes elongated by abdominal distention, the sutures come under undue tension, with a significant risk of breakage, pull-through, or knot failure. All of these complications were demonstrated to be preventable by placing stitches every 1 cm apart and with sufficient generosity of suture material that the total suture used equals at least four times the wound length. Of equal importance was the inclusion of a wide (2 cm) margin of fascia and the medial border of the muscle layer in the suture closure. This study and others suggest that the sutures should be approximated loosely in order to permit as much as 30% increase in the length of the incision due to abdominal distention during the postoperative period. Therefore, large, loose sutures are preferable to tight, forceful suture ligatures that cause ischemia of the margins of the incision and that may result in suture pull-through, breakage, or knot failure.

The inherent strength of the tissue has been related to various factors, including vitamin C deficiency, protein deficiency, anemia, wound infection, and the age of the patient. Unquestionably, major surgical wounds have a higher disruption rate in the elderly patient than in the young, a finding that has been observed by many surgeons. In addition, inflammation disrupts collagen deposition in a wound, with separation of tissue by the accumulation of purulent exudate. Such inflammatory response weakens the fascial suture line and produces necrosis of absorbable suture and allows permanent suture to pull through the fascial edge of the incision. Patients with a chronic disease, notably an advanced neoplasm, are known to have poor wound healing due to limitation of collagen deposition and fibroblastic activity. Surgery through a previous operative site is known to produce a weaker scar due to limitation of blood supply and diminished fibroblastic activity. Obesity is a common feature in most reports of wound disruption and is related to the amount of tension on the suture line. Frequency of wound infection is also increased in such patients. The thickness of the subcutaneous fat layer undoubtedly has a direct bearing on wound infection and failure of healing. Pitkin reported the incidence of abdominal wound infection or separation to be increased sevenfold in 300 obese women in comparison to a matched control group of normal weight subjects. Hematoma formation in the incision is a frequent cause of poor healing and produces an excellent nidus for sepsis. It is frequently associated with wound disruption and evisceration and is one of the preventable factors in such complications.

One of the most striking findings in most large series of wound dehiscence is the association of infection and mechanical factors, including pulmonary complications and abdominal distention. In the study by Guiney and associates, 87% of their cases experienced one or more of such complications in contrast to a 15% occurrence in a control group. Excessive vomiting and coughing, abdominal distention, and hiccups have been implicated as causative factors in increasing tension on the suture line. Many surgeons have championed the use of tension (stay) sutures to support the suture line, in such cases, particularly where tension and strain are increased. Although many believe that retention sutures help prevent dehiscence, there are those who either are uncertain about the merits of retention sutures or consider the retention suture merely as a safeguard against evisceration. We prefer to use the stay suture as a method of avoiding expulsion of the bowel through the completely separated abdominal wound should an evisceration occur. By this method, the wound edges are held firmly together but with the stay sutures anchored through the anterior rectus fascia and without producing ischemia to the suture line. When used, the stay sutures should be left in place for 10 to 14 days in high-risk patients.

Diagnosis

Evisceration must be recognized early and treated promptly, since the mortality rate has been reported to be as high as 15% to 20%. It is true that some cases of evisceration occur entirely without symptoms and are discovered on routine inspection of the incision. However, the majority of cases present symptoms and signs that at least call for investigation. Dehiscence usually occurs within the fifth to the eighth postoperative day and is associated with infection in more than half of the cases. The patient is frequently conscious of something "giving way." One of the most common signs, in our experience, is the presence of a watery, serosanguineous drainage from the incision, which should alert the astute clinician to the possibility of an impending evisceration. When such drainage occurs in the presence of discomfort in the region of the incision, disruption should be strongly suspected. When the evisceration is discovered, a sterile towel should be placed over the incision and a tight adhesive bandage applied for temporary control of the protrusion of the bowel through the incisional site.

Treatment

Immediate closure of the disrupted incision is indicated. Because this complication may be life-threatening, delay in secondary closure is not recommended, since the patient's condition will not improve until the incision is reapproximated. Secondary closure after evisceration is best accomplished by through-and-through sutures of an inert material, preferably No. 2 nylon sutures (Fig. 9–13A). Prior to closure, the wound should be cleansed thoroughly at the operating table under general anesthesia, and gentle debridement should be accomplished where needed. The intestines should be manipulated as little as possible when being replaced in the peritoneal cavity. The wound is cultured for aerobic and anaerobic bacteria, and antibiotic sensitivities are obtained. The sutures are placed through the entire thickness of the abdominal wall, including the peritoneum, as demonstrated in Figure 9–13B. Current statistics show that

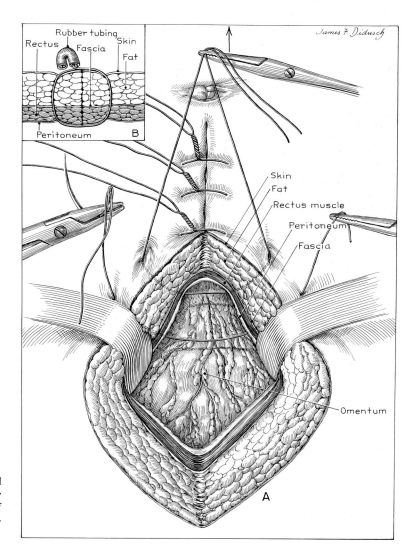

FIG. 9–13 Secondary closure of disrupted wound with through-and-through silver-wire or preferably, No. 2 nylon sutures. (*A*) Method of closure. (*B*) Suture twisted tight and approximating the wound edges.

the incidence of secondary incisional hernia is decreased by closure of the fascial margins, loosely, with interrupted sutures of a delayed-absorbable suture material that include a wide margin of fascia and the inner border of the abdominal musculature. In recent years, we have found through-and-through nylon sutures to be as effective and inert as silver wire sutures but less discomforting and traumatic to the wound. After being inserted, the sutures are held with clamps but are not tied before all are placed. This procedure pulls the abdominal wall away from the viscera and guards against injury to the bowel. The stay sutures are placed about 2 cm apart. When the sutures are closed by tying, the skin and abdominal muscles are well approximated, but if more careful approximation is desirable, interrupted black silk or delayed-absorbable sutures may be placed between the stay sutures.

A broad-spectrum antibiotic is initiated and modified according to the bacteriology and antibiotic sensitivity. Postoperatively, the patient is treated with a nasogastric tube for decompression of the bowel, and intravenous fluid replacement is maintained until bowel function returns to normal and oral feedings are well tolerated. The sutures are left in place until healing appears to be complete, which usually requires approximately 14 to 21 days. We frequently discharge the patient to her home and remove the sutures sometime later when healing is complete.

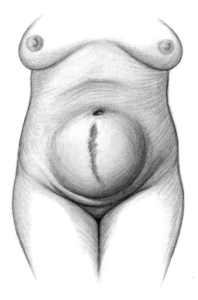

FIG. 9–14 Ventral hernia in a low midline incision.

INCISIONAL HERNIA

An incisional hernia is caused by incomplete healing of the operative wound in which the peritoneum remains intact while the fascial margins and adjacent muscles separate, leaving a defect beneath the subcutaneous fat into which the bowel may herniate. Most cases of ventral hernia follow an incisional infection with impairment of both fibroblastic activity and the synthesis of collagen during the active phase of wound healing. Increased intra-abdominal pressure from coughing and vomiting, along with necrosis of the fascial margins, permits the sutures to pull through the edge of the fascia. These changes result in separation of the wound edges and failure of fibroblastic bridging of the fascia. This complication occurs more frequently in the lower abdominal incision because of the anatomical deficit of a posterior fascial sheath beneath the rectus in the area inferior to the semicircular line. Ventral hernias occur following low midline incisions in approximately 0.5% to 1% of all gynecologic surgery; the incidence increases to approximately 10% after a wound infection, while after dehiscence and reclosure, the chance of hernia formation increases to 25%.

The etiologic factors related to poor healing and hernia formation are similar to those for wound dehiscence. Instead of complete dehiscence and evisceration of the wound, hernia formation results from incomplete dehiscence in which the peritoneum, subcutaneous fat and skin remain intact.

Although the initial fascial defect may be small, the size of the resultant hernia may assume varying proportions and may occasionally involve the entire length of the lower abdominal wall. The size of the hernia depends on the mobility of the bowel and omentum and the final aperature in the ventral defect. A large amount of small bowel and omentum can escape from a very small fascial defect into an easily expandable subcutaneous space. The smaller the fascial defect through which small bowel has herniated, the greater the frequency of incarceration and infarction.

Diagnosis

The diagnosis of a ventral hernia is not difficult in view of the fact that the abdominal wall is always distended in such cases (Fig. 9–14) and the patient complains of lower abdominal discomfort. Occasionally, the patient will observe peristalsis of the bowel beneath the skin and will note the regression of the mass while in the recumbent position with recurrence of the abdominal distention while erect.

The hernia is more noticeable on coughing and straining and may increase in size with time because of either enlargement of the hernial ring or incorporation of additional segments of bowel in the hernial sac. It is rare that a ventral hernia will produce acute symptoms of visceral torsion and infarction, and, therefore, the repair of the hernia is usually on an elective basis.

Treatment

The principles of ventral hernia repair include: (1) dissection of the hernial sac from the subcutaneous fat, rectus fascia, and peritoneal margin; (2) excision of the redundant hernial (peritoneal) sac; and (3) closure of the abdominal wound, using a layer-for-layer closure, an overlap repair of the rectus fascia, or the placement of a synthetic mesh prosthesis (Marlex).

The low midline incisional scar is excised and the underlying subcutaneous fat is mobilized free from the adjacent hernial sac. Sharp dissection is used to separate the skin and underlying fat widely from the margins of the hernial sac (Fig. 9–15A). It is important to defer opening the sac until the boundaries of the hernia have been delineated and dissected, as this aids in identifying the various tissue planes. To identify the margins of the fascial ring, it is advisable to open the sac and separate any underlying bowel from the peritoneal surface of the sac (Fig. 9–15B). Frequently, loops of small bowel and adherent omentum obscure the true identity of the sac, and many pockets of the peritoneal lining are formed by fibrous bands that anchor the bowel to the peritoneum. After releasing the omentum and bowel, with particular attention given to hemostasis, it is important to determine if the hernial defect can be adequately closed with the adjacent fascia prior to excising the lining of the sac. If there is adequate fascial tissue remaining following the dissection, either a layer-for-layer or an "overlap" fascial closure should be done. If there is inadequate fascia available to close, the defect must be bridged with a polyethylene mesh (Marlex) prosthesis. Most incisional hernias, however, can be closed without the use of a mesh support. When there has been failure of an initial hernial repair, when the hernial defect is so large that the edges cannot be approximated adequately, or when the tissues of the abdominal wall are quite attenuated, the use of a mesh prosthesis is strongly advisable.

The layer-for-layer closure is accomplished after closure of the peritoneum as the initial layer. The fascial margins of the anterior rectus sheath are then sutured with either a nonabsorbable No. 0 silk suture or a delayed-absorbable suture of poly-glactin material (Fig. 9–15C). Interrupted far-near, near-far pulley sutures (modified Smead–Jones) that include the inner margin of the abdominal musculature are placed in order to avoid subsequent pull-through of the suture from the edge of the incision. These sutures serve as internal stay sutures and increase the tensile strength of the wound while healing occurs.

If there is adequate fascial margin of good strength, a "vest-over-pants" closure will give extra support to the defect and will produce a double-layer closure of the fascia (Fig. 9–15D). It is necessary to separate the peritoneum and posterior rectus sheath from the hernial margins to permit an overlap of the anterior fascia. The peritoneum is closed separately with a continuous suture of No. 2-0 plain or chromic catgut. The anterior rectus sheath of the hernial margins is separated widely on each side of the wound. Horizontal mattress sutures of a delayed-absorbable or permanent suture material are placed 3 cm to 4 cm distant from the fascial edge and pass through only the free margin of the opposite fascia before returning to the distal portion of the anterior fascia (Fig. 9–15D). The sutures are held untied until all have been placed. When the sutures are tied, the free fascial margin is drawn firmly beneath the opposite fascial layer, producing a double support to the hernial closure. The remaining free fascial margin is sutured to the fascial surface (Fig. 9–15E) to complete the double layer closure.

When closure of the fascial margins is complete, perforated drainage tubes are inserted beneath the skin flaps and sutured to the anterior rectus fascia with fine catgut for subsequent drainage. Although Penrose drains provide a satisfactory method for wound drainage, perforated plastic tubes or rubber catheters give a better conduit for removal of serum by negative suction pressure in a potentially infected site.

LARGE HERNIAS

In repairing a ventral hernia with a large fascial defect and poor abdominal tissue, it may be necessary to reinforce the hernial defect with a polyethylene prosthetic mesh (Marlex). In using a Marlex mesh, it is important to dissect the hernial sac as previously described and to carefully define the layers of the abdominal wall (Fig. 9–16A). Because of the placement of a foreign body in the abdominal incision, meticulous hemostasis is essential. The implanted mesh must completely bridge the entire defect with adequate margins for suturing to the adjacent rectus muscles.

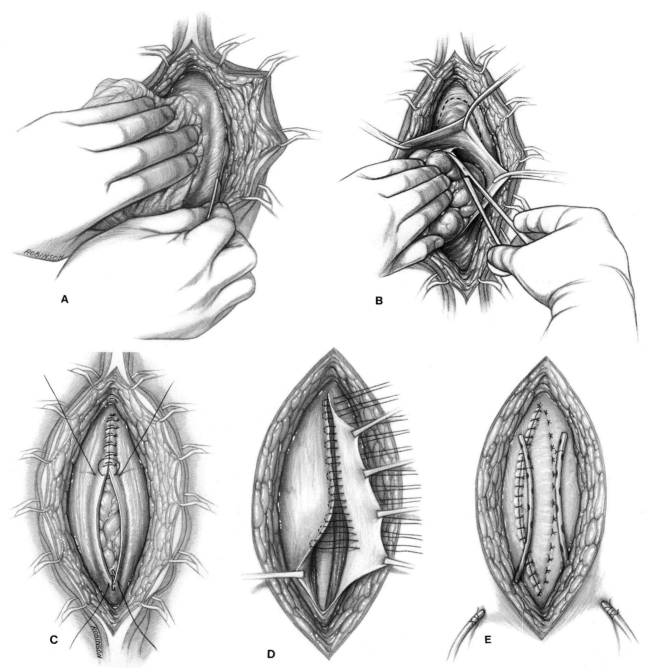

FIG. 9–15 Repair of ventral hernia. (*A*) Wide dissection of subcutaneous fat from lateral boundaries of ventral hernia. (*B*) Hernial sac opened and adherent bowel and omentum released from the peritoneal surface. Note the superior margin of the fascial defect (*dotted line*). (*C*) Layer-for-layer closure of midline ventral hernia. Redundant hernial sac has been excised and fascial margins are sutured by far-near, near-far technique. Crown stitch is demonstrated at lower pole, showing anchoring of apex of defect to lateral fascial margins. When possible, the peritoneum is closed as a separate layer. (*D*) Vest-over-pants technique of midline hernia repair. The peritoneum is separated from hernia and closed. Anterior rectus fascia dissected widely; horizontal mattress sutures are placed distant from fascial edge and passed through the opposite fascial margin. When the sutures are tied, fascial margins are drawn firmly beneath opposite layer, producing a double fascial layer closure of hernia. (*E*) Completion of pants-over-vest closure of midline ventral hernia showing suture of free margin of the fascial flap to the underlying fascial surface. Perforated plastic drainage tubes are sutured to the fascia to permit adequate drainage.

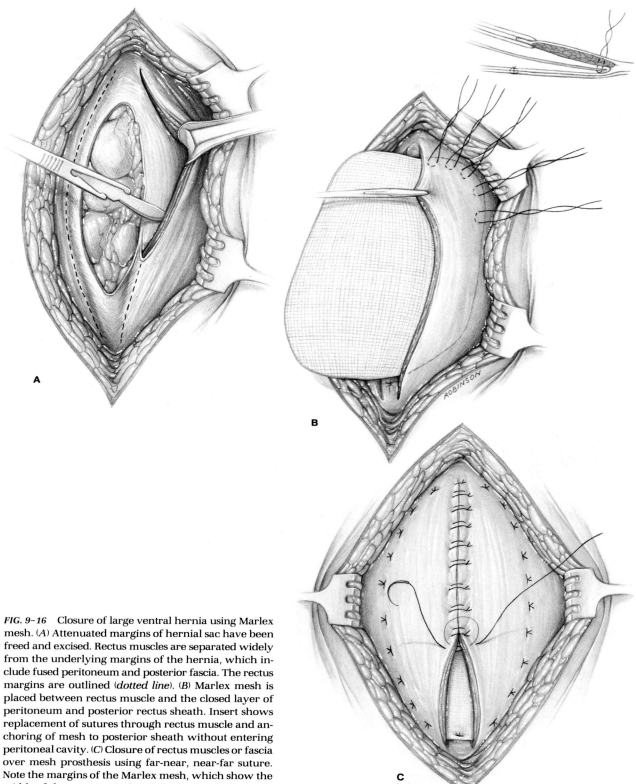

FIG. 9–16 Closure of large ventral hernia using Marlex mesh. (*A*) Attenuated margins of hernial sac have been freed and excised. Rectus muscles are separated widely from the underlying margins of the hernia, which include fused peritoneum and posterior fascia. The rectus margins are outlined (*dotted line*). (*B*) Marlex mesh is placed between rectus muscle and the closed layer of peritoneum and posterior rectus sheath. Insert shows replacement of sutures through rectus muscle and anchoring of mesh to posterior sheath without entering peritoneal cavity. (*C*) Closure of rectus muscles or fascia over mesh prosthesis using far-near, near-far suture. Note the margins of the Marlex mesh, which show the width of the permanent hernial support.

After the hernial sac is removed and the margins of the fascial defect are freed, the rectus muscle is freed from the underlying posterior fascial sheath and peritoneum (Fig. 9–16A). The fascia and peritoneum beneath the rectus muscle should be dissected widely around the margins of the defect to permit closure of the peritoneum without tension. A large rectangular piece of Marlex mesh is then inserted between the rectus muscle and the closed peritoneum (Fig. 9–16B). The mesh should be maintained under slight tension; therefore, the lateral sutures that anchor the mesh to the fascia should be strategically placed so that the mesh does not buckle when the overlying rectus muscles are approximated in the midline. Nonabsorbable No. 0 Tevdek sutures are used to anchor the mesh to the rectus abdominis muscle. Closure of the rectus fascia over the mesh is then attempted as far as possible, using the far-near, near-far closure technique (Fig. 9–16C). If the rectus muscles or fascia cannot be approximated in the midline, the attenuated hernial sac is utilized to bridge the gap and cover the underlying Marlex mesh. In this case, the margins of the hernial sac are preserved so that they can be sutured to the lateral margins of the anterior rectus fascia. Alternatively, when the peritoneum and posterior fascia cannot be separated from the margins of the hernia, the mesh may be placed on the anterior surface of the rectus and abdominal muscles and beneath the anterior fascia, rather than posteriorly. Although it is preferable to place the mesh beneath the abdominal muscles to prevent infection from the incision, placement beneath the anterior fascia has proven to be much easier and anatomically quite satisfactory.

Drainage tubes or catheters are placed longitudinally on either side of the fascial incision, and the subcutaneous fat and skin are closed separately. Suction is applied to the drainage tubes to give negative pressure beneath the skin and prevent elevation of the skin flaps by serum or blood. The drains may be removed by the fifth day, but must be left in place until there has been complete cessation of incisional drainage.

Postoperatively, the patient is ambulated on the day following surgery without prolonged bed rest. It is advisable, however, that the abdominal incision be protected from excessive stress and strain of coughing, vomiting, and retching. An elastic binder is helpful. If the bowel becomes distended, it should be decompressed immediately with a nasogastric tube until normal bowel function has returned. Prophylactic antibiotics are frequently employed perioperatively to prevent secondary infection in the operative site. Antibiotics are particularly indicated for patients in whom a polyethylene mesh has been employed for closure of a large hernial defect.

Panniculectomy and Abdominoplasty

The morbidly obese patient with a large, protruding panniculus of the lower abdominal wall presents a major technical problem and a surgical risk for pelvic surgery. Not only is the operative procedure technically difficult because exposure of the surgical field is limited when operating through a large panniculus, but wound healing is also seriously compromised. The increased incidence of wound infection and hematoma formation and the potential for development of a ventral hernia puts the obese patient in the high-risk category for both significant complications following pelvic surgery. In the past, surgical treatment of symptomatic pelvic disease was frequently not used in such patients, and alternative methods, frequently less effective, were adopted.

With the current sophistication of anesthesia techniques, the intensive care monitoring of the postoperative patient, and the medical control of cardiopulmonary reserve, the obese patient has become a less serious risk and a more frequent surgical candidate. To alleviate the anatomical problem of surgical exposure and to reduce the frequency of postoperative wound complications, panniculectomy and abdominoplasty have become more common procedures when performed as a part of major abdominal surgery.

Panniculectomy was first described by Demars and Marx in 1890 as reported by Elbaz and Flageul. Howard Kelly (1910) was among the first of a list of surgeons to recommend removal of a large panniculus at the time of pelvic surgery, remarking that, for cosmetic purposes alone, the procedure was warranted. The procedure then fell into oblivion for the next 50 years, until a resurgence of interest developed in the field of plastic and reconstructive surgery. During the past two decades, there have been many descriptions and reports on the subject of abdominal panniculectomy but few have emerged from the gynecologic literature until the experience from the Mayo Clinic was reviewed by Pratt and Irons in 1978. This large series included 126 panniculectomies performed during a 20-year period, of which 85 were done specifically to facilitate exposure to the surgical field. A modified transverse elliptic incision was used for most cases and "V"-shaped wedges of tissue were removed from the angles of the incision to reduce the redundant skin. Although 34.5% of the patients had some degree of postoperative morbidity, the average hospital stay was only 14 days.

INDICATIONS

The major indication for panniculectomy is abdominal obesity with an accumulation of fat that produces a protuberant abdominal wall that extends over the symphysis pubis and the upper thighs. The degree of abdominal obesity may be accentuated by short stature and loss of subcutaneous tissue support from advanced age. Although there are no absolute indications for this procedure based on weight alone, morbid obesity is usually defined as a weight of more than twice the ideal body weight as derived from the Metropolitan Life Insurance tables on desirable weight. Such patients are usually greater than 115 kg in weight. Women in this weight category are usually found to have a large abdominal panniculus when examined in the erect position. Excision is recommended for this group of patients when pelvic surgery by the abdominal route is indicated, particularly in those who are physically inconvenienced by the weight and size of the abdominal fat pad. The patient must also be counseled and must become strongly motivated to a weight-reduction program, as it is impractical to perform an extensive abdominoplastic procedure in a patient who makes no change in her nutritional habits. If the surgical procedure is not urgent, it should be deferred temporarily until there is clinical evidence of a weight loss of approximately 40% to 50% of the optimal weight loss that is planned. Although the panniculectomy may remove as much as 35.5 kg (Meyerowitz et al., 1973), the purpose of the preoperative weight loss is to establish a normal eating pattern prior to the operation.

Patients who have a large diastasis recti in association with the panniculus are also candidates for this procedure, at which time plication of the rectus fascia should be done, either directly or using a vest-over-pants, layered technique. In many instances, the rectus abdominoplasty is of as much cosmetic and therapeutic benefit to the patient as is the panniculectomy. When both anatomical conditions coexist, the panniculectomy alone will not give a satisfactory surgical result.

TECHNIQUE

Of the various operative techniques available for panniculectomy and abdominoplasty, the elliptical transverse incision, originally described by Kelly, has proven to be the procedure of choice in our experience. We have found two modifications of the transverse panniculectomy to be useful. The most common procedure includes an elliptical "watermelon" incision (Fig. 9–17A) extending from the lateral aspect of the lumbar regions to approx-

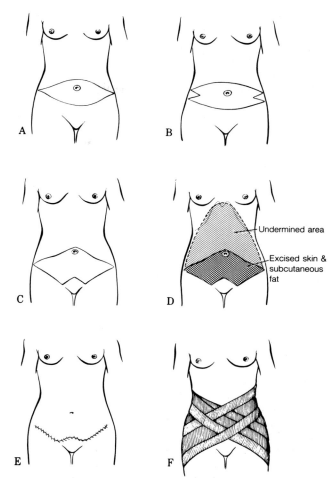

FIG. 9–17 Panniculectomy incisions. Elliptical transverse incision extending from region of iliac crest (*A*) extends above and below umbilicus. (*B*) V-shaped incision in lateral angles eliminates folds of skin in abdominal wall. (*C*) W-shaped incision over the mons pubis extends along the inguinal ligament to the iliac crest. (*D*) The upper incision passes above the umbilicus. Wide mobilization of the upper skin flap is carried to the sternum and rib margins. (*E*) After removal of panniculus and skin, the upper skin flap is sutured without tension to the lower skin margin. (*F*) A firm elastic dressing is crisscrossed over the abdominal wall for abdominal support and to prevent seroma formation.

imately 3 cm to 4 cm above the umbilicus. If the patient requests the preservation of the umbilicus, it can be excised and transplanted to the upper pedicle of skin. Inferiorly, the transverse incision follows the concave skin fold that separates the overhanging panniculus from the suprapubic skin. The underlying fat is excised deeply in a slightly wedged manner, with the deep portion of the fat extending outward and slightly beyond the skin margin to avoid ischemia of the incision. Meticulous attention must be given to absolute hemostasis, a time-consuming procedure, to avoid postoperative hematoma formation and infection. We do not recommend the excessive use of cautery, which produces a favorable environment for bacterial growth in devitalized tissue. The lateral angles of the incision may require separate "V" incisions to avoid the unsightly folds of redundant fat (19-17B). When these V-shaped wedges are closed, the angle of the incision is converted into a Y-shaped configuration, which eliminates the excessive skin in the lateral aspects of the abdominal wall. Following the removal of the large panniculus, the abdomen may be opened either transversely or vertically. If an abdominoplasty is required to approximate the widely separated rectus muscles, a midline incision is necessary. In this way, a tight closure of the rectus fascia or a vest-over-pants repair, as illustrated in Figure 9–15D, will give additional strength to the abdominal wall. If the rectus fascia is of poor quality and will not provide adequate support to the abdominal wall, a Marlex mesh graft may be inserted at the completion of the procedure, either above or below the rectus muscle (see Fig. 9–16). Alternatively, if the fascia of the rectus sheath can be plicated in the midline, wide plication and anchor of the medial margins of the rectus muscle at the closure of the procedure will close the diastasis and give a firm abdominal wall.

A second type of transverse panniculectomy is a "W" technique, initially described by Regnault in 1972 and shown in Figure 9–17C. The incision is outlined prior to the operative procedure in the form of a W over the symphysis pubis, inside the hairline. The incision is started in the center of the mons pubis and extends laterally and downward on each side to the inguinal fold near the external inguinal ring. The line then follows above the inguinal ligament in the panniculus skin crease to the region of the iliac crest on each side of the pelvis. The upper margin of the incision is drawn above the umbilicus to the upper margin of the redundant fat. If the umbilicus is to be relocated, the new umbilical site is drawn in the upper skin flap before the incision is made and is transposed to the upper skin flap after the incision is closed. The panniculus is excised prior to the pelvic operation in the manner described.

At the completion of the panniculectomy, the abdomen is opened either vertically or transversely in accordance with the surgeon's preference as wide exposure of the anterior abdominal wall is produced. It has been our preference to use a vertical incision through the linea alba since this provides an opportunity to plicate the rectus fascia or to perform a layered, vest-over-pants closure of the abdominal wall. In closing the W-shaped incision of Regnault after the abdominal or pelvic operation is completed, the upper flap of the abdominal skin is mobilized superficial to the fascia as far as necessary to the region of the xiphoid process and to the inferior margin of the costochondral junctions of the rib cage (Fig. 9–17D). Here it is particularly important to re-emphasize the necessity for meticulous ligation and control of all small bleeding vessels. A thin layer of fat is left attached to the fascia to facilitate the postoperative absorption of serous fluid. As shown in Figure 9–17E, the upper skin flap is sutured to the W-shaped, pubic skin margins, using interrupted sutures of No. 2-0 delayed-absorbable sutures for the subcutaneous fat. Multiple fine sutures are used to anchor the skin flap to the abdominal wall to prevent seroma formation and loculation. Suction drainage is always used beneath the upper skin flap, employing a small Silastic or a polyethylene catheter that is brought out through separate lateral stab wounds above the suture line. If the upper skin flap will not reach the pubic skin without excessive tension, the patient is placed in a slightly jack-knife position on the operating table by having the back elevated and the legs maintained in a straight-horizontal position. When the skin margins have been approximated over the pubis and along the inguinal ligament, additional V-shaped incisions can be taken from the lateral angles of the incision if there is redundant skin present.

The skin is closed following either procedure with interrupted vertical mattress sutures of No 3-0 silk. Alternatively, we have used inert skin staples or a removable fine subcuticular suture to approximate the skin margins. Skin staples can be left in place without the risk of infection until the skin incision has shown adequate healing. The new umbilicus is placed in the skin flap by making a 2-cm horizontal incision in the center of the flap, about 2 cm below the waistline. Fine interrupted No. 2-0 or No. 3-0 subcuticular sutures are used to anchor the fat of the incision to the transplanted umbilicus, and the skin is approximated with No. 3-0 silk vertical mattress sutures. A firm elastoplast tape dressing is applied under tension over the abdominal wall in a crisscross manner, beginning at the rib cage and extending to the thighs (Fig. 9–17F). This abdominal support will relieve tension on the suture line and will also prevent seroma and hematoma formation beneath the skin flaps.

Bibliography

Baggish MS, Lee WK: Abdominal wound disruption. Obstet Gynecol 46:530, 1975

Beck, WC, Collette TS: False faith in the surgeon's gown and drape. Am J Surg 83:152, 1952

Borkowf HI: Bacterial gangrene associated with pelvic surgery. Clin Obstet Gynecol 16:40, 1973

Cherney LS: A modified transverse incision for low abdominal operations. Surg Gynecol Obstet 72:92, 1941

Cole WR, Bernard HR: Inadequacies of present methods of surgical skin preparation. Arch Surg 89:215, 1964

Cullen TS, Brödel M: Lesions of the rectus abdominis muscle simulating an acute intra-abdominal condition. Bull J Hopkins Hosp 61:295, 1937

Elbaz JS, Flageul G: Plastic Surgery of the Abdomen, p 42. New York, Masson, 1979

Everett HS, Mattingly RF: Urinary tract injuries resulting from pelvic surgery. Am J Obstet Gynecol 71:502, 1956

Fletcher HS, Joseph WL: Bleeding into the rectus abdominis muscle. Int Surg 58:97, 1973

Goligher JC, Irvin TT, Johnston D, et al: A controlled clinical trial of three methods of closure of laparotomy wounds. Brit J Surg 62:823, 1975

Guillou PJ, Hall TJ, Donaldson DR, et al: Vertical abdominal incisions: A choice? Br J Surg 67:395, 1980

Guiney EJ, Morris PJ, Donaldson GA: Wound dehiscence. Arch Surg 92:47, 1966

Halpren SL: Quick Reference to Clinical Nutrition. Philadelphia, JB Lippincott, 1979

Haxton H, Clegg J, Lord M: A comparison of catgut and polyglycolic acid sutures in human abdominal wounds. Abdom Surg 16:239, 1974

Helmkamp BF: Abdominal wound dehiscence. Am J Obstet Gynecol 128:803, 1977

Hudson AR, Hunter GA, Waddell JP: Iatrogenic femoral nerve injuries. Can J Surg 22:62, 1979

Hunt TK: Physiology of repair. In Wound Healing. First International Symposium on Wound Healing. Rotterdam, April 1974. Montreux, Foundation for International Cooperation in the Medical Sciences, 1975

Irvin TT, Koffman CG, Duthie HL: Layer closure of laparotomy wounds with absorbable and non-absorbable suture materials. Brit J Surg 63:793, 1976

Jenkins TPN: The burst abdomen: A mechanical approach. Br J Surg 63:873, 1976

Keill RH, Keitzer WF, Nichols WK, et al: Abdominal wound dehiscence. Arch Surg 106:573, 1973

Kelly HA: Excision of the fat of the abdominal wall: Lipectomy. Surg Gynecol Obstet 10:229, 1910

Kirk RM: Effect of method of opening and closing the abdomen on incidence of wound bursting. Lancet 2:352, 1972

Masterson BJ: Wound healing in gynecologic surgery. In Mas-

terson BJ (ed): Manual of Gynecologic Surgery. New York, Springer-Verlag, 1979

Maylard AE: Direction of abdominal incisions. Br Med J 2:895, 1907

Meyerowitz BR, Gruber RP, Laub DR: Massive abdominal panniculectomy. JAMA 225:408, 1973

Morrow CP, Hernandez WL, Townsend DE, et al: Pelvic celiotomy in the obese patient. Am J Obstet Gynecol 127:335, 1977

Mowat J, Bonnar J: Abdominal wound dehiscence after cesarean section. Br Med J 2:256, 1971

Moylan JA, Kennedy BV: The importance of gown and drape barriers in the prevention of wound infection. Surg Gynecol Obstet 151:465, 1980

Peterson AF, Rosenberg A, Alatary SO: Comparative evaluation of surgical scrub preparations. Surg Gynecol Obstet 146:63, 1978

Pfannenstiel HJ: Uber die Vortheile des suprasymphysaren Fascienguerschnitt fur die gynaekologischen Koeliotomien. Samml Klin Vortr Gynaekol (Leipzig) Nr 268, 97:1735, 1900

Pitkin RM: Abdominal hysterectomy in obese women. Surg Gynecol Obstet 142:532, 1976

Pratt JH: Wound healing: Evisceration. Clin Obstet Gynecol 16:126, 1973

Pratt JH, Irons GB: Panniculectomy and abdominoplasty. Am J Obstet Gynecol 132:165, 1978

Regnault P: Abdominoplasty by the W technique. Plast Reconstr Surg 55:265, 1975

————: Abdominal lipectomy, a low W incision. Internatl J Anesth Plast Surg 1972

Rollins RA, Corcoran JJ, Gibbs CE: Treatment of gynecologic wound complications. Obstet Gynecol 28:268, 1966

Savage RC: Abdominoplasty combined with other surgical procedures. Plast Reconstr Surg 70:437, 1982

Sloan GA: A new upper abdominal incision. Surg Gynecol Obstet 45:678, 1927

Tera H, Aberg C: The strength of suture knots after one week in vitro. Acta Chir Scand 142:301, 1976

————: Tissue strength of sutures involved in musculo-aponeurotic layer sutures in laparotomy incision. Acta Chir Scand 142:349, 1976

Usher FS: The repair of incisional and inguinal hernias. Surg Gynecol Obstet 131:525, 1970

Van Winkle W, Jr, Hastings JC, Barker E et al: Effect of suture materials on healing skin wounds. Surg Gynecol Obstet 140:7, 1975

Wallace D, Hernandez W, Schlaerth, et al: Prevention of abdominal wound disruption utilizing the Smead–Jones closure technique. Obstet Gynecol 56:226, 1980

Chapter 10

Benign and Malignant Diseases of the Breast

George W. Mitchell, M.D.

Anatomy

The breast occupies the space between the third and seventh ribs and between the sternum and the midaxillary line (Fig. 10–1). Breast tissue may also extend into the anterior axillary fold along the margin of the insertion of the pectoralis major muscle. Beneath the breast is a thin layer of fibrous connective tissue through which lymphatic extensions pervade the underlying muscles. The glandular tissue lies on this pectoral fascia and, to a lesser extent, on a similar layer overlying the serratus anterior muscle. Both the ducts and the acini are enveloped in a rich interlocking network of lymphatics that communicate with the larger interlobular channels. Major lymphatic channels from the outer quadrants of the breast extend along the course of the axillary vein and, from the inner, descend through the intercostal spaces to the chain accompanying the internal mammary vessels. Supraclavicular extensions are present but relatively minor. In the axilla, palpable lymph nodes are characterized as being at Level 1, 2, or 3, depending on whether they are located just medial to the latissimus dorsi, at the level of the pectoralis minor, or at the sternoclavicular junction (Fig. 10–2). The blood supply is from three sources: the anterior aortic intercostal arteries, the internal mammary artery, and the thoracoacromial trunk of the axillary artery. These considerations are important in the clinical examination of the breast and in understanding the spread of infection or carcinoma.

The areola is a circular pigmented patch of skin, 3 cm to 5 cm in diameter, overlying the center of the breast and surrounding the nipple. On its surface are many small, rounded elevations indicating the presence of sebaceous glands, which lubricate the nipple during lactation. Infection in these glands is common, especially during nursing, when the superficial integument is liable to abrasions. The nipple consists of erectile tissue surrounding the ductal network that delivers milk at the time of lactation. Both nipple and areola are rich in blood vessels and lymphatics. Beneath the skin is a fatty subcutaneous tissue investing the glandular parenchyma of the breast and dividing it into partitions that assist in supporting both glandular and fatty elements. This connective tissue also forms a network for blood vessels and lymphatics and maintains breast contour. The parenchyma consists of a dozen or more separate, irregular lobes radiating from the nipple and lying close to the undersurface of the corium throughout the breast. This close proximity to the skin makes it difficult to excise all breast tissue while leaving the skin intact. Each lobe has its own excretory duct converging toward a main channel close to the surface of the nipple. The lobes are further subdivided by connective tissue into lobules, and the lobules into alveoli, the functional secreting units. As the ducts approach the nipple, they enlarge, forming a sinus, or reservoir, that temporarily holds the secretions of the gland (Fig. 10–3). Each duct is surrounded by a column of connective tissue that connects directly with the overlying skin. Enlarging tumors within the lobules exert downward pressure on this relatively rigid periductal connective tissue, causing localized skin retraction.

Fatty tissue makes up a large part of the bulk of the breast, and for this reason breast size may bear little relation to function. A shriveled breast with redundant skin may still contain adequate glandular tissue in a woman in the reproductive age group.

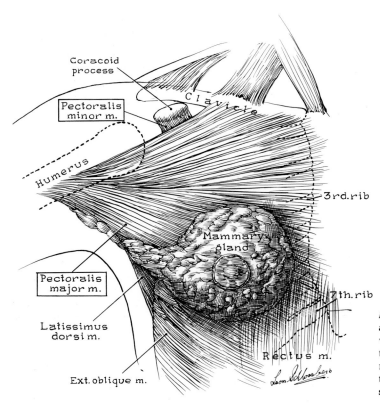

FIG. 10-1 Topography of the breast. The breast lies approximately over the midportion of the hemithorax with the tail extending toward the axilla. Ramifications also penetrate the interstices of the underlying muscle. These extensions and the close adherence of the skin to subcutaneous breast tissue make complete subcutaneous mastectomy nearly impossible.

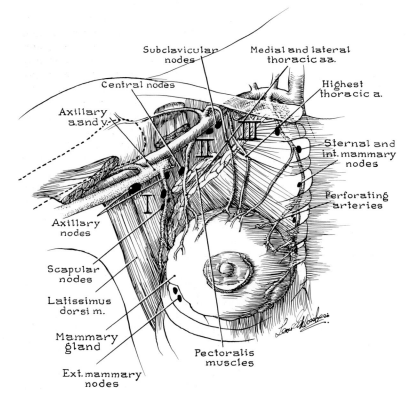

FIG. 10-2 Lymphatics and blood supply of the breast. Lymphatic drainage from the outer half of the breast is first to the axillary nodes shown here at Levels 1, 2, and 3. Medial lesions are more likely to metastasize first to the internal mammary chain.

Conversely, very large breasts offer no assurance of good function.

The breasts of prepubertal children consist entirely of ducts and connective tissue. At puberty, rudimentary gland buds increase in size and proliferate, the first manifestation being a symmetrical palpable enlargement or bud beneath the nipple. Full development requires about 4 years.

During the reproductive years, the amount of fatty tissue increases along with the development of the lobular structure, and the proportion of fat to glandular tissue has a significant effect on the size and consistency of the breast and the clarity of mammographic studies. Fat offers a translucent background against which abnormal x-ray images can be seen to better advantage. Postmenopausally, the lobules and ducts undergo atrophy, leading to sagging, while the size of the breast depends almost solely on the amount of adipose tissue.

At puberty, the development of glandular tissue, the growth of the duct system, and the pigmentation of the areola and nipple are influenced by the rise in estrogen levels. Progesterone affects the growth of the alveolar portion of the breast lobule. Prolactin also makes a contribution to this process, but the specific nature of its activity is not well understood. During pregnancy the breasts undergo a very active increase in size because of the secretion of large amounts of estrogen, progesterone, and lactogen by the placenta. Prolactin levels increase sharply, possibly as a result of the increase in estrogen. Postpartum prolactin inhibiting hormone, produced by the hypothalamus, depresses prolactin secretion and consequent lactation, but suckling suppresses its formation and allows prolactin to remain at a functional level until nursing stops. Suckling also causes the posterior pituitary to release oxytocin, which, by contracting perialveolar myoepithelial cells, moves the milk along into the large ductal lacunae from which it is ejected through the nipple.

The Breast Examination

Examination of the female breast should be a routine part of the physical examination of gynecologic patients. Previous examination by family practitioners, internists, or surgeons in no way alters this obligation or obviates the need to be thorough. The gynecologist has both a professional obligation to the patient and an obligation to protect himself legally by avoiding errors of omission. Sufficient time, not less than 3 minutes, depending on the size of the breast, should be set aside for this purpose.

The breasts are first inspected while the patient is seated on the edge of the table without encum-

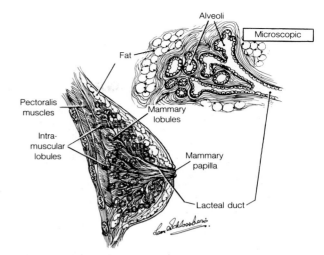

FIG. 10–3 Internal structure of the breast. The breast is a large apocrine gland. The secreting parenchyma is composed of lobules containing acini, fat, and fibrous tissue. The ducts drain centrally toward large lacunae located directly beneath the nipple. These act as reservoirs until they receive the impetus for ejection.

bering clothing or drapes and with her hands clasped behind her head and her shoulders retracted. The presence of skin lesions, striae, erythema, increased vascularity or abnormal development is noted. Inverted nipples are significant only when they have developed secondarily, and this change is usually unilateral. Secondary inversion of the nipple or dimpling of the skin over any part of the breast suggests the possibility of an underlying malignancy even if no mass is palpable.

The skin of the breast is subject to the same types of disease as the skin elsewhere on the body. Small lesions, such as nevi, warts, papillomas, hemangiomas, keratoses, and furuncles, that seem obviously minor may have a more serious connotation to the patient and should be noted in the record on a breast diagram. More serious lesions, such as melanoma and Paget's disease (which has a characteristic eczematoid appearance), must be biopsied, as must every abnormality when there is a reasonable doubt about the diagnosis.

Pendulous breasts often conceal beneath their inferior margins an erythematous reaction to chafing, referred to as intertrigo, which may become widespread, indurated, and even ulcerated. Chafe marks along the inner and outer sides of the breast or deep strap marks on the shoulders indicate the use of a bra which does not fit properly or is drawn too tight.

The left breast is often slightly larger than the right, but marked asymmetry sometimes occurs.

Anomalies of this type can cause reclusive behavior and distressing neuroses, and appropriate counseling and plastic surgery are indicated in such cases. Variations in the size of normal breasts are a cause of concern to many women and should not be treated casually. Women whose breasts are seriously underdeveloped are candidates for augmentation mammoplasty. Women whose breasts are within the normal range should be discouraged from having surgery.

Breast growth depends upon the presence of adequate numbers of steroid receptors as well as normal cyclic estrogen and progesterone production and is difficult to predict in any individual case. The mammary hypertrophy of adolescents or women in early adult life and the fatty, heavy breasts of the perimenopausal and postmenopausal years may cause distressing psychological problems as well as discomfort in neck, back, and shoulders from the abnormal weight. Reduction mammoplasties afford great relief to these women.

The seated patient next places her hands on her hips and assumes a more relaxed position. The examiner palpates the breasts (Fig. 10–4A) by gently squeezing them between the hands, with the fingers perpendicular to the rib cage and with outward traction on the breast to permit accurate evaluation of the tissue close to the chest wall (Fig. 10–4B) and also by pressing the breast tissue against the underlying muscle with the flats of the second, third, and fourth fingers (Fig. 10–4C).

With the patient still in the seated position, the lymph nodes in the anterior cervical and supraclavicular and infraclavicular areas are palpated. The examiner then takes the patient's left hand in his left hand and brings her left arm across the front of her chest to relax the pectoralis major muscle while he feels beneath its insertion, in the high midaxilla, and along the border of the latissimus dorsi for enlarged nodes. A similar examination is done on the right side, and palpable nodes are charted according to estimated level.

The patient is then placed supine on the examining table with a pillow under the shoulder on the side to be examined. First one arm and then the other is extended above her head while the breast tissue is pressed against the chest wall with the flats of the examiner's middle fingers, proceeding clock-

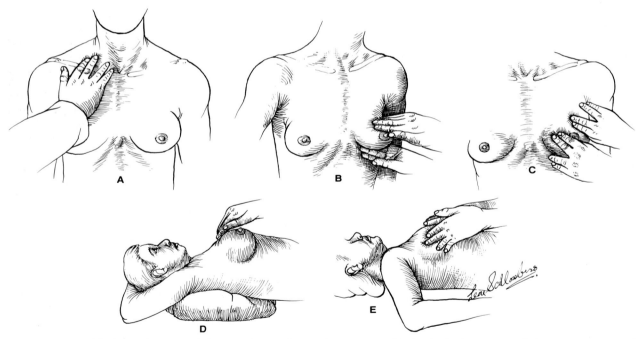

FIG. 10–4 (*A*) With the patient seated the examiner palpates the supra- and infraclavicular areas and the anterior cervical chain for enlarged nodes. (*B*) With the patient seated the examiner squeezes the breast between the fingers of both hands while pulling it outward in order to palpate lesions close to the chest wall. (*C*) With the patient seated the examiner palpates the breast tissue with the flats of the fingers of both hands in a clockwise direction, leaving no area untouched. (*D*) With the patient supine and the arm extended in order to flatten the breast, the tissue is palpated with the fingers by pressing it gently against the chest wall, again using a plan that will cover the entire breast, including the axillary tail. (*E*) The procedure is repeated with the patient's arm at her side to relax the pectoral muscles.

wise around the full circumference of the breast at its perimeter and gradually moving in toward the areola (Fig. 10–4D). The major ductal system beneath the nipple is reached last. The examination is repeated after the patient has lowered her arms to her sides (Fig. 10–4E). Some experts recommend routine "milking" of the breasts from each quadrant toward the nipple in an attempt to express secretion, but others feel that this is unnecessary in the absence of a history of nipple discharge. When there is such a history, an attempt should be made to determine from which part of the breast the discharge originates or whether it is general and stemming from a systemic cause rather than a local lesion.

Nipple Discharge

Lactation may persist for many months following the cessation of nursing, and in such instances prolactin levels tend to remain above normal. In instances unrelated to pregnancy, lactation is referred to as galactorrhea and may be due to a variety of causes, many of which have in common high-normal or elevated prolactin levels. The causes of galactorrhea and nipple discharge that are related to local conditions are listed in Causes of Nipple Discharge.

CAUSES OF NIPPLE DISCHARGE

Galactorrhea	*Other Types*
Pregnancy and childbirth	Cancer
Neonatal	Intraductal papilloma
Breast manipulation	Ductal ectasia
Surgery	Gross cystic change
Stress	Infection
Drugs*	
Sellar tumors	
Hypothyroidism	
Chronic renal disease	

---

* Phenothiazines, rauwolfia alkaloids, tricyclic antidepressants, methyldopa, oral contraceptives

Among the more common causes of galactorrhea are breast manipulation, sucking, or some form of athleticism such as jogging. Improperly fitting garments may compress or inadequately support the breasts, causing discharge. Reflex stimulation of thoracic nerves T–2 through T–6 as a result of surgical procedures or trauma may signal the hypothalamus to release prolactin into the blood. The possibility that pituitary micro- or macroadenomas (Forbes–Albright syndrome) may be secreting ele-

vated levels of prolactin must be ruled out, and a serum prolactin level and a CT scan of the brain should be obtained for this purpose. The pressure of extrasellar tumors may produce similar effects.

Some women with galactorrhea may have normal ovulatory function, but the abnormal secretion may be associated with other manifestations of an endocrine disorder, including postpartum amenorrhea (Chiari–Frommel syndrome) and amenorrhea that is not pregnancy-related (Ahumada–Del Castillo syndrome). Galactorrhea has also been known to occur following hysterectomy and myomectomy and as a result of psychic stimuli. The mechanism in these cases is unclear.

Since prolactin inhibiting factor is thought to be dopamine or a dopamine analogue, it is to be expected that dopamine antagonists would increase prolactin secretion and occasionally produce lactation. A broad range of drugs used for diverse medical conditions may have this effect. Defects in the synthesis of prolactin inhibiting factor or in receptor binding may also be caused by drug administration. Chronic renal disease and hypothyroidism may be associated with elevated prolactin levels mediated through the prolactin inhibiting factor (PIF) system.

Other nipple secretions occur in a wide variety of colors and consistencies and are usually due to local disease. From a surgical viewpoint, a frankly bloody or brownish discharge, especially one that is unilateral, is the most significant. A discharge of this type is often first noted by the patient and should be confirmed at the time of examination. A sample should be checked microscopically for red blood cells. Cytologic evaluation of the fluid is often unsatisfactory because of its relatively acellular composition, but specimens should initially be sent to the cytology laboratory. They should be taken directly from the nipple on a frosted or albumin-coated slide and fixed carefully to avoid washing away the cells. In the diagnosis of cancer, the incidence of false-negative cytologic reports is between 15% and 20% and, if atypical changes are included, the incidence of false-positive reports is approximately 20%. Because of this inaccuracy, the presence of a discharge containing blood necessitates surgical exploration of the breast ductal system with biopsy or resection of suspicious lesions regardless of the absence of a palpable mass. Usually an intraductal papilloma is found, and in about 30% of cases atypical cells or malignant changes will be present.

The breast may be the site of acute or chronic infection. Abscesses are rare and usually develop during the puerperium or as a result of trauma and hematoma formation. Occasionally, bacterial flora, particularly *Staphylococcus aureus*, may be introduced through the nipple and give rise to disseminated breast disease. Collections of pearly or yellow pus may drain through the duct system to the nipple, but such drainage is often not adequate, and incision and drainage is required. Because of the possibility of an associated carcinoma, biopsy of the abscess wall should be done at this time. In cases of widely disseminated acute infection, subcutaneous excision of large portions or all of the breast tissue under antibiotic coverage may be necessary, preserving the skin for the insertion of a prosthesis at a later date.

Chronic infection, as is found with ductal ectasia, is common during the perimenopausal and menopausal years. The ductal changes are caused by the inspissation of secreted material, with the development of intraductal and interstitial infiltration of round cells and atrophy of the epithelium. The nipple discharge is characteristically pale yellow, sticky, and bilateral. Usually, there is no mass or tenderness present, but the breast feels lumpy. Conservative management is indicated, and it is important to advise the patient to wear a carefully fitted garment and to avoid undue constraint or friction.

Diagnosis

Women should be instructed to perform monthly examinations of their breasts postmenstrually, when the breast is least engorged. Patience, repetition, reassurance, and visual aids are required to indoctrinate many fearful patients, and these can often best be offered by female office attendants. The office examination previously described should be repeated yearly or more often, depending upon the assessed degree of risk for breast cancer. Factors affecting risk are listed in Risk Factors Predisposing to Breast Carcinoma. The differential diagnosis between benign and malignant disease depends on the patient's age, the symptoms, and the findings on palpation. Although no absolute generalizations can be made, carcinomas tend to be irregular, firm, nontender, and occasionally fixed to the skin or underlying muscle. Pain is seldom a feature except in the very late stages. Benign lesions such as cysts and fibroadenomas are more likely to be smooth, well-defined, and relatively mobile. The breasts of women with fibrocystic change are often lumpy and tender, especially in the upper outer quadrants, and the changes tend to vary with the menstrual cycle. Degrees of discomfort up to severe pain may be present. The presence of one or more enlarged, firm lymph nodes in the axilla associated with an ipsilateral breast mass strongly suggests the likelihood of carcinoma, but axillary lymphadenopathy may also be caused by lesions of the hand, arm, and adjacent thorax, especially those due to trauma.

RISK FACTORS PREDISPOSING TO BREAST CARCINOMA

Data Good

Family history: first degree premenopausal relative
Advancing age
Carcinoma in other breast
Precancerous mastopathy
Early puberty
Late age at first childbirth
Late menopause
Western culture
Irradiation
Other carcinoma (colon, uterus, ovary)

Data Doubtful

Exogenous estrogens
Nutrition
Obesity
Breastfeeding
High parity

DIAGNOSTIC AIDS

Diagnostic aids available to the clinician are listed in Diagnostic Aids in the Management of Breast Disease. Of these, x-ray mammography is by far the most accurate and the only one that can diagnose breast cancer before it is palpable. Evaluation of the breast by x-ray techniques, both for screening and for diagnosis, is now well established. Because

DIAGNOSTIC AIDS IN THE MANAGEMENT OF BREAST DISEASE

1. Mammography
    Standard
        Magnification
    Xeroradiography
    Duct injection
2. Thermography
    Tele (infrared)
    Brachy (liquid crystal)
3. Ultrasonography
    B scan
    Real time
4. Diaphanography
5. Nuclear magnetic resonance

of concern about the theoretical carcinogenic effect of cumulative diagnostic x-rays on the breast and the knowledge that the danger is inherently greater the earlier in life the exposure occurs, there is some difference of opinion as to the age at which screening of asymptomatic women should begin. However, most authorities agree that women over the age of 35 should have two or three baseline mammograms, or more in the presence of risk factors, and that those over 50 should be screened yearly. Xeroradiography, a later extension of the standard technique, also uses x-rays, but has the advantage that vascular markings and microcalcifications stand out more clearly. To the radiologist who is expert in interpretation of breast films, however, it is not superior to the older method. In both instances, experience is of the utmost importance in the accurate interpretation of breast x-rays, and high-intensity light sources and magnification have been used to refine the technique further. On balance, the carcinogenic effect of x-ray exposure is less important than the potential for saving lives by early diagnosis. This is particularly true of older women, since the benefit of early diagnosis in this age group is better demonstrated than for younger women and since their shorter actuarial life expectancy provides less time for the development of cancer due to the x-ray exposure. Modern equipment uses dosages of less than 0.5 rads skin dose for the superior and lateral views ordinarily obtained for screening, and patients should be instructed to obtain their films in institutions where low dosages are routine and where radiologists specializing in mammography are available.

Mammographic screening is highly accurate, with a false-negative rate of less than 10%. In screening, 45% of all cancers are detected only by mammography. The other 55% are discovered on physical examination, but physical examination is positive alone in only 10% of cases. For this reason, accurate screening requires both mammography and palpation of the breast, and biopsies should be done if either of these examinations is positive. Mammography should always precede biopsy to rule out the possibility of other disease in the same or contralateral breast. The diagnosis is made on the presence of a mass with specific characteristics suggesting cancer (Fig. 10–5A) or on the basis of a localized cluster of microcalcifications (Fig. 10–5B).

For the diagnosis of symptomatic breasts, mammography is indicated in many different situations (Table 10–1). When cancer is suspected, mammography should be done regardless of the patient's age. Questionable but probably benign shadows should be rechecked in from 3 to 6 months to determine whether there has been any progression

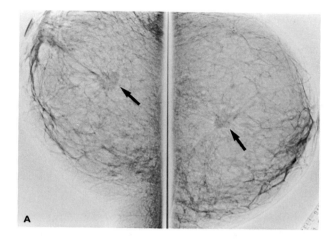

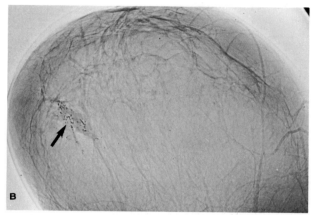

FIG. 10–5 (A) Xeroradiogram showing a dense irregular lesion in the upper outer quadrant with projections into the surrounding breast tissue characteristic of carcinoma. (B) Xeroradiogram showing the translucent breast of a postmenopausal woman with a cluster of calcifications in the lower inner quadrant characteristic of carcinoma.

of the process. A change in the diameter or contour of such a shadow or a further separation of microcalcifications is an indication for biopsy. A thermogram suggesting malignant change should be followed by the more definitive mammography before biopsy is performed. Whenever a patient believes that she has felt a lump in her breast, it is advisable to order a mammogram even if the lump cannot be palpated by the examining physician. Differences in opinion by two or more physicians regarding what can or cannot be felt should be resolved by mammography. Patients with large or very dense breasts that are difficult to palpate should have spaced sequential mammograms to detect subtle changes in shadow patterns. The fact that dense breasts are relatively difficult to interpret by

TABLE 10–1   *Indications for Mammography, by Age*

AGE	INDICATION
SCREENING MAMMOGRAPHY	
<25	None
25–35	Baseline if high risk
35–49	Baseline and biannual examination
	Annual examination if high risk
>50	Annual examination
DIAGNOSTIC MAMMOGRAPHY	
<25	Suspected cancer
>25	Dominant mass
	Discrete thickening
	Undiagnosed symptoms
	Change in previous lesion
	Positive thermography
	Patient request
	Large breasts
	Discrepancy in opinions
	Prebiopsy evaluation

x-ray, as they are by physical examination, does not obviate the need to obtain regular films.

In recent years, radiologists have attempted to classify the parenchymal patterns noted on breast x-rays according to the likelihood that cancer will develop in those breasts. The term *dysplasia* has been used increasingly to denote deviations from the normal that have serious implications for the future. It is important to understand that dysplasia, in this context, covers a broad range of histopathologic entities, particularly in the realm of so-called fibrocystic disease, and cannot be equated with a specific cellular change. Many of the studies contributing to the development of a taxonomy for premalignant mammographic patterns have been retrospective and on selected populations, but they indicate the possible presence of a high-risk category that must be closely followed.

The search for a screening technique for breast cancer that is noninvasive and cost-effective has led to significant advances in the technique of thermography. The basic principle on which this type of assessment depends is that disease states, and cancer in particular, tend to generate relatively increased amounts of heat, presumably because of intensified cellular metabolism. Beginning about 25 years ago, the patterns of heat waves emanating from the breast were detected by sensors that were hand-held above the skin and that recorded variations in the infrared range. This method, referred to as telethermometry, has undergone many technical improvements since its inception, and efforts have been made to reduce background interference

by lowering the patient's temperature prior to the test. Electronic imaging of this type is reasonably reliable, but it requires rather elaborate apparatus and experienced interpretation, usually available only in large institutions.

More recently, many thermographers have resorted to an innovation known as liquid crystal thermography, a type of brachythermometry, in the course of which the breasts are pressed directly against a thermosensitive plate lined with cholesteric crystals. The resulting thermographic film depicts the skin of the breast in contrasting colors that represent the underlying thermal pattern. The equipment with which this is accomplished is less expensive than that required for telethermometry and has been widely advertised for use in free-standing breast clinics and private offices. It appears to be a helpful tool, but much remains to be learned about the range of its reliability, especially in the category of nonpalpable or minimal breast cancer.

Thermography, in general, has the disadvantage of a higher degree of inaccuracy than mammography, particularly in the false-positive range, leading to overdiagnosis and unnecessary biopsies in some instances. New modifications offer hope of improved specificity, but the criteria for accuracy comparable to mammography have not been met to date in any long-range, well-controlled prospective studies.

Ultrasonography accurately depicts the difference between solid and cystic masses. Its accuracy in diagnosing early malignant disease in the breast is being subjected to extensive trials. Like thermography, it has been suggested as an adjunct to mammography, since combinations of the two modalities have been shown in some reports to be better than either alone, but it is not available for this purpose in many institutions. Fiberoptic transillumination to map the breast (diaphanography) is increasing in popularity, but randomized, controlled studies proving its efficacy have not been published. The delineation of soft tissue lesions by nuclear magnetic resonance holds hope for the future, but, to date, this technique has not been widely tested for efficacy in the diagnosis of breast disease. Before great reliance can be placed on screening techniques other than mammography, rigid clinical trials will be necessary. For diagnosis, mammography is the essential adjunct to physical examination.

Pathology

The term fibrocystic disease, formerly referred to as chronic cystic mastitis, includes a spectrum of conditions in which may be listed microcysts (less than 2 mm in diameter), macrocysts (greater than 2 mm in diameter) (Fig. 10–6), fibroadenomas, papillomas, and adenosis, all of which may be subject to hyperplastic epithelial changes with or without atypical cells. The universality of occurrence of microcystic disease (60%–90% of the female population) and the fact that both it and its macrocystic counterpart are subject to the cyclic changes of ovarian hormone production suggests that, at least in the subclinical variants, the process is physiologic rather than pathologic. Approximately 60% of all breast biopsies will be diagnosed in one of these categories. There would be no real significance to the term fibrocystic disease were it not for the anxiety-provoking discomfort and lumpiness imparted to the breast, especially premenstrually; the difficulty in distinguishing it from a so-called dominant mass; and the alleged positive relationship to the future development of cancer. The evidence that fibrocystic changes constitute a precancerous mastopathy consists largely of retrospective data of questionable statistical validity, especially since it has been shown that these changes will appear in up to 90% of all biopsies, whether or not cancer was present in addition. This also applies to the atypical hyperplastic changes that have not been demonstrated as necessarily progressing to invasive disease.

There is evidence to suggest that some forms of fibrocystic mastopathy, such as the proliferative intraductal lesions, may have more potential for the development of subsequent malignancy than others. Papillomas tend to develop in the larger subareolar ducts, whereas papillomatosis occurs in the medium-sized or smaller ductal ramifications and the nonproliferating forms of fibrocystic change, the micro- and macrocysts, arise in the terminal lobules and ducts. In younger women with fibrocystic change, there may be proliferation of both glandular and stromal tissue, forming firm masses that, on biopsy, are referred to as sclerosing adenosis. Histologically, this variant may be difficult to distinguish from carcinoma, but it has little malignant propensity. In older women, there may be a tendency for an increase in the fibrous elements at the expense of the glands, which can impart a feeling of firmness to the breast and occasionally suggests discrete masses.

Atypical hyperplasias, both lobular and ductal, may be difficult to separate histologically from carcinoma *in situ* and even from early invasive carcinoma. It seems likely that in some cases there is a progressive linear relationship between these changes and the eventual development of malignant disease. A diagnosis of atypical hyperplasia or carcinoma *in situ* by the pathologist necessitates careful study of the biopsy specimen and serious consid-

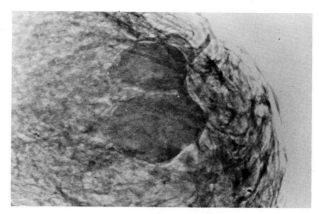

FIG. 10–6 Xeroradiogram showing two smooth, rounded shadows in the relatively dense breast of a premenopausal woman. These are characteristic of cysts but could be mistaken for fibroadenomas.

eration of the risk factors involved in allowing such patients to continue without more definitive treatment. In some series, the progression of lobular carcinoma *in situ* to invasive carcinoma is as high as 20%, and, since the duration of the follow-up is critical in this assessment, the figure may be higher. Because it is impossible to predict which women with lobular neoplasia will eventually develop invasive carcinoma, prophylactic mastectomy, on one or both sides, has frequently been advised. A policy of observation and regularly repeated mammography for patients with this disease process seems indicated, since, even when invasion occurs, lymph node metastases are uncommon and the prognosis is favorable.

By contrast, carcinoma *in situ* occurring in intraductal papillomas should, in the present state of our knowledge, probably be considered as definitely malignant and should be treated appropriately, either by mastectomy or wide excision plus axillary lymph node sampling. Because of the possibility of bilateral involvement, the opposite breast should be reexamined two or three times yearly with mammograms.

Medical Treatment

Breast symptoms, other than nipple secretion, consist chiefly of lumpiness and discomfort related to swelling and vascular engorgement, especially premenstrually. Since, in most women, these complaints are not caused by disease and are endurable, reassurance is the most important form of therapy. For those with more severe or unduly prolonged pain, a variety of medical regimens is available.

For years it has been known that small doses of androgens by mouth or by injection will relieve breast pain and soreness. Not only do these drugs have an undesirable virilizing effect in some women if taken over a long period, but the idea of taking male hormones, regardless of side effects, is abhorrent to many. More recently, it has been shown that small doses of an impeded androgen, Danocrine, will inhibit the development of fibrocystic changes that produce breast discomfort. Dosages in the range of 100 mg/day to 400 mg/day for 6 months are usually effective and do not cause amenorrhea, hirsutism, or acne in most patients. The favorable result is often maintained for months to years after discontinuance of the drug.

Oral contraceptives have been used to create a balanced menstrual cycle with lower amounts of circulating estrogen and progesterone and, consequently, less stimulation of breast tissue. For those who wish to avoid pregnancy and who are not at risk for the possible undesirable side effects of oral contraceptives, this is an acceptable method of treatment of cyclic mastalgia. No cause and effect relationship between the use of oral contraceptives and the subsequent development of carcinoma of the breast has been established, nor is it clear that the use of these drugs is protective against subsequent disease.

Studies attempting to equate the histologic changes of fibrocystic disease with an increase in estrogen and progesterone receptors have been inconclusive, but Minton has stated that there is a buildup of cyclic adenosine monophosphate (c-AMP) and guanosine monophosphate (c-GMP) in fibrocystic breast tissue, presumably as a result of an enzymatic failure to permit proper metabolic clearance. He postulated that this enzyme, phosphodiesterase, is inhibited by high levels of circulating methyl xanthines, which are commonly ingested in coffee, tea, and cocoa. Abstention from these beverages should permit free action of the enzyme, the reduction of cyclic AMP and GMP and amelioration of breast swelling and soreness. Clinical trials of this theory have been conducted with largely favorable results, but the clinical trials have not been conducted in a way to create confidence in the statistical results. Nevertheless, dietary regimens shunning coffee, tea, and cocoa have been adopted by many women with subjectively satisfactory effects.

Vitamin E has been recommended for the relief of breast symptoms, first by Abrams and more recently by London. Neither the clinical trials that have been conducted nor the scientific explanation, which postulates that the vitamin alters the metabolic pathway from pregnenolone to pregnandiol so that a 17-ketosteroid with androgenic action is produced, are convincing, but the possible placebo effect cannot be discounted.

Of great importance in the control of breast symptomatology is the support, or lack of it, in the everyday garments used. The weight of heavy breasts not properly supported exacerbates discomfort, and constriction, which interferes with proper circulation, also increases disability. Consultation and advice about this factor is best given by female office personnel familiar with the problems of fitting and with the manufacturers of special clothing.

Office Surgery

Discrete or dominant lumps in the breast must be surgically investigated. When the mass is rounded, well circumscribed, smooth and 1 cm or more in diameter, aspiration should be attempted first. With the patient lying supine in a relaxed position, well prepared by prior instruction, the mass is stabilized between the thumb and first two fingers of the left hand (Fig. 10–7). Some surgeons prefer to use local anesthesia and some do not, but in the former instance a small intradermal weal of 1% lidocaine is raised over the lesion with a No. 25 hypodermic needle, and, through this, deeper injections are made circumferentially around its perimeter. A No. 18 or No. 20 needle attached to a 20 cc syringe is passed tangentially into the mass, and aspiration is attempted. If the lesion is cystic, the fluid obtained usually flows freely into the syringe and is of a brownish color. All of this fluid should be sent to the laboratory for cytologic evaluation, although it is usually acellular and nondiagnostic. If no fluid is obtained after several attempts, the needle is withdrawn and whatever is available at its tip should be blown onto a clean slide and fixed for cytologic analysis.

Any cyst smaller than 1 cm in diameter is difficult to aspirate and should be treated by open biopsy, especially if it is the first such lesion. If the diagnosis of fibrocystic change has previously been made histologically, the question of whether re-biopsy is indicated becomes a matter of experience and judgment. The needle should always be inserted at an angle of 30 or 40 degrees rather than perpendicular to the chest wall to avoid inadvertent perforation of the pleura.

When a solid, probably benign, mass is encountered, excision biopsy is usually indicated. In some institutions where the pathology departments have developed skills in interpreting aspiration specimens, a multiple aspiration technique is attempted. With or without local anesthesia, a No. 22 needle, attached to a 20 cc syringe contained within a specially designed handle that permits the maintenance

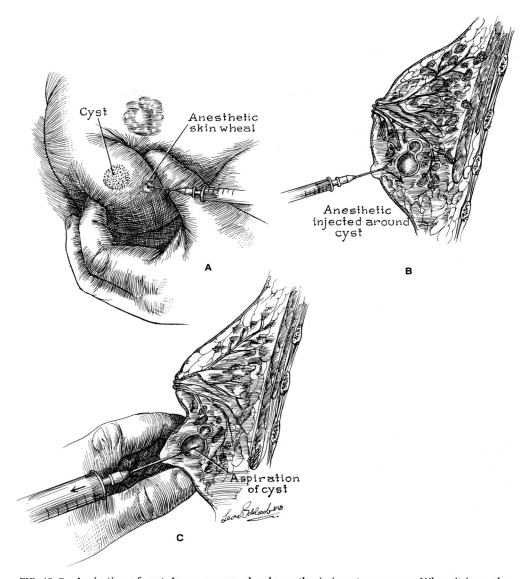

FIG. 10-7 Aspiration of cyst. In many cases local anesthesia is not necessary. When it is used, a small intradermal weal is raised over the cyst (*A*) and from this area the anesthesia is injected along the estimated path of the aspirating needle (*B*). (*C*) The portion of the breast containing the cyst is stabilized with the left hand while a No. 18 or No. 20 needle is passed into the cyst along a line tangential to the surface of the thorax in order to avoid penetration of the pleura. Fluid obtained is sent for cytologic interpretation.

of a constant vacuum within the syringe, is passed through the mass in several different planes in order to sample all of its ramifications (Fig. 10–8). The resultant aspirate, mostly in the needle, is blown onto a clean glass slide, fixed, and sent to the laboratory. A report positive for malignancy has a 90% accuracy, but most surgeons do not perform definitive surgery without a subsequent open biopsy. A negative report cannot be considered final.

Tiny biopsy specimens can be obtained by the percutaneous passage of a trocar containing a cutting needle (Fig. 10–9). Because of the size of the sheath and the necessity to push the cutting face into the breast tissue, local anesthesia is desirable. Specimens so obtained are examined histologically, but, because of their small size, may not be representative, and a negative report cannot be relied upon.

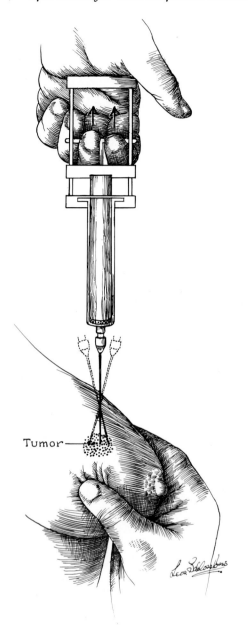

FIG. 10–8 Percutaneous needle aspiration of solid tumors. Using local anesthesia, a skinny needle (No. 22) is passed repeatedly through the lesion in different planes and directions while constant suction is maintained by means of the attached syringe holder. The aspirate is ejected on a slide and sent to Cytology. A high degree of accuracy in diagnosis is possible, but the result is not definitive.

Open biopsy is indicated whenever there is a secondarily retracted nipple or bloody discharge, a discrete mass, a dominant projection from an area of fibrocystic change, or a positive mammogram. Prior to surgery, mammograms should always be done to rule out other lesions in the same or other breast. Most biopsies should be done in the office, clinic, or ambulatory surgical area of a hospital under local anesthesia. The evidence indicates that a delay of a few days between diagnostic biopsy and a subsequent definitive surgical procedure does not adversely affect the prognosis, and patient acceptance of ambulatory surgery, which permits full discussion of the problem prior to major surgery, is much greater. Counseling of the patient and the patient's spouse or other member of the family is most important in securing the understanding that leads to good cooperation during the procedure. Each step of the operation is outlined, and the patient is reassured that nothing further will be done without consultation.

The patient should come to the minor surgical operating room having had nothing by mouth since the night before and accompanied by an interested second party. She is placed supine on the operating table with her arms at her side or with the arm on the affected side at right angles to the body, which stretches the pectoral muscles and may help to make the lesion more accessible. A pillow under the shoulder provides better exposure. If the patient is nervous, analgesic drugs such as meperidine 50 mg and diazepam 5 mg may be given intravenously a few minutes before starting.

The location of the incision is important, for cosmetic reasons if the lesion is benign and to keep it out of the line of a later mastectomy incision if the lesion is malignant. When the lesion is beneath the areola or within 3 cm or 4 cm of its outer margin, the incision is made along the areolar edge, not including more than one-half the circumference to avoid compromising its blood supply. For lesions further toward the periphery, a curved incision 3 cm or 4 cm long is made parallel to the areolar margin and medial to the lesion to permit its being more easily encompassed in any subsequent dissection, thus avoiding possible dissemination of tumor cells from the biopsy site (Fig. 10–10A). An intradermal weal is made with 1% lidocaine just below the inferior pole of the proposed incision and carried up along the areolar margin to a point above the upper pole (Fig. 10–10B). Using a longer needle at several points along the weal, the area around the lesion is infiltrated with anesthetic solution. If a nonpalpable intraductal papilloma is suspected, the major ductal system beneath the nipple is infiltrated. When the lesion is further out, it is best to delineate the proposed incision with a marking pencil after careful palpation has indicated proper placement.

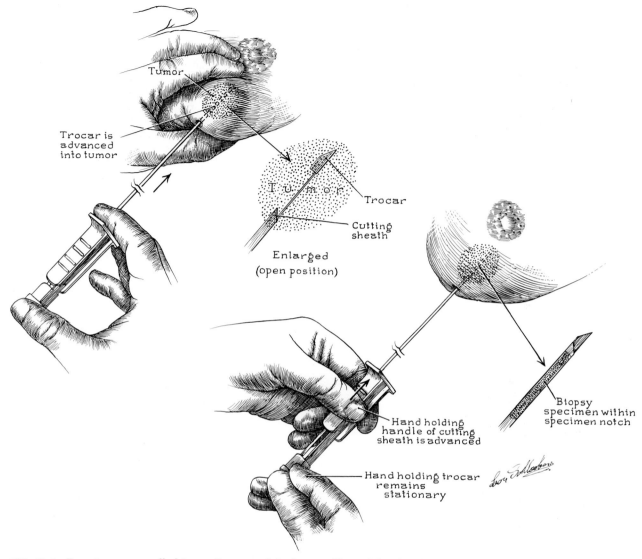

FIG. 10-9 Percutaneous needle biopsy. Because of the large caliber of the sheath to be passed, local anesthesia is usually necessary. A number of instruments are available for this purpose. The sheath is passed tangentially to the surface of the solid lesion and then directly engaged. The trocar is pushed well into the lesion and then withdrawn into the sheath bringing a small core of tumor tissue. Bleeding following this procedure can usually be controlled by pressure.

Using a No. 15 blade, the 3 cm to 5 cm incision is carried down through the dermis and the subcutaneous fat to the lobular tissue of the breast. The skin margins are slightly undercut and held back on fine hooks to facilitate exposure (Fig. 10–10C). Hemostasis by ligature is preferable to cautery, since too-free use of cautery may obscure the topography in a small opening. The location of the lesion is identified with the forefinger. If it is not directly beneath the incision, it is necessary to tunnel bluntly with scissors, pushing and spreading, to the desired location while upward and lateral traction is maintained on the margins of the dissection. With a finger on the lesion, the surgeon will usually have a better understanding of its size, consistency, and mobility and will be able to assess its structure with a fair degree of accuracy. Lesions less than 5 cm in diameter and probably malignant should be sharply excised with a surrounding margin of normal tissue (Fig. 10–10D). Larger malignant tumors should be

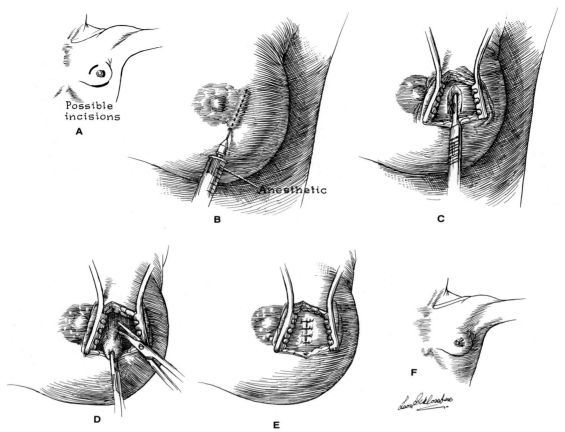

FIG. 10–10 Open biopsy. (*A*) For cosmetic reasons circumareolar incisions are preferable when the lesion is thought to be within 2 cm or 3 cm of the areola. Not more than one-half of the areolar margin should be incised. A curved incision parallel to the areola is made over lesions further out from the center. When malignant disease is strongly suspected, the surgeon should attempt to avoid the probable path of the subsequent mastectomy incision. (*B*) An intradermal weal is raised along the path of the proposed incision using 1% lidocaine and a hypodermic (No. 25) needle. From the weal, deeper injections of anesthetic are made around the circumference of the lesion and beneath it. (*C*) The incision is carried down through the dense subcutaneous tissue and into the lobule containing the lesion. Self-retaining retractors are helpful when an assistant is not available. (*D*) If the lesion is small or easily mobilized, it should be sharply dissected and excised with a thin margin of adjacent tissue. (*E*) The lobular defect is sutured with fine absorbable suture material if the closure places no tension on the overlying skin. Bleeding is controlled with absorbable ligatures or electrocoagulation. Absolute hemostasis is essential. (*F*) The skin is closed with interrupted No. 5-0 silk or nylon sutures. Drainage is seldom necessary. A pressure dressing for 24 hours is desirable if a significant amount of dead space has been left behind.

sampled by a representative V-shaped wedge of tissue, since total excision might require a difficult operation with significant blood loss (Fig. 10–11). Should the original biopsy prove negative on frozen section, additional biopsies, either with the knife or with a cutting needle, must be taken. Large cysts are often dark blue, and these may be aspirated and a piece of the wall taken for histologic verification. The giant fibroadenomas occasionally seen in adolescence and early adult life should be completely excised because of their low potential for malignancy.

Once the judgment has been made to excise the lesion, the surgeon places a small self-retaining retractor in the wound and grasps the tissue immediately overlying the lesion with Allis clamp or tooth forceps. Minor bleeding, which can obscure the field, must be controlled at each step. Although it

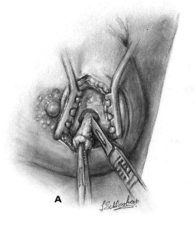
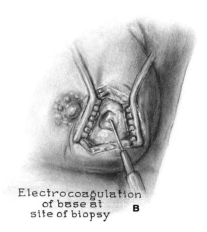

Electrocoagulation
of base at
site of biopsy **B**

FIG. 10–11 Incisional biopsy. (*A*) When a large (greater than 5 cm) or very adherent lesion is encountered, especially when carcinoma is strongly suspected, a wedge of tissue of approximately 1 cc in volume is excised from the exposed surface of the tumor and sent for frozen section. The base of the incision is usually coagulated to control bleeding. If the first pathology report is negative, additional biopsies may be necessary.

is possible to perform the operation alone, an assistant is very helpful in keeping the field clear and providing countertraction. Maintaining traction on the tissue to be resected, the surgeon proceeds to enucleate it with small curved scissors (see Fig. 10–10D). Blunt dissection is of little help when there are no well-defined tissue planes. Frequent pauses are necessary to evaluate the scope of the dissection and thus avoid cutting into the lesion or removing too much normal lobular tissue. The clamp raising the lesion is shifted around its periphery as the dissection progresses to provide better exposure of the underside.

After removal of the tumor, the lobular defect is closed with fine absorbable suture material, taking care that these sutures do not cause retraction or dimpling of the overlying skin (Fig. 10–10E). If any part of this closure involves tension on the suture, it is best to omit it. All bleeding must be controlled before the defect is closed. When the dead space left in the breast after excision is large, no effort should be made to obliterate it with subcutaneous sutures, since they are almost certain to cause distortion. Such dead space will probably lead to the accumulation of serous fluid postoperatively. In the absence of infection, the wound is closed without drainage, using a subcuticular stitch of fine absorbable suture material and interrupted No. 5-0 nylon in the skin (Fig. 10–10F). A pressure dressing for the first 24 hours is desirable, but may not be necessary in relatively minor cases. The sutures should be removed in not more than 6 days to prevent scarring and Steri-strips should be applied as necessary.

When the bloody nipple discharge suggests the likelihood of one or more intraductal papillomas, sharp dissection is carried medially from a circumareolar incision placed in the breast quadrant that

pressure tests have indicated is most likely to be the source of the bleeding. Directly beneath the nipple, the main ducts are encountered and placed on traction with a small hook (Fig. 10–12). The ducts are followed down until the lesion is encountered, usually not more than 3 or 4 cm from the surface. Papillomas are dark red and soft, and may be multiple. A generous portion of the duct system around the diseased area is resected, and the severed ends

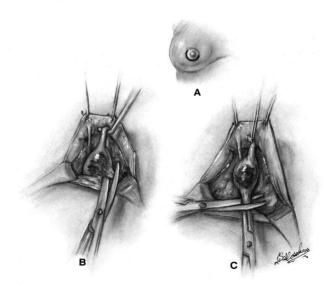

FIG. 10–12 Ductal exploration and resection of papilloma. (*A*) The incision is circumareolar and toward the quadrant most likely to be the site of the lesion. (*B*) With traction on the main duct, peripheral branches are dissected out until lesion is identified. (*C*) The duct system above and below the lesion is clamped, and the portion containing the lesion is excised.

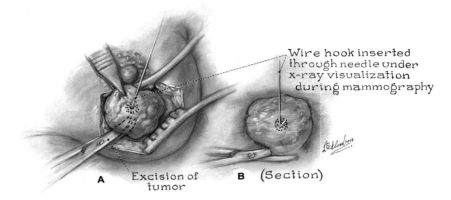

FIG. 10-13 Directed biopsy of nonpalpable lesions. (*A*) The incision has been directed downward to the insertion of the flexible hook in the vicinity of the lesion, and an appropriate volume of tissue around it is being undermined. (*B*) The lesion with at least 1 cc of surrounding tissue is resected and sent to Radiology for verification and then to Pathology. If the lesion is not identified in the specimen by x-ray, an additional volume of tissue must be resected.

are ligated (Fig. 10–12B, C). Usually, there is a relatively small defect that need not be closed, and care must be taken not to cause retraction of the nipple by suturing. Inverting the nipple and scraping all ductal tissue from the undersurface has been advocated but seems unnecessary in most cases.

Nonpalpable lesions noted on mammograms must be investigated. Often these consist of clusters of tiny calcifications that may represent the earliest stage of a malignant process and that may, therefore, have the best possible prognosis if resected early. The procedure must be done in cooperation with a radiologist interested in breast disease. Under continuous x-ray visualization, the radiologist inserts a special needle until the tip is in close proximity to the lesion. A fine wire with a reverse hook on one end is passed through the needle and beyond it and is then pulled back until the hook engages near the lesion. The needle is withdrawn. The wire is stabilized at the skin level with tape, and the patient is carefully removed to the operating room on a stretcher. Under these circumstances, some surgeons prefer general anesthesia, but in most instances the operation can be done with local. The incision is made as previously noted, but subcutaneously the dissection is directed toward the wire and carried down toward its tip. A block of tissue 2 cm or more in diameter is resected from the area under suspicion and sent back to the radiologist, who x-rays it again to determine whether the suspicious calcifications are present (Fig. 10–13). If they are, the tissue is sent to the pathologist, but if they are not, the surgeon must repeat the biopsies until successful.

All the tissue removed, including fat, must be sent to the pathologist. It is the pathologist's duty to see that a portion of the specimen is sent to the laboratory for assay of estrogen and progesterone receptors, but it is not safe to assume that this will happen. Formerly, an assay of estrogen receptors

alone was considered sufficient, but recent evidence indicates that progesterone receptors are an even better marker of hormone dependence and that the two together are superior to either alone. The remaining tissue is divided into blocks so that representative frozen sections can be taken from each area. The report should be available within 20 minutes once it has reached the laboratory and should be better than 99% accurate.

After receiving the report, the surgeon can discuss modalities of future treatment and their pros and cons with the patient and her spouse or counselor. The possible complications of the biopsy procedure are also discussed. These include skin ecchymoses, hemorrhage, seromas, and infection. Ecchymoses clear within a few days, but acute hemorrhage requires immediate reopening of the wound. Chronic accumulation of blood and serous fluid, forming an enlarging pocket, may require evacuation through the wound and constant drainage but often can be reduced by percutaneous needle aspiration. Pain is seldom a factor postoperatively, and no convalescence or loss of working time is usually necessary.

Hospital Procedures

Several different approaches to augmentation mammoplasty are currently used. The incision may be made beneath the breast along the skin attachment to the chest wall or in a circumareolar position at the pigmented border. The latter leaves a more nearly invisible scar, but both are cosmetically satisfactory. Through either incision, the prosthesis, usually a nonreactive plastic envelope filled with silicone gel, may be placed between the breast tissue and the anterior surface of the pectoralis major muscle. This location provides a good contour for the breast, but has the disadvantage in some cases of the late development of a fibrotic periprosthetic capsule that gradually puckers the external outline of the breast and may cause discomfort. To avoid this long-term complication, some surgeons split the muscle fibers of the pectoralis major and insert the prosthesis beneath it. This provides excellent long-term stability, but the protrusion of the breast above it is less accentuated and therefore less natural in appearance. All modifications of technique are subject to the short-term risks of hemorrhage and infection, which may require removal of the prosthesis, and the long-term risk of displacement. Sensation is usually preserved and lactation may occur following pregnancy, but nursing should not be recommended.

Women at serious risk for the development of breast cancer as a result of a bad family history or the presence of precancerous mastopathy and those who have the type of dense breasts that make both physical examination and mammography less definitive may have subcutaneous mastectomy and the insertion of a prosthesis recommended as a prophylactic measure. Because of the close attachment of the breast tissue to the skin, the presence of the axillary tail, and the possibility that there are extensions of breast tissue beyond its observed perimeter and into the pectoral muscle, the operation is often incomplete, and carcinomas have been reported in the residual breast tissue. Silicone implants are most commonly used following resection, but subcutaneous Dacron screens or shields have also been employed. Postoperatively, there is usually loss of sensation as well as loss of function, and complications can include skin necrosis over the prosthesis. Indications for this procedure remain poorly defined, but lately have been extended by some to include patients with severe breast pain and those with a high level of anxiety concerning cancer. It seems reasonable at present to restrict the operation to individuals in the very high risk group.

Reduction mammoplasties must be carefully tailored to the size and degree of ptosis of the breast to be reconstructed, and for this reason many different types of plastic procedures have been devised to fit the various special circumstances. All have the disadvantage of a clearly visible scar, usually transverse, across the remolded breast, and, because of the necessity to resect large areas of skin with resultant tension on the closure, these scars are likely to stretch with time, and keloid formation is not unusual. A variety of ingeniously placed incisions have been devised to hide and reduce the scarring, many of which require relocation of the nipple, areola, and a portion of the surrounding skin. In some instances, it has been possible to resect pie-shaped sections of breast tissue without affecting function in young people afflicted with severe mammary hypertrophy. The goal of forming a saucer-shaped or conical breast of normal volume is usually realized, but complications in the healing process are not uncommon. The operations are done in the hospital under general anesthesia and require several days convalescence.

Until 10 years ago, the Halsted type of radical mastectomy was the standard treatment for breast cancer against which all other modalities were measured, and it still has its adherents. With the gradual realization that local control of the disease is only one factor in determining the success of treatment and that systemic spread accounts for a preponderance of the failures, there has been a step-by-step reduction in the extent of surgery, to the point where some surgeons feel that the pendulum has swung too far the other way. A broad spectrum of operations is being performed by surgeons with widely divergent opinions about the scope of surgery necessary for different stages of disease. The TNM staging taxonomy recommended by the American Joint Committee for Cancer Staging and End Results Reporting in 1978 has gained increasing popularity and is now used by most cancer centers. T1 tumors, less than 2 cm in diameter, are those usually selected for lesser procedures such as lumpectomy (tylectomy) and quadrantectomy, which in practice conform to what their names suggest. The removal of a large pie-shaped wedge of the breast (quadrantectomy) is an attempt to get a wider tumor-free margin around the primary lesion than can be obtained with a simple lumpectomy, but without plastic reconstruction the cosmetic effect is not pleasing. It is customary on most large services to perform a concomitant resection of the lymph nodes at levels I and II, whether or not they are palpable, as a form of surgical staging that may determine future adjunctive therapy. Operations less than total mastectomy are usually followed by local irradiation, either from external sources or implanted radioisotopes like iridium, which produces a certain amount of fibrosis but permits the retention of a reasonably normal breast contour. Results from these simple operations have been widely publicized as equal in effectiveness to mastectomy, and the female public has been quick to appreciate any alteration in traditional methods that will provide improved retention of their femininity, but published reports deal largely with early cases selected for lesser procedures. Continuing trials of less radical surgery are certainly indicated on the basis of current evidence, however.

The modified radical mastectomy differs from the Halsted type, in that the pectoralis major and minor muscles are usually preserved, providing better arm motion and thoracic outline and reducing the incidence of postoperative lymphedema of the arm. It is probably the procedure most frequently used today for breast cancer. The Madden variant permits retention of the pectoralis minor and, by retracting both pectoralis muscles medially, the resection of lymph nodes to level II. The Patey operation, which is done with the arm on the affected side fully extended above the head rather than at a right angle to the body, requires resection of the pectoralis minor for better exposure, which facilitates resection of the more medial lymph nodes. Since the available data do not indicate that resection for cure of lymph nodes involved by tumor improves the prognosis, it has been suggested that simple mastectomy might serve the same purpose.

Following all types of mastectomy, radiotherapy to the chest wall, the internal mammary lymph nodes, and sometimes the dissected axilla has been customary for patients whose final pathologic report indicates the presence of lymph node metastases. This traditional approach is now in transition, since radiotherapy has not been found effective in controlling lymph node metastases or hematogenous spread, and there is some question about its efficacy in preventing chest wall recurrences.

Reconstruction procedures following modified radical and simple mastectomies have become increasingly common. These are done either at the time of mastectomy or after healing, but preferably prior to irradiation. The original line of incision about the breast, which is usually obliquely downward from the axilla to the origin of the rectus muscle, or horizontally from axilla to sternum, may be somewht modified if it is known beforehand that reconstruction is desired, so long as the modification does not compromise adequate envelopment of the tumor. It may be possible thus to save skin in an uninvolved area, which would be helpful in the secondary procedure. For those who feel that an external prosthesis is adequate for their self-image, many different types of garments are available in medical supply and department stores.

Since the radical mastectomy and its extensions—designed to remove tumor-bearing lymph nodes in the chest, neck and clavicular areas, followed by external irradiation—failed to improve survival rates during an entire generation, it became evident that a better prognosis would have to be achieved by a systemic attack on micrometastases, presumed to exist at the time of surgery, but not definable by current x-ray or laboratory studies. Before the advent of modern chemotherapy, it was well known that breast cancers were sensitive to changes in their hormonal environment, and the first attempt at systemic control was combined radical mastectomy and prophylactic oophorectomy. Although imperfect in their planning by today's standards, early reports suggested that oophorectomy prolonged the time to first recurrence but did not affect long-term survival. Another school of thought advocated therapeutic oophorectomy at the time of first recurrence, and the estrogen sensitivity of the tumor was assessed by the administration of estrogens to determine whether the patient's symptoms improved or became worse. A beneficial response to oophorectomy was often followed by adrenalectomy or even hypophysectomy, and these surgical procedures, either singly or in combination, were given extensive clinical trials by various groups, often with conflicting interpretation of results.

Beginning with the alkylating agents, chemotherapy was used prophylactically following mastectomy in the late 1950s without discernible benefit. From that time, new drugs, as they became available, have been tried both prophylactically and therapeutically in various combinations with some improvement in results in the latter group, but no breakthrough in the former until recently, when well-controlled studies here and abroad demonstrated that a relatively prolonged disease-free interval could be achieved in premenopausal patients having one or more positive axillary lymph nodes. Single agents did not prove as effective as combinations in high dosage administered early. There was no similar advantage for postmenopausal women.

Many questions remain to be answered regarding the routine use of adjuvant chemotherapy for breast cancer, not the least of which is whether women should be treated whether or not they have positive lymph nodes. The optimum combination of drugs has yet to be determined, as have the size of the dose and the duration of treatment. The role of estrogens, androgens, progestins, and antiestrogens is not clearly defined, but manipulation of the hormonal milieu is likely to be effective only in patients with known positive receptor sites and in those who are premenopausal, or postmenopausal for less than 5 years. Hormonal treatment, whether ablative or additive, also works better in those who have had a long disease-free interval or in whom the metastases are largely confined to bone. It is possible that hormonal therapy should be combined with chemotherapy, but there are no data to indicate when or how this should be attempted. It is reasonably clear that hormonal therapy alone should not be used prophylactically or therapeutically as the first-line choice in all instances just because it is well tolerated. Stem cell assays have not provided the answer to the proper selection of chemotherapeutic agents, and, for the present, it will continue to be necessary to make judgments regarding appropriate treatment on an individual basis.

Bibliography

American Joint Committee for Cancer Staging and End-Results Reporting: Staging of Cancer of the Breast: Manual for Staging of Cancer, pp. 101–108. Chicago, Whiting Press, 1978

Barnes AB: Current Concepts: Diagnosis and treatment of abnormal breast secretions. N Engl J Med 275:1184, 1966

Beale S, Lisper H, Palm B: A psychological study of patients seeking augmentation mammaplasty. Br J Psychiatry 136:133, 1980

Biggs TM, Cukier J, Worthing LF: Augmentation mammaplasty: A review of 18 years. Plast Reconstr Surg 69:445, 1982

Bolsen B: Ultrasound breast scanning: (only) A complement to mammography? JAMA 248:1025, 1982

Bonadonna G, Valagussa P: Dose-response effect of adjuvant chemotherapy in breast cancer. N Engl J Med 304:10, 1981

Brinton LA, Hoover R, Fraumeni JF, Jr: Epidemiology of minimal breast cancer. JAMA 249:483, 1983

Carlsen E: Transillumination light scanning. Diagn Imaging 51:1, 1982

Carter SK: Adjuvant chemotherapy of breast cancer. N Engl J Med 304:45, 1981

Clark GM, McGuire WL, Hubay CA, et al: Progesterone receptors as a prognostic factor in stage II breast cancer. N Engl J Med 309:1343, 1983

Cole–Beuglet C: Sonographic manifestations of malignant breast disease. In Raymond HW, Swiebel WJ (eds): Seminars in Ultrasound, pp. 51–57. New York, Grune and Stratton, 1982

Croll J, Kotevich J, Tabrett M: The diagnosis of benign disease and the exclusion of malignancy in patients with breast symptoms. In Raymond HW, Swiebel WJ (eds): Seminars in Ultrasound, pp. 38–50. New York, Grune and Stratton, 1982

Foster RS, Jr, Lang SP, Costanza MC, et al: Breast self-examination practices and breast-cancer stage. N Engl J Med 299:265, 1978

Goldwyn RM: Subcutaneous mastectomy. N Engl J Med 297:503, 1977

Golinger RC: Hormones and the pathophysiology of fibrocystic mastopathy. Surg Gynecol Obstet 146:273, 1978

Greenwald P, Nasca PC, Lawrence CE, et al: Estimated effect of breast self-examination and routine physician examinations on breast-cancer mortality. N Engl J Med 299:271, 1978

Gruber RP, Friedman GD: Periareolar subpectoral augmentation mammaplasty. Plast Reconstr Surg 67:453, 1981

Haagensen CD, Bodian C, Haagensen DE, Jr: Breast Carcinoma. Risk and Detection. Philadelphia, WB Saunders, 1981

Handley RS: The conservative radical mastectomy of Patey: 10-year results in 425 patients. Breast Dis Breast 2:16, 1976

Harper P, Kelly–Fry E: Ultrasound visualization of the breast in symptomatic patients. Radiology 137:465, 1980

Henderson IC: Breast Cancer Management Progress and Prospects, pp. 3–31. Wayne, New Jersey, Lederle Laboratories, 1982

Hindle WH, Navin J: Breast aspiration cytology: A neglected gynecologic procedure. Am J Obstet Gynecol 146:482, 1983

Jones WD, III, Reed ML: What you should know about reconstructive breast surgery. Contemp Obstet Gynecol 22:177, 1983

Kleinberg DL, Noel GL, Frantz AG: Galactorrhea: A study of 235 cases, including 48 with pituitary tumors. N Engl J Med 296:589, 1977

Koivuniemi AP: Fine-needle aspiration biopsy of the breast. Ann Clin Res 8:272, 1976

LiVolsi VA, Stadel BV, Kelsey JL, et al: Fibrocystic breast disease in oral-contraceptive users: A histopathological evaluation of epithelial atypia. N Engl J Med 299:381, 1978

Love SM, Gelman RS, Silen W: Fibrocystic "disease" of the breast: A nondisease? N Engl J Med 307:1010, 1982

Letterman G, Schurter M: The effects of mammary hypertrophy on the skeletal system. Ann Plast Surg 5:425, 1980

London RS, Solomon DM, London ED, et al: Mammary dysplasia: Clinical response and urinary excretions of 11-deoxy-17-ketosteroids and pregnanediol following α-tocopherol therapy. Breast Dis Breast 4:19, 1976

Mahler D, Hauben DJ: Retromammary versus retropectoral breast augmentation: A comparative study. Ann Plast Surg 8:370, 1982

Marchac D, de Olarte G: Reduction mammaplasty and correction of ptosis with a short-inframammary scar. Plast Reconstr Surg 69:45, 1982

McGuire WL, De La Garza M, Chamness GC: Evaluation of estrogen receptor assays in human breast cancer tissue. Cancer Res 37:637, 1977

McSwain GR, Valicenti JF, Jr, O'Brien PH: Cytologic evaluation of breast cysts. Surg Gynecol Obstet 146:921, 1978

Minton JP, Abou-Issa H, Reiches N, et al: Clinical and biochemical studies on methylxanthine-related fibrocystic breast disease. Surgery 90:299, 1981

Mitchell GW, Jr: The gynecologist and breast disease. Clin Obstet Gynecol 20:865, 1977

Mitchell GW, Jr, Homer MJ: Outpatient breast biopsies on a gynecologic service. Am J Obstet Gynecol 144:127, 1982

Moskowitz M: Clinical examination of the breasts by non-physicians: A viable screening option? Cancer 44:311, 1979

Moskowitz M: Mammography in medical practice. JAMA 240:1898, 1978

Moskowitz M, Fig SA, Cole–Beuglet C, et al: Evaluation of new imaging procedures for breast cancer: Proper process. Am J Roentgenol 140:591, 1983

Moskowitz M, Fox SH, Brun del Re R, et al: The potential value of liquid-crystal thermography in detecting significant mastopathy. Radiology 140:659, 1981

Moxley JH, III, Allegra JC, Henney J, et al: Treatment of primary breast cancer. JAMA 244:797, 1980

Nezhat C, Asch RH, Greenblatt RB: Danazol for benign breast disease. Am J Obstet Gynecol 137:604, 1980

Original Contributions: The Centers for Disease Control, Cancer and Steroid Hormone Study. Long-term oral contraceptive use and the risk of breast cancer. JAMA 249:1591, 1983

Parkes D: Drug therapy—Bromocriptine. N Engl J Med 301:873, 1979

Puga FJ, Welch JS, Bisel HF: Therapeutic oophorectomy in disseminated carcinoma of the breast. Arch Surg 111:877, 1976

Rimsten A, Stenkvist B, Johanson H, et al: The diagnostic accuracy of palpation and fine-needle biopsy and an evaluation of their combined use in the diagnosis of breast lesions. Ann Surg 182:1, 1975

Ross RJ, Thompson JS, Kim K, et al: Nuclear magnetic resonance imaging and evaluation of human breast tissue: Preliminary clinical trials. Radiology 143:195, 1982

Schneck CD, Lehman DA: Sonographic anatomy of the breast. In Raymond HW, Swiebel WJ (eds): Seminars in Ultrasound, pp. 13–33. New York, Grune and Stratton, 1982

Schwartz GF, Marchant D (eds): Breast Disease Diagnosis and Treatment. Miami, Florida, Symposia Specialists, 1981

Senn HJ: Current status and indications for adjuvant therapy in breast cancer. Cancer Chemother Pharmacol 8:139, 1982

Snyder RE, Watson RC, Cruz N: Graphic stress telethermometry (GST^tm). Am J Diag Gynecol Obstet 1:197, 1979

Speroff L: The breast as an endocrine target organ. Contemp Obstet Gynecol 9:69, 1977

Veronesi U, Saccozzi R, Del Vecchio, M, et al: Comparing radical mastectomy with quadrantectomy, axillary dissection, and radiotherapy in patients with small cancers of the breast. N Engl J Med 305:6, 1981

Walker GM, Foster RS, Jr, McKegney CP, et al: Breast biopsy. Arch Surg 113:942, 1978

Willett WC, MacMahon B: Diet and cancer: An overview. Part II. N Engl J Med 310:697, 1984

Wolfe JN: Breast patterns as an index of risk for developing breast cancer. Am J Roentgenol 126:1130, 1976

Wolfe JN: Current status of xeroradiography. Breast Dis Breast 2:17, 1976

Chapter 11

Leiomyomata Uteri and Abdominal Hysterectomy for Benign Disease

LEIOMYOMATA UTERI

A leiomyoma is a benign tumor composed mainly of smooth muscle cells but containing varying amounts of fibrous connective tissue. The tumor is well circumscribed but not encapsulated. Various terms used to refer to the tumor include *fibromyoma, myofibroma, leiomyofibroma, fibroleiomyoma, myoma, fibroma,* and *fibroid,* the last designation being the most commonly used and the least accurate. The term *leiomyoma* is preferred as a reasonably accurate one that emphasizes the origin of this tumor from smooth muscle cells and the predominance of the smooth muscle component. The tissue culture work of Miller and Ludovici suggested an origin from smooth muscle cells. The studies of Linder and Gartler and of Townsend and associates suggest a unicellular origin for leiomyomata.

Leiomyomata are the most common tumors of the uterus and female pelvis. It is impossible to determine their true incidence accurately, although the incidence frequently quoted of 50% found at postmortem examinations seems reasonable. Leiomyomata are responsible for approximately one-third of all hospital admissions to gynecology services. It is well recognized that the incidence is much greater in the black race than in the white. In a careful study of leiomyomata among women in Augusta, Georgia, Torpin and associates found the incidence among black women to be three and one-third times that among white women. There is no explanation for this racial difference. Leiomyomata also are larger and occur at a younger age in black women. Indeed, we have removed a large intramural leiomyoma that had undergone acute degeneration from a 14-year-old black girl in whom the tumor had enlarged the uterus to the level of the umbilicus. In black women, leiomyomata are not uncommon before 30 years of age. However, they are uncommon in either race before 20 years of age.

The growth of leiomyomata is dependent on estrogen production. The tumors thrive during the years of greatest ovarian activity. Following the menopause, with regression of ovarian estrogen secretion, growth of leiomyomata usually ceases. Actual regression in the tumor size may occur. There are rare instances, however, of postmenopausal growth of benign leiomyomata, suggesting the possibility of postmenopausal estrogen production either in the ovary or elsewhere. Woodruff has demonstrated the production of estrogen from postmenopausal ovarian stroma in a variety of presumably inactive ovarian tumors, including mucinous cysts and Brenner tumors. However, where uterine leiomyomata grow after the menopause, one should think first of the possibility of malignant change in the leiomyoma itself.

The observation that leiomyomata frequently show significant enlargement during pregnancy provides further clinical evidence of the relation of estrogen to the growth of these tumors, although admittedly a better blood supply during pregnancy might also encourage their growth. During the past two decades, furthermore, there has been a striking increase in the occurrence of large leiomyomata among young women of all racial backgrounds who have taken oral contraceptives that contain estrogen. Although growth of uterine leiomyomata is not invariably stimulated, oral contraceptives containing estrogen should be prescribed with caution in women with these tumors.

Scientific investigators have been intrigued by the observation that leiomyomata develop during the reproductive years, grow during pregnancy, and regress following the menopause. Nelson, Lipschutz and others have produced multiple leiomyomata artificially on the serosal surface of the uterus and other peritoneal surfaces in guinea pigs given prolonged estrogen injections. Spellacy found that levels of plasma estradiol were the same in patients with and without leiomyomata. However, Wilson and associates found a significantly higher concentration of estrogen receptors in leiomyomata than in myometrium. Farber and associates reported that these tumors bind approximately 20% more estradiol per milligram of cytoplasmic protein than does the normal myometrium of the same organ. This observation was not uniformly true for all leiomyomata, suggesting that different cellular components within a leiomyoma may be associated with different biologic activity. Otubu and associates found the concentration of estradiol to be significantly higher in leiomyomata than in the myometrium, especially in the proliferative phase of the menstrual cycle. Soules and McCarty reported that leiomyomata had more estrogen receptors than normal uterine tissues in the first phase (days 1–9) and second phase (days 10–18) of the menstrual cycle. Gabb and Stone found that the ability to convert estradiol to estrone was similar in leiomyomata and myometrium. However, Polow and associates found significantly lower conversion of estradiol into estrone in leiomyomata than in myometrium. This difference in conversion rate could result in a relative accumulation of estrogen in a leiomyoma, resulting in a hyperestrogenic state within the tumor and surrounding tissues. The enzyme 17-β-hydroxy dehydrogenase accelerates the conversion of estradiol to estrone. Leiomyomata have a low concentration of 17-β-hydroxy dehydrogenase, resulting in a relative accumulation of estradiol in leiomyomatous tissue.

Other abnormalities in endocrine function have also been suggested. Ylikorkala and associates found that pituitary function may be abnormal in women with leiomyomata. Patients with leiomyomata had a low follicle-stimulating hormone level and a diminished follicle-stimulating hormone response to pituitary gonadotropin-releasing hormone. There was an excessive prolactin response to thyrotropin releasing hormone. Spellacy found that the peak levels of human growth hormone reached during a hypoglycemic test were twice as high in patients with leiomyomata as in the control group. Reddy and Rose suggest the possibility that 5-α-reduced androgens may play a role in the pathophysiology of uterine leiomyomata, since a significant increase in 5-α-reductase has been found in leiomyoma tissue

as compared to myometrium and endometrium. When the pathogenesis of leiomyomata is clearly understood, it may be possible to control their growth with medical/endocrine therapy. Influenced by the experimental investigations of Lipschutz and associates, Goodman in 1946 treated patients with uterine leiomyomata with progesterone and noted a decrease in tumor size in all patients. However, Segaloff and associates reported no effect in their study. Goldzieher and associates produced histologic evidence of extensive degenerative changes in leiomyomata by administration of high-dosage progestin therapy (medrogestrone in high doses for 21 days). Filicori and associates have reported the regression of a uterine leiomyoma following long-term administration of a long-acting luteinizing hormone-releasing hormone agonist given to suppress ovarian estrogen secretion. Coutinho successfully used a potent 19-norsteroid antiestrogen/antiprogesterone to treat excessive uterine bleeding in 16 patients with uterine leiomyomata. A reduction in the size of the tumors was noted. Thus, effective medical/endocrine therapy may be possible in the near future.

To treat patients with uterine leiomyomata properly, the gynecologic surgeon must be familiar with their pathology, growth characteristics, and clinical features. Leiomyomata may be single, but the vast majority are multiple. They develop most commonly in the uterine corpus and much less often in the cervix. Rarely, they may develop in the round ligaments. Since they arise in the myometrium, they are all interstitial or intramural in the beginning. As they enlarge, they may remain intramural, but growth often extends in an internal or external direction. Thus, the tumor becomes subserous or submucous in location. A subserous tumor may become pedunculated and occasionally parasitic, receiving its blood supply from another source, usually the omentum. A submucous tumor may also become pedunculated and may gradually dilate the endocervical canal and protrude through the cervical os. Indeed, it may descend through the vagina. Rarely, chronic uterine inversion may result if the prolapsing submucous leiomyoma is attached to the top of the endometrial cavity.

In general, subserous leiomyomata contain more fibrous tissue than submucous leiomyomata. On the other hand, submucous leiomyomata contain more smooth muscle tissue than subserous leiomyomata. Sarcomatous change is more common in submucous tumors.

The typical uterine leiomyoma is a firm multinodular structure of variable size. The largest tumor, reported by Hunt in 1888, weighed over 65 kg. Tumors of 4 kg to 5 kg are not rare, but most are smaller. At the operating table, leiomyomata appear as nodular tumors of different sizes that distort the uterus in various ways, depending on their size and direction of growth. Growth between the leaves of the broad ligament and origin from the cervix may make surgical removal difficult. Subserous and subserous pedunculated tumors as well as intraligamentous tumors may create problems in diagnosis since they are difficult to distinguish from tumors arising from the adnexal organs. When tumors cause symmetrical enlargement of the uterus, they may be mistaken for a pregnant uterus on bimanual examination.

The normal leiomyoma, on section, appears pinkish-white and gray glistening. It is firm, and there is a whorl-like arrangement of the muscle and the fibrous tissue. The most common change is hyaline degeneration. The cut surface of a hyalinized area is smooth and homogeneous and does not show the whorl-like arrangement of the rest of the leiomyoma. Almost all leiomyomas, except the smallest, have scattered areas of hyaline degeneration. Eventually these may become liquified and form cystic cavities filled with clear liquid or gelatinous material. Sometimes the cystic change is so great that the leiomyoma becomes a mere shell and is a truly cystic tumor. Softness of a tumor does not necessarily indicate cystic degeneration. Fleshy leiomyomata may be equally soft.

Over time, with continued diminished blood supply and ischemic necrosis of tissue, calcium phosphates and carbonates are deposited. Their presence is evidence of a continuum of degenerative changes. The calcium may be deposited in varying amounts. If it is deposited at the periphery of the tumor, the leiomyoma may resemble a calcified cyst. Other calcified leiomyomata may show an irregular or diffuse distribution throughout with a honeycomb or mulberry appearance. When the degenerative change is advanced, the leiomyoma may become solidly calcified. Such calcified tumors have been called "wombstones." Calcified leiomyomata are seen most often in elderly women, in blacks, and in women who have pedunculated subserous tumors. They are easily seen radiographically.

Leiomyomata may undergo changes as a result of infection. Submucous leiomyomata are most commonly infected when they protrude into the uterine cavity or especially into the vagina. The pedunculated submucous leiomyoma thins out the endometrium as it grows downward, and eventually the surface becomes ulcerated and infected. An intramural leiomyoma in an involuting puerperal uterus may also become infected in association with endometritis. Microscopic abscesses are frequently found and gross abscesses occasionally oc-

cur, particularly if the leiomyoma descends as low as the cervical canal. Such infections are usually streptococcal and may be very virulent. *Bacteroides fragilis* infections also occur. Parametritis, peritonitis, and even septicemia may result.

Necrosis of a leiomyoma is caused by interference with its blood supply. Occasionally a pedunculated subserous leiomyoma twists, and if an operation is not done immediately, infarction results. Necrosis sometimes occurs in the center of a large tumor simply as a result of poor circulation. Necrotic leiomyomata are dark and hemorrhagic in the interior. Eventually the tissue breaks down completely. So-called red or carneous degeneration is seen occasionally, especially in association with pregnancy. This condition is thought to result from poor circulation of blood through a rapidly growing tumor. Thrombosis and extravasation of blood are responsible for the reddish discoloration.

On occasions, fat occurs in leiomyomata as true fatty degeneration. The cut surface may be given a yellowish discoloration. Still more rarely, a deposit of true fat may form a fibrolipoma. However, the presence of fat in a leiomyoma is quite rare. Indeed, if fat is seen grossly or microscopically in a curettage specimen, one should not assume that it represents fatty degeneration of a leiomyoma. One should assume that the uterus has been perforated and fragments of fats have been curetted from the mesentery or omentum.

Finally, the most important change in a leiomyoma is sarcomatous degeneration. Fortunately it is rare. There is much variation in the reported incidence of sarcoma in leiomyomata. The incidence given by Novak is 0.7%. However, a review of 13,000 myomas by Montague, Swartz, and Woodruff at Johns Hopkins revealed 38 cases of malignant change, the incidence of sarcoma thus being 0.29%. Corscaden and Singh indicated by their study that the true incidence of sarcoma developing within uterine leiomyomata is no more than 0.13%, and probably as low as 0.04%. It should be remembered that since most women with uterine leiomyomata do not undergo surgical removal, the true incidence of sarcoma in leiomyomata is probably much less than one per 1000 (0.1%). The difficulty in defining the true incidence of sarcomatous change is understandable if one is familiar with the histology of leiomyomata. Very cellular leiomyomata are relatively common, and at first glance they suggest sarcoma; however, they lack a significant number of mitotic figures, and patients from whom such tumors are removed all remain well. The misinterpretation of the histologic picture of this type of cellular leiomyoma undoubtedly accounts for the increased incidence of leiomyosarcoma reported by some. On cutting leiomyomata in the operating room, the surgeon will find that sarcomatous areas have a somewhat characteristic appearance, although the histologic diagnosis certainly cannot be made by gross examination. A sarcoma is apt to occur in a rather large leiomyoma and toward the center of the tumor, where the blood supply is poorest. Instead of being firm fibrous tissue, which grates when scraped with a knife blade, the tissue is soft and homogenous. Cullen has described it as resembling raw pork. Later, as necrosis of the malignant tissue occurs, it becomes more friable and hemorrhagic.

It has been difficult to understand uterine leiomyosarcoma because pathologists do not agree on the criteria necessary for diagnosis. Some pathologists rely on the mitotic count. All tumors with less than five mitotic figures per 10 high-power fields are considered benign. All tumors with more than 10 mitotic figures per 10 high-power fields are called malignant. Those in between may be called "smooth muscle tumors of uncertain malignant potential." Other pathologists believe the mitotic count may have some significance but choose to rely instead on the presence of nuclear hyperchromatism, nuclear pleomorphism, or the presence of giant cells and other bizarre cell forms to make the diagnosis. Corscaden and Singh believe that no combination of histologic features is reliable and that only smooth muscle tumors that metastasize or recur are definitely malignant. We believe all of these features should be taken into consideration in diagnosis and prognosis. When the tumor is confined to the uterus, both mitotic and histologic grade are important in diagnosis and prognosis. A poor prognosis is associated with high mitotic counts and extremely atypical and anaplastic cytologic features. Tumors that show obvious evidence of blood vessel invasion or spread to contiguous organs are rarely cured. The extent of the disease at the time of initial diagnosis is of even greater significance. In other words, when the diagnosis is suspected for the first time by the pathologist when he examines routine sections from a uterine leiomyoma, the patient will almost always survive. On the other hand, if the diagnosis is made preoperatively by the gynecologist or is suspected during the operative procedure because of invasion of surrounding organs, the prognosis is extremely grave.

An unusual atypical smooth muscle tumor of the uterus was first described in the stomach by Martin and associates in 1960. Variously called uterine bizarre leiomyoma, leiomyoblastoma, clear-cell leiomyoma, and plexiform tumorlet, these atypical smooth tumors probably all belong together. The term *epithelioid leiomyoma* was adopted by WHO.

Kurman and Norris have proposed that this term be used for all atypical leiomyomata. Histologically, the characteristic feature is the mixture of rounded polygonal cells and multinucleated giant cells present in epithelioid clear-cell and plexiform patterns. Clinically, most of these tumors are benign. They may rarely exhibit malignant potential. Malignancy is difficult to predict from histologic criteria, since some metastases have occurred from tumors that demonstrated very few mitoses. Kurman and Norris have suggested, however, that epithelioid neoplasms having more than five mitotic figures per 10 high-power fields should be called epithelioid leiomyosarcomas, and that the term epithelioid leiomyoma should be applied when there is a lower level of mitotic activity. Although combination therapy (surgery plus radiation therapy or chemotherapy) may not be indicated for a patient with an epithelioid leiomyoma, follow-up should be considered essential, as emphasized by Klunder and associates.

An unusual benign form of leiomyomata uteri, intravenous leiomyomatosis, was first recognized at the turn of the century and has been reported sporadically since then. About 50 cases have been reported to date, according to Bahary and associates. Marshall and Morris presented the first detailed report of this entity in the American literature in 1959. The characteristic feature of this peculiar smooth muscle tumor is the extension of the polypoid intravascular projections into the veins of the parametrium and broad ligaments. Although there may be some difficulty in distinguishing such lesions from low-grade sarcoma, they are distinctly different histologically from stromatosis uteri, since the intravenous plugs are mainly smooth muscle in origin. In 1966, Edwards and Peacock collected 32 cases of intravenous leiomyomatosis, including two cases of their own, and reviewed the clinical experience with this condition. In roughly 50% of the cases, the intravenous tumor was confined to the parametrium, and in 75%, it extended no further than the veins of the broad ligament. The observations of Edwards and Peacock suggest that the severed intravenous extensions are probably incapable of independent parasitic existence and remain dormant after removal of the uterus, although the cases presented by Bahary and associates tend to refute this idea. Total surgical excision of the tumor should be attempted for successful therapy. Some patients have survived for many years after incomplete resection of the tumor. A review of 14 cases of this rare uterine tumor from the files of the Armed Forces Institute of Pathology (AFIP) has been reported by Norris and Parmley. In this series, in two of three patients with incomplete resection who had a recurrence, the recurrent tumor was excised surgically and the patients were alive and free of disease 5 and 11 years after operation. They conclude that this tumor behaves clinically like a benign neoplasm, although its wormlike extensions may involve uterine, vaginal, ovarian, and iliac veins. The uterine veins in the broad ligaments are the most frequent sites of extension. The mitotic index is quite low, with the most active lesions showing only one mitosis per 15 high-power fields. The material from the AFIP provides histologic evidence consistent with both theories of origin of intravenous leiomyomatosis, namely, that it may be the result of unusual vascular invasion from a leiomyoma or may arise *de novo* from the wall of veins within the myometrium.

Extension of benign leiomyomatosis up the vena cava and into the right atrium has been reported in at least six cases, with fatal outcome in three. All reported cases have occurred in women. Tierney and associates reported that substantial quantities of cytoplasmic estradiol and progesterone receptors were found in the right atrial tumor removed from a patient with intravenous leiomyomatosis. Their patient was treated with the anti-estrogen tamoxifen because of residual tumor in the vena cava that could be estrogen-dependent. Irey and Norris have presented evidence that female reproductive steroids can produce intimal proliferation of veins in predisposed persons. Interestingly, of 30 patients with leiomyomata and leiomyosarcomas of the vena cava reviewed by Wray and Dawkins, 80% were female. Both intravenous leiomyomatosis and benign metastasizing leiomyoma have been reported to metastasize to the lung. As suggested by Banner and associates, by Horstmann and associates, and by Evans and associates, oophorectomy may be indicated in patients with these conditions, again because of the possibility that these tumors may be estrogen-dependent or that estrogens may have the ability to stimulate their development, whether in a uterine or extra-uterine location and whether they appear to be endothelial or mesenchymal in origin.

The possibility of metastases from a histologically benign uterine leiomyoma has been discussed by Idelson and Davids and by Clark and Weed. When such a case comes up, it is usually settled by finding a sarcomatous component in the leiomyoma or by finding evidence of intravenous leiomyomatosis. However, about 12 cases have now been reported in which a benign uterine leiomyoma metastasized. Idelson and Davids' case showed metastases to the aortic lymph nodes. The patient reported by Cramer and associates had metastatic tumor to the omentum, ovary, periaortic lymph node, and the lung. In each location the histology and estrogen receptor content of the tumor resembled that of a benign leiomyoma. The recommended treatment consists of surgical removal with castration and little or no estrogen replacement.

Leiomyomatosis peritonealis disseminata is sometimes confused with intravenous leiomyomatosis. However, only subperitoneal surfaces of the uterus and other pelvic and abdominal viscera are involved with leiomyomatosis peritonealis disseminata, and invasion of the lumen of blood vessels does not occur. Only about 15 cases have been reported, according to Pearce. All occurred in patients in the reproductive years who often had large uterine leiomyomata and were usually pregnant or taking oral contraceptives. The condition is likely to be confused with a disseminated intra-abdominal malignancy, but it is entirely benign histologically and clinically. Parmley and associates have demonstrated the histologic similarities of this peritoneal lesion to the decidual change of the mesothelium in the pelvis and propose that the condition represents a benign reparative process in which fibroblasts replace soft peritoneal decidua. They suggest that this fibrocytic reaction occurs during pregnancy and especially in the postpartum period, resulting in nodules with a pseudoleiomyomatous pattern. Similar findings have been noted in patients with endometriosis treated with prolonged Enovid therapy. These findings indicate that prolonged and continuous stimulation of subperitoneal decidua by either endogenous or exogenous estrogen and progesterone is important in the pathogenesis of this condition. Parmley and associates suggest that the condition is more appropriately called disseminated fibrosing deciduosis. Goldberg and associates, on the other hand, on the basis of electron microscopy studies, believe that the tumors arise from smooth muscles of small blood vessels. This has been confirmed by Ceccacci and associates. It has been possible to show a continuum from fibroblastic cells through myofibroblasts to leiomyocytes. Although the cell of origin of this tumor is still controversial, the tumor is benign and the acceptable treatment to date is total abdominal hysterectomy and bilateral salpingo-oophorectomy. Should this tumor occur in the omentum, an omentectomy should also be performed to define more clearly the histologic nature of the lesion.

In attempting to distinguish between benign and malignant disease in a patient with uterine leiomyomata who also has unusual clinical findings, it is appropriate to keep the above entities (intravenous leiomyomatosis, atypical bizarre leiomyoma, benign metastasizing leiomyoma, and disseminated intraperitoneal leiomyomatosis) in mind. Although they all have features similar to malignant disease, they are almost always benign and amenable to treatment. One should also remember that benign uterine leiomyomata have been associated with pseudo-Meigs' syndrome in a few cases. Meigs reported five cases in 1954. In these cases, the ascites does not reappear following removal of the uterine leiomyomata.

Asymptomatic Leiomyomata

Most leiomyomata are asymptomatic. Untold numbers of such symptomless leiomyomata are removed surgically when they would have been better left undisturbed. The incidence of malignancy in leiomyomata is less than 0.1%, which is lower than the operative mortality rate of hysterectomy in the average hospital; therefore, unless there is some reason to suspect malignant change, the danger of the operation may exceed the danger of malignancy. A history of rapid growth, particularly postmenopausal growth, does indicate removal, however, even when the tumor produces no symptoms. Signs of rapid enlargement are important in all patients, but are even more ominous in older patients. In younger patients, the most common reason for rapid enlargement of a uterus with leiomyomata is pregnancy. If pregnancy can be ruled out, a leiomyosarcoma may be suspected.

Small leiomyomata that are quite asymptomatic need only to be observed from time to time, with pelvic examinations perhaps every 6 to 12 months. In the beginning, frequent observation may be indicated to determine the growth rate. Such tumors may remain remarkably constant in size for years. If small leiomyomata are discovered late in menstrual life, it is unusual for symptoms to appear or for surgical treatment to be required. Larger tumors may also be watched safely, but if a policy of watchful waiting is adopted, one should be very sure of the nature of the tumors. If there is uncertainty of the uterine or ovarian origin of a tumor, as may well be the case when the tumor fills the whole pelvis or when a pedunculated tumor is felt in the adnexal region, special diagnostic procedures may be indicated. Pelvic examination by an experienced gynecologist can usually clear up the uncertainty. In difficult cases, an examination under anesthesia may be necessary. Laparoscopy may be of great value in determining the nature of an adnexal mass. Before resorting to invasive techniques, however, noninvasive special diagnostic procedures should be done. These include x-ray studies of the abdomen and pelvis, ultrasonography, and computed tomography. The characteristic calcification in a leiomyoma may be seen on x-ray. The ultra-

sonographic and computed tomographic features of uterine leiomyomata have been well described. Unfortunately, mistakes in the interpretation can still be made. Tada and associates reported that 5% of patients diagnosed as having uterine leiomyomata by computed tomography actually had an ovarian tumor at operation. Therefore, if uncertainty about the diagnosis persists, laparoscopy or laparotomy should be performed.

When large asymptomatic leiomyomata occur in young women who have had their families or in whom childbearing is not important, a recommendation for removal should be made. Such tumors, with many years to grow before the menopause, are bound to require surgical removal eventually; hence, it is better to remove them when the patient is relatively young and a good operative risk. Such tumors should generally be 12 weeks or larger gestational size.

There is no uniform size of an asymptomatic leiomyomatous uterus that can be used as an indication for hysterectomy. When size is the only significant indication for surgery in an asymptomatic patient, the location of the tumors is more important than the total uterine mass. When the leiomyomata are located in the cornual area or the lateral wall of the uterus and obscure the anatomy of the adnexa and broad ligament, the risk of error in the early recognition of an ovarian tumor is great. In such cases one must carefully weigh the advantages of the conservative approach to the management of uterine leiomyomata. When adnexal tumors are present, it is critical that the origin of these tumors be confirmed. The diagnostic studies mentioned earlier should be done to establish clearly that the tumors are of uterine origin before it is decided to follow the patient conservatively. It is unacceptable to wait to see if an adnexal tumor enlarges before identifying the site of origin of the mass as either uterine or ovarian. Ovarian carcinoma remains the most lethal disease of the female reproductive tract and the most difficult to diagnose. Every diagnostic and therapeutic effort must be made to avoid errors in the clinical evaluation of pelvic neoplasms. However, in women who are approaching the menopause, relatively large uterine leiomyomata may be kept under observation with the knowledge that after the menopause they will not increase in size and may actually regress somewhat.

If one elects to observe a patient with a relatively large asymptomatic uterine leiomyoma, it is a good rule to obtain an intravenous urogram. Everett and Sturgess showed many years ago that not uncommonly there is evidence of pressure at the pelvic brim so that hydroureter and hydronephrosis develop. It is usually the symmetrically enlarged uterus with intramural leiomyomata that extend near or above the umbilicus and encroach on the pelvic brim that compresses the ureters, in the same way as a symmetrically enlarged gravid uterus. The irregularly enlarged uterus with subserous tumors usually does not produce pressure on the ureters. The process is usually painless, even when hydronephrosis has occurred. Pyelographic evidence of kidney damage may be the determining factor in a decision to operate on a patient with an entirely asymptomatic leiomyoma (Fig. 11–1).

After the menopause, asymptomatic leiomyomata generally should be left undisturbed. Here again the gynecologist must be absolutely certain that an ovarian neoplasm is ruled out. Also, the appearance of even the slightest trace of vaginal bleeding should make one suspect cervical or endometrial malignancy or the possibility of sarcomatous change in the leiomyoma. Careful pelvic examination, Papanicolaou smear, and evaluation of the cervix by colposcopy or biopsy and fractional curettage should be done. If the bleeding remains unexplained and the presence of atrophic vaginitis or the use of exogenous estrogens has been excluded, the leiomyomatous uterus should be removed because of the danger of sarcomatous change.

Signs and Symptoms Necessitating Treatment

Less than 50% of patients with uterine leiomyomata will have symptoms. Symptoms may be single or multiple and will depend on the location, size, and number of tumors present. A clinical and pathologic study of 298 patients with uterine leiomyomata by Persaud and Arjoon revealed no significant relationship between the presenting symptoms and the presence of degenerative changes in the tumors. Some form of degeneration was demonstrated in 65% of the specimens, with hyaline degeneration accounting for 63% of all types of degeneration. Hyaline degeneration produces no characteristic symptoms. Symptoms, especially pain and fever, may be present in some patients with red degeneration of a leiomyoma during pregnancy, with torsion and infarction of a subserous pedunculated leiomyoma, or with an infected leiomyoma.

ABNORMAL BLEEDING

It is surprising but not unusual to find patients even with large uterine leiomyomata who have a history of normal menstruation. Such patients should be questioned carefully about recent slight increases in the amount and duration of menstrual flow. Some patients with a history of normal menstruation will be found to have iron deficiency anemia from a gradual increase in menstrual blood loss that even the patient has not recognized. If a patient with uterine leiomyomata is to be followed, she should be asked to monitor her menstrual blood loss carefully and given instructions to keep a menstrual calendar and monthly record of the number of pads or tampons used each day. Objective measurement of the amount of menstrual blood loss using the method of Hallberg and Nilsson may be helpful in doubtful cases (see Chapter 21). Iron depletion may not be evident by laboratory determinations unless one does an iron stain of the bone marrow or serum ferritin levels.

Abnormal bleeding occurs in about one-third of patients with symptomatic uterine leiomyomata and commonly indicates the necessity for treatment. The menstrual flow is usually heavy (menorrhagia), but may also be prolonged (metrorrhagia) or both (menometrorrhagia). Submucous, intramural, and subserous tumors may cause abnormal bleeding, but there is a distinct clinical impression that bleeding is more common and more severe in the pres-

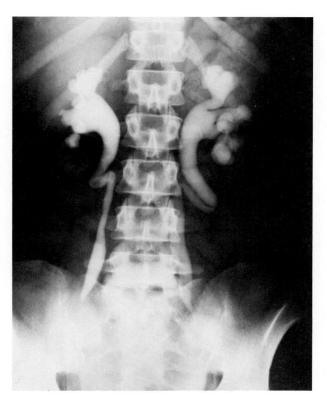

FIG. 11–1 Bilateral ureteral obstruction and dilatation from pressure of large leiomyomata.

ence of submucous tumors. The pedunculated sub-mucous leiomyoma bleeds freely at menstruation and may also bleed between periods as a result of passive congestion, necrosis, and ulceration of the surface of the tumor (Fig. 11–2). With these changes there is usually a constant, thin, blood-tinged discharge in addition to the menorrhagia. An intra-mural tumor that is just beginning to encroach on the uterine cavity can also be responsible for men-orrhagia. Intramural leiomyomata near the serosal surface and pedunculated subserous tumors can occasionally be associated with abnormal bleeding. When bleeding occurs with such tumors, however, one should search for some other lesion to account for it. The mere presence of leiomyomata in a woman who has abnormal uterine bleeding is not proof that the leiomyomata are causing the bleeding. This fact is important, particularly where there

is intermenstrual bleeding. When a patient with leiomyomata has intermenstrual bleeding, before proceeding with the treatment of the leiomyomata, it is a rule on our service to examine and study the cervix carefully with special diagnostic procedures and to curette the uterine cavity. If an endometrial or cervical malignancy is detected, the treatment of the leiomyomata will need to be altered.

There are several mechanisms by which leio-myomata may cause abnormal bleeding, although a specific mechanism may not be apparent in a particular patient. According to Seghal and Haskins, the surface area of the endometrial cavity in a nor-mal uterus is 15 cm^2. The surface area of the en-dometrial cavity in the presence of leiomyomata may exceed 200 cm^2. A correlation could be dem-onstrated between the severity of the bleeding and the area of endometrial surface. In addition to an

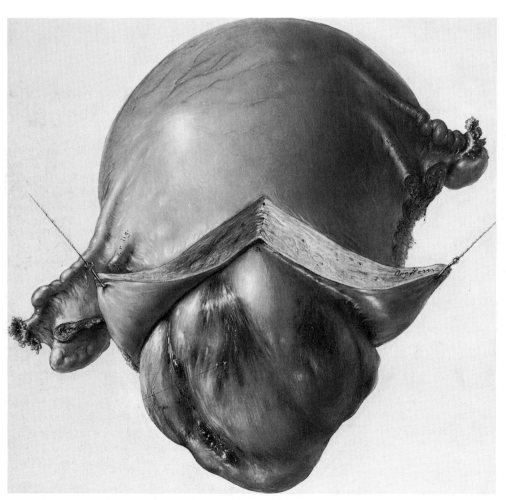

FIG. 11–2 Pedunculated submucous myoma showing necrosis and ulceration.

increased surface area, the endometrium may demonstrate a local hyperestrogenic picture in areas immediately adjacent to submucous tumors, and endometrial hyperplasia and endometrial polyps are commonly found. Deligdish and Lowenthal noted a broad spectrum of histologic abnormalities in the endometrium associated with leiomyomata, ranging from atrophy to hyperplasia. Thinning and ulceration of the endometrial surface may be present over large submucous tumors; smaller ones may show slight thinning without ulceration. The presence of leiomyomata may interfere with myometrial contractility and the contractility of the spiral arterioles in the basalis portion of the endometrium. Miller and Ludovici suggested that anovulation and dysfunctional uterine bleeding are more frequent in the presence of uterine leiomyomata.

Sampson in 1913 was the first to study the blood supply of uterine leiomyomata and its effect on uterine bleeding. More recent studies have been done by Faulkner and by Farrer-Brown and associates. The most prominent and important change is the presence of endometrial venule ectasia. Tumors that are strategically located in the myometrium may cause obstruction and proximal congestion of veins in the myometrium and endometrium. Thrombosis and sloughing of these large dilated venous channels within the endometrium will produce heavy bleeding.

In most cases, when bleeding occurs postmenopausally and leiomyomata are discovered on bimanual examination, the bleeding is due to some other factor, such as cervical or endometrial abnormalities, atrophic vaginitis, or exogenous estrogen, and the leiomyomata are purely incidental. However, the postmenopausal leiomyoma *can* be responsible for the bleeding. Leiomyomata that did not bleed during the menstrual life of the patient have been found to migrate to a submucous position in later years. This occurs because after the menopause the myometrium atrophies and the uterine wall becomes thinner. Leiomyomata also shrink somewhat, but not as much as the surrounding myometrium. Thus, a leiomyoma that was intramural before the menopause may work itself into a submucous position after the menopause, become ulcerated, and bleed. It must be emphasized again that postmenopausal growth of uterine leiomyomata may indicate malignant change, especially if associated with postmenopausal bleeding. Although we have, rarely, observed postmenopausal growth in a leiomyoma without finding malignancy in the tumor, whenever there is enlargement of the leiomyoma after the menopause one should seriously consider the possibility of sarcomatous change and remove it.

PRESSURE

Evidence of pressure on nearby pelvic viscera is also an indication for treatment. The urinary bladder suffers most often from such pressure, giving rise to frequency of urination (Fig. 11–3). Although this symptom is common with large leiomyomata, one frequently finds the pelvis filled with leiomyomata without any urinary frequency. Occasionally, acute retention of urine or overflow incontinence results from a leiomyoma and necessitates surgical intervention. These effects may occur as a result of rapid interior growth of the leiomyoma with compression of the urethra and bladder neck against the pubic bone. More frequently, a tumor of the size of a 3-months' pregnancy may become incarcerated in the cul-de-sac, wedging the cervix forward against the urethra and obstructing the flow of urine from the urethra. A large pedunculated submucous tumor may fill and distend the vagina and press the urethra against the symphysis and cause urinary retention.

As pointed out by Mattingly, one may expect to encounter many women who have uterine leio-

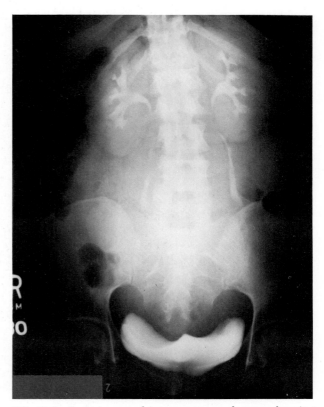

FIG. 11–3 Cystogram and intravenous pyelogram showing distortion of the bladder by pressure from a leiomyoma.

myomata of significant size and in addition have protrusion of the bladder base and posterior urethra through a widened levator muscle hiatus and a weakened urogenital diaphragm. Both conditions are relatively frequent. In addition to the usual symptoms produced by the leiomyomata, socially disabling stress urinary incontinence may be present. When the anterior wall of the uterus is greatly distorted by the presence of these tumors, pressure against the bladder can cause urinary frequency. If anatomical pressure equalization incontinence is also present, it may be aggravated by the increased intravesical pressure caused by the leiomyomata. It should be emphasized that the presence of anatomical stress urinary incontinence has no etiologic relationship to the uterine enlargement due to leiomyomata.

Silent ureteral obstruction from pressure against the pelvic brim is an uncommon complication of uterine enlargement from multiple large leiomyomata. Such an asymptomatic anatomical change occurs more frequently with a symmetrically enlarged leiomyomatous uterus that becomes large enough to fill the pelvis and compress the ureter against the pelvic side walls. Although an infrequent complication, the obstruction can occur in either ureter, depending on the location of the uterine tumors. If there has been no infection or parenchymal damage of the kidney, this anatomical alteration is completely reversible with removal of the uterus and relief of the pressure against the ureter. However, if urinary tract obstruction from leiomyomata has been neglected, uremia may result. Removal of the tumor and relief of obstruction is necessary to restore kidney function. Chronic bladder neck obstruction from uterine leiomyomata can be so severe as to cause a remarkable increase in the thickness of the bladder wall and enlargement of the bladder resembling that seen in men with urethral obstruction from prostatic enlargement. Indeed, in these neglected cases, the bladder may fill the entire lower abdominal wall so that an incision above the umbilicus is required to enter the peritoneal cavity to remove the tumor without injury to the bladder.

The bowel is less apt to show symptoms from pressure than the bladder, but constipation can be caused and aggravated by pressure against the rectum. Small intestines can become entwined with subserous pedunculated tumors and cause intermittent intestinal obstruction.

PAIN

Abdominal and pelvic pain or discomfort is present in about one-third of patients with symptomatic uterine leiomyomata and is a frequent reason for operative intervention. There are several causes for pain with leiomyomata. However, the usual hyaline or cystic degeneration of these tumors does not produce symptoms. In rare instances, pedunculated subserous leiomyomata twist and give rise to a clinical picture of acute abdominal pain much like that seen with a twisted ovarian tumor. These tumors twist more often during pregnancy and after the menopause. Acute carneous or red degeneration of a leiomyoma may occur at any period of reproductive life, although pain from this form of degeneration is more common during pregnancy. Dysmenorrhea, acquired in the fourth or fifth decade, may be the outstanding symptom of the growth of leiomyomata. A common symptom complex resulting from leiomyomata at this time of life is menstrual pain coupled with increased menstrual flow. Diffuse adenomyosis may also cause these symptoms, and the differentiation of this condition from a symmetrically enlarged intramural leiomyoma may be extremely difficult. The differentiation is chiefly academic, for in either case surgery is indicated if the symptoms are of sufficient severity.

Not infrequently, patients who have uterine leiomyomata and pain will be found to have concomitant pelvic disease such as ovarian pathology, pelvic inflammatory disease, tubal pregnancy, endometriosis, or urinary tract or intestinal pathology, including appendicitis. One must be careful to rule out other pathology that may be obscured by uterine leiomyomata.

DISTORTION

Distortion of the abdomen due to large tumors may justify their removal. Tumors of such size frequently give rise to other symptoms also, so that there is ample reason for surgical interference. When no other symptom is present, one is justified in removing the tumors if the abdominal distortion is of such proportions as to be distasteful to the patient.

RAPID GROWTH

Evidence of rapid growth of uterine leiomyomata, as observed by the same examiner or as confirmed by ultrasonography, is an indication for surgical intervention. Such rapid growth in a premenopausal patient is only rarely due to sarcoma. It may be due to pregnancy or to the use of oral contraceptives containing estrogens. In the latter case, these drugs should be discontinued and an alternative method of contraception prescribed. In the postmenopausal patient, however, growth of a uterine leiomyoma is highly suggestive of a malignancy. The malignancy may be a sarcomatous change in the leiomyoma itself, a sarcoma or carcinoma in the endometrium causing uterine enlargement, or an ovarian neoplasm whose estrogen secretion is stimulating enlargement of the leiomyoma, or whose growth may be mistaken for rapid enlargement of uterine leiomyomata. Although malignancy is not invariably found, the chances in its favor are so great that one must proceed on the assumption that it exists and do dilatation and curettage followed by immediate removal of the enlarged uterus.

Rapid growth of a leiomyomatous uterus is difficult to define in exact terms. Buttram and Reiter have arbitrarily defined it as a gain of 6 weeks or more in gestational size within a year or less. Although this definition could apply in premenopausal women, it might be disastrous to wait for this amount of growth in a postmenopausal woman. It is important to have a definite method of documenting uterine size at periodic intervals. Repeated sounding of the uterine cavity may be of some benefit, although leiomyomatous growth is not always accompanied by concomitant enlargement of the uterine cavity. It is more valuable to document the size of specific leiomyomata or the total uterine size in terms of centimeters or grams of uterine weight than in terms of gestational size of the uterus, although the latter method has gained wide popularity. Changes in a patient's weight may make evaluation of growth more difficult. A uterine leiomyoma may erroneously appear to be growing in a patient who is dieting and losing weight when actually the tumor is simply more easily felt. Conversely, in a patient who is gaining weight rapidly, the tumor will be more difficult to feel and may appear to be getting smaller. Ultrasonography is a much more objective way of establishing the size of a uterine leiomyoma in the beginning and, when indicated, of evaluating its rate of growth.

Although leiomyomata can increase dramatically in size during pregnancy, most commonly there is no appreciable growth. Winer–Muram and associates studied 89 pregnant women with uterine leiomyomata documented by ultrasonography examination. In 83 of the patients there was no demonstrable increase in the size of the leiomyomata. In six patients there was an increase in size up to 4 cm.

SPONTANEOUS ABORTION AND OTHER PREGNANCY-RELATED PROBLEMS

Uterine leiomyomata are associated with a significantly increased risk of spontaneous abortion. In a collected series of patients undergoing myomectomy, Buttram and Reiter reported that 41% had spontaneous abortions. This was reduced to 19% after myomectomy. Various mechanisms have been proposed to explain the occurrence of spontaneous abortion from uteri with leiomyomata. These include disturbances in uterine blood flow, alterations in blood supply to the endometrium, uterine irritability, rapid growth or degeneration of leiomyomata during pregnancy, difficulty in enlargement of the uterine cavity, and interference with proper implantation and placental growth by poorly developed endometrium or by subjacent leiomyomata. Implantation in thin, poorly vascularized endometrium over a submucous leiomyoma is doomed to failure, since proper growth and development of the embryo and placenta is impossible. Matsunaga and Shiota have found a twofold increase in the number of malformed embryos recovered from patients with uterine leiomyomata having artificial termination of pregnancy. Uterine leiomyomata may be associated with premature delivery, stillbirth, and interstitial pregnancy, as in the case reported by Starks, although we are unaware of good statistics regarding these associations. Muram and associates have followed patients with leiomyomata through pregnancy with ultrasonography. When there was a close proximity of a leiomyoma to the placental site, an increased incidence of pregnancy-related complications was seen. These were mainly bleeding complications, but pain, premature delivery, and postpartum hemorrhage also occurred. It should be emphasized that factors responsible for spontaneous abortion in patients without uterine leiomyomata may also be responsible for spontaneous abortion in patients with leiomyomata.

Pregnancy may cause a remarkable growth of leiomyomata in the same way that the myometrium undergoes hypertrophy in pregnancy. Red or carneous degeneration of leiomyomata during pregnancy is associated with pain, tenderness over the tumor, low-grade fever, and leukocytosis. Management should be expectant with analgesic medications and bedrest. If premature uterine contractions occur, β-mimetics may be given. Pain will usually subside within a few days. Operation is not indicated unless it is necessary to rule out other problems that require surgery for relief, but differentiation from appendicitis, placental abruption, twisted ovarian cyst, and other problems may be difficult. Following delivery, leiomyomata will involute and generally return to their prepregnancy size by the third postpartum month.

Torsion with infarction of subserous pedunculated leiomyomata is more common in pregnancy. A leiomyoma may interfere with labor and delivery by causing an abnormal presentation, by causing dysfunctional labor, or by obstructing the pelvis. A submucous leiomyoma in the lower uterine segment may entrap the placenta, necessitating manual removal. Indeed, furious postpartum hemorrhage can result if a submucous leiomyoma is disturbed at delivery or by exploration of the uterine cavity. Immediate hysterectomy will be necessary to control the bleeding.

Of course, the majority of patients with uterine leiomyomata will have no difficulty conceiving and will carry their pregnancies to term without complications. The only problem encountered may be a difficulty in estimating gestational age from uterine size because of the presence of leiomyomata.

INFERTILITY

When asymptomatic leiomyomata are discovered in young women, the question of the relation of such tumors to sterility and pregnancy usually arises. A number of factors may be responsible for infertility in a patient with uterine leiomyomata. Anovulatory cycles may be more frequent. There may be interference with sperm transport because of distortion and an increased surface area within the uterine cavity, impingement of leiomyomata on the endocervical canal or interstitial portion of the fallopian tube, or interference with prostaglandin-induced uterine contractions, which are thought to enhance sperm migration. Endometrial changes (atrophy, ulceration, focal hyperplasia, and polyps) and vascular alterations (venous congestion, venule ectasia, impaired blood flow), and enlargement of the uterine cavity may be present. The high incidence of menorrhagia may also contribute to infertility. Since uterine leiomyomata occur in later reproductive years, relatively greater difficulty accomplishing conception can be expected in older couples.

The finding of small leiomyomata in sterile women is not an indication for immediate myomectomy. Very often, an infertile patient with uterine leiomyomata will be found to have some other cause for infertility. Tubal inflammatory disease with associated pelvic adhesions is especially common in patients with uterine leiomyomata. Both marital partners should have a complete infertility investigation, and the leiomyomata should be disregarded for at least a while. The ultimate decision about the disposal of the tumors depends on their size and location. Usually, small subserous leiomyomata cannot reasonably be considered a factor in infertility. Even if the woman fails to become pregnant, removal of small, subserous leiomyomata is not justified. When leiomyomata are intramural or submucous and of significant size, they may well be factors in causing the infertility, and a myomectomy may be rewarded with a subsequent pregnancy.

When the finding of asymptomatic leiomyomata in women who expect to undergo pregnancy is totally unsuspected, it may be a severe shock to the patient. The greatest tact is required in presenting the problem to the patient, and the best of surgical and obstetric judgment is needed to arrive at the right solution. Should she be discouraged from attempting to become pregnant with the realization that her chances of complications are increased? Should a myomectomy be advised before pregnancy is attempted? If the risk of myomectomy is taken then one must also take the risk that the surgeon might be forced for technical reasons to perform a hysterectomy when attempting the myomectomy. Should she be permitted to become pregnant, go to term, and then have a cesarean section hysterectomy at term? Such questions cannot be answered by any stereotyped rule. Each case presents its own problems, and the answers are not entirely dependent upon the physical condition of the pelvis. The patient's age, her general physical condition, and, most important, her own desires, must all be considered before a final decision is made.

MISCELLANEOUS SIGNS AND SYMPTOMS

A variety of other unusual problems may be associated with uterine leiomyomata and may require treatment. Ascites and uterine inversion have already been mentioned. Sudden intraperitoneal hemorrhage may result from rupture of a dilated vein beneath the serosal surface of a subserous leiomyoma. Although leiomyomata are more often associated with iron deficiency anemia from chronic uterine blood loss, occasionally patients present with polycythemia. Islands of extramedullary erythropoiesis have been found in leiomyomata. Arteriovenous shunts within the tumors have been found and could be etiologically important in polycythemia. If the tumor obstructs the ureters and causes back pressure on the renal parenchyma, erythropoiesis could be stimulated. Weiss and other investigators have found marked erythropoietin activity within uterine leiomyomata. The polycythemia in these cases is cured by hysterectomy.

Choice of Treatment

Uterine leiomyomata are successfully treated surgically. However, abnormal bleeding from a leiomyomatous uterus may be controlled by ovarian irradiation if the patient is not a suitable surgical candidate. As will be explained, surgery is much preferred over irradiation as a method of treatment.

SURGICAL TREATMENT

Surgery is the definitive treatment for uterine leiomyomata when they are producing the significant signs and symptoms described earlier. When indicated, surgical treatment is quite satisfactory, since the mortality and morbidity of hysterectomy and myomectomy in better clinics is low. Surgery may be tailored to the needs and characteristics of the patient and can include myomectomy, total abdominal hysterectomy, and total vaginal hysterectomy. Surgery offers the advantage of conservation of ovarian function or the treatment of ovarian pathology if required. It also permits corrective vaginal plastic surgery when indicated. In patients with small symptomatic leiomyomata, vaginal hysterectomy is often the operation of choice. Although we do not advocate removal of very large tumors by morcellation from the vaginal route, vaginal hysterectomy is an extremely useful procedure when dealing with small tumors. The advantages and the contraindications for hysterectomy and for myomectomy in relation to leiomyomata are discussed later.

IRRADIATION TREATMENT

Since the growth of uterine leiomyomata depends on the presence of ovarian function, their growth can be stopped with irradiation of the ovaries. Ovarian irradiation should be reserved for those very few patients requiring treatment when their general condition contraindicates surgery. With recent advances in the management of medical conditions that affect high-risk patients with symptomatic leiomyomata and with modern anesthesia techniques, the risks for surgery have decreased significantly, and ovarian irradiation is now rarely required. Occasionally, a patient with uterine bleeding has a leiomyoma that should be removed surgically, but she steadfastly refuses operation. In such a case, irradiation castration is definitely the second-best method of treatment.

The technique of ovarian irradiation may vary. Generally, 200 rad is administered each day for 10 days through lower abdominal ports. A total mid-pelvic dose of 2000 rad is given to a patient with hormonally active ovaries. In the patient approaching menopause, a total ovarian irradiation dosage of 500 to 700 rad in one or two treatments may be sufficient to eliminate hormonal function. Intra-uterine radium may also be used and has the added advantage of a local effect on the endometrium. However, it has the disadvantage of potentially causing infection in submucous leiomyomata.

There are definite disadvantages to this form of therapy. It has been suggested that pelvic malignancies, especially mixed mesodermal sarcomas of the uterus, are more common in patients who have had pelvic irradiation for benign conditions many years previously, although this is difficult to prove with certainty. It is our clinical impression that the symptoms of an irradiation-induced menopause are, in general, more severe than those of the natural menopause. Indeed, loss of ovarian function in a young woman is a definite disadvantage, especially since substitution hormonal therapy would not be possible. In all patients who are irradiated, preliminary curettage should be done. In high-risk patients, anesthesia may be difficult or contraindicated for curettage. Finally, one does not have the opportunity to assess the pathology in the uterus and pelvis if an operation is not done. Significant pathology, such as uterine leiomyosarcoma, may be overlooked, especially in a patient whose uterus has been growing rapidly. Unfortunately, patients treated with irradiation may still require surgery at a later date for persistence or recurrence of signs or symptoms. However, irradiation offers an alternative to surgery for significant uterine bleeding from a leiomyomatous uterus for which surgery is definitely considered contraindicated because of the patient's medical condition.

Abdominal Myomectomy

The earliest operations for removal of leiomyomata uteri were myomectomies. The first myomectomy was done by Amussat in France in 1840. In 1845, W. L. Atlee performed the first successful myomectomy. It was done vaginally. Many of the earliest myomectomies consisted of removal of pedunculated tumors. In 1898, Alexander, of Liverpool, reported successfully removing 25 tumors from a single uterus. Howard A. Kelly, Charles Noble, and William Mayo wrote about myomectomy and practiced it extensively in this country during the early part of this century. They are given credit for emphasizing the importance of conservation of reproductive and menstrual function for young women with leiomyomata uteri. Victor Bonney, of London, and Isidor Rubin, of New York, were among the most enthusiastic for this procedure in the past generation. For example, Bonney removed 225 tumors from one uterus. This enthusiasm for the removal of multiple leiomyomata greatly exceeds our own, although occasionally the performance of multiple myomectomies for a large number of leiomyomas is indicated when the preservation of the uterus is of extreme importance to the patient.

INDICATIONS AND CONTRAINDICATIONS

It is difficult to lay down absolute criteria for the removal of or the saving of the uterus in patients with leiomyomata uteri, but certain advantages and disadvantages are clinically evident. Usually, the preservation of menstruation is not critical unless future childbearing is desired. Despite this, many women feel that the preservation of menstruation is essential to health, youth, and sexual life. While a simple explanation will convince many of them of their error, no explanation will suffice to satisfy others. The possibility of removal of the uterus should be discussed freely with the patient, for an understanding of the attitude of the patient will greatly aid the surgeon in making a decision at the operating table. Full, written, and duly witnessed permission from the patient to do whatever is surgically necessary is essential so that the gynecologist may be free to exercise the best surgical judgment. Because of technical reasons, discoverable only at operation, it is often difficult to be sure before operation that myomectomy is possible or wise. Should the removal of the uterus become necessary in the woman who is very desirous of retaining it, she will feel more kindly toward the surgeon and will have less difficulty in becoming mentally adjusted to its loss if she has been told previously of the possibility of hysterectomy. A preoperative hysterosalpingogram and a careful ultrasonography examination of the uterus may aid in assessing the size and location of the leiomyomata and may assist the gynecologist in advising the patient.

The greatest reason for considering myomectomy is the patient's desire for future childbearing. In general, the younger the patient the greater the role this plays. The problem actually presents itself more often during the middle thirties, since leiomyomata more commonly give rise to symptoms in the fourth decade of life than in the third.

It is obviously impossible, for technical reasons, to make a definite rule concerning myomectomy, but the more intense the desire of the woman for children, the more one is justified in extending the indications for myomectomy. If a woman with a leiomyomatous uterus is interested in attempting pregnancy now and is asymptomatic, she may try to conceive without particular regard to the size of the uterus unless it is very large. Her pregnancy could be uneventful and successful. If she had an operation first, she might develop pelvic adhesions that could cause infertility. It was concluded by

Berkeley and associates that myomectomy itself may decrease fertility, probably through adhesion formation. On the other hand, if a woman is 30 years old, thinks she may be interested in conceiving some time in the future but not now, and has a leiomyomatous uterus 10 to 12 weeks' gestation size or larger, a myomectomy should be advised even though no symptoms are present. These tumors will continue to grow and will be more likely to produce symptoms. Also, when they become larger, there will be greater technical difficulties in performing a myomectomy.

Myomectomy is occasionally justified in a woman over 35. It is rarely a reasonable procedure when she is past 40. Only in cases of late marriage in which childbearing is greatly desired should myomectomy be considered in the late thirties or early forties.

Myomectomy for relief of infertility is rarely indicated. The infertility in a patient with leiomyomata is usually attributable to such other causes as pelvic adhesive disease or tubal obstruction. Before undertaking to do myomectomy as a primary procedure, every other cause of infertility must be corrected and there must seem to be a potential relationship between the infertility and the size and location of the myomata. It is more reasonable to suspect that the infertility is caused by leiomyomata if there is distortion of the endocervical canal, obstruction or elongation of the fallopian tube, enlargement of the uterine cavity, or leiomyomata in a submucous location. A myomectomy cannot be justified for relief of infertility if only a small solitary subserous or intramural myoma is located in the uterine wall. The same statements can be made for the indications for myomectomy in patients who have had several spontaneous abortions.

In Brown, Chamberlain, and TeLinde's series, 172 married women were followed for two or more years following myomectomy. Seventy-four, or 42.5%, became pregnant, and 64 women delivered a total of 111 living children. Certainly some of these women practiced contraception, so it is probable that the 42.5% is not a true index of the pregnancy potential. In this series there were eight patients whose primary complaint was repeated abortions, and who had no apparent abnormality other than leiomyomata. Myomectomy was done primarily for the indication of repeated abortion. All of these patients became pregnant following the surgery. However, only four went to term with living infants; the other four pregnancies terminated in abortion, prematurity, or stillbirth. In a more recent series from Johns Hopkins Hospital, Babaknia, Rock, and Jones reported on 34 patients with primary infertility and 12 with secondary infertility who had no detectable pathology other than leiomyomata. After myomectomy, 38% of patients with primary infertility and 50% of those with secondary infertility had full term pregnancies.

Ingersoll and Malone treated 75 patients for infertility with myomectomy, approximately half of whom subsequently became pregnant, most within two years following surgery. Unfortunately, the incidence of abortion following myomectomy in this series is not available. In a similar series from the Chelsea Hospital it was 38%, as reported by Loeffler and Nobel. Baines reported a much lower pregnancy rate than most studies, with only 18 of 100 infertile patients achieving a pregnancy after myomectomy. This may have been related to the high incidence of pelvic inflammatory disease in his study group.

In 1983, Berkeley and associates reported the experience with myomectomy at Yale. Of 50 patients undergoing myomectomy, 25 subsequently conceived. Of the total 36 pregnancies, 24 resulted in full term deliveries and three resulted in premature but viable deliveries. However, only 16% of infertile patients with a normal infertility evaluation conceived. They concluded that myomectomy may be unjustified in women with otherwise negative infertility evaluations. In the total group of 50 patients, the average number of myomas removed was 4.6 per patient. In patients who subsequently conceived, the average was 3.2 per patient, while in those who tried to become pregnant and failed, the average was six. The average length of time from operation to conception was 20 months.

Buttram and Reiter in 1981 reported their own experience with myomectomy as well as accounts collected from the medical literature. In a collected series of 285 patients with leiomyomata and menorrhagia, 230 (81%) showed a reduction or resolution of the heavy bleeding after myomectomy. Of 76 patients in whom all causes of infertility except leiomyomata had been ruled out, 41 (54%) conceived following myomectomy. In 1941 collected cases in which preoperative and postoperative abortion rates were recorded, the spontaneous abortion rate was reduced from 41% to 19% by myomectomy.

There are few absolute contraindications to myomectomy. Malignancy of any type in the uterus or the ovaries excludes myomectomy. If it is certain that the tubes are closed, or if they have been removed previously, there is no justification for myomectomy. Under such circumstances, the retained uterus is useless; also, it is often a source of future trouble. Occasionally, one has the impression by pelvic examination that the uterus is symmetrically enlarged with leiomyomata only to find at operation that no distinct tumor is present. Instead, there is diffuse leiomyomatosis, diffuse myometrial hypertrophy, or diffuse adenomyosis of the uterine wall. In this situation, myomectomy cannot be done. Preoperative ultrasonography may be helpful in excluding these conditions.

A uterus that is the site of a large number of leiomyomata is better removed than subjected to multiple myomectomies. In the experience of Buttram and Reiter, myomectomy was successful in relieving infertility only in patients whose uterus was judged preoperatively to be of 8 weeks' gestational size or less. Many authors, notably Rubin and Bonney, report the removal of large numbers of leiomyomata from one patient. It is difficult for us to believe that the removal of such a large number of leiomyomata is ever justifiable; a uterus that is the site of many visible leiomyomata usually contains many invisible seed tumors that will continue to enlarge and eventually give trouble. Perhaps the necessity of producing an heir to a throne might justify such a procedure, but it would hardly seem good surgical judgment under ordinary circumstances. Furthermore, a multiply scarred uterus is a high-risk organ in which to carry a fetus to term and usually requires abdominal delivery should a term-size pregnancy occur. Our choice of management of a patient with leiomyomata is outlined in Figure 11–4.

If pregnancy occurs following myomectomy, the method of delivery becomes a problem. Cases of uterine rupture after myomectomy are rare. However, it is our belief that the obstetrician should be exceedingly cautious in permitting subsequent vaginal delivery. If the removal of a large leiomyoma or multiple leiomyomata involves major segments of the myometrium and multiple incisions, and especially if the uterine cavity has been entered, cesarean section for delivery at term should be recommended. On the other hand, if only a few small myomas have been removed from the uterine wall and the endometrial cavity has not been invaded, vaginal delivery may be allowed. The recommendation regarding whether or not to do an elective cesarean section for delivery should be made at the time the myomectomy is done. In defense of this attitude, one must remember that many of these women are elderly for childbirth and that this may be their last chance to have a child. However, in most cases a history of myomectomy is not an indication for cesarean section because rupture of the uterus through a myomectomy scar is rare. In the series from Johns Hopkins analyzed by Brown and associates, the method of delivery of 120 term infants was vaginal in 96 cases and by cesarean section in 24. None of the uteri ruptured. The rule has been to perform cesarean section if the uterine cavity

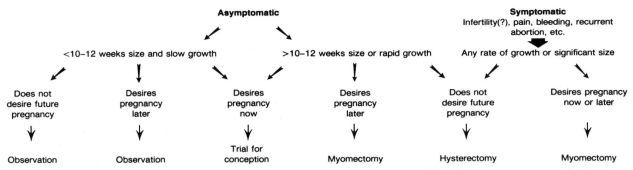

FIG. 11-4 Management of nonpregnant patients with uterine leiomyomata (Modified from Buttram VC and Reiter RC: Uterine leiomyomata: Etiology, symptomatology, and management. Fertil Steril 36: 433. 1981. Reproduced with permission of the publisher, The American Fertility Society.)

was entered at the time of myomectomy or if there was reason to believe, by the postoperative course, that the myomectomy wound was infected. Although this may be an excessively cautious attitude, it appears to be a safe one in this infertile group.

When considering myomectomy, the patient will wish to know about the possibility of further surgery and it is well to have definite facts to give her. Of course, the longer the cases are followed, the more recurrences there will be. Of the 176 cases followed by Brown for 5 or more years, 31.3% had recurrent leiomyomata, and hysterectomy became necessary in 16.5% of these cases. Hysterectomy became necessary for other causes in an additional 4.3%. Thus, over 20% of the women on whom myomectomy was done required a later hysterectomy. Ingersoll's experience was similar in that hysterectomy for recurrent leiomyomata was required in 20% of the cases. In the Chelsea series, the reoperation rate requiring hysterectomy for recurrent leiomyomata was 27%. According to Malone, when myomectomy was done for a solitary tumor, 11% of patients subsequently required hysterectomy for recurrence of tumors. When a multiple myomectomy was required, 26% were later reoperated on because of recurrence of leiomyomata. In the series from the Mayo Clinic reported by Brown and associates, hysterectomy was necessary in 32% of myomectomy patients followed for from 5 to 20 years.

Even though a patient who has had a myomectomy for infertility may not become pregnant and may need to have a hysterectomy because of recurrence of the leiomyomata, this does not necessarily mean that the myomectomy should not have been done in the first place. Many patients will indicate that even though pregnancy did not follow after the myomectomy, they were still very pleased that a conservative operation was done initially. To such women, the wish to maintain the possibility of having children, although remote, is sufficient justification for myomectomy.

Myomectomy carries a slightly greater mortality than hysterectomy for benign disease. However, if a surgeon uses reasonable judgment in selecting cases, myomectomy should carry no greater mortality than a hysterectomy. Myomectomy should always be considered a major procedure, since it carries with it the possibility of major complications, especially if the myomectomy is extensive. The most serious complication is postoperative hemorrhage. Since the bleeding comes from the site of incisions in the uterine corpus, the bleeding is intraperitoneal and occult. Such bleeding may be insidious and its detection may require more frequent postoperative evaluations of the hematocrit and vital signs. Postoperative fever is also more common following myomectomy.

Several special circumstances indicating myomectomy should be mentioned. The twisting or the necrosis of a pedunculated leiomyomata during pregnancy is a special indication for myomectomy. Although such complications are rare, the performance of a successful myomectomy without interruption of the pregnancy is a surgical feat of supreme importance to the patient. Only when the patient experiences repeated attacks of acute pain, vomiting, or fever should myomectomy be considered during pregnancy. Sedation should first be given an adequate trial. When myomectomy becomes a necessity, most authors believe that it should be done after the third month of pregnancy, when the uterus is less irritable and placental function is well established. However, the time of the onset of the symptoms may not give the gynecologist the choice of selecting the time for operation. If the pain is in the right lower abdominal quadrant and the differential diagnosis includes acute appendicitis, prompt surgical intervention may be required. Fortunately, myomectomy is rarely necessary during pregnancy. It should only be undertaken for a symptomatic pedunculated or superficial leiomyoma. Deep myometrial dissection should be avoided, and inadvertent entry into the endometrial cavity is almost certain to result in premature labor or abortion.

Myomectomy at delivery in conjunction with a cesarean section is contraindicated except under the most favorable circumstances. For example, if there is a pedunculated subserous leiomyoma attached to the uterus with a small pedicle, ligation of the pedicle and excision of the leiomyoma may be done easily. However, the removal of intramural leiomyomata from the pregnant uterus is inadvisable because of the recognized difficulty in controlling blood loss.

Another special condition is the presence of a submucous leiomyoma prolapsed through a dilated cervix and into the vagina. Such leiomyomata are frequently infected and necrotic because of exposure to vaginal bacteria and poor blood supply. We consider abdominal hysterectomy contraindicated in the presence of a prolapsed submucous leiomyoma. There are two important reasons for this. First, the lower uterine segment, cervix, and upper vagina will be quite broad and dilated and the paracervical tissue will be indurated because of infection. The ureters, therefore, will be at increased risk of injury if an abdominal hysterectomy is attempted. Second, if an abdominal hysterectomy is done, contamination of the peritoneal cavity by the infected leiomyoma tissue is unavoidable, increasing the risk of postoperative peritonitis. Rather than abdominal hysterectomy, a vaginal myomectomy should be performed first. In some cases, the prolapsed leiomyoma can simply be twisted off. In other cases, the pedicle can be clamped and ligated. If the size of the prolapsed submucous leiomyoma precludes access to the pedicle, morcellation of the leiomyoma can be done first. Postoperative bleeding is usually not a problem because the blood supply through the pedicle is limited. Vigorous traction must not be applied to a prolapsed submucous leiomyoma because of the possibility of uterine inversion. Several months following vaginal myomectomy, when the cervix has involuted and the infection has subsided, the patient may be reevaluated for abdominal hysterectomy. Sometimes abdominal hysterectomy will not be required because the most symptomatic leiomyoma or the only leiomyoma will have already been removed by vaginal myomectomy. Following vaginal myomectomy, each patient should be individually evaluated for the need for abdominal hysterectomy.

Neuwirth has described resection of submucous leiomyomata under hysteroscopic control in 28 patients. Seventeen patients returned to normal menses, and five patients subsequently had a total of eight pregnancies with five living children. This method of managing patients with submucous leiomyomata should be limited to experts in hysteroscopy technique.

TECHNIQUE OF ABDOMINAL MYOMECTOMY

Before abdominal myomectomy is performed, the patient should have ultrasonography to attempt localization of the leiomyomata and assess their individual size. A hysterosalpingogram should be done to assess patency of the fallopian tubes and proximity of the interstitial portion of the tubes to the leiomyomata. Encroachment on the uterine cavity can also be seen. After induction of anesthesia, the patient is placed in Crawford stirrups and a careful pelvic examination under anesthesia is done. Preparation and draping are carried out to allow access to the vagina and cervix in case it is necessary to place an instrument through the cervix and into the endometrial cavity during the procedure. Cervical dilatation should be done to facilitate postoperative drainage from the endometrial cavity. Abdominal myomectomy, especially multiple and extensive myomectomy, requires adequate exposure through the abdominal incision. A Maylard incision is preferred. A Pfannenstiel incision may be used for the removal of a small solitary myoma. After the peritoneal cavity is entered, the abdomen is explored as usual. Adhesions in the pelvis are released or removed and the intestines are placed in the upper abdomen and held there with packs. The operation is performed according to microsurgical techniques and principles. For example, the laparotomy packs that are used to hold the intestine in the upper abdomen are placed in plastic bags to reduce microscopic trauma to peritoneal surfaces. The operative field is kept moist and free of clots with a solution of Ringer's lactate containing Decadron and heparin. Very fine instruments and sutures are used and tissue is handled gently in order to avoid unnecessary trauma.

At this point in the operative procedure, one should pause and evaluate the size, location, and number of leiomyomas present. Their proximity to the endocervical canal, uterine vessels, and fallopian tubes should be determined. One must decide if myomectomy is still feasible, how the leiomyomata will be removed and in what sequence, and how the uterus will be reconstructed.

The blood supply of the myometrium, especially in young women, is abundant. Multiple myomectomy, especially the removal of several intramural leiomyomata, can be associated with considerable loss of blood. Several techniques have been devised to control excessive blood loss during myomectomy. Bonney designed an adjustable clamp that could be placed around the cervix to occlude the uterine arteries. Rubin recommended the use of a tourniquet placed tightly around the lower uterine segment. Lock described the use of curved ring forcep clamps applied bilaterally across the infundibulopelvic ligaments and the lower portion of the broad ligaments to incorporate the uterine arteries and veins. Jones and Andrews and also Ingersoll and Malone use an oxytocin or vasopressor solution for intramyometrial infiltration around the tumor.

Our preference in performing extensive myomectomy is to use a tourniquet around the lower uterine segment and around each infundibulopelvic ligament. A small opening is made in the avascular portion of the broad ligament lateral to the lower uterine segment taking care not to injure the uterine vessels. A 0.25-in Penrose drain is placed around the cervix. Using the same broad ligament hole, Penrose drains are also placed around the infundibulopelvic ligaments (Fig. 11–5A). These tourniquets are not tied until the operating team is ready to perform the myomectomy. When they are tied, they must be tied tightly enough to occlude the arterial supply to the uterus. If the tourniquets only occlude the venous return but not the arterial supply, the blood loss will be increased. When everything is in readiness and the operative approach has been decided, hypotensive anesthesia is induced and the tourniquets are tied tightly. A sterile doptone may be used to confirm disappearance of blood flow through the uterine artery. The combined use of hypotensive anesthesia and tourniquets will keep blood loss to a minimum. However, it is also important that the operating team work swiftly with the dissection and suturing. Rubin and Ranney and Frederick mentioned the accumulation of a histamine-like substance within the uterus if uterine circulation is obstructed. They have suggested that the release of this substance into the circulation may cause postoperative shock. To our knowledge, there is no evidence to support this idea. We have left tourniquets on for 30 minutes without evidence of postoperative shock. However, we do believe the operation should be done as quickly as possible.

If the myomectomy is a simple one, tourniquets and hypotensive anesthesia may not be necessary. Substantial blood loss can be avoided simply by performing the operative procedure rapidly while exerting direct pressure on bleeding tissue until hemostasis can be achieved with sutures. Large bleeding vessels in the myoma bed may be individually ligated.

Only a minimal number of incisions to remove all leiomyomata should be made. If possible, removal of all leiomyomata should be accomplished through a single incision in the anterior uterine corpus (Fig. 11–5B–D). Even intramural leiomyomata in the posterior uterine wall can sometimes be removed through this incision. Incisions in the posterior uterine wall may be necessary, however, if one is removing a large posterior-wall leiomyoma. Methods for removing myomas through a single anterior incision have been described by Bonney. The linear or elliptical incision in the superficial myometrium should be carried into the underlying leiomyoma. The leiomyoma is then grasped with a single tooth tenaculum or a Lahey thyroid clamp for traction. The plane of cleavage between the leiomyoma and the surrounding myometrium can be easily identified. Sharp dissection with the scapel or Metzenbaum scissors, or blunt dissection with the finger or knife handle will be required to enucleate the leiomyoma from its bed. Sometimes the leiomyoma is larger than expected. It may then be necessary to extend the incision or to remove the tumor by morcellation. Other adjacent tumors should be removed through the same incision. Any entry into the endometrial cavity should be noted, and a special attempt should be made to close it with sutures placed only in the myometrium. No. 2-0 delayed-absorbable sutures are used to repair the defects in the myometrium, if possible. Dead space must be closed and hemostasis must be satisfactory. Several layers of interrupted, figure-of-eight, or purse-string sutures may be required (Fig. 11–5E). One must be careful to avoid occlusion of the uterine vessels and of the interstitial portion of the fallopian tubes. There is a tendency to excise too much excess myometrium. This should also be avoided. The serosa of the uterus should be carefully repaired (Fig. 11–5F).

Several ingenious techniques for removing leiomyomata and for repairing the defects have been described by Bonney. For example, Bonney's hood can be used to remove a large leiomyoma in the uterine fundus. The leiomyoma is first exposed through an elliptical incision made transversely across the anterior fundus, taking care to avoid the interstitial portion of the fallopian tube (Fig. 11–6A, B). After the primary tumor is removed (Fig. 11–6,C) other leiomyomata may also be removed through the same incision. Excess myometrium is trimmed away (Fig. 11–6D). Interrupted sutures obliterate the dead space, approximate the myometrium, and accomplish satisfactory hemostasis (Fig. 11–6E). The sutures are placed in such a way that the posterior flap is folded over the anterior uterine wall, thus fashioning Bonney's hood (Fig. 11–6F).

In closing a myomectomy incision, the security of the closure comes from sutures placed in the myometrium. These sutures and knots should not

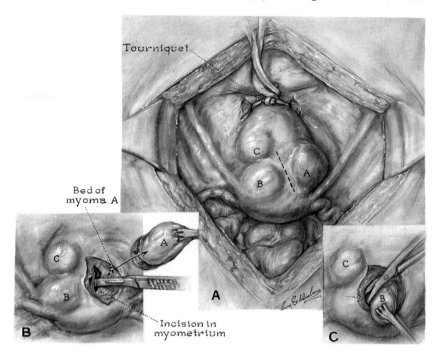

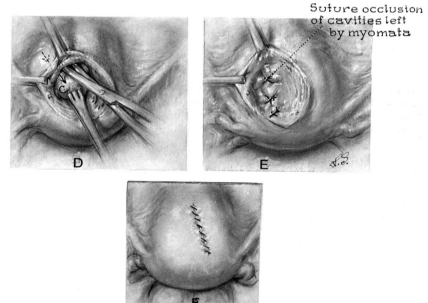

FIG. 11–5 Technique of multiple myomectomy. (*A*) A tourniquet is tied tightly around the lower uterine segment to occlude the uterine arteries. A single incision in the anterior uterine wall is outlined. All leiomyomata can be removed through this single incision. (*B*) Leiomyoma *A* has been removed. (*C, D*) Leiomyomata *B* and *C* are removed through the same incision. (*E*) Using No. 2-0 delayed-absorbable sutures, the myometrium is approximated, the dead space is obliterated, and hemostasis is secured. (*F*) The serosa of the uterus is approximated carefully with No. 5-0 delayed-absorbable continuous suture, placed subserosally if possible. The tourniquets are removed, and the defects in the broad ligament are also closed with fine sutures.

be exposed. The serosal edge should be carefully approximated with a continuous No. 5-0 delayed-absorbable suture that is placed subserosally if possible (Fig. 11–6G). Surgical loupes may be helpful in placing this suture. Free grafts of peritoneum or omentum are not used to cover myomectomy incisions.

The tourniquets are removed, the hypotensive anesthesia is reversed, and the uterus is carefully inspected for evidence of bleeding. Additional sutures for hemostasis are sometimes required. The broad-ligament defects are closed both anteriorly and posteriorly with fine sutures. If a uterine suspension is needed, a modified Coffey or modified Gilliam technique is employed. The anterior position of the uterine corpus can be maintained better if

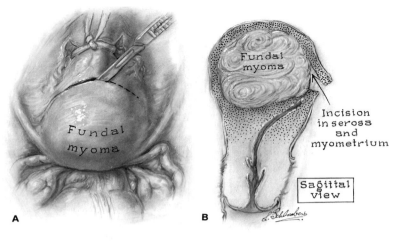

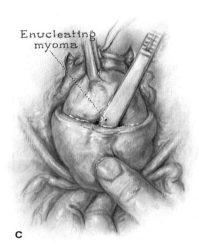

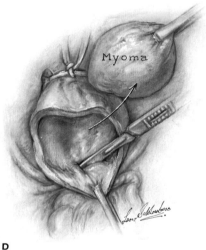

FIG. 11-6 Technique of myomectomy using Bonney's hood. (*A*) A tourniquet has been tied tightly around the lower uterine segment to occlude the uterine arteries. A transverse incision is made in the anterior uterine wall over the leiomyoma. (*B*) Sagittal view of the location of the incision over the leiomyoma. (*C*) By blunt and sharp dissection the leiomyoma is enucleated from its bed. (*D*) Excess hypertrophied myometrium may be trimmed away.

the uterosacral ligaments are approximated in the midline behind the cervix. Before the incision is closed, one may leave in a solution of high molecular weight dextran, in the hope of inhibiting the formation of postoperative adhesions.

Perioperative antimicrobial prophylaxis is indicated with myomectomy. Preferably, the operation should be performed in the follicular phase of the menstrual cycle to reduce blood loss, to reduce the chance of encountering an unknown or unsuspected pregnancy, and to reduce the problems encountered when a fresh corpus luteum is traumatized.

ABDOMINAL HYSTERECTOMY FOR BENIGN DISEASE

The first abdominal hysterectomy was performed by Heath in 1843 in Manchester, England, according to Pratt. In his textbook of operative gynecology, published in 1901, Howard A. Kelly reviewed the history of the development of abdominal hysterectomy in the United States. Burnham performed the first successful abdominal hysterectomy for leiomyomata in 1853. Stimson, who published his results in 1889, was the first to practice systematic ligation of the ovarian and uterine vessels preliminary to hysterectomy.

Hysterectomy has become the most common major operation performed in the United States. According to Dicker and associates, who studied data from the National Center for Health Statistics, 3.5 million women aged 15 to 44 years underwent hysterectomy between 1970 and 1978. As many as 800,000 hysterectomies have been recorded in a single year. By 1978, 19% of women aged 40 to 44 had undergone hysterectomy. In recent years, the number and the rate have declined. In 1980, the hysterectomy rate was 7.6 per 1000 women aged 15 to

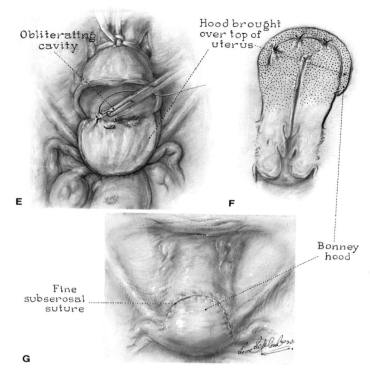

FIG. 11-6 *(continued)* *(E, F)* The hood is formed by folding the posterior flap over the anterior uterine wall and obliterating the dead space beneath with sutures, being careful not to place sutures too close to the interstitial segment of the fallopian tubes. *(G)* The serosa is approximated with continuous No. 5-0 delayed-absorbable suture. The broad ligament defects are repaired.

44 years, the lowest level since 1971. In the same year, approximately one of every 60 women in the age group 35 to 44 years had a hysterectomy. As might be expected, accusations of unnecessary hysterectomies have come from many sources. Considerable concern has been expressed that the operation is overused and not always done for proper indications. Studies suggest that the increase in the number of hysterectomies is explained largely by its liberal use as a prophylaxis against uterine cancer, as a method of sterilization, and as a method of treating mild symptoms of pelvic relaxation and menopausal menorrhagia. With the development of more accurate diagnostic procedures, and with the discovery of more effective non-surgical methods of therapy, it can be expected that fewer unnecessary hysterectomies will be performed.

The surgical mortality rate from hysterectomy in most medical centers is below 0.1%. However, morbidity continues to be a problem, and sometimes serious postoperative complications develop. It should be emphasized that the ability to perform several hundred hysterectomies with no mortality and few complications is not *ipso facto* evidence that gynecology is being practiced correctly. In addition to a low morbidity and mortality rate, one must also be concerned that only patients with proper indications are chosen for hysterectomy.

Two general strategies have been used to reduce the number of "unnecessary" hysterectomies. One is the surveillance of hysterectomies by tissue committees or special peer review groups. The experience in Saskatchawan reported by Dyck and associates indicates the effectiveness of this approach. The second strategy requires that a second opinion be obtained before elective surgery is done. A competent gynecologist who has followed a patient for several years, has kept careful records of findings and treatment, and has the patient's full confidence is probably able to make the most accurate judgment about the necessity for hysterectomy. In many circumstances, however, a second opinion should be sought before the decision is final, especially if there is the slightest doubt or question about the necessity of hysterectomy. An additional benefit accrues if a patient has a serious complication following hysterectomy, since it is good to have the opinion of another physician that the operation was indicated. Whenever the patient requests consultation with another physician, the request should be honored.

The ease with which the average hysterectomy may be done has proven both a blessing and a curse to modern womankind. There is no doubt that a hysterectomy done with proper indication may restore a woman to health and even save her life. Hysterectomy must never be done, however, without proper indications. In the final analysis, one might remember that the indications for surgical procedures, including hysterectomy, fall into three broad categories: to save life, to relieve suffering, and to correct significant deformity interfering with function. According to Taylor, hysterectomies should be done for only two reasons: when the preservation of the uterus constitutes a threat to the patient's life greater than the threat of the operation, and when there are disabling symptoms for which there is not equally successful treatment. Various appropriate indications for abdominal hysterectomy are discussed throughout this text. However, mention should be made of some inappropriate indications for abdominal hysterectomy.

In our judgment, hysterectomy is not appropriate solely as a means of surgical sterilization. The studies of Laros and Work and others substantiate our belief that the risk of complications following hysterectomy is greater than the risk of complications following tubal ligation. When requested and indicated, sterilization should usually be accomplished by tubal ligation. Hysterectomy for sterilization should be done only if significant uterine disease or symptoms are present. For example, a 30-year-old patient who requests surgical sterilization and is found to have an 8- to 10-week size leiomyomatous uterus and recurrent menorrhagia is a candidate for a hysterectomy rather than a tubal ligation. However, in a patient with normal reproductive organs, hysterectomy is not indicated simply for permanent contraception.

Hysterectomy should not be done to relieve chronic pelvic pain in the absence of organic pelvic pathology. Instead, relief should be obtained by conservative measures. Several consultants, including a psychiatrist, may be required to diagnose the cause of the patient's symptoms. A laparoscopic examination of the pelvis is essential when the origin of the pelvic discomfort is not clinically evident.

According to a study by Cole and Berlin, if all women in the United States had a hysterectomy at age 35, the life expectancy of the total group would be increased by only 2 months. Even though the uterus is one of the most common sites for the development of cancer in women, hysterectomy on all women after childbearing is completed is not a proper solution to the uterine cancer problem. Furthermore, hysterectomy is not indicated in menopausal patients simply to allow estrogens to be administered without risk of developing endometrial hyperplasia or neoplasia, or to prevent annoying episodes of uterine bleeding. Hysterectomy is not indicated to treat chronic cervicitis, leukorrhea, primary dysmenorrhea, or premenstrual tension.

The indications for hysterectomy that are appropriate for women in general are also appropriate for women who have had a previous tubal ligation. A hysterectomy for primary uterine disease or symptoms does not become more indicated because of a history of previous tubal ligation.

A hysterectomy is not the appropriate treatment for abnormal vaginal or cervical cytology. Additional studies are indicated to determine the reason for the abnormality. Mild or moderate cervical dysplasia is not an indication for hysterectomy. Only in the most severe degrees of cervical dysplasia, bordering on *in situ* carcinoma, in a patient nearing the menopause would hysterectomy be considered an appropriate alternative method of treatment. A single episode of postmenopausal bleeding is also not an indication for hysterectomy. It is an indication for careful pelvic examination and curettage. Rarely will the combination of several questionable indications constitute adequate justification for hysterectomy.

Terminology

The only suitable terms to modify the word *hysterectomy* are *total* or *subtotal* and *vaginal* or *abdominal*. Removal of the adnexal organs should be separately specified as bilateral or unilateral and as salpingectomy, oophorectomy, or salpingo-oophorectomy. Terms that are confusing or inappropriate include: *panhysterectomy, complete hysterectomy, incomplete hysterectomy, supravaginal hysterectomy,* and *supracervical hysterectomy.*

Total vs. Subtotal Abdominal Hysterectomy for Benign Conditions of the Uterus

Abdominal hysterectomy, both total and subtotal, has become a relatively safe operation in the hands of a competent gynecologist. There has been a uniform shift toward total hysterectomy in recent decades. In 1946, Miller reported 69% subtotal and 31% total hysterectomies. Johnson reported on 1246 abdominal hysterectomies done on the Tulane service at Charity Hospital between 1952 and 1954. None was a subtotal hysterectomy. In the past two decades, total hysterectomy has been accepted as the preferred method of removal of the uterus. In our clinics, over 99% of all abdominal hysterectomies are total. In a recent series of 4341 abdominal hysterectomies at Grady Memorial Hospital only 40 (0.9%) were subtotal. At the Milwaukee County Medical Complex, the cervix is retained in less than 0.5% of all cases undergoing an abdominal hysterectomy.

In our opinion, this trend toward total hysterectomy is justified, although we do not believe that it should be mandatory in every case.

In weighing the two procedures, one should balance the advantages of removal of the cervix against the possibilities of an increased morbidity and mortality for the total operation. To some extent, this is difficult to do because subtotal abdominal hysterectomy is now performed only in patients with very serious pelvic disease. Therefore, as one might expect, postoperative mortality and morbidity from subtotal abdominal hysterectomy is higher than for total abdominal hysterectomy, but for reasons that have nothing to do with differences in the operative technique. The advantages of removal of the cervix are principally that its removal eliminates it as a possible source of a troublesome discharge or bleeding and also as a site where carcinoma may develop. The incidence of the development of carcinoma is no greater in the retained stump than in the cervix of the intact uterus. Since the incidence of cervical carcinoma in a cervix that has had repeated cytologic evaluation is extremely low, the major disadvantage of the retained cervix is the requirement for continued cytologic follow-up. While there is a recognized false negative rate of vaginal cytology of approximately 10% to 15%, repeated cytologic study and clinical evaluation of the cervix reduces the risk of cancer to a negligible figure. Therefore, the rationale for the removal of the cervix must be based on the disease process that necessitates the hysterectomy and on the risk of complications that may result from attempting to remove the cervix from its anatomical location between the bladder above, the rectum below, and the ureters on each side.

The operator may perform a subtotal amputation of the uterine corpus quickly when he encounters operative difficulty or is informed by the anesthesiologist that the patient's condition is critical. The indications for subtotal hysterectomy should be based solely on the surgical risk of this added procedure, since the current indications for removal of the uterus are for a total hysterectomy. Subtotal hysterectomy is performed in such cases as severe pelvic inflammatory disease, advanced endometriosis, ovarian cancer, and other conditions in which pelvic anatomy cannot be clearly defined. Even in these circumstances, an experienced gynecologist can usually remove the cervix without danger of injury to surrounding structures. The surgical risk of removing the cervix should be significant before it is decided to retain the cervix. Although the number of patients with carcinoma developing in a cervical stump has been reduced significantly in recent years, it is unfortunate that there are still women who die of this disease when it could have been avoided by spending a few extra minutes to do a total rather than subtotal hysterectomy. Although there is a minimal increase in the risk of vesicovaginal or rectovaginal fistula and ureteral injury with removal of the cervix, none of these complications should occur, especially in the absence of significant pelvic disease, if proper surgical technique is used. This potential risk should not be a deterrent to removing the cervix at the time of abdominal hysterectomy. We are definitely not inclined to advise against total hysterectomy because of studies that purport to show that orgasm is less disturbed by subtotal hysterectomy.

Stated briefly, only when the danger of removing the cervix exceeds the danger of leaving it in should the subtotal operation be done. Since these conditions are uncommon, the cervix is usually removed when an abdominal hysterectomy is performed.

Ovarian Management at Hysterectomy for Benign Disease

The first procedure for oophorectomy was performed by Ephraim MacDowell in 1809. The operation was done for a large ovarian cystoma and was definitely indicated. In the 19th century, the removal of normal ovaries was practiced widely for various inappropriate indications, including insanity and convulsive disorders. The history of oophorectomy has been reviewed by Longo. Although the original procedure was known as the Battey operation, Battey himself performed fewer oophorectomies than others and cautioned that the operation was being performed too frequently and for indications that were too general. Enthusiasm for the operation waned as reports of a 25% mortality rate and only 25% success rate in relieving symptoms began to appear in the medical literature. By the turn of the century, many textbooks of gynecology did not mention Battey's operation.

In the early twentieth century, as ovarian physiology began to be understood, an era of ovarian conservation began. At the same time, however, the concept of prophylactic surgery (as in prophylactic removal of the appendix and cervix) was gaining acceptance. Gynecologic surgeons, frustrated mostly by the difficulty of diagnosing and curing ovarian cancer, debated the merits of prophylactic removal of normal ovaries in premenopausal and postmenopausal women at the time of hysterectomy.

There are still no uniformly acceptable and established criteria for removal or retention of normal ovaries at the time of abdominal hysterectomy. Although a surprisingly large number of gynecologists leave in ovaries in postmenopausal women according to Randall, most advocate routine prophylactic oophorectomy at the time of abdominal hysterectomy in the menopausal or postmenopausal patient. Most gynecologists also advocate ovarian conservation in premenopausal women younger than 40 years of age at the time of abdominal hysterectomy. However, according to the study by Dicker and associates of the National Center for Health Statistics Data for 1970 through 1978, almost 50% of women aged 40 to 44 years undergoing abdominal hysterectomy had a concurrent bilateral oophorectomy. It is not known how many of these oophorectomies were done for primary or associated ovarian pathology and how many were prophylactic to prevent ovarian cancer. Most of the controversy involves the establishment of an arbitrary age during the fifth decade when prophylactic oophorectomy will be practiced.

When normal ovaries are conserved at the time of abdominal hysterectomy in premenopausal women, normal hormonal function will continue unaltered in a cyclic fashion in almost all until the natural age of the menopause, at which time they will cease to produce 17-β estradiol and progesterone. Burford and Diddle and TeLinde and Wharton showed that in the Macacus rhesus and irus monkeys, normal ovarian function continues after hysterectomy with no evidence of altered arrangement of the follicular or corpus luteum development, maturation, or regression and no evidence of detectable changes in the ovarian stroma. Bancroft–Livingston and Randall and associates, using vaginal cytology, concluded that ovaries conserved after hysterectomy may continue to function for more than 15 years after hysterectomy. Since the ovary may not be the only source of estrogen affecting vaginal cytology, it has been necessary to confirm these findings with endocrine assays. Beavis and associates studied 69 patients who had partial or total ovarian conservation at the time of hysterectomy at age 25 to 48 years. Ovarian function was monitored by weekly urinary estrogen and pregnanediol determinations for periods of 4 to 6 weeks at intervals for up to 2.5 years. In the group with total conservation of the ovaries, ovarian function continued normally until the expected time of the menopause. In a study of premenopausal patients who had had radical surgery for cervical carcinoma, in whom the ovaries were conserved, Thompson and coworkers found normal estrogen values in all patients and also evidence of continued ovulation in young women. Cyclic ovarian function continued until the expected menopausal age, and patients

were spared the physical and psychological discomfort of a premature and acute surgical menopause.

If the ovary is to be conserved when hysterectomy is done, every attempt should be made to preserve its blood supply. The infundibulopelvic ligament containing the ovarian vessels must not be twisted or stretched. Clamps that are used to separate the ovary from the uterus should be placed as close to the uterine corpus as possible so that the arcade of vessels in the mesosalpinx that supply the ovary will not be interfered with (Fig. 11–7). Normal tubes should be left with the ovary. Attempts to remove the tube could interfere with ovarian blood supply. One might even elect to leave in a small hydrosalpinx, since its removal might jeopardize the blood supply to its companion ovary.

The blood supply to the ovary has been the subject of too few investigations. The general opinion is that the uterine artery supplies the medial half of the ovary and the medial two-thirds of the fallopian tube, the rest of the blood supply coming from the ovarian artery. The distribution of these arteries, however, shows great variation according to the studies of Borell and Fernstrom, ranging from cases in which the ovarian artery supplies the entire tube and ovary to cases in which the blood supply of these organs is solely derived from the uterine artery. If a significant portion of the blood supply to the ovary is derived from the uterine artery, continued normal ovarian function might not be possible after a hysterectomy because of inadequate blood supply.

A permanent disturbance of blood flow to the ovary at the time of hysterectomy may explain the occurrence of the so-called residual ovary syndrome. Interest in the residual ovary or residual adnexal syndrome began in 1955 with a report by Grogan and Duncan that 19 (5.1%) of 391 patients who had abdominal hysterectomy with ovarian conservation subsequently required removal of the ovaries because of an adnexal mass, severe pain, dyspareunia, or generalized pelvic discomfort. Another 20 patients developed similar problems of a less severe degree that did not require surgery. Grogan and Duncan stated that the interest of the patient was best served by prophylactic castration, mostly because of the frequency with which such conserved ovaries would subsequently show problems. In 1975, Christ and Lotze reported 202 (3.3%) cases of the residual ovary syndrome among 6188 patients with hysterectomy and ovarian conservation. Ranney and Abu–Ghazaleh conserved ovarian tissue in 1557 of 2153 patients (72%) who had a hysterectomy. Fourteen patients (0.9%) required a second operation to remove the conserved ovaries. Of 922 patients

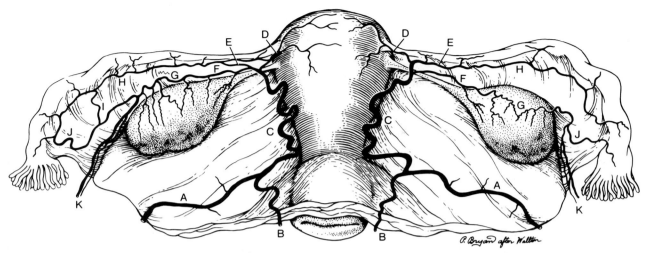

FIG. 11–7 Normal uterus and adnexa with schematic representation of the usual ovarian and uterine artery branches. Many variations exist.

A = Uterine artery in parametrium
B = Cervico-vaginal branch
C = Uterine artery along
   lateral margin of the uterus
D = Fundal branch
E = Medial tubal branch

F = Medial ovarian branch
G = Ovarian arcade
H = Tubal arcade
I = Lateral tubal branch
J = Infundibular branch
K = Ovarian artery

who had one or both ovaries conserved at the time of abdominal hysterectomy at Grady Memorial Hospital, Funt and associates reported that 13 patients (1.4%) required subsequent reoperation for pathology of the conserved adnexal tissue. These and other data suggest that 1% to 2% of patients who have one or both ovaries conserved at the time of hysterectomy will subsequently require operation for a problem with an ovary or tube. The pathology in the few residual adnexa requiring removal will usually show nothing more than a physiologic cyst, a small hydrosalpinx, or adhesions. The management of patients with physiologic cysts of the ovary remains the same whether the patient has had a previous hysterectomy or not.

The major risk of ovarian conservation at the time of hysterectomy is the risk that ovarian cancer, an admittedly devastating disease, will develop subsequently. Ovarian cancer remains one of the most lethal tumors of the female reproductive tract. Currently, in the United States about 11,000 women die each year from this disease alone. The ovary is hidden in the pelvis and is difficult to assess critically on pelvic examination. Few early warning signals accompany ovarian cancer, and in more than 60% of cases the cancer has spread beyond the boundaries of the ovarian capsule and beyond a reasonably curable stage at the time of its detection. Although there is no evidence to suggest that retained ovaries have a greater risk of neoplasia than do ovaries attached to an intact uterus, the gynecologist must accept the responsibility of assuring the patient that the continued hormonal function of the ovary has greater importance to the patient than the small risk of subsequent ovarian neoplasm.

Counseller and associates at the Mayo Clinic studied 1500 patients with ovarian cancer and found that 4.5% had previously undergone hysterectomy for benign disease. Terz and colleagues found an incidence of 5.1% and Fagan and coworkers reported an incidence of 7.5%. Among 200 patients with ovarian carcinoma in a study at the Johns Hopkins Hospital, 15 (almost 8%) had previously experienced a pelvic laparotomy. None of these patients would have developed ovarian cancer had the ovaries been removed at laparotomy. However, it should be noted that in many of the patients studied, the hysterectomy was performed vaginally. For reasons of technical difficulty the routine removal of normal ovaries is done less frequently with a vaginal than with an abdominal hysterectomy. In many cases, the vaginal hysterectomy was performed when the patient was younger than 40 years of age, an age when gynecologists would agree that normal ovaries should be retained. As shown in Table 11–1, ovarian cancer among hysterectomy patients with retained ovaries is very uncommon, occurring in approximately 0.1% of such cases.

TABLE 11-1 *Ovarian Cancer in Retained Ovaries*

STUDY (YEAR)	NUMBER OF HYSTERECTOMIES	CANCER IN RETAINED OVARIES	PERCENT
Randall (1963)	915	2	0.2
Gevaerts (1962)	300	0	0.0
Reycraft (1955)	4,500	9	0.2
Funck–Brentano (1958)	580	1	0.2
Whitelaw (1959)	1,215	0	0.0
Ranney (1977)	2,136	4	0.2
Funt (1977)	992	0	0.0
Total	10,638	16	0.1

Randall and Gerhardt, basing their assessment on the statistics of the health departments of the states of Connecticut and New York (excluding New York City), have calculated the probability of a 40-year-old woman developing cancer of the ovary is 0.9%. That probability remains at 0.9% until the woman reaches her 45th year, after which it begins to decline (0.82% at age 50; 0.7% after age 60; and 0.3% after age 70). Data from Randall's study would indicate that of the women over 50, 15 out of 1000 (1.5%) will develop an ovarian neoplasm. Of these, 9 (60%) will be malignant and 6 (40%) will be benign. Randall has further stated that if, in the 15 per 1000 women who had a pelvic laparotomy, both normal ovaries were removed, the incidence of ovarian cancer might be reduced from 9 cases to 7 cases per 1000 women. Hollenbeck concluded that prophylactic oophorectomy might conceivably save three patients from ovarian cancer if it were done routinely in 10,000 women who have a hysterectomy, although this question may require a complex equation for statistical validity. The conclusion is that, since the incidence of ovarian cancer after hysterectomy is 0.1% of all females, even universally practiced prophylactic oophorectomy would not reduce the incidence significantly. Even Grogan and Duncan, who were early advocates of oophorectomy, expressed the belief that prophylactic oophorectomy cannot be justified on the basis of its effect in reducing the incidence of ovarian malignancy. Some surgeons are of the opinion that the problem of ovarian cancer subsequent to hysterectomy can be solved by conservation of only one ovary instead of two, apparently feeling that the incidence of subsequent ovarian cancer will be reduced by 50%. There is no statistical data to support this view. Realistically, to retain one ovary is to retain 100% of the malignant potential of both ovaries. It has been shown that the incidence of anovulatory cycles increases and that menopause occurs at an earlier age if only one ovary is conserved. When it comes to the question of conservation of normal ovarian function, two normal ovaries are better than one. By conserving two normal ovaries, the incidence of subsequent ovarian cancer is not known to be increased.

After hysterectomy, of course, the role of the ovaries in the process of reproduction is irrelevant. However, the ovaries of premenopausal women play an active role in many basic metabolic processes throughout the body through secretion of estrogen, progesterone, and androgens. Ovarian hormones influence protein, calcium, bone, potassium, and carbohydrate metabolism, among others. The absence of ovarian function over a period of years has been implicated in the pathogenesis of osteoporosis, coronary artery disease, and cerebrovascular accidents. There is evidence from bone densitometry and other studies that patients with premature castration of more than ten years before expected menopause have a higher incidence of osteoporosis and coronary artery disease. Yet, there are many other interrelated factors that influence the development of these diseases. The extent to which long-term estrogen replacement therapy with or without progesterone may avert these problems in the premenopausal woman who has had bilateral oophorectomy is not completely determined. Even though it is considered desirable to give cyclic estrogen and progesterone replacement therapy to women who have been castrated, such therapy is not always well tolerated or without adverse side effects. Some premenopausal women tolerate an artificial menopause with few symptoms. Indeed, deNeef and Hollenbeck reported that only 50% of premenopausal women subjected to bilateral oophorectomy experienced menopausal symptoms. However, it is our experience that many premenopausal women undergo great discomfort, both physical and emotional, as a result of acute surgical castration. Low-dose cyclic replacement therapy appears to be safe and well tolerated by most premenopausal castrated women and is indicated to delay the appearance of osteoporosis and atrophy of the mucosa of the vagina and lower urinary tract. However, there are definite risks involved. Although as yet unproven, the risk of breast cancer may be slightly increased if benign breast lesions develop during estrogen treatment. Hypertension may develop in some patients, although the risk ratio is low and the hypertension should subside if estrogen treatment is discontinued. In the Boston Collaborative Drug Surveillance Program, the risk ratio for gallbladder disease in postmenopausal women who were users of conjugated estrogens was 2.5. The annual incidence of gallbladder disease for estrogen users was 218 per 100,000. For non-users it was 87 per 100,000. In the premenopausal woman who has had a hysterectomy and bilateral salpingo-oophorectomy, low-dose cyclic estrogen may be given so long as the patient understands and accepts her increased risk for gallbladder disease, the blood pressure is checked periodically, the breast examination is performed frequently, and estrogen treatment is discontinued if hypertension or breast tumors appear. The extent to which the adverse effect of long-term estrogen replacement treatment can be eliminated by the simultaneous use of progesterone has yet to be determined. Gambrell reports that the incidence of breast cancer is lower in estrogen-progestogen users (67.3:100,000) than in untreated women (342.3:100,000). The question of ovarian hormonal replacement for the surgically castrated premenopausal woman is a complicated one. Such replacement is not always well tolerated and certainly cannot and should not be depended upon to replace the useful function of normal ovaries to such an extent that premenopausal patients can be routinely castrated when abdominal hysterectomy is done.

Although we cannot subscribe to routine castration of premenopausal women undergoing abdominal hysterectomy, we cannot conceive of a good reason to conserve the ovaries of a woman who is menopausal or postmenopausal. Ovarian function after the menopause does not justify preservation of the ovary. Even though many menopausal and postmenopausal women have cytologic evidence of estrogen effect in the vaginal mucosa, it is clear that the ovary is not the source of the estrogen. Estradiol production rates are not significantly altered by removal of postmenopausal ovaries, according to Barlow and associates. Similarly, estrone production rates in postmenopausal women with intact ovaries and in those whose ovaries have been removed were found to be comparable by Siiteri and MacDonald. On the basis of differences in ovarian vein and peripheral vein concentrations, Judd and associates concluded that the postmenopausal ovary continues to secrete a large amount of testosterone and a moderate amount of androstenedione, but only minimal ovarian estrogen secretion was found. According to studies by Mikhail, Greenblatt and coworkers, and Vermeullen, the adrenal cortex is almost the exclusive source of plasma estradiol, estrone, and progesterone and is the most important source of plasma dehydroepiandrosterone in postmenopausal women. On the basis of these and other confirmatory investigations, it is concluded that there is no logical reason for conservation of ovaries at the time of abdominal hysterectomy in menopausal and postmenopausal women. Bilateral oophorectomy does eliminate the small chance of ovarian neoplasia developing subsequently, and it does not seem to cause the same psychological disturbance as in younger women.

The decision to remove the normal ovaries of a premenopausal woman who is undergoing hysterectomy or to conserve their function, presents a difficult choice for the thoughtful gynecologic surgeon. It is difficult to believe that we help a premenopausal woman in any way, either physically or psychologically, by removing her normal ovaries. Our evaluation of the available evidence suggests that the grossly normal ovaries of premenopausal women should be conserved when hysterectomy is done. We do not subscribe to their removal at some arbitrary age in the fifth decade. Although a decision to leave in or remove the ovaries should be based on an assessment of their functional status rather than on some arbitrary age, prophylactic oophorectomy is advised at the time of abdominal hysterectomy in women who are within 1 or 2 years of the mean age of menopause (age 51). Normal ovaries should always be removed when abdominal hysterectomy is done on the postmenopausal woman.

In this matter of removing or retaining ovaries, there are exceptions to any general rules. For example, Allen and Hertig found a family history of malignancy in 12.5% of their patients with cancer of the ovary. Counseller and associates found a family history of malignancy in 19% of patients with cancer of the ovary. Families in which women have an especially high genetic risk of ovarian cancer have been described by Lynch and associates, Fraumeni and associates, Lurain and Piver, and others. In such families one often encounters women with early-onset ovarian carcinoma as well as one or more of the cardinal tumors of the family cancer syndrome, namely, endometrial, breast, and colonic carcinoma. O'Brien and associates and others have concluded that primary carcinoma of the ovary is five times more frequent among women with previous carcinoma of the colon and rectum. A similar increase in the frequency of ovarian malignancy has been found in patients with breast carcinoma. Ovarian neoplasia is more common in the presence of the Peutz–Jeghers syndrome.* Therefore, bilateral prophylactic oophorectomy should be done when hysterectomy is indicated in premenopausal patients with the Peutz–Jeghers syndrome; with a personal history of breast, colon, or rectal cancer; or with a strong family history of ovarian cancer. Unfortunately, prophylactic oophorectomy in women who have a high genetic risk for ovarian malignancy will not always accomplish the protection desired. Tobacman and associates have reported performing prophylactic oophorectomy in 28 female members of 16 families at high risk for ovarian carcinoma. Three of these women subsequently developed disseminated intra-abdominal malignancy indistinguishable histopathologically from ovarian carcinoma. These authors suggest that in cancer-prone families, the susceptible tissue is not limited to the ovary but also includes other derivatives of the celomic epithelium, from which primary peritoneal neoplasms may arise following prophylactic oophorectomy. Woodruff has hypothesized that ovarian cancer with intra-abdominal spread may actually represent multicentric neoplasia derived from the embryonic mesothelium or celomic epithelium. The peritoneum and the germinal epithelium of the ovary have a common embryologic origin.

With few exceptions, both ovaries should be removed in postmenopausal and premenopausal patients with endometrial and ovarian malignancy. Young women who have radical abdominal hysterectomy and bilateral lymphadenectomy for early invasive cervical cancer may have both normal ovaries conserved. When an ovary is severely involved by a tumor, cyst, infection, adhesions, or endometriosis, or when its blood supply is compromised, it should be removed. If an ovarian cystectomy is done, the ovary should be meticulously repaired with fine suture material to eliminate interstitial dead space and minimize adhesions. If more than two-thirds of the ovarian parenchyma has been removed, the entire ovary should be removed. During vaginal hysterectomy, the ovaries are examined but generally are not removed vaginally in the premenopausal patient. If the ovaries are accessible, the same guidelines for prophylactic oophorectomy should apply to the menopausal and postmenopausal patient at the time of vaginal hysterectomy. If it is important to remove the ovaries because of gross pathology or to resect an ovarian lesion, it should usually be done through an abdominal incision.

If a bilateral oophorectomy is done, whether for prophylactic reasons or because of pathology of the ovaries or uterus, the ovaries should be removed completely. If a remnant of ovarian parenchyma is left remaining in a premenopausal woman, especially if it is left in an extraperitoneal location, it may eventually cause symptoms such as pelvic pain or dyspareunia. A tender mass may be palpable on the pelvic side wall. Ureteral obstruction may be found on intravenous pyelography, as discussed by Phillips and McGahan. Plasma follicle-stimulating hormone, luteinizing hormone, and estrogen levels will confirm the presence of functioning ovarian tissue. Symmonds and Pettit reviewed their experience with twenty cases of ovarian remnants at the Mayo Clinic and described the difficult technical problems encountered in operative removal. The ovarian remnant syndrome is more likely to follow a difficult abdominal hysterectomy and bilateral salpingo-oophorectomy for extensive pelvic endometriosis or pelvic inflammatory disease.

In spite of these exceptions, the golden rule of pelvic surgery is the conservation of useful organ function. And the conservation of both normal ovaries in premenopausal women at the time of abdominal hysterectomy does represent conservation of useful function, in our opinion.

The Technique of Total Abdominal Hysterectomy for Benign Disease

The technique of abdominal hysterectomy presented here was originally described by Richardson in 1929. We regard Richardson's technique as classic, and we include some of his original illustrations to emphasize the important and time-honored features of the procedure.

Abdominal hysterectomy for benign disease is done most often for leiomyomata. The great variation in size and shape of the uterus with leiomyomata makes it necessary to deviate from any standard surgical technique and, frequently, to improvise as one proceeds. Also, the complication of adnexal disease may prevent the carrying out of a uniform procedure. However, the gynecologic surgeon should have some standard plan that can be modified as may become necessary in the course of the operation. Such a standard operative technique is presented here. Although we present this procedure of abdominal hysterectomy as it might be done in the surgical treatment of leiomyomata

---

* Peutz–Jeghers syndrome is characterized by generalized multiple polyposis of the intestinal tract associated with melanin spots of the lips, buccal mucosa, and fingers. It is inherited by autosomal dominance.

uteri, this method is also used for the surgical treatment of other benign pelvic disease, including pelvic endometriosis, pelvic inflammatory disease, adnexal tumors, and other benign pathology.

The patient should be properly prepared for operation. After satisfactory general anesthesia is obtained, an indwelling urethral catheter is placed in the bladder and left in for continuous bladder drainage. Keeping the bladder empty will facilitate exposure, and the amount of urine output can be measured. A careful pelvic examination under anesthesia, including a bimanual rectovaginal abdominal examination, is always performed. The vaginal preparation prior to hysterectomy is a most important part of the procedure. Although we do not routinely use vaginal suppositories containing antibiotics prior to surgery, we do prescribe a povidone-iodine (Betadine) vaginal douche the evening before surgery. The vaginal preparation at surgery is a thorough povidone-iodine scrub, with particular emphasis placed on the intravaginal cleansing of the vaginal fornices using soaked sponges on long sponge forceps. Although it is impossible to sterilize all the rugal folds of the vagina, it is important to render this area surgically clean prior to the procedure. Dry sponges should be used to remove excess solution from the vagina. Special attention should be paid to cleansing the depths of the umbilicus with cotton tip applicators during the abdominal preparation.

To facilitate the operative procedure and to avoid injury to vital structures, adequate exposure through a lower abdominal incision is mandatory. In cases of benign disease, however, the lower abdominal transverse Maylard incision may be preferred. The exposure with a true or modified Pfannenstiel incision is usually not adequate for the performance of abdominal hysterectomy.

After the incision is made, the upper abdomen is explored. Standing on the patient's right side, the operator inserts the right hand into the the upper abdomen. The right kidney, liver, gallbladder, pancreas, stomach, left kidney, and para-aortic lymph nodes are palpated in sequence, and abnormalities are noted. Some type of self-retaining retractor is inserted to expose the pelvic contents. The O'Connor–O'Sullivan or Balfour self-retaining retractors may be used. However, we prefer to use the Bookwalter self-retaining retractor. Adhesions must be released before the intestines can be placed in the upper abdomen and held there with packs. Restoration of pelvic anatomy by release of adhesions will facilitate the operative procedure.

At this point in the procedure, one should pause and make an assessment of the nature and extent of pelvic pathology; of the anatomical relationships,

with particular reference to the ureters, bladder, and rectum; and of the operative procedure to be performed.

The Ochsner clamp (also called Kocher clamp), both straight and curved, is commonly used throughout in performing abdominal hysterectomy. The Masterson clamp was specially designed for hysterectomy. We have found it to be satisfactory. Although a modest Trendelenburg position may be helpful, an exaggerated or steep Trendelenburg position should be avoided.

The operation usually begins with the round ligaments. Even in patients with very extensive pathology and distorted anatomy, the round ligaments can usually be identified. Following the round ligaments medially will always lead to the uterine corpus. One of the round ligaments is grasped with a curved Ochsner clamp near the uterine cornu, cut with the scalpel or scissors, and ligated a short distance distal to the clamp with No. 0 delayed-absorbable suture (Fig. 11–8). Thus, the anterior leaf of the broad ligament is opened. The anterior leaf of the broad ligament is incised to the point of reflection of the bladder peritoneum on the uterus (Fig. 11–9). The posterior leaf of the broad ligament is pushed forward with the surgeon's fingers (Fig. 11–10). This portion of the broad ligament is quite avascular. It is incised with the scissors, thus making a window in the broad ligament.

If the tubes and ovaries are to be conserved, the tube and the ovarian ligament are triply clamped

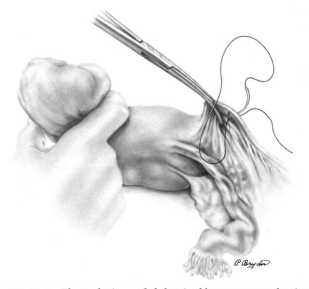

FIG. 11–8 The technique of abdominal hysterectomy begins with the round ligament. The ligament is clamped, ligated with a transfixion suture, and cut. The broad ligament is opened.

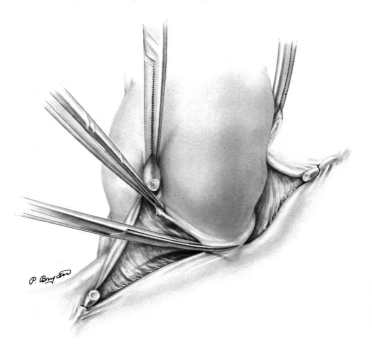

FIG. 11–9 Abdominal hysterectomy. The anterior leaf of the broad ligament is incised to the point where the bladder peritoneum is reflected onto the anterior lower uterine isthmus in the midline. To avoid unnecessary blood loss, the bladder is not dissected away from the uterus at this point.

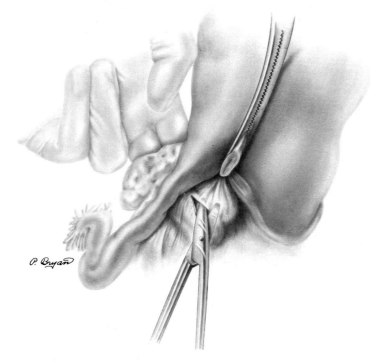

FIG. 11–10 Abdominal hysterectomy. Two fingers push the posterior leaf of the broad ligament forward. An incision is made to develop a window in the broad ligament.

(Fig. 11–11). The clamps should be placed as close to the uterine corpus as possible so that blood vessels in the mesosalpinx and mesovarium will not be interfered with. The clamp closest the uterus is to control back bleeding and to provide traction on the uterus; therefore, the incision with the scapel

is made between it and the middle clamp. Thus, the ovarian vessels are doubly clamped as they extend from the uterine artery and vein. Double clamping of the ovarian vessels is our usual routine and we believe that it is an excellent precaution. It prevents slipping and retraction of the cut vessels

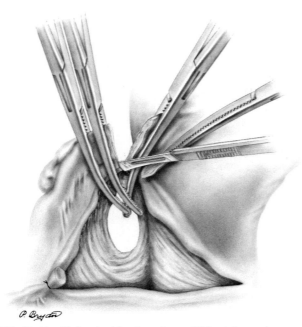

FIG. 11–11 Abdominal hysterectomy. If the tube and ovary are to be conserved, three Ochsner clamps are placed across the tube and utero-ovarian ligament as close to the uterus as possible. An incision is made between the middle and the medial clamp.

with the formation of a broad ligament hematoma. Further, the ligation must be in the nature of a mass tie, and the crushing of the tissues by means of the second clamp affords a groove in which to tie the first ligature. The second (lateral) clamp on the cut pedicle is removed as a free tie ligature is tied, and the proximal clamp is kept in place. A free tie ligature of No. 0 delayed-absorbable suture is used initially to avoid trauma to the vessels in the vascular pedicle. These vessels must be ligated first so that the pedicle may be secured again distally with a transfixion suture. A No. 0 delayed-absorbable suture is placed in front of the first ligature in the center of the pedicle beneath the remaining clamp, passing the free ends of the suture around the tip and heel of the clamp before tying. The clamp is then removed (Fig. 11–12). There are instances in which the double clamp technique cannot be used, but when it is feasible we believe it to be a worthwhile precaution.

If the tube and the ovary are to be removed with the uterus, the infundibulopelvic portion of the broad ligament is clamped with three curved Ochsner clamps (Fig. 11–13). One should locate the ureter before placing clamps on the infundibulopelvic ligament. The tip of each clamp is placed through the open window in the broad ligament. The ligament

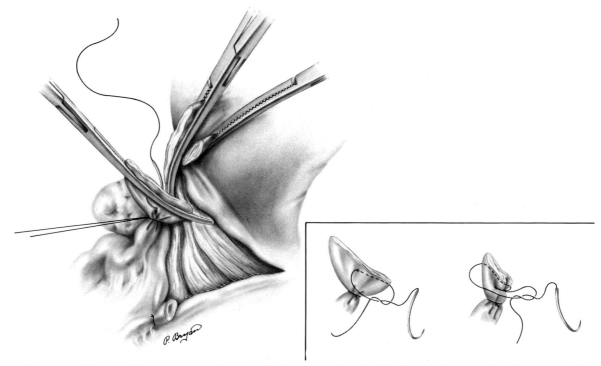

FIG. 11–12 Abdominal hysterectomy. The lateral clamp is replaced with a free tie that completely surrounds the pedicle and occludes the vessels. The middle clamp is replaced by a transfixion suture ligature that is tied securely around both sides of the pedicle.

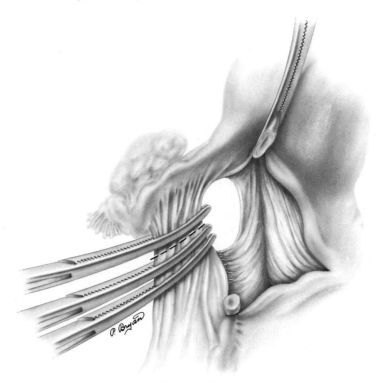

FIG. 11–13 Abdominal hysterectomy. If the tube and ovary are to be removed, three Ochsner clamps are placed across the infundibulopelvic ligament, using the window in the broad ligament. After the ureter is located, the lateral-most clamp is placed first. The ligament is incised at the dotted line, and the pedicle is doubly ligated with No. 0 delayed-absorbable suture as illustrated in Fig. 11–12.

is divided, and double ligation of the ovarian vessels by No. 0 delayed-absorbable ligature is carried out. The initial ligature around the distal clamp on the cut pedicle is a free tie, while the second tie is a transfixion suture placed distal to the first tie through the center of the tissue behind the remaining clamp. In general, it is good policy to ligate the clamped ovarian vessels as they are cut rather than to leave all the clamps on the pedicles until after the uterus is removed. Likewise, sutures used to ligate pedicles are cut and are not held.

Clamping, cutting, and ligating of the round ligament, the uterine end of the tube, and ovarian ligament or of the infundibulopelvic ligament are carried out in the same manner on the opposite side.

The midline reflection of the bladder peritoneum onto the uterus is then freed by extending the incision in the anterior leaf of the broad ligament. It is technically easier to incise and free the bladder peritoneum from the lower portion of the uterus by continuing the dissection of the anterior leaf of the broad ligament when each round ligament is cut rather than by initiating the dissection in the midline. This provides a free margin of peritoneum to incise toward the midportion of the lower uterine segment on each side of the uterus where the incisions meet. A subperitoneal tissue plane is easily obtained by sliding the Metzenbaum scissors, with

the curvature facing upward, beneath the peritoneum prior to incising the peritoneum. If the dissection is made just through the peritoneum, a good line of cleavage is entered; if the cut goes too deeply, bleeding will be encountered. At this point, the bladder should be separated from the lower uterine segment and upper cervix by careful sharp dissection of the fascial fibers beneath the bladder wall (Fig. 11–14). Complete mobilization of the bladder away from the cervix and upper anterior vaginal wall will be needed eventually. However, to avoid unnecessary blood loss, this complete dissection and mobilization may be done later. Using a sponge on a sponge forceps to push the bladder down may cause unnecessary trauma to the bladder musculature, especially if the bladder is unusually adherent to the cervix. Usually, the bladder can be dissected away and displaced into the lower pelvis quite easily, but if it is adherent, it should be surgically released with Metzenbaum scissors and not bluntly forced.

The posterior leaf of the broad ligament is cut on either side parallel with the lateral side of the uterus down to the point of origin of the uterosacral ligaments behind the cervix (Fig. 11–15). Incising the anterior and posterior broad ligament peritoneum will allow the uterine vessels to be exposed and skeletonized before they are clamped.

Before clamping and cutting the uterine vessels,

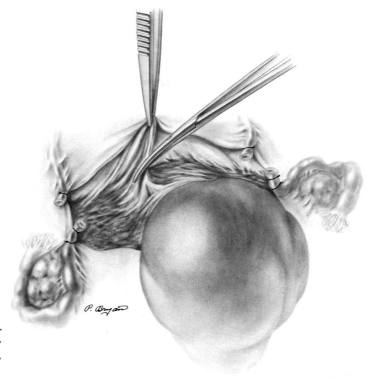

FIG. 11-14 Abdominal hysterectomy. The bladder must be mobilized inferiorly by sharp dissection away from the cervix. In order to avoid unnecessary bleeding, this step may be done in stages as necessary.

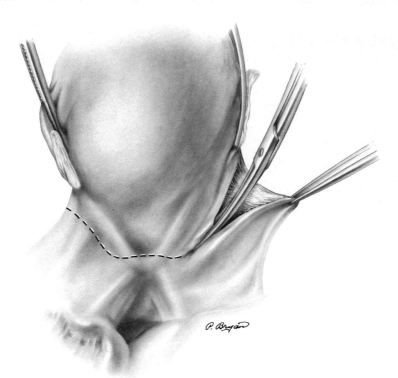

FIG. 11-15 Abdominal hysterectomy. The posterior leaf of the broad ligament is incised down to the point where the uterosacral ligaments join the cervix, as illustrated by the dotted lines. Dissection across the back of the cervix can be delayed until later to avoid unnecessary bleeding.

it is always advisable to palpate the lower portion of the pelvic ureters as they course beneath the uterine artery, lateral to the internal cervical os, and pass medially through the base of the broad ligament to enter the trigone of the bladder. With wide mobilization and displacement of the bladder base from the cervix, and with traction on the uterine corpus, the ureters are usually 1.5 cm to 2.0 cm lateral and inferior to the point of clamping of the uterine vessels. However, they may be displaced by pelvic disease and induration of paracervical tissue, particularly in the presence of endometriosis and pelvic inflammatory disease, and should be identified before the clamps are placed in this vulnerable area.

The uterine vessels are completely skeletonized and exposed and are then triply clamped bilaterally with curved Ochsner clamps (Fig. 11–16). It is desirable to have these clamps slide off the edge of the cervix. It is important to remember three rules in clamping uterine vessels: first, the lowest clamp is placed initially; second, this clamp is placed at the level of the internal cervical os; and third, it is placed at right angles to the lower uterine segment. If one places clamps on uterine vessels in this way, injury to the ureter should be avoided.

The upper clamp is intended to prevent back bleeding from the uterus, while the two lower clamps doubly occlude the uterine vessels. The vessels are cut with the scalpel between the upper and middle clamps and freed from the uterus by extending the incision around the tip of the middle clamp. This separates the vessels from the uterus and permits direct ligation of the vascular pedicles. This step also provides access to the upper portion of the cardinal ligament. Care should be taken to avoid incising the tissue beyond the tip of the lowest clamp because doing so could permit bleeding from collateral vessels that are not included in the clamp. The sutures must be placed precisely in the angle of the incision and the tip of the clamp to be certain that all of the vessels in the clamp are secured by the ligature.

The uterine vessels are doubly ligated with No. 0 delayed-absorbable suture with ligation of the tissue within the lowest clamp initially. Each suture is placed into the fascia at the tip of each clamp. As the first suture is tied, the clamp is removed; if the bite of tissue is large, it may be well to loosen the middle clamp slightly and then reclose the ratchet to permit the tissue to be compressed tightly by the ligature. As the second ligature is placed and tied, the middle clamp is removed. Double clamping is of great value here, for if only one clamp is used and the tissue slips out of the ligature and retracts, the uterine vessels must be caught again in the pres-

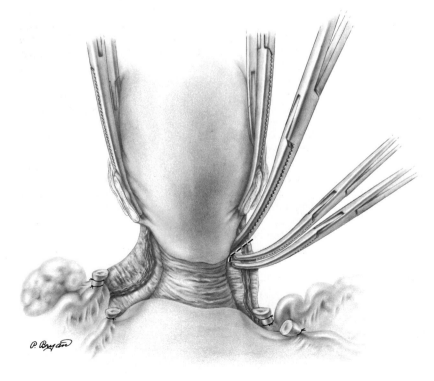

FIG. 11–16 Abdominal hysterectomy. After the uterine vessels are skeletonized, they are triply clamped and cut along the dotted lines. To avoid clamping the ureter, the lowest clamp is placed first, at the level of the internal cervical os and at right angles to the lower uterine isthmus. The lowest two clamps are replaced by No. 0 delayed-absorbable suture ligatures.

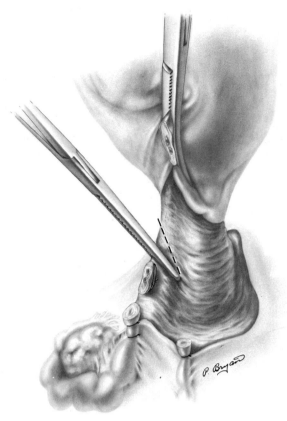

FIG. 11–17   Total abdominal hysterectomy. If a total hysterectomy is to be done, the uterine vessels are dropped away by placing an Ochsner clamp across the upper cardinal ligament between the uterine vessels and the lower uterine isthmus. The tissue is cut and ligated.

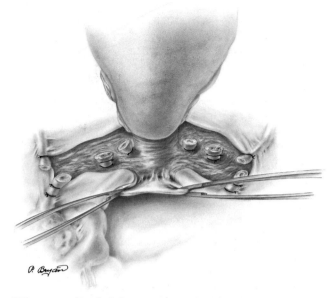

FIG. 11–18   Total abdominal hysterectomy. A flap of peritoneum is dissected from the cervix posteriorly. This will allow the uterosacral ligaments to be isolated and the rectovaginal space to be entered behind the cervix.

ence of bleeding. Attempts at clamping retracted uterine vessels in the base of the broad ligament may result in injury to the ureter.

Following ligation of the uterine vessels, a straight Ochsner clamp may be placed between the uterine vessels and the side of the uterus (Fig. 11–17). The tissue clamped is the uppermost part of the cardinal ligament. The incision is made in such a way that a fringe of tissue remains distal to the clamp. This will enhance the security of its ligation and will allow the uterine vessel pedicle to drop further laterally.

The uterus is pulled forward and upward to expose and stretch the uterosacral ligaments posteriorly. The incisions in the posterior peritoneum of the broad ligaments are carried transversely through the uterine reflection of the cul-de-sac peritoneum between the attachments of the two uterosacral ligaments. The peritoneal flap is mobilized

initially from its attachment to the cervix and posterior vaginal fornix with the Metzenbaum scissors (Fig. 11–18). Each uterosacral ligament is clamped with a curved Ochsner clamp, with particular care being taken to avoid the pelvic portion of the ureter as it courses along the base of the broad ligament. The anterior rectal wall must also be avoided. The uterosacral ligaments are then clamped, incised, and ligated with No. 0 delayed-absorbable suture (Fig. 11–19). Continued sharp and blunt dissection inferiorly in the center of the cul de sac between the ligated uterosacral ligaments will develop a plane between the cervix and vagina anteriorly and the anterior rectal wall posteriorly. This is the entrance to the rectovaginal space (Fig. 11–20). Usually there is no bleeding if a proper loose areolar plane is entered and care is taken to avoid extensive lateral dissection where the hemorrhoidal vessels insert into the rectum (Fig. 11–21).

At this point, dissection of the bladder base away from the anterior vaginal wall must be completed (Fig. 11–22). Inadequate dissection and mobilization of the bladder is one of the most frequent causes of inadvertent injury to the bladder wall. Bladder injury may result in a vesicovaginal fistula if the injury is not recognized and repaired at the time of surgery. With the uterus under firm traction, the two index fingers or the thumb and index finger

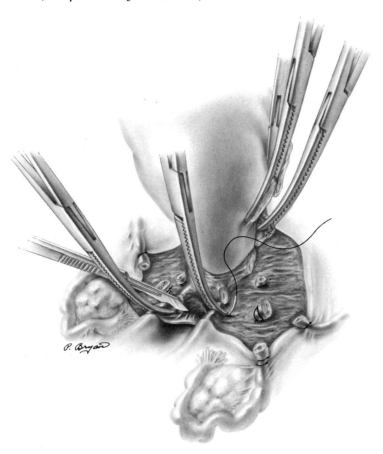

P. Bryan

FIG. 11-19 Total abdominal hysterectomy. The uterosacral ligaments are clamped, cut, and ligated adjacent to the cervix. Each clamp is replaced by a No. 0 delayed-absorbable suture.

from the same hand may be readily opposed below the cervix, and further dissection of the base of the bladder anteriorly and the rectum posteriorly can be accomplished if needed (Fig. 11–23).

It is important to call particular attention to the pubovesicocervical fascia, which was originally described by Richardson in 1929 and reviewed by Jaszczak and Evans. This fascia contains many small arteries and venous plexuses that provide collateral circulation to the base of the bladder, cervix, and upper vagina. It is part of the endopelvic fascia that surrounds the cervix and blends with the cardinal ligament, the uterosacral ligament, and the broad ligament and extends to the lateral pelvic wall. To avoid these vessels and to provide protection to the base of the bladder and the adjacent ureter, a T-shaped or V-shaped incision is made in the fascia anterior to the cervix just below the level of the internal cervical os and the ligated uterine vessels. As the edges of the fascia retract laterally, a pale avascular area of the anterior surface of the cervix and vagina can be seen. Care should be taken to avoid incising too deeply into the cervix as this will

produce additional bleeding, the loose fascial plane will be missed, and the dissection will be difficult and bloody. The blunt end of the scalpel is useful in dissecting the loosened fibers of the pubovesicocervical fascia from the cervix. The dissection can be continued with a sponge forceps until the fascia has been reflected far laterally off the anterior surface of the cervix and upper vagina. As this dissection progresses, the whitish fascial plane of the vagina comes into view and gives clear evidence to the operator that the plane of dissection is correct. Dissection of the remaining portion of the cardinal ligament is carried out by placing straight Ochsner clamps inside the cut edges of the pubovesicocervical fascia (Fig. 11–24). Usually two or three bites are required on either side of the cervix until the pale white tissue of the vaginal wall representing the lateral vaginal fornix is identified. Occasionally, the lateral fornix is entered when the lower portion of the cardinal ligament is incised, clearly defining the vaginal apex. The anterior and posterior walls of the vagina may be clamped together at each lateral vaginal angle as shown in Figure 11–25, using an

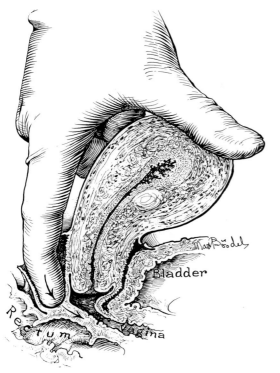

FIG. 11-20 Total abdominal hysterectomy. A sagittal view showing the bladder dissection completed and indicating depth and direction of the posterior dissection into the rectovaginal space. (Richardson EH: A simplified technic for abdominal panhysterectomy. Surg Gynecol Obstet 48:248, 1929.)

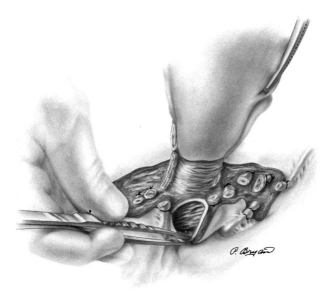

FIG. 11-21 Total abdominal hysterectomy. Dissection between the ligated uterosacral ligaments behind the cervix will enter the rectovaginal space. This step is also illustrated in Fig. 11-20.

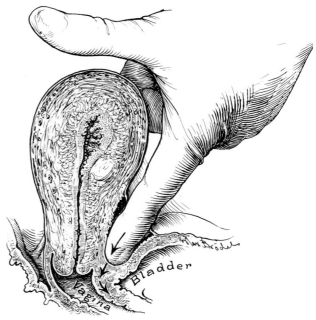

FIG. 11-22 Total abdominal hysterectomy. A sagittal view showing depth and direction of the vesicocervicovaginal dissection. This step serves to displace the bladder and the ureters still further away from the danger zone. (Richardson EH: A simplified technic for abdominal panhysterectomy. Surg Gynecol Obstet 48;248, 1929.)

Ochsner clamp, or the uterus may be removed by a circumferential incision in the vagina close to the cervix, being certain that the entire cervix is removed with the uterine corpus (Fig. 11-26). As the anterior, posterior, and lateral angles of the vagina are opened, straight Ochsner clamps are used to secure the vaginal margins. Ochsner clamps on the lateral vaginal angles are replaced with transfixion sutures (Fig. 11-27).

The original Richardson technique utilized routine vaginal drainage, which was a major contribution to this procedure. Although we formerly practiced tight closure of the vaginal vault for most of our cases, the open cuff technique has recently regained popularity as a method of extraperitoneal drainage. When the vaginal vault is left open, the incidence of cuff cellulitis, abscess, and hematoma is reduced. It has been our experience that the open cuff does remain patent for a sufficient length of time to serve as a useful conduit for serum or blood that may accumulate gradually above the vaginal vault. However, if better drainage is required for a longer time, we have found the addition of a small Penrose drain as described by Richardson to be more effective than the open cuff technique alone.

After the vaginal angle clamps have been replaced

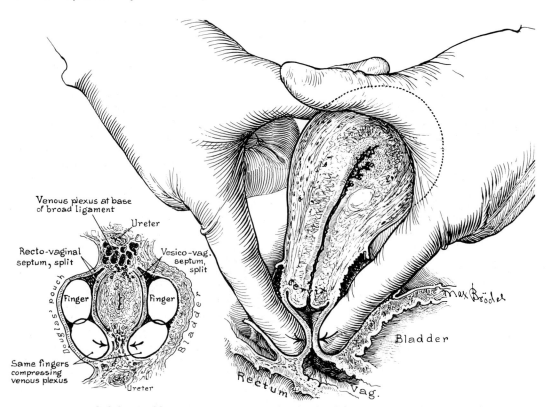

FIG. 11-23 Total abdominal hysterectomy. Testing the depth of the anterior and posterior dissections. The inset shows the method of segregating the vascular plexus on each side into a narrow zone adjacent to the basal segment of the broad ligament. (Richardson EH: A simplified technic for abdominal pan-hysterectomy. Surg Gynecol Obstet 48:248, 1929.)

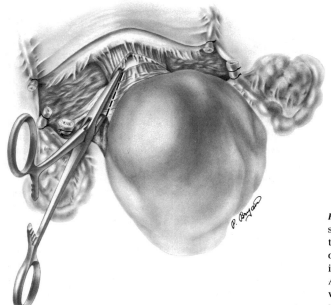

FIG. 11-24 Total abdominal hysterectomy. A T-shaped or V-shaped incision is made in the pubovesicocervical fascia anterior to the cervix. Straight Ochsner clamps are placed across the cardinal ligaments lateral to the cervix and inside the fascia in such a way that the fascia is actually peeled off the cervix. An incision is made at the dotted line and the clamp is replaced with a No. 0 delayed-absorbable suture. Several bites may be needed in each cardinal ligament.

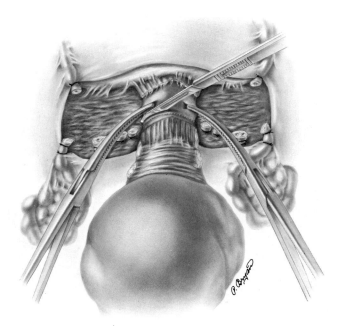

FIG. 11-25 Total abdominal hysterectomy. After one determines with certainty that the bladder and rectum have been completely dissected away from the vagina, curved Ochsner clamps are placed across the vaginal angles and the uterus is removed by incising the vagina below the cervix.

with transfixion sutures, the free margin of the vagina is reefed with a continuous locking suture of No. 2-0 delayed-absorbable suture (Fig. 11–27). Alternatively, the vaginal vault may be sutured closed (Fig. 11–28).

Because of the possibility of vaginal vault prolapse or enterocele in subsequent years after abdominal hysterectomy, careful attention must be paid to the support of the vaginal vault. A new step may be added to the standard Richardson technique at this point. It is the performance of a posterior culde-plasty as illustrated in Fig. 11–29. A No. 0 delayed-absorbable suture is passed first through the uterosacral ligament on one side. The suture then passes in and out of the posterior vaginal fornix and through the uterosacral ligament on the opposite side (Fig. 11–30). When tied, this suture approximates the uterosacral ligaments behind the vagina and pulls the posterior vaginal fornix in a posterior direction. More than one suture may be used if the posterior fornix appears unduly relaxed. Care must be taken to avoid the ureters when placing the sutures in the uterosacral ligaments.

Additional suspension of the vaginal vault is combined with a peritonization suture. This technique places the free margins of the vascular pedicles beneath the peritoneum so that any postoperative

bleeding will be contained retroperitoneally in the base of the pelvis. The technique uses a continuous No. 0 delayed-absorbable suture that first pierces the anterior vaginal wall and passes through the ligated pedicle of the angle of the vagina and the free margin of the cardinal ligament, staying distal to the original cardinal ligament ligature (Fig. 11–31). The suture then passes through the anterior bladder peritoneum near the round ligament, continues through the free margin of the round ligament and the remaining edge of the anterior leaf of the broad ligament; incorporates the free margin of the infundibulopelvic pelvic ligament or utero-ovarian ligament and continues posteriorly along the cut edge of the posterior leaf of the broad ligament, incorporating the uterosacral ligament; and, finally, pierces the posterior edge of the vaginal wall near the midline (Fig. 11–31). A similar suture is placed on the opposite side of the pelvis, and both ligatures are tied firmly in the midline. These sutures accomplish vaginal vault suspension and peritonization on each side. If the ovaries have been preserved, an alternative suspension is used in which the tip of the broad ligament is closed separately with a purse-string suture of No. 3-0 delayed-absorbable suture and the free margin of the pedicle is buried beneath the peritoneum. By this technique, the ovaries are retained high against the pelvic wall and are not anchored to the vaginal vault. This is advised in order to avoid subsequent dyspareunia and to avoid overstretching of the ovarian vessels with possible thrombosis, ischemia, and cystic change of the ovary.

Peritonization is completed by suturing the bladder peritoneum to the cul-de-sac peritoneum with No. 3-0 delayed-absorbable suture. This suture is initiated near the angle of the vagina where the anterior peritoneum is pierced, and the peritoneum over the round ligament and infundibulopelvic ligament is picked up before the cul-de-sac peritoneum is sutured (Fig. 11–32). The suture is tied, which ensures that the vascular pedicles remain beneath the peritoneum, and is then continued to the opposite angle of the vagina as a continuous suture, approximating the bladder and cul-de-sac peritoneum. If preferred, interrupted No. 3-0 delayed-absorbable sutures may be used.

In our hands, this technique of total abdominal hysterectomy has proven to be superior to any thus far described. It is logically planned to ensure complete hemostasis, to keep the pelvis free of interfering clamps at all times, and to utilize all ligamentous supports for the vagina. Basically, it is quite similar to the original Richardson procedure and has been modified only minimally from its original description.

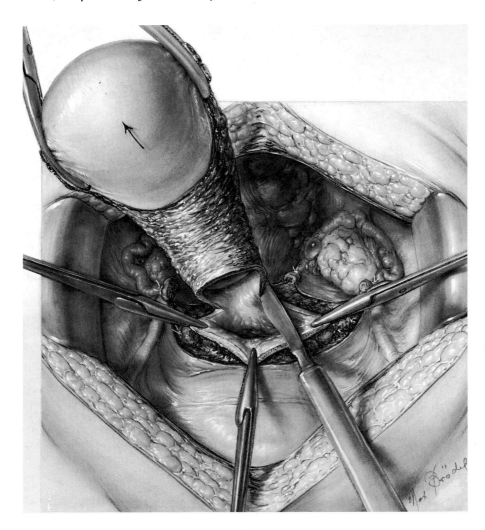

FIG. 11-26 Total abdominal hysterectomy. The dissection completed, the amputation across the vaginal vault is shown here. This should be done as closely as possible to the cervix in order to avoid shortening the vagina. The four quadrants of the vaginal vault are held with straight Ochsner clamps for subsequent placement of sutures. (Richardson EH: A simplified technic for abdominal panhysterectomy. Surg Gynecol Obstet 48:248, 1929.)

Recently, one of us (JDT) has performed all abdominal hysterectomies with patients placed in the Crawford stirrups. With proper preparation and draping, the vaginal orifice is available for the purpose of allowing a determination of ureteral integrity before the incision is closed. Five cc of Indigo carmine is injected intravenously. Approximately 200 cc of clear sterile saline is instilled into the bladder through the Foley catheter, and the catheter is removed. A cystoscope is placed in the bladder. Within 4 to 5 minutes, the blue dye will be seen spurting from both ureteral orifices. The procedure is very easy, takes very little time, and provides reassurance that both ureters are functioning normally. The urethral catheter is replaced but is removed early in the morning of the first postoperative day.

Subtotal Hysterectomy

The technique of a subtotal abdominal hysterectomy is identical to that for a total abdominal hysterectomy until ligation of the uterine arteries has been performed. In the usual subtotal hysterectomy, the bladder need not be freed extensively from the cervix. Bleeding is prevented by avoiding unnecessary dissection of the bladder from the cervix; although where a very low amputation of the cervix is desired, freeing of the bladder must be carried out as low as necessary to perform the amputation. Following ligation of the uterine arteries, the corpus is amputated as indicated by the dotted line in Figure 11-33. The level of this amputation should always be below the internal cervical os in order to avoid bothersome cyclic menstrual bleeding from rem-

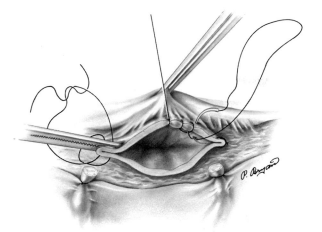

FIG. 11-27 Total abdominal hysterectomy. The clamps on the lateral vaginal angles are replaced by No. 0 delayed-absorbable transfixion sutures. A No. 2-0 delayed-absorbable continuous locking suture is placed around the vaginal margin. Again, the bladder must be completely mobilized and retracted inferiorly. An alternative method, closing the vagina, is illustrated in Fig. 11-28.

nants of endometrium. It is well to make a V-shaped cut in the cervical stroma and endocervix. This facilitates the closure of the stump and ensures that the endometrium has been removed as well as much of the endocervical canal. The cervical stump is then closed, using figure-of-eight sutures of No. 0 delayed-absorbable suture, as illustrated in Fig. 11-

34A,B. A cutting needle may facilitate placement of this suture, although it is usually not necessary. The cervical stump is suspended by suturing the various ligaments to it as described for a total hysterectomy. Figure 11–34C shows this step when the adnexa on both sides have been saved. The suture is first placed through the anterior surface of the cervix. It then picks up the anterior peritoneum and the round ligament. A bite or two is taken in the peritoneum between the round ligament and the tube. The tube to which the ovarian ligament has been tied is next included. One or two bites are taken in the posterior leaf of the broad ligament. In picking up the broad ligament, one should be careful to include only the peritoneal edge under vision because of the risk of kinking or ligating the ureter with the suture if wide bites are taken. Finally, a bite is taken in the posterior surface of the cervix. An assistant grasps the ends of the round ligament and the tube and the suspension suture is tied over them. This suture not only suspends the cervix, but also partially peritonizes the pelvis.

If the adnexa have been removed, the suspension and the peritonization are done somewhat differently. The infundibulopelvic ligament may be sufficiently mobile to be brought down to the cervix without tension, but often it is not. In such cases, the leaves of the tip of the broad ligament may be closed separately with a continuous No. 3-0 delayed-absorbable suture as previously described and the stump of the infundibulopelvic ligament buried beneath the peritoneum by a purse-string suture.

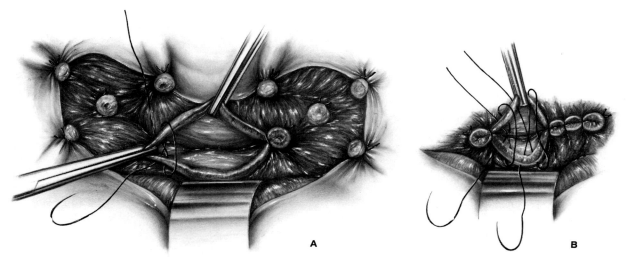

FIG. 11-28 Total abdominal hysterectomy. (*A*) The uterus has been removed by the open technique, with straight Ochsner clamps being placed on the anterior, lateral, and posterior vaginal margins. Figure-of-eight sutures are placed in each angle of the vagina and carefully tied behind the clamps to secure the vaginal vessels. (*B*) The vaginal vault is closed with figure-of-eight sutures, the last sutures placed in the midline for traction.

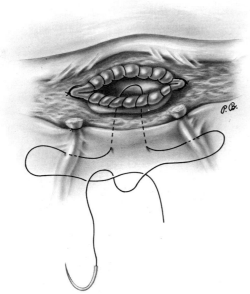

FIG. 11-29 Total abdominal hysterectomy. Taking care to avoid the ureters, No. 0 delayed-absorbable suture is passed through both uterosacral ligaments and the posterior vaginal fornix.

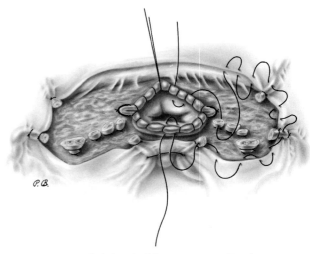

FIG. 11-31 Total abdominal hysterectomy. Further suspension and reperitonization of the pelvis is accomplished by a continuous No. 0 delayed-absorbable suture that includes the anterior vagina, the cardinal ligament, the anterior edge of broad ligament peritoneum, the round ligament, the utero-ovarian or infundibulopelvic ligament, the posterior edge of broad ligament peritoneum, the uterosacral ligament, and the posterior vagina. A similar suture is placed on the opposite side.

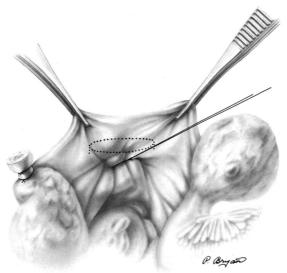

FIG. 11-30 Total abdominal hysterectomy. When the posterior culdeplasty suture is tied, the posterior vaginal fornix is pulled in a more natural direction toward the sacrum.

The peritonization of the cervical stump is carried out by suturing the edge of the bladder peritoneum to the cul-de-sac peritoneum using either interrupted or continuous No. 3-0 delayed-absorbable sutures. To ensure that the cut ends of the ligaments and the tubes are covered, it is often desirable to pick up the structures at the angles of the vagina with the suture as indicated in Figure 11-34D, to cause them to invert beneath the peritoneum.

Complications of Abdominal Hysterectomy

Serious morbidity and occasional mortality still occur from abdominal hysterectomy. According to the study of Dicker and associates, women who undergo vaginal hysterectomy experience significantly fewer complications than women who undergo abdominal hysterectomy. This is almost certainly a consequence of the fact that patients with the most serious pelvic disease are generally operated upon abdominally. Abdominal hysterectomy places the urinary tract and intestinal tract at greater risk of injury and also involves making an incision in the abdominal wall. Vaginal hysterectomy, on the other hand, is often associated with anterior and posterior colporrhaphy. Although the complications of vaginal and abdominal hysterectomy are often compared, the operations are not comparable and are not done for comparable pathology.

Some complications of abdominal hysterectomy, such as injuries to the urinary tract, are discussed in other chapters.

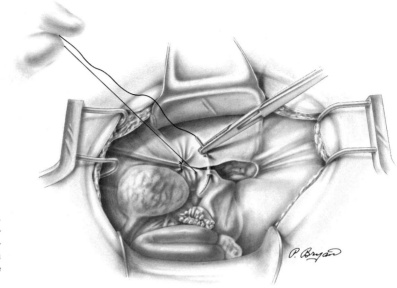

FIG. 11-32 Total abdominal hysterectomy. Reperitonization is completed with a continuous No. 3-0 delayed-absorbable suture that approximates the edge of the bladder peritoneum to the edge of the cul-de-sac peritoneum. The ovaries should be left laterally.

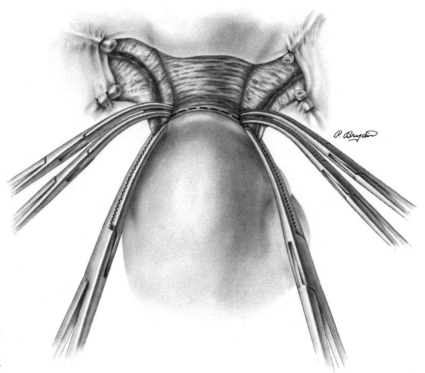

FIG. 11-33 Subtotal abdominal hysterectomy. If a subtotal hysterectomy is to be done, the uterine corpus can be amputated by cutting across the cervix at the level of the internal os, as shown by the dotted line.

MORTALITY

Of 1283 women who underwent abdominal hysterectomy in the 1982 study by Dicker and associates, only one died postoperatively. She had a deep venous thrombosis and died of complications of venography. Of 4283 abdominal hysterectomies for benign disease reported by Amirikia and Evans, seven preventable postoperative deaths occurred (0.16%), including three from pulmonary embolus,

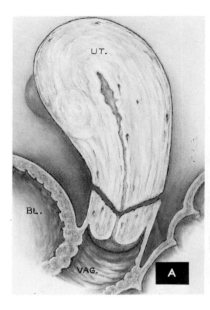

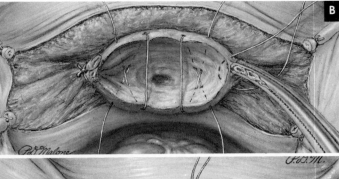

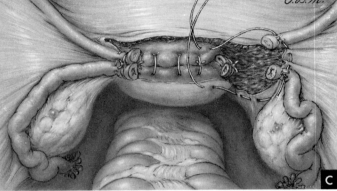

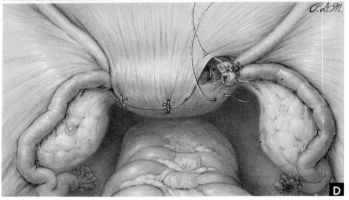

FIG. 11-34 Subtotal abdominal hysterectomy. (*A*) Method of coning out cervix to facilitate closing. (*B*) Method of ligating the uterine vessels and suturing the cervix. (*C*) Method of suspending the cervix and partial peritonization. (*D*) Peritonization is completed by suturing the bladder peritoneum to the posterior surface of the cervix.

two from infection, and one from postoperative shock and pulmonary edema. Some of the patients who died were seriously ill preoperatively. White reports a large series in which the incidence of operative death after hysterectomy was 0.7%. The incidence of mortality for hysterectomy in 1970, as performed in hospitals that participated in a Professional Activity Study, was reported as only 0.2% by Ledger and Child.

From the above figures and others, it would seem that death following abdominal hysterectomy occurs infrequently, perhaps one or two deaths per 1000 hysterectomies. However, this could amount to as many as 600 to 1200 hysterectomy-related deaths each year in the United States.

Operative deaths related to hysterectomy are rarely discussed in the current medical literature. There is no question that the risk of death from major pelvic surgery has been reduced considerably in the past quarter century. This is mostly the result of careful preoperative preparation of the patient, improvement in diagnosis and management of cardiovascular–pulmonary–metabolic problems, control of postoperative sepsis, skillful anesthesia, and skillful surgery. Nevertheless, a residual mortality risk for major pelvic surgery still exists. And the risk is not limited to the elderly or the seriously ill. The major causes of postoperative death today include cardiac arrest, pulmonary embolus, and sepsis, with occasional cases of postoperative hemorrhage, intestinal obstruction, and subarachnoid hemorrhage. Although the mortality rate is low, it is still high enough to demand that patients have proper indications for hysterectomy before the operation is performed. Our own clinical experience is similar to that of Gray, with an incidence of death of 0.4%.

POSTOPERATIVE INFECTION

Both major and minor infections can occur following elective abdominal hysterectomy for benign disease, even if no evidence of acute or chronic infection is found at operation. Febrile morbidity is the most frequent complication of abdominal hysterectomy, being reported in as many as 30% to 50% of cases. Major infections include pelvic cellulitis, infected hematoma or abscess above the vaginal cuff, abdominal wound infection, and adnexal infections. Diagnosis is made by finding tenderness and induration or a mass on palpation of the affected area in a febrile postoperative patient who complains of increasing lower abdominal pain. Gently probing the vaginal cuff or abdominal incision may yield pus, which should be cultured for both anaerobic and aerobic bacteria. In a recent study from Parkland Memorial Hospital, Hemsell and associates reported the results of cultures from the vaginal cuff or the abdominal incision of women with major infection after abdominal hysterectomy. Included in the list of aerobic bacteria cultured were the following: *Streptococcus* (4 species), *Streptococcus fecalis, Staphylococcus* (2 species), *Escherichia coli, Enterobacter* (3 species), *Klebsiella pneumoniae*, and *Proteus mirabilis*. The list of anaerobic bacteria included: *Pepto-streptococcus* (3 species), *Streptococcus intermedius, Peptococcus magnus, Gaffkya anaerobia, Clostridium* (5 species), *Bacteroides* (4 species), and *Fusobacterium nucleatum*. Usually three organisms were identified in each site of infection. Both anaerobic and aerobic organisms were isolated from one half of the sites. Aerobes only were recovered from 45% and anaerobes only from 5% of the infection sites. The lower percentage of anaerobes found, compared to other studies, may be a reflection of the great difficulty in correctly transferring anaerobic cultures from the patient to the microbiology laboratory. As many as 90% of infected gynecologic sites have yielded positive anaerobic cultures in other studies, with recovery of an average of five organisms per site. Gynecologic infections, including

postoperative infections, are polymicrobial mixed aerobic–anaerobic infections, and must be treated accordingly. The bacteria recovered from gynecologic sites of postoperative infection are the same as those found in the lower genital tract and lower intestinal tract of normal asymptomatic women. In other words, postoperative infections following abdominal hysterectomy are usually caused by bacteria that are endogenous to the patient.

The age of the patient is an important factor that is related to postoperative infections. The highest incidence of postoperative infections seems to occur in women under 40 years of age. Earlier reports suggested that vaginal hysterectomy was more commonly associated with postoperative infectious morbidity than abdominal hysterectomy. Recent studies have shown a higher rate of infection following abdominal hysterectomy. One should logically expect a higher rate with abdominal hysterectomy, since the operation involves making two incisions: one in the abdominal wall and one in the vagina. Medically indigent patients have a higher rate of postoperative infections than private patients, probably reflecting a diminished host resistance to infection among indigent women as well as the generally more serious nature of their illness and the presence of malnutrition, anemia, and other complicating problems. Surgical factors and techniques are important. The lack of hemostasis undoubtedly facilitates the growth of bacteria in traumatized tissue. The well-vascularized pelvic tissues, especially of young premenopausal women, tend to bleed more at surgery. Blood provides an excellent culture medium for bacterial contaminants in the operative site, and the operative site in abdominal hysterectomy is always contaminated with vaginal and cervical bacteria in spite of careful preoperative preparation and other technical measures to reduce the amount of contamination. A recent surgical procedure such as a recent dilatation and curettage or cervical conization may increase the amount of bacterial contamination at the time of abdominal hysterectomy. Bacteria can proliferate in surgically traumatized tissue in the cervix and uterine cavity. To avoid the increased risk of serious postoperative infection in a patient who is having an abdominal hysterectomy following cervical conization, the hysterectomy should either be done within 48 hours or be delayed until the cervix has healed completely, usually after 6 weeks.

The closed cuff method of abdominal hysterectomy deserves special emphasis. After the cervix is removed from the vagina, if one sutures the vaginal edges together to close the vaginal apex below and also closes the peritoneum above, one creates a closed space in between containing traumatized tissues, suture material, and the ends of ligated pedicles, which will become necrotic. Blood and serum accumulate in this space in surprisingly large amounts. Swartz suctioned an average of 40 ml (range 10–200 ml) of serosanguineous fluid from the post-hysterectomy retroperitoneal space above the vagina. This space is always contaminated with bacteria from the vagina. The oxygen content within the space will be reduced by the action of aerobic bacteria. To allow this space free drainage, the vaginal apex should be left open so that the possibility of infection will be decreased. In Gray's report of more than 2000 abdominal hysterectomies performed by one surgeon, the incidence of febrile morbidity was 18.2%. It was his conclusion that the open cuff technique of abdominal hysterectomy greatly decreased the incidence of this complication because it provided easy egress for serum and blood that may become secondarily infected and form a nidus for a cuff cellulitis or abscess.

The standard definition of febrile morbidity is a temperature elevation of 100.4° on any 2 of the first 10 postoperative days, excluding the first 24 hours. Although this definition is frequently used in studies of postoperative infectious morbidity, an elevated temperature alone does not reflect the true incidence of significant infection. Ledger has suggested using an alternative definition, such as a fever index. However, the presence of postoperative fever is an important sign indicating infection. The infection should be confirmed by a positive culture from the site of sepsis, such as the operative site in the pelvis, the abdominal incision, the lung, and, frequently, the kidney. It is important to take the temperature every 4 hours, day and night, in a patient who has had a recent abdominal hysterectomy. If the temperature is not taken, the earliest stage of a developing infection may be missed.

When a patient develops fever postoperatively, an evaluation to determine the cause must be made. Although infection in the operative site is by far the most common explanation for postoperative fever, one should look for other causes as well. Pulmonary atelectasis is associated with fever, tachypnea, tachycardia, and crackling lung rales. It is a more common problem in the first 24 hours following surgery and usually responds to deep breathing, coughing, tracheal–bronchial toilet, and incentive spirometry. Antibiotics are not usually required if the patient can clear her secretions. Although urinary tract infection can be diagnosed frequently in the postoperative patient, partly because of bladder catheterizations, they are not usually the source of fever. The urine should be examined microscopically and cultured, and the patient should be examined for costovertebral angle tenderness.

Thrombophlebitis may be associated with postoperative fever. The lower extremities should be examined carefully and special diagnostic procedures, such as ^{125}I scans, fibrinogen, or doppler ultrasound studies should be done when indicated. Most temperature elevations in the first 72 hours are self-limited, resolve spontaneously, and do not require antibiotics. They are due to tissue injury and a low-grade infection in the operative site. If the patient is feeling well and looks good, specific therapy may not be required. In other words, treat the patient—not the fever. If a collection of pus can be drained from the abdominal incision or vaginal cuff, the infection may subside without antibiotics. If cellulitis of pelvic or abdominal wall tissues is present, as determined by careful examination including pelvic, rectal, and speculum examination, antibiotics may be required. Any material taken from the operative site should be cultured aerobically and anaerobically and antimicrobial sensitivity studies done. However, antibiotics may be necessary before the culture results are available. In cases of serious postoperative pelvic infection, assumed to be caused by a mixture of anaerobic and aerobic organisms, a broad-spectrum antibiotic regimen must be used. Bacteroides fragilis is one of the more common anaerobic bacteria found in the pelvis, although special requirements for anaerobic culture are a prerequisite in confirming its presence. Unfortunately, the Bacteroides organism is not susceptible to penicillin in the usual therapeutic levels and is insensitive to the cephalosporins and aminoglycosides. The organism responds best to chloramphenicol, clindamycin, or intravenous metronidazol. For serious postoperative pelvic infections, we have used a combination of ampicillin, gentamycin, and intravenous metronidazol or a combination of cefoxitin and intravenous metronidazol.

Many clinical studies have demonstrated the benefits of perioperative antimicrobial prophylaxis with major pelvic surgery. Allen and associates reported the successful reduction of post-hysterectomy febrile morbidity noted in 41% of patients with abdominal hysterectomy to 14.1% when cephaloridine was given prophylactically, beginning the day of surgery and continuing for 5 days postoperatively. They found no difference in the incidence of postoperative infections when surgery was performed by an experienced or relatively inexperienced surgeon, an observation that has not been supported by most other reports. Ledger has been responsible principally for championing the short-term use of cephaloridine for reducing the febrile morbidity rate following hysterectomy, principally vaginal hysterectomy, and has advocated its short-term use for 24 hours, giving 1 g intramuscularly 2 hours prior to surgery, 1 g intramuscularly during surgery, and 1 g intramuscularly 6 hours following surgery. Further studies showed that an even shorter peri-operative regimen could also be effective, as was reported by Holman and associates. The total dose of cefazolin or placebo was 1.5 g, given as three divided doses. On the day of operation, patients were given 1.5 g of either cefazolin or placebo according to the following schedule: the first dose of 0.5 g was given intramuscularly on call to the operating room; the second dose of 0.5 g was given intramuscularly or intravenously on return from the recovery room; the third dose of 0.5 g was given intramuscularly or intravenously 6 hours after the second dose. In premenopausal patients, 19% of the cefazolin group who had abdominal hysterectomy had evidence of infection compared to 71% of the placebo group, and 10% of the cefazolin group who had vaginal hysterectomies had evidence of infection compared to 37% of the placebo group. In postmenopausal patients undergoing abdominal hysterectomy, cefazolin reduced the incidence of postoperative infection compared to placebo, but the difference was not significant (20% compared to 37%). There is no evidence that antibiotics used in this manner cause an increase in the incidence of infection with bacteria resistant to antibiotics. A great economic benefit has been a reduction in the hospital stay required for postoperative recovery. If there is evidence of infection found at operation, such as salpingitis, or if there is unusual bacterial contamination of the operative field from other sources, antibiotics may be continued after operation for several days as indicated. The most important principle in the use of antibiotics for prophylaxis against infection is that the drug must be in the patient's tissues at the time the incision is made. However, no course of antibiotic therapy can equal the benefit of precision in aseptic surgical technique and adequate hemostasis in reducing the incidence of postoperative pelvic infection.

Ledger and Willson have described the development of postoperative adnexal abscesses following hysterectomy with ovarian conservation in premenopausal women. It is proposed that the close proximity of the ovarian pedicle to the vaginal cuff may predispose to the development of these abscesses. The presence of a fresh corpus luteum at the time of operation or ovulation in the postoperative period may expose the ovarian stroma to bacterial invasion from the infected vaginal cuff.

Evidence of such an adnexal infection usually appears after the patient has been discharged from the hospital. The patient is febrile. A mass is palpable high in the pelvis or may be seen on ultrasound examination. Systemic antibiotics may not be effective. Operative intervention with removal of the abscess may be required. Fortunately, this postoperative complication is unusual.

POSTOPERATIVE HEMORRHAGE

The most common serious post-hysterectomy complication is bleeding. Fortunately, serious bleeding does not occur frequently. In a series of 2421 consecutive hysterectomies reported by Gray, bleeding was sufficient to require resuturing in 0.3% of cases. White reported that 2% of 600 hysterectomy patients had postoperative intra-abdominal hemorrhage of 3000 ml or greater, mostly following vaginal hysterectomy. This incidence is high in our experience. Intraperitoneal hemorrhage, which is occult, is far more dangerous, since its detection may be delayed. On the other hand, when pedicles are covered with peritoneum and the vaginal cuff is left open, postoperative bleeding may be more apparent coming through the vagina. Although it is easier to control intraoperative hemorrhage during an abdominal than during a vaginal hysterectomy, most of the bleeding occurs postoperatively and is usually related either to faulty surgical technique or to technical difficulties during the ligation of the vascular pedicles of the broad ligament. This is why our technique of abdominal hysterectomy emphasizes double ligation of the infundibulopelvic ligaments, utero-ovarian ligaments and fallopian tubes, and uterine vessels. We also believe that ligation with delayed-absorbable sutures is more secure than ligation with catgut sutures. In White's series, 1.3% of the cases developed profound hypovolemic shock, which emphasizes the rapidity and significance of post-hysterectomy hemorrhage. When profuse bleeding does occur, it may start suddenly and assume alarming proportions in a remarkably short time so that quick action is imperative. It cannot be assumed that the patient who spends a few hours in the recovery room without evidence of bleeding or hypotension is secure from the risk of postoperative hemorrhage. If there is a small unsecured vessel bleeding into the peritoneal cavity, the occult hemorrhage may not produce clinical signs of hypovolemia for several hours. Patients must be observed closely for at least 24 hours postoperatively. Postoperative hematocrits should be obtained routinely when the operation is completed, on the morning of the first postoperative day, and at any other time when there is the slightest suggestion of intraperitoneal bleeding or hypovolemia.

Bleeding that occurs directly after the operation is usually due to improper suturing of the angles of the vaginal cuff and should be attended to immediately by returning the patient to the operating room and suturing the cuff per vaginam. Such bleeding is usually transvaginal and evident immediately. However, some may be intra-abdominal, especially if the peritoneum has not been securely closed over the pedicles. In connection with this complication, it is important to reemphasize the rationale of the closure of the angles of the vagina. To ensure adequate ligation of the vaginal arteries and veins that arise from the hypogastric vessels, the vaginal angle suture must be placed following abdominal hysterectomy so that the free ends of the ligature are tied around the lateral margin of the vaginal cuff. Techniques for securing the vaginal angle are shown in Figure 11–27 and Figure 11–28A. If one of these techniques of anatomical closure of the vascular angles of the vagina is used, it is unusual to have postoperative bleeding after a total abdominal hysterectomy.

Post-hysterectomy bleeding most frequently occurs from the seventh to the fourteenth postoperative day. At this time, catgut sutures may partially dissolve and lose their tensile strength. Also, edematous vaginal tissue may slough and separate and cut through tightly tied suture material. We believe that this type of bleeding is quite unavoidable and will occur regardless of the method of closure of the vaginal vault. In reviewing 2421 cases of abdominal hysterectomy with three different methods of closure of the vaginal vault, Gray found no essential difference in the incidence of postoperative hemorrhage.

NECROTIZING FASCIITIS

This disease, which was first described during the Civil War by Joseph Jones, a Confederate army surgeon, is a rare postoperative complication of pelvic surgery, usually resulting from an incisional infection that involves the fascia of the anterior abdominal wall. Although the classic description of this disease was given by Meleney in 1924, who applied the term *streptococcal gangrene*, this lethal disease is more appropriately termed *necrotizing fasciitis*, since the essential feature of the disease is an extensive necrosis of the superficial fascia.

This entity has been reviewed in detail by Borkowf, who found that unless the disease is diagnosed early, before extensive fascial necrosis occurs, a 50% mortality rate is not uncommon. The predominant organism in most reported series is a β-hemolytic streptococcus, although mixed infections with enteric organisms, including *E. coli, proteus,* and *pseudomonas* bacteria are quite common. *Clostridium welchii* infection is seen rarely following pelvic surgery. When present, a clostridial wound infection usually occurs after an appendectomy or following contamination of the incision by intestinal contents. The toxic effects of the organisms are responsible for the rapid spread of necrotizing fasciitis, although there is current evidence of the presence of a mucoprotein moiety of the streptococcal cell wall that is specifically related to fascial spread of the organisms.

The disease is usually initiated by localized infection of the abdominal or vulvar incision, which rapidly becomes tense and shiny with purplish discoloration of the skin, followed by blisters and bullae that contain a brownish fluid. Necrosis of the nerves in the skin produce rapid anesthesia to the area, which is an ominous clinical sign. Often hyperbilirubinemia is seen as a result of red blood cell hemolysis and various degrees of hepatic dysfunction. The clinical picture tends to deteriorate rapidly unless there is early control of the bacterial infection and wide surgical debridement of the abdominal fascia. This radical removal of a large segment of the abdominal wall, including fat, fascia, and underlying abdominal wall musculature, must be done in an effort to remove the area of infection in order to permit high-dose, broad-spectrum, systemic antibiotics to control the hematogenous spread of the infection. The use of hyperbaric oxygen has not proven to be useful in these conditions, except in the early phase of a clostridial infection, where there have been scattered reports of success with its use.

This complication of pelvic surgery remains as one of the more lethal and difficult clinical problems to control. The morbidity and mortality from necrotizing fasciitis remain distressingly high and are directly related to the age of the patient, the presence of associated disease process, and, more important, the time interval from the onset of the infection to the recognition and institution of therapy.

OTHER COMPLICATIONS

Although infrequently discussed in modern textbooks, the formation of vaginal vault granulation tissue following total abdominal hysterectomy is not uncommon: some degree of this healing process occurs in more than 50% of the cases. Howkins and Williams found the incidence of granulation tissue to be lowest when the vaginal vault was closed using plain catgut, where the incidence was 26% as compared to 44% in cases where the vault was closed with chromic catgut suture. Greenhalf compared the various techniques of closure of the vaginal vault and found that the incidence of granulation tissue was not related to the type of catgut used if the vault was closed, but when the vault was left open, the incidence was somewhat lower when plain catgut was used. Because of better suture security, we prefer to use delayed-absorbable suture material rather than catgut when placing a continuous locked hemostatic suture around the vaginal margin. If the vaginal apex is left open for drainage, the incidence of granulation tissue is usually found to be higher when patients return for their 6 weeks postoperative examination. A vaginal vault that has been left open must heal by secondary intention and therefore one might expect the incidence of granulation tissue to be higher. Some surgeons object to leaving the vaginal cuff open because of the higher incidence of granulation tissue formation. Fifty percent or more or all patients will develop granulation tissue at the vaginal vault following abdominal hysterectomy, regardless of whether the cuff is closed or left open and regardless of the method of suturing. The basic cause of the phenomenon is the inversion of the vaginal epithelium between the margins of the vaginal vault closure. This is made clearly evident by the rarity of the condition following a vaginal hysterectomy in which the vaginal epithelium is everted and healing occurs by apposition of the submucosal tissues. The problem is easily managed by light cauterization of the granulation sites in the vaginal vault, usually by silver nitrate chemical cautery and occasionally by electrocautery. Vaginal douches with hot water may stimulate the final phases of healing. In general, we have found no difficulty in rapid healing of the vault, with no sequelae from the minimal granulation tissue that does occur. The major complaint is temporary vaginal discharge, although the tissue may produce spotting after coitus if complete epithelialization has not occurred.

Post-hysterectomy prolapse of the fallopian tube may sometimes be confused with granulation tissue. Although rare, it probably occurs more commonly than reported. The subject has been reviewed by Sumathy and Baucom and also by Thompson. In a 1975 review by Sumathy and Baucom, 35 cases of post-hysterectomy fallopian tube prolapse were reported. Eight followed abdominal surgery. In order for the fallopian tube to prolapse, a communication must exist between the peritoneal cavity and the vagina. In other words, the operative technique employed in performing the hysterectomy did not result in secure closure of the peritoneum over the vaginal vault. In some cases, it appears that the de-

velopment of a hematoma or abscess in the vaginal apex may have facilitated prolapse of the tube. Patients complain of profuse watery vaginal discharge, pelvic discomfort, and even postcoital bleeding. One may assume that the tissue seen at the vaginal apex is simply granulation tissue. However, if there is considerable discomfort when attempts are made to remove the tissue, or if it is especially resistant to local treatment, a diagnosis of prolapse of the fallopian tube may be made. A dissection in the operating room under anesthesia is usually needed to remove it. The tubes should be ligated as high as possible and the defect in the vaginal vault closed. This can usually be accomplished transvaginally.

Late complications following hysterectomy are unusual. The psychological impact of hysterectomy has been the subject of many studies. The incidence of depression and sexual dysfunction and other emotional difficulties may be increased after hysterectomy. Some patients may require special psychiatric counseling. This subject is discussed more fully in Chapter 2.

Post-hysterectomy prolapse of the vaginal vault is discussed in Chapter 24. This late complication of hysterectomy can be minimized by employing an operative technique that provides proper support to the vaginal vault and posterior vaginal fornix.

Bibliography

LEIOMYOMATA UTERI

Amussat JZ, quoted by Rubin IC: Progress in myomectomy. Am J Obstet Gynecol 44:197, 1942

Ariel IM, Trinidad S: Pulmonary metastases from a uterine "leiomyoma." Am J Obstet Gynecol 94:110, 1966

Babaknia A, Rock JA, Jones HW, Jr: Pregnancy success following abdominal myomectomy for infertility. Fertil Steril 30:644, 1978

Bahary CM, Gorodeski IG, Nilly M, et al: Intravascular leiomyomatosis. Obstet Gynecol 59:735, 1982

Baines REM: Problems associated with myomectomy in Cape Town. S Afr Med J 45:668, 1971

Banner AS, Carrington CB, Emory WB, et al: Efficacy of oophorectomy in lymphangio-leiomyomatosis and benign metastasizing leiomyoma. New Engl J Med 305:204, 1981

Beacham WD, Webster HD, Lawson EH, et al: Uterine and/or ovarian tumors weighing 25 pounds or more. Am J Obstet Gynecol 109:1153, 1971

Berkeley AS, deCherney AH, Polan ML: Abdominal myomectomy and subsequent fertility. Surg Gynecol Obstet 156:319, 1983

Bonney V: Abdominal myomectomy. In Berkeley AS, Bonney V: A Textbook of Gynaecological Surgery, 5th ed. New York, Paul B Hoeber, 1948.

Bonney V: The technic and results of myomectomy. Lancet 220:171, 1931

Brown AB, Chamberlain R, TeLinde RW: Myomectomy. Am J Obstet Gynecol 71:759, 1956

Brown JM, Malkasian GD, Symmonds RE: Abdominal myomectomy. Am J Obstet Gynecol 99:126, 1967

Buttram VC, Reiter RC: Uterine leiomyomata: Etiology, symptomatology, and management. Fertil Steril 36:433, 1981

Ceccacci L, Jacobs J, Powell A: Leiomyomatosis peritonealis disseminata: Report of a case in a non-pregnant woman. Am J Obstet Gynecol 144:105, 1982

Clark DH, Weed JC: Metastasizing leiomyoma: A case report. Am J Obstet Gynecol 127:672, 1977

Cole P, Berlin J: Elective hysterectomy. Obstet Gynecol 129:117, 1977

Corscaden JA, Singh BP: Leiomyosarcoma of the uterus. Am J Obstet Gynecol 75:149, 1958

Cramer SF, Meyer JS, Kraner JF, et al: Metastasizing leiomyoma of the uterus: S-phase fraction, estrogen receptor, and ultrastructure. Cancer 45:932, 1980

Degligdish L, Loewenthal M: Endometrial changes associated with myomata of the uterus. J Clin Pathol 23:677, 1970

Edwards DR, Peacock JF: Intravenous leiomyomatosis of the uterus (2 cases). Obstet Gynecol 27:176, 1966

Evans AT, Symmonds RE, Gaffey TA: Recurrent pelvic intravenous leiomyomatosis. Obstet Gynecol 57:260, 1981

Everett HS, Sturgis WJ: The effect of some common gynecological disorders upon the urinary tract. Urol Cutan Rev 44:638, 1940

Farber M, Conrad S, Heinrichs WL, et al: Estradiol binding by fibroid tumors and normal myometrium. Obstet Gynecol 40:479, 1972

Farrer-Brown G, Beilby JOW, Tarbit MH: Venous changes in the endometrium of myomatous uteri. Obstet Gynecol 38:743, 1971

———: The vascular patterns in myomatous uteri. J Obstet Gynecol Brit Comm 77:967, 1970

Faulkner RL: The blood vessels of the myomatous uterus. Am J Obstet Gynecol 47:185, 1944

Feeney JG, Basu SB: Bacteroides infection in fibroids during the puerperium. Br Med J 2:1038, 1979

Filicori M, Hall DA, Loughlin JS, et al: A conservative approach to the management of uterine leiomyoma: Pituitary desensitization by a luteinizing hormone-releasing hormone analogue. Am J Obstet Gynecol 147:726, 1983

Gabb RG, Stone GM: Uptake and metabolism of tritiated oestradiol and oestrone by human endometrial and myometrial tissue in vitro. J Endocrinology Great Britain 62:109, 1974

Gal D, Buchsbaum HJ, Voet R, et al: Massive ascites with uterine leiomyomas and ovarian vein thrombosis. Am J Obstet Gynecol 144:729, 1982

Garcia CR, Tureck RW: Submucosal leiomyomas and infertility. 42:16, 1984

Gilbert HA, Kagan AR, Lagasse L: The value of radiation therapy in uterine sarcoma. Obstet Gynecol 45:84, 1975

Goldberg MF, Hurt G, Frable WJ: Leiomyomatosis peritonealis disseminata. Obstet Gynecol 49:46s, 1977

Goldzieher JW, Maqueo M, Ricaud L, et al: Induction of degenerative changes in uterine myomas by high-dosage progestin therapy. Am J Obstet Gynecol 96:1078, 1966

Goodman AL: Progesterone therapy in uterine fibromyoma. J Clin Endocrin Metabol 6:402, 1946

Horstmann JP, Pietra GG, Harman JA, et al: Spontaneous regression of pulmonary leiomyomas during pregnancy. Cancer 39:314, 1977

Hunt SH: Fibroid weighing one hundred and forty pounds. Am J Obstet 21:62, 1888

Idelson MG, Davids AM: Metastasis of uterine fibroleiomyomata. Obstet Gynecol 21:78, 1963

Ingersoll FM, Malone LJ: Myomectomy: An alternative to hysterectomy. Arch Surg 100:557, 1970

Irey NS, Norris HJ: Intimal vascular lesions associated with female reproductive steroids. Arch Pathol 96:227, 1973

Jones HW, Jr, Andrew MC: Congenital anomalies and infertility. Ridley JH (ed): Gynecologic Surgery, 2nd ed. Baltimore, Williams and Wilkins, 1981

Kelly HA, Cullen TS: Myomata of the Uterus. Philadelphia, WB Saunders, 1907

Klunder KB, Svanholm H, Frimodt-Moller PC: Uterine bizarre leiomyoma. Acta Obstet Gynecol Scand 61:121, 1982

Kurman RJ, Norris HJ: Mesenchymal tumors of the uterus. VI. Epithelioid smooth muscle tumors including leiomyoblastoma and clear cell leiomyoma. Cancer 37:1853, 1976

Lapan B, Solomon L: Diffuse leiomyomatosis of the uterus precluding myomectomy. Obstet Gynecol 53:825, 1979

Lipschutz A, Murillo R, Vargas L: Antitumorigenic action of progesterone. Lancet 2:420, 1939

Lipschutz A: Experimental fibroids and the antifibromatogenic action of steroid hormones. JAMA 120:171, 1942

Lock FR: Multiple myomectomy. Am J Obstet Gynecol 104:642, 1969

Loeffler FE, Noble AD: Myomectomy at the Chelsea Hospital for Women. J Obstet Gynaecol Br Commonw 77:167, 1970

Malone LJ, Ingersoll, FM: Myomectomy in infertility. In Bermen SG, Kistner RW (eds): Progress Infertility. Boston, Little, Brown Co. 1975

Marshall JF, Morris DS: Intravenous leiomyomatosis of the uterus and pelvis: Case report. Ann Surg 149:126, 1959

Martin JF, Bazin P, Feroldi J, et al: Tumeurs myoides intramurales de l'estomac. Considerations microscopiques apropos de 6 cas. Ann Anat Pathol 5:484, 1960

Matsunaga E, Shiota K: Ectopic pregnancy and myoma uteri: Teratogenic effects and maternal characteristics. Teratology 21:61, 1980

Mattingly RF: Large myomata uteri and stress urinary incontinence. In Nichols DH (ed): Clinical Problems, Injuries, and Complications of Gynecologic Surgery, Baltimore, Williams and Wilkins, 1983

Meigs JV: Pelvic tumors other than fibromas of the ovary with ascites and hydrothorax. Obstet Gynecol 3:471, 1954

Mayo WJ: Some observations on the operation of abdominal myomectomy for myomata of the uterus. Surg Gynecol Obstet 12:97, 1911

Miller NF, Ludovici PP: On the origin and development of uterine fibroids. Am J Obstet Gynecol 70:720, 1955

Montague A, Swartz DP, Woodruff JD: Sarcoma arising in leiomyoma of uterus: Factors influencing prognosis. Am J Obstet Gynecol 92:421, 1965

Muram D, Gillieson MS, Walters JH: Myomas of the uterus in pregnancy: Ultrasonographic follow-up. Am J Obstet Gynecol 138:16, 1980

Nelson WO: Endometrial and myometrial changes including fibromyomatous nodules, induced in the uterus of the guinea pig by the prolonged administration of oestrogenic hormone. Anat Rec 68:99, 1937

Neuwirth RS: Hysteroscopic management of symptomatic submucous fibroids. Obstet Gynecol 62:509, 1983

Norris HJ, Parmley T: Mesenchymal tumors of the uterus versus intravenous leiomyomatosis: A clinical and pathologic study of 14 cases. Cancer 36:2164, 1975

Novak ER: Benign and malignant changes in uterine myomas. Clin Obstet Gynecol 1:421, 1958

Otubu JA, Buttram VC, Besch NF, et al: Unconjugated steroids in leiomyomas and tumor bearing myometrium. Am J Obstet Gynecol 143:130, 1982

Parmley TH, Woodruff JD, Winn, K: Histogenesis of leiomyomatosis peritonealis disseminata (disseminated fibrosing deciduosis). Obstet Gynecol 46:511, 1975

Pearce PH: Leiomyomatosis peritonealis disseminata. Am J Obstet Gynecol 144:133, 1982

Persaud V, Arjoon PD: Uterine leiomyoma: Incidence of degenerative change and a correlation of associated symptoms. Obstet Gynecol 35:432, 1970

Pollow K, Geilfub J, Boquoi E, et al: Estrogen and Progesterone binding proteins in normal human myometrium. J Clin Chem Clin Biochem 16:503, 1978

Ranney B, Federick I: The occasional need for myomectomy. Obstet Gynecol 53:437, 1979

Reddy VV, Rose LI: Δ⁴-3-Ketosteroid 5α-oxidoreductase in human uterine leiomyoma. Am J Obstet Gynecol 135:415, 1979

Riley P: Treatment of prolapsed submucous fibroids. S Afr Med J 62:22, 1982

Rubin IC: Uterine fibromyomas and sterility. Clin Obstet Gynecol 1:501, 1958

Rubin I: Progress in myomectomy. Surgical measures and diagnostic aids favoring lower morbidity and mortality. Am J Obstet Gynecol 44:196, 1942

Sampson JA: The influence of myomata on the blood supply of the uterus with special reference to abnormal uterine bleeding. Surg Gynecol Obstet 16:144, 1913

Segaloff A, Weed JC, Sternberg WH, et al: The progesterone therapy of human uterine leiomyomas. J Clin Endocrin Metabol 9:1273, 1949

Sehgal N, Haskins AL: The mechanism of uterine bleeding in the presence of fibromyomas. Am J Surg 26:21, 1960

Singhabhandhu B, et al: Giant leiomyoma of the uterus: Report of a case and review of the literature. Am Surg 39:391, 1973

Soules MR, McCarty KS, Jr: Leiomyomas: Steroid receptor content: Variations within normal menstrual cycles. Am J Obstet Gynecol 143:6, 1982

Spellacy WN, LeMaire WJ, Buhi WC, et al: Plasma growth hormone and estradiol levels in women with uterine myomas. Obstet Gynecol 40:829, 1972

Starks GC: Unilateral twin interstitial ectopic pregnancy, a case report. J Reprod Med 25:79, 1980

Tada S, Tsukioka M, Ishii C, et al: Computed tomographic features of uterine myoma. J Computer Assisted Tomography 5:866, 1981

Tierney WN, Ehrlich CE, Bailey JC, et al: Intravenous leiomyomatosis of the uterus with extension into the heart. Am J Med 69:471, 1980

Torpin R, Pond E, Peoples WJ: The etiologic and pathologic factors in a series of 1,741 fibromyomas of the uterus. Am J Obstet Gynecol 44:569, 1942

Townsend DE, Sparkes RS, Baluda MC, et al: Unicellular histogenesis of uterine leiomyomas as determined by electrophoresis of glucose-6-phosphate dehydrogenase. Am J Obstet Gynecol 107:1168, 1970

Weiss DB, Aldor A, Aboulafia Y: Erythrocytosis due to erythropoietin-producing uterine fibromyoma. Am J Obstet Gynecol 122:358, 1975

Wilson EA, Yang F, Rees ED: Estradiol and progesterone binding in uterine leiomyomata and in normal uterine tissues. Obstet Gynecol 55:20, 1980

Winer–Muram HT, Muram D, Gillieson MS, et al: Uterine myomas in pregnancy. Can Med Assoc J 128:949, 1983

Wray RC, Jr, Dawkins H: Primary smooth muscle tumors of the inferior vena cava. Ann Surg 174:1009, 1971

Ylikorkala O, Kauppila A, Rajala T: Pituitary gonadotrophins and prolactin in patients with endometrial cancer, fibroids or ovarian tumours. Brit J Obstet Gynaecol 86:901, 1979

ABDOMINAL HYSTERECTOMY FOR BENIGN DISEASE

Allan MS, Hertig AT: Carcinoma of the ovary. Am J Obstet Gynecol 58:640, 1949

Allen JL, Rampone JF, Wheeless CR: Use of prophylactic antibiotics in elective major gynecologic operations. Obstet Gynecol 39:218, 1972

Amirikia H, Evans TN: Ten-year review of hysterectomies: Trends, indications, and risks. Am J Obstet Gynecol 134:431, 1979

Annegers JF, Strom H, Decker DG, et al: Ovarian cancer, incidence and care-control study. Cancer 43:723, 1979

Atlee WL: Case of successful extirpation of a fibrous tumor of the peritoneal surface of the uterus by the peritoneal section. Am J Med Sc 9:26, 1845

Bancroft–Livingston G: Ovarian survival following hysterectomy. J Obstet Gynaecol Br Commonw 61:628, 1954

Barlow JJ, Emerson K, Saxena BB: Estradiol production after ovariectomy for carcinoma of the breast. N Engl J Med 280:633, 1969

Beathard GA, Guchian JC: Necrotizing fasciitis due to group beta hemolytic streptococcus. Arch Intern Med 126:63, 1967

Beavis ELG, Brown JB, Smith MA: Ovarian function after hysterectomy with conservation of the ovaries in premenopausal women. J Obstet Gynaecol Br Commonw 76:969, 1969

Bjoro K: Klimakteriet. In Bjoro K, Kolstad P (eds): Gynaekologi Oslo, Universitetsforlaget, 1979

Borell V, Fernstrom I: The adnexal branches of the uterine artery. An arteriographic study in human subjects. Acta Radiol 40:561, 1953

Borkowf HI: Bacterial gangrene associated with pelvic surgery. Clin Obstet Gynecol 16:40, 1973

Boston University Medical Center: Surgically confirmed gallbladder disease, venous thromboembolism, and breast tumors in relation to postmenopausal estrogen therapy. A report from the Boston Collaborative Drug Surveillance Program. N Engl J Med 290:15, 1974

Burford TH, Diddle AW: Effect of total hysterectomy upon the ovary of the Macacus Rhesus. Surg Gynecol Obstet 62:701, 1936

Burke JF: The effective period of preventive antibiotic action in experimental incisions and dermal lesions. Surgery 50:161, 1960

Centerwall BS: Premenopausal hysterectomy and cardiovascular disease. Am J Obstet Gynecol 139:58, 1981

Christ JE, Lotze EC: The residual ovary syndrome. Obstet Gynecol 46:551, 1975

Christian DD: Ovarian tumors: An extension of the Peutz–Jegher's syndrome. Am J Obstet Gynecol 111:529, 1971

Cole P, Berlin J: Elective hysterectomy. Obstet Gynecol 129:117, 1977

Counseller VS, Hunt W, Haigler FH: Carcinoma of the ovary following hysterectomy. Am J Obstet Gynecol 69:538, 1955

Defore WW, et al: Necrotizing fasciitis: A persistent surgical problem. J Am Coll Emerg Phys 6:2, 1977

deNeef JC, Hollenbeck ZJR: The fate of ovaries preserved at the time of hysterectomy. Am J Obstet Gynecol 96:1088, 1966

Dicker RC, Scally MJ, Greenspan JR, et al: Hysterectomy among women of reproductive age: Trends in the United States, 1970–1978. JAMA, 248:323, 1982

Dyck FJ, Murphy FA, Murphy JK, et al: Effect of surveillance on the number of hysterectomies in the province of Saskatchewan. N Engl J Med 296:1326, 1977

Fernstrom I: The normal anatomy of the uterine artery. Acta Radiologica Supp 122:21, 1955

Fraumeni JF, Jr, Grundy GW, Creagan ET, et al: Six families prone to ovarian cancer. Cancer 36:364, 1975

Funk-Brentano P: The remaining ovary after hysterectomy. Rev Franç Gynec Obstet 53:217, 1958

Funt MI, Benigno BB, Thompson JD: The residual adnexa—asset or liability? Am J Obstet Gynecol 129:251, 1977

Gambrell RD, Maier RC, Ganders BI: Decreased incidence of breast cancer in postmenopausal estrogen–progestogen users. Obstet Gynecol 62:435, 1983

Gerhard G: Sur les variations d'origine et de nombre des arteres genitales, spermatiques ou ovariennes de l'homme. Compt Rend Soc Biol 74:778, 1913

Gertman PM, Stackpole DA, Levenson DK, et al: Second opinions for elective surgery. N Engl J Med 302:1169, 1980

Gevaerts PO: Abdominale totale uterus extirpatie of supravaginalis uterus amputatie. Leiden, Holland, thesis, 1963

Grammatikati J: Experimentelle Untersuchungen uber das weitere Schicksal der Ovarien und Tuben nach der Totalexstirpation des Uterus bei Kaninchen. Centralblatt fur Gynakologie 7:105, 1889

Graves WP: Gynecology, 4th ed. Philadelphia, WB Saunders, 1928
———: Transplantation and retention of ovarian tissue after hysterectomy. Surg Gynecol Obstet 25:315, 1917

Gray LA: Open cuff method of abdominal hysterectomy. Obstet Gynecol 46:42, 1975

Greenblatt RB, Colle ML, Mahesh VB: Ovarian and adrenal steroid production in the postmenopausal woman. Obstet Gynecol 47:383, 1976

Greenhalf JO: Vaginal vault granulation tissue following total abdominal hysterectomy. Br J Clin Pract 6:247, 1967

Grodin JM, Siiteri PI, MacDonald PC: Source of estrogen production in postmenopausal women. J Endocrinol Metabol 36:207, 1973

Grogan RH: Reappraisal of residual ovaries. Am J Obstet Gynecol 97:124, 1967

Grogan RH, Duncan CJ: Ovarian salvage in routine abdominal hysterectomy. Am J Obstet Gynecol 70:1277, 1955

Hemsell DL, Reisch J, Nobles B, et al: Prevention of major infection after elective abdominal hysterectomy: Individual determination required. Am J Obstet Gynecol 147:520, 1983

Hollenbeck ZJR: Ovarian cancer: Prophylactic oophorectomy. Ann Surg 21:442, 1955

Holman JF, McGowan JE, Thompson JD: Perioperative antibiotics in major elective gynecologic surgery. So Med J 71:417, 1978

Howkins J, Williams DK: Vault granulations after total abdominal hysterectomy. J Obstet Gynaecol Br Commonw 75:84, 1968

Janson PO, Jansson I: The acute effect of hysterectomy on ovarian blood flow. Am J Obstet Gynecol 127:349, 1977

Jaszczak SE, Evans TN: Intrafascial abdominal and vaginal hysterectomy: A reappraisal. Obstet Gynecol 59:435, 1982

Johansson BW, et al: On some late effects of bilateral oophorectomy in the age range 15–30 years. Acta Obstet Gynecol Scand 54:449, 1975

Johnson CG, Moll CF, Post L: An analysis of 6,891 hysterectomies for benign pelvic disease. Am J Obstet Gynecol 71:515, 1956

Jones J: Investigations on the nature, causes, and treatment of hospital gangrene as it prevailed in the Confederate armies 1861–1865. In Surgical Memoirs of the War of Rebellion. Sanitary Commission, NY, 1871

Judd HL, Judd GE, Lucas WE, et al: Endocrine function of the postmenopausal ovary: Concentration of androgens and estrogens in ovarian and peripheral vein blood. J Clin Endocrinol Metabol 39:1020, 1974

Kelly HA: Operative Gynecology. New York, Appleton, 1898
———: Conservatism in ovariotomy. JAMA 26:249, 1896
———: Operative Gynecology, vol 2. New York, D Appleton and Company, 1901

Kelly HA, Noble CP: Gynecology and Abdominal Surgery, vol 1. Philadelphia, WB Saunders, 1907

Krailo MD, Pike MC: Estimation of the distribution of age at natural menopause from prevalence data. Am J Epidemiol 117:356, 1983

Laros RK, Jr, Work BA: Female sterilization. 3. Vaginal hysterectomy. Am J Obstet Gynecol 122:693, 1975

Ledger WJ: Bacteriologic and clinical classification of anaerobic soft tissue infections in obstetrics and gynecology. Am J Obstet Gynecol 123:111, 1975

Ledger WJ, Campbell C, Taylor D, et al: Adnexal abscess as a late complication of pelvic operations. Surg Gynecol Obstet 129:973, 1969

Ledger WJ, Child MA: The hospital care of patients undergoing hysterectomy. An analysis of 12,026 patients from the Professional Activity Study. Am J Obstet Gynecol 117:423, 1973

Ledger WJ, Gee C, Lewis WP: Guidelines for antibiotic prophylaxis in gynecology. Am J Obstet Gynecol 121:1038, 1975

Ledger WJ, Sweet RI, Headington JT: Prophylactic cephaloridine in the prevention of postoperative pelvic infections in premenopausal women undergoing vaginal hysterectomy. Am J Obstet Gynecol 115:766, 1973

Longo LD: The rise and fall of Battey's operation: A fashion in surgery. Bulletin of the History of Medicine 53(2):244, 1979

Lurain JR, Piver MS: Familial ovarian cancer. Gynecol Oncol 8:185, 1979

Lynch HT, Lynch PM: Tumor variation in the cancer family syndrome: Ovarian cancer. Am J Surg 138:439, 1979

Lynch HT, Albano WA, Lynch JF, et al: Surveillance and management of patients at high genetic risk for ovarian carcinoma. Obstet Gynecol 59:589, 1982

Lynch HT, Harris RE, Guirgis HA, et al: Familial association of breast/ovarian carcinoma. Cancer 41:1543, 1978

MacMahon B, Worcester J: Age at menopause, United States 1960–1962. Washington, D.C.: National Center for Health Statistics, 1966. (Vital and health statistics, Series II: Data from the National Health Survey, no 19), (DHEW Publication no (HSM) 66-1000)

Mattingly RF, Huang HY: Steroidogenesis in the menopausal and postmenopausal ovary. Am J Obstet Gynecol 103:679, 1969

McCall ML, Keatty EC, Thompson JD: Conservation of ovarian tissue in the treatment of carcinoma of the cervix with radical surgery. Am J Obstet Gynecol 75:590, 1958

Meleney FL: Hemolytic streptococcal gangrene. Arch Surg 9:317, 1924

Mikhail G: Hormone secretion by the human ovaries. Gynecol Invest 1:5, 1970

Miller NF: Hysterectomy: Therapeutic necessity or surgical racket? Am J Obstet Gynecol 51:804, 1946

Mocquot P, Rouvillois C: La vascularisation arterielle de l'ovarie etudié en vue de la chirurgie conservatrice. J Chir 51:161, 1938

Norris HJ, Taylor HB: Postirradiation sarcomas of the uterus. Obstet Gynecol 26:689, 1965

Novak ER: Ovulation after fifty. Obstet Gynecol 36:903, 1970

Novak ER, Williams TJ: Autopsy comparison of cardiovascular changes in castrated and normal women. Am J Obstet Gynecol 80:863, 1960

Novak ER, Woodruff JD: Novak's Gynecologic and Obstetric Pathology, 7th ed. Philadelphia, WB Saunders, 1974

O'Brien PH, Newton BB, Metcalf JS, et al: Oophorectomy in women with carcinoma of the colon and rectum. Surg Gynecol Obstet 153:827, 1981

Ohm MJ, Galask RP: The effect of antibiotic prophylaxis on patients undergoing total abdominal hysterectomy. I. Effect on morbidity. Am J Obstet Gynecol 125:442, 1976

Paloucek FP, Randall CL, Graham JB, et al: Cancer and its relation to abnormal vaginal bleeding and radiation. Obstet Gynecol 21:530, 1963

Phillips HE, McGahan JP: Ovarian remnant syndrome. Radiology 142:487, 1982

Pratt JH, Jefferies JA: The retained cervical stump: A 25-year experience. Obstet Gynecol 48:711, 1976

Randall CL, Birtch PK, Harkins JL: Ovarian function after the menopause. Am J Obstet Gynecol 74:719, 1957

Randall CL, Gerhardt PR: The probability of occurrence of the more common types of gynecologic malignancies. Am J Obstet Gynecol 68:1378, 1954

Randall CL, Hall DW, Armenia CS: Pathology in the preserved ovary after unilateral oophorectomy. Am J Obstet Gynecol 84:1233, 1962

Randall CL, Paloucek F: The frequency of oophorectomy at the time of hysterectomy. Am J Obstet Gynecol 100:716, 1968

Ranney B, Abu–Ghazaleh S: The future function and fortune of ovarian tissue which is retained in vivo during hysterectomy. Am J Obstet Gynecol 128:626, 1977

Rea WJ, Wyrick WJ: Necrotizing fasciitis. Ann Surg 172:954, 1970

Richardson EH: A simplified technic for abdominal panhysterectomy. Surg Gynecol Obstet 48:248, 1929

————: The effect of hysterectomy upon ovarian function. Trans Am Gynecol Soc 43:114, 1918

Sattin RW, Rubin GL, Hughes JM: Hysterectomy among women of reproductive age, United States Update for 1979–1980. CDC Morbidity and Mortality Weekly Report, 32:155, 1983

Shoemaker ES, Forney JP, MacDonald PC: Estrogen treatment of postmenopausal women: Benefits and risks. JAMA 238:1524, 1977

Sitteri PK, MacDonald PC: Role of extraglandular estrone in human endocrinology. In Greep RO (ed): Handbook of Physiology: The Female Reproductive System, vol 2. Bethesda, Am Physiol Soc 1973

Stimson LA: On some modifications in the technique of abdominal surgery, limiting the use of the *ligature en masse*. Trans Am Surg Assoc 7:5, 1889

Stone SC, Dickey RF, Mickal A: The acute effect of hysterectomy on ovarian function. Am J Obstet Gynecol 121:193, 1975

Sumathy V, Baucom K: Prolapse of fallopian tube following abdominal hysterectomy. Report of 3 cases. Int J Gynaecol Obstet 13:273, 1975

Swartz WH: Prophylaxis of minor febrile and major infectious morbidity following hysterectomy. Obstet Gynecol 54:184, 1979

Symmonds RE, Pettit PDM: Ovarian remnant syndrome. Obstet Gynecol 54:174, 1979

Taylor HC: Discussion of paper by D'Esopo. Am J Obstet Gynecol 83:113, 1962

TeLinde RW, Wharton LR, Jr: Ovarian function following pelvic operation: An experiment on monkeys. Am J Obstet Gynecol 80:844, 1960

Terz JJ, Barber HRK, Brunschwig A: The incidence of carcinoma in the retained ovary. Am J Surg 113:511, 1967

Thompson JD, Caputo TA, Franklin EW, et al: The surgical management of invasive cancer of the cervix in pregnancy. Am J Obstet Gynecol 121:853, 1975

Thompson JD: Fallopian tube prolapse after abdominal hysterectomy. Aust NZ J Obstet Gynecol 20:187, 1980

Tobacman JK, Tucker MA, Kase R: Intra-abdominal carcinomatosis after prophylactic oophorectomy in ovarian cancer-prone families. Lancet 2:795, 1982

Vermeullen A: The hormonal activity of the postmenopausal ovary. J Clin Endocrinol Metabol 42:247, 1976

White SC, Wartel LJ, Wade ME: Comparison of abdominal and vaginal hysterectomies: A review of 600 operations. Obstet Gynecol 37:530, 1971

Whitelaw RG: Ovarian activity following hysterectomy. J Obstet Gynecol Brit Emp 65:917, 1958

————: Pathology and the conserved ovary. J Obstet Gynecol Brit Emp 66:413, 1959

Willett W, Stampfer MJ, Bain C, et al: Cigarette smoking, relative weight, and menopause. Am J Epidemiol 117:651, 1983

Woodruff JD: The pathogenesis of ovarian neoplasia. Johns Hopkins Med J 144:117, 1979

Wynder EL, Dodo H, Barber HRK: Epidemiology of cancer of the ovary. Cancer 23:352, 1969

Chapter 12

Endometriosis

Tiffany J. Williams, M.D.

Sampson's description of endometriosis in 1921 has been little improved upon. He described endometriosis as the

> presence of ectopic tissue which possesses the histological structure and function of the uterine mucosa. It also includes the abnormal conditions which may result not only from the invasion of organs and other structures by this tissue but also from its relation to menstruation.

Although benign, endometriosis possesses the unique ability to invade tissues and to disseminate or metastasize by hematogenous or lymphatic routes or by direct implantation. These attributes are essentially characteristic of malignancy.

Endometriosis can be divided into two distinct clinical and pathologic types that frequently appear as entirely different diseases. One is *adenomyosis*, or internal endometriosis, which is characterized by invasion of the myometrium by endometrium from within the uterine cavity. The other condition is *external endometriosis*, in which tissues outside the uterus are affected or the uterine serosa is involved from without rather than by direct extension from the mucosa.

Adenomyosis

Adenomyosis may have two distinct forms, diffuse and local. Diffuse adenomyosis involves the walls of the uterus to various degrees (Fig. 12–1). Although usually quite diffuse, it may be relatively localized, but it is not encapsulated. The uterus itself is usually somewhat enlarged, rarely more than twice normal size, and is more or less symmetrical. Cut section of the uterine wall reveals a coarse trabecular pattern of interlacing musculature and fibrous tissue with small islands of endometrium that are often dark and hemorrhagic. In contrast, an adenomyoma is localized disease in the uterine wall; it is encapsulated much as an ordinary intramural leiomyoma. It is located mainly within the wall of the uterus but may project into the uterine cavity, becoming a submucous adenomyoma (Fig. 12–2).

The most generally accepted theory holds that endometrial tissue in the myometrium is of müllerian origin and is a direct downgrowth from the endometrium of the uterine cavity. Cullen showed by serial section a direct continuity between the basalis portion of the endometrium and the endometrial islands within the areas of adenomyosis. In some instances, endometrial extensions could be followed throughout the full thickness of the myometrium to the serosal surface of the uterus.

These intramural islands generally have the histologic appearance of the basalis of the endometrium, and usually respond to estrogen stimulation with a proliferative pattern or, occasionally, one of cystic hyperplasia. The progestational effect on ectopic endometrium is less predictable. Secretory changes in the glands are uncommon, whereas in pregnancy a decidual reaction of the stroma is common. Ectopic endometrial tissue, like that of the uterine endometrium, may be hormone-sensitive, and in the absence of hormonal stimulation, it will become atrophic after the menopause. Although such ectopic endometrium may be estrogen-dependent and may undergo a cystic type of hyperplasia, adenomyosis rarely shows any atypical type of hyperplasia and even more uncommonly becomes malignant.

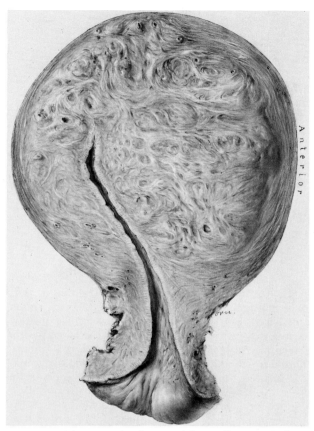

FIG. 12-1 Adenomyosis of uterus (after Cullen). Typical example with complete involvement of both anterior and posterior walls. At examination, such a uterus is moderately enlarged, usually symmetrical, and very firm to palpation.

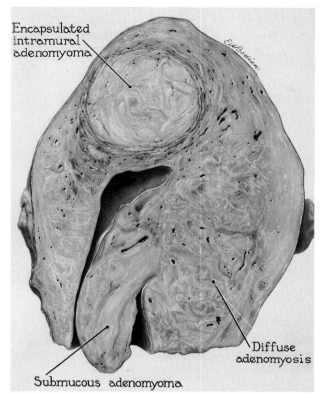

FIG. 12-2 Uterus showing three types of adenomyomatous growth: encapsulated intramural adenomyoma, submucous adenomyoma, and diffuse adenomyosis of walls.

The reported incidence of adenomyosis varies widely from one institution to another, since it is fundamentally a pathologic diagnosis. The frequency, which varies between 8% and 27%, depends not only on the criteria used for diagnosis but also on the thoroughness with which the removed uterus is studied. A rigid criterion has been suggested by Benson and Sneeden; namely, that the area must extend into the myometrium at least 2 low-power fields (8 mm) from the basalis. The incidence reaches its peak in the fifth decade. Infertility is not common with this form of the disease, and many patients are multiparous. About 12% of them have coexisting external endometriosis.

SYMPTOMS

Adenomyosis is often an incidental pathologic finding and may be entirely asymptomatic. When in-

volvement of the myometrium is extensive, pain and abnormal uterine bleeding, usually in the form of menorrhagia, are likely, probably because the enlarged uterine cavity has an increased surface area. Also, extensive involvement of the uterine wall may interfere with the normal uterine muscular contractility and allow excessive bleeding. Pain, when present, is usually associated with menstruation and is often severe, crampy, or knifelike. This dysmenorrheic pattern probably results from bleeding within the deep-lying islands of endometrium. The pathologic basis for these symptoms is shown in Figure 12-3. The histologic features of the endometrial glands and stroma that characterize these lesions are shown in Figure 12-4. The hormonal effects of pregnancy on endometriosis are shown in Figures 12-5 and 12-6.

PELVIC FINDINGS

The uterus may be very firm and is usually enlarged. Generally, it is not more than twice its normal size.

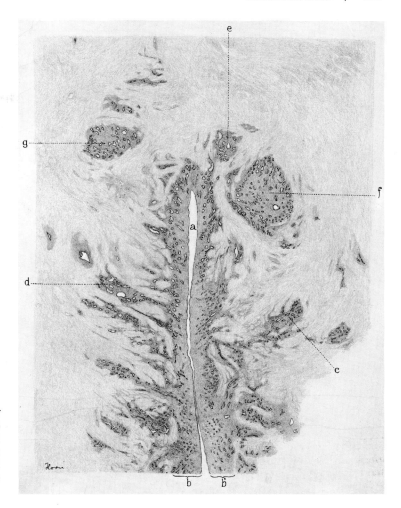

FIG. 12-3 Section through central portion of uterus with adenomyosis. (*a*) Uterine cavity. (*b*) Endometrium of cavity. (*c* to *g*) Islands of displaced endometrium into which hemorrhage occurs at time of menstruation. Poor drainage of menstrual blood with increased tension explains severe menstrual pain.

With the diffuse type of adenomyosis, which is more common, the enlargement is likely to be symmetrical. Accordingly, the uterus is a rather globular structure. When an encapsulated adenomyoma is present, the uterus may be irregular or asymmetrical, much like it is when fibroids are present. At times, particularly during menstruation, the enlarged uterus is tender to palpation.

DIAGNOSIS

Adenomyosis should always be suspected in a woman with dysmenorrhea and menorrhagia of increasing severity in the fourth or fifth decade, particularly if the uterus is symmetrically enlarged, firm, and tender. It is difficult to be certain of the diagnosis, since functional uterine bleeding and multiple small leiomyomas may have similar findings.

TREATMENT

An exact preoperative diagnosis is often difficult to make, and it may be largely of only academic interest anyway. Only in the rare instance when excessive myometrium is removed by the curette or a polypoid submucous adenomyoma is found can the diagnosis be confirmed without the uterus as a surgical specimen. Curettage does not aid in establishing the diagnosis and is ineffectual as treatment, even though it may be required because of abnormal bleeding. Cyclic hormonal therapy is likewise of little aid in treatment.

The need for surgery, therefore, is based on continued menorrhagia and dysmenorrhea, not on whether the uterus is thought to be normal in size or whether it contains adenomyosis or a leiomyoma. The definitive treatment is hysterectomy. The vaginal route is preferred if the size of the uterus per-

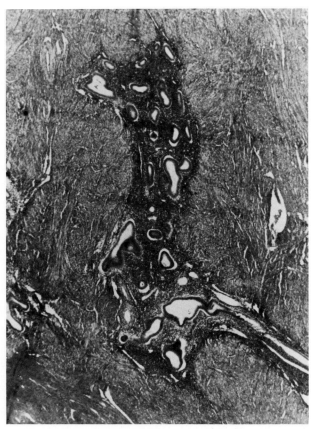

FIG. 12–4 Area of adenomyosis. Compact stroma and proliferative, slightly hyperplastic glands surrounded by hypertrophied myometrium.

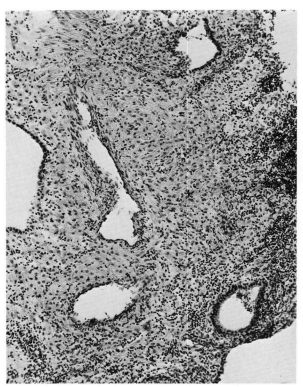

FIG. 12–5 Adenomyosis in pregnancy showing decidual reaction. Note that glands still show proliferative pattern not reacting to increased progesterone stimulation.

mits and no other pelvic abnormalities are present. At times, in a younger patient who wants to retain her reproductive capability, excision of an encapsulated adenomyoma should be considered. This situation arises infrequently, since adenomyosis is generally diffuse and usually occurs in multiparous women no longer interested in childbearing.

External Endometriosis

The term *endometriosis* more commonly refers to the external form, in which the ectopic endometrial tissue grows outside the uterus. The condition is more likely to be clinically symptomatic than are many cases of adenomyosis, in which there is minimal myometrial extension and few symptoms. Infertility, symptoms, or diagnostic problems are presented to the gynecologist.

Since the first descriptions in the latter part of the 19th century, endometriosis has been recorded

with increasing frequency. Increased clinical awareness, better education in gynecologic pathology, and the recent availability of laparoscopy have led to more frequent recognition and diagnosis. It is also probable, however, that the disease is actually increasing in frequency. In 1977, Williams and Pratt, in reporting a prospective study involving 1000 consecutive celiotomies for benign disease, documented a 50% incidence of endometriosis. Although this figure may be biased by the type of patients referred to the Mayo Clinic, the diagnosis of endometriosis is more commonly made in high-income patients than in the indigent. The difference in observed frequency may prove to be more closely related to the patient's ability to pay for specialty medical care than to a true difference in the occurrence of the disease based on socioeconomic factors.

There seems to be little question that pregnancy decreases the incidence of endometriosis and confers some protection on the parous woman. Often, 5 or more years pass after a patient's last pregnancy before symptomatic endometriosis. is discovered. Whether those benefits result from the hormones of pregnancy or the cervical dilatation at delivery is not certain.

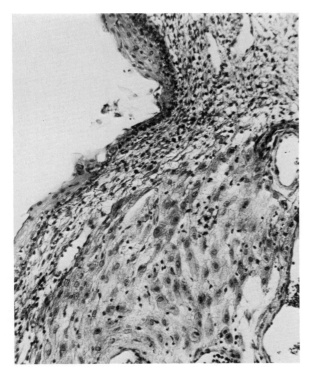

FIG. 12–6 Adenomyosis in pregnancy. Decidual change in stromal cells along with glandular changes.

Although it has been widely believed that endometriosis is rare among black women, Chatman found a 22.7% incidence among black women undergoing diagnostic laparoscopy. Among poor African women, Ekwempu and Harrison reported an 8% incidence in hysterectomy specimens. Miyazawa found a 10% incidence among Oriental women and a 5% incidence for non-Oriental patients. Recent studies have also documented endometriosis in teenagers despite previous data suggesting that the condition occurs primarily in the middle decades of life.

The ectopic endometrium, wherever it may be, depends on ovarian hormones for its maintenance and for various degrees of stimulation. Scott and Wharton, in studies on endometriosis in castrated rhesus monkeys, showed that estrogen was important in maintaining active endometrial implants and that when estrogen-primed implants were subjected to progesterone-induced withdrawal bleeding, implants became more active. Each implant may then respond to these hormonal stimuli as though it were a miniature uterus. Frequently, the response to progesterone is minimal, and in this respect the implants resemble the basalis portion of the uterine endometrium. But response varies greatly, depending on the distribution of estrogen and progesterone receptors. In the same patient, some areas may show a good progestational response while others show none. The implants, however, are usually capable of local withdrawal bleeding regardless of their histologic pattern and degree of progestational response.

In pregnancy or with progestogen therapy, implants may show a marked decidual reaction of the stroma (see Figs. 12–5 and 12–6). This response, too, is not entirely predictable. Because of the decidual reaction of the implants and the absence of menstruation, the general impression had been that endometriosis improves during pregnancy. This concept was questioned by McArthur and Ulfelder, who, in a review of reported cases, found that pregnancy had nearly similar effects of regression and progression on endometriosis.

Laboratory studies involving the cytosol estrogen and progesterone receptors have shown a difference between the receptors present in endometriosis and those in the endometrium itself. Bergqvist and associates found markedly lower receptor content for estrogen in endometriotic tissue. Data on the cytoplasmic progesterone receptors for endometriosis were conflicting. The conclusion, however, was that a functional difference existed between the endometriotic tissue and endometrium. Jänne and associates documented similar findings. These data are in accord with the often favorable but variable response noted to hormonal treatment of endometriosis.

The fact that endometriosis is dependent on ovarian hormones generally confines its clinical importance to the reproductive era of a woman's life. It has not been reported before menarche, and the implants become atrophic after the menopause. Endometriosis has its peak incidence in the fourth decade. Scott and associates found that 49.5% of their cases were in this age group and that 83.1% occurred before age 40. Thus, the classic patient with endometriosis is a nulliparous, high-income woman in her fourth decade of life.

DISTRIBUTION AND GROSS PATHOLOGY

Endometrial implants and growths have been described in a variety of places, primarily within the pelvis. Ovarian disease is noted most frequently. The incidence seems to decrease as the centrifugal distance from the uterus increases. The distribution is illustrated in Figure 12–7 diagrammatically. The numerical incidence of endometriosis in the various pelvic and other abdominoperineal structures is shown in Table 12–1. In addition to these common sites, some rare locations have been reported, in-

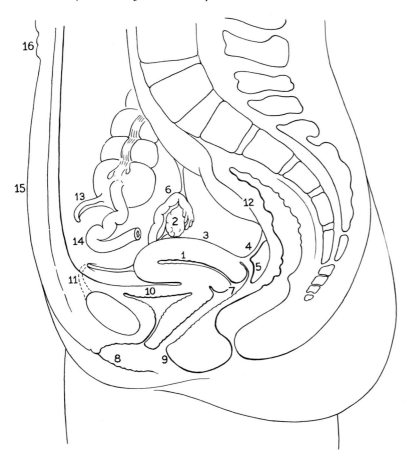

FIG. 12-7 Schematic drawing of sites of endometriosis (numbered, beginning with the ovary, in approximate order of frequency): (*1*) Adenomyosis site. (*2*) Ovary. (*3*) Serous surface of uterus. (*4*) Uterosacral ligament. (*5*) Cul-de-sac. (*6*) Tube. (*7*) Cervix. (*8*) Vulva. (*9*) Perineum. (*10*) Bladder. (*11*) Extraperitoneal portion of round ligament. (*12*) Rectosigmoid. (*13*) Appendix. (*14*) Ileum. (*15*) Abdominal scar. (*16*) Umbilicus.

cluding the extensor carpi radialis muscle and the thigh.

OVARY. The lesions encountered on the ovary vary in size from tiny spots to masses larger than 10 cm in diameter. The small superficial lesions are more often noted on the surface of the ovary; they vary from dusky red to brownish black, depending on the state of preservation of the contained blood (Fig. 12–8). The larger cysts often have a rather thick wall and the dull white of the ovarian cortex; where the capsule is thinned, the dark chocolate-colored contents may darken the wall to brown or almost black (Fig. 12–9).

The cysts characteristically perforate when the pressure resulting from intracystic hemorrhage becomes sufficiently great. Organization of the extruded blood seals over the defect in the cyst wall, and blood then accumulates anew within the cavity until perforation again takes place. This discharge of blood and subsequent organization result in adhesions about the ovary to the parietal peritoneum of the posterior leaf of the broad ligament.

The peritoneum, irritated by this blood, becomes hyperemic and thickened. When the peritoneal cavity is opened after recent rupture, the characteristic finding is old blood lying free within the cavity. Usually it is scanty, but in rare instances, as much as 100 ml to 200 ml may be present. When the cyst is dissected free, the point or points of previous perforations are inevitably entered, and the cyst contents spill. Generally, the material is a thick brown fluid, from which the name *chocolate cyst* has been derived, but it may be very thick, tenacious, and almost black. German authors have called these *tar cysts*, and, indeed, the contents may resemble tar more than chocolate.

UTERUS. The presumptive diagnosis is endometrial cyst if, when an adherent ovary or ovarian cyst is dissected free, chocolate or tarry substance appears. This rule is not invariable, since hemorrhage into the corpora lutea and also into other types of ovarian cysts may give a similar picture. But the tissue in the wall of the cyst is that of the friable corpus luteum rather than of the more fi-

TABLE 12–1 Location of External Endometriosis

TYPE	SITE	NUMBER	PERCENT*
	Ovary—one	285	55.2
Ovarian	Ovary—both	127	24.6
Superficial and small spots on serosa	Diffuse scattered pelvic	171	33.1
	Uterine surface	73	14.1
	Tubal surface	71	13.7
	Posterior cul-de-sac	24	4.7
	Uterosacral ligaments	19	3.7
	Anterior cul-de-sac	11	2.1
	Omentum	3	0.6
	Round ligaments	2	0.4
	Broad ligaments	1	0.2
	Small intestine	1	0.2
	Appendix	7	1.4
Intra-abdominal nodules	Rectovaginal septum	8	1.6
	Rectovaginal septum with rectosigmoid involvement	20	3.9
	Rectovaginal septum with vaginal extension	9	1.8
	Sigmoidal	4	0.8
	Anterior cul-de-sac	2	0.4
	Anterior cul-de-sac with bladder involvement	5	1.0
	Tube	8	1.6
	Broad ligament	4	0.8
	Round ligament	3	0.6
Extraperitoneal	Cervix	13	2.5
	Inguinal	4	0.8
	Umbilical	4	0.8
	Incisional—ventral	4	0.8
	Incisional—vulval	1	0.2

* Total amounts to over 100% because of multiple lesions.

brotic endometrioma. In addition, the blood in a corpus luteum hematoma is much more apt to form a clot than to remain a thick fluid as in an endometrial cyst. Hemorrhage into any cystadenoma may give a chocolate color to the contents; but the blood, becoming mixed with the contents, is not usually sufficient to alter the consistency of the original fluid content.

Rupture and leakage are assumed to occur frequently, and the secondary irritation is thought to be responsible for some of the symptoms. However, this may not be the case. Of 325 patients with endometriosis who were studied by Williams, 277 had endometriosis on the ovary and 132 had endometrioma. In eight of these patients, leakage or rupture was found at the time of surgery. Only one of these patients had pain that could have been attributed to that leakage. Abdominal pain associated with rupture of an endometrial cyst is generally thought to be caused by a peritoneal reaction to hemolyzed blood. Next to the ovary, the uterus is involved most

frequently. The serosal surface of the uterus is often the site of multiple implants. They are usually very small, but on occasion they can form dark vesicles up to 4 mm or 5 mm in diameter (Fig. 12–8). Where the endometrial lesion occurs on these serosal surfaces, there is likely to be a characteristic puckering or scarring of the adjacent serosa about the small, dark lesion. Implants on the anterior surface of the uterus sometimes cause adhesions between it and the peritoneal surface of the bladder or any other adjacent structure. There may be invasion of the bladder extending through the entire thickness of the vesical wall (Fig. 12–10).

The lesions of endometriosis are more common on the posterior surface of the uterus, especially on the lower and more dependent portion. The cul-de-sac is a favorite place for endometrial implants. Accordingly, the posterior wall of the vagina and the cervix may become densely adherent to the anterior rectal wall and completely obliterate the cul-de-sac. The uterosacral ligaments on either side

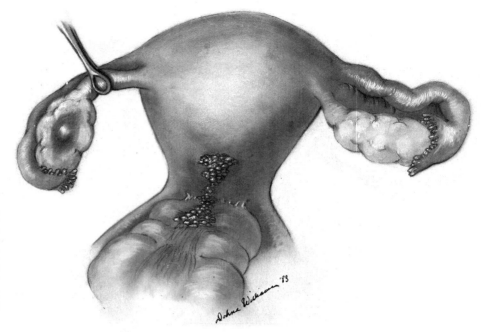

FIG. 12–8 Typical picture of old pelvic endometriosis. Ovary, uterosacral ligament, posterior surface of uterus, and rectal wall are involved. An atraumatic small ring forceps (Williams' clamp) as shown on the left utero-ovarian ligament, is used for traction when necessary.

of the cul-de-sac are commonly involved with the endometriosis, which forms small, puckered, shotty nodules along the course of the ligaments. Downward extension of the invasive endometrial process from the cul-de-sac and the uterosacral regions proceeds into the rectovaginal septum. Here, the endometriosis can involve the anterior rectal wall and, at times, penetrate the mucosa of the posterior vaginal vault. This growth may be not only palpable but also visible as a dark nodular mass posterior to the cervix (Fig. 12–11).

ROUND LIGAMENTS. Small endometrial implants may occur on the serosal surface of the round ligaments at any place within the peritoneal cavity. A lesion of special interest was described by Cullen in 1896. In this lesion the extraperitoneal portion of the round ligament is involved in an endometriotic process, forming a nodule in the region of

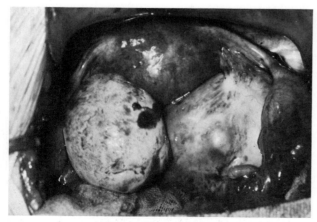

FIG. 12–9 Typical bilateral endometrial cysts of ovary almost completely destroying ovarian tissue. Old blood is disseminated on pelvic peritoneum as well.

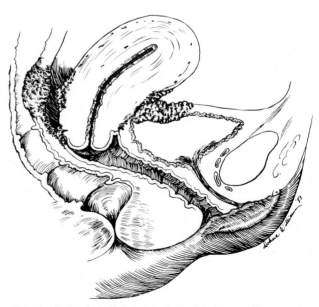

FIG. 12–10 Endometriosis involving bladder wall, posterior uterus, uterosacral ligaments, and rectosigmoid colon.

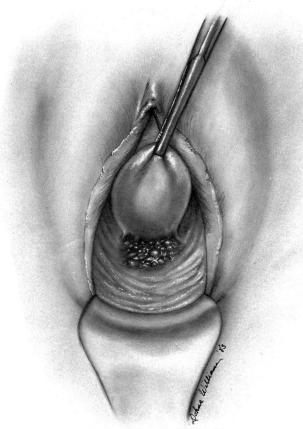

FIG. 12–11 Endometriotic lesions in posterior vaginal fornix extending from cul-de-sac endometriosis.

the inguinal ring. Such a nodule may vary from 1 cm to 3 cm in diameter and usually blends diffusely into the surrounding adipose tissue. These round ligament growths show hypertrophy of the adjacent smooth muscle along with islands of glands and stroma. The tissues may be darkened by evidence of old or recent hemorrhage. The inguinal mass is usually associated with pain, and there may also be cyclic enlargement. The pain may mimic that of musculoskeletal conditions, although there is no direct bony involvement and excision is curative.

COLON. In addition to involvement of the anterior rectal wall and invasion of the rectovaginal septum, a prominent lesion in the upper rectum or sigmoid is not uncommon. Such lesions usually result in a thickening and proliferation of the muscularis of the bowel. The degree of involvement may be great enough that encroachment on the bowel lumen produces partial or even complete obstruction.

Usually, the invasion extends through the serosa to the muscularis, but the mucosa is not directly involved by the endometriosis. This is an important diagnostic point in the differentiation of endometriosis from carcinoma of the bowel. In the latter, since the carcinoma arises from the mucosa, barium enema and proctoscopy are very helpful. Endometriosis, however, can involve the full thickness of the intestinal wall and even produce polypoid growths within the bowel lumen. Cyclic bleeding usually occurs, and the diagnosis can be made by proctoscopy or sigmoidoscopy with a biopsy of the lesion. If these have not been done, it may be difficult to distinguish bowel endometriosis from carcinoma at surgery. Endometriosis elsewhere in the pelvis generally gives a clue to the bowel lesion. Even if there is no actual involvement of the mucosa by the endometriosis, cyclic hematochezia may occur, and careful inspection of the mucosa reveals a defect contiguous with the adjacent endometriosis. It must be remembered that endometriosis is the third most common benign tumor of the colon.

In a study by Williams of 325 consecutive cases of endometriosis in which the female genital tract was involved, the intestinal tract was found to have endometriosis in 41% of cases. The sigmoid was involved in 84% and the ileum in only 9%. Obstructive symptoms, however, were far more frequent with ileal endometriosis (25% of cases) than with colonic (6%).

The appendix, cecum, and ileum are frequently involved in the process of endometriosis but rarely to the degree seen in the sigmoid and rectum. In the appendix, involvement is usually an incidental pathologic finding with appendectomy. However, the marked decidual reaction and changes that occur with pregnancy may result in spontaneous perforation of the appendix and the signs and symptoms of acute abdominal distress. Similar complications have been reported with endometriosis involving the colon, but these are merely curiosities that must be kept in mind. An extensive growth of endometriosis on an appendix is illustrated in Figure 12–12.

A loop of ileum may be adherent in the pelvis, producing angulation and obstruction, either partial or complete. The gross appearance of the lesion is usually typical of endometriosis. Biopsy of the lesion, however, may be necessary to establish the benignity of the implant. Bowel resection or excision of the involved area should be done if obstruction is present or if the caliber of the lumen shows compromise. Under such circumstances, castration alone is not adequate treatment, since subsequent fibrosis may further narrow the bowel lumen. The sequelae of intestinal endometriosis may not appear until the patient is postmenopausal. Although the endometriosis may have become inactive, the resulting

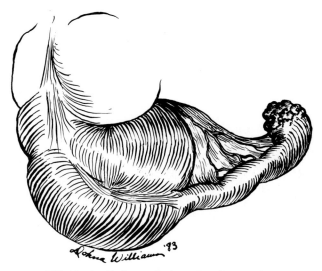

FIG. 12–12 Endometriosis at tip of appendix.

cicatrization leads to a decrease in the bowel lumen and to symptoms of obstruction.

BLADDER. The urinary tract is involved less frequently than the bowel. Peritoneal implants on the bladder may infiltrate partially or completely into the bladder wall, where they cause symptoms of vesical irritability and, occasionally, hematuria.

Vesical endometriosis may occur by direct implantation after vaginal hysterotomy for abortion. The frequency of this complication is so high that in Sweden, vaginal hysterotomy has been discontinued as a method of midtrimester interruption of pregnancy.

Cytologic evaluation may show endometrial cells, but the diagnosis usually requires cystoscopy and biopsy. Cystography may document a filling defect, but it, like ultrasound, is nonspecific. Segmental resection of the lesion is preferable to attempts at hormone management.

URETER. A more serious situation arises when the ureter is compressed by an endometrial cyst or is directly invaded by endometriosis in the pelvis. Either of these leads to ureteral obstruction and subsequent loss of renal function (Fig. 12–13). Early diagnosis and treatment are required to avoid loss of the kidney. Scarring and continued obstruction require not only definitive surgery with castration but also excision of the diseased ureter with anastomosis or implantation into the bladder.

KIDNEY. Ten cases of renal endometriosis have been reported. This condition may result from passage of fragments of endometrium up the ureter or, more likely, by lymphatic or vascular metastasis along or in the ureteral wall. The symptom is vague flank discomfort, occasionally with hematuria.

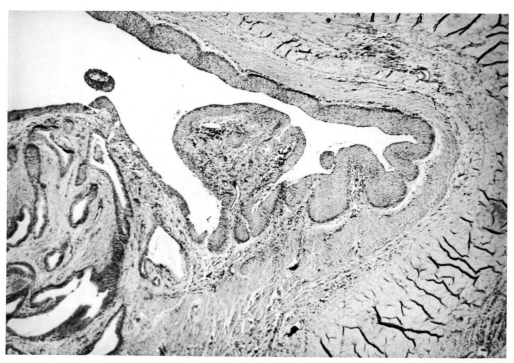

FIG. 12–13 Compression and invasion of ureteral wall by endometriosis.

Roentgenograms indicate an expansive lesion suggesting a diagnosis of malignancy.

INCISIONAL SCARS. Scars from operations are occasionally the sites of endometriotic implantation. Perineal, vaginal, or vulvar scars, particularly episiotomies, colporrhaphies, and Bartholin's gland excisions, are likely areas for involvement by endometriosis. Perhaps the hormonal effects of pregnancy on the endometrium produce adverse conditions for implantation and growth. Otherwise, one could expect nearly all episiotomies to be sites of endometriosis.

Where an incisional scar becomes a site of endometriosis, there is frequently a history of delayed wound healing. The growths appear as either deeply lying or subcutaneous nodules infiltrating the fat, fascia, and muscle. Bleeding into the tissues at the time of menstruation may cause cyclic local pain, tenderness, and discoloration of the tissues; however, the nodule may lie too deep for detection of any color change through the skin. If the nodule is very superficial, cyclic bleeding or ulceration may be apparent.

In most instances, incisional endometriomas have followed surgical procedures that violated the uterine cavity and allowed the lining endometrium to be transplanted. Wespi suggested the frequency might approach 5% among patients having cesarean section or hysterectomy. Chatterjee reported an incidence of 1% of scar endometriosis among patients having hysterectomy and described associated pelvic endometriosis in 24% of 17 patients. Indeed, endometriosis has been recorded along the needle tracts after amniocentesis or saline injection for abortion.

Careful flushing and irrigation of the abdomen and of the incision during closure should minimize the chance of contamination when incision into the uterine cavity is required. Metroplasty and myomectomy as well as cesarean section and hysterotomy increase the risk of incisional endometriosis. Episiotomy scars and cervical and vaginal lacerations also serve as implantation sites after delivery. The number is significantly elevated when curettage is done after delivery. Paull and Tedeschi reported 15 instances in 2,208 deliveries when curettage was carried out and none in 13,800 without curettage.

Management, usually best carried out by local excision, is both diagnostic and curative. The use of various hormone regimens may be proper if it is necessary to avoid surgery. However, it must be remembered that malignancy can occur in each area of ectopic endometriosis, and histologic confirmation of the tentative diagnosis is preferable.

UMBILICUS. Endometriosis involving the umbilicus accounts for about 1% of cases. It presents the problem of differential diagnosis from metastatic cancer. Here, the endometrial tissue infiltrates the surrounding tissues and, with hemorrhage, forms bluish nodules, sometimes visible through the skin (Fig. 12–14). There may be little or no associated pelvic endometriosis, and the symptoms may be cyclic, related to the periods, or completely absent save for an umbilical mass.

THORAX. In 1981, Foster and associates tabulated 65 cases of thoracic endometriosis. They described two categories of involvement, the pleura and the lung parenchyma. These areas of involvement presented different findings. In patients with pleural disease, there was pain with right-sided pneumothorax or pleural effusion in 93% of the cases. These instances were believed to be secondary to tubal regurgitation and transport through diaphragmatic defects to give implantation onto the pleura. The authors pointed out that a preponderance of defects in the right diaphragm correlated with this local predominance of endometriosis. They found that women with pleural endometriosis were younger than those having parenchymal disease. Previous pelvic surgery was more common among women who had parenchymal endometriosis; however, pelvic endometriosis was found more often in those with pleural disease. Cases involving the pleura produced pleuritic pain or pleural effusions, whereas those involving the lung parenchyma produced hemoptysis rather than the pleuritic symptoms.

Catamenial pneumothorax or hemoptysis should alert the physician to the possibility of thoracic en-

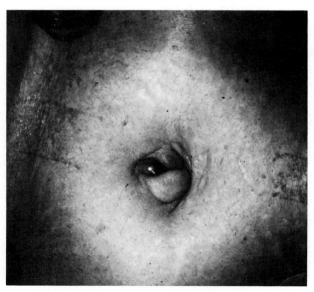

FIG. 12–14 Endometriosis of umbilicus.

dometriosis. The chest roentgenogram is usually of little value in the diagnosis; however, cytology, aspiration biopsy, and pleuroscopy may be used to confirm it. Massive effusion and bleeding may occur, but they suggest even more the possibility of a malignancy.

HISTOLOGY

Endometriosis in its different sites may present a variety of histologic patterns. In many instances, particularly when the location is the ovary, there are typical glands with an abundance of characteristic endometrial stroma (Fig. 12–15). In large chocolate cysts, the epithelium lining the cavity may be thinned by pressure, often to the point of being unrecognizable. Indeed, in some areas the epithelium may be entirely lacking. Stromal cells may be scanty in many of the lesions, and one may be forced to search diligently for enough stroma to identify the tissue. In many such situations, hemosiderin phagocytosis may be the most prominent feature.

When endometriosis grows in a setting of smooth muscle, such as on the round ligament or on the surface of the uterus or the bowel, it seems to stimulate the proliferation of the smooth muscle. The muscular components may grow in whorls between bits of endometrial tissue, so that histologically the growth resembles that of adenomyosis.

In many instances, the glands and the stroma go through the same cyclic changes as the endometrium in its normal site. During pregnancy, a full decidual reaction is frequently noted, and such responsive endometriosis seems common in the ovary (Figs. 12–5 and 12–6). The typical cyclic menstrual changes are not seen universally, and the histologic pattern of the ectopic tissue may be purely proliferative with no progestational change. In some instances, the typical pattern of hyperplasia is present. This is usually cystic, and adenomatous or atypical change is infrequent.

In some cysts, the epithelial lining resembles tubal epithelium, with ciliated and nonciliated cells. Sampson and Everett described this, and the former suggested the term *endosalpingosis*. Some cysts have been seen in which one part of the wall is lined by typical endometrium and another part by epithelium of the tubal type.

HISTOGENESIS

The classic reports of Cullen and Russell identified ectopic endometrial tissue as müllerian in origin. These lesions show all variations of response to the ovarian hormones characteristic of endometrium in its normal site. Cullen and Russell believed that the ectopic endometrial tissue was the result of misplaced embryonic müllerian rests but made no attempt to explain the mechanism by which the endometrial tissue was disseminated.

Not until 1921, with Sampson's contribution, did gynecologists begin to seriously study the histogenesis of this disease. The problem has not been solved completely by any single theory. The theory generally considered Sampson's most important contribution holds that the menstrual endometrium flows in a retrograde manner through the tubes and implants itself to proliferate and grow in the pelvic viscera.

Sampson briefly stated his implantation theory as follows:

> Ovarian and other forms of peritoneal endometriosis arise from the implantation of bits of müllerian mucosa, of either uterine or tubal origin, which, having been carried with menstrual blood escaping through patent tubes into the peritoneal cavity, have lodged on the surfaces of the various pelvic structures. The ectopic mucosa in these implants, regardless of their size or situation, may become additional foci for the spread of the endometriosis by direct extension and also by the implantation of bits of müllerian tissue which escape from them during their reaction to menstruation. The latter phenomenon is most spectacular in the ovary where ectopic endometrial cavities may attain a much larger size than elsewhere, forming the well-known endometrial cysts of that organ.

Sampson originally believed that the ovary acted as an incubator or hotbed for the development of implants on the peritoneum and that it might even impart greater virulence to the müllerian epithelium growing in it. He based this belief on the finding that, in the cases he studied up to 1922, the endometriosis seemed to be more extensive and more invasive in cases associated with endometrial cysts of the ovary. However, the study of more material showed him that extensive pelvic endometriosis may occur without ovarian involvement; hence, he later considered unwarranted his earlier suggestion that the ovary imparts greater virulence to the müllerian epithelium.

Sampson deliberately operated on many patients during menstruation and frequently observed blood coming from the ends of the tubes. This observation was substantiated by many gynecologists, and it was suggested that retroposition of the uterus would augment this flow. It seems more likely, however, that the retroposition so commonly noted with endometriosis is the effect of scarring pulling the uterus into the cul-de-sac. Sampson fixed and sectioned fallopian tubes with blood in them and demonstrated endometrial tissue; he believed this endometrial mucosa to be viable (Fig. 12–16).

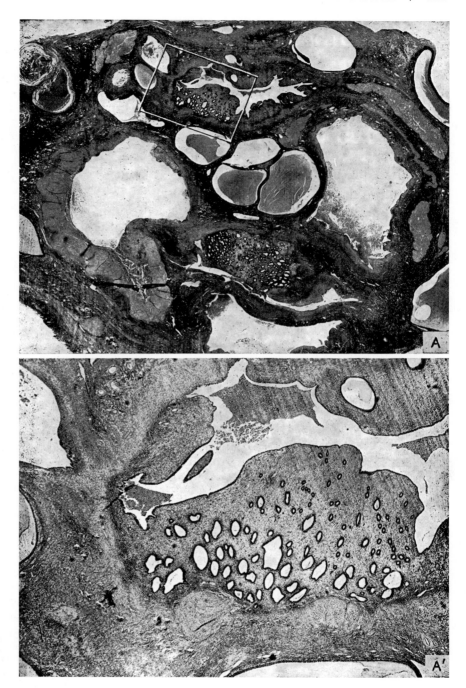

FIG. 12–15 Multiple endometrial cysts of ovary. (A) Lower-power section of most of ovary. (A') Higher-power section of one area of cyst wall.

Sampson's theory is undoubtedly the most widely accepted explanation of the phenomenon of pelvic endometriosis. Repeated observation at the operating table has shown that endometrial cysts of the ovary are associated with pelvic adhesions that may be the result of organization of old blood. If one couples this observation with the fact that many of these adhesions, when sectioned, show endometrial tissue, it is difficult to escape the conclusion that the peritoneal endometrial plaques are implants from the bloody contents of cysts. The question is whether the endometrial-lined cysts of the ovaries are the result of implantation of bits of cast-off menstrual endometrium that traveled through the tube.

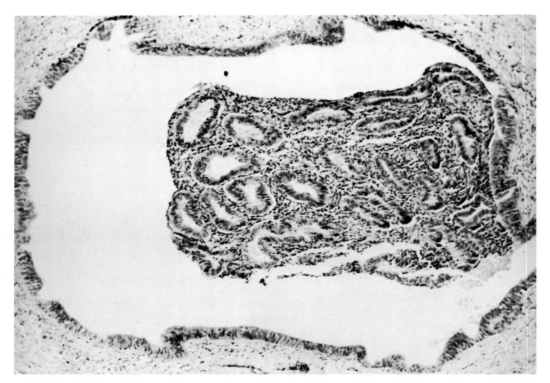

FIG. 12–16 Fragment of shed endometrium within lumen of human fallopian tube.

Although experimental studies have shown beyond doubt that endometrium taken from the uterine lining and transplanted into the pelvic cavity or other areas will grow, until recently no unimpeachable experiments had been done to show whether the cast-off particles of menstrual endometrium were capable of implantation and growth. Therein lies the crux of the entire Sampson theory, for, as Sampson himself recognized, if endometrium passed into the peritoneal cavity is always dead, the implantation theory is also dead. Even the opponents of Sampson's theory admitted that if it could be shown that cast-off menstrual endometrium is viable, Sampson's hypothesis would be greatly strengthened.

Novak summarized objections that have been raised to Sampson's theory:

(1) Retrograde menstruation, although it may occur, is a rarely observed phenomenon, in contrast to the great frequency of endometriosis; (2) it is difficult to believe that endometrium thrown off in the uterus could enter the small uterine orifice of the tube, travel outward against the current, and still be capable of implanting itself and growing on the pelvic structures; (3) endometrium thrown off at menstruation is already degenerated or dead, so that it is not easy to conceive of its taking root in the peritoneum; (4) such experiments as those of Jacobson, showing that endometrium can grow in the peritoneum, have dealt with the normal, healthy endometrium of animals; (5) experiments such as those of Heim in monkeys, in which a uteroabdominal fistula was created, all failed to show any development of endometrium despite the fact that the menstrual blood was emptied freely into the abdomen; and (6) Sampson's theory could not explain endometriosis in some locations, such as the umbilicus.

Most of those who have been reluctant to accept Sampson's theory have championed that of Iwanoff and of Meyer in one of its modifications. These two investigators independently presented the idea that aberrant endometrium originates from abnormal differentiation of the coelomic epithelium, from which all the genital mucous membrane arises. This theory in its various modifications suggests that the pelvic peritoneum under certain stimuli, inflammatory or hormonal, may develop into endometrial-like tissue. It has not seemed logical that inflammation can be such a stimulus. Pelvic endometriosis is least likely to be found in patients who have pelvic inflammatory disease, and the converse is also true. Intraperitoneal injection of blood during menstruation also does not seem to incite endometriosis, and although Merrill was able to produce structures similar to endometrial glands outside of Millipore filters, true endometriosis with typical endometrial glands and stroma has not been produced outside of the filters. It therefore seems quite clear that although coelomic metaplasia may occur and may explain some cases of pelvic endometriosis or endometriosis elsewhere in the body, it has yet to be demonstrated experimentally and proved. No factor, be it hormonal, inflammatory, or exogenous, has been shown as yet to incite the development of typical endometriosis.

Halban's theory of dissemination through the lymphatic system appears to be relevant in only a few cases of endometriosis. The usual pelvic lesions of endometriosis do not follow the paths of the lymphatics. Endometrium has been found occasionally in the pelvic lymph nodes at operation, as reported by Javert, but does not usually produce clinical endometriosis. Dissemination through the lymphatic system, however, appears to be the best explanation for endometriosis of the umbilicus, since Scott and Wharton have shown in rhesus monkeys that lymphatics of the anterior wall may drain from the pelvis to the umbilicus.

Desquamated human endometrium was grown successfully on tissue culture by Keettel and Stein. The cultured cells had the appearance of fibroblasts and epithelial cells. In short, all these studies have given strong support to Sampson's theory of retrograde menstruation and implantation and have shown not only that menstruating endometrium is viable but also that it is capable of growing and causing endometriosis.

Scott and associates reported experimental work demonstrating that desquamated menstrual endometrium is capable of growth. The uterus of each of 10 rhesus monkeys was divided from its vaginal attachment and rotated on its ovarian axis to allow intraperitoneal menstruation to occur; the menstrual flow spilled in the cul-de-sac or up toward the diaphragm (Fig. 12–17). In 6 of the 10 animals, typical areas of endometriosis developed within the peritoneal cavity. Growing endometrium was found from 75 to 963 days after the reversal operation. The other four animals did not survive. The uterus of another monkey was rotated 90°, and the cervix was brought through the anterior abdominal wall so that menstruation could occur at this site (Fig. 12–18). The uterus subsequently retracted, leaving a sinus tract in the anterior abdominal wall. Endometriosis was found in this sinus tract. In two additional animals, the rotated cervix was implanted into the rectus muscle so that menstruation could occur in an area entirely free from the peritoneum or from tissue arising from the coelomic epithelium.

Endometriosis was found adjacent to the reversed cervix within 12 to 19 months after the original operation.

It had been suggested that, by itself, blood originating from the rupture of ovarian follicles or corpora lutea or escaping from the fimbriae of fallopian tubes during menstruation might incite metaplasia of the peritoneum and produce endometriosis. To test this possibility, Scott and associates injected venous blood obtained during episodes of menstruation into the peritoneal cavities of four monkeys; in no instance did endometriosis develop.

In 1958, Ridley and Edwards documented similar findings in women. For 12 hours, they collected the menstrual flow in eight women through cervical cannulas. This material was centrifuged, and the sediment was injected into the rectus muscle of the same patient, who in each case was to have an abdominal operation 90 to 180 days after the single injection. Six of these patients did not have endometriosis in the injection site at laparotomy, one had a definite area of endometriosis 175 days after injection, and the eighth patient had an area suggestive of endometriosis at 110 days.

Four women accidentally provided a natural clinical experiment. Three of them had a noncommunicating horn of a double uterus. In these women, the only exit of the menstrual flow from the noncommunicating horn was through the fallopian tube, and endometriosis developed in each woman in the ovary on the side of the rudimentary horn. The fourth patient was an unmarried woman of 40 in whom dysmenorrhea and eventually amenorrhea developed, but with recurring monthly pain. Examination showed the upper vagina to be obliterated completely by adhesions, and laparotomy showed endometriosis of the posterior surface of the uterus and cul-de-sac. Such situations can occur as a complication of cervical agenesis with functioning endometrium and ovarian tissue. Endometriosis can occur from the retrograde flow, although this anomaly is very rare. Cervical stenosis as a complication of dilatation and curettage may also produce such a situation (Fig. 12–19).

The experiments mentioned above give no support to the theory of serosal metaplasia but give more or less conclusive support to Sampson's theory of retrograde menstruation. However, this theory does not explain the occurrence of endometriosis at the umbilicus. Because of the lymphatic drainage from the pelvic region to the umbilicus through the route to the urachus and obliterated hypogastric vessels, it would seem likely that endometrial particles are deposited in the umbilicus by way of the lymphatic channels. This hypothesis is strengthened by the results of one of Scott and associates' exper-

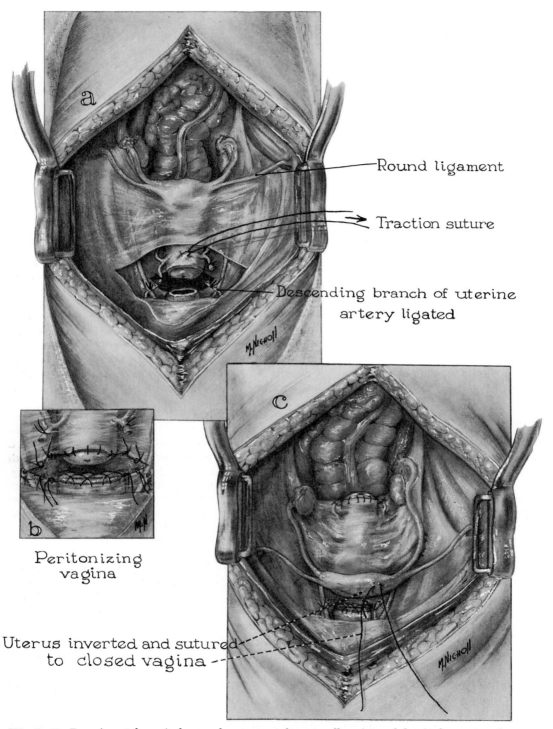

Round ligament

Traction suture

Descending branch of uterine artery ligated

Peritonizing vagina

Uterus inverted and sutured to closed vagina

FIG. 12–17 Experimental surgical procedure on monkeys to allow intra-abdominal menstruation. Entire uterus is separated from vagina and rotated through 180° to allow menstruation into peritoneal cavity.

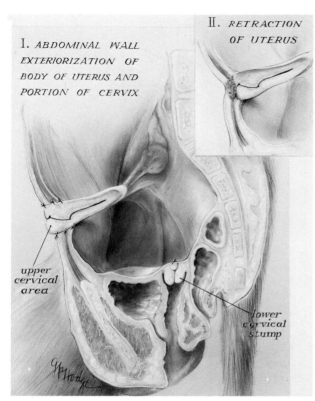

I. *ABDOMINAL WALL EXTERIORIZATION OF BODY OF UTERUS AND PORTION OF CERVIX*

II. *RETRACTION OF UTERUS*

upper cervical area

lower cervical stump

FIG. 12–18 Uterus, except for distal portion of cervix, was brought out through anterior abdominal wall. *Inset* shows retraction of uterus and scarring in anterior abdominal wall.

iments. Extensive endometriosis of the pelvis developed in a monkey and completely obstructed one ureter. An autopsy revealed endometriosis in the nonfunctioning kidney, probably the result of deposits of endometrial particles from the pelvis by way of the periureteral lymphatics. The rare occurrence of endometriosis in the lung, forearm, and thigh is certainly not explained by natural flow, and the only possible route would seem to be hematogenous. It is of historical interest that Sampson in the early days of his histologic studies believed that endometrial particles could be disseminated through the bloodstream, and indeed this is the only way in which some instances of endometriosis can be explained. If malignant cells can be shed into the bloodstream by uterine manipulation, it is surprising that more instances of distant endometriosis are not appreciated.

SYMPTOMS

Pain

Pain is the most constant single symptom of endometriosis. Scott and associates found pain, exclusive of dysmenorrhea, to be present in 57.6% of 243 patients operated on primarily for endometriosis. On the other hand, in the prospective study by Williams and Pratt, pain exclusive of dysmenorrhea occurred in 6% of all patients with endometriosis and in 8% of patients without endometriosis. Dysmenorrhea, however, was present in 17% of patients with endometriosis but in only 8% of those without endometriosis.

Despite the frequency of pain in patients with endometriosis, many women with extensive endometriosis report not even the slightest discomfort. Conversely, some women with only a few small endometrial implants in the pelvis complain of very severe pain. Since the lesions vary so much in size, number, and location, it is quite natural that the pain arising from them should vary in both location and nature, but the pain is chiefly in the lower

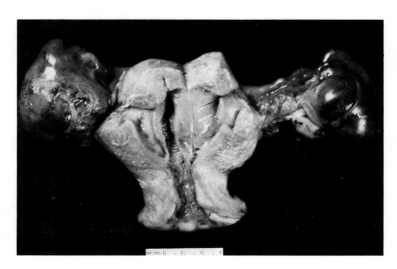

FIG. 12–19 Bilateral endometrial cysts 1 year after dilatation and curettage. Scarring and stenosis can be seen at internal os. Patient had cyclic monthly pain despite amenorrhea.

abdomen. The pain may be either unilateral or bilateral, but it is more often diffuse and tends to be aggravated premenstrually or menstrually, leaving residual postmenstrual pelvic soreness.

Endometrial cysts are inclined to rupture or leak some of their entrapped blood into the peritoneal cavity. Leakage may occur suddenly and dramatically or intermittently. In either case, the blood may produce a chemical peritonitis, with severe pain, rebound tenderness, and all other signs of peritoneal irritation. On the other hand, patients have had documented rupture of an ovarian endometrial cyst with absolutely no related signs or symptoms.

DYSMENORRHEA. Dysmenorrhea is a common symptom of endometriosis. Although acquired dysmenorrhea is usually thought to be characteristic of this disease, an analysis of the cases of endometriosis does not substantiate this pattern. In their study of 243 patients with endometriosis, Scott and associates found that 51.4% had had nonprogressive dysmenorrhea and only 9.1% acquired dysmenorrhea—probably coinciding with the development of endometriosis. The prospective evaluation of Williams and Pratt documented that dysmenorrhea as a symptom was nearly twice as likely in patients with endometriosis as in those without endometriosis. Therefore, this combination of symptoms, pain and dysmenorrhea, should alert the gynecologist to the possibility of endometriosis.

DYSPAREUNIA. Involvement of the cul-de-sac or the uterosacral ligaments or both may lead to dyspareunia and possibly to low backache. Dyspareunia was recorded by Williams and Pratt in about 6% of patients with endometriosis but in only 1% of those without. Along with dysmenorrhea and the various pain symptoms, dyspareunia is significant for endometriosis.

CYCLIC PAIN. When endometriosis involves a scar in the abdominal wall, umbilicus, inguinal region, or perineum, there usually is a nodule that undergoes painful swelling at intervals corresponding to menstruation. If these lesions are superficial, there may be a bluish discoloration from hemorrhage into the tissues and, at times, cyclic external bleeding if there is a break in the epithelium. Hematuria, generally cyclic, as well as dysuria, has been noted with bladder involvement.

When the anterior rectal wall is involved, rectal pressure and painful defecation are common. With invasion of the mucosa of the sigmoid or rectum, bleeding per rectum and diarrhea can occur at menstruation. With more extensive bowel infiltration, intestinal obstruction may result (Fig. 12–20). Even though there may be no overt mucosal involvement, careful examination of the colon will

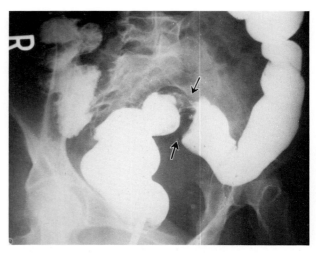

FIG. 12–20 Barium enema in patient with obstructive lesion (*arrows*) due to endometriosis. Lesion was resected by surgeon who believed it to be carcinoma.

reveal a communication from the lumen to the endometrioma in patients with cyclic rectal bleeding.

The disparity between the extent of the endometriosis and the severity of the pain remains without adequate explanation. Sturgis and Call suggested that superficial implants may expand more easily with hormonal stimulation, whereas the deeper islands of ectopic endometrium tend to be encased in fibrous tissue that makes distention more difficult and more painful. This is logical and may be a valid assumption, but supporting evidence is not convincing.

Abnormal Uterine Bleeding

Abnormal uterine bleeding is often associated with endometriosis. It may be menorrhagia or metrorrhagia, or both. Scott and associates encountered abnormal bleeding in 26.6% of patients operated on primarily for endometriosis. In further study of these patients, some associated lesions were found that obviously explained the bleeding. This reduced the incidence of abnormal bleeding with no cause other than endometriosis to 14.4%. The menorrhagia and, in some instances, the metrorrhagia may result from ovarian dysfunction secondary to ovarian involvement. At laparotomy, one frequently finds old blood in the peritoneal cavity, and the intermenstrual spotting could be due to the escape of the chocolate contents of the ovarian cysts into the abdomen and out through the uterus by way of the tubes in an antegrade fashion. The prospective evaluation reported by Williams and Pratt found that among these consecutive patients, the frequency of menorrhagia was identical among those with and without endometriosis. Of patients treated by resection of endometriosis, 14% had menometrorrhagia; 12% of the control group had the symptoms. When hysterectomy was carried out as treatment, menorrhagia was present as a symptom in 42% of both those with and those without endometriosis. Therefore, the belief is that there is *no* increase in this symptom complex of menometrorrhagia among patients with endometriosis.

Infertility

Infertility is another common and important symptom in endometriosis. Among all couples, the infertility rate is generally estimated to be approximately 10%. With endometriosis, it is generally conceded that this rate is much higher. At the Johns Hopkins Hospital, the absolute sterility rate was 33.3% and the relative sterility rate was 46%. Counseller reported rates of 32.1% and 48.9%, respectively. Haydon reported a 53% relative infertility rate.

The cause of infertility may or may not be apparent. Clinical investigators believe that about 30% of patients with infertility have endometriosis as the only predominant cause. Tubal occlusion may occur, but most women with pelvic endometriosis have patent tubes unless peritubal adhesions have caused angulation and obstruction. Extensive destruction of ovarian tissue or replacement by endometrial cysts may interfere with ovulation, and extensive periovarian adhesions can prevent the normal egress of the ovum. In addition, the numerous pelvic adhesions probably interfere with ovum pickup and prevent the normal migration of the ovum from the ovary to the uterus through the tube.

Although impossible to prove, it seems likely that the hemolyzed peritoneal blood entering the tubal lumen could interfere with the action of the tubal epithelial cilia in propelling the ovum. Dyspareunia is known to limit sexual exposure. These theories aside, however, there still are many instances in which minimal endometriosis appears to cause infertility without any apparent mechanical or endocrine abnormality. Conversely, endometriosis does not preclude pregnancy. Many women with endometriosis have had several pregnancies. Prostaglandins have been implicated in this relationship between endometriosis and infertility. Rock and associates, however, found no significant difference in either the amount of peritoneal fluid present or in the concentration of prostaglandins with or without endometriosis. At this point, the question and its significance remain unresolved.

Kaunitz and Di Sant'Agnese considered the possibility of a relationship between unruptured luteinized follicles and endometriosis and infertility. They thought that with the unruptured follicle, progesterone levels were lower, and they suggested that higher levels would kill endometrial cells. The net result of unruptured follicles would then be low levels of progestational hormones; hence, endometriosis and the subsequent decrease in fertility would be present. Thus, the endometriosis would be the consequence of the ovulation defect and its resultant infertility and not the cause of infertility.

DIAGNOSIS

The symptoms described should always suggest endometriosis, but any or most of them may be present with other pelvic conditions. There is *no* history sufficiently typical of endometriosis to justify the diagnosis on this basis alone, and a gynecologist operating without confirmatory pelvic findings will often find grossly normal pelvic organs.

If a cystic hemorrhagic nodule is visible at the umbilicus, in an abdominal scar, in the perineum, or in the vaginal vault, the diagnosis of endometriosis can be made with relative certainty, particularly if there is cyclicity to the signs and symptoms. In the usual case of intra-abdominal endometriosis, the diagnosis must be aided by bimanual examination. The finding of adherent adnexa during the menstrual years in a woman in whom venereal, tubercular, or other infection can be excluded with reasonable certainty should cause one to consider endometriosis. Shotty induration in the cul-de-sac, in the uterosacral ligaments, or on the posterior surface of an adherent retroposed uterus is the single most suggestive pelvic finding of endometriosis. These nodular areas are frequently tender, particularly just before menstruation. When these findings are coupled with an enlarged ovary or an adherent ovarian cyst, the diagnosis is almost a certainty, within the 85th percentile of accuracy. Carcinoma of the ovary can reproduce most of these findings, except that the nodules of metastatic carcinoma in the cul-de-sac usually are not tender, particularly if examined during the cyclic changes.

When the rectovaginal septum is involved, the pelvic and rectal findings may simulate carcinoma of the bowel or the induration and scarring of diverticulitis. With cancer, however, the rectal examination should suggest a mucosal component that is uncommon with endometriosis. In diverticulitis, the mass usually has a popcorn-like feeling, and the nodularity is less tender except during acute flare-up of the inflammation. At this time, induration is likely to be a significant finding along with a more diffuse tenderness and with evidence of peritoneal irritation. Bluish cysts in the posterior vaginal vault may be very helpful in deciding in favor of endometriosis (see Fig. 12–11). Moreover, they are in a readily accessible biopsy site for pathologic confirmation of the diagnosis. Histologic confirmation of the diagnosis is mandatory along with continued follow-up, since the rectovaginal septum is the second most common site of malignancy in endometriosis. If the rectal mucosa is involved, colon roentgenograms are helpful, and proctoscopy with biopsy of the lesion establishes the diagnosis.

There remains a group of women who have severe pelvic pain and other symptoms suggestive of endometriosis but who lack definitive pelvic findings on examination. If the cul-de-sac is free from adhesions, culdoscopy is a very helpful procedure, particularly in extremely obese women. Since the cul-de-sac, however, is often involved in endometriosis and since infertility is a symptom in many women with endometriosis, laparoscopy is a much more practical approach to the diagnosis of endometriosis. In the infertile patient and in the patient with severe pelvic pain and few, if any, findings on pelvic examination, ovarian endometriosis, peritubal adhesions, and endometriosis in the cul-de-sac can easily be seen and biopsy documentation obtained by the laparoscope. In some instances, small areas of endometriosis may be fulgurated through the laparoscope. Women with minimal degrees of symptomatic endometriosis can then be differentiated from those whose symptoms are psychosomatic and in whom there is a complete absence of findings for organic disease.

Other noninvasive tests, such as computed tomography and ultrasound, have been recommended. Our experience has been that such tests are not helpful in making a diagnosis. They may document and record the size and position of such ovarian enlargements but cannot be definitive. Figure 12–21 shows a scan from the patient in Figure 12–9.

STAGING

One of the difficulties in the management of endometriosis is the evaluation of various treatments. The protean nature of the condition not only in symptoms but also in extent of disease complicates the selection of appropriate therapy.

In an attempt to simplify and organize the different classifications of endometriosis, the American Fertility Society devised a staging form that grades the extent of the disease into mild, moderate, and severe (Fig. 12–22). This form can be filled out easily at the time of surgery, and point scores can be ap-

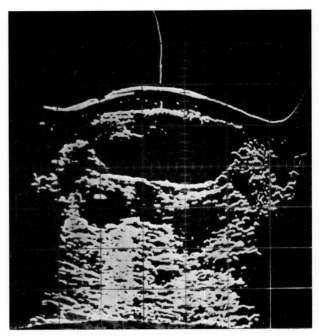

FIG. 12–21 Ultrasound study in patient with pelvic masses (same patient as in Fig. 12–9). Although echoes are seen within ovarian cysts and may be from clotted blood, malignancy cannot be excluded.

plied to different areas and amounts of endometriosis. Although the areas and numerical equivalents have been arbitrarily stated, they can serve as a guide and can be revised in the future as more information becomes available. On the basis of such accurate data, prospective information can be obtained and the true relationship of endometriosis to infertility can be assessed.

The pelvic organs should be inspected in a routine fashion so that all areas are evaluated in the same way each time. Point scores are assigned based on the numbers of lesions and bilaterality. The uterine implants are considered peritoneal. The size of lesions and organs of involvement are weighed to determine the severity and, hence, the stage of disease. It is recommended that a standardized approach and staging be used so that data on different therapeutic approaches and successes can be compared.

TREATMENT

Since endometriosis is generally a benign process that becomes quiescent with the menopause, its presence is not necessarily an indication for surgery. The need for treatment depends on the severity and type of symptoms, the extent of the disease,

Patient's name _____

Stage I   (Mild)   1–5
Stage II   (Moderate)   6–15
Stage III (Severe)   16–30
Stage IV   (Extensive)   31–54

Total _____

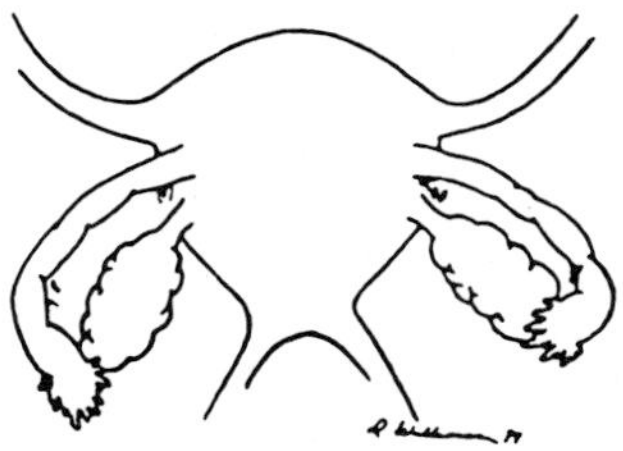

			< 1 cm	1–3 cm	> 3 cm
PERITONEUM	ENDOMETRIOSIS		< 1 cm	1–3 cm	> 3 cm
			1	2	3
	ADHESIONS		filmy	dense w/partial cul-de-sac obliteration	dense w/complete cul-de-sac obliteration
			1	2	3
OVARY	ENDOMETRIOSIS		< 1 cm	1–3 cm	> 3 cm or ruptured endometrioma
		R	2	4	6
		L	2	4	6
	ADHESIONS		filmy	dense w/partial ovarian enclosure	dense w/complete ovarian enclosure
		R	2	4	6
		L	2	4	6
TUBE	ENDOMETRIOSIS		< 1 cm	> 1 cm	tubal occlusion
		R	2	4	6
		L	2	4	6
	ADHESIONS		filmy	dense w/tubal distortion	dense w/tubal enclosure
		R	2	4	6
		L	2	4	6

FIG. 12–22 American Fertility Society classification of endometriosis. (From the American Fertility Society: Classification of Endometriosis. Fertil Steril 32:633, 1979. Reproduced with permission of the publisher, The American Fertility Society.)

the age and the general physical condition of the patient, the patient's desire to preserve childbearing function, the psychological evaluation of the patient, and the presence or absence of other disease in the reproductive tract. In the absence of palpable pelvic disease, particularly in the adnexal area, exploratory celiotomy on the basis of symptoms alone is rarely required. Moderately extensive but asymptomatic endometriosis may not require treatment, provided that the diagnosis is certain.

Four courses are available for the management of endometriosis: observation, hormonal therapy, surgery, and irradiation.

Observation

In the absence of any significant symptoms and in the absence of an adnexal mass that might suggest an ovarian neoplasm, observation is the treatment of choice for endometriosis. Analgesics can be used satisfactorily to control dysmenorrhea and pelvic discomfort. If infertility is an important factor, active treatment is sometimes indicated. Garcia and David, however, recorded that even among patients with infertility and mild to moderate degrees of endometriosis, a relatively high percentage were able to conceive without operative intervention.

Hormonal Therapy

Suppression of ovulation and menstruation, either by pregnancy or by the use of exogenous hormones, has been observed to alleviate symptoms and at times to bring about clinical improvement. Estrogens, progestogens, and androgens have been used. Danazol (Danocrine), an antigonadotropin and a derivative of a 17α-ethinyl testosterone, has also been shown to be effective in the treatment of endometriosis.

Hormonal therapy has been used rather extensively. Estrogens were the first endocrine preparations used. Estrogens in sufficient doses both inhibit ovulation and suppress menstruation. They do not induce a pseudopregnancy state, at least from the histologic aspect of the endometrium. If estrogens are used, diethylstilbestrol is the drug of choice. Karnaky recommended starting at 0.5 g daily for 3 days and then increasing the dose rather rapidly to suppress breakthrough bleeding. Frequently, doses of 100 mg daily are reached, ultimately to produce a period of amenorrhea for a total time of 3 to 6 months. General experience has shown this method of treatment to be unsatisfactory. The diethylstilbestrol causes nausea and, frequently, severe bleeding. Furthermore, it appears to effect at best only temporary symptomatic relief and is not in any sense a cure. The areas of ectopic endometrium not only do not regress but also may frequently show areas of cystic hyperplasia, as one would expect. In general, this form of therapy is rarely used and has few advocates.

Androgens, usually oral methyltestosterone, also may be used to treat endometriosis. When sublingual doses of 10 mg daily are used, ovulation and menstruation can be suppressed, but mild hirsutism may occur when the monthly dose reaches or exceeds 300 mg. Patients usually are not treated for more than 3 to 6 months because of the potential, if not actual, virilizing effects of this hormone. Another dosage schedule of 5 mg daily for up to 6 months may be efficacious. At this dosage level, there is usually menstruation and sometimes ovulation. Pelvic pain has been relieved at least temporarily, Hammond and associates reporting 75% success but with subsequent recurrence. Pregnancies can occur after such therapy, but usually additional surgical treatment is required. Histologically, the endometriosis appears to be unaffected, and the mechanism whereby this form of treatment achieves its results is not clear. Although androgens appear to achieve short-term palliation, one cannot use them for prolonged therapy, and hence this form of therapy has definite limitations.

The most popular form of hormonal treatment has been the use of the progestational agents. These synthetic progesterone-like steroids are frequently combined with an estrogen, such as mestranol or ethinyl estradiol. Some are given parenterally (hydroxyprogesterone caproate and medroxyprogesterone acetate), but most are taken orally, the most frequently used being norethynodrel and norethindrone.

Any of the currently used contraceptive pills combining a progesterone and an estrogen may be used to suppress ovulation and produce amenorrhea. The preparation selected should be started at a minimal dosage, doubled at the end of 4 weeks, and increased thereafter by one pill monthly (or weekly, if necessary) for at least 12 months, not only to suppress ovulation but also to suppress breakthrough bleeding until amenorrhea and anovulation have been achieved. In fact, dosage may be continued for 2 or 3 years, if need be. In addition to amenorrhea and anovulation, a pseudopregnancy stage with decidual reaction involving the uterine endometrium and the ectopic endometrium can be achieved. In 110 patients, Kistner reported an improvement rate of 83%, with remissions as long as 52 months and a 47% pregnancy rate in those trying to conceive. Despite these impressive results, en-

dometrial implants often become active after the cessation of the pseudopregnancy. The patients to be treated by progestogens must be selected carefully, and permanent cure should not be expected. The prime indication for this mode of treatment appears to be symptomatic endometriosis recurrent after surgery.

About 15% of users of these hormones discontinue the medication because of the side effects, which are usually those of early pregnancy. Another 15% or more of patients have an initial response level and then an apparent loss of effect. Overall, about a 50% success rate with progestational components seems to be a reasonable expectation in alleviation of symptoms or in allowing subsequent pregnancy. Moghissi and Boyce reported a 90% pregnancy success rate with this type of treatment when other factors were excluded.

Danazol is expensive and has a high incidence of side effects. Barbieri and associates quoted an 85% incidence; they also recorded a 46% pregnancy rate and 33% recurrence. Greenblatt thought the side effects were less significant, but the pregnancy rate was lower (30%) and the recurrence rate was identical. Currently, danazol seems to be the medication of choice when there is moderate disease and surgery is not required.

Hormonal therapy does not appear to be indicated in women having adnexal masses, since no one can be certain that the adnexal masses are, indeed, endometriosis rather than ovarian malignancies. Further, hormonal therapy will not cause an established endometrial cyst to regress. Since all forms of hormonal therapy, with the exception of low-dose testosterone therapy, inhibit ovulation during the course of therapy, this form of treatment delays the desired result of pregnancy. Neither estrogen nor progestin therapy is indicated in older women who have a limited time remaining to achieve pregnancy. Such hormonal manipulation, however, seems particularly useful in women approaching the menopause. In them, temporizations can be obtained in anticipation of spontaneous improvement with menopause. A summary of results of hormonal therapy in the treatment of infertile patients with endometriosis is given in Table 12–2.

Surgery

An operation may be considered conservative when the reproductive potential is retained, semiconservative when the reproductive ability is eliminated but ovarian function is retained, and radical or definitive when ovarian function is ablated along with the uterus, which is the source of the endometriosis.

Surgery is still considered the best form of therapy in most cases of symptomatic endometriosis. Defin-

TABLE 12-2 *Pregnancy of Patients with Endometriosis After Hormonal Therapy*

HORMONAL AGENT	REFERENCE (YEAR)	INFERTILE PATIENTS	PATIENTS ACHIEVING PREGNANCY	RATE OF PREGNANCY (%)
Stilbestrol	Karnaky (1948)	37	5	14
	Haskins and Woolf (1955)	15	3	20
Total		52	8	15
Progestins	Riva, et al (1961)	83	4	5
	Kistner (1962)	38	18	47
	Kistner (1965)	22	11	50
	Williams (1967)	11	8	73
	Andrews and Larsen (1974)	31	8	26
Total		185	49	26
Methyltestosterone	Hirst (1947)	19	2	11
	Creadick (1950)	25	5	20
	Preston and Campbell (1953)	80	48	60
	Katayama, et al (1976)	64	12	19
Total		188	67	36
Danazol	Friedlander (1973)	22	9	41
	Greenblatt, et al (1974)	21	9	43
Total		43	18	42

From Katayama KP, Manuel M, Jones HW Jr, et al: Methyltestosterone treatment of infertility associated with pelvic endometriosis. Fertil Steril 27:83, 1976. Reproduced with permission of the publisher, The American Fertility Society.

itive treatment consisting of abdominal hysterectomy and bilateral salpingo-oophorectomy is preferred in women with extensive endometriosis involving the pelvic structures and both ovaries, particularly if the patient is over 40 years of age and past the reproductive years. As pointed out by Garcia and Mastroianni, there is little place for "geriatric" infertility surgery in the woman over 40 years of age. When infertility surgery is planned because of endometriosis, a complete infertility evaluation is required preoperatively for both partners, and the risks, benefits, and alternatives must be thoroughly discussed. Unfortunately, there are younger women, a few in their twenties, whose ovaries have been so destroyed by endometriosis that little or no functional ovarian tissue can be salvaged. They must be subjected to the same procedure, and so must patients who require a second laparotomy for recurrent endometriosis. The removal of all ovarian tissue is curative. One should not hesitate to use estrogens for menopausal symptoms in younger women after such procedures. Theoretically, estrogens can reactivate endometriosis, but the occurrence has been less than 5% in the reported cases. The variation in the estrogen receptors found in endometriosis could explain this discrepancy.

CONSERVATIVE SURGERY. Many women with endometriosis are quite young and want to retain their ability to reproduce or, when infertility is a problem, to enhance fertility. In the latter situation, a thorough infertility study must be done to exclude other causes before the lack of pregnancy is attributed to endometriosis alone. When this has been done, or when there are other symptoms of endometriosis sufficient to require treatment, conservative surgery is advised. This generally consists of a celiotomy with the intent of destroying by resection or fulguration all areas of endometriosis. Large endometrial implants or endometrial cysts of the ovaries are managed by resection. The smaller superficial implants may be fulgurated, and the many adhesions characteristic of endometriosis, involving the cul-de-sac, posterior surface of the uterus, and adnexa, are lysed and excised. It is particularly important in problems of infertility to release any peritubal and periovarian adhesions that might interfere with ovum transport. To prevent the uterus from becoming readherent on the cul-de-sac, uterine suspension is performed, and frequently an ovarian suspension as well (Fig. 12-23). Optical augmentation by loupes or the operating microscope enables one to find areas of endometriosis that might otherwise escape detection.

An important step in these conservative procedures is a presacral neurectomy. This should be done in all cases in which dysmenorrhea is present and perhaps in all instances of infertility, for should further endometriosis develop, this procedure may prevent it from becoming symptomatic. Prevention

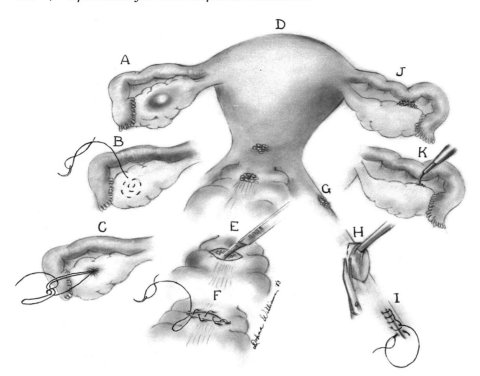

FIG. 12–23 Conservative surgery for endometriosis. Endometrioma of ovary (*A*) with excision and purse string concentric closure of defect (*B* and *C*). Posterior uterus and cul-de-sac endometriosis (*D*) with excision (*E*) and inverting baseball stitch closure of serosa (*F*). Uterosacral endometrium (*G*) with sharp dissection (*H*) and continuous lock suture closure (*I*). Tubo-ovarian endometriosis (*J*) with microcautery excision and destruction (*K*).

of dyspareunia by such procedures may reduce abstinence and increase chances for pregnancy. Data on this possibility, however, are inconclusive, so that presacral neurectomy appears to be indicated only for relief of pain.

Figure 12–24 shows the anatomy of the presacral dissection. After the bowel is packed well into the upper abdomen, the rectosigmoid is drawn to the left. A midline incision is made in the posterior parietal peritoneum beginning from a point in the hollow of the sacrum opposite the third or fourth sacral vertebra to a point 1 cm or 2 cm above the bifurcation of the aorta. The retroperitoneal exposure is made by placing stay sutures on the edges of the peritoneum or by holding the edges apart with Allis clamps. Usually, exposure of the right ureter and the inferior mesenteric vessels is accomplished easily. Beginning above the bifurcation of the aorta, usually a single nerve trunk network can be seen as it passes over the bifurcation and divides into right and left nerve bundles. The nerve trunk should be transected completely from the lower end of the aorta and the proximal portion of the common iliac vessels. The proximal, cephalic end of the nerve bundle should be ligated, but the distal pelvic end of the nerve trunk should be retracted with firm tension and the entire plexus with its left and right nerve trunks should be dissected thoroughly from the presacral region. By careful re-traction of the sigmoid mesentery and the inferior mesenteric vessels by means of a narrow Deaver retractor, the entire plexus can be visualized with the left and right pelvic ureters serving as the lateral margins of the dissection. The blunt dissection is continued along the medial aspect of the right ureter, with removal of all retroperitoneal connective tissue and nerve fibers from the presacral space to the region of the medial aspect of the left ureter. The nerve bundles are transected at the level of the third sacral vertebra, and the distal ends are ligated. Blunt dissection is best for this and minimizes bleeding. Two distinct layers of nerve-connective tissue are usually recognized during the dissection. The upper layer must be dissected free from the peritoneum, and the deeper layer, which contains the main nerve trunks, is dissected from the vessels and the presacral ligament. Bleeding must be meticulously controlled by fine ties or electrocautery. The operator must avoid injury to the inferior mesenteric artery and its superior hemorrhoidal branch. Protection can be accomplished best by retracting the vessels within the sigmoid mesentery away from the operating field. The middle sacral artery, which is closely attached to the bony structures, emerging onto the sacrum from beneath the left common iliac vein, usually escapes injury with careful blunt dissection. In order to avoid injury, the middle sacral artery and vein can be ligated

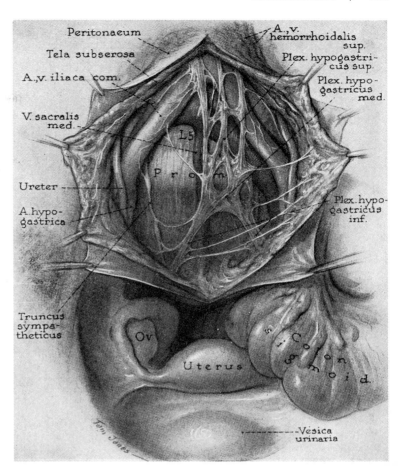

FIG. 12–24 Presacral nerves, in relation to peritoneal tissues. Anterior view of pelvis. Removal of the peritoneum and the retroperitoneal tissues, demonstrating the relation of the more prominent autonomic nerves to the pelvic anatomy. (Curtis AH, Anson BJ, Ashley FL, et al: The anatomy of the pelvic autonomic nerves in relation to gynecology. Surg Gynecol Obstet 75:743, 1942.)

initially or clipped with small vascular clips either before the presacral space is dissected or as soon as these vessels come into operative view during the procedure. If they should be injured, usually bleeding can be controlled easily by exerting firm pressure directly against the adjacent bony structures and secondarily occluding them with small vascular clips. On rare occasions, it may be necessary to place Gelfoam or microfibrillar collagen (Avitene) in the retroperitoneal space to control oozing. This carries the risk of continued bleeding, and a pelvic hematoma may occur. After removal of the connective tissue and the nerve tissue, hemostasis is assured and the peritoneal margins are approximated with a continuous suture of nonreactive material such as polyglactin.

If low back pain is the predominant symptom, it is advisable to include a resection of the uterosacral ligaments and Frankenhauser's plexus as a part of the operative procedure. This is done by grasping each uterosacral ligament as it emerges from the posterior aspect of the lower uterine segment, with a Babcock or an Allis clamp. Care should be taken to identify the lower portion of the pelvic ureter, which should be lateral to the uterosacral ligament but can be dangerously close to it when pelvic endometriosis has involved the cul-de-sac. The ligament should be divided completely with resection of approximately 0.5 cm to 1 cm. The free ends are ligated with permanent suture but are not approximated, in order to avoid regeneration of nerve fibers. The sacral portion of the uterosacral ligament may be sutured to the posterior surface of the cervix to avoid retrodisplacement of the uterus following surgery. However, in most instances the shortened ligaments cannot be made to reach the cervix and are left to retract beneath the pelvic peritoneum. The operative defect is then closed by approximating the cul-de-sac peritoneum to the back of the cervix, taking particular care to avoid damage to the adjacent pelvic ureter. The success of this procedure is related to the amount of nerve fiber that is removed in the resected uterosacral ligament; therefore, the procedure should be thorough, even if the resected ligament is not long enough to reapproximate to the posterior cervix for support of the uterus.

With conservative surgery, there is always the risk of recurrence of endometriosis. The risk, however, seems to be relatively small. Gray noted a 4% rate and Scott and Burt found a 2.7% rate, whereas McCoy and Bradford reported a 21% rate. In contrast, these authors reported pregnancy rates of 51%, 64.1%, and 63%, respectively. These figures are considerably better than those recorded with progestogen therapy. In general, an overall 40% to 50% pregnancy rate can be expected, as opposed to a 10% to 12% recurrence rate of endometriosis that is likely to require an additional operation. Studies by Buttram and others showed that the stage of the disease is correlated with the success rates of pregnancy from surgery. Surgery, since it can not only remove the endometriosis but also correct the mechanical problems caused by it, remains the logical choice in the treatment of infertility, particularly as the patient's age increases. For a very young patient, a trial of medical management may be appropriate. In a 30-year-old woman, such an attempt may waste valuable time.

Some women with symptomatic endometriosis are in a category between those treated conservatively and those requiring a complete and definitive procedure. These women, usually in their middle to late thirties, have completed their childbearing but want to avoid premature menopause. In these women, Cashman's concept of removal of the uterus and other areas of pelvic endometriosis with preservation of some ovarian tissue has much to recommend it. Such a procedure may seem illogical, since the retention of ovarian function might permit continued activity and, therefore, symptoms from any residual endometriosis. This problem, however, arises infrequently, as shown by Scott and associates, who found that only 4.1% of such patients later required further surgery. This concept is further supported by the data of Williams and Pratt, which showed that subsequent surgery for endometriosis was required in 6%. In comparison, the figures were 16% in patients having resection only and 0% in those with complete operations. Hammond and associates, however, found need for further surgery in 60% of patients.

DEFINITIVE SURGERY. Removal of the uterus eliminates not only dysmenorrhea but also any possible abnormal bleeding. In addition, it removes the main source of the ectopic endometrium. Endometrial implants themselves probably can spread to cause daughter implants, but spreading may not occur very often.

When endometriosis causes ureteral or bowel obstruction, release of the obstruction is essential, since the problem is mechanical and neither hormonal therapy nor castration relieves it. In fact, the fibrosis and scarring after castration may aggravate the obstruction. This accounts for the fact that bowel obstruction secondary to endometriosis may be encountered in the postmenopausal patient.

If the kidney has normal function, the ureter should be released from its adhesions. Scarring involving the ureteral wall usually shows evidence of proximal dilatation from obstruction. In such cases, the obstructed region must be resected, and a ureteroureteral anastomosis should be done to preserve kidney function. If the kidney has no function on the involved side and the other kidney has normal function, nephrectomy may be necessary. There is little excuse, however, for allowing endometriosis to progress to this extent. In instances of obstruction, total abdominal hysterotomy and bilateral salpingo-oophorectomy are recommended along with release or excision of the damaged ureter.

When there is extensive endometriotic involvement of the bowel wall, stenosis of the bowel lumen may occur. For this reason, obstructive lesions of the intestinal tract due to endometriosis, wherever they may occur, should be treated by resection and reestablishment of bowel continuity by an anastomosis. This treatment is appropriate when small bowel is involved and when the colon is compromised. When only the anterior wall of the rectosigmoid is extensively involved, a wedge resection of this segment of bowel with approximation of the normal bowel wall is sufficient to preserve and restore an adequate bowel lumen.

If the history or findings on physical examination suggest partial obstruction or endometriosis involving the bowel, preoperative roentgenographic and endoscopic examinations should be done. It is wise to plan early admission to the hospital for preoperative bowel preparation when findings suggest intestinal involvement with endometriosis. However, even if the surgeon is surprised at the time of operation, resection should be carried out as indicated. Careful surgical techniques minimize complications even in the absence of bowel preparation, and an incomplete operation should not be performed.

Other endometrial lesions involving the bladder wall, peritoneal surfaces, or rectovaginal septum may be removed and ovarian conservation practiced if justifiable. Endometriotic lesions involving abdominal or other scars of the umbilicus, the vulva, or the inguinal regions are infiltrating and should be excised by a wide margin so that no endometrial remnants are left to cause further problems.

It should be stressed that surgery for endometriosis can be very difficult. The adhesions may be extremely dense, often much more so than the usual inflammatory or postoperative type of scar. Sharp dissection is often necessary, especially in freeing the uterus from the anterior rectal wall. Fortunately, the rectal wall is often thickened by fibrosis so that perforation is rare. Nevertheless, in making the dissection, it is better to err by leaving a bit of uterine tissue on the rectum than by inadvertently perforating it.

Another point to be stressed is that resection of part of an ovary is worthwhile in young women. Generally, with other ovarian tumors, a complete oophorectomy is preferable to resection if the opposite ovary is normal. This dictum does not apply in endometriosis, in which bilateral ovarian involvement occurs in about 25% of the cases.

As mentioned earlier, optical augmentation helps identify areas of endometriosis requiring excision. In addition, more complete excision or destruction is possible with minimal trauma to adjacent tissues. Fine, nonreactive sutures, such as those made of polyglutanic and polyglycolic acids, are recommended. Catgut sutures have little place in conservative surgery on the pelvic organs.

Microcautery is a helpful adjunct to sharp surgical dissection and removal of areas of endometriosis. The CO_2 laser speeds the destruction of endometriosis by vaporization. Care is still essential, however, to protect other pelvic organs.

Kistner and others have used progestogen therapy before proposed exploration for endometriosis and also after conservative surgery. Preoperative hormonal therapy is thought to make the dissection easier and the implants easier to find and softer from the decidual reaction. Although our policy has been not to use this combined treatment preoperatively, it may be considered unless there is an ovarian mass or evidence of urinary or intestinal obstruction. Since the possibility always exists that the ovarian mass may be carcinoma rather than an endometrial cyst, exploration should not be delayed by attempts at hormonal manipulation. Also, such preoperative treatment may mask areas of endometriosis that might otherwise be found and excised; hence, an incomplete surgical procedure may result.

Ranney gave these reasons for not using preoperative progestational treatment: (1) Increased friability of tissues interferes with clear dissection, (2) increased bleeding increases blood loss and slows surgery, and (3) softening of tissues affects accurate palpation and delineation of the borders of the lesion.

Danazol given preoperatively may not have vascular and softening effects on tissues but may very well mask lesions. Batt and Naples found the conception rate to be lower and the stillbirth rate to be higher after preoperatively administered danazol. For preoperative medication as a routine, the disadvantages seem to outweigh the advantages.

Generally, we do not advocate hormonal therapy after conservative surgery, particularly in patients with infertility. Both the surgeon and the patient are usually concerned that she become pregnant as soon after surgery as reasonable, and we see no advantage in delaying this by progestogen-induced anovulation. As is true for tubal reconstructive surgery, conception is highest during the first 6 months after conservative surgery, before the reestablishment of peritubal adhesions. Indeed, the data by Andrews and Larsen and others show definitely that the pregnancy rate is less when surgery is combined with postoperatively administered hormones than when surgery alone is used. With danazol, however, as reported by Wheeler and Malinak, some improvement in the pregnancy rate does appear to take place. Among patients with severe endometriosis, the pregnancy rate was 30% when surgery alone was carried out and 79% when danazol was given postoperatively. Our policy with patients having severe endometriosis and conservative surgery has been to consider a 3-month course of danazol after the operation, particularly if there is concern about the completeness of the surgery. This approach has been recommended by Buttram.

Because of the significant concerns of infertile women with endometriosis, some patients request a second conservative operation for the condition. Schenken and Malinak found that only 12% of patients so managed were able to achieve pregnancy, and this has been our experience as well.

Irradiation

Castration by external irradiation treats endometriosis quite effectively. There are, however, very limited indications for this now rarely used method of treatment. One suitable circumstance is symptomatic endometriosis, recurrent after and proved by operation, in a patient who is too poor a medical risk for definitive surgical treatment. Another acceptable reason is continued symptoms despite complete surgery. In some cases, ovarian remnants may persist and be responsible for continued pain. When this situation persists even after appropriate reoperation for the residual ovary syndrome, radiation may be quite effective. This is particularly true when no pelvic masses can be found on roentgenography, ultrasound, or computed tomography scan and hormone assay supports the presence of functioning ovarian tissue.

MALIGNANCY IN ENDOMETRIOSIS

Ectopic endometrium may become malignant in rare instances but has no more, and perhaps less, proclivity to do so than endometrium within the uterine cavity.

In 1925, Sampson, in reporting seven cases of ovarian carcinoma of possible endometrial origin, outlined the criteria to establish such a diagnosis: (1) Benign and malignant tissues must coexist in the same ovary and have the same histologic relationship to each other as that in carcinoma of the body of the uterus. (2) The carcinoma must arise in the benign tissue and not invade it from some other source. (3) Additional supportive evidence includes the presence of tissue resembling endometrial stroma about characteristic epithelial glands and the finding of old hemorrhage rather than fresh.

Among 516 cases of endometriosis reported by Scott and associates, there were only 8 cases of ovarian malignancy. Three of these were papillary serous cystadenocarcinomas, two were epidermoid carcinomas arising in dermoid cysts, and one was a granulosa cell tumor. The remaining two cases were adenocarcinomas; in neither could the transition from benign endometriosis to carcinoma be shown, but the histologic features of each tumor suggested that it might be of endometrial origin. In 1957, Thompson collected 20 reported cases of ovarian malignancy arising in ovarian endometriosis. Most of these malignant tumors were adenocarcinoma (one was a carcinosarcoma). Thompson also reported 17 cases of ovarian adenoacanthoma, 7 of which definitely arose from endometriosis. Other, sporadic cases have been reported since that time, and it is thought that malignancy is an uncommon complication of endometriosis.

There have been many reports, however, of ovarian carcinomas with microscopic features of uterine endometrial carcinoma. These have been designated by the name *endometrioid carcinoma,* and they may or may not be associated with or originate from endometriosis. Although the World Health Organization histologic classification includes the category of endometrioid carcinoma, this does not presuppose that the tumors arise from endometriosis but is merely descriptive of the microscopic findings.

There are also very unusual instances of extraovarian malignancy arising in endometriosis in the rectovaginal septum. Dockerty and associates described two cases in 1954, and Lash and Rubenstone reported one case in 1959. The rectovaginal septum is the second most common site of malignancy arising from endometriosis. Even though a diagnosis of endometriosis is made, careful follow-up is required because of this association. Interestingly, the use of exogenous estrogens has been common among most of the reported cases of endometrial rectovaginal malignancy. Endometriosis in the rectovaginal septum may be a further relative contraindication to estrogen treatment.

It seems justifiable to conclude that endometriosis is capable of malignant change, but the incidence is extremely low and is of little significance in the clinical management of patients with this condition. Of greater clinical importance is the common finding of considerable enlargement of one or both ovaries in a patient with obvious endometriosis. The much more likely possibility of a coexisting ovarian malignancy unrelated to endometriosis must be considered, and exploratory celiotomy is then indicated even though the patient may have absolutely no symptoms.

Bibliography

Allen E: Endometrial transplantation. Am J Obstet Gynecol 23:343, 1932

Andrews WC, Larsen GD: Endometriosis: Treatment with hormonal pseudopregnancy and/or operation. Am J Obstet Gynecol 118:643, 1974

Barbieri RL, Evans S, Kistner RW: Danazol in the treatment of endometriosis: Analysis of 100 cases with a 4-year follow-up. Fertil Steril 37:737, 1982

Batt RE, Naples JD: Conservative surgery for endometriosis in the infertile couple. Curr Probl Obstet Gynecol 6:45, 1982

Benson RC, Sneeden VD: Adenomyosis: A reappraisal of symptomatology. Am J Obstet Gynecol 76:1044, 1958

Bergqvist A, Rannevik G, Thorell J: Estrogen and progesterone cytosol receptor concentration in endometriotic tissue and intrauterine endometrium. Acta Obstet Gynecol Scand (Suppl) 101:53, 1981

Buttram VC Jr: Conservative surgery for endometriosis in the infertile female: A study of 206 patients with implications for both medical and surgical therapy. Fertil Steril 31:117, 1979

Caffier P: Uber Endometriumexplantation: Bisherige Ergebnisse, Wachstumsmechanik und Kritik. Zentralbl Gynakol 52:63, 1928

Cashman BZ: Hysterectomy with preservation of ovarian tissue in the treatment of endometriosis. Am J Obstet Gynecol 49:484, 1945

Chatman DL: Endometriosis and the black woman. J Reprod Med 16:303, 1976

Chatman DL, Ward AB: Endometriosis in adolescents. J Reprod Med 27:156, 1982

Chatterjee SK: Scar endometriosis: A clinicopathologic study of 17 cases. Obstet Gynecol 56:81, 1980

Creadick RN: Non-surgical treatment of endometriosis: Preliminary report on use of methyl testosterone. N Carolina Med J 11:576, 1950

Cullen TS: Adeno-myoma of the round ligament. Johns Hopkins Hosp Bull 7:112, 1896

———: Adeno-myoma uteri diffusum benignum. Johns Hopkins Hosp Rep 6:133, 1897

————: Adenomyoma of the Uterus. Philadelphia, WB Saunders Company, 1908

————: Adenomyoma of rectovaginal septum. JAMA 62:835, 1914

————: The distribution of adenomyomas containing uterine mucosa. Arch Surg 1:215, 1920

Counseller VS: Surgical procedures involved in the treatment of endometriosis. Surg Gynecol Obstet 89:322, 1949

Curtis AH, Anson BJ, Ashley FL, et al: The anatomy of the pelvic autonomic nerves in relation to gynecology. Surg Gynecol Obstet 75:743, 1942

Dmowski WP, Cohen MR: Treatment of endometriosis with antigonadotropin, Danazol: A laparoscopic and histologic evaluation. Obstet Gynecol 46:147, 1975

Dockerty MB, Pratt JH, Decker DG: Primary adenocarcinoma of the rectovaginal septum probably arising from endometriosis: Report of two cases. Cancer 7:898, 1954

Ekwempu CC, Harrison KA: Endometriosis among the Hausa/Fulani population of Nigeria. Trop Geogr Med 31:201, 1979

Everett HS: Probable tubal origin of endometriosis. Am J Obstet Gynecol 22:1, 1931

Ferrari BT, Shollenbarger DR: Abdominal wall endometriosis following hypertonic saline abortion. JAMA 238:56, 1977

Foster DC, Stern JL, Buscema J, Rock JA, Woodruff JD: Pleural and parenchymal pulmonary endometriosis. Obstet Gynecol 58:552, 1981

Friedlander RL: The treatment of endometriosis with Danazol. J Reprod Med 10:197, 1973

Furman WR, Wang KP, Summer WR, Terry PB: Catamenial pneumothorax: Evaluation by fiberoptic pleuroscopy. Am Rev Respir Dis 121:137, 1980

García C-R, David SS: Pelvic endometriosis: Infertility and pelvic pain. Am J Obstet Gynecol 129:740, 1977

Garcia C-R, Mastroianni L Jr: Microsurgery for treatment of adnexal disease. Fertil Steril 34:413, 1980

Goodall JR: A Study of Endometriosis, Endosalpingiosis, Endocervicosis, and Peritoneo-Ovarian Sclerosis: A Clinical and Pathologic Study. Philadelphia, JB Lippincott, 1943

Goodman JD, Macchia RJ, Macasaet MA, Schneider M: Endometriosis of the urinary bladder: Sonographic findings. AJR 135:625, 1980

Granberg I, Willems JS: Endometriosis of lung and pleura diagnosed by aspiration biopsy. Acta Cytol 21:295, 1977

Gray LA: The management of endometriosis involving the bowel. Clin Obstet Gynecol 9:309, 1966

————: Endometriosis of the bowel: Role of bowel resection, superficial excision and oophorectomy in treatment. Ann Surg 177:580, 1973

Greenblatt RB (ed): Recent advances in endometriosis. Exerpta Medica International Congress Series No 368, 1975

Greenblatt RB, Tzingounis V: Danazol treatment of endometriosis: long-term follow-up. Fertil Steril 32:518, 1979

Halban J: Hysteroadenosis metastatica (die lymphogene Genese der sog. Adenofibromatosis heterotopica). Wien Klin Wochenschr 37:1205, 1924

Hammond MG, Hammond CB, Parker RT: Conservative treatment of endometriosis externa: The effects of methyltestosterone therapy. Fertil Steril 29:651, 1978

Harbitz HF: Clinical pathogenetic and experimental investigation of endometriosis especially regarding the localisation in the abdominal wall (laparotomy scars) with a contribution to the study of experimental transplantation of endometrium. Acta Chir Scand 74 Suppl 30:1, 1934

Haskins AL, Woolf RB: Stilbestrol-induced hyperhormonal amenorrhea for the treatment of pelvic endometriosis. Obstet Gynecol 5:113, 1955

Haydon GB: A study of 569 cases of endometriosis. Am J Obstet Gynecol 43:704, 1942

Heim K: Ergebnisse. Ber Gesamte Gynakol 17:641, 1930

Heneghan MA, Teixidor HS: Pleuroperitoneal endometriosis. AJR 133:727, 1979

Hirsch EF, Jones HO: The behavior of the epithelium in explants of human endometrium. Am J Obstet Gynecol 25:37, 1933

Hirst JC: Conservative treatment and therapeutic test of endometriosis by androgens. Am J Obstet Gynecol 53:483, 1947

Hobbs JE, Bortnick AR: Endometriosis of the lungs: An experimental and clinical study. Am J Obstet Gynecol 40:832, 1940

Irani S, Atkinson L, Cabaniss C, Danovitch SH: Pleuroperitoneal endometriosis. Obstet Gynecol 47 (Suppl 1):72, 1976

Iwanoff NS: Drüsiges cystenhaltiges uterusfibromyom complicirt durch sarcom und carcinom (adenofibromyoma cysticum sarcomatodes carcinomatosum). Monatsschr Geburtsh Gynak 7:295, 1898

Jacobson VC: The autotransplantation of endometrial tissue in the rabbit. Arch Surg 5:281, 1922

Jacobson VC: Intraperitoneal transplantation of endometrial tissue. Arch Pathol Lab Med 1:169, 1926

Jänne O, Kauppila A, Kokko E, et al: Estrogen and progestin receptors in endometriosis lesions: Comparison with endometrial tissue. Am J Obstet Gynecol 141:562, 1981

Javert CT: Observations on pathology and spread of endometriosis based on theory of benign metastasis. Am J Obstet Gynecol 62:477, 1951

Karnaky KJ: The use of stilbestrol for endometriosis: Preliminary report. South Med J 41:1109, 1948

Katayama KP, Manuel M, Jones HW Jr, et al: Methyltestosterone treatment of infertility associated with pelvic endometriosis. Fertil Steril 27:83, 1976

Kaunitz A, Di Sant'Agnese PA: Needle tract endometriosis: An unusual complication of amniocentesis. Obstet Gynecol 54:753, 1979

Keettel WC, Stein RJ: The viability of the cast-off menstrual endometrium. Am J Obstet Gynecol 61:440, 1951

King WLM: Metastatic endometriosis in abdominal scars. Can J Surg 22:579, 1979

Kistner RW: Conservative treatment of endometriosis. New Physician 11, 259, 1962

Kistner RW: The effects of new synthetic progestogens on endometriosis in the human female. Fertil Steril 16:61, 1965

Kistner RW: Current status of the hormonal treatment of endometriosis. Clin Obstet Gynecol 9:271, 1966

Koninckx PR, Ide P, Vandenbroucke W, et al: New aspects of the pathophysiology of endometriosis and associated infertility. J Reprod Med 24:257, 1980

Langmade CF: Pelvic endometriosis and ureteral obstruction. Am J Obstet Gynecol 122:463, 1975

Lash SR, Rubenstone AI: Adenocarcinoma of the rectovaginal septum probably arising from endometriosis. Am J Obstet Gynecol 78:299, 1959

Long ME, Taylor HC, Jr: Endometrioid carcinoma of the ovary. Am J Obstet Gynecol 90:936, 1964

Madsen H, Hansen P, Andersen OP: Endometrioid carcinoma in an operation scar. Acta Obstet Gynecol Scand 59:475, 1980

Markee JE: Menstruation in intraocular endometrial transplants in the rhesus monkey. In Contributions of Embryology, No 177. Washington, DC, Carnegie Institution of Washington (Publication No. 518), 1940 p 221

Maslow LA, Learner A: Endometriosis of kidney. J Urol 64:564, 1950

Mathur BB, Shah BS, Bhende YM: Adenomyosis uteri: A pathologic study of 290 cases. Am J Obstet Gynecol 84:1820, 1962

McArthur JW, Ulfelder H: The effect of pregnancy upon endometriosis. Obstet Gynecol Surv 20:709, 1965

McCoy JB, Bradford WZ: Surgical treatment of endometriosis with conservation of reproductive potential. Am J Obstet Gynecol 87:394, 1963

Meigs JV: Endometriosis: Etiologic role of marriage age and parity; conservative treatment. Obstet Gynecol 2:46, 1953

Merrill JA: Endometrial induction of endometriosis across Millipore filters. Am J Obstet Gynecol 94:780, 1966

Meyer R: Ueber eine adenomatöse Wucherung der Serosa in einer Bauchnarbe. Ztschr Geburtsh Gynakol 49:32, 1903

Meyer R: Uber entzündliche heterotope epithelwucherungen im weiblichen genitalgebiete und über eine bis in die wurzel des mesocolon ausgedehnte benigne wuocherung des darmepithels. Virchows Arch Pathol Anat 195:487, 1909

Miyazawa K: Incidence of endometriosis among Japanese women. Obstet Gynecol 48:407, 1976

Moghissi KS, Boyce CR: Management of endometriosis with oral medroxyprogesterone acetate. Obstet Gynecol 47:265, 1976

Novak E: The significance of uterine mucosa in the fallopian tube, with a discussion of the origin of aberrant endometrium. Am J Obstet Gynecol 12:484, 1926

Novak E: Gynecological and Obstetrical Pathology: With Clinical and Endocrine Relations. Philadelphia, WB Saunders Company, 1940

Novak E: Adenoacanthoma of ovary arising from endometrial cyst: With report of a case. J Mt Sinai Hosp 14:529, 1947

Paull T, Tedeschi LG: Perineal endometriosis at the site of episiotomy scar. Obstet Gynecol 40:28, 1972

Pellegrini VD Jr, Pasternak HS, Macaulay WP: Endometrioma of the pubis: A differential in the diagnosis of hip pain; a report of two cases. J Bone Joint Surg (Am) 63:1333, 1981

Preston SN, Campbell HB: Pelvic endometriosis: Treatment with methyl testosterone. Obstet Gynecol 2:152, 1953

Punnonen R, Klemi P, Nikkanen V: Recurrent endometriosis. Gynecol Obstet Invest 11:307, 1980

Ranney B: The prevention, inhibition, palliation, and treatment of endometriosis. Am J Obstet Gynecol 123:778, 1975

Ridley JH: The histogenesis of endometriosis: A review of facts and fancies. Obstet Gynecol Surv 23:1, 1968

Ridley JH, Edwards IK: Experimental endometriosis in the human. Am J Obstet Gynecol 76:783, 1958

Riva HL, Wilson JH, Kawasaki DM: Effect of norethynodrel on endometriosis. Am J Obstet Gynecol 82:109, 1961

Rock JA, Dubin NH, Ghodgaonkar RB, et al: Cul-de-sac fluid in women with endometriosis: Fluid volume and prostanoid concentration during the proliferative phase of the cycle—days 8 to 12. Fertil Steril 37:747, 1982

Russell WW: Aberrant portions of the Müllerian duct found in an ovary. Johns Hopkins Hosp Bull 10:8, 1899

Sampson JA: Perforating hemorrhagic (chocolate) cysts of the ovary: Their importance and especially their relation to pelvic adenomas of endometrial type ("adenomyoma" of the uterus, rectovaginal septum, sigmoid, etc.). Arch Surg 3:245, 1921

Sampson JA: The life history of ovarian hematomas (hemorrhagic cysts) of endometrial (Müllerian) type. Am J Obstet Gynecol 4:451, 1922

Sampson JA: Endometrial carcinoma of the ovary, arising in endometrial tissue of that organ. Arch Surg 10:1, 1925

Sampson JA: Peritoneal endometriosis due to menstrual dissemination of endometrial tissue into peritoneal cavity. Am J Obstet Gynecol 14:422, 1927

Sampson JA: Endometriosis following salpingectomy. Am J Obstet Gynecol 16:461, 1928

Sampson JA: The development of the implantation theory for the origin of peritoneal endometriosis. Am J Obstet Gynecol 40:549, 1940

Schenken RS, Malinak LR: Reoperation after initial treatment of endometriosis with conservative surgery. Am J Obstet Gynecol 131:416, 1978

Schneider V, Smith MJV, Frable WJ: Urinary cytology in endometriosis of the bladder. Acta Cytol 24:30, 1980

Scott RB, Burt JH: Clinical experimental endometriosis: Fifteen years experience at University Hospitals of Cleveland. South Med J 55:129, 1962

Scott RB, Te Linde RW: External Endometriosis—the scourge of the private patient. Ann Surg 131:697, 1950

Scott RB, Te Linde RW, Wharton LR, Jr: Further studies on experimental endometriosis. Am J Obstet Gynecol 66:1082, 1953

Scott RB, Wharton LR, Jr: The effects of excessive amounts of diethylstilbestrol on experimental endometriosis in monkeys. Am J Obstet Gynecol 69:573, 1955

————: The effect of testosterone on experimental endometriosis in rhesus monkeys. Am J Obstet Gynecol 78:1020, 1959

————: Effects of progesterone and norethindrone on experimental endometriosis in monkeys. Am J Obstet Gynecol 84:867, 1962

Stanley KE Jr, Utz DC, Dockerty MB: Clinically significant endometriosis of the urinary tract. Surg Gynecol Obstet 120:491, 1965

Strasser EJ, Davis RM: Extraperitoneal inguinal endometriosis. Am Surg 43:421, 1977

Sturgis SH, Call BJ: Endometriosis peritonei: Relationship of pain to functional activity. Am J Obstet Gynecol 68:1421, 1954

Sully L: Endometrioma of the perineum associated with episiotomy scars. Scott Med J 22:307, 1977

Te Linde RW, Scott RB: Experimental endometriosis. Am J Obstet Gynecol 60:1147, 1950

Thompson JD: Primary ovarian adenoacanthoma: Its relationship to endometriosis. Obstet Gynecol 9:403, 1957

Traut HF: Adult human endometrium in tissue culture. Surg Gynecol Obstet 47:334, 1928

Von Recklinghausen FD: Die Adenomyome und Cystadenome der Uterus- und Tubenwandung: Ihre Abkunft von Resten des Wolff' schen Körpers. Berlin, August Hirschwald, 1896

Weinstein BB, Weed JC, Collins CG, et al: The effect of diethylstilbestrol diproprionate on endometrial transplants. Endocrinology 27:903, 1940

Wespi HJ, Kletzhändler M: Uber Narbenendometriosen. Mschr Geburtsh Gynakol 111:169, 1940

Wheeler JM, Malinak LR: Postoperative Danazol therapy in infertility patients with severe endometriosis. Fertil Steril 36:460, 1981

Williams BFP: Conservative management of endometriosis: follow-up observations of progestin therapy. Obstet Gynecol 30:76, 1967

Williams HE, Barsky S, Storino W: Umbilical endometrioma (silent type). Arch Dermatol 112:1435, 1976

Williams TJ: The role of surgery in the management of endometriosis. Mayo Clin Proc 50:198, 1975

Williams TJ, Pratt JH: Endometriosis in 1,000 consecutive celiotomies: Incidence and management. Am J Obstet Gynecol 129:245, 1977

Wryens RG, Randall LM: Endometriosis in postoperative scars. Proc Staff Meet Mayo Clin 16:817, 1941

Chapter 13

Pelvic Inflammatory Disease

Until the mid-nineteenth century, there was little knowledge of the pathology of infections within the pelvis. Recamier, a French gynecologist, was the first to practice vaginal drainage of pelvic abscess between 1830 and 1840. The practice was picked up by Wells and Savage of England and by Sims and Emmett in the United States. Lawson Tait performed the first abdominal removal of a tubo-ovarian abscess in 1872. After this, evidence accumulated rapidly that the pelvic abscess was primarily an infection in the fallopian tube. The etiology and pathogenesis of various forms of pelvic infection evolved gradually. The organism responsible for gonococcal infection was discovered by Neisser in 1879. In 1886, Westermark demonstrated *Neisseria gonorrhoeae* organisms in exudate from the tube. In 1894, Westheim demonstrated these organisms invading tubal tissues. In 1921, Curtis isolated Neisseria organisms from the endometrium and the tubes. And in 1946, Falk demonstrated that access of the organism to the fallopian tube could be prevented by cornual resection of the tube. Since the beginning of the antibiotic era in 1942 with the discovery of penicillin, studies of pelvic infections have concentrated on microbial etiology, effective antimicrobial therapy, the indications for surgery, identification of asymptomatic carriers, and the importance of the control of pelvic infections to the public's health.

It is estimated that 500,000 to 700,000 women are treated each year in the United States for acute salpingitis. Gonorrhea is the most commonly reported communicable disease in this country. In the last two decades, teenagers have participated in the sexual revolution in increasing numbers, beginning at a younger and younger age. In 1981, over 250,000 cases of gonorrhea were reported among U.S. teenagers. The actual number of infections is probably at least double the number reported; thus, an estimated one-half million cases of gonorrhea occur in teenagers each year. According to projections by the Centers for Disease Control, approximately 1 of every 61 female teenagers contracted gonorrhea in 1983. Evidence suggests that the number of new cases reported has leveled off in the past few years. However, the continued high incidence of gonorrhea, especially among teenagers, means that American gynecologists will continue to see the significant morbidity associated with the late sequelae of this disease for many years to come. Approximately 15% of women with untreated endocervical gonorrhea will develop salpingitis. Almost 250,000 women, accounting for as many as one-fifth of the gynecologic admissions to some large public hospitals, are admitted with acute salpingitis, tubo-ovarian abscess, or pelvic abscess. Approximately 115,000 operations are done each year for pelvic inflammatory disease. Although mortality is low, considerable morbidity is experienced by these patients. After salpingitis, the risk for ectopic pregnancy may be increased tenfold. The risk of infertility is also increased. Salpingitis is responsible for 20% or more of all infertility cases. In addition to gonorrhea, salpingitis resulting from the use of intrauterine devices and from legal pregnancy terminations has increased.

Etiology, Terminology, and Grading of Pelvic Inflammatory Disease

TYPES OF PELVIC INFECTION

Sexually transmitted infections. Agents include:

Neisseria gonorrhoeae
Chlamydia trachomatis
Urea urealyticum, mycoplasma hominis, and other mycoplasma
Actinomycosis
Other aerobic and anaerobic bacteria
Other nonbacterial agents

Infections caused by the introduction of foreign material into the uterus. Etiologies include:

Intrauterine device use
Hysterosalpingogram
Tubal insufflation
Dilatation and curettage
Pregnancy interruption

Pelvic infections following major gynecologic surgery
Puerperal and postabortal infections
Suppurative pelvic thrombophlebitis
Pyometra
Infections in the pelvis due to primary pathology in the gastrointestinal tract
Tuberculosis
Tropical infections

Some types of pelvic infection, such as postabortal and postoperative infections, are discussed in other chapters. Those pelvic infections caused primarily by sexually transmitted agents and by tuberculosis will be discussed in this chapter. Discussions of septic pelvic thrombophlebitis and septic shock are also included in this chapter.

Many physicians use the term *pelvic inflammatory disease* (PID) to describe a variety of infections in the pelvis: acute or chronic, surgical, venereal, tuberculous, and others. The term is nonspecific and is inaccurate in that an inflammation does not necessarily result from infection. Different clinical criteria to diagnose pelvic inflammatory disease are used by clinicians and by investigators, which often results in confusing and contradictory conclusions. Whenever possible, the term pelvic inflammatory disease should be replaced by more appropriate and descriptive terminology, such as *acute salpingo-oophoritis, pyosalpinx with pelvic peritonitis, acute tubo-ovarian abscess,* and other more acceptable terms.

A system for grading salpingitis by clinical examination has been suggested by Hager and associates. A modified version of this system is used in this chapter.

GRADING OF ACUTE PELVIC INFLAMMATORY DISEASE BY CLINICAL EXAMINATION

Grade I
Uncomplicated salpingitis or salpingo oophoritis, unilateral or bilateral
A. Without pelvic peritonitis
B. With pelvic peritonitis
Grade II
Complicated salpingitis, salpingo-oophoritis, pyosalpinx, or tubo-ovarian abscess, with inflammatory adnexal mass(es), unilateral or bilateral
A. Without pelvic peritonitis
B. With pelvic peritonitis
Grade III
Large (≥8 cm in diameter) tubo-ovarian or pelvic abscess(es), spread of infection to upper abdomen, or ruptured tubo-ovarian abscess

A schematic representation of the progressive and recurrent nature of pelvic inflammatory disease is presented in Figure 13–1.

Contraception and Pelvic Inflammatory Disease

In 1980, Senanayake and Kramer reviewed 16 published reports of the relationship between intrauterine device use and acute pelvic infection. All 16 studies found that the use of an intrauterine device increased the risk of pelvic infection. Ory found that intrauterine device users have a three- to five-fold increased risk of pelvic infection, and the risk is higher for young women. The risk is greatest for women with many sexual partners and in a population with a high incidence of sexually transmitted diseases. Unfortunately, we have seen many young women with serious pelvic infections associated with intrauterine device use. Because of this, our policy is to restrict the use of intrauterine contraceptive devices to older women who have completed their families and have a stable marital relationship. All patients who have an intrauterine device are carefully instructed to report immediately any abnormal vaginal discharge or lower abdominal discomfort, especially when associated with fever. Such patients should be carefully evaluated for possible pelvic infection. If the slightest suspicion is present, antibiotics should be administered, the device should be removed, and follow-up examinations should be performed to be certain the infection has cleared. Although the normal uterine cavity is sterile, bacteria often can be cultured from a uterine cavity that contains an intrauterine device with a tail. The bacteria cultured

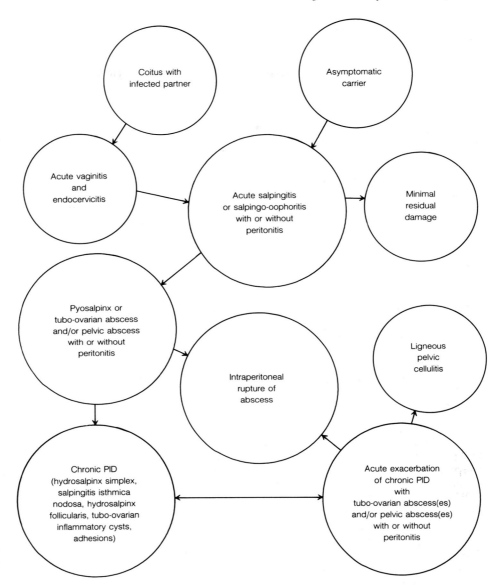

FIG. 13-1 Sequential development of pelvic inflammatory disease.

will be similar to those in the vagina. The tail of an intrauterine device facilitates access of vaginal bacteria to the uterine cavity. If the device does not have a tail, the uterine cavity will be sterile. Bacteria carried intermittently into the uterus by sperm, especially in mid–menstrual cycle, may ascend into the fallopian tubes and cause salpingitis, sometimes subclinical. This chronic residue of infection in the fallopian tubes can result later in infertility or tubal pregnancy.

Senanayake and Kramer have analyzed reports comparing the relative risks of pelvic inflammatory disease in users and nonusers of the oral contraceptive pill. With one exception, these studies show

that the risk of pelvic inflammatory disease among users is 0.3 to 0.9 times that for nonusers, indicating that this method of contraception has a protective effect. The mechanism of protection is not known. Eschenbach has theorized that the increased density of the cervical mucous plug caused by the oral contraceptive pill may inhibit the entry of bacteria into the uterus.

The relationship between use of the barrier contraceptive method and pelvic inflammatory disease has been studied by Kelaghan and associates and others. It was found that condoms, diaphragms, and chemical barrier methods provide significant protection. The prevention of pelvic inflammatory disease and its sequelae is one of the most important noncontraceptive benefits of barrier methods of contraception. They should be prescribed for women with pelvic inflammatory disease, even those women whose infection has caused sterility from bilateral tubal occlusion, to reduce the possibility of recurrent infection.

Acute Salpingitis

MICROBIAL ETIOLOGY OF ACUTE SALPINGITIS

Sophisticated studies by Sweet, Monif, Chow, Cunningham, Eschenbach, Mardh, Westrom, their associates, and many others have produced important new information about the bacterial etiology of acute salpingitis (Grade I disease).

Neisseria gonorrhoeae has an important role in causing acute salpingitis in some populations. For example, it can be isolated from 80% of inner-city U.S. women with acute salpingitis. However, in other U.S. women the number of positive endocervical cultures for *N. gonorrhoeae* with acute salpingitis is lower, and the organism is present in only 10% to 20% of Scandinavian women with acute salpingitis.

The presence of *N. gonorrhoeae* in an endocervical culture is not absolute proof that the organism has also caused salpingitis. Fallopian tube cultures obtained by laparoscopy and peritoneal fluid cultures obtained by culdocentesis and laparoscopy have shown a poor correlation with cultures obtained from the endocervix. The isolation of *N. gonorrhoeae* is dependent on the stage of infection. As demonstrated by Curtis in 1921, the organism is present when the fallopian tube is acutely inflamed but is not found in patients who have been afebrile for 14 days. Sweet and associates found *N. gonorrhoeae* in 70% of patients presenting within 24 hours of the onset of symptoms. After 48 hours, *N. gonorrhoeae* was found in only 19% of patients. *N. gonorrhoeae* is isolated less frequently in older women with salpingitis and in women who have recurrent infections. Even among women with positive cultures for *N. gonorrhoeae*, other bacteria may also be cultured from the fallopian tubes and peritoneal fluid.

The pathogenesis of salpingitis with *N. gonorrhoeae* is not completely understood. Sexual transmission between infected partners is well documented. The organism remains localized in the cervix for a varying period. It may gain access to the uterine cavity during mid-cycle when the cervical mucus is thin and penetrable by sperm and micro-organisms. The organism(s) may flourish in the uterine cavity during menstruation, since menstrual blood is an excellent culture medium. Inoculation of the fallopian tubes may be facilitated by retrograde menstruation. Women who are amenorrheic rarely develop this problem. The cervical mucus mechanical barrier is more impenetrable in anovulatory women. This barrier may be temporarily lost, however, during menstruation, even in anovulatory cycles. Different types of gonococci vary in their ability to cause salpingitis and migration of the organism to the fallopian tube during menses is facilitated by the absence of a bactericidal antibody against *N. gonorrhoeae*.

Presence of the gonococcus in the fallopian tube causes an intense inflammatory reaction. Elaboration of an endotoxin damages cells of the endosalpinx, causing a loss of cilia. The fallopian tube becomes erythematous and swollen. A purulent exudate develops in the tubal lumen. This exudate has ready access to the peritoneal cavity, and explains the common association of pelvic peritonitis. The inflammatory process spreads to adjacent surfaces of the ovary, omentum, and bowel, causing adhesions to form between these structures. Adhesions also form between the mucosal folds of the endosalpinx within the tube and at the fimbriated end, resulting in complete or partial closure of the tubal lumen.

The findings of Cunningham, Eschenbach, Sweet, and their coworkers demonstrate clearly the polymicrobial etiology of acute pelvic inflammatory disease. Cunningham and associates studied peritoneal fluid obtained by culdocentesis in 133 women with acute pelvic inflammatory disease. *N. gonorrhoeae* was isolated from the lower genital tract in over half of these women and cultured from the peritoneal fluid in 22%. *N. gonorrhoeae* and other organisms were recovered from 32%. Non-gonococcal organisms alone were recovered in 46%. These investigators believe that *N. gonorrhoeae* initiates most cases of pelvic inflammatory disease and that suprainfection with non-gonococcal organisms, which occurs later, may interfere with the recovery of gonococci. Chow, Monif, and others agree with this concept.

Eschenbach's studies confirmed this work and showed that mixed anaerobic and aerobic bacterial peritoneal infection was common in non-gonococcal pelvic disease. The most common species recovered in his studies were *Bacteroides fragilis*, peptostreptococci, and peptococci. Eschenbach proposed that tuboperitoneal gonococcal infection probably causes pelvic inflammatory disease in most patients with cervical gonococcal infection, whereas polymicrobial tuboperitoneal infection probably causes most non-gonococcal cases.

Sweet and associates found the gonococcus and anaerobic bacteria, either alone or together, in the fallopian tube in the initial episodes of salpingitis. Their findings suggest that the gonococcus may be important in initiating acute salpingitis in some patients and in establishing conditions that will facilitate subsequent invasion by other organisms present in the cervix and vagina. However, their findings also suggest an important primary role for mixed aerobic and anaerobic bacteria in the pathogenesis of acute salpingitis. A mixed anaerobic and aerobic infection causes more tubal destruction and subsequent infertility and is less likely to show a prompt and complete response to antibiotics.

Chlamydia trachomatis has received recent attention as an important agent in the microbial etiology of acute salpingitis. This intracellular bacterium has been found to cause at least 40% of acute salpingitis in Scandinavia and 20% of acute salpingitis in the United States. However, although there is evidence to support *C. trachomatis* as a major factor in acute salpingitis in Scandinavia, studies by Thompson, Eschenbach, and Sweet and their respective associates suggest that the organism may not be as important in the microbiologic etiology of acute salpingitis in the United States.

Acute fibrinous perihepatitis associated with salpingitis was originally described with *N. gonorrhoeae* infections and is called the Fitz-Hugh-Curtis syndrome. It has been reported recently with *C. trachomatis* infections of the fallopian tube. In fact, Wang and associates found the Fitz-Hugh-Curtis syndrome more frequently with *C. trachomatis* than with *N. gonorrhoeae*. Acute fibrinous perihepatitis may be suspected in patients with acute salpingitis who have right upper quadrant pain and tenderness. The pain may be pleuritic in nature and aggravated by deep inspiration. Acute fibrinous perihepatitis may be asymptomatic, being detected only by laparoscopy. The most plausible explanation for the occurrence of perihepatitis in patients with acute salpingitis is lymphatic transport. It is possible that the infection can spread from the fallopian tube to the surface of the liver by way of the peritoneal cavity in patients with peritonitis.

Mycoplasmas are the smallest known free-living organisms. They lack a cell wall. Three mycoplasmas have been implicated in acute salpingitis: *M. hominis*, *U. urealyticum*, and *M. fermentans*. These organisms can be isolated from the cervix, cul-de-sac fluid, and fallopian tubes in patients with acute salpingitis. Serologic evidence also suggests that acute salpingitis can be caused by mycoplasma. The role of the genital tract mycoplasma in acute salpingitis remains unclear due to the difficulty in determining whether these organisms cause tissue damage in the fallopian tube.

Actinomyces israelii is a gram-positive, non–acid-fast, anaerobic bacterium. It is classified as transitional between true bacteria and the complex fungi. Pelvic actinomycosis was formerly considered a rare disease, most often secondary to a primary infection in the intestinal tract, but foreign bodies in the genital tract have also been associated with actinomycosis infection. Recently, *A. israelii* infections have been noted in patients with an intrauterine contraceptive device. A few patients have had very serious and even fatal infections. Although an infection with this organism may be acute, more frequently it runs a subacute, indolent course. In most cases, diagnosis has been based on histologic identification of the organism in cytology smears or tissue sections.

CLINICAL FEATURES AND DIAGNOSIS OF ACUTE SALPINGITIS

The clinical presentation of acute salpingitis may vary from being nearly asymptomatic to showing obvious evidence of serious pelvic infection. The average patient with acute salpingitis will have an illness of moderate severity.

Since sexually transmitted infections of the lower genital tract almost always follow direct sexual contact, it is important to determine if the patient has had recent sexual activity. Although the risk of transmission of the disease to the female from an infected male is approximately 80% to 90%, only 10% to 20% of the infected cases become clinically manifest as endometritis, salpingitis, and pelvic peritonitis. It is of clinical interest that the spectrum of primary infection sites of sexually transmitted venereal disease has broadened in recent years, with gonorrheal infections of the rectum and pharynx occurring with increasing frequency. The incidence of anal gonorrhea in women with positive *N. gonorrhoeae* cultures from the cervix varies between 30% and 60%. Pharyngeal infections are detected in women examined in venereal disease clinics in 3% to 11% of cases. Consequently, in a patient with the common symptom of acute pelvic pain, identification of other glandular sites of infection, namely the vestibular glands of the vagina and urethra, the anal crypts, and the pharynx are of as much clinical importance as the endocervix. The diagnostic accuracy of cultures for *N. gonorrhoeae* is improved significantly when two sterile swabs are cultured from the endocervical and anal canals, approaching

99% as reported by Dans. Newer developments in microbiology techniques have provided a better growth potential for and a greater accuracy in detection of the gonococcus. A gram stain of cervical secretions may show intracellular gram-negative diplococci resembling, but not necessarily diagnostic of, *N. gonorrhoeae.*

In obtaining a cervical culture for *N. gonorrhoeae,* it is important to clean the cervix lightly with a sponge and to leave the sterile swab in the endocervical canal for at least 30 seconds. A second swab should also be used to increase the rate of detection of this fastidious organism. Culture of the anal canal may be obtained by applying a sterile swab well above the anal sphincter in order to remain in contact with the rectal crypts for at least 30 seconds. Culture of the urethra is also advised, and whenever a reddened pharynx is present, this site should be cultured as well. A carrier medium is less effective than direct plating of the culture material on modified Thayer-Martin media (modified Thayer-Martin VCN media), but should this not be available, a transport medium such as Stewart's or Transgrow medium should be used with early inoculation of the material on the culture media in the laboratory. It is essential that all patients who are found to have acute gonorrhea should have a serologic test for syphilis as a part of the diagnostic evaluation. A gram stain of a smear of endocervical discharge should be made. If examined by an experienced technician, it may show gram-negative intracellular diplococci. The average physician will identify the organism on smear in less than 50% of the cases that ultimately prove to have a positive cervical culture. Technicians are more likely to be adept in identifying this organism than physicians.

Cultures for *C. trachomatis* require sophisticated microbiologic resources that are not commonly available. If routine aerobic and anaerobic cultures are taken from the endocervix and vagina, a multitude of bacteria characteristically found in these locations will be reported. This information is not clinically useful.

The onset of symptoms of acute salpingitis will usually follow within 2 weeks of sexual exposure and just after the menstrual flow has ceased. Although initial location of this disease is usually confined to the endocervix with the production of increased cervical discharge, the spread of infection to the endometrium and tubes is commonly associated with the onset of menstruation. Menstruation itself may provide a method of spread of this ascending disease through the reflux of menstrual blood into the oviduct. The localized endometritis produces irregular endometrial shedding, prolongation of bleeding, and intermenstrual bleeding.

These local endometrial tissue reactions produce a wide variety of menstrual irregularities as a common clinical feature of this acute event. Endosalpingitis is clinically evident by the gradual onset of lower abdominal discomfort that becomes progressively acute until pelvic peritonitis ensues and spreads to the upper abdomen.

Although many patients with acute salpingitis may present with symptoms of urinary frequency, urgency, and dysuria, cystitis is rare. Usually the symptoms are associated with a urethritis. However, urinary tract symptoms may be the only reason the patient seeks medical treatment. A urine culture and antibiotic sensitivity studies should be done to differentiate a true bacterial cystitis from gonococcal urethritis.

Abdominal examination of the patient reveals generalized direct tenderness in both lower quadrants with occasional rebound tenderness demonstrating pelvic peritonitis. The uterus also may be quite tender on manipulation, which is an important clinical sign. The adnexa are exquisitely tender, which makes the pelvis difficult to truly evaluate for the presence or absence of an adnexal mass. Since the differential diagnosis of the patient with acute pelvic and abdominal pain must include acute salpingitis, ectopic pregnancy, acute appendicitis, and other causes of pelvic pain, an accurate assessment of the adnexa is important. It is not necessary for acute salpingitis patients to have bilateral adnexal tenderness. The infection may be less severe or even absent on one side, especially in patients with an intrauterine device in place.

Usually, the picture of bilateral pelvic peritonitis is helpful in identifying an acute salpingitis infection, which is often associated with a higher temperature and white cell blood count than is seen in a patient with an ectopic pregnancy or appendicitis. Rectal examination of the cul-de-sac produces exquisite tenderness from peritonitis, which, in the absence of palpable fluid in the pelvis, is helpful in differentiating inflammatory disease from a ruptured tubal pregnancy. Hematoperitoneum in the presence of a ruptured tubal pregnancy may cause referred shoulder pain, which is usually absent with acute salpingitis except in the rare case of the Fitz-Hugh-Curtis syndrome of fibrinous perihepatitis.

The laboratory data are also helpful, but not necessarily diagnostic. The white blood cell count may be elevated with a shift to the left, while the erythrocyte sedimentation rate may be normal or slightly elevated. A serum pregnancy test is quite accurate and should always be performed to rule out the diagnosis of an ectopic pregnancy.

If pelvic findings remain unclear, a laparoscopic examination of the pelvis is commonly employed.

The clinical diagnosis of salpingitis has been proved erroneous in many clinics by the use of laparoscopy. During the 1960s, a series of laparoscopic studies by Falk, Westrom, and Jacobson resulted in a revision of the clinical characteristics of salpingitis and the problems of differential diagnosis of acute pelvic disease. Laparoscopy offers an excellent means of diagnosis of acute salpingitis whenever the diagnosis is uncertain, especially since a rapid and accurate diagnosis must be made if the serious late sequelae of acute salpingitis are to be prevented by the early use of effective antibiotic therapy. Ledger has discussed the risk/benefit ratio of laparoscopy when acute salpingitis is suspected. He suggests that it be used more frequently, especially in patients whose illness is severe enough to require hospitalization. Laparoscopy has a major disadvantage of requiring anesthesia and an operating room. In many large public hospitals, laparoscopy for the large number of patients seen daily with suspected acute salpingitis would be difficult. Therefore, a more convenient outpatient procedure such as microscopic examination of peritoneal fluid obtained by culdocentesis should be developed.

TREATMENT OF ACUTE SALPINGITIS

The primary treatment of acute salpingitis is medical. Unfortunately, considerable long-term morbidity and sequelae may result if the treatment is delayed, inadequate, or ineffective. According to Eschenbach, 15% of patients will develop chronic pain; 20% to 25% will have subsequent attacks of pelvic infection; infertility will result in 10% to 15% with one episode of acute salpingitis, 25% to 35% with two episodes, and 50% to 75% with three episodes; and 7% of patients will have an ectopic pregnancy with the first subsequent pregnancy. Inadequate treatment may result in progression of the disease to more serious stages. Because outpatient treatment regimes have a failure rate of up to 20%, and to avoid late sequelae, the majority of patients with pelvic inflammatory disease should be hospitalized for intravenous antibiotic therapy. If that is not possible, those who receive outpatient treatment must be followed very closely. If there is no response to ambulatory therapy within 48 hours or if the disease is judged to be more severe before that time, prompt admission to the hospital should be arranged in an effort to prevent the serious sequelae of acute salpingitis with parenteral antibiotics. Hospitalization is also advisable if an intrauterine device is present; if an adnexal mass suggestive of a pyosalpinx or tubo-ovarian abscess is suspected; if a complicating medical disease such as diabetes is present; if pregnancy is diagnosed; if peritonitis is present; or if the patient's cooperation in taking medication and returning for follow-up is difficult to obtain. This may be a special problem for adolescents with acute salpingitis. All adolescents with salpingitis should be hospitalized. When the diagnosis of acute salpingitis is questionable, hospitalization for laparoscopy may also be desirable.

The Centers for Disease Control guidelines for the ambulatory treatment of patients with acute salpingitis were published in 1982. One of the following combination regimes is recommended by the CDC: Initially, the patient may receive cefoxitin, 2.0 g IM; or amoxicillin, 3.0 g by mouth; or ampicillin, 3.5 g by mouth; or aqueous procaine penicillin G, 4.8 million units IM at two sites. Probenecid 1.0 g should be given by mouth with each drug chosen for initial therapy. After the initial drug is administered, doxycycline, 100 mg, is given by mouth twice daily for 10 to 14 days. Alternatively, one may prescribe tetracycline hydrochloride 500 mg by mouth four times daily.

When patients are hospitalized for treatment of acute salpingitis, one may use a two- or three-drug parenteral broad-spectrum antibiotic regime as described for the treatment of patients with acute pelvic abscess. The recent recovery of both aerobic and anaerobic bacteria from the pelves of patients with acute salpingitis has indicated the need for a wider spectrum of antibiotic coverage. We currently have the best results on our service with a combination of intravenous penicillin or ampicillin, clindamycin and gentamicin. Alternatively, a combination of cefoxitin and metronidazole, both given intravenously, has given good results.

Acute Pelvic Abscess

Patients whose acute salpingitis has progressed or recurred may be found to have an acute pelvic abscess (Grade II disease); either bilateral or unilateral tubo-ovarian abscess; or an extratubal collection of pus in the pelvis, usually located in the cul-de-sac. Such patients are usually in the third or fourth decade of life, although we have seen large pelvic abscesses in girls as young as 13. A pelvic abscess in a postmenopausal woman is usually associated with disease of the intestinal tract such as a ruptured appendix or a ruptured sigmoid diverticulum. One-third of the patients are nulliparous but many will have been pregnant within the previous 2 years. One-third will have a history of pelvic inflammatory disease, and some will have a history of previous hospitalization for pelvic abscess. Many will have received antibiotics recently for acute salpingitis. Of 100 patients with pelvic inflammatory disease studied by Goldenberg, 42% had been treated on an outpatient basis within 2 weeks of hospitalization. Bilateral lower abdominal pain and tenderness, anorexia, and fever were present for several days.

On examination, the patient with acute pelvic abscess appears ill. She may walk slowly with a hand placed over her lower abdomen and her abdomen flexed. Abdominal distention and direct and rebound tenderness in the lower abdominal quadrants are present. The pelvic examination must be done carefully because of acute pelvic tenderness. Even the slightest motion of the cervix may cause extreme pain. Tissues in the cul-de-sac and on each side of the uterus feel firm and indurated. An irregular, tender, fixed, inflammatory mass may be felt on one or both sides of the pelvis. The outline and dimensions of the mass are sometimes indistinct. The mass is usually composed centrally of an infection in and around the fallopian tube and ovary, with components of intestine, mesentery, and omentum surrounding it. The mass may be relatively small or may extend out of the pelvis into the lower abdomen. It may extend into the cul-de-sac and appear to dissect the rectovaginal septum on rectovaginal examination. The temperature, pulse, white blood cell count, and erythrocyte sedimentation rate are usually elevated. Even in the face of dehydration, anemia is frequently found. Anemia is common in patients who have had a chronic abscess for many weeks. An abdominal x-ray is helpful to assess the degree of intestinal distention and to serve as a baseline should intestinal obstruction develop. Pelvic ultrasonography may give additional objective evidence of the size of the pelvic abscess. Repeat ultrasonography examinations during the course of medical management also will allow a more objective evaluation of the response if an abscess or inflammatory mass is seen. Taylor and colleagues reported excellent results with grey-scale ultrasonography in the detection and localization of abdominal and pelvic abscesses. Studies by Koehler and Moss, Halber and associates, and others have demonstrated the value of computerized tomography in diagnosing intra-abdominal and pelvic abscesses.

Patients with an acute pelvic abscess, usually an acute exacerbation of chronic pelvic inflammatory disease with bilateral tubo-ovarian abscesses, should be admitted to the hospital for management. They should be placed at bedrest with the head elevated in a semi-Fowler's position. Intravenous fluid, electrolyte replacement and blood transfusions should be given as needed. In the presence of a pelvic abscess, anemia usually will not respond to oral iron replacement. Suction through a nasogastric tube or a long intestinal tube should be used as indicated,

depending on the degree of abdominal distention. Other complicating medical problems should be considered. For example, response to treatment will be inadequate if the patient has diabetes that is not well controlled. The rate of intrauterine device use in our patients with acute pelvic abscess is twice the rate among women seeking contraception in the Family Planning Program of our hospital. This is consistent with the role of the intrauterine device in increasing the risk of acquiring salpingitis. It may also be an indication that patients with salpingitis who have an intrauterine device in place may not respond to antibiotics. If an intrauterine device is present in a patient with an acute pelvic abscess, it should be removed, but one should probably wait for several hours after intravenous antibiotics are started to avoid septicemia.

Appropriate intravenous antibiotics must be administered to patients with an acute pelvic abscess. When antibiotics are used to treat an infection, the microorganisms causing the infection are identified from a smear or culture, their sensitivity to a variety of antibiotics is tested, and the correct antibiotics are chosen based upon these laboratory data. In the case of an acute pelvic abscess, a culture of the cervix will not be helpful. There is little correlation between microorganisms found in the cervix and microorganisms found in the pelvic abscess. A culture of fluid obtained from the cul-de-sac also will not be helpful, since, as shown by Sweet, contamination by microorganisms of the vagina is common. Needle aspiration of the cul-de-sac in a patient with an acute pelvic abscess could also rupture the abscess wall, resulting in spillage of the infected exudate into the general peritoneal cavity. Even if culture material could be obtained, sophisticated microbiologic laboratory facilities and several days are required to identify all of the organisms causing the infection and to test their sensitivity to antibiotics. The polymicrobial etiology of acute pelvic abscess is well known. Etiologic agents include *N. gonorrhoeae*, *C. trachomatis*, anaerobic bacteria (which include Bacteroides and gram-positive cocci), facultative gram-negative rods (such as *E. coli*), *A. israelii*, *M. hominis*, and *Ureaplasma urealyticum*. In the individual patient, it is impossible to differentiate among these agents at the time a treatment regime is chosen. No single antibiotic is active against the entire spectrum of pathogens (Table 13–1). Therefore, antibiotic treatment regimes should be chosen that are active against the broadest range of these pathogens. Several antimicrobial combinations do provide a broad spectrum of activity against the major pathogens *in vitro* and have also been found to be fairly effective in clinical use. Landers and Sweet report a greater success when the drug re-

TABLE 13-1 *Bacterial Susceptibilities to Antibiotic Agents used in Gynecology*

DRUG	ANAEROBES		AEROBES					
	Peptococci Peptostreptococci Bacteriodes species	Bacteroides fragilis	Enterococci	Enterobacteriaceae E. Coli Klebsiella Proteus Enterobacter	Non-Enterococcal Streptococci	Staphylococcus aureus	Neisseria gonorrhoeae	CHLAMYDIA TRACHOMATIS
Penicillin	++++	—	++ (only in combination with aminoglycoside)	—	++++	+ (rare susceptible strain)	++++ (Some strains highly resistant due to B-lactamose production.)	—
Ampicillin	++++	—	+++ (better in combination with aminoglycoside)	++	++++	+ (rare susceptible strain)	++++ (Some strains minimally resistant due to chromosomal resistance.)	—
Carbenicillin ⎤ Ticarcillin ⎦	++++	++	+ / —	+++	++++	+ (rare susceptible strain)	++++	—
Piperacillin	++++	++ to +++	++ (better in combination with aminoglycoside)	+++ to ++++	++++	+ (rare susceptible strain)	++++	—
Cephalothin ⎤ Cefazolin ⎦	+++	—	—	+++	++++	++++	++	—
Cephamandole	++++	—	—	+++	++++	++++	++	—
Cefoxitin	++++	+++ to ++++	—	+++	++++	+++	++++	—
Moxalactam	++++	+++ to ++++	—	++++	+++	+ to ++	++++	?
Cefotaxime	++++	++	—	++++	+++ to ++++	++	++++	?
Clindamycin	++++	++++	—	—	—	+++ to +++	—	—
Chloramphenicol	++++	++++	—	+++	++++	+++	++++ (Not used because of toxicity)	±
Metronidazole	+	++++	—	—	—	—	—	—
Doxycycline or Minocycline	+++	++ to +++	+	++	+++	++	++++ (rare resistance)	++++ (Erythromycin is an acceptable alternative)
Aminoglycosides	—	—	(only in combination with Penicillin G, Ampicillin, or Piperacillin)	++++	—	++ to +++	±	±

Courtesy of Jonas Shulman, MD, Director, Division of Infectious Diseases, Department of Medicine, Emory University School of Medicine

— Not effective

± variable

+ to ++++ (Estimate of susceptibilities of strains in most hospitals (++++ being most susceptible; + being least susceptible)

gime includes clindamycin. For several years, we have used a three-drug regime consisting of intravenous ampicillin, clindamycin, and gentamicin with good results. If response is inadequate, chloramphenicol has been substituted with success. The Centers for Disease Control has listed several other combination regimes with broad activity against the major pathogens in this disease. They include the following: doxycycline plus cefoxitin, clindamycin plus gentamicin or tobramycin, and doxycycline plus metronidazole. We have had a satisfactory experience with doxycycline plus metronidazole, which has the additional advantage of being less expensive.

Patients must be followed carefully for evidence of response. Abdominal and pelvic examinations should be done each day. A scoring sheet (Fig. 13–2) is used as an index of disease severity, progression, or response. Its use will assist the physician in determining whether patients are responding to treatment, require a change in antibiotics, or require surgical intervention. Careful observations must be made for signs indicating possible rupture of the pelvic abscess.

Although antibiotics are effective in treating an acute pelvic abscess, surgical drainage is more so. Drainage of a pelvic abscess through a posterior colpotomy incision or through a gridiron incision in one or both lower abdominal quadrants will bring about a rapid improvement in the patient's condition. Occasionally, an abscess too high in the cul-de-sac to drain through a posterior colpotomy incision will drain spontaneously through the rectum and the patient's condition will improve dramatically. One should not attempt a posterior colpotomy when the abscess has drained spontaneously into the rectum because of the possibility of creating a rectovaginal fistula. A pelvic abscess never drains

through the vagina spontaneously unless the patient has had a previous posterior colpotomy for a pelvic abscess. Under these circumstances, the recurrent abscess may dissect along the tract of the previous posterior colpotomy and eventually drain spontaneously through the vagina.

If the diagnosis of acute pelvic abscess is uncertain, laparoscopy or laparotomy may be required. Although laparoscopy may be a satisfactory procedure for diagnosis in patients with acute salpingitis, more severe forms of pelvic infection may make laparoscopy more difficult, more hazardous, and less satisfactory as a diagnostic procedure. There may be adhesions that make insertion of the trocar or laparoscope difficult or impossible and cause similar problems with visualization of the pelvic organs. In cases in which the diagnosis of acute unruptured pelvic abscess is questionable, a diagnostic laparotomy may be required.

Conservative medical management with intravenous broad-spectrum antibiotics and drainage of the abscess when possible has resulted in a satisfactory resolution of acute pelvic abscesses in the majority of patients, as reported by Franklin and associates. Our experience confirms that conservative management is the treatment of choice except in cases of questionable diagnosis, suspected rupture, or failure of the abscess to respond to initial conservative management. Use of the severity score sheet will allow a more objective evaluation of the patient's response. If the patient has not shown an improvement of greater than 30% in the severity score by the 3rd or 4th day of treatment, a change of antibiotics or surgical intervention is usually necessary. When medical management is successful, however, ovarian function is conserved even though tubal function may be destroyed by the infection and most patients will remain infertile. We

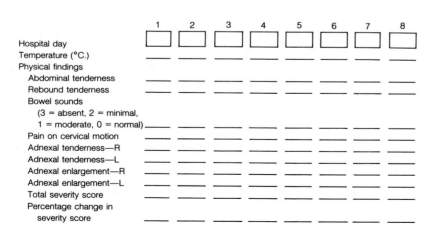

FIG. 13-2 Scoring system for evaluating the severity of pelvic inflammatory disease and for progression or response to treatment. (For each finding, 0 = absent, 1 = minimal, 2 = moderate, 3 = marked)

were surprised to find that of the 97 patients treated conservatively, 10 subsequently became pregnant with no reported ectopic pregnancies. One patient had two successful pregnancies after colpotomy drainage of 500 ml of purulent material. Rivlin reported that 5 of 40 potentially fertile patients (12.5%) had successful pregnancies at a later date following vaginal drainage of a pelvic abscess. These must be patients with a unilateral tubo-ovarian abscess that does not involve the opposite fallopian tube.

When there has been an adequate response to therapy, oral antibiotics may be continued as an outpatient procedure. Doxycycline is given by mouth for at least 2 weeks. Patients are seen frequently for evaluation of continued response. It has been suggested that the use of oral contraceptive pills to prevent ovulation and to cause the formation of a thick cervical mucous plug may help prevent recurrent infections. To our knowledge, their effectiveness has not been evaluated clinically. Also important in reducing the risk of recurrence of the pelvic infection is the examination of all sexual partners of the patient for evidence of sexually transmitted disease agents. Those affected should be treated promptly with a regime effective against uncomplicated gonococcal and chlamydial infection.

If a patient has required hospitalization on several occasions for acute exacerbation of pelvic inflammatory disease with bilateral tubo-ovarian abscesses to the point where she is more often sick than well, definitive surgical intervention may be indicated. The operation should be done when the infection is quiescent. The surgery may still be difficult, but complications will be less frequent than when patients are operated on in the acute phase of the infection. The timing of the operative intervention is important. There should be complete absorption of the inflammatory exudate surrounding the focus of infection. Bimanual examination should be possible without producing a marked or persistent febrile response. We suggest that definitive surgery should be delayed for 2 to 3 months following the recent exacerbation for more complete resolution of the infection. Ideally, the patient should have a normal erythrocyte sedimentation rate, white blood cell count, and hematocrit and a relatively non-tender pelvis.

Conservative medical management of acute unruptured pelvic abscess is not uniformly accepted. Kaplan and associates recommend a more aggressive management in patients who exhibit either no clinical response or only partial response after 24 to 72 hours of medical management. This more aggressive surgical approach, which includes a total abdominal hysterectomy and bilateral salpingo-oophorectomy, is thought to reduce the protracted period of intensive medical therapy in a group of patients who may eventually require surgery. They noted that conservative management of their cases usually resulted in protracted periods of intensive care and repeated hospital admissions, and rarely in subsequent pregnancies. However, Kaplan's surgical treatment was associated with six incidences of injury to the bowel and additional postoperative complications. Unfortunately, patients with acute pelvic abscess are frequently young, and future childbearing is often desired, even though it may be impossible. Conservation of ovarian function for these young women is an important benefit of medical management. Some differences in the percentage of patients responding to conservative management in different studies might be explained by differences in the predominant microorganisms causing the infection and their sensitivity to the antibiotics used.

Older studies of the management of patients with pelvic abscess, which emphasize the early use of surgery, are no longer pertinent, since modern antibiotic drugs were not then available. Collins and Jansen in 1959 had an early failure rate for conservative medical therapy of 10%. However, 113 of their 174 patients required later surgery, a late failure rate of 65%. In 1980, Ginsburg and associates reviewed 160 patients treated for tubo-ovarian abscess during the years 1969 to 1979. The early failure rate with broad-spectrum antibiotics was 31% whereas the late failure rate was 21%. In an averaged follow-up period of 25.5 months, 48% required no surgery later. Our recent experience is similar.

Johnson reported on long-term follow-up of patients with tubo-ovarian abscesses who were successfully treated with conservative medical therapy. Of 37 patients followed for 5 to 10 years, only two patients required surgery for recurrent pelvic abscess. Twenty-three pregnancies and 17 term deliveries occurred in nine patients. The results indicate the value of such therapy.

When complicating medical diseases such as diabetes are present, when the abscess is large (8 cm or more in diameter), and when the patient is perimenopausal with a history of repeated acute exacerbations of infection, response to medical therapy may not be satisfactory. When an acute pelvic abscess does not respond to intensive medical therapy, posterior colpotomy, extraperitoneal abdominal drainage, or laparotomy with or without hysterectomy may be necessary. In patients who have extensive bilateral adnexal disease where tubo-ovarian conservation is not feasible, or in patients past the reproductive age, we feel the operation of choice is total abdominal hysterectomy and bilateral salpingo-oophorectomy.

SURGICAL MANAGEMENT OF ACUTE PELVIC ABSCESS

Posterior Colpotomy

Wharton has described various techniques of vaginal drainage of pelvic abscess. Today, posterior colpotomy is done to evacuate pus and to establish drainage from a pelvic abscess that presents in the cul-de-sac.

Ideally, there are three requirements for colpotomy drainage of a pelvic abscess: the abscess must be midline or nearly so; it should dissect the rectovaginal septum to assure the surgeon that the drainage will be extraperitoneal and that pus will not be disseminated transperitoneally; and it should be cystic or fluctuant to assure adequate drainage. Occasionally a cul-de-sac abscess may be successfully drained without dissecting the septum. However, the serosal surface of the abscess should be adherent to the cul-de-sac peritoneum. Ultrasonography may be helpful in locating the pockets of pus.

TECHNIQUE OF POSTERIOR COLPOTOMY. After adequate anesthesia, the patient is placed in the lithotomy position. The posterior lip of the cervix is grasped with a tenaculum and drawn down and forward. It is essential that a thorough examination of the pelvis be made under anesthesia so that the operator will have in mind the size and position of the mass that is to be drained.

The vaginal mucosa of the posterior vaginal fornix is incised just below the reflection of the vaginal mucosa onto the cervix, and the transverse incision is widened with a pair of long scissors (Figure 13–3A). The incision must be large enough to allow adequate exploration and drainage of the abscess cavity. The cul-de-sac peritoneum and abscess wall are punctured with a long Kelly clamp (Figure 13–3B). As the abscess wall is perforated, there is a definite sensation of puncturing a cystic cavity. If blood or pus is present, this is soon seen in the upper vagina. The jaws of the clamp are spread, and the flow of liquid from the cul-de-sac is increased. A sample of the purulent exudate is sent to the microbiology laboratory for appropriate culture and sensitivity. A direct smear for gram stain is also made from the pus and examined for predominating organisms.

There may be more than one compartment in an abscess cavity. It is desirable to insert a finger in the cavity and explore. Fibrous adhesions within the cavity can be gently broken. If another abscess

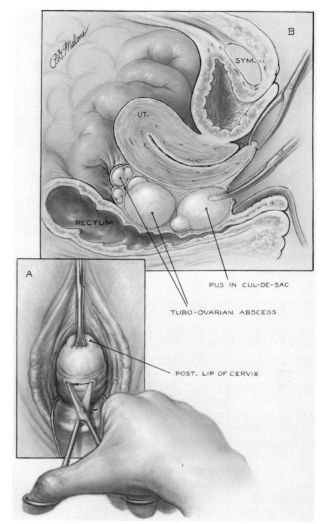

FIG. 13–3 Posterior colpotomy. (*A*) A transverse incision is made through the vaginal mucosa at the junction of the posterior vaginal fornix with the cervix. (*B*) A Kelly clamp is thrust through the abscess wall.

wall is felt, often it may be punctured safely under the guidance of the finger. Exploration and manipulation should be done carefully in order to avoid intraperitoneal rupture of the abscess or perforation of the bowel. To allow adequate drainage, the vaginal incision should be at least 2 cm wide. If pus has been obtained, two Penrose drains are inserted into the abscess cavity and anchored with fine absorbable suture to permit easy removal. These are left for several days or longer. The importance of prolonged drainage is emphasized by Wharton. A suture or two may be required to control bleeding from the vaginal mucosa.

Extraperitoneal Abdominal Drainage

An unruptured pelvic abscess that fails to present in the cul-de-sac may occasionally require abdominal drainage for control of a septic clinical course. Occasionally, a puerperal infection may progress into a parametritis and tubo-ovarian abscess that remains localized in the region of the broad ligament. A gridiron or stab wound incision in the lower quadrant of the abdomen provides an excellent retroperitoneal approach to the pelvic abscess. Care must be taken in directing a long Kelly clamp beneath the peritoneum into the pelvis to avoid trauma to the iliac vessels and the ureter, which cross the pelvic brim in this region. The drain is placed deep into the abscess cavity in order to avoid displacement by movement of the patient (Fig. 13–4).

Exploratory Laparotomy

A lower abdominal transverse Maylard incision is ideal for exploratory laparotomy, since it affords good exposure to the lateral adnexal pelvic organs. Pelvic adhesions should be released and the bowel should be packed off before the pelvic dissection commences. Free pus will often be spilled and the upper abdomen should be isolated from this, if possible. When a ruptured abscess is encountered, the exudate is collected and sent immediately to the laboratory for anaerobic and aerobic cultures and antimicrobial sensitivity studies. The easiest way to collect the material for anaerobic culture is simply to collect it in an airtight syringe and to submit a small piece of the abscess wall in an airtight container. The easiest place to begin the dissection is with the round ligament, since that is the most con-

sistently available landmark. Following the round ligament medially will always lead to the uterine corpus. Variations in the usual technique for the operation may be required because of extensive disease, dense adhesions, and distorted anatomy. For example, it is sometimes convenient to perform the central dissection first; that is, a subtotal hysterectomy. This will allow more space and adequate exposure to do the required adnexal surgery. Tubo-ovarian inflammatory masses may be found densely adherent in the cul-de-sac, behind the uterus, to the posterior surface of the broad ligament, and to the lateral pelvic sidewall. There is risk of injury to the ureters, sigmoid, rectum, and small intestines. The method of dissection used will depend on the nature of the adhesions. Soft, fresh adhesions can be broken gently and easily with finger dissection. Dense fibrotic adhesions must be carefully dissected and cut with scissors. The dissection may be especially difficult and risky if pelvic tissues are intensely indurated, as in ligneous pelvic cellulitis. If the infundibulopelvic ligament can be clamped, cut, and securely ligated, one may gain access to the lateral retroperitoneal space and identify the ureter. This will facilitate a safe dissection of the abscess wall away from the ureter. In cases with extensive disease involving one or both adnexa, we have found the use of preoperative ureteral catheterization to be helpful in identifying the location of the pelvic ureters.

When both adnexa must be removed, a hysterectomy should be performed. In some cases, only a subtotal hysterectomy is feasible. In others, the cervix may be excised following removal of the adnexa. The vaginal vault is left open for drainage. A Penrose drain may be inserted to be removed several days later. Suspension of the vaginal vault and reperitonization of the pelvis is accomplished in the usual manner, if possible. A routine closure of the abdominal incision is performed. Jackson–Pratt suction drains are often placed above the fascia and brought out through a separate incision.

Formerly, it was standard practice to do a bilateral salpingo-oophorectomy in almost all patients who had a laparotomy for acute pelvic abscess. This practice was based on the belief that the disease is almost always severe in both adnexa. Recently, studies have suggested that as many as 25% to 50% of patients will have a relatively normal tube and ovary on one side. This may be true especially of patients whose infection is associated with intrauterine device use. Golde and associates reported that 37 of 85 patients (44%) with tubo-ovarian abscesses confirmed at operation had unilateral abscesses. Of the 37 patients with unilateral abscesses, 20 were using an intrauterine contraceptive device.

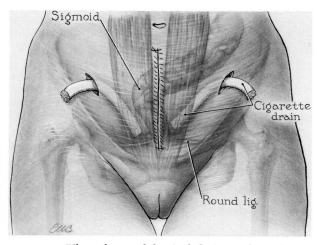

FIG. 13–4 Bilateral transabdominal drainage through stab wounds.

The studies of Landers and Sweet, Hager and Majmudar, and Ginsburg and coworkers also found a higher percentage than previously expected of unilateral adnexal disease. As a consequence of these findings, conservative adnexal surgery should be performed if possible. We have no hesitation in leaving in a relatively normal tube and ovary at the time of hysterectomy with removal of the opposite adnexa for acute pelvic abscess, including adnexa with a small hydrosalpinx and peri-ovarian adhesions. Since the uterus is also removed, and the continuity between the tube and the lower genital tract is interrupted, there is no risk of a new infection. If a strictly unilateral pelvic abscess is found at laparotomy in a young woman, removal of the affected tube and ovary only, leaving in the uterus and the opposite adnexa, is acceptable in a patient who wishes to preserve fertility, even if *in vitro* fertilization techniques are required to accomplish pregnancy. However, it should be recognized that such a patient does have a risk of recurrent tubo-ovarian abscess. It is especially important that her sexual partner(s) be examined and receive treatment when indicated.

In summary, patients with acute pelvic abscess should be hospitalized for treatment with parenteral broad-spectrum antibiotics. Surgery is indicated if the abscess presents for extraperitoneal drainage; if the diagnosis is uncertain; if intraperitoneal rupture is diagnosed or suspected; or if the patient fails to respond to medical management.

Ruptured Tubo-Ovarian Abscess

Of all the complications that can result from chronic pelvic inflammatory disease, intra-abdominal rupture of a tubo-ovarian abscess (grade 3 disease) is the most life-threatening. The mortality from this complication is due to septic shock and from the complications of generalized peritonitis and should not exceed 10% in patients with warm shock.

Abscesses may rupture spontaneously or as the result of bimanual examination or accidental trauma. Bacteriologic study of the contents of the abscess has historically been unrewarding; a specific organism has been isolated in less than 50% of the cases. The gonococcus is rarely identified in a pelvic abscess. Only recently have careful aerobic and anaerobic cultures demonstrated the frequent presence of a mixed infection that includes anaerobic organisms. As reviewed by McNamara and Mead, the results of three separate studies demonstrated 31 positive isolates of anaerobes in 39 patients with a pelvic abscess.

DIAGNOSIS OF RUPTURED TUBO-OVARIAN ABSCESS

The major clinical symptom of ruptured tubo-ovarian abscess is acute, progressive pelvic pain, which is usually so severe that the patient can accurately identify the time and place of its occurrence. In the series from the Johns Hopkins Hospital reported by Vemeeren and TeLinde, the average age of patients with a ruptured tubo-ovarian abscess was 33 years, which is at least 10 years greater than the average age of patients with acute pelvic inflammatory disease. Approximately 2% of these patients are postmenopausal. To our knowledge, only two cases of ruptured tubo-ovarian abscess in a pregnant patient have been reported. Often, there is a history of recurrent attacks of pelvic inflammatory disease, with a sudden increase in the severity and extent of abdominal pain during a recent exacerbation. On examination, the patient will appear seriously ill and dehydrated. The abdomen will be distended and quiet with diminished or absent bowel sounds. There are signs of generalized peritonitis, and shifting dullness may be noted. A pelvic mass is palpable in over 50% of cases. Tachycardia is common. Shock may be present or may develop while the patient is under observation. The temperature is usually over 101°F but can also be normal. The leukocyte count is likely to be over 15,000 but also may be normal. A culdocentesis is a valuable diagnostic aid and was positive for purulent material in 70% of cases in the Mickal and Sellmann series.

TREATMENT OF RUPTURED TUBO-OVARIAN ABSCESS

The longer the delay in the operative treatment of ruptured tubo-ovarian abscess, the higher is the primary mortality. In the Vermeeren and Te Linde series from the Johns Hopkins Hospital, death occurred less than 90 hours after the time of rupture in 88% of fatal cases, both operative and non-operative.

The treatment of patients with ruptured tubo-ovarian abscess may be divided into three phases: the preoperative, the operative, and the postoperative.

PREOPERATIVE PHASE. Operation should be undertaken after rapid but adequate preoperative preparation. The patients should be typed and cross-matched with 1500 ml blood. Monitoring of central venous pressure is essential for proper evaluation of the hemodynamics of this condition because many patients will be dehydrated, in shock, and also anemic. Variable amounts of fluid, sometimes tremendous, will have been lost into the peritoneal cavity and intestinal tract because of peritonitis. Emergency blood chemistry determinations are obtained and intravenous fluids are started immediately, including Ringer's lactate or normal saline. Vigorous broad-spectrum intravenous antibiotic therapy should be instituted. An indwelling urethral catheter is used to monitor fluid intake with hourly urine output. Generally, it is advantageous to insert a Cantor or Miller–Abbott intestinal tube before operation. Combating shock is a primary concern throughout treatment. When the patient has been properly prepared, immediate surgery should be undertaken.

OPERATIVE PHASE. Blood transfusion should be started before surgery. The anesthetic of choice depends on the preference and experience of the anesthesiologist and the medical condition of the patient.

The operation should be performed as rapidly as possible. Since access to the upper abdomen may be required, a lower midline incision should be done. It can be extended above the umbilicus if necessary. The patient should not be put in the Trendelenburg position until the abdomen is packed off, and no more of a dependent position should be used than is needed to prevent further dissemination of pus into the upper abdomen. The operation of choice is removal of the free pus, together with the abscess, the uterus, the tubes, and usually the ovaries. Only occasionally is it possible to leave the opposite ovary in the patient with a ruptured pelvic abscess. If rupture has occurred from a strictly unilateral tubo-ovarian abscess, with a relatively normal tube and ovary on the opposite side, a unilateral salpingo-oophorectomy may be done, especially if the patient is young. However, the risk of a recurrent abscess in the opposite ovary will be high if the uterus is also left in place. When the uterus is removed along with the tubo-ovarian abscess, the risk of recurrent abscess in the opposite adnexa is reduced. When hysterectomy is performed, usually a total hysterectomy can be done. However, even in the best surgical hands, a subtotal hysterectomy is faster than a total one and is sometimes justified. It is probable that the mortality rate would be increased if one insisted on always doing a total hysterectomy. Although we believe firmly in total hysterectomy, we do not believe in persisting in it when the danger of total hysterectomy exceeds the danger stemming from a retained cervix. Except in the young female, it is preferable to remove the corpus in these cases than to perform a unilateral adnexectomy alone. Furthermore, the opposite adnexa will be significantly involved in the majority of patients and subsequent operation may be nec-

essary if conservation of one side is practiced, as was required in 35% of Pedowitz and Bloomfield's cases.

In 1977, Rivlin and Hunt used conservative pelvic surgery combined with intra- and postoperative peritoneal lavage with antibiotics in 113 women with generalized peritonitis due to ruptured tubo-ovarian abscess. The uterus, ovaries, and tubes were retained whenever possible. Either one or both of the adnexa were retained in whole or in part and hysterectomy was performed in only four cases. All loculations of pus were opened and aggressive lavage of the peritoneal cavity with gentamicin was carried out for several days postoperatively. The mortality rate was 7.1% and further surgery was required in only 17.5%. We have had no experience with this method of management of ruptured tubo-ovarian abscess.

The pus from the abdomen should be cultured, both aerobically and anaerobically, and the organisms tested for sensitivity to the various antibiotics. If hemostasis is poor or if considerable necrotic material is left behind, there may be some benefit from peritoneal drainage with Penrose drains or hemovac suction catheters. Drains may be placed through a separate stab wound, through the cul-de-sac, or through the vaginal vault when a total hysterectomy has been done, but the drainage of free peritoneal exudate is of no therapeutic value. In either event, during closure of the abdominal incision, Jackson–Pratt suction drains may be placed above the fascia and below the subcutaneous fat. Alternatively, the incision may be left open above the fascial layer and allowed to close secondarily. To accomplish this, incisional stay sutures are placed at the end of the operation and are tightened as the incision begins to heal.

Before the incision is closed, the upper abdomen should be carefully explored for collections of pus in the subdiaphragmatic and subhepatic regions. If an upper abdominal abscess is found, it may be necessary to place a drain into the abscess cavity through the upper abdominal wall.

POSTOPERATIVE PHASE. Postoperative care should consider shock, infection, ileus, and fluid imbalances. Complications of the late postoperative period include pelvic and abdominal abscesses, intestinal obstruction, intestinal fistulas, incisional breakdown with or without evisceration, pulmonary embolus, and continued sepsis. Serious medical diseases such as uncontrolled diabetes or renal or pulmonary failure (ARDS) further complicate recovery from this potentially lethal disease.

Septic shock should be combated with whole blood, Ringer's lactate, or normal saline and, if necessary, dextran and norepinephrine intravenously (see Septic Shock in this chapter). Infection is controlled by the continued, aggressive use of broad-spectrum intravenous antibiotics until the patient can take antibiotics orally. The semi-Fowler's position may help prevent subdiaphragmatic abscess formation.

Constant intestinal suction by means of a long intestinal tube is a very important feature of postoperative care. Adynamic ileus persists postoperatively for a variable period and is best treated with the long intestinal tube.

Close attention to fluid balance and blood chemistry determinations is mandatory. Not infrequently, patients with ruptured tubo-ovarian abscess have poor kidney function. The fluid output and serum creatinine should be followed closely.

The results of the above therapeutic measures have been gratifying. Our current mortality rate for this formerly lethal disease is 3.5%.

Surgery for Chronic Pelvic Inflammatory Disease

Although the gonococcus may be responsible for initiating acute salpingitis, which is short-lived, the residual chronic salpingitis is usually due to secondary invaders, both aerobic and anaerobic or perhaps to an initial infection with *C. trachomatis*. As a result of the initial infection or from subsequent secondary exacerbations, the fimbria may become occluded and the tubes bound to the ovaries with adhesions. In addition, the bowel may become adherent to the broad ligament, and the fascia and loose connective tissue of the broad ligament may be converted into an indurated, brawny structure typical of ligneous induration. This may extend to include tissues beneath the peritoneum on the lateral pelvic sidewall where ligneous pelvic cellulitis may cause ureteral obstruction. If the chronic infection persists, serous effusion from the inflammatory process within the endosalpinx will produce a hydrosalpinx that may ignite periodically with secondary subacute pelvic infection or may progress to produce a pyosalpinx and tubo-ovarian abscess. If the chronic infection is left untreated or is treated inadequately, spontaneous intra-abdominal rupture or leakage of an old tubo-ovarian abscess may occur. In a review of this subject, Heaton and Ledger have identified this problem principally in menopausal women, with only 1.7% of patients with a tubo-ovarian abscess being postmenopausal.

The signs and symptoms of chronic pelvic inflammatory disease that most frequently require surgical treatment include: severe, persistent, and progressive pelvic pain, usually bilateral, although occasionally localized in one of the lower abdominal quadrants; repeated exacerbations of pelvic inflammatory disease requiring multiple hospitalizations and recurrent medical treatment; progressive enlargement of a tubo-ovarian inflammatory mass, especially if it cannot be distinguished from a neoplastic tumor of the ovary; severe dyspareunia related to the pelvic infection; and bilateral ureteral obstruction from ligneous pelvic cellulitis. It was formerly accepted that a history of previous colpotomy for drainage of pelvic abscess was sufficient reason in itself to justify definitive abdominal surgery later for removal of the uterus and adnexa. We have seen several patients who have become pregnant following posterior colpotomy for drainage of a cul-de-sac abscess and who have remained relatively free of symptoms for long periods. Today, previous posterior colpotomy for pelvic abscess drainage is not a sufficient indication by itself for definitive abdominal surgery.

SELECTION OF OPERATION

The final decision on the proper operation for the surgical management of chronic pelvic inflammatory disease is usually made with the abdomen opened. Consideration must be given not only to the pathologic lesions found at operation but also to the patient's age, parity, desire for children, previous history of pelvic disease, and other associated pelvic disease and symptoms. Because a knowledge of all these is essential to the best surgical judgment, the operator should be thoroughly familiar with the patient and her history.

In the surgical management of chronic pelvic inflammatory disease, the question of the removal or retention of the ovary at the time of hysterectomy and salpingectomy has been left open to conjecture and individual surgical opinion in most instances. This question was the subject of a study by Weiner and Wallach of the ovarian histology in ovaries removed from patients with pelvic inflammatory disease. They found that in 40 consecutive women who underwent oophorectomy during surgical treatment of pelvic inflammatory disease, nearly 50% of the removed ovaries were free of inflammatory disease and demonstrated normal follicular activity. The study concluded that ovarian histology was more often normal among patients who gave no history of dysfunctional uterine bleeding or who are operated on for salpingitis. Therefore, the menstrual history of such patients should be extremely helpful in the decision regarding ovarian conservation or ablation. Kirtley and Benigno have reviewed our experience with ovarian conservation at the time of surgery for pelvic inflammatory disease. In this series, 98 (82%) patients who required surgery had a total abdominal hysterectomy and bilateral salpingo-oophorectomy. In 22 patients (18%), either part or all of an ovary was retained. Of the 22 patients, 15 were available for follow-up hormonal assays. The mean follow-up time was 58 months. Cyclic ovarian function could be confirmed in all but two patients. In the two patients with ovarian failure, other significant disease processes were also present. No patient suffered a complication as a result of adnexal conservation. We believe that normal ovarian tissue should be conserved at the time of definitive surgery for pelvic inflammatory disease. A small hydrosalpinx on the same side as the normal ovary may be left in place so that ovarian blood supply will not be disturbed in any attempt to remove the tube.

As illustrated in Figure 13–5A, the release of peritubal adhesions for chronic pelvic inflammatory disease is indicated occasionally in women in whom future childbearing is desired, provided the tubes can be shown to be patent. This type of procedure, more fully discussed in Chapter 16, provides the most rewarding pregnancy rate of all types of tubal reconstructive surgery. More frequently, one tube is hopelessly closed and the opposite tube is patent after release of adhesions. In such a case, unilateral salpingectomy may be required if reconstructive surgery is not possible. Many other procedures are available in the treatment of this disease, including salpingo-oophorectomy with or without hysterectomy (Fig. 13–5B–E).

In a majority of instances of surgery for chronic pelvic inflammatory disease, total abdominal hysterectomy and bilateral salpingo-oophorectomy is necessary to remove the primary tubal pathology due to inflammatory damage of both tubes and ovaries. The total abdominal hysterectomy and bilateral salpingo-oophorectomy illustrated in Figure 13–6 was done for severe actinomycosis infection.

Should the uterus be removed and an ovary preserved, it may be preferable to leave the entire adnexa in place in the absence of active tubal infection rather than to compromise the venous drainage or the arterial blood supply to the ovary with subsequent cystic changes that may require an additional operative procedure. Once the continuity of the tubal lumen from the uterine cavity is broken, the chronically inflamed tube does not usually produce subsequent symptoms, as shown by Falk in his series of cases with cornual tubal resection. When it is considered advisable to remove both adnexa owing to the extent of the tubo-ovarian disease, a total hysterectomy is also advisable unless the uterus is hopelessly encased in pelvic scar tissue and densely adherent to the pelvic viscera. Usually the uterus can be removed without difficulty, which provides an easier opportunity to peritonize the operative site and avoid additional postoperative adhesions. However, there is a place for mature surgical judgment in this instance, and discretion will dictate whether a subtotal hysterectomy rather than a total hysterectomy is surgically advisable.

In the optimum case, especially in a young woman who wishes to establish or maintain the possibility of future fertility, conservative surgery may be desirable with the hope that pregnancy can be accomplished through *in vitro* fertilization techniques. In this situation, the uterus and one adnexa should be conserved, and the ovary should be positioned in the pelvis so an ovum may be harvested later through the laparoscope.

SALPINGECTOMY

At the time of surgery for the treatment of chronic pelvic inflammatory disease, every effort should be made to retain uninvolved organs. Unilateral salpingectomy should be considered when the oviduct is hopelessly destroyed by the disease process.

The abdomen is entered through a Maylard incision. The adhesions binding the tube are cut and the tube is freed. It is held by a Kelly clamp placed on the mesosalpinx just beneath the fimbriated end. The mesosalpinx is then clamped and cut, taking a succession of small bites as close to the tube as possible (Fig. 13–7A).

Keeping the operative trauma as far as possible from the ovary that is to be retained lessens the danger of imperiling its blood supply. Experience has shown that the ovary whose tube has been removed is more apt to become cystic than the ovary whose tube has been undisturbed. Therefore, it would seem logical to interfere as little as possible with the blood supply of the ovary by hugging the tube closely when excising it.

The tube is excised at the uterine cornu in a wedge-shaped manner as indicated by the dotted line in Figure 13–7B. A wide, figure-of-eight No. 2-0 delayed-absorbable suture is placed in the cornu before the wedge is excised and is tightened as the interstitial portion of the tube is removed. If there is palpable extension of the inflammation at the uterine cornu, the wedge may be rather large.

The wound at the cornu is closed with one or more No. 2-0 delayed-absorbable figure-of-eight sutures. The vessels in the mesosalpinx are ligated with transfixion No. 2-0 delayed-absorbable sutures. The transfixion suture has the advantage that it will not slip off the tissue when tied as the clamp is withdrawn (Fig. 13–7C).

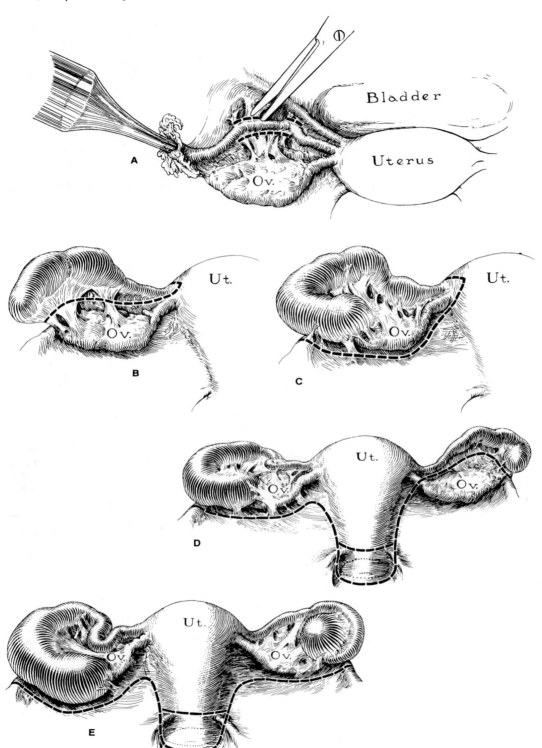

FIG. 13–5 Diagrammatic demonstration of possible operations for chronic salpingitis. (*A*) Release of peritubal adhesions. (*B*) Simple unilateral salpingectomy. (*C*) Unilateral salpingo-oophorectomy. (*D*) Bilateral salpingectomy, unilateral oophorectomy and hysterectomy, total or subtotal. (*E*) Bilateral salpingo-oophorectomy and hysterectomy, total or subtotal.

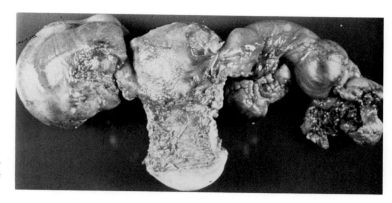

FIG. 13–6 Total abdominal hysterectomy and bilateral salpingo-oophorectomy for severe pelvic actinomycosis.

A mattress of No. 2-0 delayed-absorbable suture is taken to bring the broad and round ligaments over the cornual wound (Fig. 13–7D). This suture passes just beneath the round ligament so that the ligament will not be strangulated when the suture is drawn tight. When this suture is tied, the cornual wound is covered with the broad ligament, and to some extent the uterus is suspended in a manner similar to that used in the Coffey suspension.

Usually a second mattress or interrupted suture is necessary to cover over the mesosalpinx completely, as shown in Figure 13–7E.

SALPINGO-OOPHORECTOMY FOR CHRONIC SALPINGITIS

As in the case of salpingectomy, the abdomen is entered through a Maylard incision. The tubo-ovarian mass is first dissected free and the infundibulopelvic ligament is identified. It is doubly clamped with Ochsner clamps and a third clamp is applied to control back-bleeding (Fig. 13–8A). The ureter must be identified before the infundibulopelvic ligament is clamped.

The infundibulopelvic ligament is cut and the remainder of the broad ligament attachment of the tube and the ovary is clamped and cut. The uterine end of the tube and the ovarian ligament are excised from the uterus in a wedge-shaped manner. The ascending uterine vessels are ligated just below the cornual wound, and the cornual incision is closed with a No. 2-0 delayed-absorbable figure-of-eight suture (Fig. 13–8B).

The infundibulopelvic ligament is doubly ligated, and the vessels in the broad ligament are ligated with No. 2-0 delayed-absorbable suture. The cornual wound is peritonized, and the uterus is suspended to some degree by bringing the round and the broad ligaments over the uterine cornu with a mattress suture of No. 2-0 delayed-absorbable suture as shown in Figure 13–8C.

IDENTIFICATION OF THE URETER

Identification of the course of the ureter in a female pelvis where the pelvic anatomy has become obliterated as a result of chronic pelvic inflammatory disease is perhaps one of the most difficult and hazardous responsibilities of the gynecologist. In the surgical treatment of this disease, one frequently finds a tubo-ovarian inflammatory mass that is located between the leaves of the broad ligament and extends to the lateral pelvic wall. It is not uncommon for this ligneous induration of the thickened parietal peritoneum to obscure completely the location and course of the pelvic ureter so that dissection of the diseased adnexa produces a great surgical risk to the urinary tract and great technical skill is needed to avoid ureteral injury. Knowledge of the normal anatomical location of the pelvic ureters, as discussed in Chapter 14, is essential so that these vital structures can be identified *before* attempting to remove the adnexal masses. Ideally, such patients should have preoperative ureteral catheterization when there is clinical evidence of large, adherent adnexal masses, either benign or malignant. However, if such an anatomical problem is encountered at the time of laparotomy, the ureter may be isolated, opened, and intubated as it crosses the pelvic brim near the bifurcation of the iliac artery. Alternatively, an incision may be made in the dome of the bladder that will allow the passage of ureteral catheters.

DRAINAGE AT LAPAROTOMY FOR SALPINGITIS

Views on drainage at laparotomy for pelvic inflammatory disease have changed markedly during the past several years. Whereas drainage was an everyday occurrence in gynecologic operating rooms in the 1950s, it is used only occasionally today. Several factors are responsible for this change. Operations for acute and subacute pelvic inflammatory

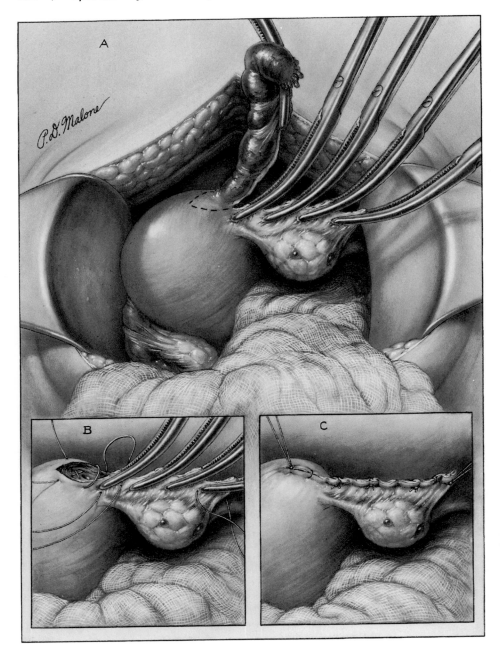

FIG. 13-7 Salpingectomy. (A) Mesosalpinx is clamped with multiple Kelly clamps and cut. Dotted line indicates cornual excision. (B) Cornual wound is closed with a figure-of-eight suture. (C) Mesosalpinx vessels are transfixed.

disease are avoided; hence, pus is encountered less frequently. Even where small pockets of pus are encountered, experience has shown that the pus may be wiped away, the peritoneum irrigated thoroughly with saline, and the abdomen closed with impunity without drainage. Antibiotic therapy has also reduced the indications for drainage. The operator is justified in depending on postoperative antibiotics to combat the infection.

Practically the only occasions when drainage in laparotomy for salpingitis is useful, aside from drainage of ruptured tubo-ovarian abscesses, are when part of a necrotic abscess wall is, through necessity, left adherent in the pelvis. When an abscess is densely adherent to the bowel wall or the region of the ureter, a thorough removal of all of the wall might result in damage to a viscus. In such cases small portions of necrotic abscess wall should

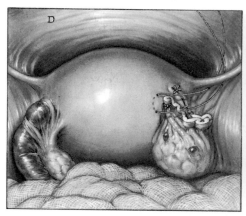
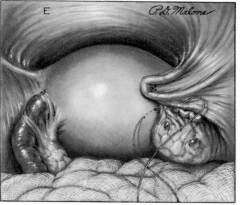

(*D*) Mattress suture is placed to cover operative area. (*E*) Round and broad ligaments cover cornual wound and mesosalpinx.

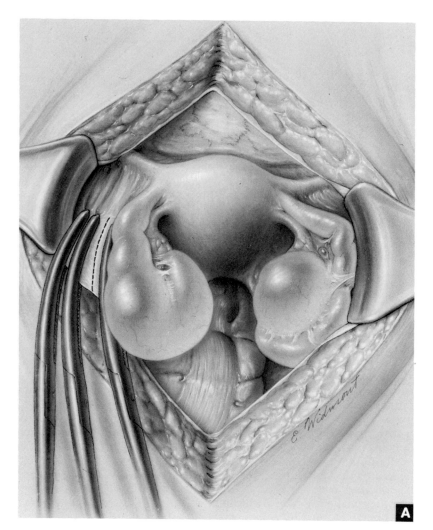

FIG. 13–8 Salpingo-oophorectomy. (*A*) The infundibulopelvic ligament is doubly clamped. Another clamp is placed to control back-bleeding. Dotted line indicates incision.

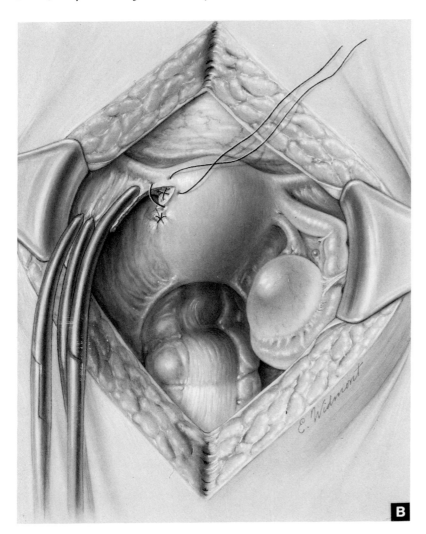

FIG. 13–8 (*Continued*) (*B*) A suture has been placed so as to ligate the ascending uterine vessels just below cornual incision. The cornual incision is being closed with a figure-of-eight of No. 2-0 delayed-absorbable suture.

be left in situ and a cigarette drain placed against the area. The ideal exit for a drain is through the cul-de-sac, as shown in Figure 13–9. Sometimes the cul-de-sac is completely obliterated by adhesions between the anterior rectal wall and the cervix. In such instances the use of the posterior vaginal vault for drainage is not feasible. When drainage is indicated under such circumstances, it should be done through a small stab wound in whichever lower quadrant is most directly above the point to be drained (see Fig. 13–4). We dislike drainage through midline incisions because of the danger of hernia formation and incisional infection. When the bowel has been entered accidentally and a perfectly satisfactory closure of healthy bowel wall effected, the abdomen is closed without drainage and the patient is placed on antibiotic therapy. If the condition of the bowel wall is such that satisfactory closure can-

not be done, temporary colostomy may be preferable to the risk of an intestinal fistula.

Septic Pelvic Thrombophlebitis

In three classic reports in 1951, Collins and associates at Charity Hospital described the pathology and clinical features of suppurative pelvic thrombophlebitis and reported their experience with its surgical management by vena caval and bilateral ovarian vein ligation. Experience at Grady Memorial Hospital and Emory University Hospital with septic pelvic thrombophlebitis and its medical management with antibiotics and heparin was reported by Josey and Cook and by Josey and Staggers.

Septic (or suppurative) pelvic thrombophlebitis is a serious but fortunately uncommon complication

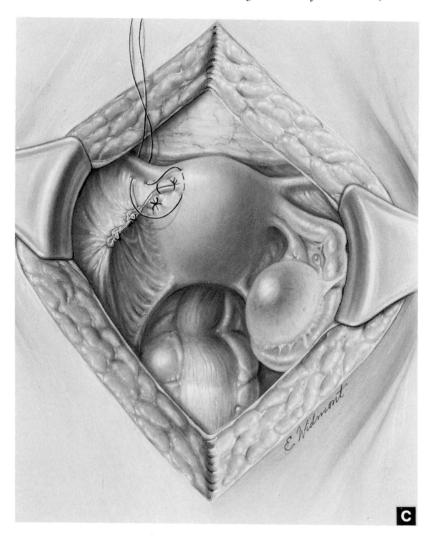

FIG. 13–8 (*Continued*) (C) The infundibulopelvic ligament and the rest of the broad ligament vessels have been ligated. Cornual wound is being covered with the round and the broad ligament by use of a mattress suture of No. 2-0 delayed-absorbable suture.

of pelvic infection. With equal frequency, both hypogastric and ovarian veins are involved. Initially, the septic process in the uterus or adnexa extends to the veins of the myometrium and broad ligament. A thrombus forms at the site of damage to the intima of the vein. Subsequently, bacteria invade the thrombus. Septic thrombi develop at multiple sites in the pelvis and may extend along the hypogastric veins into the common iliac veins and may progress into the inferior vena cava. By retrograde extension, the femoral vein may also be thrombosed. Massive infected thrombi may form in the ovarian veins and extend to the level of the renal veins. These pelvic veins are thick, enlarged, firm, and filled with infected clots. Fragments of thrombi containing bacteria may break away to form septic emboli to the lungs and other organs. The septic thrombi and emboli are the source of a bacteremia. If uncon-

trolled or unresponsive to treatment, the process may be fatal.

The clinical features of septic pelvic thrombophlebitis have been fully described, although it must be understood that only in cases where surgical exploration of the pelvis has been carried out can the diagnosis be absolutely confirmed. The disease develops most commonly in patients who have a puerperal or postabortal infection. It may also develop in patients who are septic following gynecologic operations. Few patients with tubo-ovarian abscesses will develop septic pelvic thrombophlebitis. Typically, an already septic patient will develop chills with a characteristic and erratic, high-spiking fever chart, an elevated plateau pulse, with a protracted course. The patient will appear amazingly well in spite of serious manifestations of infection. She will not complain of pain, and abdom-

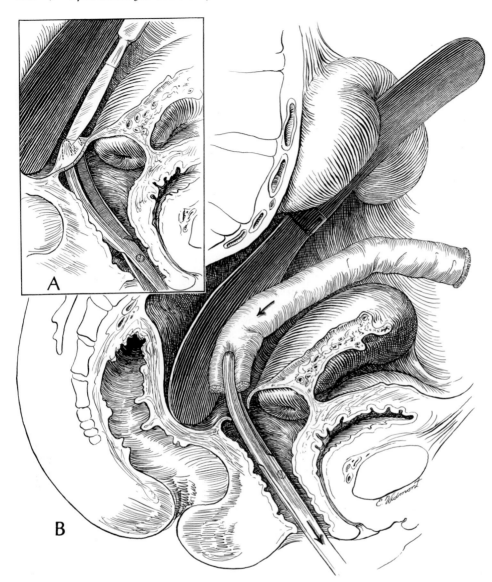

FIG. 13–9 Drainage of pelvis through cul-de-sac. (A) A long Kelly clamp is inserted into the vagina and opened slightly as the cul-de-sac is pushed upward. The scalpel incises between the jaws of the clamp. (B) Drain has been placed in the jaws of the clamp, and the clamp is withdrawn into the vagina.

inal and pelvic examination will elicit minimal tenderness. On careful pelvic examination, one may be able to feel thrombi in pelvic veins. Blood cultures may be positive for α-hemolytic streptococci, *E. coli*, anaerobic streptococci, Bacteroides species, and other bacteria. The most reliable evidence of septic pelvic thrombophlebitis is the occurrence of a septic embolism, usually to the lung, in a patient who has a pelvic infection. These septic emboli may be multiple but are not often fatal initially. Usually one has time to make the diagnosis and institute effective therapy. One of the most reliable signs of septic pelvic thrombophletibis is the failure of a patient

with pelvic sepsis to respond to antibiotics that are usually effective.

When the diagnosis of septic pelvic thrombophlebitis is made or suspected, heparin therapy should be instituted. The prompt response and improvement will often be dramatic. The temperature and pulse will quickly return to normal. The dramatic response to heparin therapy is so consistent that its absence may indicate that the patient does not have septic pelvic thrombophlebitis.

Collins and his colleagues advised immediate vena caval and bilateral ovarian vein ligation when a diagnosis of septic pelvic thrombophlebitis was made. Currently, we recommend conservative medical therapy for patients with a clinical diagnosis of septic pelvic thrombophlebitis. This should include anticoagulation with heparin. Intravenous antibiotics, preferably a combination effective against anaerobic and aerobic organisms, should be used. If used early, anticoagulation should prevent septic embolization and hasten recovery from this debilitating pyosepticemia. Surgery should be reserved for those few patients who do not respond to medical management or continue to show evidence of septic emboli. Under these circumstances, surgery may be life-saving and should be done without hesitation. The operation should include vena cava ligation or clipping plus bilateral ovarian vein ligation. The level of vessel ligation will depend on how far the thrombus has extended. Hysterectomy and removal of adnexal organs will depend on the nature and extent of the pelvic infection. Antibiotics should be continued, and adjunctive anticoagulation is recommended to inhibit further thrombus formation and propagation. When in the course of this disease a pelvic abscess is found that is amenable to drainage, it should be drained. Drainage of a pelvic abscess adds greatly to the successful resolution of pelvic infection.

Septic Shock

Between 2% and 6% of patients with septic abortion will develop septic shock. In addition, septic shock is a recognized complication of advanced pelvic neoplastic disease, ruptured tubo-ovarian abscess, chronic chorioamnionitis, and acute pyelonephritis. The elderly patient is more susceptible to bacteremic shock. This complication is usually associated with some precipitating event such as pelvic surgery, instrumentation of the urinary tract, immunosuppression, or in the case of septic abortion, secondary intrauterine infection following instrumentation. Patients with urinary tract infection, diabetes, or hepatic disease are also more susceptible to bacteremic shock. This condition is most usually caused by an endotoxin liberated by lysis of gram-negative bacteria, such as *E. coli, Bacteroides fragilis, Aerobacter aerogenes, Proteus mirabilis* or *Pseudomonas aeruginosa*. A more lethal and less common exotoxin is synthesized and excreted by *Clostridium perfringens*. *S. aureus* will also produce an exotoxin and profound septic shock. Although *E. coli* accounts for more than 50% of the cases of septic shock, almost any microorganism can cause this bacteremic disease. Many causative organisms are a part of the host's normal flora, including skin, colon, and va-

gina. Therefore, the finding of *C. perfringens* on a gram stain or culture from exudate in the vagina or cervical canal does not provide absolute evidence of a gas gangrene infection in the uterus. Since isolated intrauterine cultures are difficult to obtain without contamination, serial blood cultures, both aerobic and anaerobic, are required at 4-hour to 6-hour intervals and at the peak of a temperature rise for bacteriologic diagnosis.

In 1951, Waisbren pointed out the specific shock-like picture in patients with gram-negative bacteremia. The effect of the endotoxin produced from the degenerating bacterial cell wall was first proposed by Borden and Hall in 1951 and later confirmed by Braude and associates in 1953.

CLINICAL FEATURES OF SEPTIC SHOCK

The earliest symptoms of septic shock are rarely recognized by either the clinician or the patient. They include mild anxiety, mental confusion, and, later, disorientation. The earliest clinical signs are of respiratory distress with hyperventilation due to increased levels of norepinephrine, which may be clinically misinterpreted as atelectasis, pneumonia, possible pulmonary embolism, or even myocardial infarction. Patients may also have a transient subnormal temperature, which may coincide with a low white blood cell count. A very favorable outcome to treatment can be expected if the disease is detected at this early stage. The early clinical signs include endotoxin-induced hyperventilation associated with respiratory alkalosis, a normal or high central venous pressure, low peripheral resistance, hypotension, oliguria, and warm, dry extremities. These changes result from an increased cardiac output at the onset of this disease and a striking decline in calculated peripheral resistance, as initially documented by Blain and associates. This hyperdynamic and alkalotic state is manifested by warm extremities and is frequently called warm shock. However, progression of the shock state is typically followed by the more usual signs of hypotension, shaking chills, spiking fever frequently above 104°F, and cool, cyanotic extremities. Acidemia results as vascular perfusion fails and lactic acidosis supervenes. This late stage of endotoxic shock is described, physiologically, as stagnant shock and is due to prolonged tissue anoxia and acidosis as a result of increased venous (efferent) constriction of the capillary bed while the afferent arteriolar sphincter loses its tonicity with progressive acidosis (Fig. 13–10). These hemodynamic changes allow blood to enter the peripheral circulation, which is then trapped in the microcirculation, producing

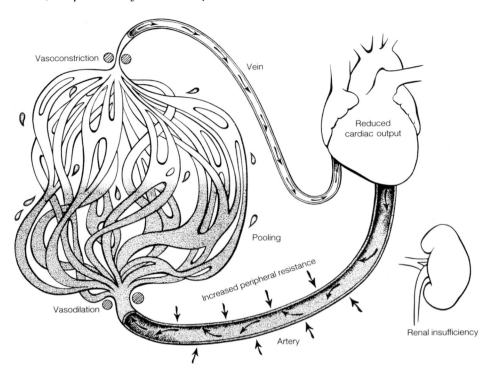

FIG. 13-10 Late (stagnant) septic shock with vasodilatation of afferent arteriole, peripheral pooling in micro circulation due to vasoconstriction of efferent capillary, tissue acidosis and reduced venous return to heart. These hemodynamic changes impair circulation to the kidney, lung, heart, brain, intestines, and other vital organs.

massive peripheral pooling and reduced venous return to the heart. The trapped blood ultimately causes the plasma to be forced into the extravascular space and interstitial tissues by the increased hydrostatic pressure. The circulating blood volume is thereby decreased and hemoconcentration occurs. Nausea, vomiting, and diarrhea, occasionally bloody, are clinical manifestations of vasospasm involving the intestinal tract. Oliguria and subsequent anuria present clinical signs of advanced vasoconstriction and renal ischemia.

When septic shock results from the exotoxin secreted by *C. perfringens,* the histotoxic effect of the gram-positive, encapsulated bacillus produces not only profound vasomotor collapse but also massive intravascular hemolysis with secondary anemia. The exotoxin also has a specific nephrotoxic effect, resulting in acute tubular necrosis and prolonged anuria that requires the use of renal dialysis. The tissue effect of gas gangrene is that of anaerobic myositis, including both skeletal and myocardial muscle. The very high mortality of advanced septic shock caused by a clostridial infection is due to cardiac arrhythmia and, finally, cardiac arrest.

PATHOPHYSIOLOGY OF SEPTIC SHOCK

Septic shock occurs in two phases. Vasodilatation occurs initially (the hyperdynamic phase) with high cardiac output and low peripheral resistance. Later, capillary leakage from the peripheral vascular bed and peripheral vascular pooling leads to hypovolemia. Advanced shock results, which is often irreversible.

The important targets of bacteremic shock are the cardiac output and the microcirculation of the peripheral capillary bed. Prior to the development of clinical shock, the endotoxemia produces an increase in cardiac output and a decline in peripheral vascular resistance, which are associated with hyperventilation and mental confusion, yet warm extremities. The duration of the warm phase varies from 30 minutes to 16 hours, and response to treatment is good. As the shock-like picture progresses, the peripheral resistance invariably increases and intense vasoconstriction results with peripheral vascular pooling, hemoconcentration, decreased venous return, and, ultimately, diminished cardiac output and lactic acidosis. The lower the cardiac output, the more likely it is that lactic acidosis will be fatal. Weil and Nishijama have shown that the cardiac output is a valuable prognostic indicator of the severity of the disease and the ultimate outcome of treatment. It is important to understand that it is the hemodynamic state of the patient prior to treatment rather than the treatment itself that influences the recovery and the mortality rates from this septic complication.

Disseminated intravascular coagulation (DIC) is a common sequela of septic shock. The effects of endotoxin on the clotting, fibrinolytic, and kinin systems are interrelated and involve the factors in the intrinsic clotting pathway. Factor XII is activated by the endotoxin, following which the extrinsic pathway may also be activated, particularly Factor VII. Plasmin (fibrinolysin) and other proteolytic enzymes are released by activated Factor XII through the kinin system. When plasmin circulates in high concentration, as in septic shock, it has an effect on several physiologic systems. Fibrin degradation products that result from excessive fibrinolysin activity play a role in the occlusion of the microcirculation and may be involved in lysis of platelets and red blood cells. Both accelerated intravascular coagulation with depletion of the circulating fibrinogen and an acceleration of the degradation of the fibrin clot lead to excessive bleeding. Since both the clotting and fibrinolytic systems may be activated by endotoxin, either thrombosis or hemorrhage may occur, depending on which system is dominant. Further, the sludging blood flow in the microcirculation caused by hypotension and peripheral pooling may activate the extrinsic coagulation pathway and accelerate the effect of various stimuli on the intrinsic pathway. As a result of these coagulation changes, multiple laboratory tests are required to document this clotting abnormality. Although the clotting time may be normal, clot retraction is poor and fibrinogen is usually decreased. Prothrombin time, which measures the extrinsic coagulation pathway, is usually prolonged as is the partial thromboplastin time (PTT) which measures the intrinsic pathway. Platelets are usually decreased and platelet adhesiveness is frequently increased. In the advanced stages of disseminated intravascular coagulation, fibrin-split products are frequently found in the blood. Euglobulin-lysis time, which measures fibrinolytic activation, is useful in determining the presence of active fibrinolysis. A shortened euglobulin-lysis time reflects excessive fibrinolytic activity.

The endotoxin produces profound effects on the microcirculation and endothelial wall that result in capillary leaks. With the increased capillary permeability in the lung, fluid collects in the interstitium and alveoli and destroys the surfactant. Respiratory distress may result from progressive pulmonary edema, atelectasis, perfusion/ventilation disturbances and finally severe hypoxemia from the development of Adult Respiratory Distress Syndrome (ARDS). As many as 25% to 50% of patients in profound septic shock will develop ARDS and among these, the mortality rate may be more than 50%.

As the shock-like state progresses, vasoconstriction increases, producing impairment of blood flow to vital organs, acidosis, peripheral vascular pooling, hemoconcentration, and decreased venous return to the heart with a diminished cardiac output. As the clinical picture worsens, the increased peripheral resistance results in a paralysis and relaxation of the afferent arterioles while the smooth muscle of the venous capillary sphincters continues to constrict. Extensive pooling of the capillary bed may progress to impairment of perfusion of the coronary and cerebral vessels at which time irreversible circulatory failure develops. The end stage of irreversible septic shock is manifested by unresponsive hypotension, progressive coma, renal failure, cardiac failure, and eventually death.

TREATMENT OF SEPTIC SHOCK

Early recognition and prompt therapy are the keys for successful outcome in the treatment of septic shock. The basic treatment protocol should have two separate objectives; initially, to control the infectious process primarily with antibiotics and second, to return the altered hemodynamic state to normal. Such therapy includes provision of adequate intravascular volume, support of vascular tone, and maintenance of cardiopulmonary function.

The treatment of shock has been discussed in detail in Chapter 6. However, there are special considerations that must be given to septic shock that differ from hemorrhagic shock. These include the use of aggressive antibiotic therapy and massive doses of glucocorticoids. Further, the Ventilation-Infusion-Pump concept of septic shock treatment (VIP) should be implemented as discussed in the treatment of hemorrhagic shock. This implies the correction of early changes of arteriovenous shunting by proper ventilation and oxygenation; adequate fluid replacement before the use of vasopressor or vasodilator agents; and clinical monitoring of cardiopulmonary status. Intravascular fluid volume expansion can be carried out rapidly in an attempt to improve venous return to the heart. Infusions of isotonic saline or Ringer's lactate at rates of 1000 ml/hr can be given to patients who do not have congestive heart failure as defined by CVP pressures equal to or less than 10 cm water or pulmonary wedge pressure less than 12 mm Hg. Patients with elevated CVP levels should receive a more gradual intravascular infusion of fluid at no more than 150 ml/30 min along with careful monitoring. Close supervision is required for the early detection of heart failure. It is our position that a Swan-Ganz catheter should always be used in patients with septic shock so that fluid replacement, pulmonary artery pressure, arterial blood gases, and cardiac output can be carefully evaluated. A standard technique of fluid challenge is recommended. Fluid is infused at rates ranging from 5 ml/min to 20 ml/min for a period of 10 minutes. If the pulmonary artery wedge or diastolic pressure increases by more than 7 mm Hg, the infusion is discontinued. If the pressure does not increase by more than 3 mm Hg after 10 minutes of fluid infusion, or if it decreases to less than the initial value over a subsequent 10-minute rest, a second challenge is administered over a 10-minute period. This "7–3 rule" has been found to be very effective in demonstrating the rapid volume replacement of patients in septic shock. Plasma volume expansion may be accelerated with the use of 5% human serum albumin, plasmanate (plasma protein fraction) or dextran 40, not to exceed 10 ml/kg/hr. For patients with anemia, the use of packed red blood cells will provide the oxygen-carrying capability without the risk of hepatitis.

Antibiotic treatment in most clinics includes high-dose penicillin, an aminoglycoside, and an anaerobic antibacterial agent. The combination of penicillin-G, sodium, 10 million units, intravenously every 4 hours, combined with tobramycin, 1.7 mg/kg of body weight every 8 hours for the first 24 hours, and 1 mg/kg every 8 hours thereafter will usually control the growth of *E. coli*, *Proteus mirabilis* and Pseudomonas microorganisms. The tobramycin dosage should be adjusted according to the creatinine level. Clindamycin, 600 mg intravenously every 8 hours is effective against anaerobes such as Bacteroides and Clostridium organisms. However, if the patient has liver disease, clindamycin is not the drug of choice; for those cases, anaerobic bacterial coverage can be achieved with metronidazole, 500 mg intravenously every 8 hours. In critical cases in which clindamycin or metronidazole have not been effective, chloramphenicol, 1 g intravenously every 6 hours may be substituted. In many clinics, only penicillin and an aminoglycoside in high dosage is given initially until the presence of anaerobic bacteria is established. Since Bacteroides occurs in no more than 10% of the cases of septic shock, this approach seems quite reasonable.

Vasoactive Drugs

Decreased perfusion of vital organs and muscles is a pathophysiologic feature of septic shock. The use of vasopressors, although tempting, is unphysiologic and may increase the hypoxemia and acidosis of the tissues rather than improve the condition. The increased peripheral resistance in advanced or late septic shock is caused by a high degree of sympathetic neuron stimulation of the vasculature, especially the precapillary arterioles. Agents with α-adrenergic activity (metaraminol, levarterenol) cause excessive vasoconstriction and have not proven particularly useful in the treatment of bacteremic shock. Although metaraminol is known to have a beneficial inotropic effect of improving coronary perfusion and cardiac output, these agents are used only if peripheral perfusion cannot be maintained by any other method.

Anti-adrenergic drugs, including α-adrenergic blocking agents and β-adrenergic stimulants, are more beneficial than potent vasoconstrictors. Chlorpromazine has had wide clinical use and is an effective α-blocker that produces splanchnic vasodilatation and improvement in urinary output. We use this drug frequently for improvement in peripheral circulation.

Dopamine (3,4-dihydroxyphenethylamine) has distinct β-adrenergic stimulatory action that increases heart contractility more than heart rate. In low doses (up to 3 μg/kg/min) dopamine can stimulate specific vascular "dopaminergic" receptors and cause dilatation of the splanchnic, mesenteric, and renal vasculature. This vascular response is beneficial in improving renal perfusion and the perfusion of other vital organs. In moderate doses (3 to 15 μg/kg/min) the dopaminergic action lessens and the primary effect is of a β_1-adrenergic agonist, affecting heart contractility more than heart rate. Large doses of dopamine (greater than 15 to 20 μg/kg/min) release more epinephrine from storage sites in the adrenergic nervous system and the drug acts as a vasoconstrictor. When used, dopamine should be initiated as a constant infusion at a rate of 3 μg/kg/min, and that infusion rate should be increased every 5 to 10 minutes until the desired effect is achieved.

Corticosteroids

Although controversial, megadoses of corticosteroids may be lifesaving in the treatment of septic shock. The improvement in cardiac output produced by the positive inotropic effect on the heart, the promotion of gluconeogenesis with enhancement of the availability of glucose to the central nervous system, and the inhibition of the intense inflammatory reaction mediated by the complement cascade and leukocyte aggregation all produce favorable effects on the patient in septic shock. Methylprednisolone, 125 mg as an initial intravenous loading dose followed by 30 mg/kg/24 hr in continuous infusion is recommended. Cavanagh recommends the use of a high dose of dexamethasone (6 mg/kg/24 hr) and reports only one maternal death in 31 patients with septic shock during the decade of 1965 to 1976. Glucosteroids decrease capillary leaks, particularly in the pulmonary-capillary bed. This is particularly beneficial in preventing interstitial edema which results in ARDS. Until there is strong clinical evidence to the contrary, it is our preference to use high doses of glucocorticoids at the earliest onset of septic shock.

Removal of Focus of Infection

When the supportive measures outlined above have been instituted, the intrauterine nidus of infection should be eliminated by a suction curettage, followed by sharp curettage at the earliest time that the patient's condition will permit. Many clinicians would attempt to evacuate the septic uterus immediately; however, we recommend that a more conservative approach should be taken, with instrumentation of the uterus being avoided until a therapeutic tissue level of antibiotics has been achieved. In general, we defer evacuation of the uterus for a period of at least 4 to 6 hours, but not more than 12 hours, following the initiation of antibiotic therapy, during which time metabolic fluid imbalance is treated. In the event that the clinical picture worsens and the hypotension becomes more progressive and refractory to treatment, evacuation of the uterus may become more immediately necessary.

In our experience, aggressive medical therapy has been effective in more than 85% of the cases. However, if the patient does not respond to any supportive measure, including curettage, or if *C. perfringens* is found in the endometrial cavity or in a blood culture, a hysterectomy may become necessary. When a rising arterial blood lactate level, progressive acidosis, deepening shock, and cardiopulmonary decompensation follow all clinical measures of management, a hysterectomy may become essential as a life-saving procedure. When suppuration has extended to the broad ligament, bilateral salpingo-oophorectomy should also be performed. In the presence of septic thrombophlebitis, both ovarian veins should be ligated prior to extirpation of the uterus and adnexa. Previously, it was our position that when any one of four life-threatening conditions was associated with septic shock, an immediate hysterectomy and adnexectomy was essential. These included: uterine perforation, *C. perfringens* infection, advanced endometritis-myometritis from long-standing infection, and the use of a corrosive toxic douche. Fortunately, these are no longer associated with bacteremic shock with great frequency. As a consequence, a more conservative treatment with high-dose multiagent antibiotic therapy is attempted before surgery is undertaken. Patients with advanced clostridial infection who fail to respond rapidly to aggressive medical therapy must not have undue delay in removing the source of exotoxin by hysterectomy; however, one or perhaps both adnexa may be saved. The use of lye as an abortifacient is rare, but when a patient is seen with a chemical toxin and shock, aggressive surgical treatment is needed.

Septic shock is a perplexing and difficult condition to treat. However, there have been major advances recently in the successful treatment of this disease. As a result, the mortality rate has been reduced to 1% to 2% in bacteremic patients without shock and to less than 10% in patients with warm shock. It remains more than 50% in patients with cold, irreversible shock. Fortunately, most cases of septic shock are diagnosed and treated before the onset of the late phase.

Pelvic Tuberculosis

Pelvic tuberculosis in the female is confined principally to the reproductive tract, particularly the endometrium and fallopian tubes. This disease has become much less frequent during recent decades and today probably accounts for less than 1% of all pelvic infections except in those cities with a large number of immigrants.

The incidence of systemic tuberculosis in the United States has declined in recent years. Because of the decrease in the systemic disease, there has been a decline in the incidence of genital tuberculosis. Pelvic tuberculosis is found in approximately 1% of infertility patients in the United States, while there is an international incidence of genital tuberculosis of 5% to 10% in infertility patients.

PATHOGENESIS OF PELVIC TUBERCULOSIS

With rare exceptions, tuberculosis of the female pelvis is secondary to a tuberculous infection elsewhere, usually the lungs. From a primary pulmonary infection, mycobacteria spread by the lymphatic system from the Ghon focus to the regional lymph nodes at the hilum of the lung and then to more distant sites. The more dramatic spread is hematogenous from the primary pulmonary complex. This produces acute miliary disease. Miliary spread of tuberculosis is more common within the first year of primary pulmonary infection. No location in the body is immune to the development of metastatic foci of infection. Patients may develop tuberculosis of the bone, meninges, kidney, epididymis, and fallopian tubes as well as other sites. At some sites of miliary spread, the lesions may remain quiescent for long periods before reactivation and further spread of the disease. Direct extension from one organ or system to an adjacent organ or system may also occur. Organs of the female reproductive tract are usually infected from a hematogenous miliary spread from a primary pulmonary lesion, from hematogenous spread from a secondary miliary site, from lymphatic spread from a primary pulmonary site to intestinal lymph nodes and then to the pelvis, or by direct extension from adjacent abdominal organs (small intestines, appendix, rectum, bladder) that are the site of tuberculosis infection.

A venereal transmission of the disease has been reported, with primary genital infection in the woman following coitus with a sexual partner who has tuberculosis of the genitourinary tract. According to Sutherland, it is not possible to prove conclusively that genitourinary tuberculosis in the male can be transmitted to the female through sexual intercourse. Since it has been shown that *Mycobacterium tuberculosis* is present in the sperm of men with urogenital tuberculosis, the possibility of transmission through intercourse to the pelvic organs of the female must be accepted, and Sutherland presents five cases in which sexual transmission of genitourinary tuberculosis from male to female presumably occurred. However, of 128 husbands of women with genital tuberculosis, only 5 (3.9%) were found to have active genitourinary tuberculosis. When tuberculosis of the vulva, vagina, and cervix is present without evidence of tuberculosis elsewhere in the body, venereal transmission should be suspected.

PATHOLOGY OF PELVIC TUBERCULOSIS

Both fallopian tubes are involved in almost all patients with pelvic tuberculosis. About one-half of patients with tuberculous salpingitis will have tuberculous endometritis. Tuberculosis of the cervix is present in 5% of cases. The vagina and vulva are rarely involved. At operation, one may find evidence of generalized tuberculous peritonitis with small greyish-white tubercles covering all peritoneal surfaces of the abdominal and pelvic organs. The mucosa of the fallopian tubes may not be involved in generalized serosal tuberculous infection. At a later stage of infection, tuberculous salpingitis may grossly resemble other forms of pelvic inflammatory disease involving the adnexa. Unless tubercles are seen, the diagnosis may not be apparent until microscopic sections are examined by the pathologist. A large pyosalpinx may contain the caseous material of a tuberculous infection but may also contain the purulent exudate of a secondary infection with other common organisms. Tubercles form in the lining of the tube. Some have caseation at the center with giant cells and epithelioid cells. A proliferation

of the mucosal lining of the fallopian tube may resemble a primary tubal carcinoma.

Tuberculous peritonitis is commonly associated with tuberculosis of the pelvis. Clinically, tuberculous peritonitis can be divided into two groups. In "wet" peritonitis, there is an outpouring of straw-colored fluid into the peritoneal cavity, producing ascites. The peritoneum of the parietal wall and viscera is covered with innumerable small tubercles (Fig. 13–11). The tubes, in addition to being covered with miliary tubercles on the serosal surface, are usually slightly enlarged and distended. In contrast to other forms of salpingitis, the fimbria may be patent. Within the tubal wall and tubal mucosa, the histology is typical of tuberculosis, with tubercle formation, multinucleated giant cells, and epithelioid reaction (Figure 13–12). In advanced cases, frank caseation is present. This pattern is more classically associated with hematogenous spread of the tuberculous organism to the peritoneal surfaces and the pelvic organs.

Another type of tuberculous peritonitis encountered in the female is the "dry" or adhesive type. Bowel adheres to bowel by innumerable dense adhesions that blend with the musculature. The muscle of the bowel is often invaded to some degree by the tuberculous process. Separation of these adhesions is extremely difficult surgically, and accidental injury to the bowel is common. The pelvic organs show evidence of tuberculous salpingitis with enlargement of the tubes, and occasionally pyosalpinges, and even tubo-ovarian abscess formation. This dry variety may represent the healed fibrotic end result of the wet ascitic pattern.

Tuberculous involvement of the myometrium is rare. Tuberculous endometritis, however, is common. Even in advanced pelvic tuberculous infections, evidence of caseation and fibrosis and calcification is rarely seen in the uterine cavity. Apparently, the uterine cavity is protected from advanced tuberculous infection by the cyclic shedding of endometrial tissue in the reproductive years. Microscopically, tubercles may be seen scattered throughout the endometrium, but they may be scanty. Tubercles are more often seen in the endometrium removed by curettage in the premenstrual phase and are more commonly located in the endometrium adjacent to the tubal ostia.

Tuberculous lesions of the cervix are rare. They may be either ulcerative or exophytic and may resemble a primary cervical malignancy or granuloma inguinale of the cervix. When there is a tuberculous lesion of the cervix, the cervical biopsy frequently will reveal tubercles.

A tuberculous infection of the ovary usually involves only the surface of the ovary and represents

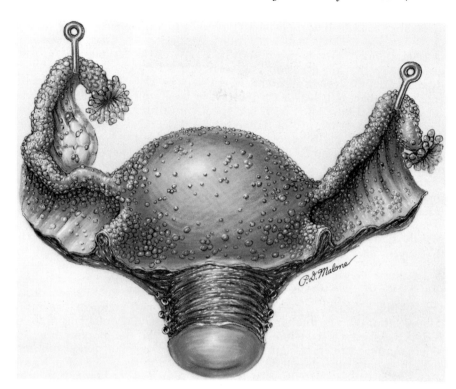

FIG. 13–11 Typical specimen of tuberculosis of reproductive organs as part of generalized tuberculous peritonitis.

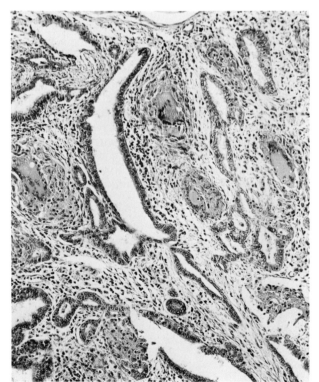

FIG. 13–12 Tuberculosis of the fallopian tube. Note the multinucleated giant cells.

simply an extension of infection in the peritoneal cavity and the adjacent fallopian tubes. The infection is usually limited to a perioophoritis. Extension of the tuberculous infection to the ovarian parenchyma may be prevented by the tunica albuginea. Tuberculous caseation may be found within the ovarian parenchyma, although this is uncommon. Presumably, it occurs as a result of hematogenous spread to the ovarian parenchyma rather than by direct extension through the ovarian capsule. However, ovulation may also allow the tubercular bacilli to gain access to the ovarian parenchyma.

CLINICAL FEATURES OF PELVIC TUBERCULOSIS

Pelvic tuberculosis occurs most frequently in patients between the ages of 20 and 40. The age incidence of gynecologic tuberculosis has changed in recent years; the proportion of patients over 40 years of age is now much higher than in the past. Falk and associates found that the incidence of pelvic tuberculosis in postmenopausal Swedish women is increasing. This was also the opinion of Sutherland who reported an investigation from Glasgow in which 26 of 701 patients (3.7%) with proved gynecologic tuberculosis were postmenopausal.

The most common clinical symptoms of pelvic tuberculosis include pelvic pain, general malaise, menstrual irregularity, and infertility. Brown and associates found that menstrual irregularity occurred in nearly 50% of patients, while amenorrhea or oligomenorrhea was prominent in 27%. A low-grade fever that on occasion may produce a fulminating septic course is noted in most cases of active or subacute disease. The failure of fever to subside with high doses of broad-spectrum antibiotics is a classic feature of pelvic tuberculosis. A clinical course that is refractory to antibiotic therapy should always alert the clinician to the possibility of tuberculosis.

Among patients with pulmonary tuberculosis, the incidence of pelvic tuberculosis generally varies between 10% and 20%. Falk and associates noted that 38% of women with genital tuberculosis had previously had tuberculosis in other organs, usually the lungs.

DIAGNOSIS OF PELVIC TUBERCULOSIS

The clinical symptoms and signs of pelvic tuberculosis should direct the clinician to the diagnosis. Today, the disease is so infrequent that it will seldom be encountered in the usual gynecologic practice and, quite naturally, the clinical index of suspicion is low. More than two-thirds of the cases will be diagnosed at the time of laparotomy performed for some other indication, or at the time of investigation for infertility or abnormal uterine bleeding. Some patients are completely asymptomatic and are found to have pelvic tuberculosis in connection with investigation for other disorders. A dilatation and curettage or endometrial biopsy will be diagnostic in many cases, especially if performed in the late premenstrual phase of the menstrual cycle. Acid-fast culture of menstrual blood is effective in detecting the organism in approximately 10% of cases, according to Overbeck. Guinea-pig inoculation with menstrual blood may be even more effective. The menstrual blood may be collected in a cervical cap. The culture or inoculation may be repeated many times before a positive result is obtained. Acid-fast stains of tissue suspected of tuberculous infection are important to confirm the diagnosis. Since some acid-fast bacilli are not tuberculous bacilli, it is important to obtain a positive culture whenever possible.

On pelvic examination, bilateral adnexal tenderness is the rule. The tenderness is usually less marked than with acute gonococcal or streptococcal infections. Occasionally, a large tuberculous tubo-ovarian abscess may be palpated on pelvic examination and even felt through the abdominal wall. The classic doughy feel of the broad ligament suggests a tuberculous inflammatory disease that is produced by a combination of thickening of the broad ligament, adherent bowel, and some ascitic fluid. On occasion, cul-de-sac nodules representing tubercles on the serosal surfaces of pelvic organs can be felt. The clinical detection of ascites is the strongest evidence obtainable in favor of pelvic tuberculosis. It was present in one-fifth of the cases reported by Brown and associates. However, other causes of ascites must be considered, including ovarian carcinoma and cirrhosis of the liver. In differentiating tuberculous salpingitis from neisserial infections, the finding of a virginal outlet in the presence of obvious tubal inflammation should lend strength to the diagnosis of pelvic tuberculosis.

The diagnosis of tuberculosis cannot be made with certainty from a hysterosalpingogram. The radiographic criteria for a suspicion of pelvic tuberculosis by hysterosalpingogram have been described by Klein and associates as follows: calcified lymph nodes or smaller, irregular calcifications in the adnexal areas; obstruction of the fallopian tube in the zone of transition between the isthmus and the ampulla; multiple constrictions along the course of the fallopian tube; endometrial adhesions or deformity or obliteration of the endometrial cavity in the absence of a history of curettage or abortion; and vascular or lymphatic extravasation of contrast material. Although a conclusive diagnosis of pelvic tuberculosis can be made only from a positive culture, these authors conclude that hysterosalpingography is a useful aid, especially in patients who are asymptomatic except for infertility.

When the diagnosis of pelvic tuberculosis cannot be made in other ways, laparoscopy has been used. Because of the possibility that numerous adhesions may be present to make visualization of the pelvic organs difficult and to make the introduction of the trocar hazardous, we believe laparoscopy should be used with particular care. If it can be done, biopsies of tubal fimbria or other suspicious areas may be examined histologically or cultured to confirm the diagnosis.

Vaginal cytology is of limited value in diagnosing tuberculosis. The cytologist must be familiar with the morphology of epithelioid cells in the vaginal smear. Only in cases of tuberculosis of the cervix may cytology be helpful. Patients with pelvic tuberculosis should also have an examination and special diagnostic procedures to rule out tuberculous infections in other sites. Chest x-ray, tuberculin skin test, intravenous pyelogram, and urine cultures for *M. tuberculosis* should be done.

TREATMENT OF PELVIC TUBERCULOSIS

Before the advent of antituberculous therapy, surgery was often used in the treatment of pelvic tuberculosis. Primary surgical treatment was technically difficult, sometimes ineffective, and associated with a high risk of fistula formation and persistent draining sinuses. With the advent of effective drug therapy, the surgical treatment for genital tuberculosis has been restricted to specific indications. Beginning first with streptomycin over 30 years ago, and later isoniazid and para-aminosalicylic acid, it became evident that many cases of pelvic tuberculosis could be cured or controlled with antituberculous drug therapy alone. There have been major advances in the antibiotic treatment of this disease, which include, principally, the use of isoniazid with rifampin, with or without ethambutol, given sometimes for a period of 2 years or longer. In 1977 and again in 1981, Sutherland analyzed the results obtained with various drug schedules.

The primary drugs that should be used to treat tuberculosis are isoniazid and rifampin. These two drugs are the most effective currently available with the lowest toxicity and should be the foundation of most drug regimes. The addition of ethambutol may not be of benefit, at least not in pulmonary tuberculosis. Severe and sometimes fatal hepatitis, which may develop even after months of treatment, has been associated with isoniazid therapy. The risk of developing hepatitis increases with age and with daily consumption of alcohol. Liver function studies should be done before treatment is started, and patients should be carefully monitored with liver function studies throughout the course of therapy and later.

The therapeutic success of modern antituberculous drug treatment regimes is difficult to assess in view of the limited number of cases available in the literature. The cure rate varies in the literature from 65% to 95%. Kardos removed the fallopian tubes from 168 patients after medical treatment for 10 months and found active tuberculosis in 35% of the surgical specimens. The experience of Sutherland suggests, however, that the results of treatment may be improved with newer drugs. The patients under treatment must be followed closely for evidence of regression or remission of the pelvic tuberculosis. Only approximately 50% of patients with genital tuberculosis have the disease in the endometrial cavity, and therefore, repeat endometrial biopsies and culture of menstrual egress will provide only limited diagnostic information. The progress of the disease can be monitored closely with the evaluation of the size of adnexal masses by pelvic examinations and ultrasonography, as well as the erythrocyte sedimentation rate, white blood cell count, and temperature response. Indefinite follow-up is probably indicated in all cases, since recurrence of the tuberculous pelvic lesion 5 and even more years after the end of drug treatment has occasionally been found.

Surgery in the management of patients with pelvic tuberculosis should be reserved for specific indications, as outlined by Schaefer and by Sutherland. In general, surgery is reserved for those patients who have failed to respond to an adequate trial of medical therapy. Our indications for the surgical treatment of pelvic tuberculosis include:

Persistence or enlargement of an adnexal mass after four to six months of antituberculous antibiotic therapy. The rare possibility of an ovarian tumor must always be considered even though pelvic tuberculosis is also present. In a 1980 report by Sutherland, the persistence or development of substantial pelvic masses was the indication for surgery in 36 of 91 women with proved tuberculosis of the genital tract treated by surgery.

Persistence of pelvic pain or recurrence of pelvic pain while on medical therapy. In Sutherland's report, 40 of 91 patients were operated on because of pain.

Primary unresponsiveness of the tuberculous infection to antibiotic therapy, as evidenced by persistent spiking temperature, leukocytosis, and elevated sedimentation rate, and evidence on biopsy of continued endometrial infection. Of the 91 women in Sutherland's report, 10 were operated upon because of persistence of endometrial tuberculosis.

Difficulty in obtaining patient cooperation for continued long-term therapy. In these cases, we are accustomed to giving a brief course of streptomycin, 0.5 g/12 hr intramuscularly for 1 week prior to surgery, and 0.5 g/24 hr in the postoperative period for 2 weeks. A persistent effort should be made to obtain the patient's cooperation for continued antituberculous therapy postoperatively. It is advisable to continue treatment for a year or longer. Isoniazid and rifampin should be used if possible. A common reason for failure of treatment is a tendency to discontinue drugs after only a few months.

The preferred surgical treatment includes total abdominal hysterectomy and bilateral salpingo-oophorectomy. However, the very nature of this inflammatory disease may make this operative procedure technically difficult, with an increased risk of injury to bowel and bladder. Consequently, in the event of a frozen pelvis from pelvic tuberculosis, it is occasionally necessary to perform only a subtotal abdominal hysterectomy and adnexectomy. Adhesions, which are invariably present and usually widespread, may make the dissection more difficult and injury more likely. However, it is usually possible to do this operation without a high incidence of bowel fistulas and other significant complications.

For young patients who are anxious to attempt future childbearing, conservative adnexectomy should be carried out only if it is possible to do so after carefully evaluating the extent of the adnexal disease and finding it minimal. It is unwise for the surgeon to be committed to a specific operative procedure prior to the time of surgery since conservative pelvic surgery for tuberculosis may constitute poor surgical judgment. The patient should be forewarned that conservative surgery will be performed only if the disease is minimal and such surgery is considered medically advisable.

Conservation of ovaries at the time of operation for pelvic tuberculosis is occasionally possible if the ovary is involved only on the surface. On the other hand, if one finds gross evidence of ovarian enlargement or other gross evidence of infection deep in the ovarian parenchyma, the ovary should be removed. Bisection of ovaries to assess the presence of disease deep in the ovarian parenchyma is not advisable.

Reactivation of silent pelvic tuberculosis following tubal reconstructive surgery has been reported by Ballon and associates and others. Reconstructive tubal surgery has no place in the management of patients who are infertile because of bilateral tubal obstruction from tuberculous salpingitis.

PREGNANCY FOLLOWING PELVIC TUBERCULOSIS

It is becoming increasingly evident from the literature, including the studies of both Schaefer and Sutherland, that only approximately 5% of patients with genital tuberculosis are capable of becoming pregnant, and only 2% will carry a pregnancy to term. It is also evident that in the presence of tuberculous tubo-ovarian abscesses, pregnancy is extremely rare and conservative treatment for the purpose of preserving fertility is unwarranted. Only when there is minimal pelvic disease without adnexal masses should conservative treatment be considered.

Bibliography

Angrish K, Verma K: Cytologic detection of tuberculosis of the uterine cervix. Acta Cytol 25:160, 1981

Ballon SC, Clewell WH, Lamb EJ: Reactivation of silent pelvic tuberculosis by reconstructive tubal surgery. Am J Obstet Gynecol 122:991, 1975

Berger GS, Keith L, Moss W: Prevalence of gonorrhea among women using various methods of contraception. Br J Vener Dis 51:307, 1975

Bircher E: Die chronische Bauchfelltuberkulose, ihre Behandlung mit Roentgenstrahlen. Zentralbl Gynakol 32:31, 1908

Blain CM, Anderson TO, Pietras RJ, et al: Hyperimmediate hemodynamic effects of gram-negative versus gram-positive bacteremia in man. Int Med 126:260, 1970

Borden GW, Hall WH: Fatal transfusion reactions from massive bacterial contamination of blood. N Engl J Med 245:760, 1951

Braude AI, Siemienski J, Williams D, Sanford J: Overwhelming bacteremic shock produced by gram-negative bacilli. A report of four cases with one recovery. Univ Mich Med Bull 19:23, 1953

Braude AI, Williams D, Siemienski J, et al: Shock-like state due to transfusion of blood contaminated with gram-negative bacilli. Arch Intern Med 92:75, 1953

Brenner RW, Gehring SW: Pelvic actinomycosis in the presence of an endocervical contraceptive device. Obstet Gynecol 29:71, 1967

Brill NE, Libman E: Pyocyaneus bacillianemia. Am J Med Sci 228:153, 1899

Brown AB, Gilbert RA, TeLinde RW: Pelvic tuberculosis. Obstet Gynecol 2:476, 1953

Burkman RT: Intrauterine device use and the risk of pelvic inflammatory disease. Am J Obstet Gynecol 138:861, 1980

Burkman RT, Schlesselman S, McCaffrey L, et al: The relationship of genital tract actinomycetes and the development of pelvic inflammatory disease. Am J Obstet Gynecol 143:585, 1982

Cavanagh D: Septic shock in pregnant or recently pregnant women. Postgrad Med 62:62, 1977

Cavanagh D, McLeod GW: Septic shock in obstetrics and gynecology: Evaluation of metaraminol therapy. Am J Obstet Gynecol 96:913, 1966

Cavanagh D, Rao PS, Comas MR: Septic shock in obstetrics and gynecology. Philadelphia, WB Saunders, 1977

Chipperfield EJ, Evans BA: Effect of local infection and oral contraception on immunoglobulin levels in cervical mucus. Infect Immun 11:215, 1975

Chow AW, Carlson C, Sorrell TC: Host defenses in acute pelvic inflammatory disease. Am J Obstet Gynecol 138:1003, 1980

Chow AW, Malkasian KL, Marshall JR, et al: The bacteriology of acute pelvic inflammatory disease. Am J Obstet Gynecol 122:876, 1975

Chow AW, Patten V, Marshall JR: Bacteriology of acute pelvic inflammatory disease. Am J Gynecol Obstet 133:362, 1979

Christy JH: Treatment of gram-negative shock. Am J Med 50:77, 1971

Collins CG: Suppurative pelvic thrombophlebitis. A study of 202 cases in which the disease was treated by ligation of the vena cava and ovarian vein. Am J Obstet Gynecol 108:681, 1970

Collins CG, Ayers WB: Suppurative pelvic thrombophlebitis. III. Surgical technique. Surgery 30:319, 1951

Collins CG, Jansen FW: Management of tubo-ovarian abscess. Clin Obstet Gynecol 2:512, 1959

Collins CG, MacCallum EA, Nelson EW, et al: Suppurative pelvic thrombophlebitis. I. Incidence, pathology, and etiology. Surgery 30:298, 1951

Collins CG, Nelson EW, Collin JH, et al: Suppurative pelvic thrombophlebitis. II. Symptomatology and diagnosis. Surgery 30:311, 1951

Cunningham FG, Hauth JC, Gilstrap LC, et al: The bacterial pathogenesis of acute pelvic inflammatory disease. Obstet Gynecol 52:161, 1978

Cunningham FG, Hauth JC, Strong JD, et al: Evaluation of

tetracycline or penicillin and ampicillin for treatment of acute pelvic inflammatory disease. N Engl J Med 296:1380, 1977

Curran JW: Economic consequences of pelvic inflammatory disease in the United States. Am J Obstet Gynecol 138:848, 1980

Curtis AH: A cause of adhesions in the right upper quadrant. JAMA 94:1221, 1930

————: Bacteriology and pathology of fallopian tubes removed at operation. Surg Gynecol Obstet 33:621, 1921

————: Chronic pelvic infections. Surg Gynecol Obstet 42:6, 1926

Dans PE: Gynecological anorectal infections. Clin Obstet Gynecol 18:103, 1975

Deane RM, Russell KP: Enterobacillary septicemia and bacterial shock in septic abortion. Am J Obstet Gynecol 79:528, 1960

Douglas GW, Beckman EM: Clinical management of septic abortion complicated by hypotension. Am J Obstet Gynecol 96:633, 1966

Duff P: Pathophysiology and management of septic shock. J Reprod Med 24:109, 1980

Durfee RB: Infections of the female genital tract. In Hoeprich PD (ed): Infectious Diseases. Hagerstown, Harper & Row, 1972

Edelman DA, Berger GS: Contraceptive practice and tubo-ovarian abscess. Am J Obstet Gynecol 138:541, 1980

Eschenbach DA: New concepts of obstetric and gynecologic infection. Arch Intern Med 142:2039, 1982

Eschenbach DA, Harnisch JP, Holmes KK: Pathogenesis of acute pelvic inflammatory disease: Role of contraception and other risk factors. Am J Obstet Gynecol 128:838, 1977

Eschenbach DA, Buchanan TM, Pollock HM, et al: Polymicrobial etiology of acute pelvic inflammatory disease. N Engl J Med 293:166, 1975

Falk HC: Cornual resection for the treatment of recurrent salpingitis. Am J Surg 81:595, 1951

————: Interpretation of the pathogenesis of pelvic infection as determined by cornual resection. Am J Obstet Gynecol 52:66, 1946

Falk V: Treatment of acute non-tuberculous salpingitis with antibiotics alone and in combination with glucocorticoids. Acta Obstet Gynecol Scand 44 (Suppl) 6:1, 1965

Falk V, Ludviksson K, Agren G: Genital tuberculosis in women. Am J Obstet Gynecol 138:974, 1980

Fine J: Intestinal circulation in shock. Gastroenterology 52:454, 1967

Fitz-Hugh T Jr: Acute gonococcic peritonitis of the right upper quadrant in women. JAMA 102:2094, 1934

Franklin EW, Hevron JE, Thompson JD: Management of the pelvic abscess. Clin Obstet Gynecol 16:66, 1973

Ginsburg DS, Stern JL, Hamod KA, et al: Tubo-ovarian abscess: A retrospective review. Am J Obstet Gynecol 138:1055, 1980

Gjonnaess H, Dalaker K, Anestad G, et al: Pelvic inflammatory disease: Etiologic studies with emphasis on chlamydial infection. Obstet Gynecol 59:550, 1982

Golde SH, Israel R, Ledger WJ: Unilateral tubo-ovarian abscess: A distinct entity. Am J Obstet Gynecol 127:807, 1977

Goldenberg H, Benigno B: Inpatient management of acute pelvic inflammator disease at Grady Memorial Hospital. Resident Research DAY, Emory University School of Medicine, unpublished material, 1976

Grimes DA: Nongonococcal pelvic inflammatory disease. Clin Obstet Gynecol 24:1227, 1981

Hager WD, Eschenbach DA, Spence MR, et al: Criteria for diagnosis and grading of salpingitis. Obstet Gynecol 61:113, 1983

Hager WD, Majmudar B: Pelvic actinomycosis in women using intrauterine contraceptive devices. Am J Obstet Gynecol 133:60, 1979

Halber MD, Daffner RH, Morgan CL, et al: Intraabdominal abscess: Current concepts in radiologic evaluation. Am J Radiol 133:9, 1979

Halbrecht I: Latent female genital tuberculosis. Int J Fertil 10:157, 1965

Hardaway RM: Syndromes of Disseminated Intravascular Coagulation: With Special Reference to Shock and Hemorrhage. Springfield, IL, Charles C Thomas, 1966

Heaton FC, Ledger WJ: Postmenopausal tubal ovarian abscess. Obstet Gynecol 47:90, 1976

Hemsell DL, Cunningham FG: Combination antimicrobial therapy for serious gynecological and obstetrical infections—obsolete? Clin Ther (Suppl A) 4:81, 1981

Henderson DN, Harkins JL, Stitt JF: Pelvic tuberculosis. Am J Obstet Gynecol 94:630, 1966

Henderson SR: Pelvic actinomycosis associated with an intrauterine device. Obstet Gynecol 41:726, 1973

Henry-Suchet J, Catalan F, Loffredo V, et al: Microbiology of specimens obtained by laparoscopy from controls and from patients with pelvic inflammatory disease or infertility with tubal obstruction: *Chlamydia trachomatis* and *Ureaplasma urealyticum.* Am J Obstet Gynecol 138:1022, 1980

Holmes KK, Eschenbach DA, Knapp JS: Salpingitis: Overview of etiology and epidemiology. Am J Obstet Gynecol 138:893, 1980

Hunt JB, Rivlin ME, Clarebout HJ: Antibiotic peritoneal lavage in severe peritonitis. S Afr Med J 49:233, 1975

Hutchins CJ: Tuberculosis of the female genital tract—a changing picture. Br J Obstet Gynaecol 84:534, 1977

Innes JA: Non-respiratory tuberculosis. J R Coll Physicians Lond 15:227, 1981

Jacob HS, Craddock PR, Hammerschmidt DE, et al: Complement-induced granulocyte aggregation: An unsuspected mechanism of disease. N Engl J Med 302:789, 1980

Jacobson L: Differential diagnosis of acute pelvic inflammatory disease. Am J Obstet Gynecol 138:1006, 1980

Jacobson L, Westrom L: Objective diagnosis of acute pelvic inflammatory disease. Am J Obstet Gynecol 105:1088, 1969

Johnson CG: Discussion of Kaplan AL, Jacobs WM, Ehresman JB: Aggressive management of pelvic abscess. Am J Obstet Gynecol 98:486, 1967

Johnston RF, Wildrich KH: "State of the Art" Review: The impact of chemotherapy on the care of patients with tuberculosis. Am Rev Resp Dis 109:636, 1974

Jones NC, Savage EW, Salem F, et al: Tuberculosis presenting as a pelvic mass. J Natl Med Assoc 73:758, 1981

Josey WE, Cook CC: Septic pelvic thrombophlebitis: Report of 17 patients treated with heparin. Obstet Gynecol 35:891, 1970

Josey WE, Staggers SR: Heparin therapy in septic pelvic thrombophlebitis: A study of 46 cases. Am J Obstet Gynecol 120:228, 1974

Kaplan AL, Jacobs WM, Ehresman JR: Aggressive management of pelvic abscess. Am J Obstet Gynecol 98:982, 1967

Kaplan RL, Sahn SA, Petty TL: Incidence and outcome of the respiratory distress syndrome in gram-negative sepsis. Arch Intern Med 1939:867, 1979

Kardos F: Late results in women with genital tuberculosis. Obstet Gynecol 29:247, 1967

Kelaghan J, Rubin GL, Ory HW, et al: Barrier-method contraceptives and pelvic inflammatory disease. JAMA 248:184, 1982

Kimball MW, Knee S: Gonococcal perihepatitis in a male. The Fitz-Hugh-Curtis syndrome. N Engl J Med 284:1082, 1970

Klein TA, Richmond JA, Mishell DR Jr: Pelvic tuberculosis. Obstet Gynecol 48:99, 1976

Koehler PR, Moss AA: Diagnosis of intra-abdominal and pelvic abscesses by computerized tomography. JAMA 244:49, 1980

Kraus GW, Yen SSC: Gonorrhea during pregnancy. Obstet Gynecol 31:258, 1968

Landers DV, Sweet RL: Tubo-ovarian abscess: Contemporary approach to management. Rev Infect Dis 5:876, 1983

Ledger WJ: Laparoscopy in the diagnosis and management of patients with suspected salpingo-oophoritis. Am J Obstet Gynecol 138:1012, 1980

Lee NC, Rubin GL, Ory HW, et al: Type of intrauterine device and the risk of pelvic inflammatory disease. Obstet Gynecol 62:1, 1983

Leff A, Lester TW, Addington WW: Tuberculosis. A chemotherapeutic triumph but a persistent socioeconomic problem. Arch Intern Med 139:1375, 1979

Lillehei RC, Longerbeam JK, Bloch JH, et al: The modern treatment of shock based on physiologic principles. Clin Pharmacol Ther 5:63, 1964

MacLean LD, Mulligan WG, McLean APH, et al: Patterns of septic shock in man, a detailed study of 56 patients. Ann Surg 166:543, 1967

Mardh P: An overview of infectious agents of salpingitis, their biology, and recent advances in methods of detection. Am J Obstet Gynecol 138:933, 1980

Mardh P, Ripa T, Svensson L, et al: *Chlamydia trachomatis* infection in patients with acute salpingitis. N Engl J Med 296:1377, 1977

McGowan L: Use of posterior colpotomy in the diagnosis and treatment of pelvic disease. Obstet Gynecol 21:108, 1963

McKay DG: Disseminated Intravascular Coagulation. An Intermediary Mechanism of Disease. New York, Paul B Hoeber, Medical, 1965

McNamara MT, Mead PB: Diagnosis and management of the pelvic abscess. J Reprod Med 17:299, 1976

Mead PB, Gump DW: Antibiotic therapy in obstetrics and gynecology. Clin Obstet Gynecol 19:109, 1976

Mickal A, Sellmann AH: Management of tubo-ovarian abscess. Clin Obstet Gynecol 12:252, 1969

Mickal A, Sellmann AH, Beebe JL: Ruptured tubo-ovarian abscesses. Am J Obstet Gynecol 100:432, 1968

Monif GRG: Clinical staging of acute bacterial salpingitis and its therapeutic ramifications. Am J Obstet Gynecol 143:489, 1982

————: Significance of polymicrobial bacterial superinfection in the therapy of gonococcal endometritis–salpingitis–peritonitis. Obstet Gynecol 55:154S, 1980

Monif GRG, Welkos SL, Baer H, et al: Cul-de-sac isolates from patients with endometritis–salpingitis–peritonitis and gonococcal endocervicitis. Am J Obstet Gynecol 126:158, 1976

Morris CA, Boxall FN, Cayton HR: Genital tract tuberculosis in subfertile women. J Med Microbiol 3:85, 1970

Morris JA: Bacteremic shock in obstetrics. In Marcus SL, Marcus CC (eds): Advances in Obstetrics and Gynecology. Baltimore, Williams & Wilkins, 1967

Nebel WA, Lucas WE: Management of tubo-ovarian abscess. Obstet Gynecol 32:382, 1968

Neuwirth RS, Friedman EA: Septic abortion. Changing concept of management. Am J Obstet Gynecol 85:24, 1963

Nickerson M: Drug therapy of shock. In Bock KD (ed): Shock, Pathogenesis, and Therapy. New York, Academic Press, 1962

Nobles ER: Bacteroides infections. Ann Surg 177:601, 1973

Ory HW: A review of the association between intrauterine devices and acute pelvic inflammatory disease. J Reprod Med 20:200, 1978

Osborne NG: The significance of mycoplasma in pelvic infection. J Reprod Med 19:39, 1977

Overbeck L: Is tuberculosis of the female urogenital tract an entity? J Obstet Gynaecol Br Comm 73:624, 1966

Pedowitz P, Bloomfield R: Ruptured adnexal abscess (tubo-ovarian) with generalized peritonitis. Am J Obstet Gynecol 88:721, 1964

Pedowitz P, Felmus LB: Ruptured adnexal abscess with generalized peritonitis. Am J Surg 83:507, 1952

Phillips LL, Skrodelis V, Quigley HR Jr: An intravascular coagulation and fibrinolysis in septic abortion. Obstet Gynecol 30:350, 1967

Reef E: Gonococcal bartholinitis. Br J Vener Dis 43:150, 1967

Rivlin ME: Clinical outcome following vaginal drainage of pelvic abscess. Obstet Gynecol 61:169, 1983

Rivlin ME, Hunt JA: Ruptured tubo-ovarian abscess: Is hysterectomy necessary? Obstet Gynecol 50:518, 1977

Rozin S: Genital tuberculosis. In Berman SJ, Kistner RW (eds): Progress in Infertility, 2nd ed. Boston, Little, Brown, & Co, 1975

Rubin GL, Ory HW, Layde PM: Oral contraceptives and pelvic inflammatory disease. Am J Obstet Gynecol 144:630, 1982

Schaefer G: Female genital tuberculosis. Clin Obstet Gynecol 19:223, 1976

Schumer W: Steroids in the treatment of clinical septic shock. Ann Surg 183:333, 1976

Senanayake P, Kramer DG: Contraception and the etiology of pelvic inflammatory disease: New perspectives. Am J Obstet Gynecol 138:852, 1980

Shafer M, Irwin CE, Sweet RL: Acute salpingitis in the adolescent female. J Pediatr 100:339, 1982

Sheagren JN: Septic shock and corticosteroids. N Engl J Med 305:456, 1981

Shubin H, Weil MH, Carlson RW: Bacterial shock. Am Heart J 94:112, 1977

Sibbald J, Anderson RR, Reid B, et al: Alveolocapillary permeability in human septic ARDS: Effect of high-dose corticosteroid therapy. Chest 79:133, 1981

Siegel JH, Fabian M: Therapeutic advantages of an inotropic vasodilator in endotoxic shock. JAMA 200:696, 1967

Simpson FF: Choice of time for operation for pelvic inflammation of tubal origin. Trans Gynecol Soc 34:161, 1909

Spence MR: The role of the gonococcus in salpingitis. J Reprod Med 19:31, 1977

Spink WW: The pathogenesis and management of shock due to infection. Arch Intern Med 106:433, 1960

Sutherland AM: Postmenopausal tuberculosis of the female genital tract. Obstet Gynecol 59:54S, 1982

————: The treatment of tuberculosis of the female genital tract with rifampicin, ethambutol, and isoniazid. Arch Gynecol 230:315, 1981

————: Surgical treatment of tuberculosis of the female genital tract. Br J Obstet Gynaecol 87:610, 1980

————: Twenty-five years experience of the drug treatment of tuberculosis of the female genital tract. Br J Obstet Gynaecol 84:881, 1977

————: The management of genital tuberculosis in women. Gazzet San 19:180, 1970

————: Treatment of genital TB in women. Bull Sloane Hosp Women 13:127, 1967

————: Latent Female Genital Tuberculosis. Basle, Karger AG, 1966

Sutherland AM, MacFarlane JR: Transmission of genito-urinary tuberculosis. Health Bull (Edinb) 40(2):87, 1982

Svensson L, Westrom L, Ripa KT, et al: Differences in some clinical and laboratory parameters in acute salpingitis related to culture and serologic findings. Am J Obstet Gynecol 138:1017, 1980

Sweet RL, Draper DL, Hadley WK: Etiology of acute salpingitis: Influence of episode number and duration of symptoms. Obstet Gynecol 58:62, 1981

Sweet RL, Draper DL, Schachter J, et al: Microbiology and pathogenesis of acute salpingitis as determined by laparoscopy: What is the appropriate site to sample? Am J Obstet Gynecol 138:985, 1980

Sweet RL, Mills J, Hadley K, et al: Use of laparoscopy to determine the microbiologic etiology of acute salpingitis. Am J Obstet Gynecol 134:68, 1979

Swenson RM, Michaelson TC, Daly JJ, et al: Anaerobic bacterial infections of the female genital tract. Obstet Gynecol 42:538, 1973

Taylor ES, MacMillan JH, Greer BE, et al: The intrauterine device and tubo-ovarian abscesses. Am J Obstet Gynecol 123:338, 1975

Thompson SE, Hager WD: Acute pelvic inflammatory disease. Sex Transm Dis 4:105, 1977

Thompson SE, Hager WD, Wong K, et al: The microbiology and therapy of acute pelvic inflammatory disease in hospitalized patients. Am J Obstet Gynecol 36:179, 1980

Toth A, O'Leary WM, Ledger W: Evidence for microbial transfer by spermatozoa. Obstet Gynecol 59:556, 1982

U. S. Department of Health and Human Services: Sexually transmitted diseases treatment guidelines 1982. MMWR (Suppl) vol 31, no 2S, 1982

Vermeeren J, TeLinde RW: Intraabdominal rupture of pelvic abscesses. Am J Obstet Gynecol 68:402, 1954

Waisbren BA: Bacteremia due to gram-negative bacilli other than salmonella. A clinical and therapeutic study. Arch Int Med 88:467, 1951

Wang S, Eschenbach D, Holmes K, et al: *Chlamydia trachomatis* infection in Fitz-Hugh-Curtis syndrome. Am J Obstet Gynecol 138:1034, 1980

Weil MH, Nishijima H: Cardiac output in bacterial shock. Am J Med 64:920, 1978

Weil MH, Shubin H, Biddle M: Shock caused by gram-negative microorganisms: Analysis of 169 cases. Ann Intern Med 60:384, 1964

Weiner S, Wallach EE: Ovarian histology in pelvic inflammatory disease. Obstet Gynecol 43:431, 1974

Westrom L: Clinical manifestations and diagnosis of pelvic inflammatory disease. J Reprod Med 28:703, 1983

————: Incidence, prevalence, and trends of acute pelvic inflammatory disease and its consequences in industrialized countries. Am J Obstet Gynecol 138:880, 1980

Wharton LR: Pelvic abscess. A study based on a series of 716 cases. Arch Surg 2:246, 1921

Wolner-Hanssen P, Mardh P, Svensson L, et al: Laparoscopy in women with chlamydial infection and pelvic pain: A comparison of patients with and without salpingitis. Obstet Gynecol 61:299, 1983

Wolner-Hanssen PW, Westrom L, Mardh PA: Perihepatitis and chlamydial salpingitis. Lancet 1:901, 1980

Wright NH, Laemmle P: Acute pelvic inflammatory disease in an indigent population. Am J Obstet Gynecol 101:979, 1968

Chapter 14

Operative Injuries of the Ureter

Injury to the pelvic ureter is one of the most serious operative complications of gynecologic surgery. Fortunately, it is uncommon, occurring on the average in between 0.1% and 1.5% of all cases of major pelvic surgery. This type of injury is associated with high morbidity, ureterovaginal fistulas, and the potential loss of kidney function. Because of the serious risk of impairment of renal function, ureteral injuries are far more troublesome than injury to either the bladder or the rectum, the other two sites of potential surgical trauma following pelvic surgery. The risk of kidney impairment stems from the fact that only one-third of all ureteral injuries are recognized at the time of surgery; the majority are identified as a result of postoperative symptomatology when ureteral obstruction or urinary leakage has occurred. Because of the close embryologic and anatomical relationship of the genital and urinary tracts, a clear understanding of the anatomy of the ureter is essential for the pelvic surgeon.

Embryology, Anatomy, and Blood Supply of the Ureters

EMBRYOLOGY

The urethra, bladder, and pelvic ureter make up the lower urinary portion of the urogenital system. At the fifth week of embryonic development, when the mesonephric duct joins with the cloaca, the ureteric bud arises from the posterolateral wall of the mesonephric duct. The ureteric bud elongates and develops into the ureter, which fuses secondarily with the developing kidney (metanephros) (Fig. 14–1). Beginning at the fourth week, the cloaca is divided by the urorectal septum, which completely separates the rectum posteriorly from the urogenital sinus anteriorly by the eighth week. The urogenital sinus later develops into the urethra, bladder, and lower portion of the vagina in the female fetus.

By virtue of their close developmental proximity, these integrated urogenital organs are subject to similar anatomical and pathologic alterations in disease. An abnormality or disease process of one system, such as congenital malformations, anatomical variants, infection, neoplasm, or injury, may affect the function of the others.

ANATOMY

In its course from the renal pelvis to the bladder, the ureter is divided anatomically into two major components: abdominal and pelvic. The ureter measures approximately 25 cm to 30 cm in length, depending on the height of the patient. In most people, the abdominal and pelvic components are approximately equal in length, 12 cm to 15 cm each. The abdominal ureter passes along the anterior surface of the psoas muscle to the pelvic inlet. The right ureter is located close to the lower portion of the vena cava where this vessel rests on the medial border of the psoas muscle. The ureters enter the pelvis by coursing over the iliac vessels at the division of the common iliac artery into the external iliac and hypogastric vessels. The pelvic ureter passes along the posterolateral pelvic wall, adjacent to the anterior border of the greater sciatic notch and slightly anterior to the hypogastric artery until it reaches deep in the pelvis at the level of the ischial spine. In this area, the ureter lies medial to the branches of the anterior division of the hypogastric

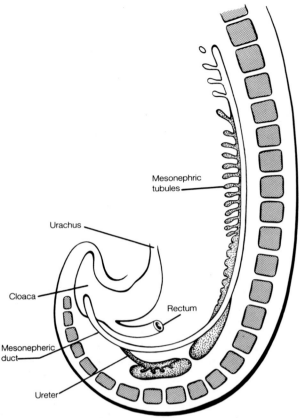

FIG. 14–1 Embryologic development of the urinary and genital systems (32 days). (Mattingly, Borkowf, 1974.)

artery and lateral to the peritoneum of the cul-de-sac of Douglas.

The retroperitoneal position of the pelvic ureter at the pelvic inlet identifies its anatomical location. The ureter tends to elevate the peritoneum as it crosses the common iliac artery at the pelvic brim and enters the upper pelvis. Here, the ureter is both visible and palpable unless the peritoneum is thickened or incorporated into a disease process. This anatomical location provides the surgeon with an easily identifiable landmark. When the peritoneum is opened on the lateral side of the ureter, the ureter's courses can be easily traced through the pelvis. Deep in the pelvis, the ureter courses along the lateral side of the uterosacral ligament to enter the base of the broad ligament (the cardinal ligament). The ureter passes beneath the uterine artery approximately 1.5 cm lateral to the cervix near the internal os lying along the anterior surface of the levator ani muscle. As the distal portion of the ureter approaches the bladder, it passes medially over the anterior fornix before entering the trigone of the bladder.

Freund and Joseph (1869) provided one of the earliest anatomical descriptions of the ureters and their normal relation to the various structures in the pelvis. These anatomists emphasized that the course of the two ureters was not always symmetrical and demonstrated that the left ureter was frequently closer to the cervix than the right. As shown by the classic study of Sampson (1904), the proximity of the ureter to either side of the cervix varies considerably with the position of the uterus in the pelvis. With displacement of the uterus to one side or the other by parametrial scarring or disease, the ureter may be drawn closer to or displaced farther from the lateral wall of the cervix near the internal os. Cinefluoroscopic studies of the topography of the pelvic ureters by Hofmeister confirmed this asymmetry of the terminal ureters and demonstrated that the average distance of the ureter from the cervix of a normal-size uterus at the level of the uterine artery was approximately 2.1 cm. The important clinical consideration for the pelvic surgeon to understand is the close approximation of the terminal ureter to the cervix and to the vaginal fornices as it passes medially to enter the bladder (Fig. 14–2). This close relationship was reemphasized by Hofmeister, who found by cinefluoroscopy during an anterior vaginal repair that the ureter was only 0.9 cm from the needle at its closest approach, in the upper one-third of the vagina.

BLOOD SUPPLY

The ureter has the advantage of a blood supply from multiple sources, which gives it preferential healing capabilities, should injury occur. The freely anastomosing arterial network supplies the superior segment of the ureter with branches from renal and ovarian arteries. The middle segment derives its blood supply directly from aortic branches and from a vessel from the common iliac artery. The pelvic ureter is nourished by multiple anastomosing vessels, including branches from the uterine, vaginal, middle hemorrhoidal, and vesical arteries. A rather constant branch arises from the hypogastric artery near its origin. The veins follow a similar intercommunicating network. Both arteries and veins can be easily demonstrated by the prominent longitudinal vessels that course within the adventitia of the ureter (Fig. 14–3). Because the blood supply to the upper and middle portions of the ureter is from its medial side, ureteral exploration or an incision into the ureter is made, preferably, along the *lateral* margin, taking care not to injure the longitudinal arteries and veins. Since the pelvic ureter derives its blood supply principally from the lateral side, it would be logical to dissect along the medial

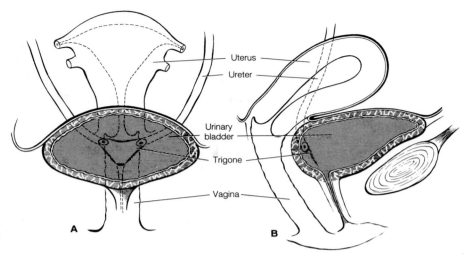

FIG. 14-2 (*A*) Anterior view of the normal anatomy of ureter and bladder. The terminal end of the ureter passes medially from the lateral pelvic wall and crosses over the anterior fornix, where it enters the trigone of the bladder, which rests on the upper one-third of the anterior vaginal wall. (*B*) Sagittal view of anatomical relationship of ureter and bladder base. Note that the ureter enters the trigone in the area of the upper one-third of the vagina.

side in an effort to produce the least vascular damage. However, because of the proximity of the branches of the hypogastric artery and vein on the medial side, the pelvic ureter is much easier to explore from its lateral side. The rich collateral blood

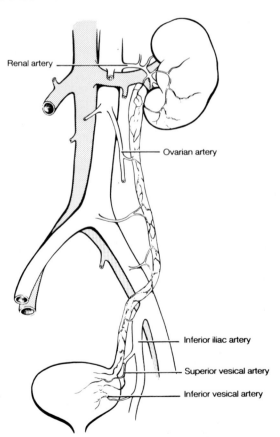

FIG. 14-3 Blood supply of the ureter.

supply permits extensive mobilization of the ureter from its retroperitoneal course as long as the longitudinal blood supply in the periureteral adventitia is unaltered.

As shown in Fig. 14–4A,B the ureteral vessels anastomose freely with each other in the surrounding adventitia. Waldeyer (1892) described this loose connective tissue adjacent to the muscular wall of the ureter, noting the longitudinal course of the small arteries and veins that intercommunicate along the entire ureter. Interference with these vessels by trauma or skeletonization of Waldeyer's sheath for more than 2 cm may produce local ischemia and subsequent necrosis or fibrosis of a segment of the ureter.

Type of Injury and Operative Procedure

Operative injury to the ureter results from one of four types of trauma: ligation, crushing, transection, or angulation with secondary obstruction. Each type of injury may be either partial or complete. As shown in Table 14–1, this complication occurs more often during the performance of a hysterectomy than any other pelvic operation. Two-thirds of ureteral injuries result from an abdominal hysterectomy as compared to one-third that occur as a complication of a vaginal hysterectomy. This difference in frequency of injury is due primarily to the fact that an abdominal hysterectomy is associated with the removal of significant pelvic disease, at which time the adjacent ureter may be damaged. In general, a vaginal hysterectomy is performed in patients with symptomatic vaginal relaxation and uterine prolapse; these patients do not have pelvic disease that would distort the location of the pelvic

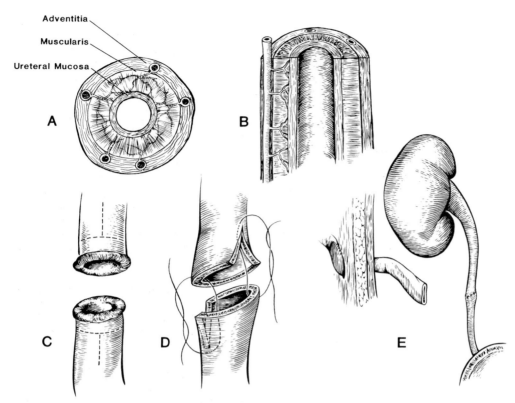

FIG. 14–4 Cross section *(A)* and sagittal *(B)* views of the longitudinal arteries and veins in the adventitia provide the important collateral circulation along the course of the ureter. *(C,D)* Ureteroureteral anastomosis. Free ends of ureter are excised to the level of visible tissue, the ends are spatulated and cut obliquely, and the spatulated margin of each end of the ureter is sutured to the opposite free margin. *(E)* Ureteral anastomosis complete with retroperitoneal drain in operative site.

ureter. A ureteral accident may occur in other pelvic operations, such as the removal of a tubo-ovarian abscess, pelvic endometriosis, intraligamentary myomata, or an adherent ovarian neoplasm.

More than any other pelvic operation, the Wertheim type of radical hysterectomy for cervical car-

TABLE 14–1 *Gynecologic Procedures Associated with Ureteral Injury**

OPERATIVE PROCEDURE	INCIDENCE OF URETERAL INJURY (PERCENT)
Abdominal hysterectomy	0.5–1.0
Vaginal hysterectomy	0.1
Radical Wertheim hysterectomy	1.0–2.0
Adnexectomy	0.1
Marshall–Marchetti–Krantz procedure	<0.1

* Data derived from current literature

cinoma has contributed to ureteral injury. The dissection of the pelvic ureters as originally done in this radical operation resulted in a high incidence of injury, even when the operation was performed by an experienced pelvic surgeon. Wertheim himself reported a 10% incidence of ureteral fistula in his original experience of 500 cases of radical hysterectomy (1900). Meigs revived interest in the Wertheim type of operation for cervical cancer in 1939 and reported a 7.2% incidence of ureteral fistula in a series of 85 cases. In a 1955 report by Liu and Meigs of 473 radical hysterectomies, the fistula rate remained essentially unchanged, at 7.4%. With more recent improvements in the technique for the Wertheim hysterectomy, the frequency of operative injury to the ureter should be only slightly above that for a nonradical hysterectomy and should be seen in no more than 1% to 2% of such cases.

Many reports have suggested that the incidence of ureteral injury has increased sharply during the past three to four decades since removal of the uterine cervix has become a standard procedure with an abdominal hysterectomy. Yet, current data do not support this view. Sampson's original report in 1902 in a review of 4086 major gynecologic procedures recorded a ureteral injury in 0.78% of patients. In 1939, Newell reported an incidence of 0.4% ureteral injuries among 3144 hysterectomies. This complication rate was similar to that found by Benson and Hinmann, who noted an injury rate of 0.58% when reviewing 6211 major gynecologic operations. In 1956, Everett and Mattingly observed an incidence of ureteral injury of 0.26% among 15,000 major pelvic operations at The Johns Hopkins Hospital. Their data showed that 60% of these complications occurred following abdominal procedures and 40% followed vaginal operations, including 500 vaginal hysterectomies. More recent reports provide similar evidence that the ureter is damaged once in every 200 to 300 major gynecologic operations for benign disease.

If unrecognized at the time of injury, ureteral damage may lead to a relatively high incidence of permanent kidney impairment. Between 1959 and 1977, Thompson reported ureteral injuries in 39 patients at the Grady Memorial Hospital in Atlanta among 9171 major gynecologic operations (0.43%). Six kidneys were lost among 23 patients (26%) where there was failure to recognize the injury at the time of surgery, the injury being discovered sometime after the original operation.

Anatomical Location of Ureteral Injury

Prevention is always better than cure; hence, a consideration of ureteral injury from this point of view deserves our attention. The best way to prevent ureteral injury is to be forewarned of any abnormal position, displacement, or existing pathologic condition prior to surgery. The following are specific indications for a preoperative intravenous pyelogram that we have found helpful.

INDICATIONS FOR PREOPERATIVE INTRAVENOUS PYELOGRAM

Previous pelvic surgery
Extensive or strategically located pelvic disease
Upcoming radical surgery or treatment of pelvic neoplasm
Suspected anomalous development of urogenital system
Unusual urinary signs and symptoms
Presence of a unilateral pelvic mass

Ureteral injury usually occurs in one of four strategic anatomical locations (Fig. 14–5): (1) in the cardinal ligament where the ureter passes beneath the uterine vessels; (2) beyond the uterine artery where the ureter lies adjacent to the anterior vaginal wall and enters the base of the bladder; (3) at or below the infundibulopelvic ligament; and, less frequently, (4) along the course of the broad ligament, including the uterosacral ligament. Injuries to the lower segment of the pelvic ureter are three times more frequent than injuries at the pelvic brim.

Of the four common sites of ureteral injury, the first is the most frequent. If the uterine vessels are clamped carefully close to the uterus, with the clamps at right angles to the internal cervical os and within the pubovesicocervical fascia, the danger of ureteral injury is reduced significantly. The danger of injury to the ureter is greatest in cases in which the vessels slip from the clamp or the ligature and reclamping is attempted quickly in the presence of profuse bleeding.

The second most common injury occurs in the distal, terminal 3 cm to 4 cm of the ureter between the uterine artery and the trigone of the bladder. In a difficult pelvic dissection where the bladder base and adjacent ureter have not been displaced adequately from the upper vagina and base of the cardinal ligament, the paracervical and paravaginal clamps or sutures may inadvertently crush or ligate the ureter as it passes medially to enter the bladder. In a total abdominal hysterectomy for benign uterine disease, ureteral injury between the uterine artery and the bladder base can be avoided by adherence to the Richardson intrafascial technique, described elsewhere in this volume. Regardless of the particular technique used in total abdominal hysterectomy, care should be taken to dissect the bladder well away from the upper vaginal wall before excising the cervix from the vaginal fornices. The surgeon should also note carefully what is included in each stitch as the vagina is sutured and suspended.

Quite differently, trauma to the distal ureter that occurs following a Wertheim hysterectomy for cervical cancer results from necrosis due to interference with the blood supply in Waldeyer's sheath, rather than from direct injury to the ureter. The important longitudinal veins and arteries provide an excellent collateral blood supply to the dissected ureter. Should these vessels be traumatized, thrombosed, or ligated in dissecting the ureter from the cardinal ligament (the web), a segment of ureter may become avascular, and stenosis or a fistula may develop. In a previously irradiated pelvis, the biologic effects of radiation cause obliterative endarteritis of the nutrient vessels of the ureter and reduce its blood supply. Any additional surgical dissection often robs the ureter of the remainder.

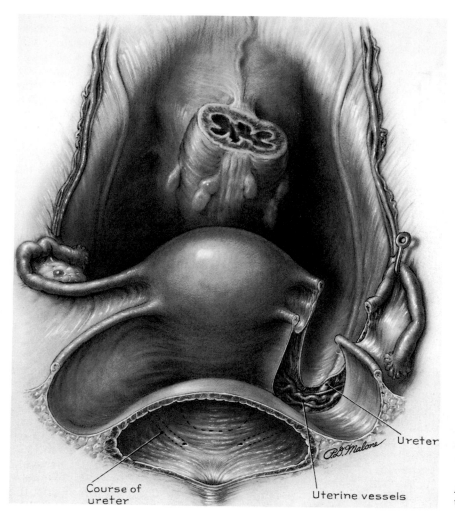

Course of ureter

Uterine vessels

Ureter

FIG. 14–5 Dissection showing relation of ureters to pelvic viscera.

The third common site of ureteral injury is at the pelvic brim. A short infundibulopelvic ligament may result from distortion of the normal anatomy by a variety of disease processes, such as a large ovarian tumor, a paraovarian cyst, pelvic endometriosis, or a large tubo-ovarian abscess. The clamp placed on the ovarian vessels in such cases may include the underlying ureter unless this is carefully identified. Prior to clamping the infundibulopelvic ligament, it is incumbent upon the surgeon to identify the location of the ureter as it enters the pelvis and to make certain that the pedicle clamp does not encroach upon the underlying ureter. If necessary, the location of this segment of the ureter should be verified by opening the peritoneum lateral to the bifurcation of the common iliac artery and reflecting the peritoneum medially until the ureter comes into full view. With this anatomical security, the distorted ovarian pedicle can be clamped safely without risk of injury to the adjacent ureter.

With large pelvic tumors, especially those that have developed between the leaves of the broad ligament, freeing the tumor from the pelvis may endanger an adherent ureter. Although the broad ligament is the least common site of ureteral injury, identification and exposure of the pelvic ureter may be necessary. When ureteral identification is desirable during the operation, it is important to locate the ureter at the pelvic brim, open the peritoneum on the lateral side of the ureter, and leave the pelvic peritoneum and the periureteral tissue attached to the ureter, for in this tissue lie the important blood vessels that supply the ureter.

When an intraligamentary fibroid, an adherent ovarian tumor, or advanced pelvic inflammatory disease suggests proximity or adherence of the disease to the pelvic wall, preoperative catheterization of the ureter(s) is both time saving and a great safety factor. By this procedure, the ureter can be identified more easily and speedily during the operation and its course can be followed throughout the pelvis without dissection and without the attendant danger of impairment of its blood supply. In the event that a catheter has not been inserted preoperatively and the broad ligament anatomy is distorted by extensive inflammation, dense adhesions from endometriosis, or other obscuring disease, the bladder dome may be opened and a catheter inserted into the ureter through the ureteral orifice. Alternatively, the ureter can be identified as it crosses the common iliac artery to enter the pelvis, the peritoneum can be opened on the lateral side, and the entire pelvic ureter can be exposed to the base of the broad ligament. The ability to skillfully trace the course of the pelvic ureter, without separating it widely from its peritoneal attachment or jeopardizing its blood supply, should be within the surgical capability and experience of every gynecologic surgeon.

Although concurrent pelvic disease and uncontrolled bleeding are commonly associated with operative injury to the ureter, of near equal frequency is the inadvertent trauma to the ureter in the absence of significant pelvic disease or bleeding complications. Unfortunately, it is in these cases that ureteral damage is unrecognized until several days or weeks following surgery. Ureteral injury is now among the most common of the complications of pelvic surgery that result in medical-legal action by the patient. So important is this complication that it is critical for a gynecologic surgeon to become "ureter conscious" and to develop a routine method of ensuring the integrity of both ureters before concluding a major operative procedure. Whether direct palpation, mobilization and inspection, ureteral catheterization, or some other means of ureteral identification, the surgeon should develop some failsafe method of evaluating the integrity of the pelvic ureter at the time of the operative procedure. An intravenous chromogen test has proven to be an effective method of providing this assurance. Prior to closing the peritoneal cavity, either abdominally or vaginally, the surgeon may quickly ascertain bilateral ureteral integrity by inspecting the ureteral orifices in the bladder trigone with a cystoscope or hysteroscope after an intravenous bolus of 5 cc of indigo carmine or methylene blue dye has been injected. If both ureters are intact, the ureteral orifices will spurt a blue-colored urine with equal pressure and frequency. This simple procedure does not require urologic consultation or special expertise in cystoscopic procedures. Any endoscopic instrument may be used if a cystoscope is not readily available, including a laparoscope or hysteroscope. Should a ureteral orifice fail to spurt dye after the patient has been adequately hydrated, the ureter should be explored along its entire pelvic course to determine if injury has occurred. It is important to keep in mind the timeless statement that has benefited many noted pelvic surgeons: It is no sin to injure the ureter during pelvic surgery, but it is a serious sin to fail to recognize it.

Treatment of Operative Ureteral Injuries

The treatment of ureteral injuries should be considered in the two groups into which they naturally fall: those recognized at the operating table and those discovered postoperatively.

INJURIES RECOGNIZED AT OPERATION

It is a regrettable fact that no more than 30% of ureteral injuries are recognized at the time of occurrence during surgery. When a clamp or a ligature is discovered on a ureter during the course of an operation, it should be removed immediately and the ureter should be inspected carefully. In many instances, damage will not have been severe enough to prevent normal function of the ureter. If the damage is slight but the operator feels uneasy about the condition of the ureter, a stab wound may be made and a cigarette drain placed extraperitoneally, adjacent to the injury site as a safety valve. The peritoneum should be closed over this site, so that if there is leakage, it will be extraperitoneal. If the operator feels uneasy about simple pelvic drainage, the prudent approach is to intubate the ureter for a period of 7 to 10 days while revascularization takes place. This can be done by means of water cystoscopy and retrograde catheterization of the ureter. This should be done at the time of surgery to make certain that the area of trauma can be bypassed by the ureteral catheter. If there is difficulty with insertion of the catheter by cystoscopy, the bladder dome should be opened and a soft, pliable Silastic catheter should be inserted through the ureteral orifice to a position in the renal pelvis well beyond the damage site of the ureter. Recent developments in indwelling ureteral stents have made temporary ureteral intubation more practical. Silicone stents that are reinforced with a fine stainless steel spring and contain small silicone projections from the catheter surface are more stable and make prolonged ureteral intubation possible.* A J-shaped stent that passes up the ureter and anchors firmly in the renal pelvis is another, newer method of ureteral intubation.

Obviously, there is room for judgment on the seriousness of the damage. If the ureter is discovered to be cut, or if extensive damage following clamping or ligation makes spontaneous healing unlikely, the operator has two choices. The severed or damaged ureter may be implanted into the bladder or a ureteroureteral anastomosis may be done. The ideal repair should preserve normal kidney function and restore continuity of the ureter. Implantation of the ureter into the bladder offers a closer approach to this ideal than ureteroureteral anastomosis. Hence, if the injury to the ureter is within 4 cm to 5 cm from the ureterovesical junction, implantation into the bladder is the preferred procedure. If the injury is in the region of the pelvic brim and too high for implantation, ureteroureteral anastomosis is our preferred treatment. However, the psoas muscle hitch procedure, in which the bladder wall is mobilized widely and the dome is anchored to the psoas muscle near the pelvic brim, affords the opportunity for direct ureterovesical anastomosis of a ureter that has been damaged within the lower half of the broad ligament.

High injuries to the ureter near the pelvic brim may also be anastomosed to the bladder dome by means of a bladder flap (Boari) procedure. Many clinics have found this technique to be useful in performing a ureteroneocystostomy on a short ureter, since a lengthy segment of a distended bladder wall can be fashioned in a tubular manner and the ureter can be brought into the end of the bladder flap in a submucosal fashion. If a submucosal implant is used with the bladder flap procedure, vesicoureteral reflux can be avoided. Others have found that the limited blood supply in a lengthy bladder flap leads to a higher risk of impairment of healing, which may result in ureteral stenosis, obstruction, or leakage. For these reasons, we prefer a ureteroureteral anastomosis in cases where the proximal and distal segments of the ureter are normal. Injuries to large segments of the pelvic ureter that leave only the upper half of the ureter intact rarely fall into the domain of the gynecologic surgeon. In such cases, a transperitoneal anastomosis to the opposite ureter has proven to be a very effective method of providing continuity to a very short ureter.

Only on rare occasions, in our opinion, is simple

* Gibbons Indwelling Ureteral Stent. Heyer-Schute Corp., Goleta, California.

ligation of the injured ureter justifiable; namely, in cases of advanced pelvic cancer where the life expectancy of the patient would not be enhanced by an extensive effort to reestablish ureterovesical or ureteroureteral continuity. In most cases of ureteral injury, a skin ureterostomy as a last resort is preferable to permanent ligation. Before deliberate ligation is done, one should have complete information concerning the normal function of the opposite kidney, preferably by a preoperative intravenous pyelogram. In the absence of such information, the damaged ureter should be anastomosed to the bladder or to the remaining segment of the pelvic ureter. If neither procedure seems reasonable, due to the patient's condition, a skin ureterostomy is an acceptable alternative. Experience has shown that ureteral ligation when the urine is uninfected usually results in an asymptomatic death of the kidney. Ligation of the ureter under these circumstances should be done with strong nonabsorbable suture.

Bilateral cutting or severe damage of the ureters is rare, and still more uncommon is the discovery of this situation at the operating table. When one is confronted with such a serious accident during an operation, ureteroureteral anastomosis or ureterovesical implantation must be done. In case the patient's condition does not permit repair of both ureters, one ureter should be repaired and the opposite ureter brought out as a skin ureteroscopy, to permit adequate function of that kidney until it can be repaired at a later date.

INJURIES UNRECOGNIZED AT OPERATION

Unilateral ureteral injury may become apparent during the postoperative period by symptoms of pyelitis and flank pain; by evidence of ureterovaginal fistula; or by appearance of a tender abdominal mass in the kidney region due to hydronephrosis. In general, a postoperative intravenous pyelogram should be obtained if any unusual clinical conditions, symptoms, or signs become evident postoperatively.

INDICATIONS FOR POSTOPERATIVE INTRAVENOUS PYELOGRAM

Loin or costovertebral angle tenderness
Unexplained or persistent fever, with or without chills
Persistent abdominal distention
Unexplained hematuria
Escape of watery fluid through vagina
Appearance of lower abdominal or pelvic mass after operation

Oliguria or elevated serum creatinine levels

Any operation with extensive pelvic disease that distorts the ureters

Questionable ureteral integrity

Complete and permanent occlusion of one ureter in the absence of infection may, on rare occasions, lead to renal atrophy without symptoms. In most instances, however, ureteral injury is accompanied by acute symptoms. The appearance of fever and costovertebral angle tenderness may indicate an acute pyelitis, but when these symptoms and signs occur following pelvic surgery, the possibility of ureteral injury should be considered and an intravenous pyelogram should be obtained. If the pyelogram shows unilateral impairment of kidney function, or hydronephrosis, ureteral catheterization by cystoscopy will confirm whether or not the ureter has been damaged. If one is fortunate enough to catheterize the ureter and bypass the obstruction, the catheter should be left in place for 14 days or longer to permit drainage of the kidney and healing of the injured ureter. If the ureteral catheter will not pass the area of obstruction, either immediate ureteral repair or a percutaneous nephrostomy should be done to preserve the kidney function. When temporary, percutaneous nephrostomy is done, surgery should be deferred for a period of 6 to 8 weeks. At that time, reexploration may be undertaken and a ureteroplastic procedure may be performed when the patient's local and general condition are such as to ensure the success of the necessary repair.

There is still controversy regarding the management of a ureteral injury when this is noted immediately, 1 week, or even 2 to 3 weeks postoperatively. Early deligation has been championed by many gynecologists and urologists, whereas others have taken a more conservative approach to this difficult complication. At present, there is some support to early deligation or reimplantation should the ureteral injury be diagnosed within the first 48 to 72 hours following surgery. However, if the diagnosis is made 2 to 3 weeks postoperatively, percutaneous nephrostomy is the treatment of choice, with definitive repair delayed until 6 to 8 weeks later. Frank contraindications to immediate ureteral repair include those cases in which extensive devascularization and injury are likely to have occurred, namely, following radical hysterectomy. In these cases, skeletonization of the distal ureter usually has occurred and extensive retroperitoneal fibrosis, cellulitis, and induration may be expected as a result of the extensive pelvic dissection. In other cases of delayed recognition, where retroperitoneal

cellulitis or abscess formation has occurred prior to diagnosis of the ureteral injury, temporary percutaneous nephrostomy and delayed ureteral repair is preferable to an attempt at immediate anastomosis. Ureteral repair should also be deferred in debilitated patients with a chronic disease process, since such patients may have poor healing of tissues.

Our conservative position on the timing of the repair of operative injuries of the ureter has been modified somewhat in recent years. In a young, healthy patient with an otherwise normal urinary tract without pelvic induration and cellulitis, immediate repair of a distal ureteral injury that requires only ureteroneocysostomy may be performed with relative safety within the first 10 to 14 days following the original surgery. The use of wide mobilization of the bladder base combined with a psoas muscle hitch procedure and a submucosal (tunnel) ureteral anastomosis has made the repair of the damaged pelvic ureter a relatively uncomplicated operation. With early ureteral repair, 3 cm to 4 cm of distal ureter can be sacrificed, if necessary, with excellent healing and anatomical results. In a report from the Grady Hospital at Emory University, among 13 cases of repair of injury to the lower ureter, 4 patients had deligation only, 5 patients had ureteroureteral anastomosis, and 4 patients had ureteroneocystostomy. All patients were operated on as soon as the diagnosis was made, usually in the immediate postoperative period. Results were satisfactory in all but one patient, who required reoperation. In this select group of healthy women in whom inadvertent injury to the terminal ureter occurred following total hysterectomy, immediate ureteral reimplantation was preferable to a 6 to 8 week delay. If there is a lengthy delay, drainage of urine from the vagina or the nephrostomy tube may prove to be a serious hardship to some patients. However, surgery should be delayed in the presence of significant pelvic infection, cellulitis, or postoperative abscess formation or in any patient with a chronic, debilitating disease in whom primary healing of the reimplanted ureter may be impaired. Broad-spectrum antibiotics that inhibit both aerobic and anaerobic bacteria have improved the resolution of pelvic cellulitis and have aided in the prompt healing of ureterovesical anastomosis. In cases in which ureteral injury has occurred near the pelvic brim and ureteroureteral anastomosis may be required, every effort should be made to delay surgery and maintain kidney drainage for 6 to 8 weeks or longer if the pelvic cellulitis has not resolved. Ureteral stenosis and obstruction are serious complications of a ureteroureteral anastomosis that can be avoided by delaying surgery until an adequate blood supply is assured and all clinical evidence of infection has resolved.

COMPLICATIONS OF URETERAL INJURY

Fistula

The appearance of urine in the vagina may give the first intimation of ureteral injury. If the ureter has been cut without ligation, the urine may appear almost immediately postoperatively. However, this is a rare complication, as transection of the ureter is usually the result of clamping the ureter within the tissue pedicle. In most instances, when a ureter has been cut or incorporated in a ligature, 10 to 14 days pass before necrosis of the wall occurs or the suture loosens from shrinkage and retraction of the pedicle. When the ureteral damage is the result of stripping the ureter of its blood supply, as in the Wertheim operation, a longer period may elapse before ischemia has progressed to the point of necrosis of the ureteral wall and fistula formation.

The classic canine experiments of Sampson (1909) provide the most descriptive information of the pathologic changes in the ureter that precede fistula formation. As described by Sampson, the most important factor is the extent of damage to the periureteral arterial plexus (Fig. 14–6). As a result of localized ischemia, a hemorrhagic infarct occurs in the ureteral wall, beginning first in the submucosa. The size of the infarct and the extent of the process depends on the severity of the ureteral trauma and circulatory impairment. These changes in the submucosa provide an anatomical explanation for the early obstruction of the ureteral lumen that makes retrograde catheterization either extremely difficult or impossible when the injury is diagnosed in the postoperative period. Although necrosis and fistula formation will usually result from the process of hemorrhagic infarction, a fistula will not occur if the necrosis is not extensive or if the ureteral wall becomes adherent to adjacent pelvic organs and develops a collateral blood supply. If a fistula does not occur, scarring and stricture are equally damaging and, if uncorrected, may produce progressive hydroureteronephrosis with impairment of renal function. Should secondary infection occur in the operative site or from within the urinary tract, bacteria may be seeded into the periureteral lymphatics and produce pyelonephritis or a perinephric abscess that will further endanger the kidney (Fig. 14–6C).

After a total hysterectomy, urine from a ureteral fistula enters the vagina through a small tract in the vault. In most cases, the appearance of the fistula is preceded by an attack of pyelitis, including a

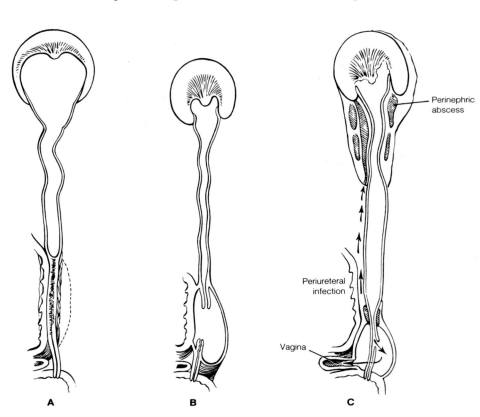

FIG. 14–6 Sampson's canine experiments showing the pathogenesis of ureteral stenosis and fistula from injury and ischemia. (*A*) Ureteral necrosis and occlusion 3 weeks following stripping of periureteral arterial-venous plexus for 1 cm. (*B*) Similar experiment in dog in which ureteral necrosis results in loss of ureteral wall with urinoma formation. (*C*) Similar experiment with necrosis of ureteral wall due to localized ischemia with secondary periureteral ascending infection and perinephric abscess formation.

A   B   C

spiking temperature and unilateral costovertebral angle tenderness. The onset of vaginal drainage afforded by the fistula may result in subsidence of pain and temperature. In other cases the evidence of pyelitis may appear after the fistula has occurred, for there is a tendency for a fistulous opening to contract and to produce ureteral obstruction. Depending on the location and extent of ureteral injury, the fistula may close spontaneously with reestablishment of the ureteral lumen. Because of this possibility, a reasonable period of expectant treatment is permissible before kidney drainage is established by nephrostomy. This conservative approach to management of a ureteral injury is quite likely to be rewarded by spontaneous healing if there is evidence of ureteral continuity by retrograde pyelography or intravenous pyelogram studies. If the policy of watchful waiting is pursued for several weeks, particularly if delayed repair of the ureter is planned, intravenous pyelogram studies should be done repeatedly at 2 to 3 week intervals, to make certain that there is adequate kidney drainage and that there is no increase in the initial degree of hydronephrosis (Fig. 14–7). If the hydronephrosis

becomes progressive, nephrostomy or surgical repair of the ureter should be done without delay. Which one of these two procedures is chosen depends on the local condition of the tissues and the general condition of the patient. The spontaneous cessation of vaginal drainage of urine may represent complete obstruction of the ureter from scar formation and is usually an ominous sign. Occasionally, the urine may be diverted elsewhere, such as into the retroperitoneal space (urinoma) or, rarely, into the peritoneal cavity, as has been reported by Hunner and Everett. Only when an intravenous pyelogram demonstrates normal kidney function with an intact ureter can the cessation of urinary drainage into the vagina be considered beneficial.

An intravenous pyelogram is one of the first studies indicated after the appearance of urine in the vagina. The objective is to show whether the fistulous tract communicates with the bladder or the ureter. The most common pyelogram abnormality that results from a ureteral injury is the impairment of kidney function and the finding of hydroureteronephrosis. A convenient way to determine whether there is also a bladder injury is to place a

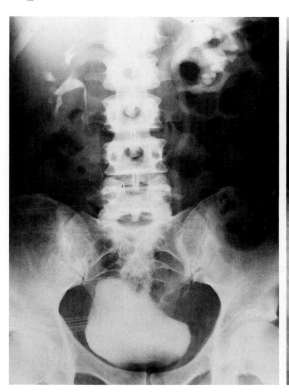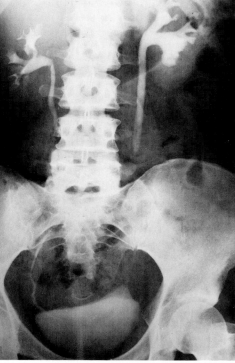

FIG. 14–7 (*Left*) Urogram taken 2 weeks after operative injury to left ureter. Hydronephrosis is stationary, but the patient is still draining urine from the vagina. Ureter was reimplanted 6 weeks after injury. (*Right*) Urogram taken 5 weeks after implantation of injured left ureter into bladder, showing ultimate result. Note the delicate caliber of the pelvic ureter.

gauze sponge or tampon into the vagina and fill the bladder with a weak solution of methylene blue. If the vaginal sponge or tampon remains free of methylene blue after ambulation, the evidence points to a ureteral fistula.

The location of the fistula can be identified more accurately by water cystoscopy, with inspection of the ureteral orifices, and by passage of a ureteral catheter on the suspect side. As a rule, the ureteral orifice will not spurt urine on the affected side and it is impossible to force the catheter past the point of injury. The impasse is usually due to the submucosal infarction, edema, and stricture formation, as explained by Sampson's experiments. If, by good fortune, the catheter is made to pass the injured area of the ureter, it should be left in the ureter for 14 days or longer, during which time the ureteral wall will usually heal. A retrograde pyelogram should be done to demonstrate an intact ureter with healing of the fistula before the catheter is removed. Before the operation for repair or implantation of the ureter that is associated with secondary kidney damage is undertaken, an intravenous pyelogram and differential kidney function studies should be done to determine beyond question the function of the kidney on the uninjured side. Knowledge of the function of the opposite kidney is invaluable to the surgeon in making a decision on how to treat the injured ureter.

Only when the final operation is undertaken, and after investigating the local conditions from within the pelvis, can one decide on the exact procedure that must be done. If the injury is at the level of the uterine vessels or within 4 cm to 5 cm from the ureterovesical junction, ureterovesical implantation is preferable to ureteroureteral anastomosis. In some instances when the shortened ureter near the pelvic brim will not quite reach the bladder, the bladder may be elongated by rolling up a flap (Boari technique). If the blood supply of the unirradiated bladder is abundant, this generally can be accomplished without fear of sloughing. However, we have not found it necessary to use the Boari method often, because the usual site of injury to the terminal ureter makes ureterovesical anastomosis a preferable procedure. In our experience, ischemia of an elongated flap and secondary stenosis of the anastomosis have produced more complications with the bladder flap procedure than with alternative techniques.

A frequently asked question is, for how long can a kidney be completely obstructed and subsequently return to normal function after relief of the obstruction? Animal experiments suggest that there is rarely any return of renal function with complete ureteral obstruction of more than 40 days. However, there is clinical evidence of recovery of renal function in the human after prolonged periods of ureteral obstruction. Three cases reported by Shapiro and Bennett showed recovery of normal renal function following apparent occlusion for periods ranging from 28 to 158 days. The major problem in defining the absence of renal function in these and other cases is the imprecision of most diagnostic techniques. While intravenous pyelograms and renograms are helpful clinical tests, they do not document the complete absence of renal function. Therefore, there have been many reports of cases of apparent renal obstruction lasting more than 100 days in which relatively normal kidney function returned after relief of the ureteral obstruction, such as those reported by Everett and Williams. Based on this information, if any evidence of renal function is present within 3 months following apparent ureteral obstruction, it is reasonable to attempt to salvage the kidney by reimplanting the ureter.

Bilateral ureteral ligation is an extremely rare operative complication that is soon apparent when the patient becomes anuric immediately following surgery. For the first 24 to 48 hours, anuria is usually the only symptom, but soon thereafter the blood urea nitrogen and creatinine levels begin to rise and the patient shows increasing signs of uremia. Back pain and bilateral costovertebral angle tenderness are usually present but are frequently obscured by the administration of postoperative analgesics. If the obstructions are unrelieved, progressive uremia and renal failure will result. If there was no evidence of kidney disease in the preoperative studies and the operative procedure was not associated with excessive blood loss or prolonged hypotension, one can be reasonably certain that anuria for 24 to 48 hours postoperatively signifies bilateral ureteral obstruction. Ureteral injury is easily demonstrated by an intravenous pyelogram, which will show evidence of either a bilateral faintly visible nephrogram or hydroureter and hydronephrosis. An intravenous pyelogram should always be obtained when the surgeon is concerned about the possibility of ureteral injury. As Sampson succinctly put it, one of the greatest aids in the diagnosis of a ureteral fistula is "the conscience of the operator." Before resorting to emergency surgery, it is our custom to attempt to insert ureteral catheters to confirm the presence of ureteral obstruction or, as is occasionally possible, to pass the catheter beyond the areas of obstruction. When one is certain that the condition exists, the earlier that treatment is instituted, the better. If discovered within 48 to 72 hours following surgery and before the patient is profoundly ill from uremia, immediate deligation is the treatment of choice in reestablishing ureteral patency. Bilateral percutaneous nephrostomies are preferable to attempting deligation or anastomosis in a seriously ill patient who is not a surgical candidate. This percutaneous procedure can be done quite easily with the aid of fluoroscopy and ultrasound, using a needle trocar (2.8 mm) and a small radiopaque catheter (1.8 mm). Nephrostomy can also be accomplished surgically through bilateral flank incisions. With both procedures, ureteral repair may be deferred for a period of 6 to 8 weeks or, if a longer period of renal recovery is required, until the patient is a good surgical candidate. With bilateral nephrostomies, the patient soon begins to pour forth quantities of urine, and the blood urea nitrogen and creatinine levels fall rapidly. Occasionally, the ureteral continuity may become spontaneously reestablished after nephrostomy or pyelostomy. If not, an additional attempt should be made to pass a ureteral catheter beyond the areas of obstruction, although such attempts usually fail. If catheterization is unsuccessful, a laparotomy should be performed 6 weeks or later after the nephrostomy, and a ureteroplastic procedure should be done. The condition of the patient will then be adequate to permit the meticulous, painstaking work that is necessary to restore normal ureteral drainage and kidney function. In cases where deligation has been successful by means of immediate reoperation, it is advisable to place a catheter in each ureter by means of water cystoscopy or direct catheterization by cystotomy at the time of surgical repair. The ureters should remain intubated for a period of 10 days to 2 weeks while the surgical trauma and ureteral edema gradually resolve. Renal function and regression of the ureteral obstruction should be followed carefully with frequent intravenous pyelogram studies (Fig. 14–8). If one or both ureters have been cut or irreparably damaged, bilateral ureterovesical anastomosis may be required.

Ureteroureteral Anastomosis

Ureteroureteral anastomosis may be done at the time of injury or at the time of subsequent repair. The procedure is usually performed for ureteral injuries that occur near or above the pelvic brim. If diagnosed and repaired at the time of injury, the intraoperative trauma is usually due to transection of the middle or upper segment of the ureter. A ureteral catheter, preferably a silicone (Silastic) tube (internal diameter 0.078 in), is threaded into the upper and the lower segments of the ureter and then into the bladder, where it is permitted to curl up

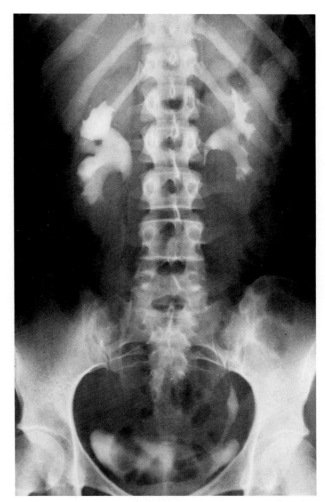

FIG. 14–8   Intravenous pyelogram taken several months after bilateral ureterovesical anastomosis, following bilateral ligation.

as shown in Figure 14–9. The Silastic tube is quite inert, soft, and pliable. It can be left in the ureter for long periods without obstructing it or creating a foreign-body reaction in the operative site. Reinforcement of the wall of the soft silicone stent with finely coiled stainless steel wire has improved the efficiency of the indwelling catheter in draining the ureter.

If the ureteral anastomosis is done at some time subsequent to the original injury, a No. 7 French whistle-tip catheter is passed into the ureter by cystoscopy until it meets the site of obstruction. By retaining the stent in the lower ureter the operator can identify the lower segment of the ureter easily at the time of operative repair. Edema and infection

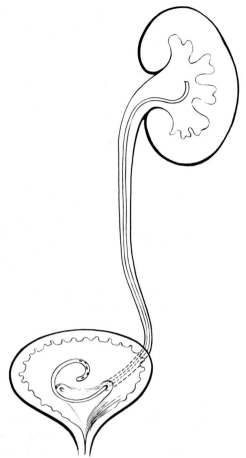

FIG. 14-9 Splinting ureteral tube (silicone, internal diameter, 0.078 in), which is threaded into renal pelvis and coiled in bladder. This is used for ureterovesical or ureteroureteral anastomosis.

in the surrounding tissues may make ureteral identification difficult without the aid of the catheter. It is our preference to repair all ureteral injuries by an abdominal, transperitoneal approach rather than by a more limited, retroperitoneal approach because the abdominal approach provides much greater exposure of the operative field. The peritoneum is incised and reflected along the lateral side of the injured ureter. The ureter is opened at the site of injury, the area of the traumatized tissue is excised (Fig. 14-4C), and a silicone (Silastic) tube is passed into the kidney pelvis. The other end of the Silastic tube is threaded through the lower ureter and into the bladder. It is removed through a cystoscope within 14 days. A silk suture placed in the bladder end of the Silastic stent will assist in identifying the free end at cystoscopy, should the

catheter need to be exteriorized or irrigated. The ureteral closure should be reasonably watertight, although too many sutures can produce a ureteral stricture. After the ureteral ends are excised to the level of viable tissue, the free ends are spatulated for 5 mm and cut obliquely to ensure a wide anastomosis site. With the ureter splinted by the Silastic tubing, the two ends are drawn together and united by four interrupted sutures of No. 4-0 chromic catgut placed through the seromuscular wall of the ureter. The sutures are tied gently and without undue tension on the anastomosis (see Fig. 14-4D). Recently, we have found the use of No. 4-0 delayed-absorbable suture to enhance the integrity of the ureteral suture line without undue scarring or stricture formation. If the ureteral wall is quite thin and attenuated, through-and-through sutures from serosa to mucosa are placed to ensure adequate approximation of the ureteral margins. Before the abdomen is closed, drainage is established extraperitoneally by use of a cigarette or Penrose drain through a small stab wound. The drain is easily placed under direct vision to a point near the site of anastomosis. Then the peritoneum is closed over the ureter. If, during the postoperative course, there is any reason to believe that the Silastic tubing is not draining adequately, the end of the tubing can be brought out through the urethra and irrigated.

This technique is suitable in the usual case, but there is a special precaution that should be taken when, owing to the condition of the ureter, it is feared that the anastomosis is not as satisfactory as one might desire. In such a case, where urinary leakage at the anastomosis seems likely, it may be desirable to leave the indwelling ureteral tubing in place for more than the usual 14 days. To further assist in decompressing the suture line, the urine may be diverted by using a T-tube for the ureteral splint, bringing one end through the upper segment of the ureter and out retroperitoneally, through the flank. Alternatively, a pyelostomy tube can be placed at the time of the ureteral procedure and exteriorized through the flank, to provide a safety valve for kidney drainage, should the ureteral tube become obstructed. If the anastomosis is satisfactory, it is our preference to use only the indwelling Silastic stent, although many gynecologists and urologists remove the stent at the completion of the procedure.

Submucosal Tunnel Ureteral Implantation

The submucosal tunnel technique has been found to be most useful in restoring the intramural anatomy of the ureter and in avoiding vesicoureteral reflux, one of the major complications of uretero-vesical anastomosis (Fig. 14–10). Although it is questionable whether minimal ureteral reflux will produce long-term renal complications, recurrent pyelonephritis in conjunction with ureteral reflux can prove to be a difficult clinical problem in the presence of a previously damaged kidney. Consequently, it is important to consider the use of a submucosal tunnel procedure to avoid this complication. It is our preference to use a transabdominal approach for the repair of all ureteral injuries, purely because of the anatomical advantage of surgical exposure. The distal ureter is carefully dissected from the site of trauma in order to preserve as much of the distal ureter as possible for anastomosis, excising all areas of devitalized tissue. Both sides of the bladder base and adjacent peritoneum are mobilized widely. If necessary, the mobilized bladder dome should be sutured to the psoas muscle near the pelvic brim to accommodate implantation of a shortened ureter (psoas muscle hitch). The submucosal tunnel to be created in the bladder for placement of the ureter, should be approximately four times as long and three times as wide as the normal ureter. In general, the tunnel should be at least 1 cm to 1.5 cm in length in order to prevent reflux with voiding. After the dome of the bladder is opened transversely, the most dependent portion of the bladder wall that will reach the ureter without undue tension is selected for the site of the submucosal tunnel (Fig. 14–11A). The tunnel is then initiated from inside of the bladder by making two small, 5-mm horizontal mucosal incisions, one approximately 1.5 cm above the other, that outline the upper and lower margins of the tunnel (Fig. 14–11B,C). The upper incision is extended through the bladder wall with a small scalpel blade and the free end of the ureter is drawn into the bladder by a traction suture. The submucosal tunnel is developed between the two mucosal incisions, following

which the ureter is guided beneath the mucosa and sutured to the margins of the lower incision, thereby establishing the submucosal implantation (Fig. 14–11D).

A mucosa-to-mucosa anastomosis of ureter to bladder is performed using interrupted No. 4-0 chromic catgut or delayed-absorbable suture over an indwelling Silastic tube (Fig. 14–11E). The Silastic tube is either left coiled in the bladder or passed through the urethra and anchored to an indwelling urethral catheter. The upper mucosal incision at the top of the tunnel is closed with two or three interrupted sutures. The anastomosis is supported with four No. 3-0 catgut or delayed-absorbable sutures placed in the muscularis of the bladder and the seromuscular layer of the ureter. The bladder wall should be anchored firmly to the musculature of the adjacent pelvic wall or psoas muscle (psoas muscle hitch) with No. 3-0 delayed-absorbable sutures to make certain that there is no tension on the suture line. The transverse incision in the dome of the bladder is closed in a double layer with No. 3-0 delayed-absorbable suture, using a continuous, through-and-through, mucosa–inner muscularis suture for the first layer and interrupted seromuscular sutures for the second layer. The operative site is then peritonized by approximating the cul-de-sac and bladder peritoneum and closing the peritoneum over the ureter. The catheter is left in the ureter for approximately 10 days. The anastomosis site should always be drained retroperitoneally, with the drain exteriorized through a stab wound that is separate from the abdominal incision.

An alternate method may be used to produce a submucosal tunnel for ureteral implantation from the external surface of the bladder wall. After the location of the ureterovesical anastomosis is established and the dome of the bladder is opened transversely, a small, 5-mm transverse muscular incision is made in the posterior wall of the bladder (Fig. 14–12A) and extended obliquely to the submucosa. After an Allis clamp is placed on either side of the incision for traction, a long Adson clamp is inserted beneath the bladder mucosa for a distance of 1.5 cm, thereby establishing a submucosal tunnel (Fig. 14–12B). The mucosa is tented slightly by elevating the tip of the clamp and a 5-mm mucosal opening is made under direct vision with a scalpel. With a small straight rubber catheter as a guide, the catheter is drawn through the tunnel and muscular wall by retracting the Adson clamp (Fig. 14–12C). At this point, the catheter is sutured to the free end of the excised ureter and the ureter is drawn through the bladder wall and tunnel by traction on the rubber catheter (Fig. 14–12D). A mucosa-to-mucosa anasto-

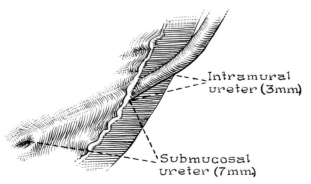

FIG. 14–10 Normal anatomy of the intramural ureter.

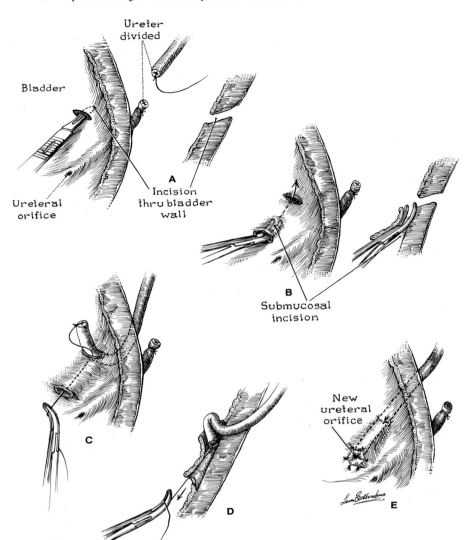

FIG. 14–11 Submucosal tunnel technique of ureterovesical implantation. (*A*) Bladder mucosa is incised above trigone at planned site of implantation; oblique incision through bladder wall made from exterior. (*B*) Adson clamp is inserted through new orifice and tunneled beneath mucosa for 1.5 cm to upper mucosal incision. (*C*) Ureter guided through bladder wall and upper mucosal orifice and gently guided through submucosal tunnel (*D*) by traction suture. (*E*) Mucosa-to-mucosa anastomosis of ureter to bladder; upper incision is closed with fine suture.

mosis of ureter to bladder is accomplished with No. 4-0 delayed-absorbable suture (Fig. 14–12E).

Direct Implantation of the Ureter Into the Bladder

Because of the associated risk of vesicoureteral reflux, direct ureter implantation into the bladder is used less frequently today, although it has served as a time-honored procedure for many surgeons and is still an effective method. It has been our experience that, in the absence of previous urinary tract infections or chronic renal disease, urinary reflux has not produced subsequent clinical problems such as recurrent ascending infection or loss of renal function. The operation is frequently referred to as the "fish-mouth" procedure because the ends of the ureter are incised and splayed on each side for approximately 5 mm to produce ureteral flaps that are sutured to the inside of the bladder wall.

The ureter is dissected free from the site of injury and mobilized from its bed for a sufficient distance to permit its implantation into the bladder without tension. Usually the bladder can be brought up to the shortened ureter if the ureter cannot be brought down to the bladder in its usual position. There is no advantage in performing the implantation retroperitoneally; hence the implantation may be done as close to the base of the bladder as possible (Fig. 14–13A).

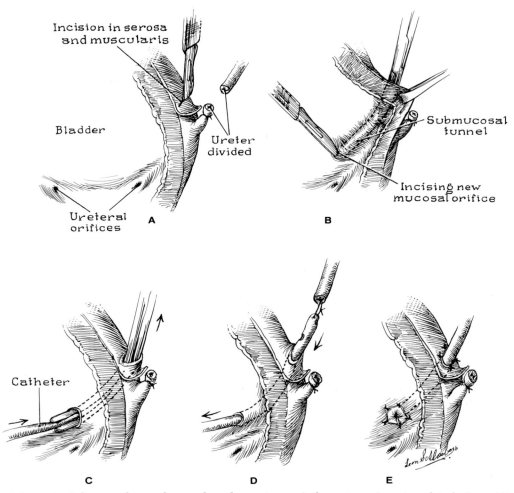

FIG. 14–12 Submucosal tunnel procedure for ureterovesical anastomosis, external technique. (A) Oblique incision through bladder wall initiated on external surface. (B) Adson clamp passed through muscular wall and beneath mucosa for 1.5 cm (tunnel formation); bladder mucosa incised over tip of clamp at site of new ureteral orifice. (C) Small, straight rubber catheter drawn through tunnel and bladder wall. (D) Catheter sutured to excised ureter; ureter guided through bladder wall and tunnel by traction on catheter. (E) Mucosa-to-mucosa anastomosis of ureter to bladder.

Each side of the lower end of the ureter is split for about 5 mm and a substantial bite is taken into each ureteral flap with No. 4-0 chromic catgut or delayed-absorbable sutures. A Silastic tube is threaded into the ureter and is used as a guide for the suture placement. A small opening is made directly through the full thickness of the bladder wall at the point selected for the implantation, preferably as close to the base of the bladder as can be done without tension. The bladder base should be freed, mobilized, and advanced to facilitate this anastomosis. The edges of the bladder opening are held with Allis clamps and the end of the catheter is introduced into the bladder. The anastomosis is per-formed by using the two traction sutures that were previously placed in the lower end of each ureteral flap. Each suture is introduced through the small opening into the lumen of the bladder and passed through the full thickness of the bladder wall, from serosa to mucosa, as shown in Figure 14–13B. The sutures are placed on opposite sides of the bladder incision so as to hold apart the slit ends of the ureter. These sutures are tied, thus drawing the ureter into the bladder and against the mucosal surface. An-choring sutures are placed in the seromuscular layer of the bladder and the adventitia of the ureter to fix the ureter to the bladder wall. These stitches pass through the edges of the incision in the bladder

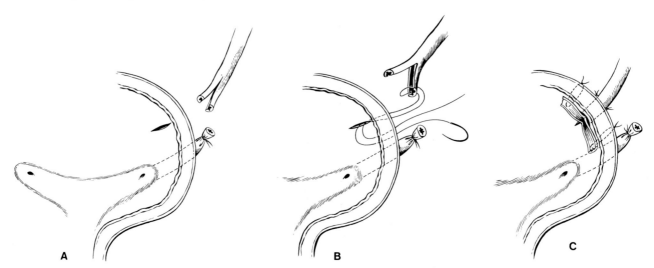

FIG. 14-13 Ureterovesical implantation, fish-mouth technique. (*A*) Excised free end of ureter is spatulated for 1 cm to 2 cm. New ureteral orifice has been made by scalpel above the trigone in position to reach excised ureter. (*B*) Each end of ureteral flap is anchored with a mattress suture of No. 4-0 delayed-absorbable suture and passed through new ureteral orifice and full thickness of bladder wall. (*C*) Bladder flaps are tied on external surface of the bladder and reinforced with seromuscular sutures in bladder wall and ureter at site of implantation.

wall and pick up the sheath of the ureter (Fig. 14-13C). Any residual opening in the bladder wall is closed with interrupted No. 3-0 delayed-absorbable sutures. The bladder wall should be anchored to the pelvic wall as close as possible to the anastomosis, to relieve the tension on the ureterovesical suture line. Ordinarily, the cul-de-sac or bladder peritoneum is advanced over the operative site to maintain the suture line beneath the peritoneum. A retroperitoneal drain is placed in the area of the anastomosis and brought through a stab wound incision in the lower abdomen.

The Silastic tubing used for splinting the anastomosis may be notched for improved drainage, coiled in the bladder, and left in place for about a week. The urethral catheter may be left in the bladder for an additional day after removal of the ureteral splint while ureteral drainage becomes well established. During the 7 days that the tubing is in place, it is irrigated only if it fails to drain freely, and then only 5 ml of 1% neomycin solution is used.

Ureterovesical Anastomosis of the Short Ureter

For the ureter that is badly traumatized within the broad ligament and where the injury is more than 5 cm above the ureterovesical junction, the technique of the psoas muscle hitch, as popularized by Harrow and others, permits ureterovesical anas-

tomosis of a shortened ureter. This procedure also avoids the necessity of a ureteroureteral anastomosis. After assessing the extent of the devitalized pelvic ureter, it is important to determine if a ureterovesical anastomosis can be performed without undue tension on the anastomosis. If the ureter does not reach the bladder wall, the lateral bladder peritoneum can be incised from each side of the inferior ramus of the pubis and the bladder base sharply dissected and mobilized from its fascial attachments to the upper vagina. To facilitate mobility of the bladder, both sides of the bladder wall should be freed from its peritoneal attachment. In so doing, the bladder wall can be extended and anchored to the psoas muscle near the pelvic brim with No. 3-0 delayed-absorbable suture to assure firm fixation (Fig. 14-14A). Care must be taken to avoid damage to the adjacent iliac vessels during this procedure.

Following the mobilization, funneling, and anchoring of the bladder wall to the psoas muscle, a ureteral anastomosis may be performed by one of the methods described above, including a direct mucosa-to-mucosa anastomosis, a "fish-mouth" procedure, or, preferably, by the submucosal tunnel procedure. A fine suture of No. 4-0 delayed-absorbable suture is used to suture the ureteral and bladder mucosa and an indwelling Silastic tube is inserted to the renal pelvis and coiled in the bladder for postoperative drainage. The angles of the bladder incision are closed with interrupted seromuscular sutures. The implant is supported by 3 or 4 an-

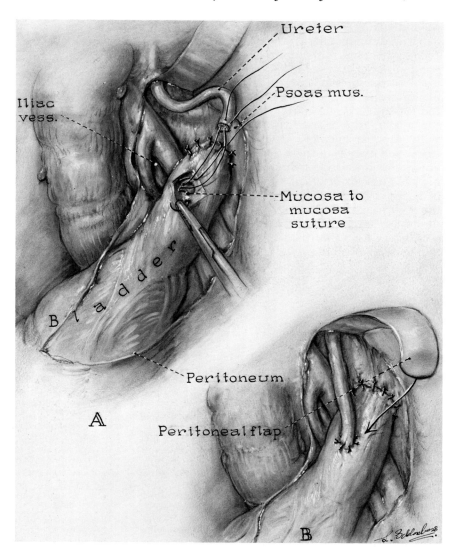

FIG. 14-14 Ureterovesical anastomosis of the short ureter–psoas muscle hitch procedure. (*A*) Bladder peritoneum is incised from lateral pelvic wall, and bladder is mobilized and anchored to psoas muscle at pelvic brim (psoas muscle hitch) near site of planned ureterovesical anastomosis. Mucosa-to-mucosa anastomosis of ureter to bladder is performed. (*B*) Ureterovesical anastomosis is reinforced with fine serosal sutures and peritoneum is advanced over anastomotic site.

choring sutures of fine, delayed-absorbable suture in the serosa-muscularis layer of the bladder and ureter (Fig. 14–14B). We have found this technique superior to the Boari bladder flap procedure, as the latter is frequently associated with reflux and is subject to ischemia with secondary stenosis or necrosis of the flap if the pedicle graft is lengthy.

Results of Ureteral Plastic Surgery

The long-term results of any type of ureterovesical anastomosis are quite good if the procedure has been performed with meticulous surgical skill. Healing will fail only when there has been an error in surgical judgment or when ischemia or irre-

versible ureteral damage has occurred at the site of anastomosis. However, vesicoureteral reflux may be associated with the "fish-mouth" anastomosis. Although recently there has been concern about the detrimental effect of reflux on the upper urinary tract, our past experience with the "fish-mouth" procedure has been extremely favorable without evidence of progressive infection or deterioration of kidney function. There is no question that the submucosal tunnel technique of implantation is more physiologic, and in the presence of chronic urinary tract infection, it is obviously preferable.

The success rate with ureteroureteral anastomosis has been improved in recent years by the careful selection of cases for this procedure and improvements in the operative technique used. In general, the indwelling Silastic catheter has helped to ensure a dry anastomotic site. The stent can be left in place for long periods until ureteral healing has been complete without creating a foreign-body effect on the anastomotic site. Only when the blood supply of the ureter has been seriously compromised or more than 1.5 cm of ureter has been resected has there been an increased risk of failure of healing with secondary fistula formation or ureteral stricture. Such cases require drainage of the kidney for an extended period of time and should probably have a T-tube drainage of the ureter from the flank or a protective pyelostomy to enhance healing of the suture line. Alternatively, a J-tube inserted in the ureter at the time of anastomosis can be firmly secured in the renal pelvis and left to drain into the bladder for long periods.

Bibliography

Benson RC, Hinmann F, Jr: Urinary tract injuries in obstetrics and gynecology. Am J Obstet Gynecol 70:467, 1955

Bergman H (ed): The Ureter. New York, Springer-Verlag, 1981

Blandy JP: Operative Urology. Oxford, Blackwell, 1978

Boari A: Chiurgia dell'uretere, con prefazione del Dott: I. Albarran, 1900, Contributo sperimentale alla plastica delle uretere. Atte Dell'a Acad Delle Science Med. E Naturali di Ferrara 14:444, Seduta 27, May, 1894

Boyce WH: Use of the internal ureteral stent in surgery of the kidney and ureter. In Boyarksy S, Gottschalk EA, Tanagho EA, et al. (eds): Urodynamics: Hydrodynamics of the Ureter and Renal Pelvis. New York, Academic Press, 1971

Bright TC, Peters PC: Ureteral injuries secondary to operative procedures. J Urol 9:22, 1977

Brudenell M: The pelvic ureter. Proc R Soc Med 70:188, 1977

Ehrlich RM, Melman A, Skinner DG: The use of vesicopsoas hitch in urologic surgery. J Urol 119:322, 1978

Everett HS, Mattingly RF: Urinary tract injuries resulting from pelvic surgery. Am J Obstet Gynecol 71:502, 1956

Everett HS, Williams TJ: Urology in the Female. In Campbell MF, Harrison JB (eds): Urology, 3rd ed. Philadelphia, WB Saunders, 1970

Flynn JT, Tiptaft RC, Woodhouse CR, et al: The early and aggressive repair of iatrogenic ureteric injuries. Brit J Urol 51:454, 1979

Freund WA, Joseph L: Ueber die Harnleiter—Gebarmutter—Fistel nebst neuen Unntersnchungen uber das normale Verhalten der Harnleiter im Weiblichen Becken. Berlin Klin Wochenschrift 6:504, 1869

Fry DE, Milholen L, Harbrecht PJ: Iatrogenic ureteral injury: Options in management. Arch Surg 118:454, 1983

Glenn JF (ed): Urologic Surgery, 3rd ed. Philadelphia, JB Lippincott, 1983

Harrow BR: A neglected maneuver for ureterovesical implantation following injury at gynecologic operation. J Urol 100:280, 1968

Hofmeister FJ: Pelvic anatomy of the ureter in relation to surgery performed through the vagina. Clin Obstet Gynecol 25:821, 1982

Hunner GL, Everett HS: Ureteroperitoneal fistula with urinary ascites and chronic peritonitis. JAMA 95:327, 1930

Kaye KW, Goldberg ME: Applied anatomy of the kidney and ureter. Urol Clin North Am 9(1):3, 1982

Lewis HY, Pierce JM: Return of function after complete ureteral obstruction of 69 days duration. J Urol 88:377, 1962

Liu W, Meigs JV: Radical hysterectomy and pelvic lymphadenectomy. Am J Obstet Gynecol 69:1, 1955

Marmar JL: The management of ureteral obstruction with silicone rubber splint catheters. J Urol 104:386, 1970

Mattingly RF, Borkowf HI: Lower urinary tract injuries in pregnancy. In Barber HK, Graber EA (eds): Surgical Disease in Pregnancy. Philadelphia, WB Saunders, 1974

Meigs JV: The Wertheim operation for carcinoma of the cervix. Am J Obstet Gynecol 49:542, 1945

Newell QU: Injury to ureters during pelvic operation. Ann Surg 109:48, 1939

Notley RG: Ureteral morphology: Anatomic and clinical considerations. Urology 12:8, 1978

————: Anatomy and Physiology of the Ureter. In Blandy JP (ed): Urology. London, Blackwell, 1976

Prout GR, Jr, Koontz WW, Jr: Partial vesical immobilization: An important adjunct to ureteroneocystostomy. J Urol 103:147, 1970

Sampson JA: Ligation and clamping of the ureter as complications of surgical operations. Am Med 4:693, 1902

————: The relation between carcinoma cervicis uteri and the ureters and its significance in the more radical operations for that disease. Johns Hopkins Med Bull 156:72, 1904

————: Ureteral fistulae as sequelae of pelvic operations. Surg Gynecol Obstet 8:479, 1909

Shapiro SR, Bennett AH: Recovery of renal function after prolonged unilateral ureteral obstruction. J Urol 115:136, 1976

Shoenwald MB, Orkin LA: Bilateral intravesical ureteral ligation. Complication of Cooper's ligament suspension. J Urol 3:787, 1974

Thompson IM: Bladder flap repair of ureteral injuries. Urol Clin North Am 4(1):51, 1977

Thompson IM, Ross G, Jr: Long-term results of bladder flap repair of ureteral injuries. J Urol 111:483, 1974

Thompson JD, Benigno BB: Vaginal repair of ureteral injuries. Am J Obstet Gynecol 3:601, 1971

Thompson RH: Ureteral injuries in pelvic surgery. Bull Dept Gyn OB Emory U 11 (No 2) 93, 1980

Van Nagell JR, Jr, Roddick JW, Jr: Vaginal hysterectomy, the ureter and excretory urography. Obstet Gynecol 39:784, 1972

Waldeyer, W: Über die sogenannte Ureterscheide (Verhandlugen der Anatomischen Gesellschaft). Anatomischer Anzeiger 9:259, 1892

Wertheim E: Zur Frag der Radikaloperation beim Uteruskrebs. Arch Gynäk 61:627, 1900

Wesolowski S: Bilateral ureteral injuries in gynaecology. Br J Urol 41:666, 1969

Chapter 15

Surgery for Anomalies of the Müllerian Ducts

Anomalies of the müllerian ducts are an unusual but interesting group of gynecologic problems. The most commonly encountered ones are the septate, bicornuate, didelphic, and unicornuate uteri and congenital absence of the vagina and uterus. Since there is some commonality of information about embryologic origin, clinical presentation and operative correction among these müllerian duct anomalies, some of the more common ones will be discussed together in this chapter.

A recent classification of anomalies of the müllerian ducts, proposed by H. W. Jones, is presented here with slight modification.

CLASSIFICATION OF MÜLLERIAN DUCT ANOMALIES

Agenesis of the müllerian ducts, partial or complete
  Obstructive
  Nonobstructive
Problems of vertical fusion of the müllerian ducts
  Obstructive
  Nonobstructive
Problems of lateral fusion of the müllerian ducts, partial or complete
  Obstructive
  Nonobstructive
Combinations and other problems

Agenesis of both müllerian ducts results in congenital absence of the vagina and usually of the uterus, a syndrome sometimes referred to as the Mayer–Rokitansky–Kuster–Hauser syndrome. Problems of vertical fusion result from a failure of the müllerian ducts to establish a proper communication with that part of the vagina formed from the urogenital sinus below. Problems of lateral fusion result in arcuate, unicornuate, bicornuate, didelphic, and septate uteri. The septate uterus results from a failure of reabsorption of the septum between the fused müllerian ducts. Problems with vertical and lateral fusion may exist together. Both obstructive and nonobstructive problems may be present in all four categories. Obstructive lesions require immediate attention to relieve the retrograde flow of trapped mucus and menstrual blood, and the increasing pressure on surrounding organs and structures. When no obstruction is present, attention may not be required immediately but will be required eventually to establish or improve reproductive or coital function.

Embryology

The reproductive organs in the female (indeed, also in the male) consist of external genitalia, gonads, and an internal duct system between the two. These three components originate embryologically from different primordia and in close association with the urinary system and hindgut. Thus, the developmental history is complex. Even in the 4 mm to 5 mm embryo, it is possible to recognize bilateral thickenings of the coelomic epithelium medial to the mesonephros (primitive kidney) in the dorsum of the coelomic cavity. These thickenings are the gonadal ridges (Fig. 15–1). At about the sixth week, in the 17 mm to 20 mm embryo, the gonad can be distinguished as either a testis or an ovary.

In the female, the labia minora and majora develop from the labioscrotal folds, which are ectodermal in origin. The phallic portion of the urogenital sinus gives rise to the urethra. The müllerian

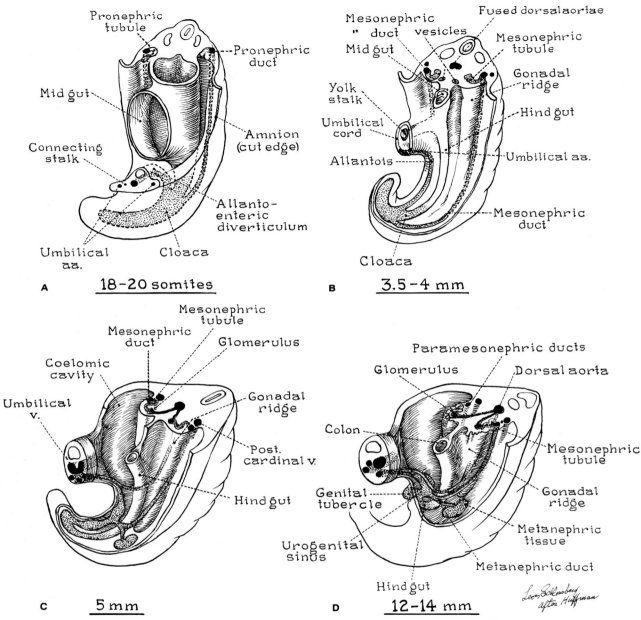

FIG. 15–1 Diagrammatic representation of the development of the female reproductive organs and structures in early embryogenesis. (*A*) At the 18 to 24 somite stage (4th week) the gonadal ridges have not yet begun to form. (*B*) In the 3.5 to 4 mm embryo (5 weeks) the gonadal ridges can be recognized as thickenings of the coelemic cavity just medial to the mesonephric tubules. Gonadal differentiation into either testis or overy does not occur until the 6th week of development. The allanto-enteric diverticulum is joined caudally to the dilated cloaca. (*C, D*) The genital tubercle and labial folds form in the region just anterior to the cloaca. The cloaca later divides into the ventral urogenital sinus and the dorsal rectum.

The development of the urinary system closely parallels that of the reproductive system. The nonfunctioning pronephric tubules shown in *A* develop to form the mesonephric ducts. The permanent kidneys eventually develop from the metanephric tissue, and the urinary collecting system develops from the metanephric ducts. The paramesonephric (müllerian) ducts are apparent by the 12 to 14 mm stage. Their subsequent development is illustrated in Figure 15-2.

(paramesonephric) duct system is stimulated to develop preferentially over the wolffian (mesonephric) duct system, which regresses in early female fetal life. The cranial parts of the wolffian ducts may persist as the epoophoron of the ovarian hilum; the caudal parts may persist as Gartner's ducts. The müllerian ducts persist and attain complete development to form the fallopian tubes, the uterine corpus and cervix, and a portion of the vagina.

About 37 days after fertilization, the müllerian ducts first appear lateral to each wolffian duct as invaginations of the dorsal coelomic epithelium. The site of origin of the invaginations remains open and ultimately forms the fimbriated end of the fallopian tubes. At their point of origin, the müllerian ducts each form a solid bud. Each bud penetrates the mesenchyme lateral and parallel to each wolffian duct. As the solid buds elongate, a lumen appears in the cranial part, beginning at each coelomic opening. The lumina extend gradually to the caudal growing tips of the ducts. Eventually, the caudal end of each müllerian duct crosses the ventral aspect of the wolffian duct. The paired müllerian ducts continue to grow in a medial and caudal direction until they eventually meet in the midline and become fused together in the urogenital septum. A septum between the two müllerian ducts gradually disappears, leaving a single uterovaginal canal lined with cuboidal epithelium. Failure of reabsorption of this septum can result in a septate uterus. The most cranial parts of the müllerian ducts remain separate and form the fallopian tubes. The caudal segments of the müllerian ducts fuse to form the uterus and part of the vagina. The cranial point of fusion is the site of the future fundus of the uterus. Variations in this site of fusion can result in an arcuate or bicornuate uterus. Complete failure of fusion can result in a didelphic uterus.

The vagina is formed from the lower end of the uterovaginal canal, developed from the müllerian ducts and the urogenital sinus (Fig. 15–2). The point of contact between the two is the müllerian tubercle. A solid vaginal cord results from proliferation of the cells at the caudal tip of the fused müllerian ducts. The cord gradually elongates to meet the bilateral endodermal evaginations (sinovaginal bulbs) from the posterior aspect of the urogenital sinus below. These sinovaginal bulbs extend cranially to fuse with the caudal end of the vaginal cord, forming the vaginal plate. Subsequently, canalization of the vaginal cord occurs, followed by epithelialization with cells derived mostly from endoderm of the urogenital sinus. Recent proposals hold that only the upper one-third of the vagina is formed from the müllerian ducts, with the lower vagina developing from the vaginal plate of the urogenital sinus. Recent studies also suggest that the vaginal canal is actually open and connected to a patent uterus and tubes, even in early embryonic life and that the vagina does not form and later become canalized from an epithelial cord of squamous cells growing upward from the urogenital sinus. Most investigators now suggest that the vagina develops under the influence of the müllerian ducts and estrogenic stimulation. There is general agreement that the vagina originates as a composite formed partly from the müllerian ducts and partly from the urogenital sinus.

At about the twentieth week, the cervix takes form as a result of a condensation of stromal cells at a specific site around the fused müllerian ducts. The mesenchyme surrounding the müllerian ducts becomes condensed early in embryonic development and eventually forms the musculature of the female genital tract. The hymen is the embryologic septum between the sinovaginal bulbs above and the urogenital sinus proper below. It is lined internally by a layer of vaginal epithelium and an external layer of epithelium derived from the urogenital sinus (both of endodermal origin) with mesoderm between the two. It is not derived from the müllerian ducts.

Anomalies in the organogenesis of the vagina are easily understood. Should there be a failure in the development of the müllerian ducts at any time between their origin from the coelomic epithelium at 5 weeks of embryonic age and their fusion with the urogenital sinus at 8 weeks, the sinovaginal bulbs will fail to proliferate from the urogenital sinus and the uterus and vagina will fail to develop. The Mayer–Rokitansky–Kuster–Hauser syndrome is the most common clinical example of this anomaly. The uterus is absent in approximately 90% of patients with congenital absence of the vagina. However, other variations in the embryologic development may be seen. For example, the uterine corpus may develop with absence of the uterine cervix and vagina. Or the uterine corpus and cervix may develop with absence of the vagina.

A transverse vaginal septum can develop in any location in the vagina, but is more common in the upper vagina at the point of junction between the vaginal plate and the caudal end of the fused müllerian ducts. This defect is caused, presumably, by a failure of absorption of the tissue that separates the two or a failure of complete fusion of the two embryologic components of the vagina.

In cases of abnormal gonadal development in which the müllerian ducts have been ineffectively suppressed, the development of ambiguous external

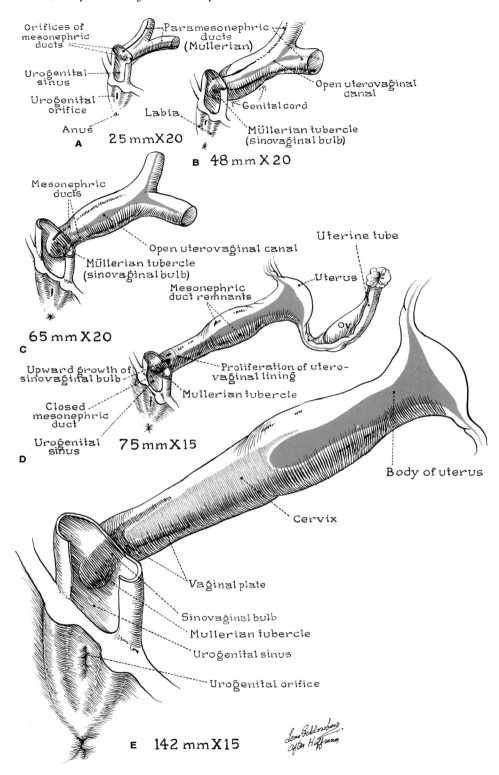

Orifices of mesonephric ducts
Paramesonephric ducts (Mullerian)
Urogenital sinus
Urogenital orifice
Anus
Labia
Open uterovaginal canal
Genital cord
Müllerian tubercle (sinovaginal bulb)
A   25 mm X 20
B   48 mm X 20

Mesonephric ducts
Open uterovaginal canal
Müllerian tubercle (sinovaginal bulb)
65 mm X 20
C

Uterine tube
Uterus
Mesonephric duct remnants
Ov.
Upward growth of sinovaginal bulb
Proliferation of uterovaginal lining
Mullerian tubercle
Closed mesonephric duct
Urogenital sinus
75 mm X 15
D

Body of uterus
Cervix
Vaginal plate
Sinovaginal bulb
Mullerian tubercle
Urogenital sinus
Urogenital orifice
E   142 mm X 15

Leon Schlossberg.
after Hoffman

genitalia will frequently be accompanied by a small rudimentary uterus or a partially developed vagina. Additionally, when there is a genetic loss of cytoplasmic receptor proteins within androgenic target cells, such as occurs in the androgen insensitivity syndrome (formerly called testicular feminization syndrome), it is understandable that the vagina will not be completely developed, since in this XY female the existing male gonads have suppressed the development of the müllerian ducts. Since these genetic male patients are seen clinically as phenotypic females without a completely formed vagina, it is important that a vagina be surgically constructed so that they may function satisfactorily sexually in their female gender role.

Congenital rectovaginal fistula, imperforate (covered) anus, hypospadias, and a variety of anatomical variants of cloacal dysgenesis may also occur. These anomalies may be associated with maldevelopment of the müllerian and mesonephric duct derivatives.

Abnormalities in the formation or fusion of the müllerian ducts can result in a variety of anomalies of the uterus and vagina—single, multiple, combined, or separate. The entirely separate origin of the ovaries from the gonadal ridges explains the infrequent association of uterovaginal anomalies with ovarian anomalies. Also, the close developmental relationship of the müllerian ducts and the wolffian ducts can explain the frequency with which anomalies of the female genital system and urinary tract are associated. Failure of development of a müllerian duct is likewise associated with failure of development of a ureteric bud from the caudal end of the wolffian duct. Thus, the entire kidney may be absent on the same side as agenesis of a müllerian duct. Depending on the time when the teratogenic influence may be operative, renal units may be absent, fused, or in unusual locations in the pelvis. Ureters may be duplicated or may open in unusual places such as the vagina or uterus. Jones has pointed out that failure of lateral fusion of the müllerian ducts with unilateral obstruction is associated consistently with absence of the kidney on the side with obstruction. Bilateral obstruction has not been observed clinically, presumably because it would be associated with bilateral renal agenesis, a condition that would not allow the embryo to develop. According to Thompson and Lynn, 40% of female patients with congenital absence of the kidney will be found to have associated genital anomalies.

Problems of Agenesis

The problems of agenesis include congenital absence of the vagina, and the Mayer–Rokitansky–Kuster–Hauser syndrome as well as variants and associated anomalies.

Congenital absence of the vagina may be partial or complete. In partial vaginal agenesis, the uterine cervix and corpus usually are both present and a small pouch of upper vagina can be found just below the cervix. In the more common complete vaginal agenesis, the entire vagina is absent, along with the uterus. The uterus is usually represented by small uterine bulbs located on each side of the pelvis next to small rudimentary fallopian tubes and normal ovaries. Rarely, with complete vaginal agenesis, the uterine corpus will form in the midline even though the cervix is absent. Such anomalies and others discussed later are clinically significant because they cause or have the potential to cause obstruction to coitus or to menstrual drainage. Although the Mayer–Rokitansky–Kuster–Hauser syndrome is the classic and most common example, absence of the vagina may be associated with a heterogeneous group of disorders with a variety of genetic, endocrine, and metabolic manifestations and associated anomalies of other body systems.

Realdus Columbus first described congenital absence of the vagina in 1559. In 1829, Mayer described congenital absence of the vagina as one of the abnormalities found in stillborn infants with multiple

FIG. 15–2 Further development of the paramesonephric (müllerian) ducts and the urogenital sinus. (A) Early development of the paramesonephric ducts. The cranial ends of the paramesonephric ducts develop first. These ends remain open to form the fimbriated end of the fallopian tubes. The paramesonephric ducts grow caudally, cross the mesonephric ducts ventrally, and (B) eventually fuse together to form the uterovaginal canal. (C) Further development caudally brings this structure into contact with the wall of the urogenital sinus, producing the müllerian tubercle. The caudal ends of the fused paramesonephric ducts form the uterine corpus and cervix. Together with the urogenital sinus, they also form the vagina. The cranial point of fusion of the paramesonephric ducts marks the location of the future uterine fundus. The fallopian tubes form from the unfused cranial parts of the paramesonephric (müllerian) ducts. The proliferation of the lining of the uterovaginal canal above and the upward growth of the sinovaginal bulb from below (D) form the vaginal plate (E), which later becomes canalized to leave an open vaginal canal. Thus, the vagina is of composite origin. The mesonephric ducts in the female degenerate but may persist into adult life as Gartner's ducts.

birth defects. Rokitansky in 1838 and Kuster in 1910 described an entity in which the vagina was absent, a small bipartite uterus was present, the ovaries were normal, and anomalies of other organ systems (renal and skeletal) were frequently observed. Hauser and associates emphasized the spectrum of associated anomalies. Pinsky suggested that congenital absence of the vagina is part of a symptom complex and not a true syndrome. Over the years, the disorder has come to be known as the Mayer–Rokitansky–Kuster–Hauser syndrome or the Rokitansky–Kuster–Hauser syndrome or simply as the Rokitansky syndrome (Fig. 15–3).

Counseller found that the condition occurred once in 4,000 female admissions to the Mayo Clinic. Evans estimated that vaginal agenesis occurred once in 10,588 female births in Michigan from 1953 to 1957.

There may be some variation in the incidence based on race. Congenital absence of the vagina is an extremely rare entity among the predominantly black gynecologic patients at Grady Memorial Hospital in Atlanta.

The individual with an absent vagina and the classic Mayer–Rokitansky–Kuster–Hauser syndrome is usually brought to the gynecologist at the age of 14 to 15 when the absence of menses gives the mother concern. Such young women have a normal complement of chromosomes (46XX) and usually have normal ovaries and secondary sex characteristics, including external genitalia. Menstruation does not appear at the usual age because the uterus is absent, but ovulation occurs regularly. Some exceptions to the rule of normal ovaries have been noted. For example, polycystic ovaries and gonadal

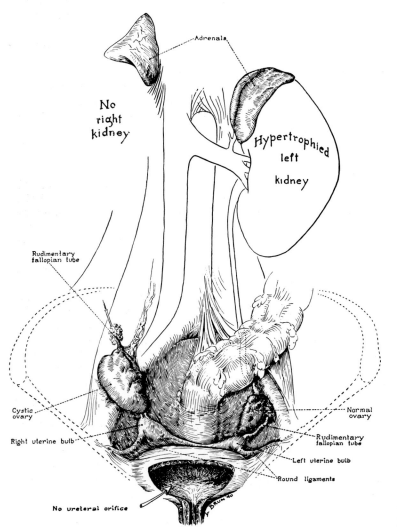

FIG. 15–3 Typical findings in a patient with Mayer–Rokitansky–Kuster–Hauser syndrome. Note absence of the right kidney and right ureteral orifice. The uterus is represented by bilateral rudimentary uterine bulbs joined by a band behind the bladder. The ovaries appear normal.

dysgenesis have been reported in patients with congenital absence of the vagina.

An exclusive genetic etiology cannot be ascribed to vaginal agenesis, since almost all patients have a normal karyotype (46XX). Also, the discordance of vaginal agenesis in three sets of monozygotic twins has been reported. The occurrence of complete vaginal agenesis in sisters with a 46XX karyotype suggests an autosomal mode of inheritance for these patients. Shokeir investigated the families of 13 unrelated females with aplasia of müllerian duct derivatives. Similarly affected females were found in 10 families. Usually there was an affected female paternal relative, suggesting female-limited autosomal dominant inheritance of a mutant gene transmitted by male relatives. Other investigators point to the variety of associated anomalies as support for the etiologic concept of variable expression of a genetic defect possibly precipitated by teratogenic exposure operative between the thirty-seventh and the forty-first gestational day, the period during which the vagina is formed. Knab has suggested that the possible etiologic factors of the Mayer–Rokitansky–Kuster–Hauser syndrome are (1) inappropriate production of müllerian regressive factor in the female embryonic gonad; (2) regional absence or deficiency of estrogen receptors limited to the lower müllerian duct; (3) arrest of müllerian duct development by a teratogenic agent; (4) mesenchymal inductive defect; (5) sporadic gene mutation. Knab believes that the teratogenic and the mutant gene etiologies are the most probable.

A significant number of patients with complete or partial vaginal agenesis will have associated anomalies of the upper müllerian duct system as well as associated anomalies of other organ systems. Complete absence of the vagina is associated with absence of the cervix and corpus in 90% to 95% of the cases. By gentle rectal examination, one can feel an absence of the midline müllerian structure that should represent the uterus. Instead one feels a smooth band (possibly a remnant of the uterosacral ligaments) that extends from one side of the pelvis to the other. In the classic Mayer–Rokitansky–Kuster–Hauser syndrome, the uterus is represented by bilateral rudimentary uterine bulbs that may vary in size, are not usually palpable, are connected to small fallopian tubes, and are located on the lateral pelvic side wall adjacent to normal ovaries. Depending on their size, these rudimentary uterine bulbs may or may not contain a cavity lined by endometrial tissue. If present, the endometrial tissue may appear immature or, rarely, may show evidence of cyclic response to ovarian hormones. The endometrial cavity does not often communicate with the peritoneal cavity since the tube may not be patent at the point of junction between the tube and the rudimentary uterine bulb. However, it is certainly possible for the endometrium to menstruate and for the endometrial cavity to communicate with the peritoneal cavity through patent fallopian tubes. A patient with a classic Mayer–Rokitansky–Kuster–Hauser syndrome has been reported who had a 4-cm endometrioma removed from the left ovary by laparotomy at the time of operation to create a vagina. Myomas have been known to form in the muscular wall. Mild dysmenorrhea has been attributed to their presence. A small myoma has been found, along with the tube and ovary, in the inguinal canal or in an inguinal hernia sac. Garcia and Jones reported one patient with some functioning endometrial tissue in one rudimentary uterine bulb. It was removed. Fore and associates reported removing rudimentary uterine bulbs containing endometrial tissue in order to relieve cyclic discomfort from cryptomenorrhea. We have two such patients in our series.

Variations in development of upper müllerian ducts in patients with congenital absence of the vagina are shown in Figure 15-4.

The potential for function from the rudimentary bulbs has been clearly demonstrated by Chakravarty and associates and by Singh and Devi. These authors have attempted to use these rudimentary uterine bulbs to reconstruct a midline uterus. The reconstructed uterus is then connected to the newly constructed vagina. A surprising number of these patients have experienced cyclic menstruation, although recurrent stenosis and obstruction of the rudimentary horns is the most common outcome of such efforts. The present author has had no experience with this technique and questions its usefulness. However, these rudimentary uterine bulbs usually are insignificant structures that cause no problems.

In incomplete or partial vaginal agenesis, the cervix and functioning uterus are usually present. The vagina is represented by a small space beneath the cervix. At the menarche, this space and the uterine cavity are likely to become greatly enlarged by a hematocolpometra caused by the accumulation of menstrual discharge. Infants with this anomaly may develop a hydrocolpometra. Evans and associates reported that among 160 patients with complete vaginal agenesis who underwent operation to create a vagina, 149 (93%) had an absent or rudimentary uterus and 11 (7%) had an anomalous uterus with functioning endometrium and cryptomenorrhea.

Fore and associates reported that 47% of patients in whom evaluation of the urinary tract was performed had associated urologic anomalies. In other studies, approximately one-third of patients with

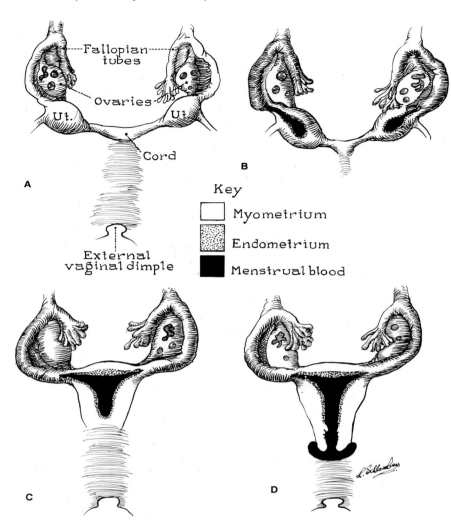

Key

☐ Myometrium

▨ Endometrium

■ Menstrual blood

FIG. 15–4 Patients with congenital absence of the vagina may show variations in the development of the upper müllerian ducts. (*A*) Bilateral rudimentary uterine bulbs without endometrium. (*B*) Bilateral rudimentary uterine bulbs with functioning endometrium. (*C*) Midline uterine corpus with functioning endometrium and absent or rudimentary cervix. (*D*) Midline uterine corpus and cervix with small upper vaginal pouch.

complete vaginal agenesis were found to have significant urinary anomalies, such as unilateral renal agenesis, unilateral or bilateral pelvic kidney, horseshoe kidney, hydronephrosis, hydroureter, and a variety of patterns of ureteral duplication. A significant number of patients with partial vaginal agenesis will also have associated urinary tract anomalies. One interesting association is the presence of a fistula between the blind upper vagina and the bladder, urethra, or a persistent urogenital sinus. The classic symptom that leads one to suspect this anomaly is the appearance of cyclic hematuria that begins after the menarche. These patients also have frequent associated anomalies of the upper urinary system, skeleton, and uterus.

Associated skeletal anomalies have been recognized since congenital absence of the vagina was first described. In a review of 574 reported cases,

Griffin and associates found a 12% incidence of skeletal abnormalities. Most of these involve the spine (wedge vertebrae, fusions, rudimentary vertebral bodies, and supernumerary vertebrae), but the limbs and ribs can also be involved. Other anomalies include syndactyly, absence of a digit, congenital heart disease, and inguinal hernias, although inguinal hernias are apparently more often present in patients with androgen insensitivity syndrome than in patients with the Mayer–Rokitansky–Kuster–Hauser syndrome.

FEATURES OF THE CLASSIC MAYER–ROKITANSKY–KUSTER–HAUSER SYNDROME

Congenital absence of the vagina (a 1 cm to 2 cm vaginal dimple may be present above the hymenal ring).

Congenital absence of the uterus (small rudimentary uterine bulbs are usually present with rudimentary fallopian tubes).

Normal ovarian function, including ovulation.

Sex of rearing female.

Phenotypic sex female (normal development of breasts, body proportions, hair distribution and external genitalia).

Genetic sex female (46XX karyotype).

Frequent association of other congenital anomalies (skeletal and especially renal).

PREOPERATIVE CONSIDERATIONS

If functioning endometrial tissue is present, symptoms from cryptomenorrhea will begin shortly after female secondary sex characteristics develop. Usually this indicates an incomplete agenesis of the vagina with a uterine cervix and corpus present above. A small vaginal space beneath the cervix will distend with menstrual blood. If this type of anomaly is recognized early, a proper operation can be performed vaginally to allow an external exit to the menstrual discharge and to preserve reproductive function. This is an obvious indication for operation.

Occasionally, older patients with the classic Mayer–Rokitansky–Kuster–Hauser syndrome consult a gynecologist, either before or after marriage, because of difficult or painful intercourse. The indication for operation in these patients is also obvious. Of all patients, they are the most satisfied with the operative results.

Most commonly, patients of 14 to 16 years of age are seen by a gynecologist because of primary amenorrhea. Regrettably, an examination may not have been done by a previous physician because the patient was "too young," but various hormonal medications may have been given with hope that menstruation would begin. An examination may have led to a mistaken diagnosis of imperforate hymen. Futile attempts to incise the hymen may have resulted in scarring of the apex of the vaginal dimple before a proper diagnosis of congenital absence of the vagina was finally made.

Formerly, it was customary to advise a delay in operating to create a vagina for these young patients until just prior to their marriage. This led to difficulties at times, particularly when complications developed that required delay in the marriage until the vagina healed completely. More recently, we have performed the procedure in the late teenage years, when it became clearly evident that the patient was emotionally mature and intellectually reliable enough to manage the vaginal form without difficulty. In essence, the operative procedure has been removed far enough from the marriage bed

that a delay in healing of the newly constructed vagina would create no unnecessary emotional trauma for the patient or her family.

Probably insufficient attention has been given to the psychological aspects of this problem. Obviously, the patient with congenital absence of the vagina cannot be made into a whole person simply by creating a perineal pouch for intercourse. Establishment of sexual function is only one concern and may be the easiest problem to correct. Evans reports that 15% of his patients have real psychiatric difficulty. He and David and associates suggest that psychiatric help should be initiated before the operation. Learning about this anomaly, especially at a young age, is a shock and is always accompanied by diminished self-esteem. Such patients may, fortunately, be encouraged by their gynecologist with the offer of appropriate surgery to establish coital function. The gynecologist may point out that functionally the patient will be like thousands of young women who have had a hysterectomy because of serious pelvic disease, and who have also satisfied by adoption their desire to be a parent.

Regardless of which operative technique is chosen, the patient must cooperate if the operation is to be successful. When a McIndoe operation is performed, patients must understand the need to wear a form continuously for several months and intermittently for several years until the vagina is no longer subject to constriction and regular intercourse is taking place. The operation should not be done until it is certain in preoperative interviews that the patient understands her essential role in its success. This is especially important when the patient is a young teenager.

A buccal smear should be done to determine the presence or absence of the chromatin body. If the chromatin body is absent, or there is a suspicion of ovarian dysgenesis, androgen insensitivity syndrome, or some aberration of the classic Mayer–Rokitansky–Kuster–Hauser syndrome, a complete chromosomal analysis should be done. Obviously, an intravenous pyelogram should be done preoperatively. This will also provide an adequate survey for anomalies of the spine. If a pelvic mass is present, one should differentiate between hematometra, hematocolpos, endometrial and other ovarian cysts, and pelvic kidney with additional special studies, including ultrasonography.

Some patients without a pelvic mass will complain of cyclic pain. This pain may be ovulatory or possibly dysmenorrhea originating in well-developed rudimentary uterine bulbs. One can differentiate between the two by asking the patient to keep a basal body temperature chart and marking the days when pelvic pain is present. Occasionally, there may be a question about whether a patient has congenital absence of the vagina or an imperforate hymen with cryptomenorrhea. This question can usually be answered simply by placing a metal catheter or similar instrument in the urethra and a finger in the rectum. If the metal instrument in the urethra can be easily felt through the anterior rectal wall, then the vagina is probably absent. On the other hand, if there is an intervening mass between the rectal finger and the instrument in the urethra, this may represent a hematocolpos behind an imperforate hymen. The hymen will bulge from the force of accumulated blood in the vagina, especially when the hematocolpos is palpable suprapubically.

METHODS OF CREATING A VAGINA

Even today there is no unanimity of opinion regarding the correct approach to the problem of vaginal agenesis. A review of some of the methods devised for the formation of a vagina is given below.

Non-surgical Methods

Simple intermittent pressure: Frank, 1938; Ingram, 1981.

Surgical Methods

Intestine
Small intestine: Sneguireff, 1892; Baldwin, 1907 (double loop of ileum)
Large intestine: Popoff, 1910, Schubert, 1911 (rectum); Wagner, 1908, Pratt, 1961 (sigmoid)
Pedunculated skin flaps
Simple labial and thigh flaps: Graves, 1921
Tubed pedicle flaps from thigh: Frank and Geist, 1927
Gracilis myocutaneous flaps: McCraw, 1976
Dissection of perineal space: Amussat, 1835
With insertion of inlay split-thickness skin graft: Abbe, 1898.
With insertion of form for continuous dilatation: Wharton, 1938.
With insertion of both inlay split-thickness skin graft and form for continuous dilatation: McIndoe, 1938.
Lined with peritoneum: Davydov, 1969.
Vulvovaginal pouch: Williams, 1964.

Non-Surgical Methods

In 1938, Robert Frank described a method of formation of an artificial vagina without operation. In 1940 he reported remarkably satisfactory results in 8 cases treated by this method. His follow-up study showed that a vagina formed in this manner remained permanent in depth and caliber, even in patients who neglected dilatation for more than a year. It has been emphasized that the pelvic floor itself may be embryologically deficient in some patients. Indeed, the ease with which some patients are able to create a vagina with intercourse alone or with other intermittent pressure techniques may be explained on this basis. Three patients have even been reported to develop enteroceles, one following coitus alone, one following a Williams vulvovaginoplasty, and one in our clinic following a McIndoe operation. This complication may develop when the vaginal mucosa is brought in close proximity to the pelvic peritoneum, but it may also be contributed to by a relative embryological weakness or absence of endopelvic fascia.

Our results in a few cases in which we attempted this method have not been very satisfactory. Great persistence and cooperation are necessary on the part of the patient, and even with complete cooperation, in some cases the cavity fails to materialize. If a patient desires to attempt this rather tedious exercise, we encourage her to do so. In case of failure, a surgical procedure can be done later.

Recently, Rock and associates at Johns Hopkins Hospital reported that an initial trial of vaginal dilatation was successful in 9 of 21 patients. Prompted by the rewarding results of Broadbent and Woolf, Ingram has described a modified Frank technique of creating a new vagina. Using dilators especially designed for use with a bicycle seat stool, Ingram was able to produce satisfactory vaginal depth and coital function in 10 of 12 patients with vaginal agenesis and 10 of 14 patients with various types of stenosis. Ingram's technique is worthwhile and deserves additional trials.

Surgical Methods

During the past three decades, experience has crystallized our ideas so that we believe there is one method of dealing with the complete vaginal absence that is superior to others in the majority of cases, namely, the Abbe–Wharton–McIndoe operation, more popularly called the McIndoe operation. In special circumstances the vulvovaginal pouch of Williams, the sigmoid transplant of Pratt, or the simple intermittent pressure technique of Frank or Ingram may be indicated.

In 1907, Baldwin used a double loop of ileum to line a space dissected between the rectum and bladder, leaving the mesentery connected to the bowel. The continuity of the intestinal tract was re-established by an end-to-end anastomosis. He reported that the new vagina was absolutely normal in every way. In 1910, Popoff constructed a vagina utilizing a portion of the rectum which was moved anteriorly. This operation was modified by Schubert in

1911. The rectum was severed above the anal sphincter and moved anteriorly to serve as the vagina. The sigmoid was sutured to the anus and the continuity of the intestinal tract was thus re-established. The high mortality and morbidity of both operations were a sobering influence and their popularity declined. Today, segments of sigmoid are used more often to create a vaginal pouch or extend vaginal length in patients who have lost vaginal function because of extensive surgery and/or irradiation for pelvic malignancy.

Less formidable procedures consisting of dissection of a space between the bladder and rectum and lining this space with flaps of skin from the labia or inner thighs were also tried. Marked scarring resulted and hair usually grew in the vagina.

Extensive plastic procedures to construct a vagina are no longer necessary or desirable and have been discarded in favor of safer procedures, unless one is faced with the problem of maintaining a vaginal canal in a patient who is having an extensive exenterative operation for pelvic malignancy. Here one may wish to consider utilizing the gracilis myocutaneous flap technique described by McCraw and associates in 1976.

The operation that is most popular today for creating a new vagina began with simple surgical attempts to create space between the bladder and the rectum. The earlier attempts were often in patients with cryptomenorrhea. However, such a space would usually constrict because of a failure to recognize the importance of prolonged continuous dilatation until the constrictive phase of healing was complete. Wharton in 1938, at the Johns Hopkins Hospital, combined an adequate dissection of the vaginal space with continuous dilatation by a balsawood form covered with a thin rubber sheath and left in the space. Rather than using a split-thickness skin graft, his operation is based on the principle that the vaginal epithelium has remarkable powers of proliferation and in a relatively short time will cover the raw surface. Recalling that a similar process occurs in the fetus when the epithelium of the sinovaginal bulbs and urogenital sinus form the vaginal canal, Wharton merely applied this same principle in the adult. This simple procedure is entirely satisfactory as long as the space is kept dilated for enough time to allow the epithelium to grow in. But occasionally, even after several years, the vault of the vagina remains without epithelial covering. Coital bleeding and leukorrhea result from the persistent granulation tissue and there is a tendency for vaginas constructed by this method to be constricted from scarring in the upper portion. In Counseller's 1948 report from the Mayo Clinic of 100 operations to construct a new vagina, 14 were done by Wharton's method with excellent results in all 14 patients. It was stated that the disadvantages of persistent granulation tissue with bleeding and leukorrhea was of no consequence. This has not been our experience.

When inlay skin grafts were first used to construct a new vagina, the results were poor because the necessity for dilatation of the new vagina was not recognized. Severe contraction, uncontrolled by continuous or intermittent dilatation, almost invariably spoiled the results. Although Heppner, Abbe, and others had preceded him by many years in utilizing a skin-covered prosthesis in neovaginal construction, it was Sir Archibald McIndoe at the Queen Victoria Hospital in England who popularized the method and gave it substantial clinical trial. He emphasized the three important principles used today in the operation for vaginal agenesis. These principles are: first, dissection of an adequate space between the rectum and the bladder; second, inlay split-thickness skin grafting; and third, the cardinal principle of continuous and prolonged dilatation during the contractile phase of healing.

Other tissues such as amnion and peritoneum have been used to line the new vaginal space, but usually without substantial success. However, Tancer and associates reported good results with human amnion. Karjalainen and associates stated that a more physiological result was achieved with an amnion graft than with a skin graft.

TECHNIQUE OF THE ABBE–WHARTON–MCINDOE OPERATION. First, a careful pelvic examination under anesthesia must be done to verify previous findings. The patient is then positioned for taking a skin graft. Because pigmentation of the donor site is likely to be different from that of the surrounding skin, for cosmetic reasons, the graft should not be taken from the thigh or hip unless for some reason it cannot be obtained from the buttocks. Patients may be asked to sunbathe in a brief bathing suit before coming to the hospital in order that its outline can be seen. Hopefully, the graft can be taken from both buttocks within these borders. The quality of the graft will determine to a great extent the success of the operation. We have found the pneumatic Reese dermatome to be the most satisfactory instrument for taking the graft. With relatively little experience and practice, the gynecologic surgeon can scarcely fail to cut a graft successfully. A graft of controlled width and thickness can be cut (Fig. 15–5). The instrument is set and checked for taking a graft approximately 0.018 inches thick and 8 cm to 9 cm wide. The total graft length should be 16 cm to 20 cm. Therefore, a graft of 8 cm to 10 cm in length will be needed from each buttock. The skin of the donor sites is prepared with an antiseptic solution (povidone iodine) which

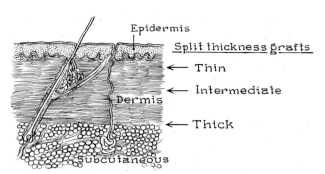

FIG. 15–5 Skin graft should be uniform in thickness. The Reese dermatome is set to take a graft approximately 0.018 inches thick. A graft that is a little too thick is better than a thin graft.

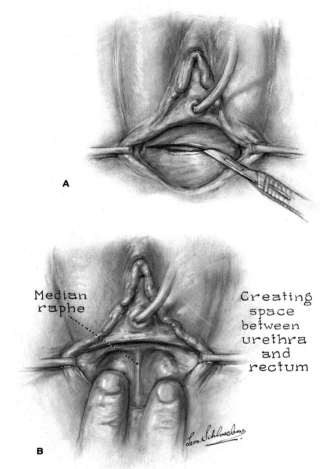

FIG. 15–6 The McIndoe procedure. (*A*) A transverse incision is made in the apex of the vaginal dimple. (*B*) A channel can usually be dissected on each side of a median raphe. The median raphe is then divided. Careful dissection will prevent injury to the bladder and rectum.

should be thoroughly washed away. It is then lubricated with mineral oil. Assistants steady and stretch the skin tight. Considerable pressure is made uniformly across the dermatome blade. The thickness of the graft must have minimal variation. A graft that is a little too thick is better than one a little too thin. There should be no breaks in the continuity of the graft. The graft is placed between two layers of moist gauze and the donor sites are dressed. Beginning 2 and 3 weeks later, the gauze dressing can be soaked and gradually removed as it separates from the healing donor sites.

The patient is placed in the lithotomy position, and a transverse incision is made through the mucosa of the vaginal vestibule as shown in Figure 15–6A. The space between the urethra and bladder anteriorly and the rectum posteriorly is dissected until the undersurface of the peritoneum is reached. This step may be made safer by placing a catheter in the urethra and sometimes a finger in the rectum to guide the dissection in the proper plane. After incising the mucosa of the vaginal vestibule transversely, one is often able to create a channel on each side of a median raphe (Fig. 15–6B). This can be started with blunt dissection and each channel can then be dilated with Hegar dilators or with finger dissection. The median raphe is divided, thus joining the two channels (Fig. 15–7). This maneuver is very helpful in dissecting an adequate space without injury to surrounding structures. To avoid subsequent narrowing of the vagina at the level of the urogenital diaphragm, we have found it helpful to incise the margin of the puborectalis muscles bilaterally along the midportion of the medial margin. Although useful in all patients, incising the puborectalis muscle is particularly important in the patient with the androgen insensitivity syndrome who has an android pelvis where the levator muscles are more taut against the pelvic diaphragm than in the patient who

has a gynecoid pelvis. We have found no difficulty with fecal incontinence in this procedure and it has significantly improved the ease with which the vaginal form can be inserted into the canal in the postoperative period. This procedure has also avoided contracture of the upper vagina because of a poorly applied form. The dissection should be carried as high as possible without entering the peritoneal cavity and without cleaning away all tissue beneath the peritoneum. A split-thickness skin graft will not take well when applied against a base of thin peritoneum. Care must be taken to ligate all bleeders. They are clamped and tied with very fine sutures. It is essential to have the vaginal cavity dry to prevent bleeding beneath the graft. Bleeding will cause the graft to separate from its bed, resulting in the inevitable fail-

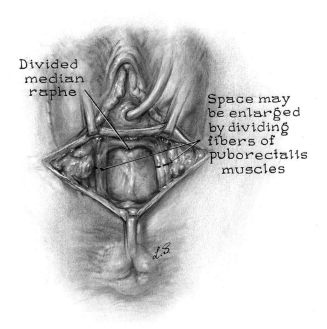

Divided median raphe

Space may be enlarged by dividing fibers of puborectalis muscles

FIG. 15-7 The McIndoe procedure. A space between the urethra and bladder anteriorly and the rectum posteriorly is dissected until the undersurface of the peritoneum is reached. Incision of the medial margin of the puborectalis muscles will enlarge the vagina laterally.

ure of the graft to implant in that area and local graft necrosis.

Formerly, the skin graft was placed over a balsa-wood form. Balsa wood has many advantages. It is inexpensive, easily available, and light, and it can be sterilized without difficulty. It can also be easily whittled in the operating room to a proper shape to fit the new vaginal space. However, we have seen a few instances in which the pressure from the form caused the skin graft to slough in places. One may also use a foam rubber form fashioned from a 6-in by 6-in block of styrofoam, trimmed approximately to the length and width of the new vagina, compressed and covered with a 0.25-in sheet of foam rubber to give a smooth external surface to the rubber form. Alternatively, one may cover a balsa-wood form with a foam rubber sheath to conform more correctly to the dimensions of the new vagina. Two rubber sheaths (condoms) are placed over the form and tied with silk about the base. The size of the form can then be tested by inserting it into the new vaginal space. The edges of the skin graft are sutured together over the form with very fine polyglycolic sutures with the outer skin surface facing the rubber sheath (Fig. 15–8). Under no circumstances should the graft be "meshed" to make it stretch farther, and the edges of the graft should be approximated me-

ticulously around the form without gaps. Granulation tissue will form at any little place where the form is not covered with skin. Contraction will occur where granulation tissue forms. The form, covered with the skin graft, is then fitted into the vaginal canal. To encourage drainage, the free edges of the graft are not sutured to the mucosal margins of the vaginal introitus. One must be careful not to have the form so large as to cause undue pressure on the urethra or rectum. A balsa-wood form should have a groove to accommodate the urethra. With a styrofoam rubber form, this is unnecessary. A suprapubic silicone catheter is placed in the bladder for drainage. If the labia are of sufficient length, the form can be held in place by suturing the labia together with two or three nonreactive sutures.

After 7 to 10 days, the form is removed and the vaginal cavity is irrigated with warm saline solution and inspected. Usually this can be done with the use of mild sedation and without an anesthetic. The cavity should be inspected carefully to determine if the graft has taken satisfactorily in all areas of the new vagina. Any undue pressure by the form should be noted and corrected. It is especially important that the form not make too much pressure superiorly against the peritoneum of the cul-de-sac. Such a constant upward pressure could result in weakness with subsequent enterocele formation. A new form is fashioned with a sterile sheath cover (condom) to fit the size of the vaginal canal and the patient is given instructions on its daily removal and reinsertion. She is advised to do so at the time of urination and defecation, but otherwise to wear the form continuously for a period of 6 weeks. The form is rinsed daily with povidone-iodine (Betadine) solution. A silicone or balsa-wood form is substituted for the original form in 6 weeks. It is much easier to remove and keep clean than a foam rubber form. However, the new vaginal cavity must be inspected frequently to detect and to prevent pressure necrosis of the skin graft. The patient is instructed to use the form during the night for the following 12 months. If there has been no change in the caliber of the vagina by that time, it is unlikely to occur later and the insertion of the form at night may be used intermittently until coitus is a frequent occurrence. However, if there is the slightest difficulty in inserting the form, the patient should be advised to use the form continuously again. Most patients are able to maintain the form in place by simply wearing a panty girdle and perineal pad. Douches are advisable while there is residual vaginal healing and discharge.

COMPLICATIONS AND RESULTS. The serious complications formerly associated with the McIndoe operation have been significantly reduced in recent

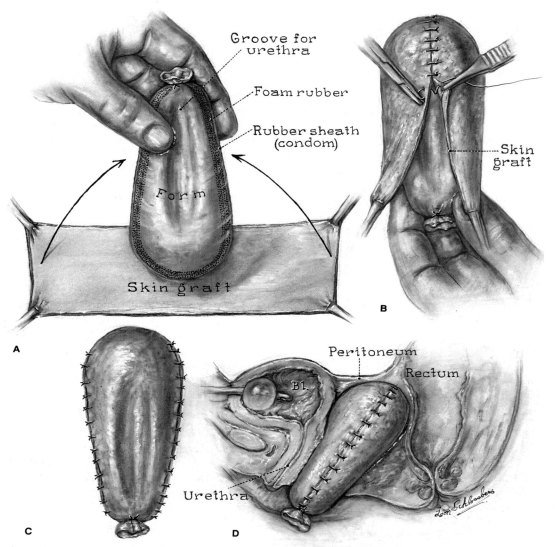

FIG. 15-8 The McIndoe procedure. (*A*) The form may be constructed of a central core of balsa wood covered by foam rubber and an outer rubber sheath (condom). A groove can be made to accommodate the urethra. The outer skin surface should be placed against the form. (*B, C*) The edges of the graft are sutured with No. 5-0 polyglycolic acid interrupted sutures. (*D*) The form should fit the new vaginal space exactly, without undue pressure at any points. The bladder may be drained suprapubically.

years by improvements in technique and greater experience. The results have also improved. Recently reported percentages of satisfactory results have ranged from 80% to 100%. Some serious complications still occur, including a 4% postoperative fistula rate (urethrovaginal, vesicovaginal, and rectovaginal). Postoperative infection, intraoperative and postoperative hemorrhage, and failure of graft take are still reported as occasional complications. Failure of graft take will often lead to the development of granulation tissue, with the possible re-

quirement for reoperation, curettement of the granulation tissue down to a healthy base, and even regrafting. The functional result is more important than the anatomical result in evaluating the success of this operation. A vagina of only 4 cm in some instances may be adequate for both husband and wife, whereas, in most cases, a shorter vagina is usually a major marital problem. Evans documented the fact that the procedure is not without complications, the most significant of which was the occurrence of vaginal infection in 17% of patients.

Between 1956 and 1975, the McIndoe operation was done on 64 patients at the Johns Hopkins Hospital as reported by Garcia and Jones. This procedure was used in 44 patients with the Mayer–Rokitansky–Kuster–Hauser syndrome; 9 male hermaphrodites, 7 patients with the testicular feminization syndrome, and 4 male transsexuals. The postoperative results have improved significantly since the balsa-wood vaginal form has been replaced by a foam rubber form during the past 10 years. In the total 20-year experience, 73% of the 64 patients had a 100% take of the graft, while in only 2 cases was there a significant area where the graft failed. Stenosis and loss of vaginal length was avoided by the use of levator incisions.

Urethrovaginal fistula has become even more infrequent since the introduction of the suprapubic catheter and the foam rubber form. The catheter is removed when the patient is voiding well and has no residual urine. In general, the patient is able to void without difficulty within the first few days following the procedure. We have found the use of prophylactic broad-spectrum antibiotics, started within 12 hours before surgery and continued for 5 days, to be of definite value in reducing the incidence of graft failures from infection in the operative site.

In the past, these patients were confined to bed for 2 weeks until the vaginal form was removed and the graft inspected. With the use of the foam rubber form, patients are ambulated gradually within 24 hours following surgery, while perineal pressure on the suture line is avoided during the first week by having the patient in either the upright or the prone position.

It is important that a McIndoe operation be done correctly the first time. If the vagina becomes constricted because of granulation tissue formation, injury to adjacent structures, or failure to use the form properly, subsequent attempts to create a satisfactory vagina will be more difficult. The first operation has the best chance of success.

There have been at least five case reports of primary malignant disease developing in a vagina created by various techniques. These were reviewed by Rotmensch and associates in 1983. Since primary carcinoma of the normally developed vagina is rare, it would seem that carcinoma in a neovagina could be a more frequent occurrence. Obviously, it would be difficult, perhaps impossible, to secure sound epidemiologic data to prove this point. However, it would be prudent to keep it in mind when advising these patients to have long-term follow-up examinations.

THE WILLIAMS VULVOVAGINOPLASTY. Although construction of a "perineal bridge" to help contain the vaginal mold was a routine part of the operation described by McIndoe, it was not subsequently adopted by others. However, Williams described a similar vulvovaginoplasty procedure in 1964 and advised that it could be used to create a vaginal canal. In 1975, he reported that the procedure was unsuccessful in only 1 of 52 patients. Feroze, Dewhurst, and Welply reported that the anatomical results were good in 22 of 26 patients. According to these authors, the advantages of the Williams operation are: (1) its technical simplicity, (2) the absence of serious local complications even when the operation is done as a repeat procedure, (3) the ease of postoperative care, (4) the absence of postoperative pain and the speed of recovery, (5) the absence of a need for dilators and the consequent applicability of the operation to patients who do not intend to have regular intercourse in the near future, and (6) the higher success rate of primary and repeat procedures. The technique is not applicable to patients who have poorly developed labia. It does result in an unusual angle of the vaginal canal, which, however, is reported to straighten out to a more normal direction with intercourse. If a very high perineum is created, urine may momentarily collect in the pouch following urination. This may give the impression of post-void incontinence. Failure of the suture line to heal primarily will result in a large area of granulation tissue and most likely an unsatisfactory result.

Obviously, if a patient has a functioning uterus, she must have a McIndoe operation to relieve the cryptomenorrhea. Also, Williams believes that if the urethral meatus is patulous, a vulvovaginoplasty should not be done because of the possibility that the urethra will be further stretched by coitus. He suggests that deficiencies in muscular and fascial tissue may be the reason that some patients with uterovaginal agenesis are able to develop a satisfactory vaginal canal with simple intermittent pressure with coitus and some are prone to develop enteroceles.

The technique of vulvovaginoplasty is illustrated in Fig. 15–9. As described by Williams, a horseshoe-shaped incision is made in the vulva. It extends across the perineum and up the medial side of the labia to the level of the external urethral meatus. The success of the operation depends on the appropriation of sufficient skin to line the new vagina. For this reason, the initial mucosal incisions are made as near the hairline as possible and approximately 4 cm from the midline. After complete mobilization, the inner skin margins are sutured together with knots tied inside the vaginal lumen. A second layer of sutures approximates subcutaneous fat and perineal muscles for support. Finally, the

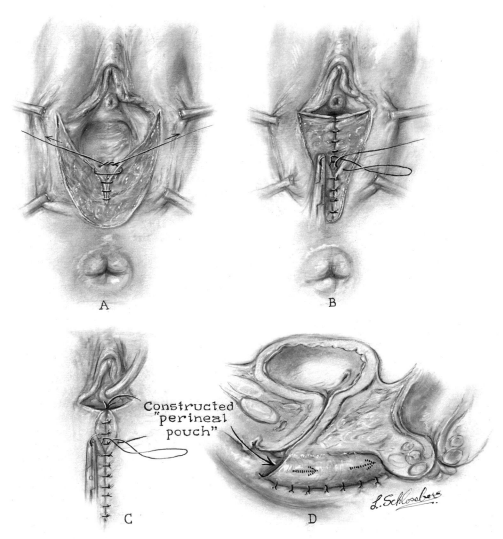

FIG. 15-9 The William's vulvovaginoplasty. No. 3-0 polyglycolic acid sutures may be used throughout to close both inner and outer skin margins and the tissue between. The entrance to the pouch should not cover the external urethral meatus.

external skin margins are approximated with interrupted sutures. If the procedure is properly done, it should be possible to insert two fingers into the pouch for a depth of 3 cm. An indwelling bladder catheter is used. The patient is confined to bed for 1 week with efforts to avoid tension on the suture line. Examinations are avoided for 6 weeks, at which time the patient is instructed to use dilators.

Capraro and Gallego have advised a modification of the above technique. They make the U-shaped incision in the skin of the labia majora at the level of the urethra or even lower. It is claimed that this modification will result in a more normal vulva to

sight and to touch, that the stagnant urine trapped in the vaginal pouch will be avoided, and that the vagina will still be satisfactory for intercourse. Other modifications have been made by Feroze and associates.

The Williams vulvovaginoplasty is a useful operation and should certainly be considered as the operation of choice in patients who may need a supplement to an unsatisfactory McIndoe operation or a supplement to a small vagina resulting from extensive surgery or radiation therapy. Rarely, a patient with a solitary kidney low in the pelvis will not have room for dissection of an adequate vaginal space. A Williams vulvovaginoplasty can be used instead. However, we continue to use the McIndoe operation as the preferred procedure in most cases.

CONGENITAL ABSENCE OF THE VAGINA WITH A FUNCTIONAL MIDLINE UTERUS

A functional midline uterus may be present in 5% to 10% of patients with congenital absence of the vagina. Cyclic menstruation with cryptomenorrhea will begin in early adolescence and soon will be associated with fairly regular monthly episodes of intense lower abdominal pain and the gradual enlargement of a lower abdominal mass. If the tubes are normally developed and patent, endometriosis from retrograde menstruation may also develop. Obviously, an operation must be done to relieve the cryptomenorrhea as soon as a proper diagnosis can be made. Unnecessary delay will result in continued suffering and further damage to the reproductive organs.

These young patients present a difficult diagnostic problem. They will all have normal female secondary sex characteristics. Karyotype and sex chromatin studies will indicate genetic females. Menses will be absent externally and cyclic lower abdominal pain will be present. An intravenous pyelogram may show urinary tract anomalies. However, they may be different from one another in one very important respect and that is whether the cervix is present or absent. Some patients will have vaginal and cervical aplasia with a functioning midline uterine corpus, and others will have aplasia of the lower two-thirds of the vagina with an upper vaginal pouch and a properly developed uterine cervix and corpus above. Ultrasonography may be helpful or confusing, but should be done. Valdes and associates have reported preoperative ultrasonography to be useful in the evaluation of two patients with atresia of the vagina and cervix. It is more helpful when it can be correlated with the findings of a careful pelvic examination under anesthesia and laparoscopy. When a small part of the upper vagina is present, a normally formed cervix and uterus will usually, but not always, be found above. Niver has reported two patients with an upper vaginal pouch who did not have a properly formed cervix. When the cervix and vagina are completely absent, laparoscopy is more likely to show a distended uterine corpus, which rarely may be bicornuate. Pelvic endometriosis and especially endometrial cysts of the ovaries may be present if the condition has remained undiagnosed for several years.

The proper operation for these patients depends on whether or not a cervix is present. Unfortunately, it may not be possible to answer this question until abdominal and vaginal exploration is carried out. If a normal cervix is found, the creation of a vagina by the McIndoe technique or the Jeffcoate vaginal advancement technique will correct the patient's problem and preserve the potential for satisfactory intercourse and normal pregnancies in the future. The operation consists of dissecting a space from below, in the same manner as in the McIndoe procedure, until the upper vaginal segment is reached. If this upper vaginal segment is still distended with menstrual blood and mucus, it is easier to identify, mobilize, and drain from below. On the other hand, if it has been previously drained and emptied through an abdominal approach, it will be more difficult to find with the dissection from below and easily confused with the bladder or rectum. During the perineal dissection, needle aspiration will help identify the location of a collection of mucus and menstrual blood. A dissection can then be made along the needle track and an incision can be made transversely in the thick inferior wall of the distended vaginal pouch. Complete drainage of the pouch is allowed. The rim of the dilated cervix and the interior of the uterine cavity can be visualized through this vaginal pouch. The walls of the vaginal pouch can sometimes be mobilized sufficiently in all directions to allow suturing to the lower vagina at the introitus, as advised by Jeffcoate. However, this technique does require extensive dissection and if there is tension on the suture line, it will pull away, leaving a gap where granulation tissue will develop and endometrial fragments may implant. Constriction of the vagina will be difficult to prevent and a subsequent operation to revise the vagina, perhaps using a skin graft, may be necessary. Therefore, if mobilization cannot be accomplished well enough to suture the edges together without tension, a skin graft should be used initially to cover the intervening space. The graft is usually sutured *in situ* in the vagina rather than sutured to a form. It is absolutely vital to the success of the operation that the new space not become constricted. To avoid this, a form must be worn for many months during the constrictive phase of healing. Recognizing the difficulty of obtaining satisfactory cooperation in wearing a form from such young adolescent girls, Andrews and Jones have designed a special lucite form that can be left in place for 6 months without removal. The form has a bulb at the upper end that should fit snugly in the upper vaginal pouch. The lower cylinder comes through the newly dissected vaginal canal. A lumen through the middle of the form provides an exit for the menstrual flow. According to Andrews and Jones, if the form is left in place for at least six months, the new canal will not only remain open but will also become completely epithelialized without a skin graft. Anesthesia may be necessary to remove the form.

When the vagina and cervix are both absent and a functioning uterine corpus is present, the management is quite different. A satisfactory vaginal canal can be created, but it is generally impossible to create a cervix with a functional endocervical canal. Many methods have been tried, mostly involving the creation of a passage through dense fibrous tissue between the uterine cavity and the vagina with placement of a stent to keep the tract open. Occasional success in maintaining an open passageway has been reported and a few patients have experienced normal cyclic menstruation. However, endocervical glands do not develop and there is no way to compensate for the absence of the cervical mucus, which plays an important role in sperm transport. Even though cyclic ovulatory menstrual periods can be achieved in a few patients, pregnancy will usually not be possible. Eventually the uterovaginal fistulous tract closes from constriction by fibrous tissue. Endometriosis may develop along the tract. Endometriosis may also develop in the ovaries and other pelvic sites because of retrograde menstruation. Recurrent and severe pelvic infection is a common problem.

Many authors have recommended that a patient with a functioning uterine corpus who has congenital absence of the cervix and vagina should have a hysterectomy as an initial procedure. This will eliminate much needless suffering from painful cryptomenorrhea, sepsis, endometriosis, and multiple operations. If a hysterectomy can be done soon enough, it may then be possible to conserve ovaries for their useful function for years to come. In spite of recommendations to the contrary by Farber, Mitchell, and Marchant, most authors agree with Geary and Weed, Maciulla and associates, Dillon and associates, Niver and associates, and Jones that a recommendation for hysterectomy as initial primary therapy in these cases seems realistic, with very few exceptions.

It should be mentioned that congenital atresia of the uterine cervix can occur as an isolated anomaly in a patient with an apparently normal vagina and a functioning uterus. Such a case has been reported by Nunley and Kitchin. The vagina was 10 cm long and large bilateral endometrial ovarian cysts were resected. It was impossible to create a satisfactory channel between the uterine cavity and the vagina and eventually a hysterectomy was necessary. The "cervix" was a fibrous cord that showed no endocervical glands microscopically. This anomaly is

rare but presents the same difficulties as mentioned above.

ACQUIRED VAGINAL INADEQUACY

Although unusual types of infection and atrophy rarely may result in closure of part of the vagina, acquired vaginal inadequacy most often results from the treatment of various gynecologic malignancies with surgery or radiation or a combination of both. The maintenance or restoration of vaginal function is now considered an important part of the treatment plan for such malignancies, especially when the patient is young and otherwise healthy. The techniques of vaginal reconstruction in gynecologic oncology have been reviewed by Magrina and Masterson, by Pratt, and by McCraw and associates.

Problems of Vertical Fusion

The problems associated with vertical fusion include transverse vaginal septum with or without obstruction. Although imperforate hymen is a vertical fusion problem, the hymen is not a derivative of the müllerian ducts (see chapter 30).

TRANSVERSE VAGINAL SEPTUM

No reliable epidemiologic data exist regarding the incidence of transverse vaginal septum. Reported incidences vary from 1 in 2,100 to 1 in 72,000. It is probably less common than congenital absence of the vagina and uterus. It has been diagnosed in newborns, infants, and older adolescent girls. Its etiology is unknown, although McKusick has suggested that in some and perhaps most cases it results from a female sex-limited autosomal recessive transmission. Obviously, there is a developmental defect in vaginal embryogenesis that leads to an incomplete fusion between the müllerian duct component and the urogenital sinus component of the vagina. This incomplete vertical fusion results in a transverse septum. The septum varies in thickness. It can be located at almost any level in the vagina. Lodi has reported that 46% occur in the upper vagina, 40% in the midvagina, and 14% in the lower vagina. In contrast to müllerian duct aplasia, transverse vaginal septum is associated with few urologic or other anomalies. Imperforate anus and bicornuate uterus may be found, as reported by Mandell and associates. The lower surface of the transverse septum is always covered by squamous epithelium. The upper surface may be covered by glandular epithelium, which is likely to be transformed into squamous epithelium by a metaplastic process after correction of the obstruction.

In neonates and young infants, imperforate transverse vaginal septum with obstruction may lead to serious and life-threatening problems caused by the compression of surrounding organs by fluid that has collected above the septum. The fluid undoubtedly comes from endocervical glands and müllerian glandular epithelium in the upper vagina that have been stimulated by the placental transfer of maternal estrogens. Continued fluid collection in infants even after the first year has also been reported and should make one consider the possibility of a fistula between the upper vagina and the urinary tract. The distended upper vagina creates a large pelvic and lower abdominal mass that may displace the bladder anteriorly; displace the ureters laterally with hydroureters and hydronephrosis; compress the rectum with associated obstipation and even intestinal obstruction; and limit diaphragmatic excursion, compress the vena cava, and produce cardiorespiratory failure. Fatalities have been reported. The hydrocolpos develops along the axis of the upper vagina and, therefore, may not cause the outlet or perineum to bulge when there is compression of the mass from above. After careful preoperative radiologic and endoscopic investigations of the infant, the septum should be removed

through a perineal approach. Jones suggests that bilateral Schuchardt incisions may be required to ensure that the septum has been removed. Because of a subsequent tendency for vaginal stenosis and reaccumulation of the fluid in the upper vagina, follow-up studies to assess the recurrence of urinary obstruction are important. Vaginal reconstruction may be required in later years to allow satisfactory menstruation and coitus.

A hydrometrocolpos may not develop until puberty. Patients with this problem will present with cyclic lower abdominal pain, no visible menstrual discharge, and gradual development of a central lower abdominal and pelvic mass. Sometimes a small tract will open in the septum, some menstrual blood will escape periodically, and symptoms will be variable. A septum large enough to allow pregnancy to occur may still cause dystocia during labor. Cyclic hematuria may be present if a communication between the bladder and upper vagina exists. The pelvic organs of a woman who had a transverse vaginal septum are shown diagrammatically in Figure 15–10. Because of the transverse vaginal septum, the woman had difficulty at the time of onset of menstruation with the development of severe cyclic pain, but no external bleeding. Finally, menstrual blood began to flow externally through the small sinus shown in Figure 15–11A. Pelvic examination

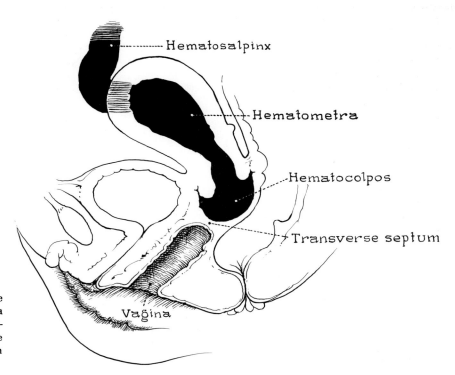

FIG. 15–10 A transverse septum at the junction of the mid and upper vagina has caused menstrual blood to accumulate above. For this condition the operation illustrated in Figure 15-11 can be done.

Hematosalpinx

Hematometra

Hematocolpos

Transverse septum

Vagina

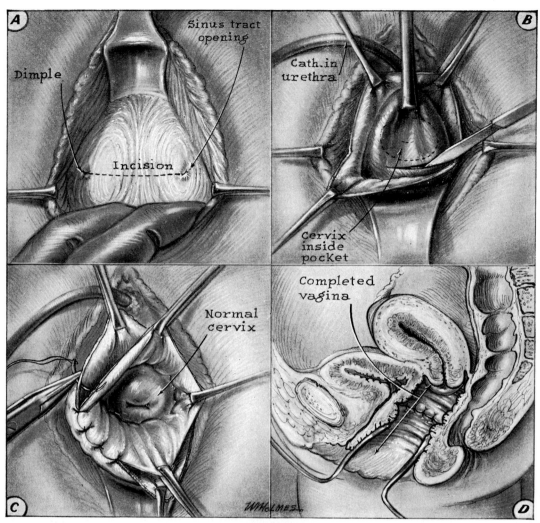

FIG. 15–11 (*A*) Upper end of a short vagina, showing sinus tract opening through which patient menstruated and incision through mucous membrane. (*B*) Areolar tissue has been dissected through to the pocket of mucosa which covered the cervix. The mucosa is being incised. (*C*) An anastomosis is being made between the lower vagina and the upper vagina. (*D*) Showing completed vagina. It is slightly shorter than normal but of normal caliber.

per rectum revealed a cervix and a normal-sized corpus. The ovaries were palpable, but adherent, probably because of organized blood from hematosalpinx and hematoperitoneum. Remarkably, the woman had little dysmenorrhea after beginning to menstruate externally. Coitus was fairly satisfactory before surgical correction, but the shortness of the vagina was something of a handicap. The operative procedure performed to correct this patient's problem is shown in Figure 15-11B,C, and D.

Rock and associates at the Johns Hopkins Hospital

reported their experience with 26 patients with complete transverse vaginal septum. Associated congenital anomalies of the urinary tract, coarctation of the aorta, atrial septal defect, and malformations of the lumbar spine were found. Vaginal patency and coital function was successfully established in all patients and 7 of 19 patients attempting pregnancy eventually had children. The incidence of endometriosis and spontaneous abortion was high. A lower pregnancy rate and more extensive endometriosis were present when the transverse septum was located high in the vagina, suggesting that retrograde flow through the uterus and fallopian tubes occurs earlier in these patients. More extensive dissection between the bladder and rectum is required to identify the upper vagina when the septum is thick and high. In five patients, an exploratory laparotomy was necessary to guide a probe through the uterine fundus and cervix and to assist in locating a high hematocolpos.

SURGICAL TECHNIQUE FOR A TRANSVERSE VAGINAL SEPTUM. A transverse incision is made through the vault of the short vagina (Fig. 15–11A). A probe can be introduced through the septum after a portion of the barrier has been separated by sharp and blunt dissection. One usually finds some areolar tissue in dissecting the space between the vagina and the rectum. Palpation of a urethral catheter anteriorly and insertion of a double-gloved finger along the anterior wall of the rectum posteriorly will provide the proper surgical guidelines so that the bladder and rectum can be avoided during this blind procedure. After the dissection is continued for a short distance, the cervix can usually be palpated, and continuity can be established with the upper segment of the vagina (Fig. 15–11B,C). The lateral margins of the excised septum are extended widely by sharp knife dissection to avoid postoperative stricture formation. The edges of the upper and the lower vaginal mucosa are undermined and mobilized enough to permit anastomosis, using interrupted delayed-absorbable sutures (Fig. 15–11C). Figure 15–11D shows the completed anastomosis with a vagina that is of normal caliber but slightly shorter than the average length. A sponge rubber vaginal form covered with a sterile latex sheath is placed in the vagina and removed in 10 days for evaluation of the healing process. The form is worn for 6 weeks until complete healing has occurred. After this, coitus is permitted. If the patient is not sexually active, a Silastic vaginal form is inserted at night until the constrictive phase of healing is complete.

If removal of a thick vaginal septum will not allow the upper and lower vaginal margins to be approximated without tension, one may consider the use of a split-thickness skin graft to bridge the gap. A lucite form described by Jones and Wheeless may be inserted and left in place for several months to permit epithelialization, thus avoiding the need for a graft. A rather ingenious but complicated Z-plasty method of bridging the gap has been described by Garcia and by Musset. A simpler flap method was described by Brenner and associates. Lees and Singer have described yet another technique that tends to avoid vaginal constriction.

Problems of Lateral Fusion

The problems associated with defects in lateral fusion include septate uterus; bicornuate uterus; didelphic uterus; unicornuate uterus; and longitudinal vaginal septum, with or without obstruction.

UNOBSTRUCTED LATERAL FUSION PROBLEMS

Double Uterus (Didelphic, Bicornuate, and Septate Uteri)

Complete failure of medial fusion of the two müllerian ducts may result in a complete duplication of the vagina, cervix, and uterus. A partial failure of fusion may result in a single vagina with a single or duplicate cervix and complete or partial duplication of the uterine corpus. A failure of disappearance of the uterine septum between the two fused müllerian ducts may result in the septum persisting inside the uterus to a variable extent while the external appearance is that of a single uterus. The septum may be so complete as to divide both the uterine cavity and endocervical canal into two equal or unequal components. More commonly, incomplete disappearance of the septum may leave only the upper uterine cavities divided. Each of these and a variety of other forms of "double uteri" have their own special clinical significance. When no obstruction is present, surgical reconstruction has been done primarily for difficulties with reproduction.

Some aspects of this subject remain controversial because information is still inaccurate or incomplete. Many reports are based on small numbers of selected patients, patients have been diagnosed to have one anomaly or another based on incomplete data, and some patients have received unification operations without preliminary studies to rule out other causes of reproductive difficulty. A comparison of results from one series to the next may be difficult because authors have used different classifications based on a variety of embryologic, anatomical, physiologic, functional or radiologic considerations. An unknown number of uterine anomalies escape detection, especially if the patient has an acceptable reproductive performance and no gynecologic difficulties.

Ruge, in 1882, first reported excision of a uterine septum in a woman who had had two abortions. She subsequently carried a pregnancy to term. Paul Strassman of Berlin and later Erwin Strassman, his son, were strong advocates of uterine unification operations. The studies of Jones and Jones have greatly improved the understanding and management of patients with uterine anomalies. Their studies began with a report in 1953 of a series that began in 1936. Updates have been published from time to time. Jones, Wheeless, Rock, Andrews, and others have joined in these reports.

If a uterine anomaly is associated with obstruction of menstrual flow, it will cause symptoms that will come to the attention of the gynecologist shortly after the menarche. Unobstructed uterine anomalies will be diagnosed later in a variety of circumstances. Young girls may notice difficulty in using tampons or later in coitus if a longitudinal vaginal septum is present. This can lead to the diagnosis of an associated uterine anomaly. A patient with an anomalous upper urinary tract on intravenous pyelogram may be found to have a uterine anomaly when referred for gynecologic evaluation. A uterine anomaly may occasionally be found when a patient complains of dysmenorrhea or menorrhagia or when a dilatation and curettage is done for abortion or some other indication. A palpable mass may be found to be a uterine anomaly when confirmed by ultrasonography, by hysterography, or by laparoscopy. As Semmens has pointed out, the diagnosis of uterine anomaly may result from the astute observation of an abnormal uterine contour during pregnancy, either in the antepartum period or at the time of abdominal or vaginal delivery. The abnormal contour is caused by a combination of fetal malpresentation and an anomalous uterus. An anomalous uterus may be diagnosed when a patient becomes pregnant in spite of the presence of an intrauterine device in the uterus. Persistent postmenopausal bleeding in spite of recent dilatation and curettage may lead to a diagnosis of an anomalous uterus. Sometimes the diagnosis is made as an incidental finding at laparotomy. However, most uterine anomalies are diagnosed as a result of hysterosalpingography to evaluate patients with infertility or reproductive loss, usually repeated spontaneous abortion.

Although some uterine anomalies may cause infertility, the vast majority of patients with uterine anomalies are able to conceive without difficulty. There is no question that uterine anomalies may be associated with a perfectly normal reproductive performance. Overall, however, the incidence of spontaneous abortion, premature birth, fetal loss, malpresentation, and cesarean section is clearly increased when a uterine anomaly is present. Unfortunately, it is not possible to predict which patients with uterine anomalies will have these problems.

The etiology of reproductive failure in patients with uterine anomalies remains unclear. Mahgoub considers that the presence of a uterine septum may lead to abortion because of diminished intrauterine space for fetal growth or because of implantation of the placenta on a poorly vascularized septum. Mizuno and associates have attached importance to the inadequacy of vascularization of the uterine septum. Associated cervical incompetence, luteal phase insufficiency, and distortion of the uterine milieu have all been implicated in the etiology of increased reproductive loss. However, it is as yet unexplained why some patients with a uterine anomaly have normal reproductive function whereas others abort early in pregnancy. Interestingly, it has been reported that the chance for a liveborn child increases with each pregnancy loss. It is unknown whether this conditioning of the uterus is due to better vascularization, better myometrial stretching and accommodation, or some other factor.

A patient with a history of three or more spontaneous abortions or premature labor should have a hysterosalpingogram to determine if structural abnormalities of the uterus are present. An abnormality will be found in about 10% of such patients. Among chronic early second-trimester aborters, the incidence may be higher. The etiology of spontaneous abortion is complex, and a complete workup should be done even when an anomalous uterus has been found. A careful history should include a detailed discussion of each previous pregnancy loss; inquiry about diethylstilbestrol exposure; drug and chemical toxicity; specific medical illnesses; and exposure to contagious diseases. A family history should place special emphasis on reproductive failures among family members of the patient and the husband. Specific medical diseases such as thyroid disease, diabetes mellitus, renal disease, and systemic lupus erythematosus should be ruled out. The possibility of infection, including such agents as *N. gonorrheae*, chlamydia, mycoplasma, toxoplasma, and Listeria, should be considered. Chromosome analysis should be done with the expectation of finding abnormalities in up to one-fourth of couples with a history of habitual abortion, and the understanding that more than 50% of spontaneous abortions have chromosomal abnormalities in the aborted tissue. Identifying such couples makes it possible to offer genetic counseling for subsequent pregnancies. Uterine leiomyomata, especially lower uterine segment and submucous leiomyomata, may cause spontaneous abortion. Basal body temperature charts, serum progesterone determinations, and endometrial biopsies timed in the luteal phase will help determine the presence of luteal phase deficiency. The cervix should be studied for incompetence. Couples with multiple etiologies for reproductive loss should have all other problems corrected before a uterine unification operation is done.

Correcting other factors first may, indeed, correct the problem of reproductive loss without a metroplasty. Rock and Jones reported seven patients with anomalous uterine development who also were found to have extrauterine factors in the etiology of their reproductive loss. These patients had had 16 pregnancies of which 5 (31%) resulted in a living child. After therapy to correct the extrauterine factor, the success rate rose to 71%. Stoot and Mastboom reported an impressive improvement in reproductive performance among uterine anomaly patients simply by improving abnormal carbohydrate metabolism.

The technique of performing hysterosalpingography to diagnose uterine anomalies is important. The hysterogram must be taken at right angles to the axis of the uterus in order that a true assessment of the deformity can be made. The study is best done under fluoroscopy. The distinction between a septate uterus and a bicornuate uterus cannot be made with hysterogram alone (Fig. 15–12). The external uterine configuration also cannot usually be determined by pelvic examination alone, but some idea of the configuration may be obtained by ultrasonography. McDonough has suggested the use of double-contour pelvic pneumoperitoneum-hysterographic studies for precise identification of müllerian malformations. Of course, laparoscopy is even more certain. One must be prepared to correct either anomaly depending on the findings at laparotomy, if the uterine corpus has not been previously visualized (Fig. 15-13).

A complete investigation should also include semen analysis, assessment of tubal patency, and an intravenous pyelogram. A variety of upper urinary tract anomalies are seen, including absence of one kidney, horseshoe kidney, pelvic kidney, duplication of the collecting system, and ectopically located ureteral orifices. The lower urinary tract (bladder and urethra) is much less often anomalous.

The percentage of full-term pregnancies in an unselected series of women with various types of double uterus who have not been operated on is unknown. For all types combined, it is probably about 25%. In patients selected for operation, it probably rises from about 5% to 10% to about 80% to 90%. Because patients with uterine anomalies who have relatively normal obstetric histories cannot be identified, there is confusion in the literature about which anomalies are more often associated with obstetric difficulties and which are relatively benign in their effect. Special diagnostic procedures to detect uterine anomalies are not usually done before reproductive performance is tested. The didelphic uterus is an exception. This anomaly can be diagnosed easily by identifying two complete cervices and perhaps a longitudinal vaginal septum as well on routine pelvic exam. A study by Heinonen in Finland of 182 women with uterine anomalies indicated that pregnancies in the septate uterus had a better fetal survival rate (86%) than complete bicornuate uteri (50%) or unicornuate (40%). These findings differ from the prevalent opinion that the septate uterus is associated with the highest reproductive loss, as proposed by Jones and Seegar-Jones.

In 1968, Capraro and associates reported seeing 85 patients with uterine anomalies between 1962 and 1966. One uterine anomaly was seen for every 645 admissions (0.145%). In only 14 (16%) of these 85 patients was metroplasty considered necessary. According to Jones and Seegar-Jones, only one-third of patients with a double uterus have important reproductive problems. Obviously, the presence of a double uterus is not in itself an indication for unification operation.

Jewelewicz has estimated the spontaneous abortion rate to be 33.8% in women with a bicornuate uterus, 22.2% in those with a septate uterus, and 34.6% in those with a unicornuate uterus. Capraro and associates found a preoperative fetal salvage rate of 33.3% for the septate uterus, 10% for the bicornuate uterus, and 0% for the didelphic uterus. Postoperatively, the fetal salvage rate was 100% for the bicornuate uterus, 80% for the septate uterus, and 66% for the didelphic uterus. The report gives the improved salvage figures after metroplasty from several previous studies.

A didelphic uterus with two hemicorpora is easily diagnosed since all patients will be found to have two hemicervices visible on speculum examination,

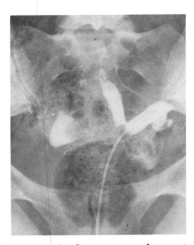

FIG. 15–12 Preoperative hysterogram demonstrating patent fallopian tubes and two uterine cavities. It is impossible to tell if this uterus is bicornuate or septate until the uterine corpus is seen.

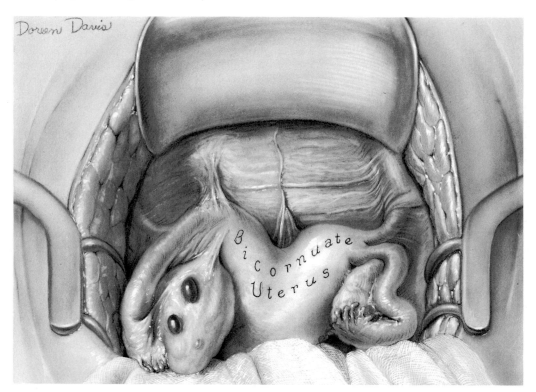

Doreen Davis

FIG. 15-13 A typical bicornuate uterus with two hemicorpora. A septate uterus has only one corpus.

and most if not all, will have a longitudinal sagittal vaginal septum. In the series reported by Heinonen and associates, all 21 patients with a didelphic uterus had a vaginal septum. Conversely, a patient with a longitudinal vaginal septum will usually, but not always, be found to have a didelphic uterus. The indication for uterine unification is related to the role of this anomaly as an etiologic factor in the reproductive loss. Of all the uterine anomalies (except an arcuate uterus), the didelphic uterus is associated with the best possibility of a successful pregnancy. However, there is still some increase in perinatal mortality, premature birth, breech presentation, and cesarean section for delivery. Heinonen and associates reported a fetal survival of 64% without metroplasty. Musich and Behrman state that the didelphic uterus was found to give the best chance for a successful pregnancy (57%) and was not considered an appropriate indication for metroplasty. Jones and Wheeless agree. However, W. S. Jones considered the didelphic uterus to give the worst obstetric outcome. In our opinion, a unification operation for a didelphic uterus is not indicated often and the results may be disappointing, especially when an attempt is made to unify the cervix. Not only is this procedure technically very

difficult in a complete didelphic anomaly, but it may also result in cervical incompetence or cervical stenosis.

Our own experience would confirm the larger experience of Jones and others that most patients who are evaluated for repeated abortion and are found to have a uterine anomaly will have a septate uterus. A few will have other anomalies, mostly bicornuate uterus. In our experience, fetal survival rates are higher after the repair of a septate uterus than after repair of other types of anomalies. Rock and Jones report that, at Johns Hopkins Hospital, of 43 patients with septate uteri selected for Jones metroplasty, 95% became pregnant postoperatively, 73% of pregnancies were carried to term, and 77% of patients had a living child.

Dysmenorrhea and abnormal and heavy menstrual bleeding have been reported to occur more frequently in patients with any form of double uterus, and to be relieved after unification operations. Capraro and associates reported several cases in which dysmenorrhea was cured by metroplasty. Erwin Strassman also believed that all cases of dysmenorrhea and menorrhagia in conjunction with uterine anomalies were relieved by unification of the two uterine cavities. In general, we believe dysmenorrhea and menorrhagia are not appropriate indications for uterine unification, and would hesitate to do the operation solely for these reasons.

There is considerable difference of opinion regarding whether or not infertility is a proper indication for metroplasty. Erwin Strassman stated that primary infertility could be cured in 60% of patients with uterine anomaly provided all other causes of infertility were excluded. Strassman reported doing eight metroplasties for "primary sterility." These operations yielded 9 pregnancies and 7 living children, although the number of patients who conceived is not given. Similar reports of small numbers of patients can be found throughout the literature. Heinonen and Pystynen indicated that uterine anomalies are rarely the reason for infertility. Nonuterine causes of infertility must be ruled out before, as a last resort, metroplasty is performed.

Certainly, a full infertility investigation must be done first to rule out other causes of infertility before the anomalous uterus is blamed. Even then, if no other cause for infertility is found and the uterus is septate or bicornuate, one may not have a proper indication for metroplasty. This question has simply not yet been answered, and the decision is therefore difficult. One has an even more difficult decision to make if an infertility patient with a septate or bicornuate uterus requires laparotomy for some other reason such as endometriosis or tubal occlusion. Should a metroplasty operation be done at the same time? Experience with such combined operations is not sufficient to answer this question. In our experience, combining metroplasty with microsurgical tubal reconstruction has been successful in two patients with infertility.

SURGICAL TECHNIQUE FOR UTERINE UNIFICATION. Two types of metroplasty operations are used as unification procedures, depending on whether one is operating on two separate hemicorpora or on a single uterine corpus with a septum (Fig. 15–14). The

Jones procedure is used for a septate uterus and the Strassman procedure is used for unification of a bicornuate and a didelphic uterus. If the Strassman transverse incision is used for a septate uterus, one may encounter difficulty with bleeding, and the postoperative configuration of the uterine cavity may show considerable deformity, as reported by Kusuda. Both procedures described here are modified from the original descriptions given by their authors, and have been adequately tested in our clinic.

The surgical technique for the modified Jones unification operation is demonstrated in Figure 15–15. The abdomen is generally opened through a transverse incision. If a unification operation only is planned, a Pfannenstiel incision is permissible. The pelvic viscera are inspected. The septate uterus may demonstrate a median raphe across the fundus, but it is surprising how often the corpus looks normal. To facilitate manipulation, a traction suture of heavy silk is placed through the top of the septum. The site of this suture will be removed when the septum is excised.

No attempt is made to stain the uterine cavity with methylene blue. The normal unstained endometrial tissue can be easily differentiated from the myometrium. We prefer not to inject the myometrium with a vasopressor solution because of the theoretical possibility of interfering with subsequent healing. For hemostasis, a tourniquet is applied at the junction of the lower uterine segment and cervix by inserting a 0.5-in Penrose drain through an avascular space in the broad ligaments just lateral to the uterine vessels on each side. The tourniquet is placed around the lower uterine segment and is tied anterior to the uterus. Since the uterine corpus receives a significant blood supply through the ovarian arteries, tourniquets should also be tied around the infundibulopelvic ligaments on each side, using the same hole in the broad ligament. All tourniquets must be tied tightly enough to occlude both the arterial supply to and the venous drainage from the uterus. If only the venous drainage is occluded, the corpus will become engorged and congested and bleeding will be increased. If the arterial supply is occluded, the uterus will blanche and the bleeding will be minimal. A sterile Doptone can be used to establish disappearance of uterine artery pulsations. The use of hypotensive anesthetic techniques in conjunction with the tourniquets will allow a uterine unification operation to be accomplished with negligible blood loss.

An outline of the septum may be drawn on the anterior and posterior serosal surface of the uterus. After experience with several cases, however, this will not be necessary. The size of the septal wedge

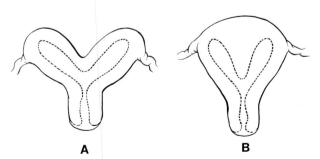

A　　　**B**

FIG. 15–14 (*A*) A bicornuate uterus. The Strassman operation should be used. (*B*) A septate uterus. The Jones or Tompkins operation should be used.

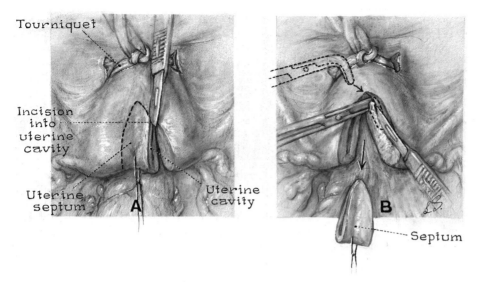

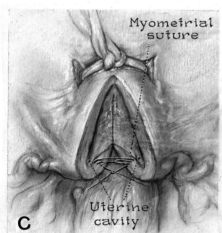

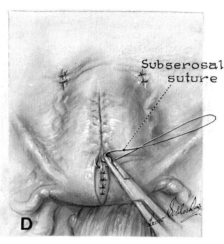

FIG. 15–15 The Jones metroplasty with modifications. (*A*) After placing tourniquets to control bleeding, the septum is excised. (*B*) The remaining septum is removed from each side. (*C*) The myometrium is reapproximated with No. 3-0 polyglycolic acid interrupted vertical figure-of-eight sutures. Avoid placing sutures too close to interstitial portion of fallopian tubes. (*D*) A continuous No. 5-0 polyglycolic acid subserosal suture is used as a final layer. Tourniquets are removed and defects in the broad ligaments are closed.

to be removed can be determined by experience, from careful palpation of the uterine corpus, from a review of the hysterosalpingogram films during the operation, and from a judgement regarding the location of the interstitial portion of the fallopian tubes. It is better to excise a wedge that is a little too small than one that is a little too large. The septum is sharply excised in a wedge with an anterior-to-posterior incision on each side of the midline fundal suture until the endometrial cavity is reached. One must be careful not to transect the endometrial cavity. The modified Jones procedure differs from the traditional Jones procedure in that a smaller wedge of septum is excised initially in the modified procedure. This prevents the excessive removal of normal endometrial and myometrial tissue and will protect the interstitial portion of the fal-

lopian tubes from being damaged by sutures that are placed too close. The remaining lateral portions of the septum are excised by inserting a clamp into the uterine cornu on each side and removing an additional small wedge of tissue. Inferiorly, the entire septum is usually excised to create a single lower uterine segment canal. However, any part of the septum that extends into the endocervical canal may be left *in situ* at the internal os to avoid the possibility of creating an incompetent cervix by its removal.

After the septum has been removed, the myometrium must be reapproximated. Many different suture techniques have been described. We prefer to use interrupted vertical figure-of-eight sutures of a delayed-absorbable polyglycolic acid suture (No. 3-0 Vicryl) with an atraumatic needle. The sutures are placed at approximately 0.5 cm intervals. The most inferior sutures approximating the lower uterine segment anteriorly and posteriorly should be placed first. After they are tied, the endocervical canal should be tested for patency. The remainder of the sutures are then placed, gradually approximating the two sides. At the uterine fundus, the sutures are placed carefully to avoid obstruction of the interstitial portion of the fallopian tubes. As the sutures are tied, the two sides of the uterus should be squeezed together to relieve tension. The sutures are cut short and the knots are covered by a running subserosal suture of fine polyglycolic acid suture (No. 5-0 Vicryl). If possible, no suture lines are exposed to the endometrial or peritoneal cavity.

It has not been considered necessary or desirable to pack the uterine cavity with iodoform gauze or to leave an intrauterine device in the uterine cavity. These methods have been advised to prevent the formation of intrauterine adhesions. Actually, adhesions in the uterine cavity form very infrequently after uterine unification.

The technique of metroplasty described above is a compromise between the classic Jones metroplasty and the Tompkins metroplasty. In the Jones operation the entire septum is removed. In the Tompkins operation, a single median incision divides the uterine corpus and septum in half. The incision is carried inferiorly until the endometrial cavity is reached. Each lateral septal half is then incised up to within 1 cm of the tubes. No septal tissue is removed. The myometrium is reapproximated, taking care not to place sutures too close to the interstitial portion of the tubes. Proponents of this technique suggest that it is simpler. It conserves all myometrial tissue and leaves the utero-tubal junction in a more normal and lateral position. Good results with this technique have been reported recently by McShane and associates.

The Strassman procedure is not easily adapted to the septate uterus, but it is the procedure of choice for unification of the two endometrial cavities of an externally divided uterus (bicornuate or didelphic) (Fig. 15–16). When there has been failure of fusion of the two müllerian ducts, inspection of the pelvic cavity will often reveal a broad peritoneal band that lies in the middle between the two lateral hemicorpora (Fig. 15–16A). This rectovesical ligament is attached anteriorly to the bladder, folds over and is attached between the uterine cornua, continues posteriorly in the cul-de-sac, and ends with its attachment to the anterior wall of the sigmoid and rectum. It is not invariably present, but when it is, one cannot help but wonder about its possible significance in the etiology of this anomaly, possibly by preventing the two müllerian ducts

from joining. It must be removed before a unification procedure can be done. Then, for hemostasis, tourniquets are used in a manner similar to that described for the modified Jones procedure. The two uterine cornua are incised on their median sides in their longitudinal axes, deeply enough to expose the uterine cavities (Fig. 15–16B). Superiorly, the incision must not be too close to the interstitial portion of the fallopian tubes. Inferiorly, the incision is carried far enough to join the two sides into a single endocervical canal. If it appears that a deeper incision will compromise the competence of the cervix, a double cervical canal may be left. If the cervix is already duplex, it should not be joined. As the incision in the myometrium releases the internal stresses in the walls of the hemicorpora, each one everts and is perfectly positioned for apposition, almost as if the original intention in embryologic development was finally to be realized. The suture technique for joining the two sides is exactly the same as for the modified Jones procedure (Fig. 15–16C,D,E). The tourniquets are removed, and the defects in the broad ligaments are closed with very fine sutures. After removal of the tourniquets, the suture line in the uterine corpus should be observed for several minutes to determine the adequacy of hemostasis. Occasionally it will be necessary to place one or two extra sutures to control bleeding.

A uterine suspension may be performed as necessary. However, in the event of pregnancy, the shortened round ligaments may produce symptoms from an enlarging uterus. Presacral neurectomy in association with uterine unification should be considered only in patients with severe dysmenorrhea or endometriosis.

The cervix should be dilated to ensure proper drainage from the uterine cavity. This can be accomplished transvaginally after the abdominal procedure or from above by inserting a dilator through the cervical canal into the vagina, to be removed later.

The operative technique employed should be consistent with the goal of maintaining or enhancing fertility and the possibility of a successful pregnancy. Tissue surfaces should be kept moist throughout the procedure; instruments should be selected and used in such a way that tissue damage is minimized; abdominal packs should be placed in plastic bags to avoid adhesions; talc should be carefully washed from gloves; meticulous aseptic technique should be used; and the appendix should not be removed. A solution of Ringer's lactate containing heparin and corticosteroid is used for peritoneal lavage throughout the procedure and is left in the peritoneal cavity prior to closing the abdomen. The

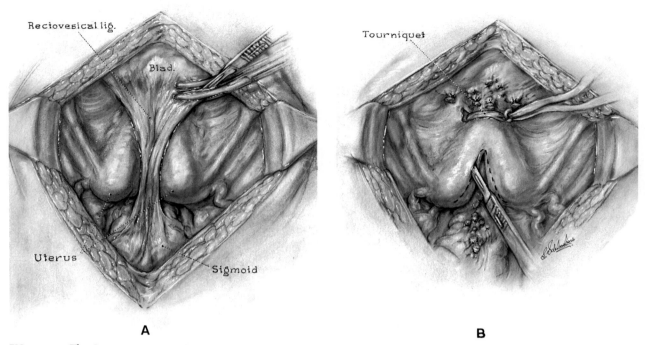

A   **B**

FIG. 15-16 The Strassman metroplasty with modifications. (*A*) If a rectovesical ligament is found, it should be removed. (*B*) An incision is made on the medial side of each hemicorpus and carried deep enough to enter the uterine cavity. The edges of the myometrium will evert to face the opposite side.

instillation of 100 ml of 32% dextran 70 is also effective in reducing postoperative adhesions. A three-dose regimen of prophylactic perioperative antibiotics is prescribed, with the first dose administered preoperatively in time for an adequate tissue concentration before the incision is made. The second dose is given in the recovery room, and the third dose is given 6 hours later.

Recently, several authors have reported on the use of hysteroscopy for resection of uterine septa. Thus, DeCherney and Polan treated 21 women with habitual abortion by transcervical resection with concomitant laparoscopic control. Hysterosalpingograms performed 4 months later were essentially normal in all cases. Sixteen of the patients subsequently carried pregnancies to term. Daly and associates and Chervenak and Neuwirth have reported similar experiences. Daly and associates have recently reported hysteroscopic resection of the uterine septum in the presence of a septate cervix. As more experience is gained, this technique could offer an alternative to abdominal metroplasty in selected patients with a septate uterus.

OTHER CONSIDERATIONS. A period of 3 months of contraception is sufficient before allowing conception. Local means of contraception (condom, diaphragm, foam) should be used assiduously during this time to avoid pregnancy. Hysterosalpingogram is not advised routinely following surgery just to evaluate the configuration of the uterine cavity or to assess tubal patency. If it is done, one usually will see a slight remaining deformity of the uterine cavity. In spite of this, the functional results are quite satisfactory. Certainly, if a patient has difficulty conceiving within the first 2 years after operation or has another spontaneous abortion or premature delivery, then a repeat hysterosalpingogram should be performed and the tubes should be evaluated with laparoscopy.

When a patient with an anomalous uterus, with or without unification, becomes pregnant, she must be watched closely for evidence of cervical incompetence, especially if a history of previous reproductive loss suggests cervical incompetence. Heinonen and associates were able to improve fetal survival from 57% to 92% by cerclage. Cervical cerclage was used mostly in patients with a partial bicornuate uterus, in whom fetal salvage was improved from 53% before cerclage to 100% afterward. Prematurity was also decreased, from 53% to 3%. The authors stress that cervical incompetence, not the uterine anomaly, is the indication for cerclage in these patients. However, the frequency with which these problems are found together suggests

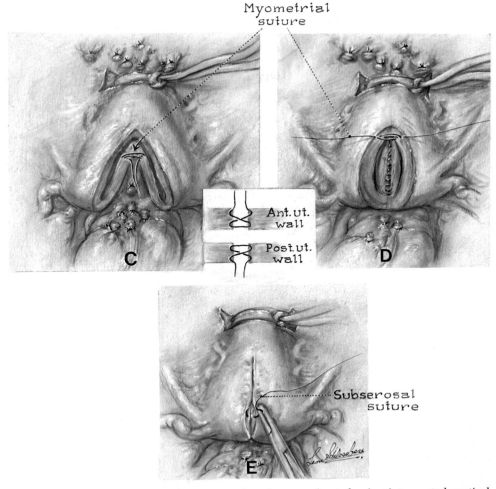

FIG. 15–16 (continued). (*C, D*) The myometrium is approximated using interrupted vertical figure-of-eight No. 3-0 polyglycolic acid sutures. Avoid placing sutures too close to the interstitial portion of the fallopian tubes. (*E*) A continuous No. 5-0 polyglycolic acid subserosal suture is used as a final layer. Tourniquets are removed and defects in the broad ligament are closed.

the importance of doing a careful evaluation for both problems. Obviously, some reproductive losses in patients with a uterine anomaly, before and after metroplasty, can be prevented by cerclage of an incompetent cervix. However, routine cerclage at the time of metroplasty is not recommended.

We do not recommend an attempt to unify a double cervix or a septate cervix because of the possibility of causing cervical incompetence. However, a double or septate cervix may adversely affect the outcome of delivery if vaginal delivery is attempted. Delivery should be by cesarean section if it appears the cervix will cause dystocia.

The scar in the myometrium following unification is as strong as, if not stronger than that following cesarean section. The biologic conditions in which healing takes place are entirely different in these two situations. Endomyometritis is a common complication following cesarean section but is not a complication of uterine unification. Of 71 known pregnancies in Strassman's collected series reported in 1952, 61 were delivered per vaginam. There were no cases of uterine rupture during pregnancy or delivery. In spite of evidence that the uterine scar heals securely after unification operations, our policy is to recommend delivery by elective cesarean section in all patients who have undergone metroplasty.

Exposure of the female fetus to diethylstilbestrol may result in significant anomalous development of the uterus, as reported by Kaufman and associates and by Haney and associates. The T-shaped uterus is the variant most commonly seen. It is associated with an increased rate of spontaneous abortion, preterm deliveries, and ectopic pregnancies. No operative procedure is indicated, but such patients must be monitored closely for evidence of dilatation and effacement of the cervix early in pregnancy. Cervical cerclage may be indicated in some patients.

Unicornuate Uterus

A unicornuate uterus may be present alone or with a rudimentary uterine horn on the opposite side. In a series reported by Heinonen and associates, 11 of 13 patients with a unicornuate uterus had a rudimentary horn and two did not. Most rudimentary horns are noncommunicating (90% according to O'Leary and O'Leary). The two sides may be connected by a fibromuscular band or there may be no connection and no communication between the two uterine cavities. As pointed out earlier, urinary tract anomalies are often associated with unicornuate uterus. On the side opposite the unicornuate uterus may be a horseshoe or a pelvic kidney, or the kidney may be hypoplastic or absent. This is especially true if there is associated müllerian duct obstruction. When all müllerian duct derivatives and the kidney are absent on one side, the ovary may also be absent, since this implies a complete failure of development of the entire urogenital ridge, including the genital ridge where the ovary forms.

According to Heinonen and associates the unicornuate uterus has the poorest fetal survival (40%) of all uterine anomalies. W. S. Jones reported similar findings. It has been suggested that the abnormal shape and insufficient muscular mass of the uterus, and a reduced uterine volume with inability to expand may explain the poor obstetric outcome.

Since most patients with a unicornuate uterus will have a noncommunicating rudimentary uterine horn on the opposite side, there is danger of pregnancy developing in the rudimentary horn from transperitoneal migration of the sperm or ovum from the opposite side. O'Leary and O'Leary found the corpus luteum to be on the side contralateral to the pregnant rudimentary horn in 8% of cases. Signs and symptoms of an ectopic pregnancy will develop, with eventual rupture of the horn if the pregnancy is not detected early. Rupture through the wall of the vascular rudimentary horn is associated with sudden and severe intraperitoneal hemorrhage and shock. Death may occur in a few minutes. It is surprising that the current mortality has decreased to 5%. According to Holden and Hart, some 350 cases of pregnancy in a rudimentary horn

have been reported since the original case report by Mauriceau in 1669.

Very little, if anything, can be done to improve the reproductive performance of patients with a unicornuate uterus. One should observe closely for cervical incompetence and do cerclage as indicated. Andrews and Jones have suggested that removal of the rudimentary uterine horn may improve the chances of a successful pregnancy, but the experience is too small to support a definite recommendation. Asymmetrical development as with unicornuate uterus and an opposing rudimentary uterine horn is not amenable to unification. It is better to remove the rudimentary horn, especially if it is noncommunicating.

Longitudinal Vaginal Septum

Failure of fusion of the lower müllerian ducts that form the vagina will result in a vagina with a longitudinal septum. Almost always, a didelphic uterus will also be present. Young patients will have difficulty using tampons. There may be difficulty with intercourse. In patients with didelphic uterus and a longitudinal vaginal septum, one uterine hemicorpus is usually better developed than the other. If intercourse consistently takes place on the vaginal side connected to the uterine hemicorpus that is less well developed, then infertility or repeated abortion could result. For these reasons, the septum should be removed in the nonpregnant state unless there is a contraindication. It can usually be done easily with reasonable precaution against injury to the urethra, bladder, and rectum.

OBSTRUCTED LATERAL FUSION PROBLEMS

One müllerian duct may develop normally and completely while the opposite müllerian duct may fail to develop or develop incompletely. On one side, a relatively normal hemiuterus with a hemicorpus connected to a hemicervix is found. On the opposite side, the cervix, musculature, uterine cavity, endometrium, fallopian tube, blood supply, and ligamentous attachments may be absent or hypoplastic to a varying degree. Obstruction to menstruation may occur at any level on this side. For example, if a rudimentary uterine horn does not communicate externally but does have an endometrial lined uterine cavity, symptoms of obstructed menstruation may begin soon after the menarche. Severe dysmenorrhea will be present. Unfortunately, cryptomenorrhea may not be thought of, since the patient will also experience cyclic menstruation from the opposite side. If the lumen of the tube communicates with the endometrial cavity of the rudimentary uterus, retrograde menstruation

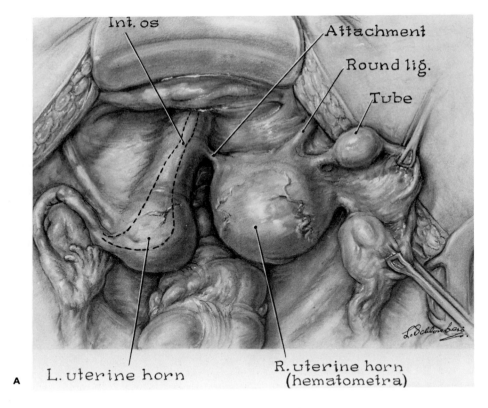

Int. os   Attachment

Round lig.

Tube

A

L. uterine horn   R. uterine horn (hematometra)

B

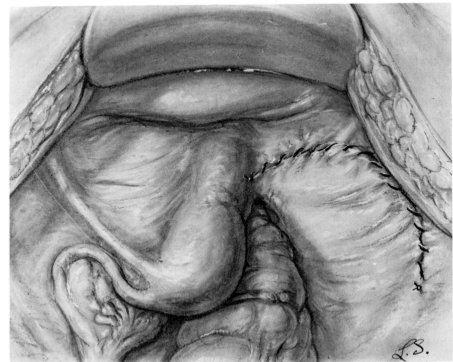

FIG. 15–17 (*A*) A noncommunicating rudimentary horn with functional endometrium and containing menstrual blood under pressure. Note the congenital abnormality of the fallopian tube, which prevented retrograde menstruation. (*B*) The same patient following excision of the rudimentary horn.

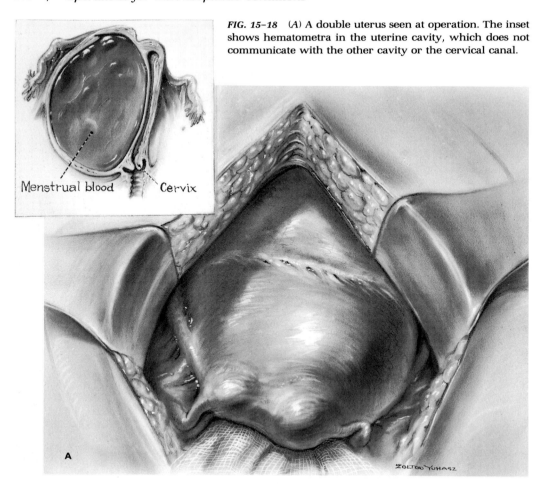

FIG. 15–18 (A) A double uterus seen at operation. The inset shows hematometra in the uterine cavity, which does not communicate with the other cavity or the cervical canal.

Menstrual blood

Cervix

A

and pelvic endometriosis will develop. It is, therefore, important to make the diagnosis as soon as possible so that reproductive potential will not be destroyed. The findings at an operation to remove an obstructed rudimentary uterine horn are illustrated in Figure 15–17. Fortunately, in this case, the fallopian tube was obstructed by an anomaly and retrograde menstruation was not possible. The fallopian tube connected to a rudimentary uterine horn may not be patent because of incomplete development.

Another example of a rare obstructed lateral fusion problem is illustrated in Figure 15–18A. A complete septum was present between two uterine cavities. One cavity communicated with a cervix and the other did not. This could represent an example of unilateral failure of cervical development. The patient complained of incapacitating dysmenorrhea that appeared shortly after the menarche and lasted 5 days. A tense cystic mass was palpable in the right half of the pelvis. The operation, described origi-

nally by Jones in the 2nd edition of this text, consisted of making an incision through the anterior wall of the cystic right portion of the uterus. It was found to contain old menstrual blood. The entire septum was excised and the uterus was reconstructed by anastomosis of the two cavities. A continuous lock-stitch was reinforced by interrupted myometrial sutures (Fig. 15–18B). The plastic reconstruction of the uterus was completed by a third layer of interrupted sutures uniting myometrium and serosa (Fig. 15–18C).

Another problem of lateral fusion with obstruction is seen when a didelphic uterus and a longitudinal vaginal septum are present with obstruction of the vagina on one side of the septum, as illustrated in Figure 15–19. A large amount of blood may accumulate in the distensible obstructed vagina while the patient continues to have cyclic menstruation from the opposite side. As time passes, sufficient old menstrual blood may accumulate to cause not only a large hematocolpos, but a hematometra, hema-

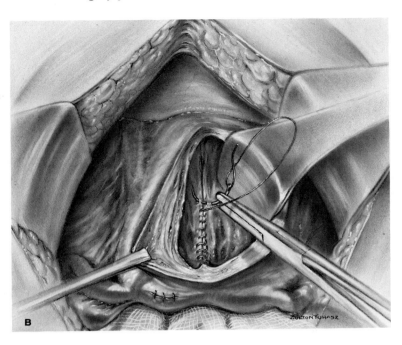

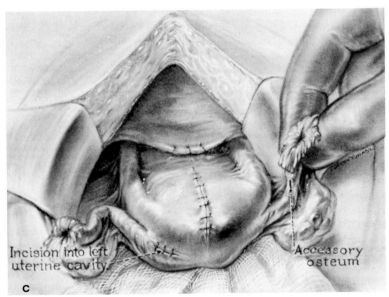

FIG. 15-18 (continued). *(B)* The septum of the double uterus has been excised and anastomosis is being made uniting the two cavities. *(C)* Anastomosis is completed. The small incision in the left uterine cavity was made before the septum was removed for the purpose of orientation.

tosalpinx, and even endometriosis. Unfortunately, the hemiuterus, tube, and ovary may be removed before it is realized that in order to allow escape of monthly menstrual flow from the obstructed side, it is only necessary to remove the septum in the divided vagina.

Rock and Jones reported 12 patients with a double uterus, unilateral vaginal obstruction, and ipsilateral renal agenesis and reviewed 71 patients previously reported in the literature. They emphasized that early accurate diagnosis followed by the excision of the obstructing vaginal septum offers complete relief while preserving reproductive capacity. Rarely, a communication may exist between the obstructed and the unobstructed vagina or between the two uterine cavities. The clinical picture will vary, depending on whether the obstruction is partial or complete.

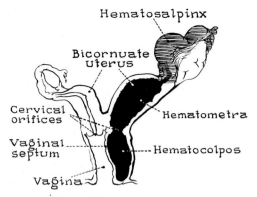

FIG. 15-19 A failure of lateral fusion with obstruction of one vagina results in a hematocolpos, hematometra, and hematosalpinx. If this anomaly can be diagnosed preoperatively, it can be solved simply by removing the vaginal septum.

Combinations and Other Problems

Müllerian duct anomalies may occur in association with a variety of other problems. For example, Stanton has reported that in a series of 70 patients with bladder exstrophy, 30 patients (43%) had reproductive tract abnormalities. He suggested that the number may actually be higher. Müllerian abnormalities included absence of the vagina; septate vagina; unicornuate, bicornuate, and didelphic uterus; and absent uterus. Fewer müllerian anomalies were seen with epispadias. Jones called attention to anomalies of the external genitalia and vagina among 30 patients with bladder exstrophy seen at the Johns Hopkins Hospital, and suggested operative techniques for correction. Operative techniques for correction of these anomalies as well as for the management of other gynecologic and obstetric problems (especially uterine prolapse) have also been discussed by Weed and McKee and by Blakely and Mills. A number of other congenital malformations of the vagina and perineum may also be associated with uterine anomalies. These rare combinations and their surgical correction, especially in children, are reported by Hendren and Donahoe and by others.

Müllerian duct anomalies are seen in patients with the McKusick–Kaufman syndrome, an autosomal recessive disorder. Other clinical findings reported in this syndrome include hydrometrocolpos, postaxial polydactyly, syndactyly, congenital heart disease, intravaginal displacement of the urethral meatus, and anorectal anomalies. Jabs and associates added an additional case to the previous twenty-eight cases reported in the literature.

Bibliography

Abbe R: New method of creating a vagina in a case of congenital absence. Medical Record 54:836, 1898

Andrews MC, Jones HW: Impaired reproductive performance of the unicornuate uterus: intrauterine growth retardation, infertility, and recurrent abortion in five cases. Am J Obstet Gynecol 144:173, 1982

Blakeley CR, Mills WG: The obstetric and gynaecological complications of bladder exstrophy and epispadias. Brit J Obstet Gynecol 88:167, 1981

Brenner P, Sedlis A, Cooperman H: Complete imperforate transverse vaginal septum. Obstet Gynecol 25:135, 1965

Broadbent TR, Woolf RM: Congenital absence of the vagina: Reconstruction without operation. Brit J Plast Surg 30:118, 1977

Capraro VJ, Chuang JT, Randall CL: Improved fetal salvage after metroplasty. Obstet Gynecol 31:97, 1968

Capraro VJ, Gallego MB: Vaginal agenesis. Am J Obstet Gynecol 124:98, 1976

Chakravarty BN: Congenital absence of the vagina and uterus—simultaneous vaginoplasty and hysteroplasty. J Obstet Gynecol India 27:627, 1977

Chakravarty BN, Gun KM, Sarkar K: Congenital absence of vagina anatomico-physiological consideration. J Obstet Gynecol India 27:621, 1977

Chervenak FA, Neuwirth RS: Hysteroscopic resection of the uterine septum. Am J Obstet Gynecol 141:351, 1981

Counseller VS: Congenital absence of the vagina. JAMA 136:861, 1948

Counseller VS, Davis CE: Atresia of the vagina. Obstet Gynecol 32:528, 1968

Daly DC, Tohan N, Walters C, et al: Hysteroscopic resection of the uterine septum in the presence of a septate cervix. Fertil Steril 39:560, 1983

Daly DC, Walters CA, Soto–Albors CE, et al: Hysteroscopic metroplasty: Surgical technique and obstetrical outcome. Fertil Steril 39:623, 1983

David A, Carvil D, Bar-David E, et al: Congenital absence of the vagina. Clinical and psychological aspects. Obstet Gynecol 46:407, 1975

Davydov SN: Colpopoiesis from the peritoneum of the uterorectal space. Obstet Gynecol (Moscow) p 55, December 12, 1969

DeCherney A, Polan ML: Hysteroscopic management of intrauterine lesions and intractable uterine bleeding. Obstet Gynecol 61:392, 1983

Dillon WP, Mudaliar NA, Wingate NB: Congenital atresia of the cervix. Obstet Gynecol 54:126, 1979

Evans TN: The artificial vagina. Am J Obstet Gynecol 99:944, 1967

Evans TN, Poland ML, Boving RL: Vaginal malformations. Am J Obstet Gynecol 141:910, 1981

Farber M, Marchant DJ: Reconstructive surgery for congenital atresia of the uterine cervix. Fertil Steril 27:1277, 1976

Farber M, Mitchell GW: Bicornuate uterus and partial atresia of the fallopian tube. Am J Obstet Gynecol 134:881, 1979

————: Surgery for congenital absence of the vagina. Obstet Gynecol 51:364, 1978

————: Surgery for congenital anomalies of müllerian ducts. Contemp Obstet Gynecol 9:63, 1977

Feroze RM, Dewhurst CJ, Welply G: Vaginoplasty at the Chelsea Hospital for women: A comparison of two techniques. Brit J Obstet Gynaecol 82:536, 1975

Fore SR, Hammond CB, Parker RT, et al: Urologic and genital anomalies in patients with congenital absence of the vagina. Obstet Gynecol 46:410, 1975

Frank RT: The formation of an artificial vagina without operation. NY State J Med 40:1669, 1940

————: The formation of an artificial vagina without operation. Am J Obstet Gynecol 35:1053, 1938

Frank RT, Geist SH: The formation of an artificial vagina by a new plastic technic. Am J Obstet Gynecol 14:712, 1927

Garcia J, Jones HW: The split thickness graft technic for vaginal agenesis. Obstet Gynecol 49:328, 1977

Garcia RF: Z-plasty for correction of congenital transverse vaginal septum. Am J Obstet Gynecol 99:1164, 1967

Geary WL, Weed JC: Congenital atresia of the uterine cervix. Obstet Gynecol 42:213, 1973

Genest D, Farber M, Mitchell GW, et al: Partial vaginal agenesis with a urinary-vaginal fistula. Obstet Gynecol 58:130–134, 1981

Graves WP: Method of constructing an artificial vagina. Surg Clin North Am 611, 1921

Griffin JE, Edwards C, Madden JD, et al: Congenital absence of the vagina. Ann Intern Med 85:224, 1976

Haney AF, Hammond CB, Soules MR, et al: Diethylstilbestrol-induced upper genital tract abnormalities. Fertil Steril 31:142, 1979

Hauser GA, Keller M, Koller T: Das Rokitansky-Kuster-Syndrom. Uterus bipartitus solidus rudimentarius cum vagina solida. Gynaecologia 151:111, 1961

Hauser GA, Schreiner WE: Das Mayer-Rokitansky-Kuster Syndrom. Schweiz Med Wochenschr 91:381, 1961

Heinonen PK: Longitudinal vaginal septum. Eur J Obstet Gynec Reprod Biol 13:253, 1982

Heinonen PK, Pystynen PP: Primary infertility and uterine anomalies. Fertil Steril 40:311, 1983

Heinonen PK, Saarikoski S, Pystynen P: Reproductive performance of women with uterine anomalies. Acta Obstet Gynecol Scand 61:157, 1982

Hendren WH, Donahoe PK: Correction of congenital abnormalities of the vagina and perineum. J Ped Surg 15:751, 1980

Holden R, Hart P: First-trimester rudimentary horn pregnancy: Preruptute ultrasound diagnosis. Obstet Gynecol (Suppl) 61:56, 1983

Ingram JM: The bicycle seat stool in the treatment of vaginal agenesis and stenosis: A preliminary report. Am J Obstet Gynecol 140:867, 1981

Jabs EW, Leonard CO, Phillips JA: New features of the McKusick-Kaufman syndrome. Birth Defects 18:161, 1982

Jeffcoate TNA: Advancement of the upper vagina in the treatment of haematocolpos and haematometra caused by vaginal aplasia. Pregnancy following the construction of an artificial vagina. J Obstet Gynaecol Brit Comm 76:961, 1969

Jewelewicz R, Husami N, Wallach EE: When uterine factors cause infertility. Contemp Obstet Gynecol 16:95, 1980

Jones HW: An anomaly of the external genitalia in female patients with exstrophy of the bladder. Am J Obstet Gynecol 117:748, 1973

————: Reproductive impairment and the malformed uterus. Fertil Steril 36:137, 1981

Jones HW, Delfs E, Seeger–Jones GE: Reproductive difficulties in double uterus: The place of plastic reconstruction. Am J Obstet Gynecol 72:865, 1956

Jones HW, Seegar–Jones GE: Double uterus as an etiological factor in repeated abortion: Indications for surgical repair. Am J Obstet Gynecol 65:325, 1953

Jones HW, Mermut S: Familial occurrence of congenital absence of the vagina. Am J Obstet Gynecol 114:1100, 1972

Jones HW, Wheeless CR: Salvage of the reproductive potential of women with anomalous development of the müllerian ducts: 1868–1968–2068. Am J Obstet Gynecol 104:348, 1969

Jones TB, Fleischer AC, Daniell JF, et al: Sonographic characteristics of congenital uterine abnormalities and associated pregnancy. J Clin Ultrasound 8:435, 1980

Jones WS: Obstetric significance of female genital anomalies. Obstet Gynecol 10:113, 1957

Karjalainen O, Myllynen L, Kajanoja P, et al: Management of vaginal agenesis. Ann Chir Gynaecol 69:37, 1980

Kaufman RH, Binder GL, Gray PM, et al: Upper genital tract changes associated with exposure in utero to diethylstilbestrol. Am J Obstet Gynecol 128:51, 1977

Knab DR: Müllerian agenesis: A review. Dept. of Gyn/Ob, Uniformed Services University School of Medicine, & Naval Hospital, Bethesda, Maryland, 1983.

Kusuda M: Infertility and metroplasty. Acta Obstet Gynecol Scand 61:407, 1982

Lees DH, Singer A: Vaginal surgery for congenital abnormalities and acquired constrictions. Clin Obstet Gynecol 25:883, 1982

Lodi A: Contributo clinico statistico sulle malformazioni della vagina osservate nella clinica Obstetrica e Ginecologica di Milano dal 1906 al 1950. Annali di Obstetricia Ginecologia, Medicina Perinatale 73:1246, 1951

Maciulla GJ, Heine MW, Christian CD: Functional endometrial tissue with vaginal agenesis. J Reprod Med 21:373, 1978

Magrina JF, Masterson BJ: Vaginal reconstruction in gynecological oncology: A review of techniques. Obstet Gynecol Survey 36:1, 1981

Mahgoub SE: Unification of a septate uterus: Mahgoub's operation. Int J Gynaecol Obstet 15:400, 1978

Mandell J, Stevens PS, Lucey DT: Diagnosis and management of hydrometrocolpos in infancy. J Urol 120:262, 1978

McCraw JB, Massey FM, Shanklin KD, et al: Vaginal reconstruction with gracilis myocutaneous flaps. Plast Reconstr Surg 58:176, 1976

McDonough PG, Tho PT: Use of pelvic pneumoperitoneum: A critical assessment of 12 years experience. South Med J 67:517, 1974

McIndoe A: The treatment of congenital absence and obliterative conditions of the vagina. Br J Plast Surg 2:254, 1950

McIndoe AH, Banister JB: An operation for the cure of congenital absence of the vagina. J Obstet Gynaecol Br Empire 45:490, 1938

McKusick VA: Transverse vaginal septum (hydrometrocolpos). Birth Defects 7:326, 1971

McKusick VA, Bauer RL, Koop CE, et al: Hydrometrocolpos as a simply inherited malformation. JAMA 189:119, 1964

McKusick VA, Weilbaccher RG, Gragg GW: Recessive inheritance of a congenital malformation syndrome. JAMA 204:111, 1968

McShane PM, Reilly RJ, Schiff I: Pregnancy outcomes following Tompkins metroplasty. Fertil Steril 40:190, 1983

Mizuno K, Koike K, Ando K, et al: Significance of Jones-Jones operation on double uterus: Vascularity and dating of endometrium in uterine septum. Jap J Fertil Steril 23:9, 1978

Musich JR, Behrman SJ: Obstetric outcome before and after metroplasty in women with uterine anomalies. Obstet Gynecol 52:63, 1978

Musset R: Traitement chirurgical des cloisans transversales due vagin d'origine congenitale par la plastie en "Z" a l'Hopital Lariboisiere. Gynec et Obstet 55:382, 1956

Niver DH, Barrette G, Jewelewicz R: Congenital atresia of the uterine cervix and vagina—three cases. Fertil Steril 33:25, 1980

Nunley WC, Kitchin JD: Congenital atresia of the uterine cervix with pelvic endometriosis. Arch Surg 115:757, 1980

O'Leary JL, O'Leary JA: Rudimentary horn pregnancy. Obstet Gynecol 22:371, 1963

Pinsky L: A community of human malformation syndromes involving the müllerian ducts, distal extremities, urinary tract, and ears. Teratology 9:65, 1974

Pratt JH: Vaginal atresia corrected by use of small and large bowel. Clin Obstet Gynecol 15:639, 1972

Rock JA, Jones HW: The clinical management of the double uterus. Fertil Steril 28:798, 1977

————: The double uterus associated with an obstructed hemivagina and ipsilateral renal agenesis. Am J Obstet Gynecol 138:339, 1980

Rock JA, Reeves LA, Retto H, et al: Success following vaginal creation for müllerian agenesis. Fertil Steril 39:809, 1983

Rock JA, Zacur HA: The clinical management of repeated early pregnancy wastage. Fertil Steril 39:123, 1983

Rock JA, Zacur HA, Dlugi AM, et al: Pregnancy success following surgical correction of imperforate hymen and complete transverse vaginal septum. Obstet Gynecol 59:448, 1982

Rotmensch J, Rosensheim N, Dillon M, et al: Carcinoma arising in the neovagina: Case report and review of the literature. Obstet Gynecol 61:534, 1983

Semmens JP: Abdominal contour in the third trimester: An aid to diagnosis of uterine anomalies. Obstet Gynecol 25:779, 1965

Shokeir MHK: Aplasia of the müllerian system: Evidence for probably sex-limited autosomal dominant inheritance. Birth Defects 14:147, 1978

Singh KJ, Devi L: Hysteroplasty and vaginoplasty for reconstruction of the uterus. Int J Gynaecol Obstet 17:457, 1980

Stanton SL: Gynecologic complications of epispadias and bladder exstrophy. Am J Obstet Gynecol 119:749, 1974

Stoot JE, Mastboom JL: Restriction on the indications for metroplasty. Acta Europaea Fertil 8:79, 1977

Strassmann EO: Operations for double uterus and endometrial atresia. Clin Obstet Gynecol 4:240, 1961

————: Plastic unification of double uterus. Am J Obstet Gynecol 64:25, 1952

Strassmann P: Die operative vereinigung eines doppelten uterus. Zentrbl Gynaek 31:1322, 1907

Tancer ML, Katz M, Veridiano NP: Vaginal epithelialization with human amnion. Obstet Gynecol 54:345, 1979

Thompson DP, Lynn HB: Genital anomalies associated with solitary kidney. Mayo Clin Proc 41:538, 1966

Thompson JD, Wharton LR, TeLinde RW: Congenital absence of the vagina. Am J Obstet Gynecol 74:397, 1957

Tompkins P: Comments on the bicornuate uterus and twinning. Surg Clin North Am 42:1049, 1962

Valdes C, Malini S, Malinak L: Sonography in the surgical management of vaginal and cervical atresia. Fertil Steril 40:263, 1983

Weed JC, McKee DM: Vulvoplasty in cases of exstrophy of the bladder. Obstet Gynecol 43:512, 1974

Wharton LR: A simple method of constructing a vagina. Ann Surg 107:842, 1938

————: Congenital malformations associated with developmental defects of the female reproductive organs. Am J Obstet Gynecol 53:37, 1947

————: Further experiences in construction of the vagina. Ann Surg 111:1010, 1940

Williams EA: Congenital absence of the vagina, a simple operation for its relief. J Obstet Gynecol Br Comm 71:511, 1964

————: Uterovaginal agenesis: Ann R Coll Surg Engl 58:266, 1976

————: Vulva-vaginaplasty. Proc R Soc Med 63:40, 1970

Chapter 16

Reconstruction of the Fallopian Tube

John A. Rock, M.D.

The major physiologic functions of the human oviduct concern the process of ovum pickup and the provision of a safe conduit for a fertilized zygote to reach the uterine cavity. Tubal surgery may be required for the control of infection, neoplasia, infertility, and fertility. Since pelvic inflammatory disease, tubal pregnancy, and tubal sterilization are discussed elsewhere in this text, this chapter will discuss the remaining clinical problems that frequently require tubal surgery, concentrating on the problems associated with infertility.

In vitro fertilization has revolutionized our approach to the treatment of the infertile couple. There is now hope for the oligospermic male and the woman with severe tubal disease. Nevertheless, because of the decreased pregnancy rates and great expense of extracorporeal fertilization, the techniques have limited application. When these techniques are perfected, some of the procedures described in this text (*i.e.,* salpingostomy) may become of merely historical interest, whereas others, such as microsurgical tubolysis, will continue to be useful. The contemporary microsurgical procedures presented here were developed and found useful at The Johns Hopkins Hospital.

Tubal Factors in Infertility

The factors that most seriously, as well as most frequently, influence infertility are related to the anatomical and pathologic alterations of the fallopian tube. The ciliated lining of the fimbriae that embraces the surface of the ovary at the time of ovulation is responsible for ovum pickup prior to fertilization in the outer third of the fallopian tube.

The disease that most commonly alters the cilia and produces anatomical deformity of the tube is gonococcal endosalpingitis. Unless treated early, this infection will produce tubal occlusion at various locations from the uterine cornu to the fimbriae and may result in tubal obstruction, hydrosalpinx, or a tubo-ovarian inflammatory mass. The initial infection is usually the most damaging to the tubal mucosa and motility: recent evidence shows that the initial inoculum of the gonococcus may be accompanied to the tube by secondary infection from staphylococcus, streptococcus, or coliform organisms, which can result in chronic and irreversible tubal damage. Furthermore, chlamydial infection may be subclinical and equally devastating to the oviduct. Although the fallopian tube may not be completely obstructed as a result of such infections, fusion of the fimbriated appendages or impairment of ciliary activity may produce infertility by interference with ovum pickup and transport. Peritubal scarring from pelvic endometriosis or from other causes of extrapelvic infection (appendicitis or diverticulitis) may produce similar interference in tubal motility. Peritubal adhesions and impaired tubal motility explain an infertility rate of approximately 30% among patients with endometriosis even when there is demonstrable evidence of tubal patency.

Because tubal factors are among the major causes of infertility, tubal function studies should be carried out early in the investigation of the infertile couple. The remainder of the infertility evaluation should also be completed, since in approximately 15% of infertility cases two or more factors are involved. Basically, three methods of observing tubal function are currently available, namely, tubal insufflation (Rubin's test), hysterosalpingography, and pelvic endoscopy (peritoneoscopy).

Special Diagnostic Studies

TUBAL INSUFFLATION

Tubal insufflation was first described by Rubin in 1920 and although there have been modifications of the original technique, this test rightfully bears his name, the Rubin's test. The procedure uses an endocervical cannula connected by rubber tubing to a mercury manometer and a source of carbon dioxide. The rate of gas flow through the system is gradually increased to approximately 30 ml/min to 60 ml/min. The cervix may be submerged in sterile water in the upper vagina in order to detect any leakage of the gas from the cervical canal. Tubal patency may be determined by: (1) a direct-writing record of the rise and rapid fall of the gas pressure; (2) by auscultation of the lower abdomen for the sound of gas passing from the tubes into the peritoneal cavity; and (3) by direct visualization of the pressure changes on a mercury manometer. Although normal fallopian tubes demonstrate patency by the rapid escape of gas at pressures below 100 mm Hg, the test is still considered to be in the normal range if patency is demonstrated below 180 mm Hg. At higher pressures, however, there is a higher incidence of partial tubal obstruction. At pressures of 200 mm Hg without demonstrable patency, the test is considered to be negative and the tubes are either in spasm at the cornu or are pathologically obstructed. However, this test is considered only one of several methods of evaluating tubal patency, and a negative Rubin's test cannot be interpreted as conclusive evidence of tubal obstruction, as has been stressed repeatedly by Stallworthy and others. A study by Sweeney and Gepfert documented this fact by reporting a 50% pregnancy rate ultimately in patients whose tubal insufflation tests had recorded pressures of greater than 180 mm Hg. The Rubin's test can only be interpreted as a study of gross tubal function and must be either repeated or combined with other studies for final evaluation of tubal patency. The use of a smooth muscle relaxant, such as inhaled amyl nitrite, or a mild sedative such as Valium, 10 mg prior to any tubal function test, may be helpful in decreasing tubal spasm.

In general, the tubal insufflation should preferably be performed before midcycle, about the 10th day, to avoid the risk of transporting particles of endometrium through the tube, which would be possible if the test were performed during the late secretory phase.

HYSTEROSALPINGOGRAPHY

Hysterosalpingography is a permanent, visual record of the presence or absence of tubal patency and was first described by both Cary and Rubin in 1914. This test is always performed in the evaluation of an infertile patient, regardless of the results of the tubal insufflation study, because it serves as a permanent radiographic record that can be compared with subsequent tubal studies. If an oil-base dye is used, the study should not be performed in the latter part of the cycle because extravasation of oil into pelvic veins and lymphatics is increased when the vascularity of the endometrium and uterus is increased. Lipiodol, which made its appearance in 1922, was later abandoned by Rubin because of the occurrence of oil granuloma and lipoid salpingitis. Rubin noticed some persistence of oily media after hysterosalpingography in two-thirds of the cases in one of the earliest studies he conducted. However, less than half of the cases of lipoid salpingitis reported by Elliott and associates could be attributed to oily contrast media; the remainder were thought to be caused by the ascent of oily media placed in the vagina periodically by the patient. The current use of a water-soluble opaque medium avoids such complications. Although the rapid absorption and drainage of the dye prevents the use of delayed 24-hour x-ray study of the tubes, we have not found this to be a particular disadvantage.

As is true of the tubal insufflation study, interpretation of a hysterosalpingogram must be done with some reservation. Not only is peritoneal spill important, but free dissemination of the dye throughout the pelvis suggests the absence of peritubal adhesions. The presence of rugal folds in the preoperative salpingogram is a favorable prognostic sign for postoperative pregnancy. Young and co-workers from the Boston Hospital for Women found a 60.7% pregnancy rate in cases with good rugal markings and a 7.3% pregnancy rate where such markings were absent.

Altemus and associates believe that the complications and shortcomings of conventional hysterography can be overcome by supplementing the study with fluoroscopic visualization of the uterus and tubes, employing image intensification. A 30-second fluoroscopic exposure is equivalent in irradiation to one conventional radiographic exposure by most modern fluoroscopic units, and can avoid the necessity for multiple films when uterine or tubal filling is inadequate. This technique also avoids excessive venous or lymphatic injection when the dye is visualized in the myometrium. Fluoroscopy has been incorporated as a part of the technique of hysterosalpingography in our clinic and has been found to be useful.

The best evidence to date of the clinical unreliability of a negative hysterosalpingogram study is the work of Hutchins, who compared the accuracy of hysterosalpingography to that of laparoscopy with retrograde dye studies. This is one of the few current studies using general anesthesia for both procedures, which were performed at different times on the same group of infertile patients. The use of an anesthetic eliminates the complication of uterotubal spasm, which frequently produces erroneous results. The study clearly demonstrated this problem, as shown by the finding that 45 of 62 patients (73%) with proximal tubal occlusion on hysterosalpingogram had laparoscopic evidence of normal oviducts with demonstrable patency by methylene blue insufflation. Although other studies also have questioned the reliability of evidence for cornual obstruction provided by hysterosalpingography, Hutchins's study supports our view that an infertile patient should have a minimum of three separate tubal studies before the diagnosis of tubal occlusion can be established. Many comparative studies have found only a 50% to 60% agreement between laparoscopy and hysterosalpingography.

PERITONEOSCOPY

Peritoneoscopy, usually by laparoscopy, is important in the assessment of fallopian tubes in cases of prolonged infertility. It is particularly useful when there is a discrepancy between the tubal insufflation study and hysterosalpingogram.

The main information provided by a Rubin's test and hysterosalpingogram concerns tubal patency or obstruction, whereas direct visualization of the adnexa with the laparoscope provides an excellent opportunity for evaluation of tubal patency and motility, peritubal adhesions, and other pelvic disease, such as possible endometriosis or unsuspected ovarian pathology. By inserting a uterine cannula through the cervical canal, indigo carmine or methylene blue dye may be instilled into the uterine cavity with direct observation of the presence or absence of intraperitoneal spill of dye from the fimbriated end of the tubes. Of all the tubal function studies, laparoscopy is the most difficult to perform (since we prefer to conduct this procedure during anesthesia in order to have the opportunity to evaluate the pelvis thoroughly); yet it is perhaps the

most informative. Open laparoscopy allows the evaluation of patients following previous abdominal surgery. It is our policy to evaluate the pelvis by laparoscopy prior to considering definitive surgery for correction of tubal disease.

Laparoscopy provides the same information about tubal function as culdoscopy except that the approach is through the abdominal wall rather than the cul-de-sac. It has the advantage of providing a direct view of the fallopian tubes from the anterior surface of the broad ligament and consequently provides a more complete view of the entire oviduct as well as the cul-de-sac and pelvic viscera than can be observed through the cul-de-sac. We are convinced now that the laparoscopic view of the pelvis through an infraumbilical puncture site with or without the aid of an additional probe inserted through a separate puncture site in the lower abdomen has enhanced the view of the pelvis considerably and has greatly improved our understanding of the extent of tubal abnormalities and pelvic disease. A more complete discussion of the use of laparoscopy is presented in Chapter 17.

Microsurgery

Microsurgery is usually defined as surgery requiring the use of an operating microscope; however, Gomel defines the approach broadly to include surgery performed under magnification provided by loupes, hood, or microscope. In general, there is agreement that microsurgery represents the philosophy of a gentle operative technique using fine needles and sutures, delicate instruments, constant irrigation, and precise hemostasis with minimal electrodesiccation of tissue.

Magnification techniques for tubal surgery in gynecology were introduced by Swolin, who used either loupes or the operating microscope for salpingolysis and salpingostomy. Reports by Winston and by Gomel suggested improved pregnancy success following reversal of sterilization procedures in which an operating microscope was used for magnification. Similar results have been obtained with loupes or the hood.

Microsurgery is an acquired skill whose execution requires a magnification system, delicate microinstruments, and fine microsutures. Although each component may be modified to meet the operational requirements of a particular surgeon, certain general features are constant. Foremost is the execution of delicate and precise manual movements, which are governed by hand coordination and visual acuity. The small operative field and the vertical plane of vision requires microinstruments. Instrument manipulation is controlled by a precise, graded pinch closure between index finger and thumb, as the instrument is supported on the first, web space. Methods for knot tying and instrument handling are acquired by laboratory training. The time required to obtain these skills may vary. There are several laboratory manuals outlining specific training schedules, including ones by Acland, Buncke and associates, and Rock.

MAGNIFICATION

Magnification of the operative field may be provided by the microscope, operating hood, or binocular lenses. Magnification may range from ×1 to ×20, depending upon the optical system. The major difficulties with the hood and the binocular lenses have been the excessive weight and short focal length required to obtain an acceptable magnification. In the past few years, however, modifications involving the use of lighter materials have obviated the weight problem. Lens adjustments have increased the focal lengths, allowing for comfortable working distances and a wider and greater depth of field of vision. At present, binocular lenses may be selected with magnifications between ×2 and ×6. Proper lighting can be provided by a fiber-optic cable covered by a sterile plastic sheath.

The operating microscope offers the advantages of a wider range of magnification and a coaxial light system. In general, the range of magnification is dependent on the magnification coefficient of the eyepiece and the focal length of the objective. Eyepieces of ×10 magnification and objective lengths of 250 mm provide a magnification ranging from ×3.6 to ×16. A manual zoom system for the control of magnification and focusing, photographic attachments, and an assistance binocular observation system are available to assist the microsurgeon.

A difference of opinion regarding the therapeutic benefit derived by using the various systems appears to focus on the importance of the source and amount of magnification necessary for accurate control of hemostasis and the placement of fine suture. Our observations support the belief that a magnification greater than ×6 is, in most instances, unnecessary. However, there is general agreement that magnification greater than ×4 to ×6 is critical in anastomosis of the cornual-isthmic portions of the tube.

INSTRUMENTATION

A variety of specialized instruments are available to aid the microsurgeon; however, a basic set of microinstruments includes only jeweler's forceps, spring-handled scissors, and needle holder (Fig.

16–1). In general, instruments should facilitate though minimize hand movement; that is, the needle holders with rounded handles reduce hand movements when placing a 4 mm to 6 mm needle through tissue. Locks are usually cumbersome and may impede a smooth motion when tying knots.

Microelectrode monopolar or bipolar cautery is useful in obtaining hemostasis with minimal tissue trauma. Constant irrigation may be provided by a bulb-tipped syringe or intravenous set to which a 16 to 18 gauge polyethylene cannula is attached. Glass or plastic rods are useful for the gentle manipulation of tubes and ovaries, as well as for elevating adhesions to facilitate their lysis and excision.

SUTURE MATERIAL

Suture material with minimal reactivity should be used for oviduct approximation. Winston demon-

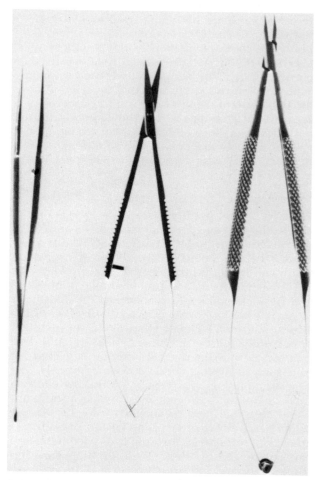

FIG. 16–1 Microsurgical instruments: *Left*, jeweler's forceps (No. 4); *center*, fine straight vascular scissors; *right*, Barroquer curved needle holder. (Jones, Rock, 1983)

strated the superiority of No. 10-0 nylon suture as compared to No. 8-0 chromic catgut in the rabbit oviduct. Stangel and associates demonstrated that No. 9-0 polyglycolic acid suture could be used for anastomosis with minimal reactivity in the muscular layers or endosalpingeal folds. Smith reported that no inflammatory reaction was found with polyglactic acid suture as compared with the use of nylon suture, after which some tissue reaction was still present at 6 months. There have been no studies to demonstrate the correlation of a particular suture material with pregnancy success.

Good surgical technique requires the use of delicate fine suture with minimal reactivity, and the general principle that the fewer sutures used, the less foreign body reaction, does apply. Use of No. 7-0 or No. 8-0 absorbable nonreactive suture with a 4 mm to 6 mm reverse cutting atroloc needle has proved adequate for our technique. This needle may be easily passed through serosa and muscularis with minimal tissue trauma or suture drag. This choice of suture is arbitrary, however; other surgeons have achieved similar success using various types of fine suture material.

MICROSURGICAL TECHNIQUES

Position of the Hands

The correct positioning of the hands allows fingertip movement without fatigue. The hands, wrists, and forearms should rest on an immovable surface. In most instances, this is the patient's upper thigh and lower abdomen. Proper hand and wrist support is essential to the proper placement of suture and tying techniques.

Instruments should be held in the writing position (Fig. 16-2). This position gives more stability than any other. The gynecologist is not required to touch the middle fingers together as does the vascular surgeon when performing vessel anastomosis; tying techniques are, in fact, more freehand. Vaginal packs are placed in the cul-de-sac to elevate the uterus and a rubber pelvic diaphragm (lid) is used to support the tubes slightly below the level of the incision.

Needle Handling and Placement

The suture should be grasped with the forceps in the left hand, which will stabilize the suture while the needle is positioned in the holder. Minor adjustments of the needle in the needle holder can be made by touching the needle with the left-handed forceps. The needle is in the stable position if it is set at 90 degrees to the axis of the tips of the forceps. The needle should be grasped just behind

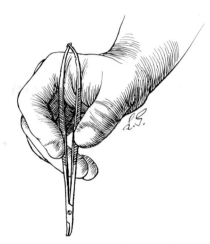

FIG. 16-2 Proper hand position for grasping a microneedle holder.

its midpoint so that the needle tip points horizontally.

The needle should pass perpendicular to the surface of the oviductal tissue. At times, this position is difficult to achieve if the tissue edge is not everted slightly to provide the distortion that is necessary. One may elevate the edge of the tissue with left-handed forceps while simultaneously placing the needle through the tissue or simply press the tubal lumen with the forceps very gently while passing the needle (Fig. 16-3A). One should avoid grasping the thickness of the tissue with the jaws of the forceps because this is a breach of atraumatic technique. The width of the bite of tissue obtained with the needle should be between two and three times the width of the needle itself. The bite in the opposite end of the tissue, which may include muscularis or serosa, should be of equal width. Once the needle has been placed through the opposite lumen, pulling the suture in one straight movement should be avoided as this can cause movement and visible distortion of the tissue and enlargement of the needle hole. One may avoid this with gentle, short pulls in line with the needle holes. Furthermore, using the tissue forceps to keep the tail of the suture in line with the exit hole avoids damage to tissue caused by angulation of the thread at the entry hole.

Knot Placement

Knot placement with delicate instruments may be a principal source of frustration for the surgeon. However, the mastering of these tying techniques until knot tying is second nature is essential so that the surgeon's thoughts may be directed exclusively toward the particulars of the anastomosis. A min-

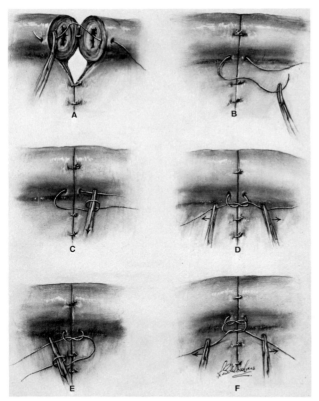

FIG. 16–3 Suture placement and knot tying with microinstruments under magnification. (*A*) Needle placement. (*B*) Grasping the thread with the right-handed forceps palm up. The suture is brought across as the hand is pronated. (*C*) Making a loop about the tip of the left-hand forceps and grasping the short end of the suture. (*D*) Tightening the first throw of the knot. (*E* and *F*) A second half-knot is placed as the sequence of movements is repeated.

imum of 100 hours of laboratory training is usually needed before these techniques are applied to the human oviduct.

Tying a knot consists of several maneuvers. First, the suture is grasped with the right-handed forceps or needle holder. Second, a loop is made with the long tail of the suture. Third, the suture is wrapped over and under the pickup tips. The short end of the thread is picked up with the left-handed forceps. Fourth, the loop is pulled off the left-handed forceps, and fifth, the knot is tightened.

With a smooth motion, one should pick up the longer length of thread with the tip of the right-handed forceps, approximately 2 cm from the suture site (Fig. 16–3B). The length of thread that lies between the forceps and the suture site is referred to as *loop length*. The suture is laid parallel to the oviduct. The suture should be taken with the hand

(palm up), and the hand is then rotated so that the suture is brought across as the hand is pronated. This first movement is critical and is often a source of error.

Once the thread has been grasped with the right hand, a single loop may be made around the top of the left-handed forceps (Fig. 16–3C). This may be accomplished by winding the forceps around the thread or the thread around the forceps. An additional loop may be made if the knot is to be placed under some tension. The loop should be well onto the tip of the left-handed forceps and loose. If not, the loop will easily fall off the tip of the forceps and an additional movement will be necessary to complete the loop.

There is usually little difficulty in grasping the short end of the suture (Fig. 16–3C). However, difficulty may be encountered if the end is too short, if the suture lies at an angle awkward for the forceps, or if the suture tip is hidden or is lying on a flat surface. If the short end is too short, it is usually because the loop length was too short, which was necessarily caused by some pulling of the suture with the right-handed forceps as the loop was made. The problem, therefore, may be avoided if one inspects the short end of the suture before making the loop. One may manipulate a flat or hidden suture end with the tips of the left-handed forceps, if necessary. One should not force the issue but stop, reanalyze the position of the suture, and, if necessary, repeat the knot placement.

Once the short end of the suture has been grasped, the loop may be pulled off the left-handed forceps, drawing the knot tight (Fig. 16–3D). The suture has been drawn too tightly if the tissue bunches together or the tissue edges are not approximated but overlap.

A second half-knot is placed as the sequence of movements is repeated in reverse (Fig. 16–E,F). One should release the short tail from the left-handed pickup and take hold of the long tail next to the right-handed forceps or needle driver. One should then reverse the thread in the distal direction, creating a U-shaped opening and thereafter lift the long tail with the pickup and wrap the suture over and under the slightly opened forceps (Fig. 16–3E). The short tail may then be grasped with the forceps or needle driver, pulled through the loop, and then tightened (Fig. 16–3F). Each knot should be square. An additional throw may be necessary if absorbable suture is used. The number of sutures to be placed about the tubal lumen for an anastomosis varies, but the general principle applies that the fewer the knots placed about the circumference of the tube, the less the tissue reaction.

The organization of an operating room surgical

team is essential. The surgical scrub nurse should be knowledgeable in microsurgical techniques and familiar with instrumentation. With careful organization of the operating theater, the best atmosphere will be provided for an efficient operation with a minimum of lost time.

TUBAL RECONSTRUCTION

Historically, the field of tubal plastic surgery has less than one century of clinical experience since the first report by Schroder in 1884 of a unilateral ampullary cuff salpingostomy. By the turn of the 20th century, most of the operative procedures that are in use today had been initiated by a few pioneers in infertility surgery. The historic details of this era are summarized in Table 16–1.

Pelvic laparotomy is usually deferred until two or more tubal function studies confirm the presence of tubal obstruction. Direct visualization of the tubes by laparoscopy and retrograde dye studies is always performed prior to laparotomy in order to evaluate the pelvic organs and fallopian tubes prior to committing the patient to a major operative procedure. The use of laparoscopy has greatly influenced our selection of patients for tubal surgery. Patients with far-advanced, irreversible, destructive disease of the tube are excluded as surgical candidates, *before* an exploratory procedure is performed. It is our feeling that many hopeless surgical cases are operated upon simply because the surgeon has performed the exploratory laparotomy before making an adequate assessment of the extent of the tubal disease. Had the surgeon known the extent of the disease before surgery, it is unlikely that the patient would have been encouraged to have the surgical procedure. This realistic approach to the more conservative

use of surgery in the treatment of irreversible tubal occlusion has greatly improved the pregnancy rates in the highly selective group of cases that are true candidates for surgery. Microsurgical tubal plastic surgery may also be performed in conjunction with a pelvic operation, primarily for relief of other symptoms, such as pelvic endometriosis or repeat ectopic pregnancy.

The carbon dioxide laser may assist the microsurgeon during tuboplasty. Opinions differ about the efficacy of the carbon dioxide laser for tuboplasty. The reported advantages include the precise vaporization of adhesions with minimal tissue damage and a consequent reduction in adhesion formation and minimal bleeding. There may be an advantage of increased ease in performing the procedure. There is, however, no evidence to suggest that the laser technique leads to an increased pregnancy success rate.

Many procedures for tubal obstruction have been described, but most of them can be included among the following procedures. In general, tubal surgery for infertility must deal with four major areas of tubal disease: (1) peritubal adhesions, for which salpingolysis is performed; (2) occlusion of the distal end of the tube, for which salpingostomy or fimbrioplasty is required; (3) segmental obstruction, for which end-to-end anastomosis has become popular in an effort to anastomose tubes that have been previously ligated; and (4) proximal tubal obstruction, which may require reimplantation.

A major difficulty in comparing different series of surgical procedures is the lack of a universally accepted classification of tubal surgery. In an attempt to arrive at a workable classification, the Ad Hoc Committee of the International Federation of Fertility and Sterility introduced a classification that

TABLE 16–1   *Historical Development of Tubal Surgery for Infertility*

AUTHOR (YEAR)	OPERATIONS	CONTRIBUTION
Schroder (1884)	1	Unilateral ampullary cuff
Skutsch (1889)	1	Bilateral ampullary cuff; first to use term *salpingostomy*
Martin (1891)	24	First reported postoperative pregnancy (aborted)
Polk (1894)	12	Described salpingolysis
Ries (1897)	1	First uterotubal implantation; first to use term *metrosalpingoanastomosis*
Gouillioud (1900)	1	First illustration of ampullary cuff salpingoneostomy with partial tubal resection
Burrage (1900)	17	Dorsal slit salpingoneostomy
Ferguson (1903)	6	Intraoperative tubal testing prior to tuboplasty
Turck (1909)	2	Term pregnancies following bilateral uterotubal implantations

From Siegler, 1975.

was modified by the same committee at the 10th World Congress of Fertility and Sterility in Madrid in July, 1980 (Table 16–2). This classification will create some uniformity in reporting results. However, before reliable success rates can be established, careful consideration must be given to all prognostic factors that may alter pregnancy outcome. For instance, a group of patients treated with a uniform technique may have varying pathogeneses and varying extents of adhesion formation. Therefore, all factors must be carefully delineated before surgical results can be critically evaluated.

TABLE 16–2 Classification of Tubal Procedures

1. Lysis of periadnexal adhesion (Salpingolysis-Ovariolysis): Classified according to adnexa with least pathology
   a. Minimal: 1 cm of tube or ovary involved
   b. Moderate: Partially surrounding tube or ovary
   c. Severe: Encapsulating peritubal and/or periovarian adhesions

2. Lysis of extra-adnexal adhesions
   a. Minimal
   b. Moderate
   c. Severe

3. Tubouterine implantation
   a. Isthmic: Implantation of isthmic segment
   b. Ampullary: Implantation of ampullary segment
   x. Combination: Different type of implantation on right and left sides

4. Tubotubal anastomosis
   a. Interstitial (intramural)–isthmic
   b. Interstitial (intramural)–ampullary
   c. Isthmic–isthmic
   d. Isthmic–ampullary
   e. Ampullary–ampullary
   f. Ampullary–infundibular (fimbrial)
   x. Combination: Different type anastomosis on right and left tubes

5. Salpingostomy (salpingoneostomy): Surgical creation of a new tubal ostium
   a. Terminal
   b. Ampullary
   c. Isthmic
   x. Combination: Different type salpingostomy on right and left tubes

6. Fimbrioplasty: Reconstruction of existent fimbriae
   a. By deagglutination and dilatation
   b. With serosal incision (for completely occluded tube)
   x. Combination: Different type fimbrioplasty on right and left tubes

7. Other reconstructive tubal operations (specify)

8. Combination of different types of operations
   a. Bipolar: For occlusion at both proximal and terminal end of tube (specify)
   b. Bilateral: Different operations on the right and left sides (specify)

From the Ad Hoc Committee of the International Federation of Fertility and Sterility. From Gomel V: Classification of operations for tubal and peritoneal factors causing infertility. Clin Obstet Gynecol 23:1259, 1980

SALPINGOLYSIS

Patients with peritubular adhesions as the sole factor responsible for infertility are not common. The incidence in our institution has been approximately 4% and has remained fairly constant. Peritubular adhesions may result from postabortal or puerperal infection, residual endosalpingitis, previous appendicitis, pelvic endometriosis, or, possibly, previous gynecologic surgery. The infundibulum is by definition uninvolved. The careful excision of adhesions about the tube will restore the normal tubo-ovarian anatomical relationships. Patients with endometriosis should not be included in this series.

Tubal surgery requires careful mobilization and elevation of the adnexa so that proper hand support may allow careful excision of adhesions. If extensive adhesion formation is present, careful, painstaking removal of individual adhesions is required. Gentle blunt dissection with the finger may allow elevation of an adnexa adhered to the pelvic sidewall onto a rubber platform after the cul-de-sac has been gently packed with a lint-free laparotomy pad. Once the adnexa are mobilized, the surgeon should carefully excise all adhesions using a fine-needle monopolar insulated microelectrode with a cutting or blended current (Fig. 16-4). Plastic or insulated metal rods are used to elevate adhesions so that their insertion and origin are clearly identified. All adhesions should be removed from the pelvis using meticulous technique, avoiding trauma to serosal surfaces.

A variety of different types of adhesions to various locations may be identified. Large fibrous avascular adhesions between ovary, fallopian tube, and small bowel are particularly difficult to remove without damage to the serosal surface. An appropriately insulated manipulator prevents accidental electrocautery to surrounding tissues. Once all adhesions are removed and the anatomy is normalized, careful inspection of the fimbriae should be performed with magnification. Often, fine adhesions involving the infundibulum are missed. Careful dissection in even the best hands often results in denuded areas that must be carefully reperitonealized with fine absorbable suture.

Postoperative pregnancy results are satisfactory following salpingolysis. Most series quote pregnancy rates ranging from 32% to 60%; our experience is similar (Table 16–3). All patients had adhesions

TABLE 16-3 *Pregnancy Success Following Salpingolysis (1961–1983)*

PARAMETER	OUTCOME
Number of patients	51
Number of patients pregnant	38 (75%)
Number with living children	32 (63%)
Number of pregnancies	49
Term	37
Spontaneous abortion	7
Premature delivery	0
Ectopic pregnancy	5

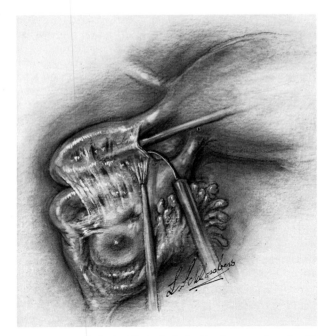

FIG. 16–4 Tubolysis. (A) Peritubal adhesions are lysed with fine-needle monopolar cautery and removed.

which were iatrogenic or inflammatory in nature. Patients with endometriosis were not included. Of patients with bilateral adhesions treated by salpingolysis, 63% conceived and delivered live-born infants. Five ectopic pregnancies were noted among the total number of pregnancies.

Recently, Gomel has advocated salpingolysis by laparoscopy. Among 92 women, 57 (62%) achieved a term pregnancy after laparoscopic lysis of adhesions. He cautions that skilled techniques are needed to avoid trauma. In selected patients, this approach may be an alternative to exploratory surgery and a microsurgical tubolysis.

SALPINGOPLASTY

Salpingoplasty, a collective term, implies a corrective procedure involving the distal portion of the oviduct (infundibulum). It may also imply the creation of a new ostium (salpingoneostomy) or fimbrioplasty through which disagglutination or dilatation of the tubal ostium is performed.

FIMBRIOPLASTY

The normal anatomy must be restored when the distal oviduct is being repaired. Tubo-ovarian relationships should be completely restored before patency is established. In particular, the fimbria ovarica and utero-ovarian ligament should be carefully identified.

Fimbrioplasty is defined as the lysis of fimbrial adhesions or dilatation of fimbrial phimosis. On occasion, a peritoneal ring of adhesions results in a relative obstruction of the distal portion of the fallopian tube such that simple lysis of these strands will uncover normal-appearing fimbriae. In most instances, periadnexal adhesions are also present. It is important to mobilize the tube and ovary prior to attempting to establish patency by fimbriolysis.

If fimbrial agglutination is found, a fine delicate mosquito forceps can be introduced into the phimotic opening of the tube and gently opened (Fig. 16–5). The forceps are gently withdrawn in the open position, causing dilatation of the tubal ostia. By repeating this procedure in several directions, even dilatation of the fimbrial os is accomplished. In some instances, a small incision of scarred tissue may be necessary. The opening may also be aided by a few sutures of No. 8-0 polyglactic acid suture to maintain established fimbrial eversion.

SALPINGONEOSTOMY

Salpingoneostomy is the creation of a new tubal ostium where the fimbrial end is totally occluded. Terminal salpingoneostomy is the procedure of choice in establishing tubal patency. Ampullary and isthmic salpingostomy are largely historical procedures that result in dismal pregnancy success rates.

Salpingoneostomy, as performed today, avoids the removal of the distal end of the tube and emphasizes the importance of maintaining the fimbriae in as nearly normal an anatomical condition as possible (Fig. 16–6). A successful salpingoneostomy requires a complete understanding of the normal tubo-ovarian relationships, specifically, the fimbria ovarica and the relationship of the shaft of the oviduct to the ovary. Although the fimbria ovarica may vary

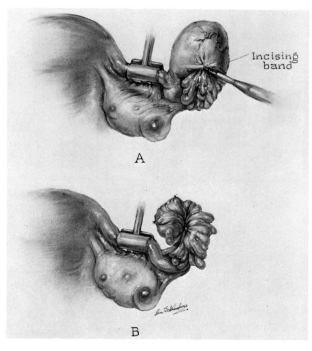

FIG. 16-5 Fimbrioplasty. (*A*) Incomplete tubal obstruction resulting from a tubal band. When the scar is removed, normal fimbriae appear. (*B*) One to three fine sutures may be needed to establish patency. (Jones, Rock, 1983)

in length, it is always present and provides a clue as to the normal axis of the oviduct. It should be clearly identified before an ostium is created.

With gentle lysis of adhesions with a monopolar insulated microelectrode, adhesions are excised and the ovaries are mobilized. The cul-de-sac may then be packed with lint-free laparotomy pads and the adnexa placed on an appropriate platform before the tubo-ovarian relationships are established. Once these relationships are established, attention is turned to the fimbria ovarica. The tubes are distended by injecting dilute methylene blue or indigo carmine dye through the fundus. Under magnification, a distinct vascular pattern that surrounds an avascular area may be easily identified. As this scar is incised with cutting cautery, colored fluid will escape (Fig. 16-6). We prefer to introduce a fine glass probe into the tube and explore the ampullary portion of the fallopian tube. On occasion, normal-appearing fimbriae may protrude through the opening. More often than not, the fimbriae are severely damaged, agglutinated, and confined to the tubal lumen. In this case, an initial incision at 6 o'clock is performed in the direction of the fimbria ovarica (Fig. 16-7D) and the edges are everted with No. 7-0 or No. 8-0 polyglactic acid suture (Fig. 16-7E,F). The mucosa is then carefully everted with a minimal number of sutures. Bleeding capillaries

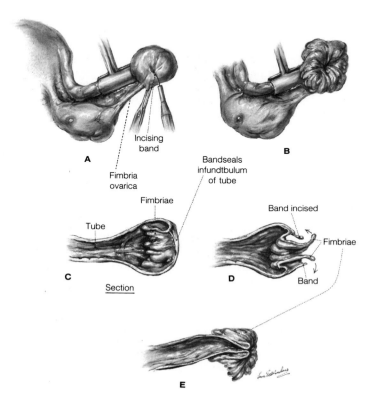

FIG. 16-6 Complete distal fimbrial obstruction without significant hydrosalpinx or fimbrial destruction. (*A*) Whitish scar is incised with electrocautery. (*B*) Fimbrial strands are revealed. Some agglutination may be noted. Delicate fine forceps may be used to dilate the phimotic os. (*C*) A cross section reveals strands by peritoneal band. (*D*) When band is incised, fimbriae are released. (*E*) Fimbriae assume their normal anatomical position. (Jones, Rock, 1983)

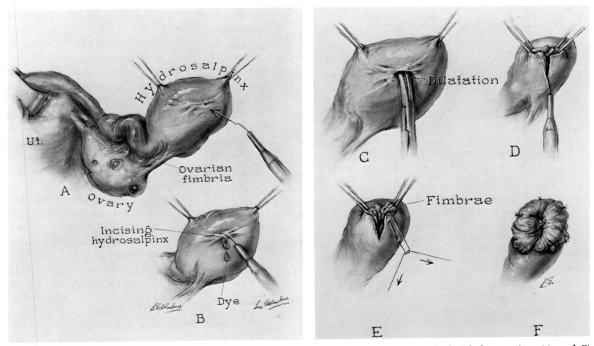

FIG. 16–7 Distal fimbrial obstruction with moderate hydrosalpinx and complete fimbrial destruction. (*A* and *B*) Whitish scar over the distended hydrosalpinx is incised, releasing indigo carmine dye. (*C*) The ostium is first dilated with a fine forceps to release trapped fimbrial strands. (*D*) If none are noted, the incision is extended down at 6 o'clock toward the fimbria ovarica. (*E* and *F*) A cuff salpingostomy is accomplished by everting the mucosa using No. 7-0 polyglactin suture. (Jones, Rock, 1983)

may be visualized by irrigation and coagulated with bipolar cautery at a low setting.

Prognostic Factors for Salpingoneostomy

There is a marked disparity among pregnancy success rates with different salpingoneostomy techniques. The disparity is probably a result of the inadequate description of surgical technique as well as of the lack of documentation of the degree of tubal disease and pelvic adhesion formation at the time of surgery. Furthermore, differences in classification systems have added to the confusion. Siegler has stressed the importance of uniformity in reporting results following salpingoneostomy to allow study comparison. In the classification of operations noted by the 9th World Congress on Fertility and Sterility, it was proposed that the term *salpingoneostomy* be used for those procedures designed to relieve distally obstructed fallopian tubes where no identifiable fimbriae could be recovered. Our classification differs in that not all patients who have complete distal fimbrial obstruction where salpingoneostomy is required have total destruction of the fimbriae. The condition of the fimbriae may vary once patency is established (Fig. 16-8). Thus,

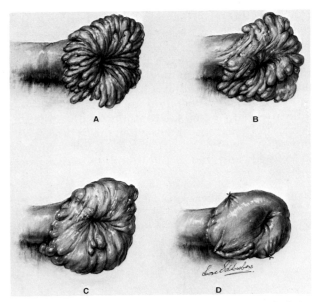

FIG. 16–8 Distal fimbrial obstruction: condition of the fimbriae following salpingostomy. (*A*) Normal-appearing fimbriae. (*B*) Some minimal fimbrial agglutination with scarring at 12 o'clock. (*C*) Fragmental fimbrial strands with rugal loss. (*D*) Few fimbriae noted with essentially smooth flattened mucosa.

TABLE 16–4 *Classification of the Extent of Tubal Disease with Distal Fimbrial Obstruction*

EXTENT OF DISEASE	FINDINGS
Mild	Absent or small hydrosalpinx ≤ 15 mm diameter
	Inverted fimbriae easily recognized when patency achieved
	No significant peritubal or periovarian adhesions
	Rugal pattern on preoperative hysterogram
Moderate	Hydrosalpinx 15–30 mm diameter
	Fragments of fimbriae not readily identified
	Periovarian or peritubular adhesions without fixation, few cul-de-sac adhesions
	Absence of a rugal pattern on preoperative hysterogram
Severe	Large hydrosalpinx ≥ 30 mm diameter
	No fimbriae
	Dense pelvic or adnexal adhesions with fixation of the ovary and tube to broad ligament, pelvic sidewall, omentum or bowel
	Obliteration of the cul-de-sac
	Frozen pelvis (adhesion formation so dense that limits of organs are difficult to define)

Adapted from Rock et al, 1978.

the condition of the fimbriae may be of prognostic value and should be taken into consideration in patients who require the creation of a new tubal ostium.

Shirodkar suggested classifying different types of hydrosalpinges on the basis on their size, the presence of peritubular adhesions, the condition of the muscular wall, the condition of the ciliary epithelium after biopsy, and the condition of the fimbriae. Pregnancy was more likely when the hydrosalpinx ranged in size between the size of the surgeon's little finger and that of the thumb, whereas preg-

nancy was noted to fall from 50% to 10% when the hydrosalpinx was larger than the surgeon's thumb. Young and coauthors demonstrated an increased pregnancy rate in patients noted to have rugae on preoperative hysterogram. A pregnancy rate of 61% when rugae were present decreased to 7% when rugae were not demonstrated. Garcia and Aller suggested a classification of tubal disease for patients with distal occlusion and a hydrosalpinx. This classification was based on the degree of periadnexal adhesion involvement. No correlation, however, was established between the extent of the disease and the pregnancy rate. Siegler summarized the opinion of most tubal surgeons when he stated: "The most favorable tubes for salpingostomy are those with a small hydrosalpinx, recoverable fimbriae, and minimal endosalpingeal adhesions."

A more practical classification system for tubal disease was formulated (Table 16–4) using factors that have been shown to influence pregnancy, specifically the size of the hydrosalpinx, the condition of the fimbriae, the presence or absence of rugae on hysterogram, and the extent of pelvic adhesion formation. Using this classification system, our experience confirms that these factors influence subsequent pregnancy success. That is, the extent of tubal disease and pelvic adhesion formation are directly related to the pregnancy rate as well as to the tubal patency rate (Table 16-5). These observations were confirmed by Rock and coauthors in a multicenter randomized clinical trial in which pregnancies occurred up to 43 months after salpingoneostomy (Fig. 16–9). This time interval has also been noted by Jansen. The delay in conception may result from a gradual regeneration of oviductal mucosal elements. This concept is supported by the work of Petrucco and Winston, who demonstrated that oviducts damaged by hydrosalpinx formation showed a highly significant decrease in both cytoplasmic and nuclear estrogen receptors compared to normal oviducts at equivalent stages of the menstrual cycle. The decrease in estrogen receptors cor-

TABLE 16–5 *Pregnancy Outcome and Tubal Patency Following Salpingoneostomy*

EXTENT OF DISEASE	PREGNANCY OUTCOME			POSTOPERATIVE HYSTEROGRAM	
	Number of Patients	Patients Pregnant	Ectopic Pregnancy	Number of Patients	Patency
Mild	15	13 (86%)	1 (6%)	7	7 (100%)
Moderate	34	9 (26%)	4 (12%)	19	14 (74%)
Severe	50	4 (8%)	1 (2%)	26	17 (65%)
Totals	99	26 (26%)	6 (6%)	52	38 (73%)

From Rock et al, 1978.

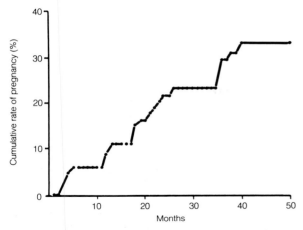

FIG. 16–9 Cumulative rate of pregnancy over 43 months after salpingoneostomy. (Jones, Rock, 1983)

related with a decrease in the percentage of ciliated cells.

The condition of the cilia on microscopic examination from biopsies of a hydrosalpinx has not been correlated with pregnancy rate. Crane and Woodruff found that microscopic changes offered a poor method of evaluating the physiologic disturbance produced by inflammatory disease in the oviduct. Recent scanning electron microscopy studies have demonstrated the pathologic alterations of the mucosal folds and secretion in patients with distal fimbrial obstruction. Vasquez and associates, using scanning electron microscopy, found a significant reduction in ciliated cells in a hydrosalpinx. With microbiopsy techniques, a correlation may be established between the condition of these elements and subsequent pregnancy success.

Additional variables may further hinder the comparison of results of different series. At this writing, the only adjunctive therapy found to be efficacious in the prevention of adhesion formation following tuboplasty is the intraperitoneal instillation of 32% high molecular weight dextran 70. The Adhesion Study Group found high molecular weight dextran to be effective in preventing adhesion formation in a randomized clinical trial. The mechanism of action of dextran includes the following. (1) The siliconizing effect of dextran is antithrombotic; that is, dextran coats raw serosal surfaces and retards peritoneal abrasions and blood clot adherence. (2) By its nonpolar properties, dextran maintains the negativity of the serosal surface and may cause repulsion of fibrinogen molecules and decrease or prevent adhesions. (3) Dextran has a mechanical effect. Tissues are held apart by a heavy fluid in the pelvis, a hydroflotation effect. Dextran establishes an osmotic gradient, increasing the volume of intraper-

itoneal fluid and thereby decreasing tissue apposition during the early stages of healing. (4) Dextran modifies the fiber network and renders it more susceptible to lysis. (5) Dextran does not alter the activity of thrombin but changes the kinetics of polymerization of fibrin monomers and yields a decreased clotting time. Whether this solution ultimately results in an increased pregnancy rate remains to be established.

Grant emphasized the need for postoperative hydrotubation to enhance fertility following salpingoneostomy. Contrary to his view, the efficacy of postoperative hydrotubation could not be demonstrated in our multicenter randomized clinical trial.

Swolin has suggested the use of second-look laparoscopy to lyse adhesions 8 days to 2 weeks postoperatively. Others have suggested waiting 6 months to perform a second-look laparoscopy to determine the existence of postoperative adhesions and to assess the surgical result. At that time, lysis of adhesions is possible, as well as retrograde dye insufflation.

Results of salpingoneostomy have been discouraging (Table 16–6). Salpingoneostomy performed with magnification has resulted in intrauterine pregnancy rates similar to those following conventional techniques, although an increased ectopic pregnancy rate has been observed. The usefulness of the operating microscope in this surgery remains to be established. Our own experience, using loupe magnification, has been similar to previously reported pregnancy rates.

END-TO-END ANASTOMOSES

The role of end-to-end anastomosis is limited primarily to reconstruction of fallopian tubes in previously sterilized patients. It is used infrequently in the conservative treatment of an *unruptured* tubal pregnancy where a small segment of the tube has been destroyed by the invading trophoblast. The request for elective sterilization has become a major medical issue in recent years, with an estimated 2.3 million tubal sterilizations and vasectomies each performed in the United States in 1975. It is clearly evident that the gynecologist will be called upon more frequently during the next decade to anastomose these ligated or fulgurated tubes in patients who have reversed their thinking on this matter and who desire further childbearing. Among all couples desiring no further children, sterilization is second in demand only to the contraceptive pill.

Prognostic Factors for End-to-End Anastomosis

SURGICAL TECHNIQUE. Microsurgery implies very delicate atraumatic surgical technique to minimize

TABLE 16–6   *Results of Salpingoneostomy*

AUTHOR (YEAR)	NUMBER OF PATIENTS	PERCENTAGE OF INTRAUTERINE PREGNANCIES	PERCENTAGE OF TERM PREGNANCIES	PERCENTAGE OF TUBAL PREGNANCIES
Conventional Surgery				
O'Brien, et al (1969)	57	25		2
Grant (1971)	103	16	12	3
Cognat and Rochet (1977)	118	24	20	4
Microsurgery				
Swolin (1975)*	33	27	27	18
Gomel (1978)*	72	30.5	29	10
Rock, et al (1978)†	99	26	18	6

* Microscope.
† Loupe, ×1 to ×2 magnification.
From Jones, Rock, 1983.

tissue damage. Prior to 1976, the Hellman technique using a polyethylene catheter and No. 5-0 suture material was practiced in our institution to reverse tubal ligation. At the Johns Hopkins Hospital, a comparison of Hellman's macrosurgical approach and our microsurgical technique revealed an increased pregnancy rate with the latter. There are, however, other variables which are thought to affect subsequent pregnancy success following reversal of sterilization.

STERILIZATION PROCEDURE.   There are several types of sterilization procedures that may be reversed. Depending on the extent of tubal destruction, different segments of tube are anastomosed. It is difficult to separate these variables when discussing sterilization procedures in general.

In our experience, a rather large amount of tube may be destroyed with tubal cautery procedures, especially when a triple-burn technique is employed. Of 48 women who underwent monopolar high-frequency diathermia, 25 conceived following tubal anastomosis and 17 of these delivered living children. Among ectopic pregnancies for the overall series of 125 patients with tubal reconstructive surgery, four of five occurred in patients following monopolar cautery.

The extent to which normal physiologic function returns to cauterized tubes is unknown, but the increased incidence of ectopic pregnancies suggests some interference with tubal transport. Damage to the oviduct cilia may extend 2 cm from the site of cautery. For these reasons, one should be certain that when the obliterated tube is excised and patency is established, healthy, well-vascularized tissue is present before proceeding with the anastomosis.

Others have reported good success following reversal of cauterized fallopian tubes. Winston reported that 55% of patients conceived after tubal cautery. Gomel has suggested that diathermic coagulation has one major advantage in that the pelvis is relatively clean and the tubes are free of adhesions. Although this may be true in some instances, it is by no means the rule. Associated tubal pathology has been observed in up to 30% of women after tubal cauterization using monopolar high-frequency diathermia at The Johns Hopkins Hospital.

As a result of the high variability in tubal destruction, preoperative laparoscopy is indicated to determine the amount of distal fallopian tube available for the anastomosis. The amount of proximal tube is not an issue. That is, if destruction of the intramural portion of the fallopian tube is noted, and there is sufficient distal tube, uterotubal implantation may be performed.

Other forms of tubal sterilization may offer higher pregnancy rates following anastomosis. In particular, anastomosis following Falope ring sterilization is associated with a pregnancy rate of more than 75%. Winston has reported no failures with clip sterilization. Similar experiences have been reported by Gomel, Grunert and associates, Patterson, and Jones and Rock.

SEGMENTS ANASTOMOSED.   At present, five varieties of tubal anastomoses have been identified, involving the isthmic, ampullary, and intramural portions of the fallopian tube. Recent reports record the highest pregnancy rates among isthmic-isthmic anastomosis in which there is no discrepancy in tubal lumen size.

Decreases in frequency of pregnancy success have been noted in intramural-isthmic, isthmic-ampullary, ampullary-ampullary, and intramural-ampullary anastomoses, respectively (Table 16–7). There are several techniques to overcome tubal lumen discrepancy in ampullary-isthmic anastomo-

TABLE 16–7   *Intrauterine Pregnancies after Tubal Anastomosis by Site of Anastomosis*

| | NUMBER OF INTRAUTERINE PREGNANCIES/NUMBER OF CASES | | | |
SITE OF ANASTOMOSIS	Winston	Rock and Jones	Silber and Cohen	Total
Intramural-isthmic	12/17	1/2	1/1	14/20 (70%)
Intramural-ampullary	13/26	0/1	7/13	20/40 (50%)
Isthmic-isthmic	12/16	24/32		36/48 (75%)
Isthmic-ampullary	15/27	38/54	6/11	59/92 (64%)
Ampullary-ampullary	8/19	12/16		20/35 (57%)
Totals	70/126	75/105	14/25	159/256 (62%)

From Jones, Rock, 1983.

ses. Comparison of pregnancy success rates among these varying techniques is difficult, although contemporary data suggest that one should expect a pregnancy rate of approximately 60%.

TUBAL LENGTH.   There is a direct relationship between pregnancy success and length of fallopian tube that may be reunited. Gomel has observed that fallopian tubes of less than 3 cm in total length were associated with a long interval between reconstructive surgery and occurrence of pregnancy. With oviducts of over 6 cm in length, pregnancy occurred within 3 to 4 cycles and not infrequently during the first month following surgery. A decreased pregnancy rate was noted in patients with fallopian tubes of less than 4 cm in length and this has also been our experience. Furthermore, we have demonstrated an increased incidence of endometriosis in women whose proximal fallopian tubes are less than 4 cm in length.

We have noted a significant incidence of associated pelvic pathology in 125 patients undergoing reversal of sterilization. Thirty percent of patients, the majority of whom underwent anastomosis after tubal cautery, were noted to have associated pelvic findings. A high incidence of endometriosis and proximal hydrosalpinges was noted in the cautery group. That is, 34 of 85 (40%) oviducts sterilized by unipolar cautery had endometriosis. There were 18 (21%) fistulas.

TIME INTERVAL FROM STERILIZATION TO ANASTOMOSIS. Associated tubal pathology increases with an increasing interval from previous sterilization. In particular, the condition of the cilia is significant in that deciliation and tubal polyps increase 4 years after sterilization. Additionally, the pregnancy rate is less among patients who have been sterilized for four years or more. The pathogenesis of these intraluminal tubal polyps has not been elucidated; however, chronic inflammation has been implicated.

When shortened oviducts are less than 4 cm in length, retrograde menstruation may result in a proximal hydrosalpinx, which predisposes to the development of endometriosis and subsequent fistulization. Furthermore, the incidence of endometriosis and fistula formation increases abruptly 3 years after previous sterilization. It is probable that these associated pathologic findings are linked with a reduced pregnancy success rate.

TUBAL VASCULARITY.   Some sterilization procedures may result in a decrease in tubal vascularity, which may result in interruption of uterotubal-ovarian blood flow. Radwanska and associates noted a decrease in progesterone production in patients who underwent reversal of sterilization. These findings were supported by those of Donnez and associates; however, Meldrum was unable to demonstrate a reduction in progesterone in a similar group of patients. Unfortunately, several types of sterilization procedures were included as a group, and no particular procedure could be identified as associated with a luteal phase deficiency. Further studies in this area are needed to confirm this possible association. In principle, however, procedures that destroy a minimal amount of the fallopian tube are less likely to interfere with the vascular supply to the fallopian tube.

Magnification of the Operative Field

There has been some controversy as to the efficacy of loupe lenses in providing adequate magnification for the reversal of sterilization—pregnancy success rates are comparable to those obtained with the operating microscope after anastomosis. Although the loupe lenses may provide sufficient magnification to perform an isthmic-isthmic, ampullary-ampullary, or ampullary-isthmic anastomosis, there is some question about the precision and accuracy of suture placement. There is little debate on the need for a microscope to obtain sufficient magnification to perform an isthmic-cornual anastomosis. A recent study by Rock and coauthors reported reversal of sterilization by microsurgery tubal anastomosis in 72 women using either loupe lenses (n = 36) or microscope (n = 36). The study design called for randomization of patients within tiers that were matched with the method of sterilization and the site of anastomosis. A significant difference between methods could not be demonstrated. The authors suggested that the results did not imply that any surgeon may use loupe lenses with comfort and confidence. The selection of magnification system is a personal choice and should not be influenced by concern over a difference in subsequent pregnancy success.

TECHNIQUE OF TUBAL ANASTOMOSIS

The endosalpinx does proliferate under the influence of estrogen, as does the endometrium. For this reason, anastomosis should be performed during the proliferative phase of the cycle. Furthermore, supplemental oral estrogen given to inhibit ovulation and prolong the proliferative phase should increase tubal secretion and promote ciliogenesis. A loupe, visor, or microscope may be used to obtain magnification. Magnification with loupe lenses ranges from ×1 to ×6, while the microscope may provide magnification from ×3 to ×20.

Isthmic-Isthmic Anastomosis

The proximal portion of the fallopian tube is identified and its occluded tip resected (Fig. 16–10). A No. 2-0 nylon suture of 100 cm (40 in) is introduced into the lumen with fine forceps. Its passage may be facilitated by the distention of the uterine cavity and the interstitial portion of the oviduct with indigo carmine dye injected through the uterine fundus, with cervical obstruction by suitable instruments, as well as by stretching the tubal stump in a superior direction. Approximately 60 cm (25 in) of No. 2-0 nylon may be threaded through the tubal lumen and be placed within the uterine cavity. The same procedure is carried out on the opposite side. There is no discrepancy in luminal size if the distal segment is truly part of the isthmus. The proximal obstructed end is resected and the No. 2-0 nylon is then passed through the oviduct and out the fimbriated end. The mesosalpinx is carefully approximated to eliminate tension at the anastomotic site. The lumina of the two ends are then approximated with No. 7-0 or No. 8-0 polyglactic acid suture on a ⅜ circle taper (BV130-4) needle. Such suture is not routinely available and must be specially ordered. No. 8-0 nylon may also be used. The needle is passed only through the muscularis of the proximal tube and through the muscularis of the distal segment (see Fig. 16–10). The sutures are tied securely, and

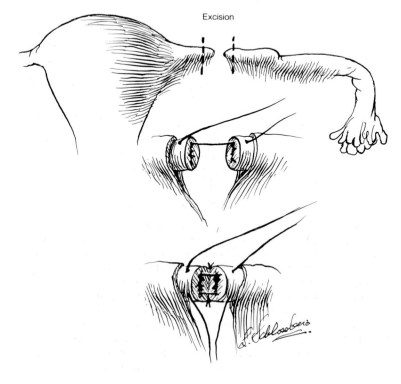

Excision

FIG. 16–10 Isthmic-isthmic anastomosis. Patency of obstructed lumina is established by excision of obstructed segment. The lumina may be approximated over a No. 2-0 nylon splint in two layers after the mesosalpinx is approximated. Three sutures are placed in the muscularis and the serosa is then approximated.

a second layer of the three additional sutures is placed to approximate the tubal serosa. The remaining portion of the No. 2-0 nylon splint extending through the fimbriated portion of the tube is cut with approximately 1 cm to 2 cm extending beyond the fimbriae. This nylon can be easily drawn into the ampulla. The nylon splints are removed through the cervix during the subsequent menses. Alternatively, the splint may be removed at the termination of the procedure. The possible benefit of leaving the nylon splint in the tube for 2 to 3 weeks postoperatively is now being addressed in a randomized clinical trial at The Johns Hopkins Hospital.

Isthmic-Ampullary Anastomosis

A No. 2-0 nylon splint is placed through the proximal isthmic portion of the tube into the uterus in a manner similar to that described above. A major difficulty is encountered in the isthmic-ampullary anastomosis because there is a large discrepancy between the diameter of the lumen in the isthmic and the ampullary portion of the tube. This discrepancy occurs as a result of a variety of sterilization procedures. In order to prevent too large an opening in the ampulla, a needle technique for opening the ampulla has been described as follows: A No. 16 Teflon obturator of an intravenous catheter set is introduced through the fimbriated end of the ampullary segment of the oviduct and advanced to the obstructed site (Fig. 16–11). The needle is inserted through the obturator, and the obstructed end is perforated by the needle and the Teflon sheath (Fig. 16–11A). After the needle is removed, the No. 2-0 nylon suture is then passed in a retrograde manner through the obturator. The mesosalpinx is approximated to reduce tension at the anastomotic site. Three to five No. 7-0 or No. 8-0 polyglactic acid sutures are placed through the serosa, muscularis, and endosalpinx of the proximal (isthmic) oviduct and then through the endosalpinx, muscularis, and serosa of the distal (ampullary) tube (Fig. 16–11B). The tip of the needle may be introduced into the ampullary lumen by being placed in the tip of the lumen of the Teflon obturator; then the tip of the obturator is withdrawn into the ampullary portion of the tube. Sutures are then tied securely (Fig. 16–11C). In some instances, a two-layer closure is possible; in those cases, an additional, second layer of suture is placed to approximate the tubal serosa.

Alternate methods of overcoming tubal discrepancy have been described by Diamond and Gomel. Winston prefers to circumcise the very tip of the ampulla over the bulbous end of a probe inserted through the fimbrial ostium. Before cutting across the mucosa, he suggests stripping back the peritoneal coat to facilitate subsequent two-layer closure.

In most instances, it has been our experience that a two-layer closure is possible using this circumcision technique. A single-layer closure, however, is necessary in the rather large lumen of the distal ampullary portion of the fallopian tube. The wall of the oviduct is quite thin, and if attempts are made to circumcise the fallopian tube, extensive bleeding occurs, as well as inadvertent widening of the oviductal lumen. This is particularly frustrating when large fronds of mucosa appear through the lumen. These fronds may be troublesome when placing suture; however, using a fine metal blunt probe, they may be pushed back into the lumen as the cardinal sutures are placed.

Ampullary-Ampullary Anastomosis

The muscularis of the ampullary region is relatively delicate. Because the lumina are quite large, a suture through all layers easily approximates to the tubal lumina (Fig. 16–12). Six or eight No. 7-0 or No. 8-0 polyglactic acid sutures are placed around the circumference of the ampulla. These sutures are placed through the serosa, muscularis, and endosalpinx in each approximating lumen. No splints are used.

Cornual-Isthmic Anastomosis

Cornual-isthmic anastomosis, on occasion, must be performed if a small proximal portion of the interstitial oviduct is occluded. A fine knife is used to core out the obstructed portion of the fallopian tube, creating a crater around the intramural tube. The isthmic portion of the fallopian tube is then approximated to the intramural portion of the fallopian tube. This is, in the author's opinion, the only procedure that requires high magnification and in which the microscope is most useful. These procedures are usually performed at a magnification of from ×10 to ×20. Hemostasis must be achieved using high-frequency fine-needle cautery. A two-layer closure is, in most instances, required. Winston has found pregnancy success rates approaching 60% with this type of anastomosis. With these improved pregnancy success rates, uterotubal implantation is only indicated when complete obliteration of the intramural portion of the fallopian tube is noted. Thus, attempts should be made to identify the amount of intramural obstruction before uterotubal implantation is considered.

Cornual-Ampullary Anastomosis

Special attention is necessary to ensure that a lumen of similar size is obtained during this anastomosis.

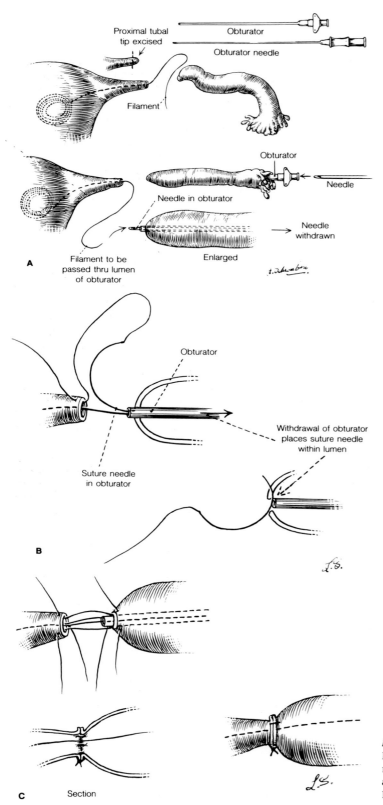

FIG. 16–11 Isthmic-ampullary anastomosis. (*A*) Method of performing isthmic-ampullary anastomosis. (*B*) Use of obturator to place needle tip within ampullary lumen. (*C*) Completed procedure. (Jones, Rock, 1983)

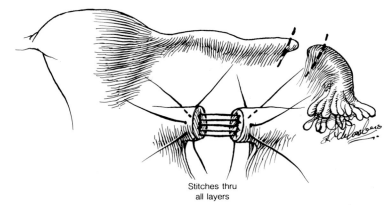

Stitches thru
all layers

FIG. 16–12 Ampullary-ampullary anastomosis. Anastomosis of these lumina requires six to eight sutures of No. 7-0 or No. 8-0 absorbable suture placed circumferentially equidistant about the oviductal lumen.

The cornual segment is prepared with a fine knife. Approximation is most difficult if the ampullary portion of the tube is transected. The catheter technique previously described for an isthmic-ampullary anastomosis or the use of a fine metal probe is essential to obtain an ampullary lumen similar in size to the cornual lumen. A two-layer closure may not be possible. Each approach should be individualized based on the side of the ampullary or cornual segment of oviduct. A No. 2-0 nylon splint placed in the uterus as previously described is useful for manipulation of the oviduct for suture placement. We have elected to leave the splint in situ for 2 to 3 weeks as the healing process is completed. In our experience, anastomosis of these segments is rare; furthermore, the techniques must stress an avoidance of lumen disparity to maximize functional success.

RESULTS OF ANASTOMOSIS

Pregnancy success after reversal of sterilization must be considered in light of the site of the anastomosis and the sterilization procedure performed. From experience with microsurgical techniques, one may expect an overall pregnancy success rate in the range of 55% to 60% live births; the ectopic pregnancy rate approaches 3% to 4% (Tables 16–8 and 16–9).

The site of anastomosis was found not to affect pregnancy success in Gomel's series of 112 patients. However, the experience of others has been to the contrary (see Table 16–7). Isthmic-isthmic anastomosis is associated with the highest pregnancy rate, whereas intramural-ampullary anastomosis has a reduced pregnancy success rate. Our own experience has noted a reduced pregnancy rate among patients requiring isthmic-ampullary anastomosis, although our procedure using a catheter technique

has resulted in an improved pregnancy rate over those achieved using macrosurgical techniques.

Monopolar cautery as a sterilization procedure may be reversed, although pregnancy success rates are diminished over those reported with the Falope ring and clip (see Table 16–9). Furthermore, tubal anastomosis following bilateral partial salpingectomy has a higher pregnancy rate than following monopolar cautery. Four of our five ectopic pregnancies subsequent to anastomosis were in patients who had received monopolar cautery. Furthermore, associated pelvic pathology in the form of proximal hydrosalpinges and endometriosis is higher in patients following monopolar high-frequency diathermy. Reversal of Falope ring or clip sterilization has been associated with excellent pregnancy success rates. Larger patient series, however, are necessary to establish the superiority of these over other reversible sterilization methods.

TABLE 16–8 Pregnancy Success Following Tubal Anastomosis Using Microsurgery Technique

AUTHOR (YEAR)	NUMBER OF CASES	LIVE BIRTHS	ECTOPIC PREGNANCIES
Silber, Cohen (1980)	25	56%	4%
Patterson (1980)	50	40%	4%
Winston (1980)	126	58%	2%
Gomel (1980)	118	64%	1%
Grunert, et al (1981)	40	57%	3%
Rock, Jones (1982)	125	50%	4%
Seiler (1983)	73	64%	2%
Totals	557	56%	3%

Adapted from Jones, Rock, 1983.

TABLE 16-9   *Pregnancy Success Following Reversal of Sterilization*
             (The Johns Hopkins Hospital, 1976–1981)

STERILIZATION METHOD	NUMBER OF PATIENTS	PATIENTS PREGNANT	TERM DELIVERY	ABORTIONS	ECTOPIC PREGNANCIES
Bilateral partial salpingectomy	17	12	9	3	0
Clip	1	1	1	0	0
Falope ring	22	18	17	1	0
Irving	6	4	2	2	0
Monopolar cautery	48	25	17	4	4
Pomeroy	31	22	17	4	1
Totals	125	82 (66%)	63 (50%)	14 (11%)	5 (4%)

From Rock, 1982.

There appear to be several variables to be considered, such as tubal polyps and endometriosis, which may only be identified after the sterilization reversal has been performed. These factors may influence subsequent pregnancy success. In particular, the tubal length, the sterilization procedures previously performed, and the segments anastomosed may have a significant bearing on subsequent pregnancy success.

The usefulness of microsurgery for the reversal of sterilization was recently emphasized in an international program to determine the reversibility of female sterilization in Asia using microsurgical technique. Rock and associates reported that 111 of 219 patients (51%) conceived following tubal anastomosis; of these, 79 had a living child. The overall cumulative probability of conception at the end of the follow-up period as determined by life table analysis was 63%. The success of this program demonstrated that sophisticated technological advances can be adopted and applied in developing countries.

Uterotubal Implantation

In the past, proximal obstruction (intramural or isthmic obstruction) has been considered an indication for uterotubal implantation. However, with the development of microsurgical techniques for cornual-isthmic anastomosis with reported pregnancy success rates in excess of 60%, uterotubal implantation is primarily reserved for patients with complete intramural obstruction. Furthermore, patients are candidates for uterotubal implantation using the posterior fundal incision technique when a short oviduct is encountered where mobilization is difficult without distortion of the tubo-ovarian relationship. Although uterotubal implantation is considered a rather gross technique, the reproductive surgeon should approach this procedure with the same attitude as when performing a tubal anastomosis. Gentle handling of tissues with fine instruments to avoid serosal trauma, the use of a delicate electrocautery needle for precise hemostasis, and the use of fine nonreactive suture will decrease postoperative adhesion formation. The use of minimal magnification ($\times 1.7$ to $\times 2.5$) assists in the placement of sutures and in obtaining accurate tissue approximation, as well as complete hemostasis. Using these precepts, the surgeon should minimize iatrogenic adhesion formation, which should improve surgical results and subsequent pregnancy success.

UTEROTUBAL JUNCTION

The length of the intramural portion of the oviduct may range from 1.5 cm to 2.5 cm. Its pathway is characterized by convolutions and abrupt changes in direction. The lumen follows a straight course through the uterine wall to the muscular layer and then angles sharply into the vascular layer. Thus, any attempt to pass a probe into the uterus may create a false passage.

The uterotubal junction may serve as a mechanical barrier and a site of sperm reserve in some species. The importance of intrinsic motility in sperm transport through the uterotubal junction is unclear. Motile sperm may be transported more efficiently than dead sperm. These observations suggest that contractions or fluid currents may play some role in sperm transport. Furthermore, the competence of the uterotubal junction varies with the hormonal environment in several species. Unfortunately, conflicting results in different species limit the application of these animal observations to humans.

If the uterotubal junction is removed in rabbits, the frequency of implantation of a fertilized ovum is decreased. However, Winston has reported intrauterine pregnancies in 11 of 16 patients after microsurgical tubocornual anastomosis (intramural-ampullary). Furthermore, pregnancy does occur in patients following uterotubal implantation where the uterotubal junction is removed. Thus, pregnancy is possible if the uterotubal junction is absent or destroyed.

DIAGNOSTIC TECHNIQUES

Proximal occlusion with abnormal fimbriae or distal fimbrial obstruction is a contraindication for uterotubal implantation. Patients with dense pelvic or adnexal adhesions with fixation of the ovary to the broad ligament or pelvic sidewall have a poor prognosis for conception after uterotubal implantation. It is therefore essential that a careful and accurate laparoscopic assessment of the pelvis be performed to aid in patient selection.

Each patient with proximal obstruction should receive a complete infertility evaluation, including documentation of ovulatory status, postcoital test, and an analysis of the husband's semen. Prior to uterotubal implantation, an evaluation of the intramural block should consist of two diagnostic tests, hysterosalpingography and laparoscopy. Errors in technique and misinterpretation of results of hysterosalpingography can account for inaccurate diagnoses with this technique. False positive laparoscopy findings of cornual obstruction may be expected in 3% of patients. In our opinion, hysterosalpingography is easy to perform with minimal risk to the patient and is superior to laparoscopy in the diagnosis of intrauterine or endometrial lesions. Therefore, hysterosalpingography and laparoscopy should be looked on, not as alternative but rather as complementary diagnostic procedures.

SURGICAL TECHNIQUES FOR UTEROTUBAL IMPLANTATION

One should make every attempt to maintain tuboovarian spatial relationships and to preserve as much fallopian tube as possible. Although the minimum length of fallopian tube necessary for conception has not been determined, preliminary results suggest that pregnancy rates following tubal reanastomosis are highest where 4 cm to 5 cm of fallopian tube are preserved.

There are three principal types of uterine incisions for the creation of a stoma for tubal implantation. Bonney advocated sharp excision of a cornual wedge prior to implantation, whereas Holden and Sovak used a reamer to make a cornual opening prior to implantation. There have been numerous modifications to these techniques, including the transverse fundal incision that enables the surgeon to visualize clearly the position of the implanted tube as it is sutured in place. Most recently, Von Csaba and associates and Peterson and associates reported uterotubal implantation through a posterior fundal incision between the utero-ovarian ligaments. Peterson and associates advocated the transverse fundal approach to overcome difficulties with mobilization of a shortened tube, where cornual implantation may distort the normal utero-ovarian relationships. Furthermore, this procedure is purported to restore some of the sphincteric action of the uterotubal junction, which cornual implantation removes.

There is controversy as to whether the isthmic or ampullary portion of the fallopian tube should be inserted into the uterus. Palmer reported a series of 118 patients who underwent uterotubal implantation, 25 of whom received an isthmic implantation. The term pregnancy rate was 10% higher with isthmic than with ampullary implantation. Unfortunately, variation in technique, histological diagnosis, and the extent of disease were not taken into consideration in these comparisons.

In a review of 52 patients who underwent uterotubal implantation at The Johns Hopkins Hospital, the term pregnancy rate was 10% higher among the 17 who received an ampullary implantation than among the 35 who received isthmic implantation. The highest pregnancy rate was observed in patients who received ampullary implantation with the reamer technique. This improved pregnancy rate was in part due to the lower reobstruction rate in these patients. Consideration must be given to the fact that fewer patients with chronic salpingitis had ampullary implantation; therefore, these observations must be stated with reservation. As larger numbers of patients accumulate, comparisons of homogeneous groups may resolve this controversy.

In light of the observation that the reobstruction rate in our series of patients was markedly decreased when the wider lumen had been implanted into the uterus, it has been our practice to sacrifice the isthmus when implanting the tube into the cornua. The posterior fundal incision technique, in our experience, has been useful in patients with excessively short tubes. Thus, the ampulla is implanted into the posterior uterus.

Ampullary Uterotubal Implantation

A generous transverse muscle-cutting abdominal incision, in most instances, will provide excellent exposure. We prefer to leave the muscles attached to the fascia so that they may be incised if further exposure is needed. The margins of the incision are then wrapped with Sof-Wick (Johnson and Johnson) low-lint laparotomy pads. Filmy adhesions may then be lysed with fine-needle electrocautery and removed. When both tubes are completely mobilized, tubal patency should be tested. If proximal obstruction is noted, the tube should be incised approximately 0.5 cm from the cornua and an attempt should be made to pass a No. 2-0 nylon suture into the uterus (Fig. 16–13A). On occasion, the suture may pass freely into the uterus, demonstrating the imprecision of our present methods for documenting proximal obstruction. If patency is established, it is our practice to insert about 60 cm (25 in) No. 2-0 nylon suture into the uterus and pass it distally through the fimbriated portion of the tube, over which a two-layer isthmic anastomosis is performed. If obstruction is noted, one may shave portions of the fallopian tube until the intramural portion of the oviduct is encountered. If this is obstructed, one should then proceed with the techniques for cornual uterotubal implantation.

Preparation of the Distal Oviduct

Our results following uterotubal implantation have suggested that the reobstruction rate is lower and the pregnancy rate higher if the ampullary portion of the fallopian tube is implanted into the uterus. Therefore, it has been our practice to sacrifice approximately 2 cm of the isthmic portion of the fallopian tube to provide a wide ampullary lumen for uterotubal implantation.

We use a Teflon ring splint to maintain tubal patency. A small monofilament nylon suture may be placed at the ring for easy extraction at a later date. A No. 28 wire guide within the Teflon splint lends rigidity and serves to prevent expulsion. A fine lacrimal duct probe to which a Teflon ring prosthesis is attached is passed through the fimbriated portion of the oviduct. The probe is then retracted, bringing the prosthesis through the lumen of the tube (Fig. 16–13B). The prosthesis must be carefully selected so that the smallest diameter is used. With an ampullary implantation, this consideration is often moot, since the lumen is quite large. The end of the oviduct to be implanted into the uterus is then split longitudinally for a distance of 0.5 cm (Fig. 16–13C). This is required with an ampullary implantation to minimize the possibility of tearing the anterior and posterior portions of the fallopian tube as each

is sutured to the wall of the uterus. By slightly bivalving the tube, the ends separate easily, avoiding tension. A suture of No. 5-0 nonreactive absorbable suture is then placed through the edge of each end (Fig. 16–13C).

Uterine Incision

A 7-mm reamer (cork borer) is used to create a uterine stoma. When the intramural portion of the fallopian tube is removed, the uterus should be grasped with the left hand so that the thumb stabilizes the posterior wall of the uterus (Fig. 16–13D). The reamer then may be precisely guided toward the uterine cavity while excising the intramural portion of the right tube as a core. A similar procedure is used to create a stoma in the left cornua.

Tubal Implantation

A fine hemostat is inserted through the uterine stoma on the left side and grasps the tip of the Teflon splint, bringing it through the uterine wall and into the uterine cavity so that the ring rests at the midportion of the cavity (Fig. 16–13E). The left oviduct is then prepared for intraluminal placement of the splint (Fig. 16–13F). A grooved needle director over which a Ferguson needle may be guided is introduced into the uterine defect so that the two No. 5-0 nonreactive absorbable sutures in the anterior tubal flap are brought out through the anterior uterine wall and the additional two sutures in the posterior tubal flap are brought out through the posterior uterine wall. These sutures are tied securely as the tube is drawn into the uterine cavity (Fig. 16–13G). The oviductal serosa may be sutured to the adjacent uterine serosa with several interrupted sutures of No. 7-0 nonreactive absorbable suture.

POSTERIOR FUNDAL UTEROTUBAL IMPLANTATION. When the fallopian tubes are shortened to 3 cm to 4 cm, we prefer a posterior fundal uterotubal implantation. The fallopian tube is mobilized to perform a posterior implantation and is prepared in the manner described for a cornual implantation. The posterior fundus is injected with a dilute solution of Pitressin (1:20 saline dilution) (Fig. 16–14A). A posterior fundal incision, approximately 4 cm long, is placed between the utero-ovarian ligaments, thus exposing the posterior uterine cavity (Fig. 16–14B). The ampullary portions of the fallopian tubes are then inserted into the uterine cavity and the nonreactive absorbable No. 5-0 suture is brought out through the uterus, superior and inferior to the transverse incision, and tied securely (Fig. 16–14C). The myometrium between the fallopian tubes is then closed in two layers, the first consisting of interrupted No. 3-0 nonreactive absorbable suture, and

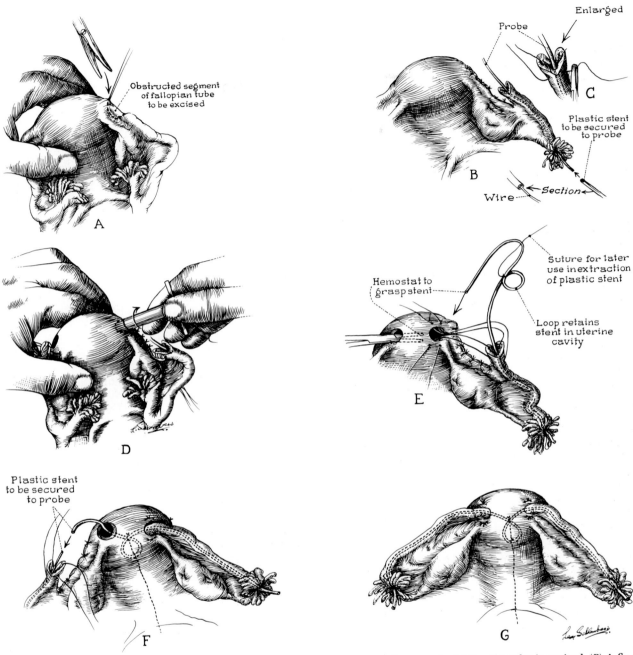

FIG. 16–13 Ampullary-uterotubal implantation. (*A*) The obstructed proximal segment of fallopian tube is excised. (*B*) A fine lacrimal duct probe to which a Teflon ring prosthesis (0.028–0.68 in internal diameter) is attached is placed through the fimbriated portion of the fallopian tube and brought through the lumen of the tube. (*C*) The end of the oviduct to be implanted into the uterus is split longitudinally for a distance of 0.5 cm. A No. 5-0 polyglactin suture is then placed through the edge of each end. (*D*) A 7-mm reamer is used to remove the intramural portion of the fallopian tube. (*E*) A fine hemostat is inserted through the uterine defect on the opposite side and the tip of the Teflon splint is grasped and brought through the uterine cavity. (*F*) The small lacrimal duct probe is then gently inserted into the fimbrial portion of the distal segment of the oviduct on the opposite side. The stent is attached to the probe and pulled through the lumen and the polyglactin sutures are then placed through the longitudinally split oviduct and brought out through the anterior and posterior walls and tied securely. (*G*) The Teflon splint is in place with both ampullary portions of the oviduct implanted into the uterine cavity. (Jones, Rock, 1983)

the second of a serosal approximation using interrupted sutures of No. 6-0 nonreactive absorbable suture (Fig. 16–14D). A peritoneal graft is then taken from the anterior abdominal wall and placed over the incision to minimize adhesion formation (Fig. 16–14E).

POSTOPERATIVE THERAPY

All patients receive prophylactic antibiotics to minimize the possibility of an acute flare of postoperative salpingitis. We have not used steroids or antihistamines postoperatively, although during the procedure the peritoneal cavity is lavaged with copious amounts of lactated Ringer's solution containing 1 gm of hydrocortisone and 5000 units of heparin. The Teflon splint is left in place for 4 months and then removed through the cervix with a Novak curet. A postoperative hysterosalpingogram is performed 2 months after the splint is removed. A second-look laparoscopy is performed if the patient has not conceived within the subsequent 13 ovulatory cycles.

COMPLICATIONS OF UTEROTUBAL IMPLANTATION

The most common complication of tubal implantation is postmenstrual irregular spotting. In most instances this will resolve without therapy and appears to be associated with the presence of the intrauterine Teflon splint. On occasion, however, progesterone therapy may be necessary to prevent this irregular shedding of endometrial tissue. Two patients developed excessive menstrual bleeding that resolved with oral contraceptive therapy while the splint was in place. One patient had a flare of chronic pelvic inflammatory disease 1 week postoperatively and was treated with intravenous antibiotic therapy. This patient conceived approximately 4 months postoperatively and delivered a term infant. Two patients (4%) developed an ectopic pregnancy in the ampullary portion of the fallopian tube. This ectopic pregnancy rate is similar to that reported by Grant and by Wirtz.

There was a rupture of the uterus as a result of the weakening of the uterine wall at the cornua in one of our patients following cornual uterotubal implantation. Thus, we have advised our patients to accept a delivery by cesarean section.

Shirodkar (1960) advocated the use of a pseudopregnancy regimen during the first 4 months following uterotubal implantation. He felt that this prevented endometriosis caused by menstrual blood spilling through the shortened tube. Endometriosis has not been observed as a complication of uterotubal implantation in our series.

FAILURE OF UTEROTUBAL IMPLANTATION

A life-table analysis of pregnancy success following uterotubal implantation reveals that the maximum cumulative rate of pregnancy is achieved approximately 48 months after surgery (Fig. 16–15). A few pregnancies occur after that time. In fact, most of the pregnancies occur within the first 18 months after surgery. Therefore, the strict definition of failure would include the failure to conceive after 48 months provided the patient has had regular ovulatory cycles and an adequate male factor. It has been our recent practice to perform diagnostic laparoscopy after 13 ovulatory cycles if the patient has not conceived. This allows us the opportunity to lyse adhesions and to directly visualize patency with insufflation of indigo carmine dye.

Failure to conceive may be the result of a variety of factors. These may be divided into two categories: postoperative obstruction and technical errors (Table 16–10). Tubal obstruction may occur due to adenomyosis or fibrosis as a result of an inflammatory reaction to the splint. Furthermore, a flare of chronic pelvic inflammatory disease or a postoperative ascending salpingitis may result in subsequent proximal or distal fimbrial obstruction. In our experience with ampullary implantation, obstruction is rare. With the use of prophylactic antibiotics, salpingitis should rarely be observed.

Technical errors may result in failure of uterotubal implantation. If careful hemostasis is not achieved, hematoma formation may result in the expulsion of the implanted tube. Furthermore, if the prosthesis is not placed within the uterine cavity, it may be subsequently expelled into the abdominal cavity, resulting in peritoneal reaction and the formation of adhesions. Proximal oviduct malposition may result if the sutures through the tips of the ampulla are tied so as to bury the tubal osium in the uterine mucosa. Furthermore, if the sutures are brought too close to the midline of the uterus, the oviduct may extend too far into the uterine cavity. More importantly, if microsurgical atraumatic technique is not used, postoperative adhesions may result.

In our most recent series, following uterotubal implantation, all 20 patients had documented tubal patency.

PATHOLOGY

Proximal cornual obstruction may result from an episode of acute salpingitis, or, less often, from salpingitis isthmica nodosa. Intramural occlusion is also observed when sterilization is accomplished by aggressive monopolar electrocautery.

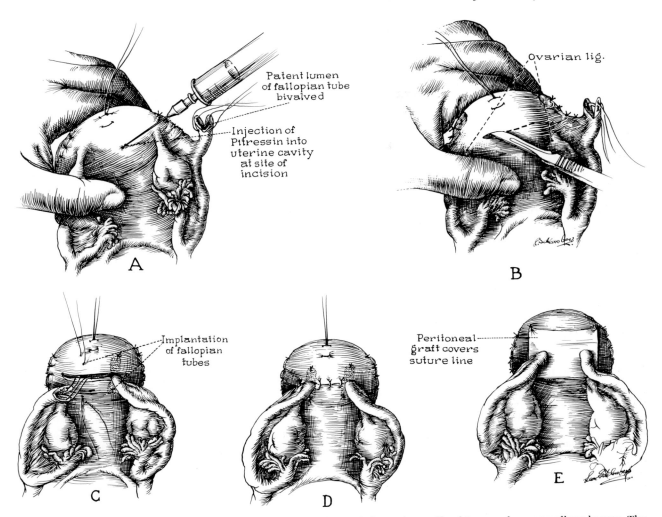

FIG. 16–14 Posterior fundal uterotubal implantation. *(A)* Sufficient isthmus is sacrificed to reveal an ampullary lumen. The tube is then split longitudinally and a suture of No. 5-0 polyglactin suture is placed through the edge of each end. The posterior uterine fundus is then injected with a dilute solution of Pitressin (1:20 saline dilution, or approximately 1 unit per ml). *(B)* A posterior fundal incision exposes the posterior uterine cavity, and the ampullary portions of the fallopian tubes are then inserted into the uterine cavity. *(C)* The polyglactin sutures are brought out above and below the transverse incision and tied securely. *(D)* Myometrium of the uterus is closed in two layers, the first consisting of interrupted No. 3-0 nonreactive absorbable suture, and the second of a serosal approximation. *(E)* A peritoneal graft taken from the anterior abdominal wall may then be placed over the incision to minimize adhesion formation. (Jones, Rock, 1983)

Histologic examination of the excised isthmic or intramural portion of the fallopian tube sometimes fails to confirm the clinical diagnosis of intramural obstruction. Grant reported histologic observations in 67 excised specimens, 87% of which were of inflammatory origin. Mucosal or interstitial involvement was found in 49 of 67 specimens. Grant suggested that obstruction in a number of instances was related to a flap-like block and, in his view, did not represent tubal spasm. Arronet and associates reported 37 specimens from 42 patients who underwent tubal implantation. They indicated that 57% of specimens were of noninflammatory origin; 57% of these patients conceived following uterotubal implantation. Thirty-eight percent of the specimens were inflammatory, and only 13% of these patients conceived postoperatively. Rock and associates reported evidence of chronic salpingitis in 21 patients (40%), five of whom (24%) conceived. Pregnancy success was higher in patients with salpingitis isthmica nodosa or intramural block due to a sterilization procedure. Moore–White reported a pregnancy rate

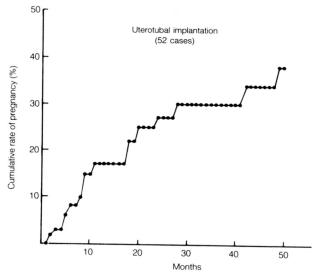

FIG. 16–15 Life-table analysis. Expectancy of pregnancy in 52 patients treated with uterotubal implantation. (Rock JA, Katayama KP, Martin EJ, Rock BM, Woodruff JD, Jones HW, Jr: Pregnancy outcome following uterotubal implantation: A comparison of the reamer and sharp cornual wedge excision technique. Fertil Steril 31:634, 1979. Reproduced with permission from the publisher, the American Fertility Society.)

TABLE 16–10 *Etiology of Failure of Techniques of Uterotubal Implantation*

Postoperative obstruction
    Tubal obstruction due to adenomyosis or fibrosis
    Flare of chronic pelvic inflammatory disease or a postoperative ascending salpingitis with subsequent proximal or distal fimbrial obstruction.

Technical errors
    Hematoma formation with expulsion of the implanted tube.
    Escape of the prosthesis into the peritoneal cavity with subsequent adhesion formation.
    Proximal oviduct malposition so that the lumen is buried in the uterine cavity.
    Lack of microsurgical atraumatic technique.

Adapted from Jones, Rock, 1983.

of 31% among patients with pure cornual obstruction. Thus, patients with chronic pelvic inflammatory disease are less likely to conceive following uterotubal implantation; this may be related to the high incidence of associated pelvic adhesion formation and fimbrial involvement at the time of uterotubal implantation.

RESULTS OF UTEROTUBAL IMPLANTATION

Successful pregnancy following uterotubal implantation is thought to depend upon the operative technique, the extent of adhesion formation, tubal pathology, and pre- and postoperative management. In addition, the postoperative tubo-ovarian relationship and the length of the oviduct may also have a bearing on pregnancy success. Comparison of results is difficult due to the lack of large homogeneous patient groups having the same etiology for proximal obstruction. Furthermore, confusion in comparisons is created by the optional use of different splinting techniques and postoperative therapy regimens. As a result, it is difficult to establish the advantage of a particular technique by a simple comparison of pregnancy success rates.

Results must be stated in terms of the nature and extent of pathologic change. Shirodkar graded the extent of disease and correlated subsequent pregnancy success. He noted pregnancy success to be approximately 40% in patients with occlusion at the cornua extending not beyond the first 2 inches of tube, leaving two-thirds of the tube for implantation. Pregnancy success dropped off markedly once the fimbriated ends of the tube were involved with adhesions. This has also been our experience. The patients with minimal or no peritubular adhesions and without involvement of the fimbriated portion of the fallopian tube were found to have the best chance for pregnancy. Once the fimbriated ends of the fallopian tube were involved or fixation of the adnexal structures was noted, the pregnancy success rate dropped to less than 10% (Table 16–11).

Although postoperative patency rates have been reported in the 70% to 90% range, the term pregnancy rate has been disappointingly low—between 0% and 48% (Tables 16–12 and 16–13). Pregnancy success following uterotubal implantation using the sharp cornual wedge technique and the reamer technique has been difficult to gauge from previous reports because the patient population is not clearly defined in age, race, parity, duration of infertility, and extent of adhesion formation. Furthermore, only two reports take into consideration the segment of fallopian tube implanted into the uterus. Palmer divided his patients into groups, categorized by whether the ampullary or isthmic portion of the fallopian tube was implanted into the uterus; however, splints were not used. Rock similarly divided patients into ampullary and isthmic categories and splints were used. Palmer found that an isthmic implantation was associated with a 4% higher pregnancy rate than an ampullary implantation (Table 16–12), while Rock found that an ampullary im-

TABLE 16–11   *Pregnancy Outcome and Tubal Patency following Uterotubal Implantation*

	PREGNANCY OUTCOME		PATENCY ON HYSTEROGRAM	
EXTENT OF DISEASE	*Number of Patients*	*Patients Pregnant*	*Number of Patients*	*Number with Patent Tubes*
Mild 　Minimal or no peritubular 　adhesions	29	11 (38%)	15	8 (53%)
Moderate 　Substantial peritubular and 　periovarian adhesions without 　fixation.	10	3 (30%)	5	5 (100%)
Severe 　Dense pelvic or adnexal adhesions 　with fixation of ovary.	13	1 (8%)	9	3 (33%)

From Rock et al, 1979.

TABLE 16–12   *Pregnancy Outcome following Uterotubal Implantation (Sharp Cornual Wedge Excision)*

AUTHOR (YEAR)	*NUMBER OF PATIENTS*	*PREGNANCY RATE*	*TERM DELIVERY*	*TECHNIQUE*
Moore-White 　(1951)	4	50%	25%	No splint
Shirodkar (1960)	25	25%	0	Fundal incision splint
Siegler (1969)	12	8%	0	Splint
Young, et al (1970)	11	9%	9%	Ring splint
Horne, et al (1973)	11	64%	46%	Ring splint
Palmer (1977)	118	44%	38%	No splint
Ampullary	93	42%	33%	
Isthmic	25	46%	43%	
Rock, et al (1979a)	26	16%	8%	Ring splint
Ampullary	20	15%	10%	
Isthmic	6	17%	0	

Adapted from Jones, Rock, 1983.

TABLE 16–13   *Pregnancy Outcome following Uterotubal Implantation (Reamer Technique)*

AUTHOR (YEAR)	*NUMBER OF PATIENTS*	*PREGNANCY RATE*	*TERM DELIVERY*	*TECHNIQUE*
Shirodkar (1960)	140	35%	0	Ring splint
Hanton, et al (1964)	22	48%	48%	No splint
Arronet, et al (1969)	37	43%	43%	Ring splint
Grant (1971)	73	34%	26%	Splint (cervical removal)
Williams (1973)	16	38%	25%	Splint
Rock (1981)	35	41%	25%	Ring splint
Ampullary	20	55%	40%	
Isthmic	15	27%	13%	

Adapted from Jones, Rock, 1983.

plantation was associated with a 28% higher pregnancy rate than an isthmic implantation (Table 16–13).

Since the report of improved pregnancy success following uterotubal implantation of the ampullary portion of the fallopian tube using the reamer technique, this technique has been used exclusively at the Johns Hopkins Hospital. Of the 20 patients so treated, 11 conceived, with term pregnancies resulting in 8 (Table 16–13). Pregnancy success following uterotubal implantation was noted to be higher in patients in whom obstruction was due to salpingitis isthmica nodosa than in those in whom intramural obstruction resulted from previous electrocauterization. Of note is the observation that the single ectopic pregnancy that occurred in a patient with intramural block was a result of chronic salpingitis. With careful patient selection, the accumulation of a large patient group may demonstrate the efficacy of the reamer technique of ampullary uterotubal implantation.

Recently, Von Csaba and associates and Peterson and associates have reported uterotubal implantation through a posterior uterofundal incision between the utero-ovarian ligaments. Von Csaba and associates reported that three of nine patients with a proximal obstruction due to pelvic inflammatory disease conceived, for a pregnancy rate of 33%. Peterson and associates reported a 50% pregnancy rate and a 77% tubal patency rate in 16 patients with obstruction after previous sterilization. We have found this posterior fundal technique particularly useful in patients with excessively shortened fallopian tubes as a consequence of vigorous electrocauterization for sterilization. The tube may be easily implanted into the posterior uterus without distorting the tubo-ovarian relationships.

Over the past decade there has been a decline in the number of uterotubal implantations performed in our institution. Diamond, in a comparison of macro- and microsurgical techniques for the repair of cornual occlusion in infertility, demonstrated that the term pregnancy rate was 4.7 times greater when microsurgery was used for anastomosing the transected ampulla or isthmus to the intramural portion of the tube. With the development of these microsurgical techniques, uterotubal implantation may be reserved for patients with intramural obstruction.

ESTES PROCEDURE

The Estes procedure is included for its historical interest only. The initial attempts to restore fertility after salpingectomy were made by Tuffier in Paris. He attempted to implant the ovary in the uterine cavity, but few pregnancies resulted from this procedure and almost all of them ended in spontaneous abortion. Occasionally, the uterus gave birth to the implanted ovary, which required surgical removal. This procedure has been almost universally abandoned, although Ghosal in India reported one case of a patient who had five pregnancies after utero-ovarian implantation. There have been no successful reports in the American literature during the past quarter of a century.

Estes reported the procedure in 1909 and later with Heitmeyer reported 4 of 50 cases (8%) who became pregnant, 2 going to term. Von Graff reported 3 pregnancies (2.5%) for ovarian transplants of all types. The major risk of a pregnancy following an Estes implantation of the ovary into the cornu of the uterus is not only of spontaneous abortion. A ruptured uterus may also occur should the patient be successful in implanting a fertilized ovum that happened to ovulate into the endometrial cavity. In view of the poor success with this procedure and the added obstetric risks that it imposes, it is our opinion that this procedure should be dropped from the armamentarium of gynecologic surgery.

Conclusions

Refined technique and the use of magnification will improve pregnancy success by reducing postoperative adhesion formation. Microsurgery, however, should not appear as a panacea for tubes with significant pathology. Although a reproductive surgeon can established patency and minimize adhesion formation, this may be of no value in the oviduct where the mucosa has been severely damaged. Over the next several years, such factors as deciliation, endometriosis, and the presence of polyps may be valuable prognostic indicators of subsequent pregnancy success. Furthermore, basic research in tubal mobility and the tubal hormonal milieu may clarify why tubal patency and pregnancy rates are significantly disparate. Finally, *in vitro* fertilization is a major therapeutic success that will afford hope to women with severe tubal damage that is not treatable by contemporary microsurgical techniques.

Bibliography

Acland RD: Microsurgery Practice Manual: Louisville, Kentucky, University of Louisville Microsurgery Laboratory, Price Institute of Surgical Research, 1977

Adhesion Study Group: Reduction of postoperative pelvic adhesions with intraperitoneal 32% dextran 70: A prospective randomized clinical trial. Fertil Steril 40:612, 1983

Altemus R, Charles D, Yoder VE: Conventional hysterosal-pingography used in the evaluation of sterility problems. Fertil Steril 18:713, 1967

Arronet GJ, Eduljee SY, O'Brien JR: A nine-year survey of fallopian tube dysfunction in human infertility: Diagnosis and therapy. Fertil Steril 20:903, 1969

Bonney V: The fruits of conservationism. J Obstet Gynecol Br Commonw 44:1, 1937

Boyd IE, Holt EM: Tubal sterility: Patency tests and results of operation. J Obstet Gynaecol Br Comm 80:142, 1973

Buncke HJ, Chater NL, Zoltans S: Manual of Microvascular Surgery. San Francisco, R. K. Davies Medical Center, Microsurgical Unit, Davis & Geck distributor, 1975

Cary WH: Note on determination of patency of the fallopian tubes by the use of collargol and x-ray shadow. Am J Obstet Gynecol 69:426, 1914

Crane M, Woodruff JD: Factors influencing the success of tuboplastic procedures. Fertil Steril 19:810, 1968

Cullen TS: A normal pregnancy following insertion of the outer half of a fallopian tube into the uterine cornu. Bull Johns Hopkins Hosp 33:344, 1922

Diamond E: A comparison of gross and microsurgical techniques for repair of cornual occlusion in infertility: A retrospective study, 1968–1978. Fertil Steril 32:370, 1979

Donnez Casanas–Roux F, Ferin J: Macroscopic and microscopic studies of fallopian tubes after laparoscopic sterilization. Contraception 20:498, 1979

Donnez J, Wauters M, Thomas K: Luteal function after tubal sterilization. Obstet Gynecol 57:65, 1981

Elliott GB, Brody H, Elliot KA: Implications of "lipoid salpingitis." Fertil Steril 16:541, 1965

Estes WL: A method of implanting ovarian tissue in order to maintain ovarian function. Penn Med J 13:610, 1909

Estes WL, Jr, Heitmeyer PL: Pregnancy following ovarian implantation. Am J Surg 24:563, 1934

Fjalbrant B: Tubal surgery. Acta Obstet Gynecol Scand 54:463, 1975

Garcia CR, Aller J: Surgical approach to tubal disease. Clin Obstet Gynecol 17:102, 1974

Ghosal KK: Ovarian function after Estes operation. J Obstet Gynecol India 16:540, 1966

Gomel V: Tubal reanastamosis by microsurgery. Fertil Steril 28:59, 1977

———: Salpingostomy by laparoscopy. J Reprod Med 18:265, 1977

———: Tubal reanastomosis by microsurgery. Fertil Steril 28:59, 1977

———: Classification of operations for tubal and peritoneal factors causing infertility. Clin Obstet Gynecol 23:1259, 1980

———: Microsurgical reversal of female sterilization: A reappraisal. Fertil Steril 33:587, 1980

———: Salpingo-ovariolysis by laparoscopy in infertility. Fertil Steril 40:607, 1983

Grant A: Infertility surgery of the oviduct. Fertil Steril 22:496, 1971

Grunert GM, Drake TS, Takaki NK: Microsurgical reanastomosis of the fallopian tubes for reversal of sterilization. Obstet Gynecol 58:148, 1981

Hafez ESE, Blandau, RJ: The Mammalian Oviduct. Chicago, University of Chicago Press, 1969

Hafez ESE, Evans TN: Human Reproduction, Conception and Contraception. Hagerstown, Harper & Row, 1973

Hanton EM, Pratt JH, Banner EA: Tubal plastic surgery at the Mayo Clinic. Am J Obstet Gynecol 89:934, 1964

Hoerenz P: Magnification: Loupes and the operating microscope. Clin Obstet Gynecol 23:1151, 1980

Holden FC, Sovak FW: Reconstruction of the oviducts: An improved technic with report of cases. Am J Obstet Gynecol 24:684, 1932

Horne HW, Jr, et al: The prevention of postoperative pelvic adhesions following conservative operative treatment for human infertility: a final 3-year follow-up report. Int J Fertil 18:190, 1973

Hutchins CJ: Laparoscopy and hysterosalpingography in the assessment of tubal patency. Obstet Gynecol 49:325, 1977

Jansen RPS: Surgery-pregnancy time intervals after salpingolysis, unilateral salpingostomy, and bilateral salpingostomy. Fertil Steril 34:222, 1980

Jessen H: Forty-five operations for sterility. Obstet Gynecol Surv 27:227, 1972

Jones HW, Jr, Rock JA: On the reanastomosis of fallopian tubes after surgical sterilization. Fertil Steril 29:702, 1978

Jones HW, Jr, Rock JA: Reparative and Constructive Surgery of the Female Generative Tract. Baltimore, Maryland, Williams and Wilkins, 1983

Keirse MJ, Vandervellen R: A comparison of hysterosalpingography and laparoscopy in the investigation of infertility. Obstet Gynecol 41:685, 1973

Kistner RW, Patton GW: Atlas of Infertility Surgery. Boston, Little, Brown, 1975

Lamb EJ, Moscovitz W: Tuboplasty for infertility. Int J Fertil 17:53, 1972

Maathuis JB, Horback JGM, Van Hall EV: A comparison of the results of hysterosalpingography and laparoscopy in the diagnosis of tube dysfunction. Fertil Steril 23:428, 1972

Meldrum D: Microsurgical tubal reanastomosis: The role of splints. Obstet Gynecol 57:613, 1981

Molumsky A: The prenatal diagnosis of hereditary diseases. Springfield, Charles C Thomas, 1973

Moore–White M: Evaluation of tubal plastic operations: Classifications of tubal disease. Int J Fertil 5:237, 1960

Mulligan WJ: Results of salpingostomy. Int J Fertil 11:424, 1966

Musick JR, Behrman, SJ: Surgical management of tubal obstruction at the uterotubal junction. Fertil Steril 40:423, 1983

O'Brien JR, Arronet GH, Eduljee SY: Operative treatment of fallopian tube pathology in human fertility. Am J Obstet Gynecol 103:520, 1969

Palmer R: Presented to the Ad Hoc Committee on Tubal Surgery Thirty-Third Annual Mtg of the American Fertility Society, Miami, 1977

Patterson P: Reversal of sterilization. Population Reports, Population, Information, Program. Vol. 8, No. 5, 1980

Peel J: Utero-tubal implantation. Proc R Soc Med 57:710, 1964

Peterson EP, Musich JR, Behrman SJ: Uterotubal implantation and obstetrics outcome after previous sterilization. Am J Obstet Gynecol 128:662, 1977

Petrucco OM, Winston RML: Presented at Tenth World Congress of Fertility and Sterility, Madrid, Spain. July 7–12, 1980

Population Reports: Reversing female sterilization, Series C, No. 8, September, 1980

Radwanska E, Berger GS, Hammond J: Luteal deficiency among women with normal menstrual cycles requesting reversal of tubal sterilization. Obstet Gynecol 54:189, 1979

Rock JA, Chang YS, Limpaphayom K, et al: Microsurgical tubal anastomosis: A controlled trial in four Asian centers. Microsurg 5:95, 1984

Rock JA: Uterotubal implantation. In Lauersen N, David S (ed): Microsurgical Techniques in Infertility. New York, Plenum Press, 1982

Rock JA, Bergquist CA, Kimball AW, Jr, et al: Comparison of

the operating microscope and loupe for microsurgical tubal anastomosis: A randomized clinical trial. Fertil Steril 41:229, 1984

Rock JA, Katayama KP, Martin EJ, et al: Factors influencing the success of salpingostomy techniques for distal fimbrial obstruction. Obstet Gynecol 52:591, 1978

Rock JA, Katayama KP, Jones HW, Jr: Tubal reanastomosis: A comparison of Hellman's approach without magnification and a microsurgical technique. In Phillips JM (ed): Microsurgery in Gynecology. Los Angeles, American Association of Gynecologic Laparoscopists, 1981

Rock JA, Katayama PK, Martin EJ, et al: Pregnancy outcome following uterotubal implantation: A comparison of the reamer and sharp cornual wedge excision techniques. Fertil Steril 31:634, 1979

Rock JA, Parmley TH, King TM, et al: Endometriosis and the development of tuboperitoneal fistulas after tubal ligation. Fertil Steril 35:16, 1981

Rock JA, Siegler AM, Meisal MB, et al: The efficacy of postoperative hydrotubation: A randomized prospective multicenter clinical trial. Fertil Steril 42:393, 1984

Roe RE, Laros RK, Jr, Work BA: Female Sterilization: I. The vaginal approach. Am J Obstet Gynecol 112:1031, 1972

Rosenberg SM, Board JA: High molecular weight dextran in human infertility surgery. Am J Obstet Gynecol 148:380, 1984

Rubin IC: Roentgendiagnostik der Uterus Tumorens mit Hilfe von Intrauterine Collargol Injectionen Vorlaeufige Mitteilung. Zentralbl Gynaekol. 38:658, 1914

Rubin IC: Non-operative determination of patency of fallopian tubes in sterility: Intrauterine inflation with oxygen and production of a subphrenic pneumoperitoneum: Preliminary report. JAMA 74:1017, 1920

Rubin IC: Retention of Lipiodol in fallopian tubes with special reference to occlusive effect in cases of permeable strictures. NY J Med 36:1089, 1936

Rubin IC: Therapeutic aspects of uterotubal insufflation in sterility. Am J Obstet Gynecol 50:621, 1945

Rutherford RN: The therapeutic value of repetitive lipiodol tubal insufflations. Western J Surg 54:145, 1948

Schroder C: Die Excision von Ovarientumoren mit Erhaltung des Ovarium. Zentralbl Gynak 8:716, 1884

Seiler JC: Factors influencing the outcome of microsurgical tubal ligation reversals. Am J Obstet Gynecol 146:292, 1983

Shirodkar VN: Contributions to Obstetrics and Gynecology. Edinburgh, E & S Livingston, 1960

Shirodkar VN: Further experiences in tuboplasty. Aust NZ J Obstet Gynecol 5:1, 1965

Shirodkar VN: Factors influencing the results of salpingostomy. Int J Fertil 2:361, 1966

Siegler AM: Salpingoplasty: Classification and report of 115 operations. Obstet Gynecol 34:339, 1969

Siegler AM (ed.): Hysterosalpingography, 2nd ed. New York, Medcom Press, 1974

Siegler AM, Perez RJ: Reconstruction of fallopian tubes in previously sterilized patients. Fertil Steril 26:383, 1975

Siegler AM: Tubal surgery for infertility. In Sciarra JJ (ed): Gynecology and Obstetrics. Hagerstown, Harper & Row, 1975

Stangel J, Settles H, Reyniak J, et al: Microsurgical anastomosis of the rabbit oviduct using 9-0 monofilament polyglycolic acid suture. Fertil Steril 30:210, 1978

Sweeney WJ III, Gepfert R: The fallopian tube. Clin Obstet Gynecol 8:32, 1965

Swolin K: 50 Fertilitatsoperationen: Literatur und Methodik. Acta Obstet Gynecol Scand 46:234, 1967

Swolin K: Die einwirkung grossen intraperitonealen dosen glukokortikoidauf diebildungvon-postoperativen adhasionen. Acta Obstet Gynecol Scand 46:119, 1967

Swolin K: Fertiltratsoperatronen, Teil I and II. Acta Obstet Gynecol Scand 46:204, 1967

Tuffier T, Letulle M: Transposition de l'ovaire avec son pedicule vasculair dans canite de l'uterus apres ablation des trompes uterine pour annexites. Bull Acad Nat Med Paris, 3(S)91:362, 1924

Umezaki C, Katayama KP, Jones HW, Jr: Pregnancy rates after reconstructive surgery on the fallopian tubes. Obstet Gynecol 43:418, 1974

Vasquez G, Winston RML, Boeckx W, et al: Tubal lesions subsequent to sterilization and their relation to fertility after attempts at reversal. Am J Obstet Gynecol 138:86, 1980

Von Csaba I, Keller G, Magy P, et al: Chirurgische Behandbing der Weiblichen Steriletat Tubenimplantation. Zentralbl Gynaekol 96:490, 1974

VonGraff E: Operative treatment of female sterility. J Iowa Med Soc 26:31, 1936

Williams GFJ: Fallopian tube surgery for reversal of sterilization. Br Med J 1:599, 1973

———: Microsurgical reanastomosis of the rabbit oviduct in its functional and pathological sequelae. Br J Obstet Gynecol 2:513, 1975

———: Microsurgical tubocornual anastomosis for reversal of sterilization. Lancet 1:284, 1977

———: Reversal of sterilization. Clin Obstet Gynecol 23:1261, 1980

———: Microsurgery and the fallopian tube: From fantasy to reality. Fertil Steril 34:521, 1981

Winston RML, Magara RA: Techniques for the improvement of microsurgical tubal anastomosis. In Microsurgery in Female Infertility. Second Clinical Colloquia on Reproduction. New York, Grune & Stratton, 1980

Wirtz JW: Experience with a method for implantation of the fallopian tubes into the uterus. Aust NZ J Obstet Gynaecol 5:7, 1965

Woodruff JD, Pauerstein CJ: The Fallopian Tube. Baltimore, Williams and Wilkins, 1969

Young PE, Egan JE, Barlow JA, et al: Reconstructive surgery for infertility at the Boston Hospital for Women. Am J Obstet Gynecol 108:1092, 1970

Chapter 17

Laparoscopy and Tubal Sterilization

Clifford R. Wheeless, M.D., and
K. Paul Katayama, M.D., Ph.D.

Laparoscopy

The first description of an instrument for visualizing the inside of the urinary bladder is generally attributed to Philip Bozzini of Frankfurt. The year was 1805, and the instrument was called a *Lichtleiter*. Not until 1929, however, was the branch of endoscopy now known as laparoscopy developed into an effective diagnostic and surgical procedure, principally by Kalk. Although laparoscopy enjoyed some success in Europe, American surgeons found the existing equipment to be inadequate and had little enthusiasm for the technique. In fact, laparoscopy was scarcely used in the United States between 1935 and 1950.

The foundation for the rebirth and modernization of laparoscopy had been well laid. Palmer, Fourestier, Gladu and Valmiere developed its techniques and the fiberoptic system of endoscopic illumination. Steptoe was doing pioneering work in England. But it took the recognition that a rapidly expanding population would soon demand a safe, simple, effective, and inexpensive method for female sterilization to revive the American medical community's interest in laparoscopy in the 1950s.

At the same time, Europeans were also looking to laparoscopy with renewed interest. They saw it as principally useful for diagnosis and for such surgical procedures as ovarian biopsy.

EQUIPMENT FOR LAPAROSCOPY

The lenses and prisms of the modern laparoscope are arranged so that the image of the field at the abdominal end of the instrument is correctly oriented when viewed through the eyepieces (Fig. 17-1A). The objective can be visualized at angles ranging from 90 to 180 degrees (Fig. 17-1B). Angles of 130 to 180 degrees are most commonly used. The actual field of view of most optic systems encompasses an angle of about 60 degrees (Fig. 17-1B). Operating procedures may be accomplished through the laparoscope by offsetting the eyepiece from the main shaft. Specially designed instruments can be passed through a small channel in the shaft. Using this system, only a single incision is necessary (Fig. 17-2). Others use a laparoscope with the eyepiece and optic system centered in the shaft and a separate, small, suprapubic incision for the manipulating probe or other instruments.

Lighting

Fiberoptic light systems have replaced the original incandescent light bulb at the end of the endoscope. A bright, 150-watt, projector-type lamp is housed in a special external device. The beam from this lamp enters the end of a cable composed of a large number of flexible glass fibers, each coated with a layer of glass having a lower index of refraction than the central fiber (Fig. 17-3). The light entering each fiber travels by multiple total reflections from the coating layer, emerging essentially undimmed at the other end of the cable.

Gas Insufflation Apparatus

A special gas insufflation apparatus is used to produce controlled pneumoperitoneum of appropriate pressure and volume. Carbon dioxide passes through a needle piercing the abdominal wall. There are two varieties of pneumoperitoneal nee-

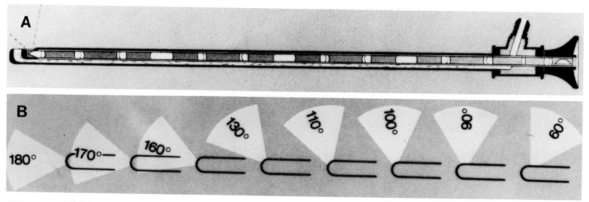

FIG. 17–1 (*A*) Diagram of the laparoscope's lens system. (*B*) Diagram of the angles of visualization obtainable with different laparoscopes. Field of view is always about 60 degress. (Courtesy of Richard Wolff Medical Instruments Corp, Rosemont, Illinois.)

dle: the Verres needle, specially designed to reduce the chance of accidental puncture of the gastrointestinal tract, and the Touey epidural anesthesia needle, readily available, inexpensive and as effective as the Verres needle. For safety, the gas flow proceeds from a large gas supply into a small gas bottle of 5 to 10 liters capacity and then through a series of gauges that monitor its flow into the patient. Pressure in the gas line to the needle is measured constantly.

Trocar

The trocar that punctures the abdominal wall and the trocar sleeve through which the laparoscope is inserted into the peritoneal cavity come in two basic models. The flapper-valve model (Fig. 17–4A) allows laparoscopic and other instruments to be inserted into or withdrawn from the abdominal cavity without escape of gas. The traditional model has a trumpet valve (Fig. 17–4B). The trocar is made of steel and has a pyramid-shaped point.

STERILIZATION OF LAPAROSCOPY INSTRUMENTS

Most endoscopic clinics throughout the world sterilize laparoscopy instruments in antiseptic solutions. The most effective solution for soaking is a combination of 10% formaldehyde and dialdehyde (Cidex). The instruments should be soaked for at least 10 minutes in the solution. Gas sterilization is also acceptable, but instruments must be ventilated for 24 hours following gas sterilization before they may be used. Steam sterilization should not be used on the laparoscope or fiberoptic cable, as it will damage the lens system and shorten the effective life of the fiberoptic cable.

INDICATIONS FOR LAPAROSCOPY

Laparoscopy offers the gynecologist the means for elucidating many undiagnosed intra-abdominal conditions without resorting to laparotomy and for carrying out many minor intra-abdominal surgical procedures. For the following discussion, the indications are divided into the categories of diagnostic laparoscopy and surgical laparoscopy.

Diagnostic Laparoscopy

Diagnostic laparoscopy is indicated where there are insufficient findings by palpation to justify laparotomy, yet the patient's symptoms and signs demand that intra-abdominal organic disease be identified or ruled out. The most common indication is infertility. In the course of determining the cause of infertility, it is often highly desirable to visualize the pelvic organs. Formerly, culdoscopy was used most frequently for this diagnostic procedure, but laparoscopy has rapidly assumed the leading role.

Endocrinologic problems, whether associated with infertility or not, are another diagnostic indication. For example, Stein–Leventhal ovaries can be visualized, measured, and biopsied when indicated. In rare instances, anomalies of müllerian or wolffian ducts may require visualization for elucidation of the specific anatomical defect. Especially when access to modern genetic and endocrinologic laboratories is not available, laparoscopy may be valuable.

The pelvic pain syndrome constitutes an important indication for diagnostic laparoscopy. The differentiation of acute pelvic inflammatory disease from acute appendicitis may avoid unnecessary laparotomy. Laparoscopy may resolve the suspicion

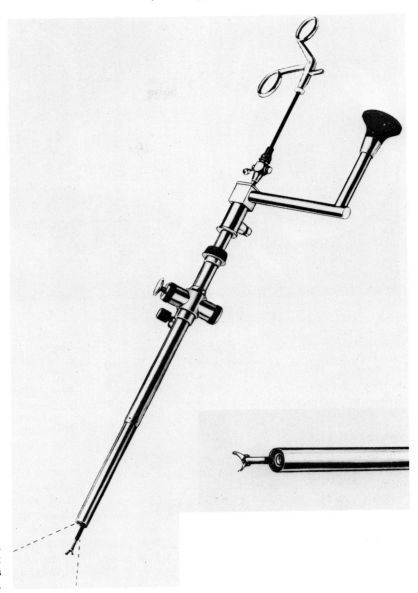

FIG. 17-2 Operating laparoscope with grasping forceps in place. Such an instrument allows intervention with rigid instruments without the necessity for a second puncture.

of an unruptured ectopic pregnancy. Laparoscopy may be helpful in confirming the suspected perforation of a uterus during dilatation and curettage or an intrauterine radium application. The perforation site can be observed, and if hemorrhage is not a significant factor, laparotomy may be avoided. Equally important, the therapeutic procedure in progress can be completed without delay. The laparoscope allows the surgeon to visualize the withdrawal of the radium applicator or the suction curette until it is no longer extrauterine; then the abortion or the radium application may often be completed safely without further damage, especially to the gastrointestinal tract.

Surgical Laparoscopy

Surgical laparoscopy is suitable for various minor intra-abdominal operative procedures. The most common is tubal sterilization. In most cases, tubal sterilization can be performed as an outpatient procedure, using local anesthesia.

Biopsy of pelvic abnormalities can sometimes be accomplished through the laparoscope. Small implants of recurrent carcinoma in the pelvis can be

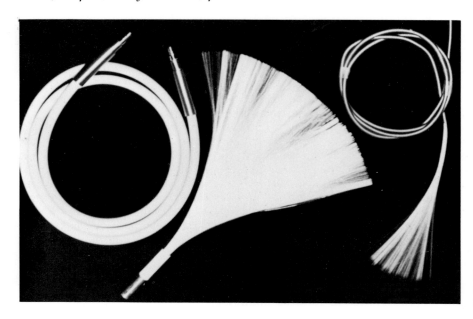

FIG. 17-3 The fiberoptic light-carrying cable with its glass fibers spread out.

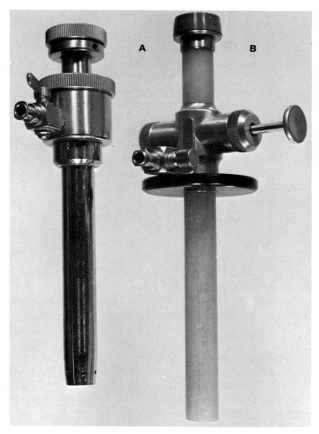

FIG. 17-4 (*A*) Trocar sleeve with flapper valve. (*B*) Trocar sleeve with trumpet valve.

biopsied easily, and ovaries have been biopsied successfully for various conditions. However, biopsy can be followed by significant morbidity, and mature judgment should be used to avoid its indiscriminate use.

In cases of infertility or chronic pelvic pain, laparoscopy permits lysis of adhesions around the tubes and ovaries. Laparoscopy also permits fulguration of endometrial implants in the pelvis. However, this should be done cautiously, using experience and good judgment, especially if the implants are on easily damaged structures such as bowel, major pelvic vessels, bladder or ureters.

Removal of a foreign body, such as an IUD that has migrated from the uterine cavity to the peritoneal cavity, can be accomplished at laparoscopy. Finally, ovum aspiration for *in vitro* fertilization is carried out with the aid of a laparoscope.

Contraindications to Laparoscopy

In the 1950s the list of contraindications to laparoscopy was lengthy. However, with improvements in equipment and experience, fewer conditions are seen as increasing the risks associated with laparoscopy, and fewer still as absolute contraindications.

Both absolute and relative contraindications to laparoscopy are associated with one of the four principal steps, namely: the creation of the pneumoperitoneum, the insertion of the trocar and sleeve, the viewing of the abdominal contents, and the performance of intra-abdominal surgical procedures. When such obvious pelvic abnormalities as large uterine masses or large ovarian tumors are present, laparoscopy prior to laparotomy is not necessary, although it is occasionally useful in differentiating an asymptomatic pedunculated fibroid from an ovarian tumor. It should be noted that most reported complications derive not from conditions that increase the risks of laparoscopy, but from inadequate training of the operating surgeons.

There are few contraindications to insertion of the pneumoperitoneum needle. However, increased intra-abdominal pressure and reabsorption of gas from the extensive surface area of the peritoneal cavity can exacerbate certain conditions. Patients with cardiorespiratory conditions are considered to be at increased risk. So are patients with hiatus hernias, which may be affected by elevation of the diaphragm under increased intra-abdominal pressure. These conditions are now considered relative contraindications. Currently, laparoscopy is performed on patients with cyanotic heart disease and severe rheumatic valvular disease. The only modification to normal procedure is the use of strict cardiac monitoring. Local anesthesia is usually used in these cases.

The hazard of inadvertently damaging the gastrointestinal tract while inserting the trocar and sleeve is increased where there is an intestinal obstruction, a history of prior abdominal surgery (especially of the bowel), or pelvic tuberculosis.

Although inserting the trocar is riskier where there are known or suspected adhesions between the abdominal wall and the intra-abdominal viscera, the risk is relative and not absolute. Nearly 18% of 6000 patients who had laparoscopic sterilization at Johns Hopkins had previous pelvic surgery.

In widespread intra-abdominal carcinomatosis, the omentum and intestines frequently adhere to the anterior abdominal wall. The increased risk is similar to that in patients with prior abdominal surgery. But in patients with advanced pelvic cancer, laparoscopy often provides incomplete information, and exploratory laparotomy is preferable. Acute peritonitis is no longer thought to be an absolute contraindication. Moreover, studies from Scandinavia as well as the experience at Johns Hopkins suggest that, in certain cases, peritonitis may actually be an indication for this diagnostic procedure.

Laparoscopy is contraindicated when it will be impossible to visualize the abdominal contents even after safe insertion of the laparoscope. The most frequent condition rendering visualization impossible is a ruptured ectopic pregnancy with massive hematoperitoneum. However, laparoscopy can be valuable in cases of suspected unruptured ectopic pregnancy. Severe pelvic inflammatory disease is another common condition that makes visualization of abdominal contents difficult. The pelvis may be totally obliterated by tubo-ovarian adhesions, and, depending on the extent of the disease, these patients may be better explored by laparotomy.

Contraindication and increased risks for laparoscopic intra-abdominal surgical procedures are essentially the same as those for intra-abdominal visualization. The absolute contraindications to laparoscopy are limited, therefore, to the following: intestinal obstruction, widespread intra-abdominal carcinomatosis, acute untreated pelvic tuberculosis, and ruptured ectopic pregnancy with massive hemorrhage. In addition, laparoscopy should not be done solely for sterilization when there is obvious extensive pelvic inflammatory disease or a history of extensive intra-abdominal gastrointestinal surgery.

ANESTHESIA FOR LAPAROSCOPY

Thus far, no single method of anesthesia has been proven superior in safety or more effective for ease of performing laparoscopy. Laparoscopy can be performed under sedation plus local anesthesia, under general anesthesia, or under regional anesthesia. In general, the choice of anesthetic will be influenced most by the surgeon's and anesthetist's experience and preferences. Occasionally, strong preferences of the patient may play a role.

Local anesthesia together with mild sedation can be quite satisfactory. The patient is placed on the operating table, without having received prior medication, and 50 mg meperidine (Demerol) plus 10 mg diazepam (Valium) are given intravenously. After the patient has been prepared and draped, a semicircle of skin around the inferior rim of the umbilicus is infiltrated with a 1% lidocaine solution. Laparoscopic sterilization using a local anesthesia has an equal or lower incidence of reported complications than laparoscopic sterilization with general anesthesia and avoids the known complications of the latter.

TECHNIQUES OF LAPAROSCOPY

Preparation of the Patient

The patient must be prepared meticulously for laparoscopy. She must have a complete gynecologic and obstetrical history and physical examination. Minimum laboratory studies should include a hematocrit and hemoglobin determination and a urinalysis. A negative Papanicolaou smear is a prerequisite for patients who desire laparoscopic sterilization.

A decision on whether to perform the operation as an outpatient or inpatient procedure must be reached. The experience at Johns Hopkins with various minor gynecologic outpatient procedures in over 150,000 patients since 1942 indicates that outpatient surgery under general anesthesia is safe if certain criteria are met. For laparoscopy, the patient should be less than 50 years of age and free of any significant medical or surgical disease. She should live within a reasonable travel distance of the hospital and she should not be allowed to travel home alone. Both outpatients and inpatients are told to take nothing by mouth after midnight of the day before surgery. No other special preparation is required.

Positioning of the Patient

A standard operating table equipped with gynecologic stirrups is used. The small Sheppard hook stirrups are ideal for laparoscopy because they can be put in a 45-degree rather than a 90-degree flexion position. The large lithotomy stirrups found in most operating rooms are poorly suited to laparoscopy because there is little support for the patient's legs in the modified lithotomy position. Obstetrical stirrups, with support of the legs at the popliteal fossa, are a good substitute for the Sheppard hook stirrups.

The patient is placed in a modified lithotomy position with the legs at a 45-degree angle to the axis of the table. If the legs are brought to a 90-degree angle the knees encroach upon the surgeon's operating field; moreover, the patient is less comfortable. In positioning the patient for laparoscopy, it is most important to be certain that her buttocks extend just over the edge of the operating table. Inattention to this point accounts for much of the difficulty that laparoscopists encounter in fully visualizing the pelvic organs. If the buttocks are not over the edge of the table, the Rubin's cannula and Jacob's tenaculum cannot be completely depressed on the cervix to move the uterus to the extended, anteflexed position that exposes the entire uterus, the fallopian tubes, the ovaries, and the cul-de-sac to full view. The operating table is tilted to approximately 15 degrees of Trendelenburg's position; this helps the pneumoperitoneum to displace the intestines out of the pelvis.

Surgical Preparation and Draping

Laparoscopy cannot be regarded as a totally sterile procedure, but good aseptic technique should be maintained, keeping the procedure as bacteria-free as possible. In the 9000 surgical laparoscopies performed at Johns Hopkins from 1968 to 1976, only 7 major pelvic infections were associated with laparoscopic sterilization, an incidence of 0.08%.

With the patient properly positioned on the table, bimanual examination and vaginal cleansing are performed. There is no need to shave the vulva. The abdominal wall is scrubbed with povidone-iodine and painted with antiseptic solution, with special attention directed to the umbilicus. The sterile sheet used for draping is one that is fenestrated in the midline to allow a surgical approach to the umbilicus and at the same time, permit the laparoscopist to manipulate the Jacob's tenaculum and Rubin's cannula protruding from the vagina. Before the procedure is started, the patient's bladder should be emptied by a catheter.

Insertion of the Needle

After bimanual examination, preparation, and draping, the operation of laparoscopy proceeds as follows. A vaginal retractor is inserted and the anterior lip of the cervix is grasped with a Jacob's tenaculum. A Rubin's cannula is inserted into the uterine cavity and is attached to the Jacob's tenaculum. The surgeon then moves to the side of the patient and anesthetizes the inferior rim of the umbilicus (if local anesthesia has been chosen). Two towel clips are placed on the inferior rim at 5 o'clock and 7 o'clock, and a 2 mm skin incision is made in the lower margin of the umbilicus.

For the pneumoperitoneum, a large-bore epidural-type needle with a slight curve at the point (Touey needle) or Verres needle is used. The Touey needle gives a more accurate measurement of the intra-abdominal gas pressure. The needle is inserted through the incision and passes down to the fascia. Then, counter-traction is applied by means of towel clips and a quick, short push plunges the needle through the abdominal fascia and peritoneum, and into the peritoneal cavity. The needle should be directed toward the center of the uterus. If it is directed vertically toward the spine, the aorta may be lacerated. In an obese patient, it is occasionally difficult to place the needle correctly. When this occurs, a needle can be passed into the peritoneal cavity through the posterior cul-de-sac, just as in culdocentesis.

There are three classic tests to ascertain whether the needle has been properly placed.

THE SYRINGE TEST. Saline solution is injected and then aspirated by means of a 30 ml syringe attached to the needle. If the solution returns to the syringe, the point of the needle is extra-peritoneal.

THE NEEDLE TEST. A few drops of saline solution are applied to the hub of the needle. When the towel clips lift the margins of the umbilicus, the drops will disappear into the needle (because of negative intra-abdominal pressure) if the needle point is in the peritoneal cavity.

OBSERVATION OF GAS PRESSURE. The most accurate method for determining proper placement of the needle is observation of the gas pressure registered by the pneumoperitoneum apparatus. With a spinal needle of about No. 17 gauge, as the needle enters the peritoneal cavity, the pressure will be approximately 10 mm Hg. If the pressure through the large-bore needle is above 15 mm Hg, something is obstructing the flow of gas (e.g., a kink in the gas tubing or an intrinsic obstruction in the pneumoperitoneum needle) or the point of the needle is in an improper space such as the omentum, bowel, or subfascial space. If an elevated pressure is observed, the flow of gas should be stopped at once, and the needle should be reinserted. Proper placement of the needle must be accomplished before gas flow can continue.

Formerly it was customary to use 3 to 4 liters of gas for the pneumoperitoneum, but under local anesthesia the patient develops discomfort or pain after about 2 liters. This amount has proven to be ample, and more need not be used no matter what the anesthesia.

Insertion of the Trocar

With the pneumoperitoneum established, the needle is withdrawn, and the umbilical incision is enlarged from 2 mm to 1 cm. The towel clips are lifted with one hand and the laparoscopic trocar and sleeve are inserted through the incision with a twisting motion. The trocar is inserted as far as the rectus fascia. The trocar and sleeve are then angled to point slightly toward the pelvis and a short, quick, stabbing motion is used to penetrate the rectus fascia and the peritoneum all at once.

Occasionally great resistance is encountered against the linea alba. When this occurs the tip of the trocar should be slid laterally. At the lateral margin of the linea alba, the trocar tip is redirected toward the hollow of the pelvis and the peritoneal cavity is entered, thus avoiding the difficulty of perforating the tough linea alba.

In order to avoid injuries to the iliac arteries, the tip of the trocar has to be aimed at the fundus of the uterus rather than the pelvic side wall. The trocar must also be sharpened for better control of the direction. After presumed entry into the peritoneal cavity, the trocar is withdrawn from its sleeve and the trumpet valve on the sleeve is depressed slightly while the surgeon listens for the sound of gas escaping from the pneumoperitoneum. This sound confirms that the trocar sleeve is properly located.

Connection of the Light Cable and Gas Hose

The fiberoptic light cable is now connected to the laparoscope and the light is turned on. The laparoscope is gently inserted into the trocar sleeve while the surgeon watches through the eyepiece. If the sleeve is in the peritoneal cavity, omentum or loops of bowel will be seen. The laparoscope should be inserted at an angle to the abdomen of approximately 15 degrees to 20 degrees. This avoids obstruction of the lens by bowel or omentum and affords an immediate view of the pelvic cavity. The laparoscope can then be advanced into the pelvis to identify the structures there.

The gas hose is now connected to the gas port on the sleeve. A small amount of gas—perhaps 1 liter to 1.5 liters—is allowed to flow into the abdomen to better displace the intestine out of the pelvis. The pelvis is then thoroughly inspected for visible gynecologic abnormalities. This inspection is facilitated by manipulating the position of the uterus by moving the Rubin's cannula and Jacob's tenaculum with one hand while holding the laparoscope with the other.

Two-Incision Technique

To visualize the entire pelvis, including the inferior aspects of ovaries, where endometriosis is often found, the two-incision technique is often necessary. The two-incision technique is also useful for operative laparoscopy, such as lysis of extensive adhesions or aspiration of the oocyte for an *in vitro* fertilization.

The puncture site for the second incision is selected by transilluminating the abdominal wall with the viewing laparoscope introduced through the subumbilical incision. An avascular area in the lower midline of the abdomen, just inside the pubic hairline and about 6 cm above the symphysis pubis, is selected, and a 6 mm incision is made in the skin. Through this, a second trocar and sleeve are inserted down to the fascia. Countertraction is then exerted with the viewing laparoscope, and the trocar and sleeve are pushed through the fascia and peritoneum, using a short, quick push. The insertion is continuously observed through the viewing laparoscope. The second trocar is then withdrawn and an operating instrument or probe is introduced.

Tubal Sterilization

Before any type of tubal sterilization procedure is performed, it is imperative that an informed consent be obtained from the patient and her husband. Although there is no legal requirement for the husband to sign a sterilization authorization, it is a good practice to obtain the signature of both husband and wife for this procedure. If there is a medical or psychiatric indication, a full medical consultation note should be included in the hospital records.

Although a considerable number of patients do request reversal of the tubal sterilization later, it is important to stress the fact that the procedure is intended to secure permanent sterilization. Additionally, the patient and her husband must have a complete explanation of the alternative methods of family planning as well as of all possible complications that have been associated with a permanent tubal sterilization procedure. These complications should include the known failure rates of the procedure and the incidence of infection, bleeding, and anesthetic complications, including pulmonary and cardiac complications. If sterilization is being considered as a puerperal operative procedure, the request for sterilization should be obtained well before the expected date of delivery.

TIMING

When cesarean section is needed, it is common and convenient to perform a sterilization procedure at the same time. However, the sterilization should not be used as an indication for cesarean section. Section carries considerably greater risks of hemorrhage, shock, and postoperative complications than does vaginal delivery followed by puerperal tubal ligation.

Puerperal sterilization is best done in the first 24 to 36 hours after delivery. We prefer to wait at least 6 hours following delivery to reduce the likelihood of bleeding and permit rest after labor. Historically, sterilization has not been recommended later then 48 hours postpartum, as bacteria are present in the uterus by this time and the postoperative course is more likely to be febrile. However, with the intraoperative use of prophylactic antibiotics for a period of 24 hours, in recent comparative studies this time limitation has proven to be less rigid. If there has been premature rupture of membranes, intrapartum fever, manual removal of the placenta, or any factor predisposing to infection and postoperative complications, the procedure should be deferred until involution is completed. One advantage of early puerperal sterilization is easy access to the uterus, which may be approached by a small incision over the fundus a short distance below the umbilicus. Another is the convenience of combining postpartal and postoperative convalescence with minimal additional hospitalization.

Interval sterilization may be done 6 weeks after delivery or at any later period in the nonpregnant individual. For the patient who is not practicing contraception, interval sterilization is best carried out during the proliferative phase of the menstrual cycle, in order to avoid so-called luteal phase pregnancy. Women with cardiac disease, marked hypertension, renal disease, or acute toxemia should not be subjected to sterilization in the labile early puerperium but should have an interval procedure when the disease has become well stabilized.

In patients of high parity with significant symptoms of pelvic support relaxation, where there is need for extensive vaginal plastic repair, the treatment of choice is a vaginal hysterectomy and vaginal repair, performed no earlier than 6 months postpartum. It is not logical to perform a tubal ligation in conjunction with a vaginal repair unless the patient is adamant in her desire to continue to menstruate and to retain her uterus. However, it is important to emphasize that the major surgical indication of vaginal hysterectomy should be repair of the symptomatic pelvic relaxation and *not* sterilization.

METHODS OF TUBAL STERILIZATION

Although many methods are available for tubal sterilization, only techniques that are used frequently will be discussed. These include laparoscopic tubal sterilization and surgical sterilization by the Pomeroy, Irving, Uchida, and Kroener methods. The most widely used laparoscopic sterilization techniques are unipolar or bipolar electrocoagulation and the spring-loaded clip (Hulka) and Silastic ring (Yoon) methods. Failure rates range from 0.2 to 2 per 100 women per year (Fig. 17–5). After reviewing 24,439 procedures, Bhiwandiwala and associates (1982) concluded that laparoscopic sterilization was safe and effective. The electrocoagulation method is associated with less pain than mechanical means, but it has a danger of serious gastrointestinal burn. It is noteworthy that a pregnancy following unipolar electrocoagulation technique sterilization is more often than not an ectopic pregnancy. This may be the result of thermal damage to the cilia and muscularis in the remainder of the fallopian tube, or it may be due to formation of a fistula at the cornu of the uterus.

Unipolar Electrocoagulation Technique

Some of the electrocoagulation forceps used in the sterilization procedures described below are shown in Fig. 17–6. The operating laparoscope is introduced into the abdominal cavity and the pelvis is thoroughly inspected for abnormalities. The electrocoagulation grasping forceps is introduced through the operative part of the laparoscope or through a

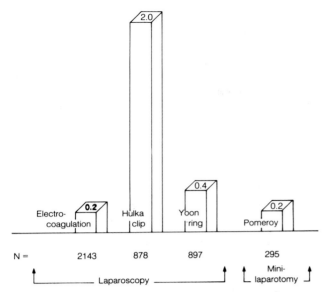

FIG. 17–5 Pregnancy failure rates per 100 women after various sterilization procedures by 12-month life-table method. (McCann M, 1978.)

grasping forceps. The fallopian tube is then traced from the uterine cornu to its fimbriated end to ensure identification. The tube is grasped approximately 5 cm from the cornu with a large bite that completely encompasses it and also includes a portion of the mesosalpinx. The tube is then moved to a safe position away from bowel and bladder.

The placement of the electrocoagulation forceps is then checked. Its insulation must be visible beyond the abdominal end of the laparoscope, so that the metal of the alligator-mouth forceps is not in contact with the metal laparoscope. By means of the foot switch the surgeon then passes electric current through the grasping forceps for approximately 5 seconds, thus thoroughly coagulating the tube. While the current is applied, the tube smokes and swells, and occasionally a popping noise is heard as fluid in the tubal lumen and tissue is released. When the tube swells and then collapses, coagulation is sufficient to permit complete destruction of a segment. The electric current is turned off and only then is the grasping forceps drawn back into the laparoscope. It is a serious error to withdraw the forceps while the electric current is on because structures in contact with the trocar sleeve or laparoscope may be burned in the process.

After proper electrocoagulation, the tensile strength of the coagulated portion of the tube is so low that the forceps can easily divide it. If hemorrhage occurs, the electrocoagulation was insufficient. In the rare instances of hemorrhage, bleeding points should be picked up with the electrocoagulation forceps and recoagulated. This is usually sufficient to control bleeding.

After the first burn and avulsion of the tube, a second burn is applied to its proximal stump, *never* to the distal stump. If the distal part is grasped at this time the current may return toward the fimbriated end of the tube, creating a spark between the fimbria and the intestine. The proximal stump

separate suprapubic puncture site. As a safety precaution, it is important that the electric cable not be attached to the grasping forceps while it is being inserted. The cable should not be attached until the surgeon is actually ready to grasp the fallopian tube.

The surgeon holds the laparoscope in one hand and manipulates the Rubin's cannula and the Jacob's tenaculum with the other. The uterus can thus be moved into a favorable position—usually anteflexed—so that the fallopian tubes, the round ligaments, and the ovaries are clearly visible. An assistant then holds the Rubin's cannula and the Jacob's tenaculum in the desired position. With the uterus thus fixed, the surgeon can move one hand to the operating laparoscope and the other to the

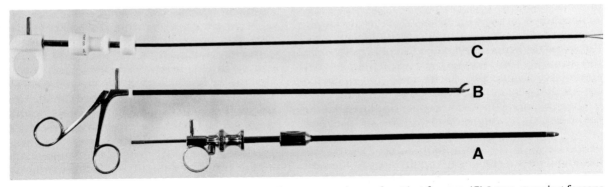

FIG. 17–6 (*A*) Palmer drill forceps. (*B*) 5 mm grasping and cutting forceps. (*C*) 3 mm grasping forceps.

is grasped in a nonburned area adjacent to the uterus, and current is applied for 3 to 4 seconds; however, the tube is not avulsed as with the first burn. If the tube is seen to be incompletely transected after the first burn and the avulsion, it should be grasped again and recoagulated with a second burn until total transection can be accomplished.

Occasionally, excessive smoke makes visualization difficult. When this occurs, the laparoscope can be withdrawn from the sleeve and the trumpet valve on the sleeve opened. This permits the smoke-filled carbon dioxide of the pneumoperitoneum to escape. A new pneumoperitoneum is then instituted.

After one tube has been coagulated and divided, the Jacob's tenaculum and Rubin's cannula are manipulated to expose the other tube, and the process is repeated. A thorough inspection should then be made for any bleeding point. The laparoscope is then withdrawn and the trumpet valve is opened to evacuate the pneumoperitoneum. It is important to evacuate the carbon dioxide completely from the peritoneal cavity, as postoperative discomfort is directly proportional to the amount of carbon dioxide remaining.

The skin incision is closed with a single suture of No. 3-0 chromic catgut. There is no need to perform any closure of the peritoneum or the rectus fascia. A small adhesive bandage is applied, and the patient is taken to the recovery room. If local anesthesia has been used, she is discharged home in 2 hours; if general anesthesia is used, after 4 hours. She is instructed in cleansing the incision and told to change the bandage daily.

Even where careful technique as described above is used, cases of fatal intestinal burns have been reported. In order to reduce the risk of thermal injury, Soderstrom recommends using only low-voltage generators with a maximum peak voltage of 600 volts and a maximum power of 100 watts. An isolated output system is more desirable than a grounded system.

When the unipolar electrode is used through an operative laparoscope, the laparoscope may act as a capacitor. The static electricity thus created in the scope can create a spark between the intestine and the scope. In order to disperse the electricity from the scope to the abdomen through the sleeve, a conductive sleeve should be used for operative scopes that accommodate unipolar electrodes.

Thermal injury most commonly occurs in the terminal ileum, although injuries to the rectosigmoid or transverse colon have been reported. Small burns of the serosa of the terminal ileum or of the rectosigmoid do not ordinarily require special therapy, but patients with such burns should be hospitalized for careful observation for 5 to 7 days. If signs and symptoms of peritonitis do develop, exploratory laparotomy must be performed.

The most serious gastrointestinal injuries are those that are not recognized at the time of surgery. Patients who sustain unrecognized injuries and who are discharged after laparoscopy reappear on the third to fifth postoperative day complaining of bilateral lower abdominal pain. At first the necrosing bowel causes symptoms similar to those of acute appendicitis; later, after perforation, the symptoms and signs are those of a ruptured appendix. There are five important principles to be observed in the management of this problem (Fig. 17–7). (1) The damaged segment of bowel should be resected rather than oversewn, and no attempt should be made to excise only the perforation site. The actual diameter of the area of thermal damage is about five times greater than it appears to be on inspection. Thus, resection of the bowel should be made at least 5 cm away from the edge of a 1 cm burn, for example. (2) All areas of electrocoagulation on fallopian tubes and uterus must be completely excised, even if hysterectomy becomes necessary, since these areas are potential sites of infection. (3) The abdomen must be thoroughly lavaged to remove all foreign matter. This principle is the one most frequently ignored in the management of these cases, with disastrous results. (4) The pelvis should be drained through the vagina. (5) Aggressive antibiotic therapy should be employed. Thermal injury and perforation of the large bowel often require exteriorization of the damaged segment of colon with reoperation in a properly prepared bowel when the tissue has healed. Resection and anastomosis of large bowel without proper preparation can result in serious complications.

Bipolar Electrocoagulation Technique

To reduce the chance of thermal injuries to the bowel and the abdominal wall, Rioux devised a technique of bipolar electrocoagulation. Whereas unipolar systems use a small active electrode and a broad-surfaced return electrode, the bipolar grasping forceps is designed so that one jaw is the active electrode and the other is the return electrode (Fig. 17–8). The mechanism allows the electric current to heat only the tissues between the jaws. When the bipolar forceps is placed through an operating scope, there is no capacitance effect, and no unpredictable sparks are generated between laparoscopic instruments and the bowel.

The technique of bipolar coagulation is similar to that of unipolar coagulation. After examination of the pelvic organs, the mobile midportion of the fal-

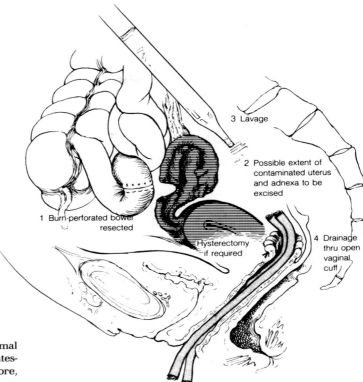

FIG. 17–7 The principles of treatment of electrothermal injury to the bowel. (Wheeless CR: Thermogastrointestinal injuries. In Phillips JM (ed): Laparoscopy. Baltimore, Williams & Wilkins, 1977.)

lopian tube is grasped with a pair of bipolar forceps and elevated free of surrounding structures. Both ends of the bipolar cord should be dry when the electrosurgery unit is attached.

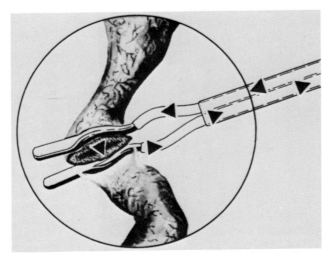

FIG. 17–8 Grasping jaw of Kleppinger bipolar forceps showing the direction of electric current (*triangles*).

If the Kleppinger bipolar forceps is used, closing the forceps handle will compress the tube and simultaneously bring the flat, duck-bill portion of the tips in contact with the mesosalpinx. Activation of the electrosurgical unit will produce almost immediate coagulation in the mesosalpinx. Within a few seconds, coagulation will extend to the tube. Complete coagulation requires application of electric current for approximately 10 seconds when a proper bipolar generator is used at a proper setting. The cauterized segment of the tube and mesosalpinx are transected with a pair of hook scissors.

Seiler and associates (1981) reported no pregnancies following bipolar laparoscopic sterilization in 232 patients. Larger series with longer follow-up periods will probably show a pregnancy rate comparable to other sterilization methods.

Even with bipolar methods, thermal burns have been observed. If this risk is to be avoided entirely, mechanical methods—a band technique or a clip technique—should be tried.

Silastic Band Technique (Yoon Band)

The laparoscopic technique for application of Silastic bands is the same as for the electrocoagulation

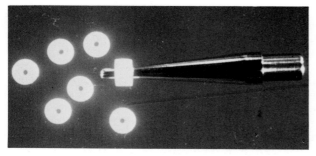

FIG. 17–9 Silastic Yoon bands for tubal sterilization.

procedure. The specially equipped laparoscope is loaded with a Silastic band, commonly called the Falope ring, (Fig. 17–9) and is inserted in standard fashion. First, each fallopian tube is identified. The tongs of the band applicator are then extended and one tube is grasped at the ampulloisthmic junction and brought into the applicator (Fig. 17–10A). Spraying 2 ml of 4% lidocaine solution on the fallopian tube before applying the band reduces the patient's immediate postoperative pain. The band is pushed over a knuckle of tube (see Fig. 17–10B). The tongs are then released and the tube is dropped into the cul-de-sac. If the two-incision technique is used, the band applicator is passed through a trocar sleeve in the second incision under observation by the viewing laparoscope in the first incision. The second tube is treated in the same manner as the first, and the abdominal incision (or incisions) is closed as described above.

Occasionally, the tube is transected. This complication is managed by grasping the transected stumps with the tongs and applying a band to each. The bleeding can also be controlled by applying the band to the bleeding point.

Spring-Loaded Clip Technique (Hulka Clip)

This spring-loaded clip consists of two small serrated Silastic jaws held together by a metal clip. Teeth at the end of the jaws lock the clip into place (Fig. 17–11). The clip is attached to the fallopian tube with an applicator. Although the failure rate with this method (2%) seems to be somewhat higher than with other laparoscopic sterilization methods, the damage to the tube may be less. For this reason, the clip technique can be used for a young woman of low parity who might wish to have a reversal of sterilization in the future.

Surgical Sterilization

IRVING METHOD. The Irving sterilization method has a very low failure rate (<0.1%) and is our procedure of choice when sterilization is in conjunction with a cesarean section. It may, however, be associated with somewhat more bleeding than the other methods.

The fallopian tube is doubly ligated with No. 2-0 chromic catgut about 3 cm from the uterine cornu and then severed. The sutures on the proximal end of the tube are left long. This tubal stump is then dissected free from the mesosalpinx and mobilized. A very small nick is made in the serosa on the posterior surface of the uterus near the cornu in as avascular an area as possible, and the musculature is penetrated with a mosquito clamp for about 1 cm, with the clamp spread sufficiently to admit the tube (Fig. 17–12A). One of the ligatures attached to

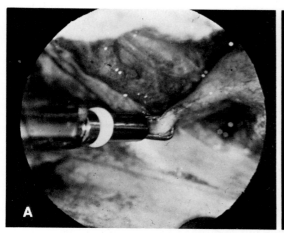
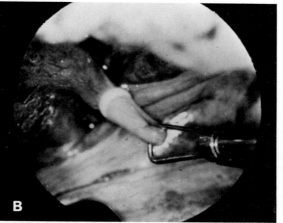

FIG. 17–10 Silastic band sterilization. (*A*) Fallopian tube held by tong forceps preparatory to applying Silastic band. (*B*) Knuckle of tube with Silastic band in place.

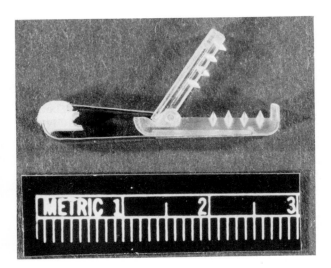

FIG. 17–11 The Hulka spring-loaded plastic clip.

the tubal stump is threaded with a round needle. Guided by a grooved director, the needle is thrust to the bottom of the pocket created by the mosquito clamp and carried out to the uterine surface. The other suture attached to the tubal stump is treated in a similar manner, bringing it to the surface of the uterus about 1 cm from the first suture (Fig. 17–12B). Traction is exerted on the sutures and the tubal stump is buried in the uterine musculature. Then the sutures are tied together. A suture of fine catgut is used to close the edges of the pocket more tightly about the tube.

According to Irving's original description of the operation, the ligated end of the distal portion of the tube is buried beneath the leaves of the broad ligament (Fig. 17–12C). The burying of this end of the tube is now considered to be optional. It gives a neat apearance but adds nothing to the effective-

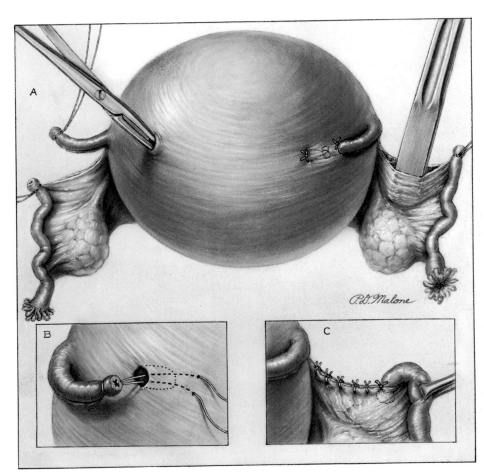

FIG. 17–12 Modified Irving sterilization. (*A*) Tubes have been cut and are being buried in musculature of posterior uterine wall. (*B*) Method of burying proximal tubal end. (*C*) Broad ligament is closed, and distal end of tube is buried.

ness of the sterilization. Furthermore, a blood vessel may be nicked occasionally during this step.

UCHIDA METHOD. The originator of this operation has had extensive experience and remarkable success. Although an excellent technique and quite similar to Irving's original description, the Uchida technique is possibly the most complex sterilization method. It is performed through a 1 cm suprapubic incision in the nonpregnant patient. Uchida used it almost exclusively as an interval sterilization procedure.

The uterine fundus is maneuvered forward by a large curette in the uterine cavity. A Babcock clamp or tubal hook is then used to deliver the tube through the small incision. At about its midpoint,

the mesosalpinx is dissected from the overlying muscular tube. This is accomplished by injecting a sufficient amount of a saline–epinephrine solution at the tubo-mesosalpingian junction to produce ballooning of the mesosalpinx (Fig. 17–13A). The avascular portion of the mesosalpinx is then incised with scissors (Fig. 17–13B). The muscular tube is grasped through this incision with a clamp and delivered into a loop, and the tube is divided. The serosa from the proximal end is stripped back by blunt dissection. A 3 cm to 5 cm segment of tube is excised, leaving only a small stump (Fig. 17–13C). This proximal stump is ligated with nonabsorbable suture and allowed to fall back between the ballooned leaves of the broad ligament. The distal stump is

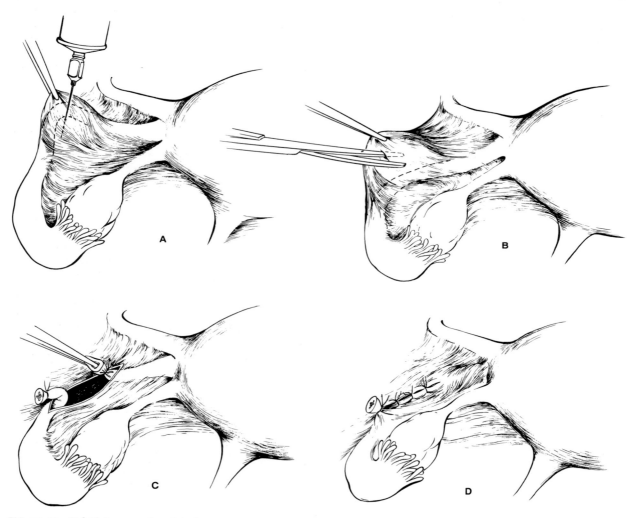

FIG. 17–13 Uchida's operation. (*A*) The mesosalpinx is ballooned with saline–epinephrine solution. (*B*) Peritoneum around tube is opened. (*C*) Tube is ligated at ampullary segment and proximal segment is buried within mesosalpinx. (*D*) Peritoneal edge of broad ligament is closed, with exteriorization of distal end of ligated tube.

then ligated and the edge of the broad ligament is closed with a suture of No. 3-0 catgut that terminates with a purse-string suture around the free end of the distal tube. The suture is tied so that the distal end of the tube projects into the abdominal cavity (Fig. 17–13D). Alternatively, the distal tube and fimbria can be removed.

POMEROY METHOD. As an interval procedure, the Pomeroy technique can be carried out through a suprapubic minilaparotomy incision or a colpotomy incision. Following delivery, it must be done through a small subumbilical vertical incision. One tube is grasped about the middle with a Babcock clamp and delivered. As the loop is held up, it is ligated with an absorbable suture (Fig. 17–14). If the tube has been crushed by a clamp prior to ligation, there is greater likelihood of failure. The loop is cut off with the scissors, as shown by the dotted line in Fig. 17–14. At the completion of the operation, the two severed ends of the tube have a tendency to retract from one another, as shown in the inset. The process is repeated on the opposite side and the incision is closed.

Fig. 17–15 shows tubes as they appeared at laparotomy some years after Pomeroy sterilization. The resected tubal ends are widely separated. If a permanent suture is used, wide separation may not take place.

KROENER METHOD. The Kroener fimbriectomy can be done through a minilaparotomy incision or a colpotomy incision. When the entire fimbria is removed the failure rate is quite low.

The fimbriated end of the oviduct is drawn into the operative field with a Babcock clamp. The mesosalpinx and outer third of the tube are clamped, doubly ligated with absorbable sutures, and excised to remove the entire fimbriated end of the tube (Fig. 17–16). After the outer third of the tube is grasped with a Heaney clamp, the initial ligature is a free tie to secure the blood vessels in the mesosalpinx. A transfixing ligature through the wall of the tube is placed between the Heaney clamp and the initial ligature to completely secure the collateral circulation and to occlude the lumen of the oviduct. The fimbriated end of the tube is then excised with scissors between the clamp and the outer ligature. This procedure excises the fimbria and a small segment of the ampullary portion of the tube to make certain that the entire functional component of the oviduct is completely removed.

SEQUELAE OF TUBAL STERILIZATION

With the increasing use of a variety of surgical methods of sterilization, certain pitfalls of these early surgical decisions are emerging. Smibert has

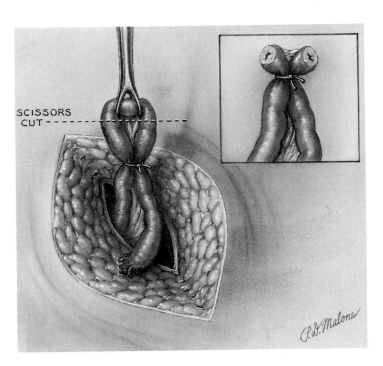

FIG. 17–14 Pomeroy tubal sterilization. The tube has been withdrawn through a short midline incision and a knuckle has been ligated. Inset shows knuckle excised with divergent ends.

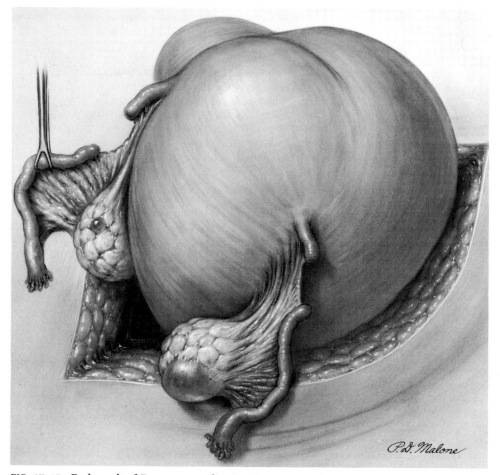

FIG. 17–15   End result of Pomeroy sterilization done 3 years before.

enumerated a wide variety of emotional conflicts stemming from elective sterilization including regret, behavioral aberrations, and frank psychoses, although Cooper and his associates found no evidence that elective sterilization increased the risk of psychiatric disturbances in their prospective study. Peel and Potts record an incidence of significant regret in less than 5% of sterilized patients. Akhter found that 5% of patients reported dissatisfaction with tubal sterilization. Dissatisfaction most often arises when an unstable marriage fails and fertility is subsequently desired with a new partner. Therefore, it is important that the marital unit be thoroughly evaluated and the motivations of sterilization be fully explored. It is mandatory that the patient have a detailed and complete understanding of the irreversible nature of the procedure before surgery is performed.

Surgical errors in which a segment of the round ligament is ligated and removed instead of the ovi-

duct have proven to be embarrassing complications when the procedure is hastily performed without adequate exploration of the entire tube. Such errors are automatically avoided by the use of the Kroener and Uchida fimbriectomy techniques, since these procedures require the identification of the fimbriated end of the tubes. Adequate pneumoperitoneum and positive identification of both the round ligament and the fimbriated end of the fallopian tube will minimize the danger of misidentification. Even if both tubes are properly ligated, 1 to 20 per 1000 women may conceive in the future. The failure rate seems to be high with a clip procedure, although this technique has the advantage of the least damage to the tubes and permits a higher rate of successful reanastomosis should the patient change her mind in the future.

McCausland reported that 51% of the pregnancies following laparoscopic tubal coagulation failures are tubal gestations. Furthermore, since the coagulation

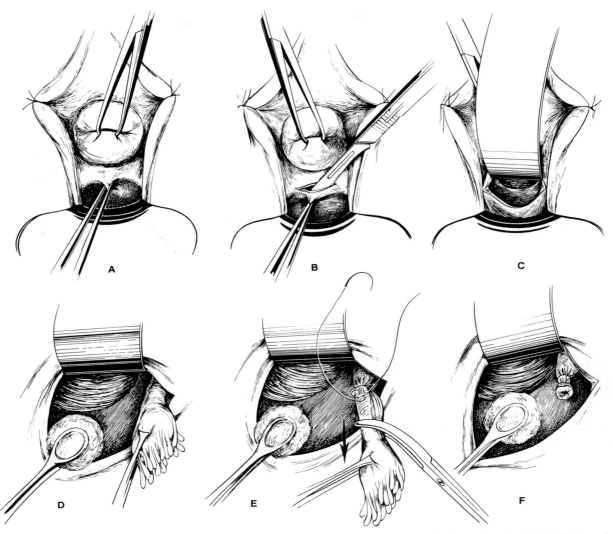

FIG. 17–16 Vaginal tubal ligation—fimbriectomy. (*A–C*) Colpotomy procedure. (*D*) The fimbriated end of tube is delivered into the vagina. (*E*) The tube is doubly ligated with a free tie and a transfixation suture followed by (*F*) fimbriectomy and removal of outer portion of ampullary portion of tube.

method carries an added risk of serious burn of intestines and other organs, this technique should be discouraged.

Several retrospective studies report a high prevalence of menstrual disturbances following female sterilization. However, a prospective study by Bhiwandiwala and associates based on 1025 cases showed that the majority of the women experienced no change in menstrual pattern following sterilization. Kwak and associates, studying the sterilized women as their own controls, also found no significant menstrual irregularity following sterilization except among those who previously had used the IUD and pill. Decreased menstrual flow was observed in the women who used an IUD prior to sterilization and an increased flow occurred in those who previously were pill users. Kasonde and Bonnar actually measured menstrual blood loss before and after tubal sterilization and concluded that the operation made no significant difference. Be that as it may, it is conceivable that extensive destruction of oviducts carried out by unipolar cauterization could interrupt the arterial or venous arcade in the broad ligament. This interference in ovarian blood flow could produce luteal phase defects or anovulation.

Poma reported a 7% incidence of subsequent hysterectomy with tubal ligation during a 7 year followup. In this regard, if there is definite evidence of pelvic pathology when permanent sterilization is planned, a hysterectomy will resolve both the pathology and the problem of future fertility.

Bibliography

Akhter MS: Vaginal versus abdominal tubal ligation. Am J Obstet Gynecol 115:401, 1973

Bhiwandiwala PP, Mumford SD, Feldblum PL: A comparison of different laparoscopic sterilization occlusion techniques in 24,439 procedures. Am J Obstet Gynecol 144:319, 1982

Cohen MR: Culdoscopy vs. peritoneoscopy. Obstet Gynecol 31:310, 1968

———: Laparoscopy, Culdoscopy and Gynecography. Philadelphia, WB Saunders, 1970

Fourestier N, Gladu A, Valmiere J: Perfectionnements a l'endoscopie medicale. Realisation bronchoscopique. Presse Med 60:1291, 1952

Gunning JE: History of laparoscopy. In Phillips JM (ed): Laparoscopy. Baltimore, Williams and Wilkins, 1977

Hulka JF, Omran KF: Comparative tubal occlusion: ring and spring loaded clips. Fertil Steril 23:633, 1972

Irving FC: A new method of insuring sterility following cesarean section. Am J Obstet Gynecol 8:335, 1924

Kalk H: Erfahrungen mit der Laparoskopie. Z Klin Med 111:303, 1929

Kampany NS: Fiber optics. In Strong J (ed): Concepts of Classical Optics. San Francisco, WH Freeman, 1958

Kasonde JM, Bonnar J: Effect of sterilization on menstrual blood loss. Br J Obstet Gynecol 83:572, 1976

Kroener WF, Jr: Surgical sterilization by fimbriectomy. Am J Obstet Gynecol 104:247, 1969

Kwak HM, Chi I, Gardner SD, et al: Menstrual pattern change in laparoscopic sterilization patients whose last pregnancy was terminated by therapeutic abortion. J Reprod Med 25:67, 1980

McCann M: Laparoscopy versus minilaparotomy. In Sciarra JJ, et al (eds): Risks, benefits, and controversies in fertility control. Maryland, Harper & Row, 1978

McCausland A: High rate of ectopic pregnancy following laparoscopic tubal coagulation failures. Am J Obstet Gynecol 136:97, 1980

Palmer R: Instrumentation et technique de la coelioscopie gynecologique. Gynecol Obstet (Paris) 46:420, 1947

Peel J, Potts M: Textbook of Contraceptive Practice. London, Cambridge University Press, 1969

Peterson EP, Behrman SJ: Laparoscopy of the infertile patient. Obstet Gynecol 36:363, 1970

Poma PA: Tubal sterilization and later hospitalization. J Reprod Med 25:272, 1980

Seiler JS, Roland M, Snyder JR, et al: Tubal sterilization by bipolar laparoscopy: Report of 232 cases. Obstet Gynecol 58:92, 1981

Smibert J: Pitfalls of Sterilization. Med J Austria 59:901, 1972

Soderstrom RM: Electrical Safety in Laparoscopy. Phillips JM (ed): Endoscopy in Gynecology, Baltimore, Md, AAGL, 1978

Steptoe PC: Laparoscopy in Gynecology. Edinburgh, E and S Livingston, 1967

Thompson BH, Wheeless CR: Gastrointestinal complications of laparoscopy sterilization. Obstet Gynecol 41:669, 1973

Uchida H: Uchida tubal sterilization. Am J Obstet Gynecol 121:153, 1975

Wheeless CR: A rapid, inexpensive and effective method of surgical sterilization by laparoscopy. Reprod Med 5:65, 1969

———: Laparoscopic sterilization: Review of 3,600 cases. Obstet Gynecol 42:751, 1973

———: Laparoscopy. Clin Obstet Gynecol 19:277, 1976

Yoon IB, Wheeless CR, King T: A preliminary report on a new laparoscopic sterilization approach: The silicone rubber band technique. Am J Obstet Gynecol 120:132, 1975

Chapter 18

Ectopic Pregnancy

Ectopic pregnancy was first recognized by Busiere in 1693, on examining the body of an executed prisoner in Paris. Gifford made a more complete report, in 1731 in England, describing the condition in which the fertilized ovum was implanted anywhere outside the uterine cavity. During the past three-and-a-half centuries, ectopic or extrauterine gestation has increased in incidence to 1 out of every 130 pregnancies, and the disorder has become one of the more serious complications of pregnancy. Ectopic pregnancy is now one of the leading causes of maternal morbidity and mortality in the United States, accounting for 12% of all maternal deaths in 1978.

Epidemiology of Ectopic Pregnancy

Although the total number of pregnancies has declined over the past decade, the rate of ectopic pregnancy has increased dramatically. The overall rate per 1000 reported pregnancies, including live births, legal induced abortions, and ectopic pregnancies, increased from 4.5 in 1970 to 9.4 in 1978 (Table 18–1).

The increase in the ectopic pregnancy rate during the period from 1970 to 1978 is much greater for nonwhite than for white women (Fig. 18–1). In 1977, an estimated 8 ectopic implantations occurred for every 1000 conceptions in white women, whereas the rate for nonwhite patients was approximately 12 in 1000. The increased ratio of extrauterine to intrauterine pregnancies is related to the rising incidence of sexually transmitted disease and to the efficacy of modern antibiotic therapy in preventing total tubal occlusion following an episode of salpingitis.

The ectopic pregnancy risk also increases with advancing age. According to Rubin and colleagues at the Centers for Disease Control (CDC), ectopic pregnancies occur in 4.5 per 1000 reported pregnancies for women aged 15 to 24 years; in 9.7 per 1000 for women aged 25 to 34; and in 15.2 per 1000 for women aged 35 to 44 years. An increased incidence of ectopic pregnancy with advancing age has been noted in other countries as well, including Great Britain and Sweden.

Although the total rate of ectopic pregnancies has increased, the number of women who die as a result of the disorder (death-to-case rate) has declined more than 70% according to a CDC survey. In 1970 the death rate was 3.5 per 1000 ectopic pregnancies, whereas in 1978 the rate had dropped to 0.9 per 1000. Since the total rate of maternal deaths has also decreased dramatically in the last decade, the deaths from ectopic pregnancy as a percentage of all maternal deaths has actually increased, from 7.8% in 1970 to 11.5% in 1978.

In summary, although a woman's chance of having an ectopic pregnancy has increased during the past decade, her risk of dying from this condition decreased at a more rapid rate. The percentage of maternal deaths from ectopic pregnancy has actually increased, and the rate is consistently higher for nonwhite women than it is for white women. A pregnant nonwhite woman at age 35 years or older has approximately a 2.6% chance that her pregnancy will be extrauterine. Among black women specifically, 3.1 out of 1000 ectopic pregnancies will result in maternal death.

TABLE 18–1   Numbers and Rates of Ectopic Pregnancies by Year, United States, 1970–1978

| | | RATES | | |
YEAR	NUMBER	Women Aged 15–44*	Live Births†	Reported Pregnancies‡
1970	17,800	4.2	4.8	4.5
1971	19,300	4.4	5.4	4.8
1972	24,500	5.5	7.5	6.3
1973	25,600	5.6	8.2	6.8
1974	26,400	5.7	8.4	6.7
1975	30,500	6.5	9.8	7.6
1976	34,600	7.2	11.0	8.3
1977	40,700	8.3	12.3	9.2
1978	42,400	8.5	12.8	9.4
Total	261,600	6.3	8.8	7.1

* Rate per 10,000 females
† Rate per 1,000 live births
‡ Rate per 1,000 reported pregnancies (live births, legal induced abortions, and ectopic pregnancies)

Etiology of Ectopic Pregnancy

TUBAL FACTORS

Both the increased incidence of sexually transmitted disease resulting in salpingitis and the efficacy of antibiotic therapy in preventing total tubal occlusion following an episode of salpingitis are related to the increasing incidence of ectopic pregnancy. Levin and associates have demonstrated that the risk of ectopic pregnancy is increased in women with a primary history of pelvic inflammatory disease. Westrom compared women with pelvic inflam-

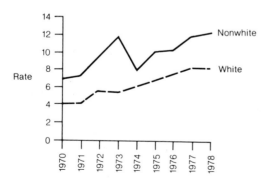

FIG. 18–1   Ectopic pregnancy rates per 1000 reported pregnancies (including live births, legal induced abortions, and ectopic pregnancies) by race and year, United States, 1970 through 1978. (Rubin GL, et al.: Ectopic pregnancy in the United States 1970 through 1978. JAMA 249, No. 13:1725, 1983. Copyright 1983, American Medical Association.)

matory disease confirmed by laparoscopy to women matched by age and parity and found a six-times greater incidence for the women with pelvic inflammatory disease, an alarming rate of one ectopic pregnancy out of every 24 gestations. Similar statistics are recognized among other high risk groups. In Jamaica, where the ectopic pregnancy rate is one in 28 deliveries, the frequency of pelvic inflammatory disease is proportionally high. Many of the patients in these studies had received antibiotic treatment for salpingitis.

Before the antibiotic era, salpingitis resulted in an acutely inflamed tube that usually became totally occluded, resulting in permanent sterility. Women who attempted pregnancy following a pelvic infection were successful less than 40% of the time. The current pregnancy rate exceeds 60% for patients who have been adequately treated with antibiotics. After an initial infection is treated appropriately with antibiotics, agglutination of the cilia may occur and synechial bands form within the tubal lumen, resulting in partial tubal obstruction. Westrom has demonstrated by laparoscopy that occlusion occurs in approximately 12.8% of patients following treatment for a single tubal infection; after two infections, in 35%; and after three or more infections, in 75% of women. Westrom found that of the patients who achieve a subsequent pregnancy after salpingitis, 4% or 5% will have an ectopic pregnancy.

RELATIONSHIP TO CONTRACEPTIVE DEVICES

Recently, use of intrauterine devices (IUDs) has been linked to the increased incidence of ectopic pregnancy, but a direct relationship has not been proven. In a summary of published reports on ectopic pregnancy, Tatum and Schmidt noted that 4% of the pregnancies that occurred with an IUD in place were ectopic. A different conclusion was reached by Ory in a collaborative multicenter case-control study of the incidence of ectopic pregnancy in the United States from 1965 through 1977 showing that the IUD did not play a significant role in the increased incidence of ectopic pregnancy.

Since the probable mode of action of an IUD is to prevent intrauterine implantation, the actual number of total conceptions with an IUD in place is difficult to identify, and the World Health Organization task force on IUDs for fertility regulation concluded that different devices could not be validly compared for their association with ectopic pregnancy. The association between IUDs and pelvic inflammatory disease may have contributed to the correlation between IUDs and ectopic pregnancy. Although the role of the IUD in the rising incidence of ectopic pregnancy cannot be proven at present, a limited cause and effect relationship probably exists.

OTHER FACTORS

Pauerstein presented a new view of the oviduct as an organ of many functions and not merely a conduit for ova and sperm. In particular, the ampullary-isthmic junction of the tube, the principal junction where the ovum is trapped, is said to be under hormonal regulation. Progesterone enhances tubal motility and the patency of the ampullary-isthmic junction. Alterations in serum and tissue concentrations of prostaglandins, catecholamines, estrogen, and progesterone could interfere in the transport of the fertilized ovum through the oviduct and could result in a tubal gestation. Hormonal factors would be particularly relevant in cases with no evidence of salpingitis. Evidence of the phenomenon has been documented by Falk and associates in a report of a very early tubal pregnancy in which the ovum was attached to a tubal fold and salpingitis was not a factor.

Transperitoneal migration of the ovum has been postulated as an additional factor in ectopic pregnancies, because the corpus luteum of pregnancy is found in the ovary on the opposite side from the gestation in 15% to 33% of reported cases. Other factors, such as peritubal adhesions from previous pelvic surgery, endometriosis, and previous microsurgery to reestablish tubal patency, also play significant roles in the incidence of ectopic gestation. For example, Winston relates that among patients of even the most experienced tuboplasty surgeons, 12% to 15% who become pregnant following tubal reconstructive surgery will have an ectopic pregnancy. The rate of ectopic pregnancies is lowest with tubal reanastomosis of previously ligated oviducts, and highest when surgery is required to repair extensive obstruction and postinflammatory distortion of the tubes. As many as 5% to 11% of all ectopic pregnancies result from tubal sterilization failures, most commonly when a fistula forms in the proximal end of the oviduct.

Sites of Ectopic Pregnancy

Approximately 95% of extrauterine implantations occur in the oviduct. The ampulla is the most common site, with approximately 55% of all tubal implantations; the isthmic portion has 20% to 25%; the infundibulum and fimbria have 17%; and the interstitial segment has 2% to 4%. Implantations occur less often in the ovary, the cornua, the cervix, and the peritoneal cavity (Fig. 18–2).

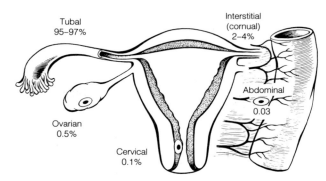

FIG. 18-2 Sites and incidence of ectopic pregnancy.

Future Reproduction and Repeat Ectopic Pregnancy

Tubal pregnancy is associated with a poor prognosis for subsequent reproduction. In most cases, an extrauterine pregnancy represents an impairment of the fertilized ovum's ability to migrate through the deep rugal folds of the oviduct as a result of altered tubal function. The morphologic abnormality is usually bilateral and irreversible and may produce repeated ectopic pregnancy, spontaneous abortion, or permanent sterility. In a 1975 study, Shoen and Nowak concluded that approximately 70% of the patients who have an ectopic first pregnancy are not able to produce a living child. As many as 30% of the patients will have a repeat ectopic pregnancy, compared to the total repeat ectopic rate of between 10% and 20%. More than half of the subsequent extrauterine pregnancies will occur within a two-year period, and 80% will occur within four years from the initial ectopic pregnancy. In reviewing the experience of the Kaiser Foundation hospitals, Hallatt reported a 9.2% incidence of repeat ectopics among 1330 women who had extrauterine pregnancies. Hallatt's figure correlates well with the overall rate for repeated ectopic pregnancies.

The potential reproductive capacity for a patient who has had an ectopic pregnancy depends on her reproductive history. If she is unfortunate enough to have had an ectopic pregnancy as a result of her first reproductive effort, the prognosis is much worse than had the complication occurred after one or more successful pregnancies.

Diagnosis of Ectopic Pregnancy

The morbidity and mortality associated with extrauterine pregnancy is directly related to the length of time before diagnosis is made. In the CDC survey, two-thirds of all patients later proven to have an ectopic pregnancy were previously seen by a physician and the diagnosis was either deferred or incorrectly assessed. The mortality rate from an ectopic pregnancy is higher in rural areas, where patients are less likely to receive early medical care.

For a successful outcome, an ectopic pregnancy must be diagnosed early. In some clinics where the complication is treated frequently, more than 50% of the cases are diagnosed and operated on before tubal rupture occurs. However, in about 85% of all cases, the symptoms that bring a patient to seek medical care are caused by a leaking or ruptured ectopic pregnancy. As many as 15% of all tubal pregnancies rupture before the first missed menstrual period, especially if a patient's periods are usually irregular.

The diagnostic record is improved somewhat in repeat ectopic pregnancies. As many as 25% to 30% of the repeat cases will be diagnosed and treated surgically prior to tubal rupture. Another difference is that with a repeat ectopic pregnancy, it is usually the patient herself who raises the question of an extrauterine pregnancy. Being suspicious, the patient seeks medical care earlier and provides a more specific medical history than does a patient experiencing her first ectopic pregnancy. The result is an earlier diagnosis and an improved chance for a successful outcome.

Some form of menstrual shedding occurs around the expected time of menses in more than 50% of women with an ectopic pregnancy, so most patients and their physicians are not aware that a pregnancy has occurred. The menstrual shedding is followed by a period of amenorrhea lasting between 6 and 10 weeks, after which the clinical symptoms of ectopic pregnancy appear.

CLASSIC SYMPTOMS: PAIN, BLEEDING, AND ADNEXAL MASS

The classic presentation of pain and uterine bleeding, with the finding of an adnexal mass has been the clinical hallmark of extrauterine pregnancy. But even classic presentations can be misleading, as Schwartz and DiPietro recently observed. Of the patients who presented with the classic symptoms, only 14% were shown to have an ectopic pregnancy. The severity of these symptoms and signs depends on the stage of the disease, but in the early stages of an ectopic gestation, symptoms are less accurate than in the more advanced stages of the reproductive process.

A discrete, unilateral mass, separate from the adjacent ovary, has been detected in less than a third of all proven ectopic pregnancies. Locating a mass

depends on many unpredictable factors, including the diagnostic skill of the examiner, the degree of pelvic peritonitis present, the presence or absence of tubal rupture, and the degree of stoicism and cooperation of the patient. If all factors are optimal, an adnexal mass can be felt in only half of the cases. More often, the clinical, physician, and patient factors combine in a normal way, so early diagnosis demands exceptional clinical acumen.

DIAGNOSTIC STUDIES

Three major improvements have made early diagnosis of extrauterine pregnancy possible: (1) the development of highly sensitive, rapid β-hCG (human chorionic gonadotropin) assays; (2) the ability to use ultrasound to evaluate the uterus and adnexa; and (3) application of laparoscopy as a diagnostic tool.

hCG Assays

Urine pregnancy tests using the slide method have a hCG sensitivity level of 1500 mIU/ml to 3500 mIU/ml (mIU = milli-International Units) (Table 18–2). The tests are frequently imprecise and have been positive in only half of the later proven cases of ectopic pregnancy, where the hCG level is often lower than the sensitivity of the urine slide test. The current availability of very sensitive and ac-

TABLE 18–2 *Qualitative Procedures for Detection of hCG*

TEST	SENSITIVITY (mIU/ml)
Tube tests	
Biocept-G (radioreceptorassay, Wampole Labs)	200*
Sensitex (Roche Labs)	250
UCG-Test (Wampole Labs)	500
Accusphere (Organon, Inc.)	750
Pregnostic (Organon, Inc.)	750
Pregnosis Placentex (Roche Labs)	1000
UCG-Lyphotest (Wampole Labs)	1250
EPT (Warner-Chilcott Labs)	1250
Slide tests	
Dri-Dot (Organon, Inc.)	1500
Pregnosis (Roche Labs)	1500
Pregnosticon (Organon, Inc.)	1500
UCG (Wampole Labs)	2000
Gravindex (Ortho Pharmaceutical Corp.)	3500

hCG = human chorionic gonadotropin.
* Biocept-G RRA can also be used as a semiquantitative test.
From Hussa RO, 1982.

curate serum pregnancy tests has resulted in an increased use of this method in the detection of an ectopic pregnancy. A radioimmunoassay for β-hCG can detect levels of hCG as low as 5 mIU/ml to 10 mIU/ml of serum. Thus, the test is approximately 400 to 500 times more sensitive than the more conventional urinary hemagglutination tests.

The β-hCG assay requires 24 hours for desired sensitivity and reliability. A semi-quantitative radioreceptor assay may be used by laboratories in which quantitative hCG assays are not available. The Bicoep-G (Wampole Labs) radioreceptor assay can be used semi-quantitatively when standardized against a qualitative method. With its lower sensitivity level of 200 mIU/ml, the radioreceptor test is positive in approximately 90% of the cases of ectopic pregnancy, compared to the β-hCG radioimmunoassay, which is positive in nearly 100% of cases.

Although helpful diagnostic guides, positive pregnancy tests cannot define the location of a pregnancy, either intrauterine or extrauterine. The tests must be used with other clinical information. Recent studies by Kadar and associates, for example, document that an intrauterine sac could be detected reliably only when the hCG level was above 6500 mIU/ml. When he compared ultrasound findings with hCG levels, Kadar was able to confirm that hCG values above 6500 mIU/ml without an intrauterine sac were almost always diagnostic of an ectopic pregnancy, but hCG values below 6500 mIU/ml without ultrasound demonstration of an intrauterine sac were more difficult to interpret. Kadar's studies also showed that the serum hCG level increases by at least 66% in a 48-hour period in 85% or more of normal pregnancies, but will increase by a value less than 66% in an ectopic pregnancy. Unfortunately, 15% of normal pregnancies have abnormal changes in hCG levels. If the patient is stable, more reliable information can be obtained by repeating the test after 48 hours.

Ultrasound

The major use of pelvic ultrasound is to document an intrauterine pregnancy by demonstrating the gestational sac and fetus. The recent application of the imaging technique to cases with a suspected ectopic pregnancy has greatly facilitated the clinical diagnosis of the disorder.

In a normal intrauterine pregnancy, a gestational sac can be seen 5 to 6 weeks from the time of the last menstrual period, while a fetus can be identified at 6 to 7 weeks. It is not until the 7th or 8th week, when the serum level of hCG reaches 13,610 mIU/ml or more, that a fetal heartbeat can be visualized by ultrasound. Recognition of the critical intra-uterine events is sufficient for ruling out a diagnosis of extrauterine pregnancy.

Diagnosis by ultrasound can be confusing. Only a few clinics have a high ultrasound accuracy rate; the normal false-negative rate varies from 2% to 35%. One problem is that a "pseudogestational" sac due to a decidual cast may be mistaken for an amniotic sac. Recently, the finding of a double-sac image, representing both the decidual lining of the uterus and the amniotic sac has been used to confirm the accuracy of a diagnosis of intrauterine pregnancy. The double-sac image can be visualized as early as 5 weeks following the last menstrual period.

Combined Studies

Just as the hCG radioimmunoassay is best used with other diagnostic tools, inconclusive ultrasound findings are best supported with hCG assays and other diagnostic techniques. The Medical College of Wisconsin has established a protocol for diagnosing and managing ectopic pregnancies (Fig. 18–3), using culdocentesis, serum hCG values, and ultrasonography.

When a patient is seen who has a clinical history suspicious for ectopic pregnancy, a culdocentesis is performed. If the test is positive for nonclotting blood, the patient is treated further by laparoscopy, laparotomy, or tubal surgery, depending on subsequent findings. If the culdocentesis is negative, a series of conservative methods of evaluation are undertaken. First a β-hCG assay is made, and if negative, ectopic pregnancy can be ruled out. When the β-hCG level is more than 6500 mIU/ml, an ultrasound is employed for diagnosis. The image will show either a gestational sac as evidence of an intrauterine pregnancy, or no gestational sac. If no gestational sac is found, the patient must be evaluated further by laparoscopy or laparotomy.

More commonly, an ectopic pregnancy will produce a low level of β-hCG from the aborting or degenerating trophoblast. If the hCG level is less than 6000 mIU/ml, further testing with ultrasound generally will not differentiate an ectopic pregnancy from a spontaneous abortion or blighted ovum. When diagnosis is uncertain, and the patient is in an unstable condition, she should be evaluated immediately by laparoscopy, and if necessary by laparotomy.

If the patient is in a stable condition, serial hCG samples should be taken at 48-hour intervals, and the assays should be correlated with the patient's initial serum value. If the hCG level increases more than 66% within a 48-hour period, the patient most probably has a normal intrauterine pregnancy, and nonsurgical care is indicated. If the increase in serial hCG levels is less than 66% of the original value, an

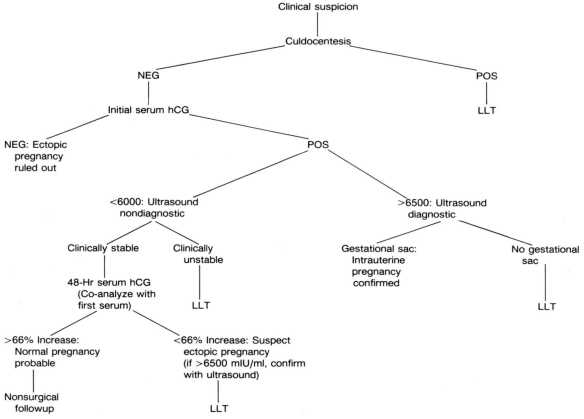

FIG. 18-3 Use of sensitive and quantitative hCG-specific radioimmunoassay and ultrasound in diagnosis of ectopic pregnancy. *LLT* = laparoscopy, laparotomy, and tuboplasty if indicated clinically. (Adapted from Hussa, 1982)

ectopic pregnancy should be suspected. Ultrasound can be used as a diagnostic support, showing a gestational sac in the adnexa or fluid in the cul-de-sac of Douglas. But as Kadar recognized, only when the hCG level is greater than 6500 mIU/ml will the sonogram be positive.

Dilatation and Curettage

Although in the past, histologic changes in the endometrium accompanying an ectopic gestation were confirmed by dilatation and curettage, more accurate measurements can be achieved with newer diagnostic studies, such as the radioimmunoassay for β-hCG, ultrasonography, and laparoscopy. If a patient is bleeding excessively and requires a dilatation and curettage, the removed material may be assessed. Decidua without chorionic villi, although it suggests the diagnosis of an ectopic pregnancy, does not provide absolute proof, since these findings also occur with a spontaneous abor-

tion. Endometrial changes provide only supportive rather than diagnostic information.

Arias–Stella Reaction

The atypical epithelial changes of the gestational endometrium were first described by Polak and Wolfe in 1924, in a case of tubal pregnancy, and were expanded upon by Arias–Stella in 1954 (Fig. 18–4). The highly controversial method of identifying these changes depends on a precise definition of a definitive cell involved in the morphologic change, together with some ill-defined physiologic events that produce the changes. Arias–Stella and others remain convinced that the histologic changes represent a progressive phenomenon resulting from exaggerated proliferative and secretory responses to the elevated hormonal levels of pregnancy. Fienberg and Lloyd disagree, maintaining that the changes are regressive and involutional and are the result of declining hormonal levels. Whatever an-

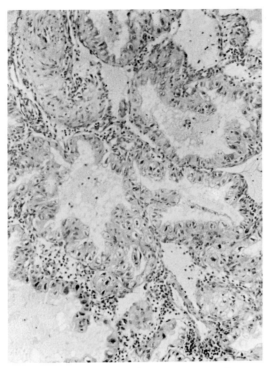

FIG. 18-4 Arias–Stella reaction in endometrial cells associated with ectopic pregnancy, showing nuclear enlargement, irregularity, and hyperchromasia with cytoplasmic vacuolation.

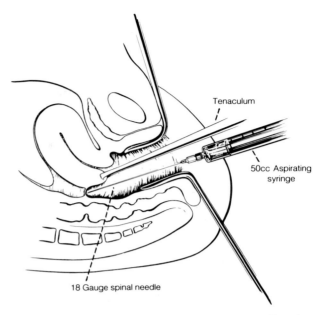

FIG. 18-5 Culdocentesis. A No. 18 gauge spinal needle is inserted through the posterior fornix and enters the cul de sac between the uterosacral ligaments.

swer is proven, the endometrial changes can be associated with normal pregnancy as well as with a spontaneous abortion or an ectopic pregnancy, so the histologic reactions have no specific value for the detection of an extrauterine pregnancy.

Culdocentesis

A culdocentesis is a useful diagnostic tool for identifying the presence of intraperitoneal bleeding. The simple procedure of inserting a No. 18 gauge spinal needle attached to a 50 ml aspirating syringe into the cul-de-sac between the uterosacral ligaments (Fig. 18–5) provides immediate and useful clinical information when unclotted blood is aspirated from the cul-de-sac. The procedure cannot be used for an absolute diagnosis, because a tubal pregnancy may not have ruptured or leaked into the peritoneal cavity. Culdocentesis can indicate the presence of free blood in the peritoneal cavity, but it cannot determine whether the blood is from an ectopic pregnancy or from some other cause of intra-abdominal bleeding. A ruptured corpus luteum hematoma or the rupture of another viscera would result in similar bleeding patterns.

The most common cause of a false-negative peritoneal aspiration is faulty technique or inexperience in the proper placement of the needle into the cul-de-sac. While some clinicians consider culdocentesis to be an invasive technique, the introduction of bacteria into the peritoneal cavity is a rare complication, even after the adjacent sigmoid colon or small bowel is inadvertently punctured.

Laparoscopy

Laparoscopy is useful when an unruptured ectopic pregnancy is suspected but the patient has no signs of intraperitoneal bleeding. Laparoscopic examination should be undertaken when a patient has a β-hCG level less than 6500 mIU/ml or a negative pelvic ultrasound. If a patient is in stable condition, the examination can be deferred for a period of 48 hours following the initial β-hCG radioimmunoassay, so that a subsequent titer can be determined. Patients who have less than a 66% increase in the β-hCG titer have a high incidence of ectopic pregnancy and should be examined by laparoscopy.

The laparoscopic technique (described in Chapter 17) is useful for diagnosis because its cold fiberoptic light provides precise visibility of the entire female reproductive tract. Laparoscopy is a great improvement over the more cumbersome and difficult technique of culdoscopy. Once the possibility of an ectopic pregnancy has been recognized, the adnexa must be visualized in order to be thoroughly evaluated before the patient can be discharged from the hospital. Laparoscopy has reduced the clinical error in diagnosing an ectopic pregnancy to less than 4% of cases, and the simpler technique has limited the need for laparotomy. When laparotomy was used to determine the presence or absence of an extrauterine pregnancy, 20% of the procedures resulted in a negative finding.

Laparoscopy is best performed using general anesthesia, because the physician is then able to perform a thorough pelvic examination before using the laparoscope. When an adnexal mass can be clearly detected and separated from the adjacent ovary, a laparotomy can be performed immediately, sparing the patient the extra procedure. In cases with extensive intraperitoneal bleeding, laparoscopy is usually unsuccessful and should not be used. Laparotomy is always required to control the source of persistent bleeding, regardless of the cause. In the case of a leaking corpus luteum hematoma, laparoscopy is particularly useful because defining the cause allows the physician to provide conservative treatment, unless the intra-abdominal bleeding persists. If a leaking corpus luteum hematoma is suspected from the clinical evidence and the patient's history, laparoscopy may not be required.

Treatment for Ectopic Pregnancy

More than 100 years have passed since Parry reported his earliest experience with the operative treatment of ectopic pregnancy among 529 patients. At that time, Parry's surgical treatment resulted in a mortality rate of 69%. Robert Lawson Tait is credited as one of the first surgeons to follow Parry's advice and to embark upon a policy of surgical treatment. Exploratory laparotomy and salpingectomy remain the definitive methods of surgical treatment of ectopic pregnancy, specifically for advanced or ruptured cases. A more conservative surgical approach has developed only during the past decade.

Some clinics today are pursuing an ultra-conservative, nonoperative course of management for unruptured tubal pregnancies. As Mashiach and associates recently explained, management consists of monitoring the absorption of the disease process with serial β-hCG assays and confirming the information with ultrasound. Ultra-conservative management can only be maintained in clinics with easily available equipment and highly reliable patients. Nonsurgical and surgical treatment show the

same results for subsequent pregnancy rates and recurrence of ectopic pregnancies.

CONSERVATIVE SURGICAL TREATMENT

The conservative management of an unruptured ectopic pregnancy usually includes one of three possible procedures: linear salpingotomy, manual expression of the pregnancy (tubal abortion), or segmental resection with or without repair. A conservative surgical approach is possible because early diagnosis of ectopic pregnancy avoids destruction of the oviduct from rupture, so surgery also attempts to maintain functioning of the tube.

Salpingotomy

Recent studies have found that in more than 50% of patients, the uninvolved tube is abnormal, usually as a result of pelvic inflammatory disease, and that 10% to 20% of patients will have a subsequent ectopic pregnancy in that tube. As many as 60% to 70% of patients who undergo salpingectomy will never have a normal pregnancy. In 1896, Howard A. Kelly was among the first to advocate conservative surgery for tubal gestation by drainage of the pregnancy per vaginam, particularly for chronic hemorrhage and formation of a pelvic hematoma. More than half a century elapsed before Stromme reported the successful use of salpingotomy to treat a patient with tubal pregnancy; the patient subsequently achieved a normal pregnancy.

In 1973, Stromme reported his more recent surgical experience with 36 cases of unruptured tubal pregnancy. Out of 21 conservative salpingotomies, five were performed on patients with only one remaining tube. Although only one term pregnancy resulted from the five single-tube procedures, Stromme's work led to the development of conservative surgical procedures during the late 1970s. Stromme's rate of 13.5% of repeat ectopic pregnancies was no higher than the rate for patients treated with radical procedures.

Since Stromme's report, much success has been achieved using the conservative salpingotomy. Even before Stromme's report, Timonen and Nieminen from Finland reported one of the largest series, 185 patients, who achieved a full-term delivery rate of 36.1% for all subsequent pregnancies. The specific benefit of this salpingotomy procedure is difficult to assess from the data, because the functional status of the opposite oviduct was not recorded. Timonen and Nieminen inserted a transabdominal polyethylene tube in the operated oviduct for 6 weeks following surgery and employed hydrotubation with 4 ml sterile fluid containing penicillin (200,000 units) and hydrocortisone (50 mg) daily during the first postoperative week. Their repeat ectopic pregnancy rate of 16% was similar to other reports.

Järvinen reported a 42% normal pregnancy rate among 43 salpingotomy patients in whom both tubes were in situ. DeCherney and Kase also had a 40% normal pregnancy rate following salpingotomy treatment of 48 patients with an unruptured ectopic pregnancy. In a later series, 8 of 16 of DeCherney's patients (50%) had normal pregnancies, and none of the 16 patients had ectopic pregnancies. Bruhat reports one of the best experiences to date with a 72% normal pregnancy rate after the salpingotomy procedure was used among a group of 25 patients. In most of the salpingotomy studies, the functional status of the uninvolved oviduct was not defined, and whether or not the subsequent pregnancy was achieved through the operated oviduct can only be conjectured.

Langer and associates did include a description of the uninvolved oviduct when they reported experiences with salpingotomy in 30 patients. Of the patients in whom the contralateral tube was grossly normal, 80% subsequently had normal pregnancies. When the contralateral tube was damaged or contained peritubal adhesions, only 11 patients, or 55%, achieved a viable pregnancy.

Among recent reports where salpingotomy was performed on a single remaining oviduct, an intrauterine pregnancy rate of approximately 50% was achieved by several investigators, but precise circumstances are difficult to define because of the incompleteness of reports. The repeat ectopic pregnancy rate in the single-tube salpingotomy patients was 20%, higher than for the series that did not report the condition of the contralateral oviduct.

In general, conservative salpingotomy is the preferred treatment for patients who are less than 35 years of age and who desire further pregnancies. For the operation to be feasible, the oviduct should be unruptured, and the patient should be in a surgically stable condition.

TECHNIQUE OF LINEAR SALPINGOTOMY. A linear salpingotomy is an ideal procedure for an unruptured tubal pregnancy, since more than 75% of these ectopic gestations occur in the outer two-thirds of the oviduct.

The procedure for linear salpingotomy starts by exposing, elevating, and stabilizing the tube. Then a linear incision is made over the distended segment of the tube (Fig. 18–6). The incision is extended through the antimesenteric wall until entry is made into the lumen of the distended oviduct. When gentle pressure is exerted from the opposite side of the tube, the products of gestation are gently expressed

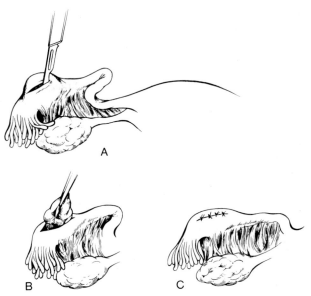

FIG. 18–6 Linear salpingotomy for unruptured tubal pregnancy. (*A*) Longitudinal incision made over distended, antimesenteric segment of tube. (*B*) Gestational products are removed with counterpressure and fine forceps. The endosalpinx is irrigated with lactate solution, removing all placental fragments from tubal mucosa. (*C*) Interrupted seromuscular sutures of No. 6-0 delayed-absorbable suture that avoid the mucosa are used to close the incision without tension. Alternatively, the margins of the incision can be sutured and left open to close by secondary healing.

from the lumen. Since a certain amount of separation of the trophoblast has usually occurred, the conceptus generally can be easily removed from the lumen. Gentle traction by forceps without teeth or suction may be used if necessary, but care should be taken to avoid trauma to the mucosa. Any remaining fragments of the anchoring trophoblast should be removed by profuse irrigation of the lumen with warm Ringer's lactate solution, as this will avoid further damage to the mucosa.

Care must be taken to provide complete hemostasis in the tubal mucosa; failure to do so results in troublesome postoperative bleeding, which leads to the formation of intraluminal adhesions. The small tubal vessels are easily identified while the tube is being irrigated, and, if necessary, loupe magnifying glasses can be used. An operating microscope is not needed, because the bleeding points can be easily identified with 2× to 4× magnification.

The mucosal margins are then closed with interrupted sutures of No. 6-0 or No. 7-0 delayed-absorbable suture, making certain that only the serosa and muscularis are approximated and without using undue tension. Care should be taken to ensure that no suture material is retained on the mucosal surface, since even a small amount can produce a secondary inflammatory reaction with subsequent adhesion formation.

Manual Expression

A fimbrial or infundibular implantation can be more expeditiously evacuated from the oviduct by gentle manual compression. Since bleeding can be a problem from residual trophoblastic elements, every effort should be made to irrigate all components of the trophoblast free from the mucosa lining. Using 2× to 4× magnification with the loupe lenses, the surgeon is able to identify the bleeding capillaries in the mucosa and coagulate them using the bipolar forceps. Fimbrial expression is associated with a rather high incidence of recurrent ectopic pregnancy, probably because the mucosa lining is damaged and the cilia in this region of the tube are lost. In some cases, a salpingotomy may be required to control the mucosal bleeding in the outer end of the tube.

Segmental Resection

Segmental resection and end-to-end reanastomosis has been proposed as an alternative treatment to salpingotomy. The procedure removes the implantation site, so it cannot be involved in a subsequent tubal pregnancy. Another objective is to restore a more normal architecture to the oviduct, a time-consuming process. The procedure requires special expertise and extensive microsurgical experience; it should not be undertaken by an inexperienced surgeon. The success of future pregnancies will depend on the skill, precision, and technique used in the procedure, and once begun the only alternative is salpingectomy. Swolin initially advocated this procedure in 1967 in Sweden. More recently, that clinic staff reported experience with 42 patients who received the segmental resection and end-to-end anastomosis. The subsequent intrauterine pregnancy rate was 23.9% and only 9.5% were able to deliver at term. A repeat ectopic pregnancy occurred in 14.3% of all pregnancies. Stangel and Gomel have found segmental resection preferable to salpingotomy for patients with an isthmic pregnancy.

The resection is best performed with loupe magnification or with the operating microscope; the microsurgical techniques used are identical to those used for primary infertility surgery. Care must be taken to avoid trauma to the very vascular oviduct: only cases with minimal bleeding should be considered for the operation. The adjacent mesosalpinx must also be removed with care to avoid the formation of a hematoma in the broad ligament.

The seromuscular sutures are placed using the operating microscope and utilizing No. 6-0 delayed-absorbable suture. The serosa is secondarily supported by interrupted sutures. Then the patency of the oviduct is tested with insufflation of the uterine cavity with indigo carmine dye.

RADICAL SURGICAL TREATMENT

Salpingectomy

When a tubal pregnancy has ruptured causing intra-abdominal hemorrhage that must be quickly controlled, total salpingectomy must be performed. Under no circumstances should a conservative operation be attempted if a patient has extensive hematoperitoneum, because the patient is in serious cardiopulmonary jeopardy.

Many recent reports in the literature advocate the combined use of a prophylactic oophorectomy with salpingectomy, but the need for an expedient procedure does not exclude conservative management of the ovary adjacent to a ruptured tube. Theoretically, the removal of the ipsilateral ovary would cause the other ovary to ovulate more frequently, favoring future pregnancy. In reality this consideration is outweighed by the fact that if the contralateral ovary were removed in a future operative procedure the patient would be castrated. The current high success rate of *in vitro* fertilization provides another reason to try to maintain functioning of both ovaries.

Total salpingectomy with partial cornual resection, the mainstay of the surgical procedures for an ectopic pregnancy, has been recently criticized for providing a residual sinus tract that allows the development of a subsequent interstitial pregnancy. The problem is not in the procedure, but in the performance. If the surgeon completely peritonizes the cornual incision, advancing the broad and round ligaments over the uterine cornua (modified Coffey suspension), complete protection is provided from a recurrent interstitial pregnancy. Too vigorous a cornual resection can also cause problems. A residual myometrial defect can cause uterine rupture, interstitial recanalization, or placental encroachment during a subsequent intrauterine pregnancy, and should be avoided by making certain the interstitial section includes less than one-half of the thickness of the cornual portion of the myometrium.

TECHNIQUE OF SALPINGECTOMY. A suprapubic Pfannenstiel incision is used. The distended tube is elevated, and the mesosalpinx is clamped with a succession of Kelly clamps as close to the tube as possible (Fig. 18–7A). The tube is then excised by cutting a small myometrial wedge at the uterine cornu (Fig. 18–7B). Care should be taken to avoid a deep incision into the myometrium. A figure-of-eight or mattress suture of No. 0 delayed-absorbable material is used to close the myometrium at the site of the wedge resection. The mesosalpinx is closed with interrupted ligatures of No. 0 delayed-absorbable suture. Complete hemostasis is essential to avoid hematoma of the broad ligament.

The fundus is held forward and the round and broad ligaments are sutured over the uterine cornu (Fig. 18–7C). The procedure, known as the modified Coffey technique of uterine suspension, accomplishes complete peritonization. Mattress sutures anchor the broad ligament to the uterus. The No. 0 delayed-absorbable suture first penetrates the broad ligament from its anterior surface, just below the round ligaments, 2 cm or 3 cm from the cornu. The next bite is taken into the fundus of the uterus, a little posterior and superior to the uterine incision. The suture is then placed through the posterior aspect of the broad ligament, about 1 cm lateral to the previous suture. When this suture is tied, the cornual incision and the mesosalpinx are peritonized (Fig. 18–7D). If there is excessive tension on this suture, or incomplete peritonization, supporting sutures may be placed in the myometrium and the round ligament to be certain that the peritonization suture will remain in place.

Interstitial Pregnancy

Interstitial pregnancy is a rare condition, accounting for no more than 2% to 4% of all tubal pregnancies. The condition occurs once for every 2500 to 5000 live births. Although many surgeons have attempted to differentiate an interstitial pregnancy from a cornual pregnancy, the two are difficult to separate anatomically and should be classified together.

The gestational sac is protected better in the interstitial portion than in the rest of the tube, so the symptoms manifest later, and the pregnancies are more advanced when they rupture. After 2 to 3 months of amenorrhea, vaginal spotting begins. The developing chorionic villi eventually erode into the blood vessels and the uterine cornu, causing a severe hemorrhage. Because the pregnancy occurs at the most richly vascularized area of the female pelvis, the junction of the uterine and ovarian vessels, rupture usually causes profound and sudden shock.

Before 1893, the only available reports on interstitial pregnancies were from autopsies, but since then, 250 cases have been reported in the literature. More experience and earlier diagnoses have reduced the mortality rate to approximately 2% to 2.5% of all interstitial and cornual pregnancies.

The diagnosis of an interstitial pregnancy is made by the critical evaluation of all the criteria used for other types of tubal pregnancy. Patients will have acute abdominal pain, intraperitoneal bleeding, a low hematocrit, and a positive serum or urine pregnancy test. Diagnostic tests include the sensitive radioimmunoassay or radioreceptor assay for β-hCG, culdocentesis, and ultrasonography.

The asymmetry of the uterus may be misinterpreted as a pregnancy in a bicornuate uterus or a myoma in a pregnant uterus instead of an interstitial pregnancy. Previous knowledge of the shape of the uterus may help to confirm or exclude the existence of a bicornuate or myomatous uterus. A firm protrusion on the uterus would suggest a myoma; a soft, tender asymmetrical enlargement suggests an interstitial pregnancy.

Because ultrasound cannot usually be used to identify the position of the pregnancy, laparoscopy is required to confirm the diagnosis. When the patient is experiencing massive intra-abdominal bleeding, an immediate laparotomy should be performed.

The etiologic factors for interstitial pregnancy are similar to those for the other types of tubal pregnancies; most important are pelvic inflammatory disease, operative trauma, and tumors. The management of the tubal stump at the time of salpingectomy is the subject of much controversy concerning a subsequent interstitial pregnancy.

Kalchman and Meltzer collected reports of 73 cases of interstitial pregnancy following total salpingectomy along with two additional cases resulting from his own surgery and another 24 cases occurring after partial salpingectomies. In Kalchmann's report, ectopic pregnancy was the original indication for 60% of the initial salpingectomies. Too vigorous a cornual resection was considered to be one of the major factors in the subsequent development of an interstitial pregnancy.

More recently Hallatt has questioned the advisability of cornual wedge resection because he feels that the technique predisposes to interstitial pregnancy and uterine rupture. Hallatt's opinion was based on four cases in a study of 123 repeat ectopic pregnancies.

Basically, a portion of the interstitial tube is removed for the purpose of avoiding a subsequent cornual pregnancy, and properly performed surgery has not resulted in interstitial pregnancies. Another problem with blaming the cornual wedge procedure for subsequent implantations is that it is impossible to determine whether a fertilized ovum entered the peritoneal side of the resected tube or if the ovum traveled to that cornu from the opposite tube.

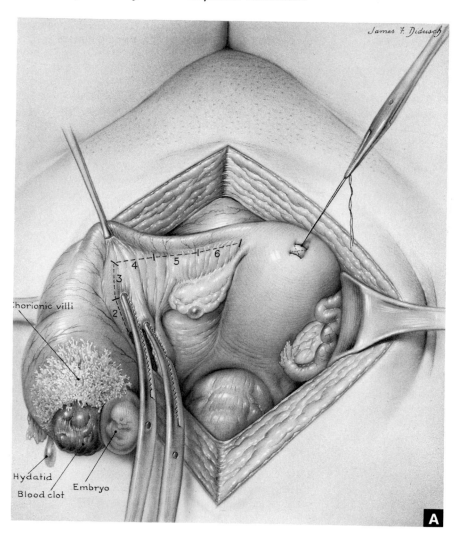

James F. Didusch

Chorionic villi

Hydatid
Blood clot
Embryo

A

FIG. 18–7 Salpingectomy for tubal pregnancy. (*A*) The tube has been delivered, and the mesosalpinx is being clamped and cut, using a succession of Kelly clamps.

TREATMENT FOR INTERSTITIAL PREGNANCY

The choice of treatment for an interstitial cornual pregnancy depends on the extent of trauma that has occurred in the uterine wall and on the interest of the patient in preserving her childbearing function. Cornual resection and repair of the defect can be performed in more than 50% of the cases, while hysterectomy is required in the remainder. Hysterectomy remains the treatment of choice for patients whose pregnancy has advanced to such a stage that repair of the cornu would be technically difficult, time consuming, and medically hazardous.

When extensive resection of the myometrium is required to preserve the uterus, particularly in a patient with extensive intra-abdominal bleeding, the surgical risk is high and the risk of the uterus rupturing in a subsequent pregnancy must be consid-

ered. Efforts to conserve the uterus are reserved for the patient under 35 with a stable surgical condition who is adamant about retaining the option of future childbearing.

Technique of Excision of Interstitial Pregnancy With Salpingo-Oophorectomy

Whenever possible the ovary should be saved, but if the ovary cannot be conserved because of rupture or involvement in the ectopic pregnancy, a salpingo-oophorectomy must be performed (Fig. 18–8). As the ascending uterine vessels are approached near the cornu, they are ligated separately with a figure-of-eight suture. The interstitial pregnancy is excised in a V-shaped manner and the myometrium is approximated with a figure-of-eight closure using No. 1 delayed-absorbable suture (Fig. 18–8B). If it becomes necessary, the round ligament can be cut

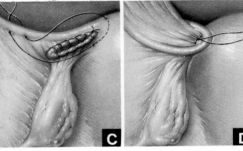

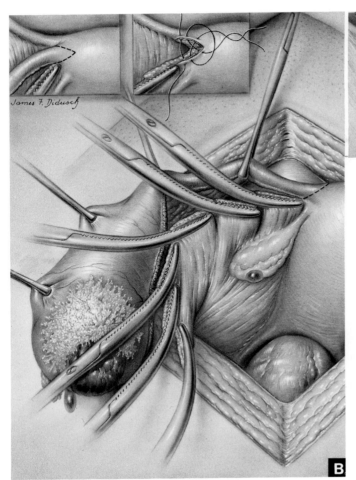

FIG. 18–7 (continued). (B) The mesosalpinx has been completely clamped and cut. The dotted line indicates the line of excision of the tube at the cornu. Insert shows the superficial wedge resection of the interstitial tube and the suture of the excised cornu. (C) The method of placing of mattress suture for peritonization is shown with anchoring of the medial portion of the broad ligament to the uterus, a little posterior and superior to the uterine incision. (D) Peritonization is completed by tying mattress sutures, which brings the broad and the round ligaments over the uterine cornu.

and resutured to the cornu and the uterine serosa using interrupted sutures (Fig. 18–8C). The round and broad ligaments are brought over the incision with mattress sutures (the modified Coffey suspension) (Fig. 18–8D). Additional interrupted sutures of No. 2-0 or No. 3-0 delayed-absorbable material may be used to secure the serosa of the round ligament to the serosa of the uterus in order to maintain the operative site in a permanent retroperitoneal position.

Ovarian Pregnancy

Because IUDs protect the endometrium and, to a certain degree, the proximal oviducts from implantation, future reports of extrauterine pregnancy may show an increased rate of ovarian involvement. Data from the Cooperative Statistical Program of the Population Council show an ovarian pregnancy in 1 out of every 9 ectopic pregnancies that occur among IUD users. Of pregnancies among IUD users, 4.3% are extrauterine.

There have been several reviews in the English-speaking literature on the subject of primary ovarian pregnancy. Boronow and associates summarized 62 cases in a review of the literature between 1950 and 1963. Campbell and associates added 91 cases to the list as of 1973, including 3 new cases of their own, and Pratt–Thomas and associates reported an additional 10 new cases in 1974. Grimes and associates summarized the major reviews in the literature and added 18 cases of primary ovarian pregnancy from the records of 6 hospitals in which the reviews extended through 1980. By combining the data from his review with four other recent reports, Grimes determined that 34 cases of primary ovarian pregnancy occurred among 236,983 deliveries, a rate of 1 ovarian pregnancy in 7,000 deliveries, approximately.

In an intrafollicular pregnancy, the second stage

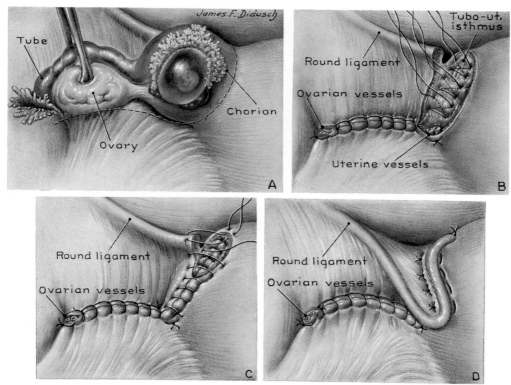

FIG. 18–8 Cornual resection of interstitial pregnancy. (*A*) Dotted line denotes line of excision. (*B*) Tube, ovary, and cornual pregnancy have been excised. Myometrium is being approximated with figure-of-eight sutures of No. 0 delayed-absorbable suture. Note that the uterine vessels have been ligated separately. (*C*) The round ligament, which was cut, is being resutured to the cornu. The ovarian vessels have been ligated, and the broad ligament has been closed with a continuous lock stitch. Serosa of the uterine wound is closed with a simple continuous stitch. (*D*) The cornual wound is covered over with the round and the broad ligaments.

of meiosis, as well as ovum capacitation and fertilization, occur within the follicle. Only 15% of cases of ovarian pregnancy are intrafollicular in origin. In an intrafollicular pregnancy, a well-preserved corpus luteum can be identified in the wall of the gestational sac. Other criteria presented by Spiegelberg for identifying an intrafollicular pregnancy are that: (1) the tube, including the fimbria ovarica, is intact and the tube is clearly separate from the ovary; (2) the gestational sac definitely occupies the normal position of the ovary; (3) the sac is connected with the uterus by the utero-ovarian ligament; and (4) ovarian tissue is unquestionably demonstrated in the wall of the sac.

DIAGNOSIS OF OVARIAN PREGNANCY

The early diagnosis of an ovarian pregnancy is one of the most difficult of all diagnoses relating to extrauterine gestation. Abdominal pain, amenorrhea, and bleeding are common manifestations of a tubal gestation, but chronic pelvic pain is the most frequent clinical manifestation of an ovarian gestation. Although an adnexal mass is palpable in as many as 60% of the patients, the mass is frequently confused with a leaking corpus luteum hematoma.

All of the criteria used for diagnosing a tubal pregnancy are helpful in diagnosing a primary ovarian pregnancy. In particular, the highly sensitive β-hCG radioimmunoassay is very effective for identifying the presence of low levels of hCG. The test can confirm the presence of a gestation process, but knowing the β-hCG level does not help determine the precise location of the gestation. One of the most common pregnancy complications to mimic an ovarian pregnancy is an incomplete spontaneous abortion with a leaking corpus luteum hematoma. In such cases, a dilatation and curettage will show the remnants of trophoblastic villi that are responsible for the low level of β-hCG.

Culdocentesis is also of assistance in confirming that an extrauterine pregnancy exists, but the technique cannot differentiate between a tubal and an ovarian gestation. A tubal pregnancy can easily be ruled out with laparoscopy, but an ovarian pregnancy is still difficult to differentiate by gross appearance from a leaking corpus luteum hematoma. Ultrasonography can be used, but only when an ovarian pregnancy is advanced does the ultrasound image show a gestational sac that would raise the clinical suspicion of an ovarian pregnancy.

A critical analysis of all of the diagnostic studies, especially the sensitive radioimmunoassay for the β-hCG, must be used in making the diagnosis. When the β-hCG is positive, ultrasonography shows no intrauterine gestational sac, and culdocentesis shows free blood in the peritoneal cavity, a laparotomy is needed in order to make a definite diagnosis.

TREATMENT FOR OVARIAN PREGNANCY

Although an ovarian pregnancy usually results in more bleeding, it is still easily confused with a leaking corpus luteum hematoma, and a safe approach is to proceed with surgical resection when either is diagnosed. Unless the diagnosis is made quite late, the ovary can be preserved by a conservative resection of the hemorrhagic portion of the gonad. Only rarely is the hemorrhage so complete that oophorectomy is required to control the bleeding. Even if the last trophoblastic villus cannot be removed in the ovarian resection, the ovary should be preserved. Any remaining trophoblastic tissue will degenerate rapidly and produce no clinical problem.

Abdominal Pregnancy

An abdominal pregnancy is perhaps the rarest, as well as the most serious, type of extrauterine gestation. Reports on the frequency of abdominal pregnancy are variable, ranging from 1 in 3,371 deliveries (Beacham, 1962) to more than 1 in 10,200 deliveries (Rahman, 1982). Strafford and Ragan reported an incidence of 1 abdominal pregnancy in 7,269 deliveries, a representative figure.

Abdominal pregnancies are classified as either primary or secondary. Most abdominal pregnancies are secondary, resulting from early tubal abortion or rupture with secondary implantation of the pregnancy into the peritoneal cavity. To be considered a primary abdominal pregnancy, the pregnancy must meet several criteria defined by Studderford in 1942: (1) Both tubes and ovaries must be in normal condition with no evidence of recent or remote injury; (2) no evidence of uteroperitoneal fistula should be found; and (3) the pregnancy must be related exclusively to the peritoneal surface and must be early enough in the gestation to eliminate the possibility of secondary implantation following primary implantation in the tube.

Friedrich and Rankin reviewed 24 cases of confirmed primary abdominal pregnancies, including a case of his own in which the gestation was less than 12 weeks in duration. Undoubtedly other isolated experiences have occurred, but none have been reported.

Secondary abdominal pregnancy results when a tubal gestation attaches itself to the other viscera as the enlarging placenta spreads through the wall of the tube or is aborted through the fimbriated end. The placenta probably retains some tubal attachment, which supplies blood for the gestation to continue developing in the new peritoneal site. Rare types of secondary abdominal pregnancies have occurred following spontaneous separation of an old cesarean section scar, following uterine perforation during a therapeutic or elective abortion, and after subtotal or total hysterectomy.

DIAGNOSIS OF ABDOMINAL PREGNANCY

The early diagnosis of an abdominal pregnancy is difficult but critical, because a catastrophic hemorrhage can result from separation of the placenta. A history of recurrent abdominal discomfort, fetal movement beneath the abdominal wall, and the presence of fetal movements high in the upper abdomen should alert the clinician to the possibility of an abdominal implantation. Other clinical clues include cessation of fetal movement, vomiting late in pregnancy, fetal malposition, and closed and uneffaced cervix.

Confirmation of the diagnosis requires demonstration of the fetus outside the uterine cavity. If the uterus can be palpated separately from the fetal parts, the abdominal pregnancy can be confirmed either by hysterosalpingography or by the failure of oxytocin to stimulate the gestational mass.

The x-ray finding of fetal small parts in the lateral position overlying the maternal spine was first noted by Weinberg and Sherwin in 1956; the finding is a fairly reliable sign of an abdominal pregnancy. An x-ray examination of the abdomen, including anterior, posterior, and lateral views, is also helpful in defining malposition of the fetus, which is most commonly found in the transverse position.

The most effective method used currently to diagnose an abdominal pregnancy is ultrasound. The ultrasound image can clearly identify the gestation as separate from the nonpregnant uterus. The use of ultrasonography should enhance the diagnostic accuracy in more than two-thirds of the cases.

Maternal mortality rates have varied in the past to 18%. Rahman reported statistics from an Arab population of a 20% maternal mortality among 10 patients with advanced abdominal pregnancy. Recent experience has been more favorable. Clark and Jones reported maternal death estimates from 4% to 10%, and in a review of 10 cases, Delke and associates had no case of maternal mortality, although morbidity was quite high. A high incidence of pelvic abscess, peritonitis, and sepsis results from the remnants of the placenta being retained.

Fetal mortality has been notoriously high, ranging from 75% to 95% of cases. Recent techniques of fetal monitoring have decreased the fetal mortality rate and have served as a diagnostic adjunct in the management of the abdominal pregnancy. Fetal assessment, including repeated sonography to measure biparietal diameter, nonstress testing, monitoring of fetal movements, and contraction stress tests, can provide clinical evidence of fetal maturity and fetal welfare. Despite the use of these diagnostic tools, fetal death occurred in 7 of the 10 cases reported by Delke, while only 3 of the 10 cases reported by Rahman resulted in fetal death. Clark and Jones reported an overall fetal salvage rate of only 11.4% in a study of 35 abdominal pregnancies.

One of the major factors in fetal survival is the condition of the fetal membranes. Should the membrane rupture, the fetus usually dies in the peritoneal cavity within a short time from respiratory distress. A very high incidence of fetal anomalies (35%–75%) also results from abdominal pregnancies, including facial and joint deformities, torticollis, and hypoplasia of the extremities. These are thought to be related to the extrauterine environment of the fetus.

Management of the placenta remains a controversial issue. Most clinicians feel the best treatment is to clamp the cord, leave the placenta in situ, close the abdomen, but allow retroperitoneal drainage if possible. The placenta can be removed after complete cessation of function, as determined by quantitative hCG titers. The placenta should be removed during laparotomy only if it is accessible and if its removal can be accomplished without excessive blood loss. When all functioning stops, the circulation has undergone fibrosis. When in doubt, leave the placenta in place and await sclerosis of its blood supply. Thompson reports leaving a placenta in the peritoneal cavity for a period of 13 years without physical harm to the patient. Methotrexate has been used on occasion to hasten trophoblastic degeneration, which is determined by serial hCG titers.

Other Forms of Ectopic Pregnancy

COMBINED PREGNANCY

Coexistent intrauterine and extrauterine pregnancies were described by Duverney in 1708. In 1966, Felbo and Fenger collected a total of 523 reported cases. More recently, Reece and associates reviewed the literature from 1966 to 1979 and provided 66 new cases, including 5 cases from the Sloane Hospital for Women, bringing the total to 589 cases reported in the recent literature. In the past, combined intrauterine and extrauterine gestations have occurred in approximately 1 in 30,000 pregnancies. The increasing incidence of ectopic pregnancies may mean that the incidence of combined pregnancy is now higher, perhaps as many as 1 in 15,000 live births.

Although the precise cause of a combined pregnancy is frequently obscured, most of the factors are the same as those associated with ectopic pregnancy. Recently the use of ovulation-inducing agents has greatly increased the incidence of multiple gestations and combined pregnancies. Berger and Taymore reported an incidence of combined pregnancy of as many as 1 in 100 stimulated patients. Still, the most common anatomical finding associated with combined pregnancies is pelvic inflammatory disease.

The combination of abdominal pain, adnexal mass, peritoneal irritation, and an enlarged uterus are the major clinical features associated with a combined pregnancy. Additional diagnostic findings include: (1) the presence of two corpora lutea found at the time of laparotomy or laparoscopy; (2) hematoperitoneum; (3) acute abdominal pain following the termination of an intrauterine pregnancy; or (4) the persistence of an enlarged uterus with amenorrhea after excision of an ectopic pregnancy. Continued enlargement of the uterus and a positive pregnancy test after treatment of an ectopic pregnancy confirms the diagnosis.

Treatment of Combined Pregnancy

The major problem in the management of a combined pregnancy concerns the timing of the termination, especially if both fetuses are alive and have reached the stage of midpregnancy. In a review of the world's literature, Reece and associates found only 13 cases in which both pregnancies reached term and in which both infants were delivered and survived the neonatal period. Although fetal mortality rates have ranged from 20% to 70% for the intrauterine pregnancy, the extrauterine gestation has a mortality rate higher than 90%. Recent experience has shown a marked improvement for the survival of the intrauterine pregnancy. Little information is available on the growth and development of infants who survive the neonatal period, but the incidence of congenital malformations and mental retardation is increased because of hypotension from the extrauterine pregnancy. Maternal mortality has also been reduced with recent aggressive medical management to a rate of 0.98%.

CERVICAL PREGNANCY

The cervix is a rare but hazardous site for placental implantation because the trophoblast can penetrate through the cervical wall and into the uterine blood supply. Cervical gestations have received little attention in the literature until recently, but an increased awareness of the condition has resulted in a number of recent reports. The number of reported cases now exceeds 300.

The criteria for the diagnosis of cervical pregnancy were established initially by Rubin in 1911: (1) There must be cervical glands opposite the placental attachment; (2) the attachment of the placenta to the cervix must be situated below the entrance of the uterine vessels or below the peritoneal re-

flection of the anterior and posterior surfaces of the uterus; and (3) fetal elements must not be present in the corpus uteri. A determination of whether Rubin's criteria were met was difficult without a complete study of the entire uterus, so Paalman and McElin proposed more practical clinical criteria for the diagnosis of this condition: (1) Uterine bleeding without cramping pain following a period of amenorrhea; (2) a soft, enlarged cervix equal to or larger than the fundus—the so-called hourglass uterus; (3) products of conception entirely confined within and firmly attached to the endocervix; (4) a closed internal cervical os; and (5) a partially opened external os.

The incidence of this rare entity varies; the Mayo Clinic reported 1 in 16,000 pregnancies. The highest incidence of 1 in 1,000 pregnancies was reported from Japan. The high incidence of elective abortion in Japan is probably a factor in the higher rates, and cervical pregnancy may increase in frequency in the United States with the increased use of elective abortion. Other investigators have found a high incidence of antecedent curettage.

Cervical gestations are frequently confused with a neoplastic process because of the marked vascularity and friable appearance of the cervix. Pro-

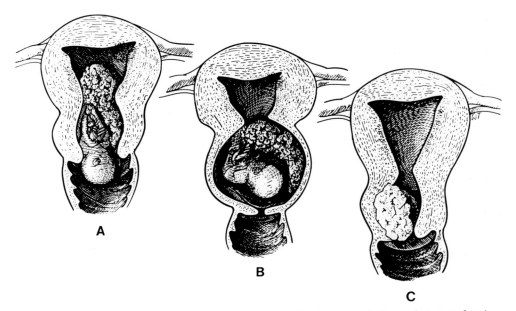

FIG. 18–9 Differential diagnosis of cervical pregnancy. (*A*) In the cervical phase of uterine abortion, the placenta is mainly within the expanded cervix, and the external and internal ora are dilated. (*B*) In a cervical abortion (abortion into the cervix) due to stenosis of the external os, spontaneous rupture of the cervical wall may cause severe hemorrhage. (*C*) Ragged, friable cervix seen in cervical pregnancy mimics that of carcinoma of the cervix. (Roth DJ, Birnbaum SJ: Cervical pregnancy: Diagnosis and management. Obstet Gynecol 42:675, 1973.)

fuse bleeding may occur if the placenta is mistaken for a tumor and a biopsy taken. The gestation is also mistaken for a spontaneous abortion with the assumption that the products of conception were retained within the cervical canal (Fig. 18–9).

The serum pregnancy test for β-hCG may be used, but the diagnosis is more firmly established with ultrasonography. The gestational sac with or without the fetus can be located below the internal cervical os. If the uterine cavity is empty, the distorted cervical canal becomes clearly visible with the ultrasound. As is true for other types of gestation, both intrauterine and extrauterine, the accuracy of ultrasound depends on the duration of the pregnancy and the experience of the ultrasonographer.

Treatment of Cervical Pregnancy

The treatment of a cervical pregnancy is surgical; the condition usually requires an abdominal hysterectomy. Since a true cervical pregnancy is incompatible with a viable fetus, the abnormal implantation will usually produce symptoms within the first trimester. Although conservative evacuation of a very early cervical pregnancy has been accomplished by a skillful dilatation and curettage, as documented by Whittle, the procedure is complicated by profuse hemorrhage, which usually necessitates an abdominal hysterectomy. Mortimer recommends that conservative measures should never be attempted if the gestation is beyond 8 weeks.

Bibliography

Adhesion Study Group: Reduction of postoperative pelvic adhesions with intraperitoneal 32% Dextran 70: A prospective randomized clinical trial. Fertil Steril 40:612, 1983

Arias–Stella J: Atypical endometrial changes associated with the presence of chorionic tissue. Arch Pathol 58:112, 1954

Ashley DJB, Lloyd MI: Coexisting ovarian and uterine pregnancy. J Obstet Gynaec Br Commonw 73:152, 1966

Auslender R, Arodi J, Pascal B, Abramovici H: Interstitial pregnancy: Early diagnosis by ultrasonography. Am J Obstet Gynecol 146:717, 1983

Aznar R, Berry CL, Cooke ID, et al: Ectopic pregnancy rates in IUD users. Brit Med J (6115):785, March 25, 1978

Barnes AB, Grover JW, Sudduth SS: Simultaneous intra- and extra-uterine pregnancy: Report of a case. Obstet Gynecol 31:50, 1968

Beacham WD, Hernquist WC, Beacham DW, et al: Abdominal pregnancy at Charity Hospital in New Orleans. Am J Obstet Gynecol 84:1257, 1962

Beral V: An epidemiological study of recent trends in ectopic pregnancy. Br J Obstet Gynaecol 82:775, 1975

Berger MJ, Taymore ML: Simultaneous intrauterine and tubal pregnancies following ovulation induction. Am J Obstet Gynecol 113(2):812, 1972

Bernstein D, Holzinger M, Ovadia J, Frishman B: Conservative treatment of cervical pregnancy. Obstet Gynecol 58:741, 1981

Boronow RC, McElin TW, West RH, et al: Ovarian pregnancy: A report of 4 cases and a 13-year survey of the English literature. Am J Obstet Gynecol 91:1095, 1965

Breen JL: A 21 year survey of 654 ectopic pregnancies. Am J Obstet Gynecol 106:1004, 1970

Bronson RA: Tubal pregnancy and infertility. Fertil Steril 28:226, 1977

Bruhat MA, Manhes H, Mage G, et al: Treatment of ectopic pregnancy by means of laparoscopy. Fertil Steril 33:411, 1980

Campbell JS, Hacquebard S, Mitton DM, et al: Acute hemoperitoneum, IUD, and occult ovarian pregnancy. Obstet Gynecol 43:438, 1974

Centers for Disease Control: Ectopic Pregnancy Surveillance, 1970–1978. July 1982

Clark AD, McMillan JA: Maternal death due to primary peritoneal pregnancy. J Obstet Gynaecol Br Commonw 81:652, 1974

Clark JFJ, Bryant W: Chronic ectopic pregnancy. J Natl Med Assoc 67:118, 1975

Clark JFJ, Jones SA: Advanced ectopic pregnancy. J Reprod Med 14:30, 1975

Cullen TS: New sign in ruptured extrauterine pregnancy. Am J Obstet Gynecol 78:457, 1918

DeCherney A, Kase N: Conservative surgical management of unruptured ectopic pregnancy. Obstet Gynecol 54:451, 1979

DeCherney AH, Romero R, Naftholin F: Surgical management of unruptured ectopic pregnancy. Fertil Steril 35:21, 1981

Delke I, Veridiano NP, Tancer ML: Abdominal pregnancy: Review of current management and addition of 10 cases. Obstet Gynecol 60:200, 1982

Dougherty RE, Diddle AW: Intrafollicular ovarian pregnancy: Management with ovarian conservation. Obstet Gynecol 33:20, 1969

Ellis RW: Ovarian pregnancy. Obstet Gynecol 14:54, 1959

Falk HC, Hassid R, Dazo EP: Tubal pregnancy: A report of a very early luminal form of imbedding. Obstet Gynecol 45:215, 1975

Felbo M, Fenger HJ: Combined extra- and intrauterine pregnancy carried to term. Acta Obstet Gynecol Scand 45:140, 1966

Felmus L, Pedowitz P: Interstitial pregnancy. Am J Obstet Gynecol 66:1271, 1981

Fienberg R, Lloyd HED: The Arias–Stella reaction in early normal pregnancy: An involutional phenomenon. Hum Pathol 5:183, 1974

Foster HW, Moore DT: Abdominal pregnancy: Report of 12 cases. Obstet Gynecol 30:249, 1967

Friedrich EG, Rankin CA: Primary pelvic peritoneal pregnancy. Obstet Gynecol 31:649, 1968

Gray CL, Ruffolo EH: Ovarian pregnancy associated with intrauterine contraceptive devices. Am J Obstet Gynecol 132:134, 1978

Grech P, D'Sa, ALM: Radiological diagnosis of advanced extrauterine pregnancy. Br J Radiol 38:848, 1965

Grimes HG, Nosal RA, Gallagher JC: Ovarian pregnancy: A series of 24 cases. Obstet Gynecol 61:174, 1983

Hall J St E: Retroperitoneal ectopic pregnancy. J Obstet Gynaecol Br Commonw 80:92, 1973

Hallatt JG: Repeat ectopic pregnancy: A study of 123 conservative cases. Am J Obstet Gynecol 122:520, 1975

Hertz RH, Timor–Tritsch I, Sokol RJ, et al: Diagnostic studies and fetal assessment in advanced extrauterine pregnancy. Obstet Gynecol (Suppl) 50:62, 1977

Holtz G, Baker ER: Inhibition of peritoneal adhesion reformation after lysis with thirty-two percent Dextran 70. Fertil Steril 34:394, 1980

Holtz G, Kling OR: Effect of surgical technique on peritoneal adhesion reformation after lysis. Fertil Steril 37:494, 1982

Hreshchyshyn MM, Naples JD, Jr, Randall CL: Amethopterin in abdominal pregnancy. Am J Obstet Gynecol 93:286, 1965

Hussa RO: Clinical utility of human chorionic gonadotropin and α-subunit measurements. Obstet Gynecol 60:1, 1982

Ishida Y, de Ungria P, Correnti NA: Ovarian pregnancy. South Med J 66:731, 1973

Järvinen PA, Nummi S, Pietila K: Conservative operative treatment of tubal pregnancy with postoperative daily hydrotubations. Acta Obstet Gynecol Scan 51:169, 1972

Jolly GF, Norman RM: Co-existing intra- and extrauterine pregnancy associated with cerebral malformation in the surviving twin. J Obstet Gynaecol Br Commonw 72:125, 1965

Kadar N, DeVore G, Romero R: Discriminatory hCG zone: Its use in the sonographic evaluation for ectopic pregnancy. Obstet Gynecol 58:156, 1981

Kalchman GG, Meltzer RM: Interstitial pregnancy following homolateral salpingectomy: Report of 2 cases and review of literature. Am J Obstet Gynecol 96:1139, 1966

Kassab AY: Concurrent ovarian and normal intrauterine pregnancy. Br J Obstet Gynaecol 82:77, 1975

Kelly HA: Operative Gynecology. Vol. II, New York, I. Appleton Co, p. 453, 1898

Kuppuswami N, Vindekilde J, Sethi CM, et al: Diagnosis and treatment of cervical pregnancy. Obstet Gynecol 61:651, 1983

Langer R, Bukovsky I, Herman A, et al: Conservative surgery for tubal pregnancy. Fertil Steril 38:427, 1982

Last PA: Pregnancy and the intrauterine contraceptive device. Contraception 9:439, 1974

————: Pregnancy and intrauterine device. Lancet 1:877, 1974

Lehfeldt H, Tietze C, Gorstein F: Ovarian pregnancy and the intrauterine device. Am J Obstet Gynecol 108:1005, 1970

Levi S, Leblicq P: The diagnostic value of ultrasonography in 342 suspected cases of ectopic pregnancy. Acta Obstet Gynecol Scand 59:29, 1980

Levin AA, Schoenbaum SC, Stubblefield PG, et al: Ectopic pregnancy and prior induced abortion. Am J Public Health 72:253, 1982

Mashiach S, Carp HJA, Serr DM: Nonoperative management of ectopic pregnancy: A preliminary report. J Reprod Med 27:127, 1982

Mastroianni L, Jr: Conservative management in ectopic pregnancy. In Garcia CR, Mastroianni L, Jr, Amelar RD, et al (eds): Current Therapy of Infertility. Trenton, NJ, BC Decker, 1983

McElin TW, Iffy L: Ectopic gestation: A consideration of new and controversial issues relating to pathogenesis and management. In Wynn RM (ed): Obstetric and Gynecological Annual. New York, Appleton–Century–Crofts, 1976

Mead PJ, Smith GL, Rubell D: Cervical implantation of an ectopic pregnancy: Two case reports. Texas Med 74:61, 1978

Mortimer CW, Aiken DA: Cervical pregnancy. J Obstet Gynaecol Br Commonw 75:741, 1968

Nylander PPS, Akande EO, Ogunbode O: Simultaneous advanced extrauterine and intrauterine pregnancy. Int J Gynecol Obstet 9:102, 1971

Ory HW: Women's health study: Ectopic pregnancy and intrauterine contraceptive devices: New perspectives. Obstet Gynecol 57:137, 1981

Paalman R, McElin T: Cervical pregnancy. Am J Obstet Gynecol 77:1261, 1959

Parente JT, Chau–Su OU, Levy J, et al: Cervical pregnancy analysis: A review and report of five cases. Obstet Gynecol 62:79, 1983

Parry JS: Extrauterine Pregnancy. Philadelphia, Lea, 1876

Pauerstein CJ, Hodgson BJ, Kramen MA: The Anatomy and Physiology of the Fallopian Tube. In Wynn RM (Ed).: Obstet Gynecol Annual Vol 3. Norwalk, Conn, Appleton-Century-Crofts, 1974

Polak JO, Wolfe SA: A further study of the origin of uterine bleeding in tubal pregnancy. Am Obstet Gynecol 8:730, 1924

Pratt–Thomas HR, White L, Messer HH: Primary ovarian pregnancy: Presentation of ten cases, including one full-term pregnancy. South Med J 67:920, 1974

Rahman MS, Al-Suleiman SA, Rahman Al-Sibai MH: Advanced abdominal pregnancy. Obstet Gynecol 59:366, 1982

Ranade V, Palermino D, Tronik B: Cervical pregnancy. Obstet Gynecol 51:502, 1978

Raskin MM: Diagnosis of cervical pregnancy by ultrasound, a case report. Am J Obstet Gynecol 130:234, 1978

Reece EA, Petrie RH, Sirmans MF, et al: Combined intrauterine and extrauterine gestations: A review. Am J Obstet Gynecol 146:323, 1983

Reeves CP, Savarese MFR: Simultaneous intra- and extra-uterine pregnancies. Obstet Gynecol 4:492, 1954

Richards S, Stempel L, Carlton B: Heterotopic pregnancy: Reappraisal of incidence. Am J Obstet Gynecol 142:928, 1982

Rimdusit P, Kasatri N: Primary ovarian pregnancy and the intrauterine contraceptive device. Obstet Gynecol (Suppl) 48:57, 1976

Rothe DJ, Birnbaum SJ: Cervical pregnancy: Diagnosis and management. Obstet Gynecol 42:675, 1973

Rubin IC: Cervical pregnancy. Surg Gynecol Obstet 13:625, 1911

Rubin GL, Peterson HB, Dorfman SF et al: Ectopic pregnancy in the United States 1970 through 1978. JAMA 249:1725, 1983

Saxena BB, Landesman R: The use of radioreceptor assay of human chorionic gonadotropin for the diagnosis and management of ectopic pregnancy. Fertil Steril 26:397, 1975

Schenker JG, Evron S: New concepts in the surgical management of tubal pregnancy and the consequent postoperative results. Fertil Steril 40:709, 1983

Schneider J, Berger CJ, Cattell C: Maternal mortality due to ectopic pregnancy: A review of 102 deaths. Obstet Gynecol 49:557, 1977

Schwartz RO, DiPietro DL: β-hCG as a diagnostic aid for suspected ectopic pregnancy. Obstet Gynecol 56:197, 1980

Scott JW, Diggory PLC, Edelman PJ: Management of cervical pregnancy with circumsuture and intracervical obturator. Br Med J 1 April:825, 1978

Seppala M, Ranta T, Rutanen EM, et al: Improved diagnosis of pregnancy-related gynaecological emergencies by rapid human chorionic gonadotropin beta-subunit assay. Brit J Obstet Gynaecol 88:138, 1981

Shoen JA, Nowak RJ: Repeat ectopic pregnancy: A 16-year clinical survey. Obstet Gynecol 45:542, 1975

Smith M, Vessey MP, Bounds W, et al: Progestogen-only oral contraception and ectopic gestation. Br Med J 4:104, 1974

Spiegelberg O: Zur Casuistik den Ovarial-Schwangenschaft. Arch Gynaek 13:73, 1878

Stangel JJ, Gomel V: Techniques in conservative surgery for tubal gestation. Clin Obstet Gynecol 23:1221, 1980

Stangel JJ, Reyniak JV, Stone ML: Conservative surgical management of tubal pregnancy. Obstet Gynecol 48:241, 1976

Strafford JC, Ragan WD: Abdominal pregnancy; Review of current management. Obstet Gynecol 50:548, 1977

Stromme WB: Salpingotomy for tubal pregnancy: Report of a successful case. Obstet Gynecol 1:472, 1953

————: Conservative surgery for ectopic pregnancy: a twenty-year review. Obstet Gynecol 41:215, 1973

Studderford WE: Primary peritoneal pregnancy. Am J Obstet Gynecol 44:487, 1942

Swolin K: Electromicrosurgery and salpingostomy: Long term results. Am J Obstet Gynecol 121:418, 1975

Swolin K, Fall M: Ectopic pregnancy. Acta Eur Fertil 3:147, 1972

Szeja ZJ, Rahaghi A, Rentz FP: Ultrasound diagnosis of cervical pregnancy. Am J Obstet Gynecol 136:416, 1980

Tait RL: Pathology and treatment of extrauterine pregnancy. Br Med J 2:317, 1884

Tatum HJ, Schmidt FH: Contraceptive and sterilization practices and extrauterine pregnancy: A realistic perspective. Fertil Steril 28:407, 1977

Thompson LR: Abdominal pregnancy at term with late removal of placenta. Am J Surg 111:272, 1966

Timonen S, Nieminen U: Tubal pregnancy, choice of operative method of treatment. Acta Obstet Scand 46:327, 1967

Varga L, Obolensky W, Scheidegger S: Ovarian pregnancy and the intrauterine device. Int J Fertil 17:142, 1972

Vessey MP, Johnson B, Doll R, et al: Outcome of pregnancy in women using an intrauterine device. Lancet 1:495, 1974

Webster A, Price JJ: Cervical pregnancy. Am J Obstet Gynecol 99:134, 1967

Weinberg A, Sherwin AS: A new sign in roentgen diagnosis of advanced ectopic pregnancy. Obstet Gynecol 7:99, 1956

Westrom L: Effect of acute pelvic inflammatory disease on fertility. Am J Obstet Gynecol 121:707, 1975

Whittle MJ: Cervical pregnancy management by local excision. Br Med J 2:795, 1976

Winston RML: Microsurgery and the fallopian tube: From fantasy to reality. Fertil Steril 34:521, 1981

Chapter 19

The Intestinal Tract in Relation to Gynecology

Larry C. Carey, M.D., and
Peter J. Fabri, M.D.

The gynecologist may encounter disease of the gastrointestinal tract in four ways. First, postoperative complications of gynecologic surgery frequently involve the intestinal tract; intestinal obstruction, adynamic ileus, and fistula formation may be imposing problems. Second, primary gastrointestinal disease may mimic pelvic disease. Acute intra-abdominal and intrapelvic disorders may be quite difficult to differentiate preoperatively; appendicitis, Meckel's diverticulum, colon diverticulitis, and volvulus may appear to be acute gynecologic disorders. Third, primary gastrointestinal disease may be encountered during pelvic surgery. Such disease includes regional enteritis, occult colon carcinoma, or colon diverticulitis. Fourth, primary gynecologic disorders may involve the gastrointestinal tract. These disorders include intestinal obstruction from tubo-ovarian abscess, endometriosis, or pelvic cancer.

The following discussion outlines the diagnosis and treatment of the more common gastrointestinal diseases that the gynecologic surgeon is likely to encounter.

Postoperative Complications Involving the Gastrointestinal Tract

INTESTINAL OBSTRUCTION

Etiologically, adhesive bands, groin hernias, or neoplasms of the bowel account for more than 80% of all intestinal obstructions. Other causes, such as intra-abdominal abscess, volvulus, intussusception, gallstone ileus, and congenital disorders, occur less frequently. Review of the recent literature shows small bowel obstruction from adhesions to be increasing, whereas small bowel obstruction from hernias is decreasing. Undoubtedly, the increasing enthusiasm for hernia repair is in part responsible for this trend, as is the increasing frequency of pelvic surgery. Intestinal obstruction caused by adhesions frequently follows gynecologic surgery, where the dependent position of the female reproductive tract provides a favorable operative site for bowel adherence and possible obstruction.

Pathophysiology

Increased understanding of the pathophysiology of intestinal obstruction has led to great improvement in survival rate. Forty years ago, mortality of 40% to 60% was not uncommon. Presently, there is a mortality rate between 10% and 20% for all patients with obstruction of the small intestine. If we could choose a single factor to alter to further reduce mortality, it would be to lessen the delay between onset of symptoms and surgical intervention. Few diseases not involving overt hemorrhage are as adversely influenced by delays in treatment as intestinal obstruction. The difference between simply dividing an adhesive band to relieve an early obstruction and resecting two feet of black, gangrenous, perforated ileum in the presence of extensive peritonitis and gram-negative shock may be as little as 12 hours in time.

Older patients have a greater tendency to ignore the discomfort of intestinal obstruction and to delay in seeking medical advice. The need for prompt action by the physician dealing with intestinal obstruction is clear. If inordinate patient delay has occurred, the need for physician haste is even greater. The adage, "One never goes to bed on intestinal obstruction," is well conceived.

Obstruction of the small intestine causes distention, which occurs as a result of fluid collection proximal to the obstruction. But of much greater importance is swallowed air. Well over 70% of the air in the gastrointestinal tract is swallowed. In his classic experiments, Wangensteen showed that animals could survive for long periods with complete small bowel obstruction if the esophagus was simultaneously ligated to prevent air swallowing. The tension on the surface of a cylinder is proportional to the diameter and intraluminal pressure (Laplace's Law). Since the veins and arteries enter the intestinal wall tangentially, the tension on them increases rapidly with distention. The veins, having the lower pressure of the two, show the effect of the increase in tension first. As they are stretched, resistance in them increases, and flow slows. Fluid rich in protein and salt begins to exude from the capillaries. Edema is the result. Intraluminal fluid accumulation increases from both decreased absorption and active secretion. Blood cells begin to escape from the capillaries, venous flow finally stops, arterial flow continues, blood accumulates in the wall and in the lumen of the bowel, gangrene occurs, intestinal integrity is lost, and peritonitis quickly follows.

The effect of increased intraluminal pressure on absorption and secretion from the human ileum was measured in volunteers who had ileostomies. Absorption of test solution was found to increase at moderate elevation of intraluminal pressures, but at pressures three or four times normal, the absorption begins to decrease. Conversely, secretion of fluids into the lumen steadily increased as the pressure rose. These findings indicate that increased secretion is the primary cause of vascular fluid loss and that decreased absorption plays a lesser role.

The total volume of daily secretions into the normal gastrointestinal tract is estimated to be about 10 liters. As much as 7 to 8 liters of fluid can easily be sequestered in the bowel with intestinal obstruction.

The important effects of nonstrangulating obstruction and its progression to peritonitis have been studied in detail by both Wangensteen and Sperling. Stagnant bowel contents in a distended loop of ileum show an increase in the number of bacteria. As long as the mucosa is intact and viable, the bacteria are harmless. However, increased intraluminal pressure for a sustained period will produce patchy areas of necrosis that allow some of the intestinal contents to escape into the peritoneal cavity. The main avenue of sepsis from intestinal obstruction is absorption from the peritoneal cavity and not the venous and lymphatic drainage system.

Diagnosis

Intestinal obstruction is characterized by sudden onset of crampy abdominal pain. Vomiting may be associated with the first symptoms and then may stop, only to start again as the obstruction persists. The pain is periodic, with pain-free intervals longer than the periods of pain. The pain is classically periumbilical.

Initial inspection of the abdomen may show little abnormality. As obstruction persists, distention will occur. In the very thin patient, loops of intestine can be seen beneath the abdominal wall, and peristalsis may be visible. The characteristic bowel sounds of obstruction are high-pitched, tinkling, or metallic and may occasionally be heard without a stethoscope. These sounds reflect the existence of the air-fluid interface. Motility with violent bursts of peristalsis occurs proximal to the obstruction. The duration of quiet intervals between bursts of peristalsis may suggest the level of obstruction; in high obstruction, the time may be 3 to 5 minutes, while in low obstruction it may be 10 to 15 minutes.

Palpation in the early stage of the disease may disclose no tenderness. As distention progresses, it is usual to find tenderness over the point of obstruction. One must remember that distended loops of bowel are painful when disturbed, so vigorous examination may produce misleading signs. The intraluminal pressure, normally 2 mm Hg to 4 mm Hg in small bowel, may reach 30 mm Hg with vigorous peristalsis. Pressures of over 30 mm Hg cause lymphatic and capillary stasis. Any evidence of peritoneal irritation should sound the alarm to consider obstruction or strangulation, and plans for operative intervention should begin. Strangulation occurs secondary to adhesive bands (60%), strangulated hernia (25%), volvulus (12%), and mesenteric thrombosis (2%).

Laboratory tests are helpful, frequently indicate hypovolemia and, specifically, plasma volume loss. An increase in the hematocrit level, with high urine osmolality and normal serum osmolality, are common findings. The presence of leukocytosis is distressing, and levels of over 15,000/mm³ after hydration suggest strangulation. Metabolic acidosis is an ominous sign and may indicate dead bowel, as may thrombocytopenia or hyponatremia.

X-ray evidence of small bowel obstruction must be interpreted in light of clinical findings. If clinical evidence points toward intestinal obstruction and x-ray examination shows distended bowel with air-fluid levels, the diagnosis is confirmed. Early in the course of the disease the roentgenograms may be of little diagnostic assistance. Lo, Evans, and Carey reported in their Milwaukee series that in only 60% of their cases was the conclusive diagnosis made preoperatively by abdominal x-ray examination. Late in intestinal obstruction, as the bowel becomes filled with fluid, air-fluid levels may be few or even absent. The importance of an upright or lateral decubitus film cannot be overstressed. Supine films of the abdomen may be of no benefit and, indeed, may be misleading. Contrast material may be helpful in distinguishing adynamic ileus from obstruction. Recent reports advocate the use of thin barium suspensions rather than the more irritating water-soluble media. If the contrast material has not reached the cecum within 6 hours, small bowel obstruction rather than ileus is likely.

Preoperative Preparation

Correction of existing hypovolemia is the keystone of preoperative preparation for surgery for small bowel obstruction. It has been shown that nearly 50% of the plasma volume and 30% of the blood volume may be sequestered in the bowel in intestinal obstruction. Blood pressure, pulse rate, clinical appearance, central venous pressure, hematocrit, urinary output, and urine and plasma osmolality are all helpful in evaluating the degree of hypovolemia. Central venous pressure and hematocrit, along with pulse and urinary output, should be monitored as fluid replacement is accomplished with balanced salt solution, whole blood, and solutions containing protein. If a specific electrolyte disturbance exists (e.g., hypochloremic alkalosis in high intestinal obstruction), it should be corrected. Usually, the loss of extracellular fluid with normal electrolyte concentration results in no apparent electrolyte disturbance. As soon as central venous pressure, pulse rate, and urinary output indicate that intravascular volume is adequately replaced, surgery should be begun.

Preoperative antibiotics are useful, especially when strangulated obstruction is suspected. Significant advances in antibiotic therapy have resulted in dramatic change in the first-line antibiotics for this situation. Any agent chosen should have a wide bacteriostatic or bactericidal spectrum of activity for both aerobic and anaerobic organisms. Recent data suggest that the parenteral administration of antibiotics with a spectrum that covers aerobic as well as anaerobic organisms increases the tolerance of the intestine to ischemia and may delay the onset of full-thickness necrosis of the intestinal wall. On the basis of this observation, most authorities would recommend preoperative broad-spectrum antibiotics for all patients as soon as a diagnosis of intestinal obstruction is made.

Operative Procedure

The incision should allow exploration of the entire abdomen. If possible, the incision should not be made over a previous one because the obstructing adhesion may be directly under a previous incision, and injury to the bowel may be difficult to avoid.

After the peritoneum has been opened, a loop of collapsed bowel should be located and followed until the point of obstruction is found. Nondistended bowel is much easier to handle and less susceptible to injury, and the point of obstruction is more easily identified in this manner. Unless the patient's condition is grave, all adhesions should be taken down and loops of bowel returned to the peritoneal cavity. Great care should be used in taking down the adhesions. Only the gloved hand should handle the intestine and the use of sponges or laparotomy pads should be avoided. Sharp dissection is the only safe method of dispensing with adhesions. The ease with which distended bowel can be torn may come as a disastrous surprise to the neophyte. If the bowel is injured, it should be repaired with interrupted No. 4-0 silk sutures. Rents in the serosa are not dangerous, and there is no need to repair serosal tears unless the mucosa is injured. In fact, current evidence suggests that repaired serosal injuries actually enhance the likelihood of postoperative adhesion formation.

Distinguishing between viable and nonviable bowel may be extremely difficult. All obviously necrotic bowel should be resected. If areas of questionable viability remain, reexploration after 24 hours may be necessary to ascertain that no necrotic intestine has been overlooked. Clinical factors such as color, peristalsis, serosal appearance, and consistency are not reliable, although brisk bleeding from the cut end of the bowel may help in determining viability. Several intraoperative adjuncts may be helpful in identifying safe margins of intestine with blood supply adequate to support an anastomosis. Doppler apparatus and intravenous fluorescein have received the greatest attention. Intraoperative use of a hand-held Doppler instrument along the antimesenteric border of the intestine will identify the sounds of characteristic arterial pulsatile flow. Areas of bowel with intact antimesenteric pulsations will have a blood supply adequate to support an intestinal anastomosis. However, some areas of bowel without audible Doppler signals may still be suitable. For this reason, the use of intravenous fluorescein is recommended in patients in whom major segments of bowel must be removed. One thousand milligrams of sterile fluorescein (1500 mg in dark-complected patients) is administered intravenously. After approximately 10 minutes, the lights in the operating room are extinguished and a Wood's lamp is used to induce fluorescence of the bowel. Patches less than 2 cm in diameter that do not demonstrate fluorescence can safely be left in place but should not be included in the areas of anastomosis. By using the fluorescein technique, the minimum amount of bowel is resected, which may make the difference in preventing a short bowel syndrome. Even with the use of Doppler and fluorescein, there should be a high index of suspicion for reinfarction. A second-look procedure should be used when there is clinical suspicion of intestinal necrosis.

Nonoperative Treatment

In general, there are three circumstances in which nonoperative treatment for intestinal obstruction should be considered. Patients with known widespread intra-abdominal cancer may sometimes be successfully treated by using intestinal intubation (Miller-Abbott or Cantòr tube). Occasionally, a patient who has had several operative procedures for intestinal obstruction and who is known to have dense intra-abdominal adhesions may also be treated best nonoperatively. Last, patients who develop obstructions in the early postoperative period are candidates for a trial of nonsurgical treatment.

If nonoperative treatment is chosen, one of the long, small intestinal tubes should be used. Our preference is the Miller-Abbott tube with a balloon containing 2 ml mercury. A nasogastric tube is passed simultaneously and connected to intermittent suction to avoid continued distention from air swallowing. The long tube is not connected to suction, since this will often interfere with its passage. Frequent roentgenograms will demonstrate the progress of the tube through the pylorus. Frequently, the mercury bag will remain in the stomach even when the patient is optimally positioned. In this circumstance, it is desirable to bring the patient to the radiology department for directed advancement of the tube with fluoroscopic control. Once the mercury bag has passed the pylorus, appropriate positioning of the patient should result in continued passage through the duodenum into the small intestine. After passing the ligament of Treitz the tube may be attached to intermittent suction. Continued use of the nasogastric tube may be beneficial, but it may be discontinued if adequate

bowel decompensation is being accomplished with the long tube.

Careful surveillance must be maintained for the previously described signs of strangulation (*i.e.*, leukocytosis, metabolic acidosis, or loss of bowel sounds). If they are discovered, operative intervention must proceed immediately.

ADYNAMIC ILEUS

Some degree of adynamic ileus occurs after every intra-abdominal operation and with any intra-abdominal inflammation. The rate of recovery of motor function depends on the extent of handling of bowel, the length of operation, the extent of chemical or bacterial peritonitis, and the underlying disease. After abdominal operations, the patient usually becomes hungry and begins to pass flatus on about the third postoperative day. If the patient is not interested in eating, denies flatus, and the abdomen is distended, further diagnostic studies may be in order. X-ray evidence of adynamic ileus shows distention of both small and large bowel with scattered air fluid levels. The treatment consists of correction of electrolyte imbalance, if present. Both low potassium and low sodium can cause bowel atony, as can hypomagnesemia or severe protein depletion. The possibility of intra-abdominal localized inflammation or a leaking anastomosis must be considered. Otherwise, nasogastric decompression, ambulation, and, occasionally, localized intestinal stimulation by rectal suppositories may be helpful. Postoperative ileus rarely fails to respond to nonoperative measures.

INTESTINAL FISTULAS

Fistula formation, one of the more difficult problems associated with intra-abdominal surgery, is often associated with a technical error in intestinal anastomosis, para-anastomotic abscess, or an anastomosis with the use of diseased bowel. Broadening the scope of gynecologic surgery to include radical pelvic dissection has greatly increased the frequency with which the gynecologist encounters fistulas of the intestinal tract. Previous irradiation damage to the intestine compounds the problem, greatly increasing the risk of fistula development.

The first priority in the management of a patient with a suspected fistula is to evaluate and control the underlying septic process. Patients with uncontrolled sepsis should undergo early operation after appropriate fluid and electrolyte replacement. Adequate drainage of abscesses and control of ongoing peritoneal soilage are essential components of the early treatment of intestinal fistulas. Only when sepsis is well controlled by antibiotics or operation can expectant management of a fistula be employed.

The severity of physiologic disturbance resulting from an intestinal fistula varies with the location of the fistula. Fistulas of the stomach, duodenum, or high jejunum may be devastating. The volume of electrolyte-rich fluids lost from such a fistula may cause life-threatening imbalance in a very short time. Distal ileal or colonic fistulas may be very well tolerated and cause no greater electrolyte disturbance than would an ileostomy or colostomy.

There are occasions when diagnosing a fistula may be very difficult. If the intestinal opening is small, drainage may be intermittent. At times, an abdominal wound infected with enteric organisms will discharge material resembling intestinal contents. In these instances the oral administration of a dye, such as brilliant blue or carmine red, may readily establish the diagnosis. Alternatively, a radiographic contrast material may be injected into the cutaneous opening through a small rubber catheter to determine whether a fistula exists. Caution should be exercised when injecting contrast material. Vigorous injection may separate the bowel from its adherence to the abdominal wall, with peritonitis resulting.

All fistulas tend to close spontaneously, but some circumstances prevent closure. The most common is the presence of some degree of obstruction distal to the fistula. This factor may play a role in the genesis of most fistulas. Malignant growth in the fistulous tract will also inhibit spontaneous closure. The presence of a foreign body in the fistulous tract will prevent healing. Chronic fistulas may remain patent because of epithelialization of the tract. Previous radiation to the involved bowel is a notorious cause for failure of fistulas to heal and may actually be one of the more absolute negative factors in fistula closure. If none of these conditions pertain, intestinal fistula closure can be anticipated. When fistulas do not close after an appropriate time interval, surgical closure becomes necessary and must be associated with correction of the factors that have prevented spontaneous closure.

The more proximal the fistula, the more urgent is the need for closure. There are measures, however, that enable control of even the most difficult fistulas. As in intestinal obstruction, the consideration of prime concern is restoration of fluid and electrolyte balance. This, on a rare occasion, may be nearly impossible without performing an enterostomy distal to the fistula. A jejunostomy distal to the duodenal fistula allows the fistula drainage to be instilled into the gastrointestinal tract and greatly facilitates the fluid and electrolyte management. Proximal suction by intestinal intubation may lessen fistulous drainage and encourage healing.

The development of intravenous nutritional support (total parenteral nutrition or TPN), has clearly emerged as a cornerstone in the management of intestinal fistulas. Whether parenteral nutrition actually hastens closure of intestinal fistulas is a matter of some debate. However, most authorities agree that appropriate use of parenteral nutrition will maintain positive nitrogen balance in fistula patients and will encourage wound healing. The improvement in nutrition with concomitant improvement in collagen synthesis may allow closure that might not otherwise occur. Even when fistulas do not close, appropriate nutritional support during the management period will result in a well-nourished patient who is capable of withstanding additional operations.

A major problem in fistula management is the care of the skin about the fistula. Gastrointestinal content, especially from the upper tract, has an ulcerative effect on skin. Enterostomal therapists have become skillful at constructing collection and drainage devices to facilitate control of the fistula drainage. A well-trained enterostomal therapist can assist in minimizing skin breakdown around the area of skin involvement. When an enterostomal therapist is not available, techniques should be developed to allow adequate control of drainage and prevent puddling in dependent areas. The great variety of methods used to protect the skin suggests that in fact no good method is available. Most effective is the total isolation of the skin from the effluent. If it is technically possible, the following procedure is used. The skin is washed and carefully dried; a square of peristomal covering (Stomadhesive) is cut so that the opening in the square approximates the opening of the fistula; the backing of the Stomadhesive is removed and, when the skin is perfectly dry, is pressed into place. Any postoperative pouch can be applied to this square so that the skin surrounding the fistula is protected. The dressing requires changing every 3 to 4 days, depending on the level of the fistula and the volume of drainage from the tract. The bag can be connected to a drainage system to assist collection and further protect the skin. The indication to change the peristomal square is leakage underneath the edge. Many of the bags are odor-proofed, and various tablets and liquids can be put into the pouch to neutralize undesirable odor.

If the fistulous opening will not permit placement of such a bag, other methods may be employed. The drainage may be partially controlled by insertion of a commercial or fabricated sump drain. The skin may be further protected by such agents as karaya powder or a paste made of zinc oxide ointment and castor oil. If severe corrosive dermatitis has occurred, use of a heat lamp and local measures will succeed in controlling the problem, but only with great effort and constant attention. Like many problems in medicine, prevention of skin irritation from an intestinal fistula is infinitely easier and more successful than treatment.

The operative management of an intestinal fistula requires superb timing and judgment as well as great technical facility. By and large, intestinal fistulas are usually attacked too soon. Unless large volumes of fluid are being lost or severe skin problems supervene, a fistula is fairly well tolerated. Most fistulas can be expected to close in 4 to 6 weeks if sepsis has been controlled and appropriate nutritional support is instituted. If a fistula has not closed by 6 weeks, the likelihood of spontaneous closure is small. Waiting an additional 4 to 6 weeks to allow complete resolution of the intra-abdominal inflammatory response, however, will make the subsequent surgical procedure considerably easier. Abdominal adhesions will become much easier to dissect and the possibility of intestinal injury will be minimized. The actual optimum time for surgical intervention is variable and should be individualized for each patient.

If possible, the fistula should be excised and the bowel resected. Occasionally, the involved bowel may be excluded from the gastrointestinal tract but not removed. This is particularly helpful in the presence of radiation enteritis or recurrent carcinoma, where attempts to resect the diseased area with primary anastomosis may be associated with major postoperative complications in a patient whose ability to tolerate the complications is poor. Bypassing the area of disease may accomplish the objective of intestinal decompression without instigating uncontrolled bleeding or multiple accidental enterostomies with recurrent postoperative fistula. Very careful surgical technique is required in reconstructing the gastrointestinal tract if recurrence of the fistula is to be avoided.

Primary Gastrointestinal Disease Mimicking Acute Gynecologic Disorders

MECKEL'S DIVERTICULUM

Meckel's diverticulum, a remnant of the vitelline duct, is a congenital abnormality of the small bowel.

The diverticulum occurs in the terminal 24 in to 48 in of the ileum. Occasionally, gastric mucosa is found in the sac, and perforation or hemorrhage may result from ulceration. These diverticula should be resected if they have caused difficulty or have a narrow neck. The technique consists simply of clamping the base and excising the pouch. Closure of the resulting defect is best accomplished with interrupted No. 3-0 catgut Lembert sutures supported by a seromuscular layer of interrupted silk (No. 2-0) sutures. Care must be taken to avoid narrowing the bowel lumen. If encountered in an asymptomatic patient, Meckel's diverticulum need not be removed. Most complications occur in young children, and the likelihood of difficulty with a Meckel's diverticulum in an adult is extremely small.

COLON DIVERTICULITIS

Occasionally, perforated diverticulitis of the sigmoid colon may be mistaken for pelvic inflammatory disease. Ordinarily these two processes occur in different age groups, but acute diverticulitis does occur in patients under 40 years of age. Discovery of acute diverticulitis of the sigmoid colon with perforation warrants special consideration. If the perforation has occurred into the free peritoneal cavity and generalized peritonitis is present, drainage of the area of perforation with several soft Penrose drains is necessary. In addition, a proximal diverting colostomy is indicated. If possible, the colostomy should be placed in the descending colon proximal to the perforation. This shortens the segment of bowel between the colostomy and the perforation. The disease may then be managed with only one subsequent procedure. If the colostomy is placed in the right colon, resection and colostomy closure must be done as separate procedures. Occasionally, an area of diverticulitis will be mobile enough that the diseased segment may be exteriorized or resected primarily with construction of an end sigmoid colostomy. When this can be done without extensive dissection in the presence of acute inflammation, it is the ideal approach; extensive dissection should be avoided when it is difficult or hazardous.

If the perforation is localized and an abscess has formed, the abscess should be drained extraperitoneally, if possible. This may require a separate flank incision, which should be done without hesitation. Proximal colostomy is necessary. Perforated diverticulitis is life-threatening if generalized peritonitis supervenes, and patients with this condition require constant attention postoperatively.

VOLVULUS

Sigmoid volvulus is of interest to the gynecologist only as it pertains to differential diagnosis. While the sudden onset of pain may resemble ovarian torsion, the presence of obstipation, abdominal distention, and the characteristic radiographic appearance (massively distended sigmoid colon, "bird-beak" in appearance on barium enema) should establish the correct diagnosis. Sigmoid volvulus is radiographically characterized by a massively dilated, gas-filled sigmoid colon that appears like an inverted horseshoe, extending up from the pelvis into the upper abdomen. Occasionally, in the mentally deficient patient, the colon may be distended and full of stool. But the characteristic x-ray picture is not present, which differentiates the two entities.

Although volvulus is generally seen in people over 60 years of age, two cases have been encountered in women under 25 in our clinic within a year. When sigmoid volvulus is diagnosed preoperatively, the problem can usually be remedied nonoperatively by careful and expeditious sigmoidoscopy or low-pressure barium enema. However, when the diagnosis is discovered at the time of a pelvic laparotomy, the surgical treatment usually consists of untwisting the loop of bowel. Colostomy may be necessary on occasion, particularly when the viability of the segment is doubtful. Use of intravenous fluorescein or Doppler apparatus as described previously may be helpful. Primary resection should never be employed unless gangrene or nonviability is documented. Furthermore, primary anastomosis is never justified in the presence of an unprepared distended colon.

Volvulus of the cecum is quite rare. It usually occurs in the very elderly and is managed by simple derotation. Fixation of the cecum to the posterolateral peritoneum (cecopexy) may prevent recurrence.

Primary Gastrointestinal Disease Encountered During Gynecologic Surgery

Among the primary gastrointestinal diseases found during the course of gynecologic surgery, colon diverticulitis has already been discussed.

REGIONAL ENTERITIS (CROHN'S DISEASE)

Regional enteritis is a granulomatous inflammatory process, usually involving the small intestine. It may be encountered occasionally by the gynecologic surgeon and is usually unexpected. This disease may occur in all age groups, but is most frequent in young adults. The usual age at onset of symptoms is late teens.

Clinically, the disease usually causes diarrhea, weight loss, and abdominal pain. Surgery is most often necessitated by either acute exacerbation of the inflammatory process or intestinal obstruction from edema and cicatrix. Fistula formation is common and in women may involve the bladder or vagina. Fistulas may also develop between the terminal ileum and the site of a previous appendectomy. When the disease is encountered unexpectedly, resection should not be performed unless obstruction is present, since medical treatment may be successful. The diseased segments appear beefy, dull purple-red, thickened, and covered with strands of thick, gray-white exudate. The mesenteric fat creeps over the serosa so that it nearly encompasses the bowel. Since skip areas are common, the extent of the disease should be thoroughly documented by examining the entire length of the bowel. Extensive clinical and laboratory investigations have been directed at identifying the etiology of this disease. Initial enthusiasm about a possible viral cause has been dampened by failure to reproduce experimental results. Consequently, regional enteritis is still an enigma, and medical treatment is less than optimal.

Definitive procedures should, where possible, be directed at resection of the diseased bowel. Usually, the terminal ileum and right colon are removed and an ileotransverse colostomy performed. Bypass procedure has been recommended but seems less satisfactory than resection in most cases, since it is attended by a higher recurrence rate.

In doing a small bowel resection for regional enteritis, there is no advantage in removing the enlarged mesenteric lymph nodes. If a dilated ureter is found near the area of the terminal ileum, no attempt should be made to free it. This will resolve with successful treatment of the small bowel. When this disease is encountered, the rule of thumb is to avoid resection unless there is perforation or obstruction. The patient should be given a trial of medical management. Only when there is no improvement with expectant management, or when a surgical complication develops, should surgical intervention be entertained. If operation is performed the appendix may be resected if the base of the cecum is not involved with disease. This eliminates any future diagnostic concern about appendicitis if right lower quadrant pain recurs. Several recent reports suggest that the incidence of enterocutaneous fistulas increases if the appendix has been removed, but the majority of patients can probably undergo appendectomy safely. This complication may be avoided by omitting an appendectomy in any case where the terminal ileum or cecum is involved with regional enteritis.

Special mention must be made of the treatment of fistulas. Enterocutaneous, enterovesical, and enterovaginal fistulas are common and present an extreme challenge to the physician or surgeon. Treatment by traditional surgical approaches is fraught with a high complication rate and almost certain recurrence. When a fistula to the vagina is identified in a patient with a history compatible with inflammatory bowel disease, careful and extensive preoperative evaluation is necessary. If regional enteritis can be diagnosed preoperatively, intense nutritional support and medical therapy should be attempted. Initial experience with parenteral nutrition support in the cure of regional enteritis has been followed by a more realistic understanding of the role of nutrition in the disease. Nutritional support is clearly essential in preparing these patients for surgery and in maintaining their general nutritional status.

Sulfasalazine and corticosteroids are the mainstay of therapy. Sulfasalazine is administered in 1 g doses four times a day and appears to have some benefit in the treatment of both acute disease and possibly in maintaining remission. It is not free of gastrointestinal side effects, however, and patient compliance may be poor. Steroids have been utilized in acute exacerbations of the disease and, in refractory patients, for long-term maintenance. Most commonly, prednisone is given in a dosage of 30 mg/ 24 hr to 60 mg/24 hr, tapered to the lowest possible dosage that will control the symptomatology. Adrenocorticotropic hormone (ACTH) has been used by some experts with comparable results. There is no good evidence, however, that ACTH is superior to prednisone. Whether prednisone or ACTH is given, the dose should be decreased to the minimum amount possible to prevent the serious and frequently irreversible consequences of long-term corticosteroid therapy.

Demonstration of very high recurrence rates following surgical resection of regional enteritis has dampened enthusiasm for prophylactic resections. Virtually all patients will develop at least radiographic recurrence of the disease if follow-up is long enough. Medical therapy is the mainstay of treatment unless complications (perforation, obstruction, bleeding, or fistula) occur.

Definitive treatment of an enterovaginal fistula must include treatment of the intra-abdominal disease. Perineal approaches to closure of the fistula are uniformly unsuccessful. As previously indicated, preoperative evaluation, optimum nutritional support, and attempts at medical management with sulfasalazine and steroids are essential. If surgical intervention becomes necessary, the intra-abdominal disease must be resected. The area of resection should include only the section of bowel that is grossly involved. Extensive resection should be avoided, with its sequela of short bowel syndrome. Considerable judgment is required in any surgical undertaking because of the chronicity and high recurrence rate. Since long-term follow-up is essential and complications frequent, it is preferable to enlist the help of a specialist in treating inflammatory bowel disease.

COLON OPERATIONS

If elective surgery that may involve colostomy is planned, the question of bowel preparation is raised. There is little controversy over the mechanical preparation. Clear liquids for 48 to 72 hours preoperatively combined with citrate of magnesium and possibly saline enemas the evening prior to operation are very effective measures.

The controversy about the use of nonabsorbable oral antibiotics seems to have been resolved. Most surgeons now use preoperative enteral, as well as parenteral antibiotics because of the demonstrated decrease in intra-abdominal complications and wound infection. Oral antibiotics should include an agent effective against aerobes (aminoglycosides) and an agent effective against anaerobes (clindamycin, third-generation cephalosporins, or metronidazole). Systemic antibiotics should be initiated prior to operation and be continued for 24 hours postoperatively.

COLON OBSTRUCTION

Etiologically, obstruction of the large intestine differs from that of the small bowel in that adhesions and hernia are uncommon causes, and tumor and inflammation are quite common. The gynecologist may encounter obstruction of the large intestine as a result of contiguous or metastatic cancer, irradiation changes in the intestine, pelvic abscess, or primary intestinal inflammatory disease. The general principles for management of large bowel obstruction are the same as those for small bowel obstruction, but there are some differences. In the presence of a competent ileocecal valve, an obstructed large bowel becomes a closed loop. A closed loop is the most dangerous of all types of intestinal obstruction.

When the large bowel is involved, the most likely site of complication is the cecum, which may perforate if over-distended. For this reason, obstruction of the colon with a competent ileocecal valve is a matter of great surgical urgency. If the ileocecal valve is incompetent, large bowel obstruction becomes, in effect, a total small bowel obstruction.

A major difference between large and small bowel obstruction is the operative management. In the large intestine, obstruction may be relieved with a relatively minor operation and the etiologic problem may be dealt with electively. Any part of the large bowel, including the cecum, may be exteriorized proximal to the point of obstruction. Prior to operation, sigmoidoscopy and barium enema under fluoroscopic observation are needed to define clearly the point of obstruction. The exception to this rule is acute obstructed or perforated diverticulitis, in which case a barium enema may be dangerous even in experienced hands.

Sigmoid colon cancer or severe diverticulitis should be managed by transverse colostomy in the right upper abdomen. If the disease is encountered through an incision that does not permit the colostomy to be done easily, the incision should be closed. A separate muscle-splitting incision is made in the right upper quadrant, and a loop of bowel exteriorized. The bowel can be opened later. If immediate decompression is required, it is best done by the insertion of a large tube into the colostomy, thus avoiding soilage of the peritoneal cavity. After the incision is sealed, in 24 to 48 hours, the colostomy can be opened safely.

RADIATION INJURY TO LARGE AND SMALL INTESTINE

Radiation therapy for malignant pelvic tumors, particularly carcinoma of the cervix, occasionally causes complications in the colon or small intestines. Although the radiation complications of colitis, proctitis, or enteritis are not common, they are definite complications. In a series of 777 patients treated for pelvic malignant disease at the Radiation Department of Hahnemann Medical College and Hospital from January 1969 to June 1973, 47 (6.1%) such complications occurred. The average dose was 6000 rad of external irradiation and 2000 rad from radium insertion. Colcock and associates indicated that bowel symptoms began to be produced at total radiation doses of approximately 4800 rad. Symptoms during or directly after irradiation therapy are common but are usually short-lived and present no significant long-term problems. Persistence of symptoms beyond 1 month after the termination of therapy strongly suggests that permanent bowel damage may be present. The most common bowel symptoms include diarrhea, abdominal pain, rectal bleeding, vomiting, and weight loss. In the analysis of the 47 patients, Colcock and associates found the following complications: small bowel obstruction in 15, large bowel stenosis in 5, rectal bleeding in 36, and proctitis in 31.

Radiation enteritis can be characterized as acute, subacute, or chronic. Acute radiation enteritis occurs during and immediately following a course of therapeutic radiation. It is caused by suppression of mucosal regeneration in the exposed area of intestine and results in malabsorption with diarrhea and occasional bleeding. This is usually a self-resolving problem and is not correlated with the subsequent occurrence of chronic symptoms.

Subacute and chronic radiation enteritis are distinguished by the delay between treatment and the onset of symptoms. Symptoms of subacute radiation damage usually occur within 3 to 6 months of radiation treatment, whereas chronic radiation enteritis may not be obvious until years after the therapy. Both abnormalities are characterized pathologically by fibrosis and endarteritis. The fibrosis results in areas of stricture and may lead to intestinal obstruction. Another finding is dense interloop adhesions that defy surgical separation. However, the pathologic manifestation that requires an attitude of extreme caution is the endarteritis, which causes obliteration of the native blood vessels of the intestine, even in areas of bowel that appear grossly normal. The characteristic appearance of chronic radiation enteritis, a marblelike bowel with telangiectatic blood vessels, is by no means a reliable indicator of radiation damage. Adjacent, grossly normal-appearing segments of intestine may also show microscopic damage. It is important to recognize that the endarteritis of radiation results in a very poor blood supply for the support of intestinal anastomosis or closure of enterotomies.

Operation should be avoided in the patient with abdominal complaints following radiation treatment unless definitive indications are present. The wary clinician will recognize the high risk associated with operation and advise his patient to use caution. When operation is necessary, however, several principles are important. First and foremost, the surgeon must recognize the significance of the endarteritis and its effect on healing of intestinal suture lines. Extreme caution should be taken to avoid injury to the bowel because of the subsequent hazards of closure. Second, the surgeon should remember that radiation damage occurs only within the area of the radiation portal. Incisions can be placed safely out of the radiated field in many cases. Extensive lysis of adhesions should be avoided, and dissection should be confined to those areas where it is necessary. Intestinal anastomosis should be performed with at least one and preferably two segments of grossly normal bowel. These can be reinforced with a tongue of omentum over the suture line to provide additional exogenous blood supply. Frequently, intestinal bypass with side-to-side anastomosis in normal bowel is preferable to extensive mobilization of irradiated intestine from the pelvis. Irradiated bowel should be regarded warily. Such an approach will be rewarded by a decrease in the incidence of intra-abdominal abscess and enterocutaneous fistula.

Rectovaginal and vesicovaginal fistulas following radiation to the pelvis are not trivial problems and should be managed by experienced personnel. Simple mobilization and closure is usually attended by major complications and is rarely successful.

When operation is necessary in the patient who has previously undergone radiation therapy, careful postoperative monitoring for signs of peritonitis is essential. When peritoneal irritation is apparent, reexploration is essential because of the high likelihood of a failed suture line.

Primary Gynecologic Diseases Affecting the Gastrointestinal Tract

TECHNIQUES OF TREATMENT FOR TUBO-OVARIAN ABSCESS, ENDOMETRIOSIS, AND PELVIC CANCER

Tubo-ovarian abscess, endometriosis, and pelvic cancer are discussed in other chapters. Each of these entities occasionally causes small bowel obstruction. It should be remembered that although endometriosis is a frequent finding in women, it rarely causes obstruction of the small bowel. Endometriosis of the small bowel tends to be limited to the serosal and muscular coats and does not usually penetrate to the mucosa. Obstruction is due to fibrosis and kinking of the bowel. When obstruction from endometriosis of the small bowel is encountered, the involved segment should be resected. As a general rule, the postoperative course is uneventful.

Open End-to-End Anastomosis

Open end-to-end anastomosis (Fig. 19–1) follows intestinal resection. Crushing clamps are placed obliquely on the intestine, with the apex on the mesenteric side. This gives some advantage in providing a large lumen at the anastomotic site and favors a good blood supply to the antimesenteric

margin. With fine needles (French eye or "pop-off" GI needles), a row of No. 3-0 silk mattress sutures is used to approximate the serosal surface. The crushing clamps are then removed, the crushed ends of the bowel are trimmed, and a mucosal layer of No. 3-0 or No. 4-0 silk sutures is placed. At the angles, the sutures become interrupted Connell sutures, with the knots on the luminal aspect. The serosal suture line is then completed with mattress or Lembert sutures. The use of continuous absorbable suture on the mucosal layer is quite acceptable. When the lumen is small, however, continuous sutures are more likely to narrow the anastomotic stoma. After the anastomosis is completed, the mesenteric rent is repaired with fine sutures. Care must be taken not to injure the blood supply to the suture line during mesentery closure.

Closed Anastomosis

Closed anastomosis (Fig. 19–2) is particularly useful in ileocolostomy construction with unprepared bowel. Four noncrushing clamps, such as Allen clamps, are placed across the unopened bowel to isolate the segment to be removed. As with all anastomoses, moist pads are used to carefully isolate the gut from the peritoneal cavity. The mesentery of the segment to be resected is divided in a wedge.

Careful placement of hemostats on the mesenteric vessels is critical. Suture ligation of these vessels is much safer than simple ligation. If a vessel is lost and retracts into the mesentery, attempts to find and control it may result in vascular damage, necessitating a greater bowel resection. The time spent carefully isolating and ligating these vessels will be well rewarded.

After the bowel to be resected has been removed, the clamps on the cut ends are approximated, and No. 3-0 silk Lembert sutures are placed through the bowel wall to include the mucosa, about 3 mm apart, around the entire circumference. The clamps are then removed, and the cut, compressed ends of bowel separated to ensure that no suture has been placed across the lumen, possibly occluding the anastomosis. The sutures are then tied. As they are tied, any needed additional stitches are placed. Patency of the lumen is assured and the mesenteric defect repaired. This anastomosis, carefully performed, is quick, safe, and assures maximum patency. For the surgeon who only occasionally performs an anastomosis, it is an excellent method. The area of greatest difficulty is at the site of mesenteric attachment to the bowel wall; by carefully dissecting the mesentery off the bowel for 5 mm, trouble can be avoided. If this is not done, the bowel wall may be missed and the sutures placed in the mesenteric fat, with disastrous results.

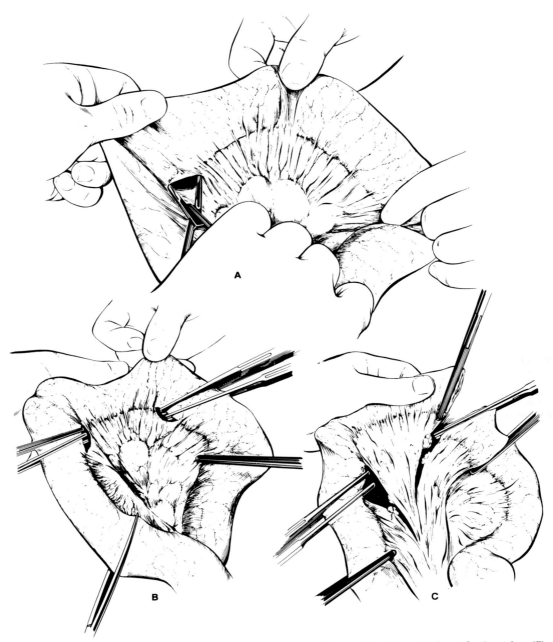

FIG. 19–1   Open end-to-end anastomosis. (*A*) The mesentery is carefully dissected from the intestine. (*B*) The resected segment is defined by clamps. Note the noncrushing clamps proximally placed to control spill. (*C*) Note the individual ligatures on the mesentery. Suture ligation of these vessels is important.

Side-to-Side Anastomosis

The side-to-side method of anastomosis (Fig. 19–3) is less popular than end-to-end. It may be quite useful in excluding a segment of the intestinal tract, as in regional enteritis. The two segments of bowel to be anastomosed are approximated with stay sutures. A distance of about 4 in between these sutures is ideal. Serosal mattress sutures of No. 3-0 silk are placed. With noncrushing clamps, the segments to be connected are isolated. This aids in controlling bleeding and also in avoiding contamination. Both

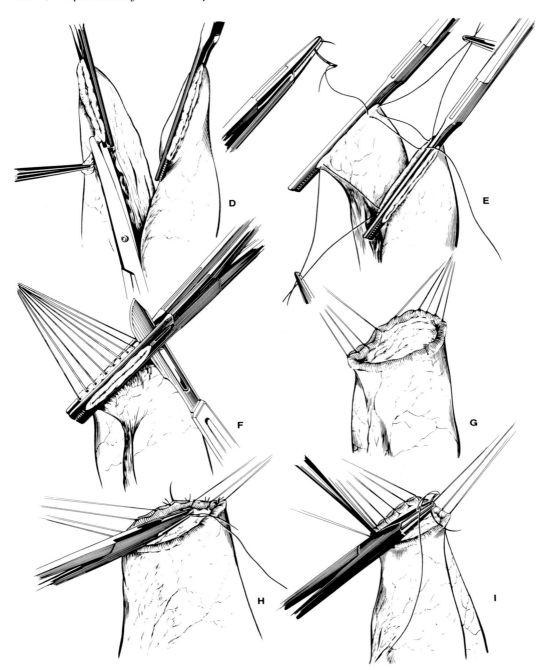

FIG. 19-1 (continued). (D) Careful dissection of the mesentery from the intestine is essential. (E) Posterior interrupted sutures are about 5 mm apart. (F) The crushed end of the bowel is trimmed away. (G, H) Note that the posterior serosal sutures are not cut until the first mucosal suture has been placed. (I) Beginning to "turn the corner."

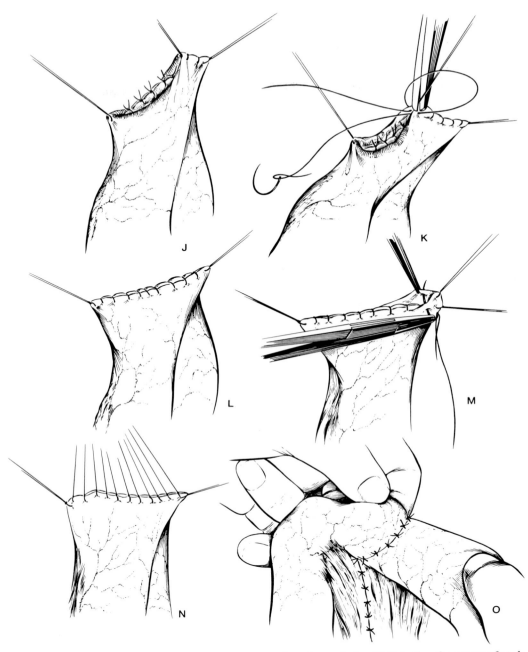

FIG. 19–1 (continued). (J) The inverting suture is continued anteriorly. (K) Note the placement of each suture before cutting the previous one. (L, M) Completion of the anterior mucosal suture line and beginning the anterior serosal one. (N, O) The anastomosis is complete and the mesenteric defect closed.

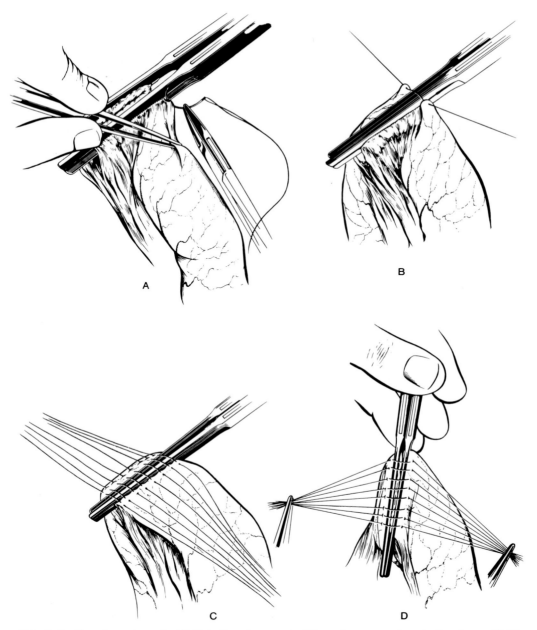

FIG. 19–2 Closed anastomosis. (*A*) Note the placement of the suture very close to the clamp. (*B*) The first suture is completed. (*C*) The row of sutures has now been placed. (*D*) The clamp on the intestine is rotated 180°.

segments of bowel are then opened with a parallel incision about 3 mm from the suture line. Mucosal sutures may be either continuous or interrupted. The larger lumen in this method makes continuous suture less hazardous. The serosal suture line is then completed as before.

An important aspect of this technique is to place the initial suture line in a perfectly straight line parallel to the long axis of the bowel. Angulation may interfere with stomal function.

Stapled Anastomosis

The development of intestinal staples has simplified the performance of anastomoses, particularly for

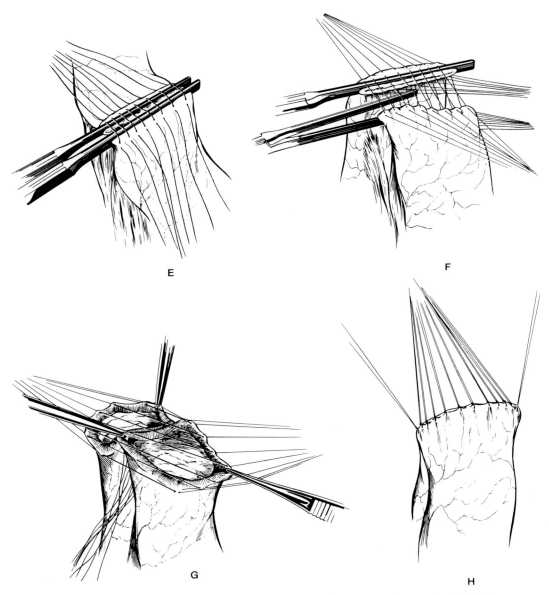

E

F

G

H

FIG. 19-2 *(continued)*. *(E)* Following rotation of the clamp, the suturing is completed. *(F)* Clamps are removed prior to tying the sutures. *(G)* The lumen is inspected to assure that no sutures have been placed across the lumen. *(H)* Sutures tied. One layer is adequate. The mesenteric defect is closed as in Fig. 19–1N, O.

the person who infrequently operates on the bowel. The three most commonly used instruments are the GIA stapler, the TA 55 or TA 90 staplers, and the EEA stapler. Each instrument is designed to perform a different function, and they are frequently used in combination.

The GIA instrument (Fig. 19–4) is designed to place two double parallel rows of metallic staples over a length of approximately 5 cm and simultaneously cut between them. This instrument can be used in a variety of settings. The most common use is in dividing the intestine. Applied across the bowel, it effectively closes both ends of the divided bowel and prevents peritoneal spillage. It can also be used

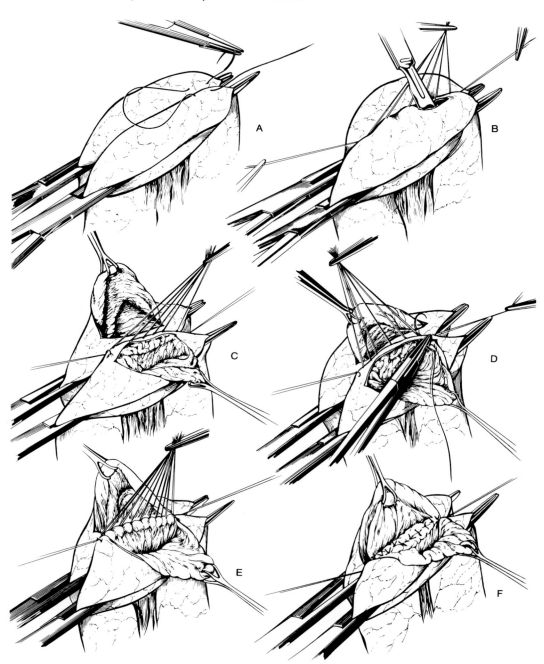

FIG. 19–3 Side-to-side anastomosis. (*A*) Horizontal mattress sutures are used on the posterior row. (*B*) The noncrushing clamps avoid spill as the bowel is opened. (*C, D*) The posterior serosal suture line is completed and the first mucosal suture is placed before cutting the serosal ones. (*E, F*) Completion of the posterior mucosal sutures.

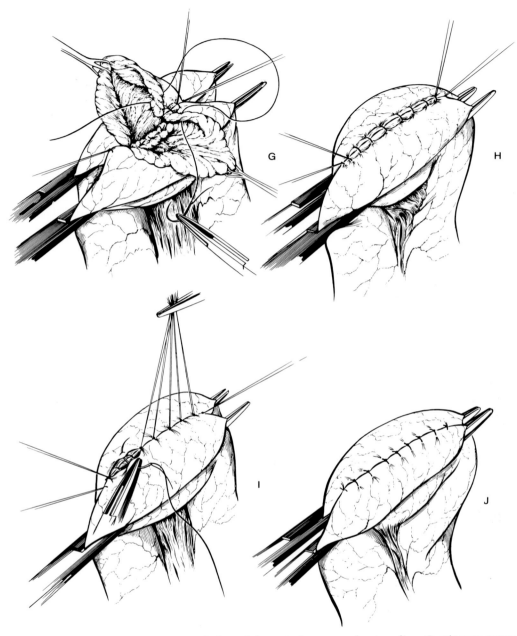

FIG. 19–3 (continued). *(G, H)* Completion of the anterior mucosal suture line. Continuous suture can be used more safely in side-to-side than in end-to-end anastomosis. *(I, J)* Completion of the anterior serosal suture line.

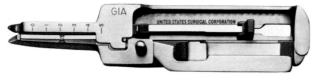

FIG. 19-4 The GIA instrument applies two double rows of staples and cuts between them. It is available in only one size.

in conjunction with the TA 55 instrument for constructing a side-to-side (functional end-to-end) anastomosis.

The TA 55 and TA 90 instruments (Fig. 19–5) apply two parallel rows of staples and are most commonly used for permanently closing the end of a segment of bowel. The two instruments differ in width of the staple line. Care must be exercised that the entire width of bowel is included within the instrument and that the open end of the instrument is effectively closed by placement of the retaining pin. After placement and firing of the TA instrument, the bowel is divided with a knife.

The EEA instrument (Fig. 19–6) performs an inverting end-to-end anastomosis. It requires an opening in an adjacent portion of bowel (enterotomy, colotomy, or anus) which usually must be closed subsequently with sutures or with a single application of a TA instrument. Purse-string sutures of polypropylene or nylon are applied over the ends of the bowel to be anastomosed. This can be accomplished with a purse-string instrument or by a simple over-and-over baseball stitch around the circumference of the intestine. After both ends of the bowel have been placed and secured around the center rod of the instrument and the purse-string sutures tied, the instrument is closed and fired. This effectively staples the two ends together and removes the excess intraluminal tissue with a circular blade. After removal of the apparatus, security of the anastomosis can be tested by removing the two circular "doughnuts" of tissue contained within the instrument. If either remnant is not a complete circle, a secure anastomosis is unlikely. The anastomosis may be reinforced, if desired, with a row of Lembert sutures.

STAPLED SIDE-TO-SIDE ANASTOMOSIS. A side-to-side anastomosis (which has been popularized as a functional end-to-end anastomosis) can be performed by a single application of the GIA instrument followed by an application of the TA 55 or TA 90 instrument. After removal (or clamping) of the appropriate section of intestine (Fig. 19–7A), the two ends of intestine are placed side-to-side and secured with stay sutures. The two arms of the GIA instrument are inserted into the open ends of the intestine, and traction is applied on the open end to seat the instrument to its maximum depth (Fig. 19–7B,C). The instrument should be applied on the antimesenteric border of both segments of intestine. The instrument is closed by squeezing the lock level into the instrument. Prior to firing the instrument, location of application should be rechecked to ensure that the instrument is fully seated and does not include the mesentery. The instrument is fired by sliding the push bar forward, stapling and dividing the tissue between the two double rows of staples. The TA 55 or TA 90 instrument is then applied to the combined ends, closed by tightening the wing nut, and fired (Fig. 19–7D,E). After the redundant tissue is trimmed with a scalpel (Fig. 19–7F), patency of the anastomosis can be confirmed by palpation. A row of Lembert

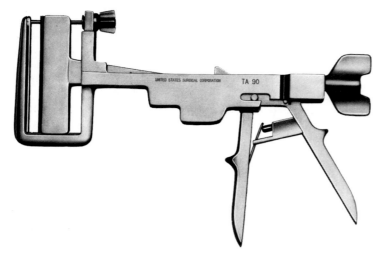

FIG. 19-5 The TA 90 is wider than the TA 55 (not shown). This instrument crushes the tissue while applying a double row of staples. It is best suited for an end closure of the intestine and is frequently reinforced with an external row of sutures.

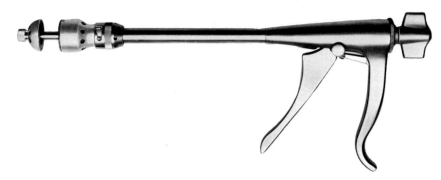

FIG. 19-6 The EEA performs an end-to-end anastomosis by applying two circular concentric rows of staples and cuts away the central redundant tissue. The distal end (opposite the pistol grip) is disposable and is available in three sizes—25 mm, 28 mm, and 31 mm. The appropriate size is determined with the assistance of the sizers that are provided with the instrument. In general, the largest size should be used.

sutures exterior to the staple line is optional but is preferred by many surgeons to take the tension off the staples.

STAPLED END-TO-END ANASTOMOSIS. An end-to-end anastomosis can be constructed quite easily with the use of the EEA instrument, and an end-to-side anastomosis can be done with the EEA and the TA 55 or TA 90 instruments. After the bowel is resected, the EEA instrument, with the end cone (anvil) removed, is inserted through a small colotomy made with a knife, approximately 5 cm from the transected end of the bowel (Fig. 19–8A). The free end of the bowel is secured around the rod with a purse-string suture. The cone (anvil) is then attached securely to the center rod. A purse-string suture of No. 3-0 polypropylene is placed on the opposite loop of intestine, either with the provided clamp (Fig. 19–8A) or with a running baseball stitch (Fig. 19–8B). The intestine is then brought over the anvil with the aid of Allis clamps. The polypropylene suture is tied and the instrument is closed by tightening the wing nut (Fig. 19–8C). The instrument is fired, which cuts out a round segment of tissue and simultaneously anastomoses the two segments of bowel. The instrument is carefully removed by turning the wing nut two or three turns and carefully extracting the instrument with a back-and-forth rotary motion (Fig. 19–8D). The colotomy site can be closed with a single application of the TA 55 or TA 90 instrument (Fig. 19–8E). Both staple lines can be reinforced with Lembert sutures if desired.

An end-to-side anastomosis can be performed in an analogous fashion by inserting the EEA *into* the open end of the colon, passing the center rod (without the anvil) through a small colotomy in the antimesenteric taenia, and securing this with a purse-string suture around the rod. The small intestine or colon is treated as in Figure 19–8A–C. After the instrument is closed and fired, the open end of the colon can be closed with a single application of the TA 90.

Enterostomy

The safest method for performing an enterostomy is shown in Figure 19–9. Two concentric purse-string sutures of No. 3-0 silk are placed in the bowel wall. A stab wound is made and a catheter inserted. The sutures are tied and the bowel is sutured to the anterior abdominal wall. Omentum may be pulled up to the catheter to assist in controlling any possible leakage.

Colostomy

Although ideally gastrointestinal continuity should be restored with an appropriate anastomosis whenever possible, there are many circumstances where a colostomy is either essential or unavoidable. Examples of an essential colostomy include an end-sigmoid colostomy following a standard proctectomy or pelvic exenteration, an ileostomy following a total proctocolectomy, an end-colostomy and oversewing of the rectum (Hartmann pouch) for an urgent sigmoid resection with unprepared bowel. A colostomy may be undesirable yet unavoidable when an injury has occurred to the colon without prior mechanical and antibiotic preparation, when incontinuity resection of the colon for pelvic disease is required, or for proximal decompression when obstruction or perforation is discovered (Fig. 19–10). Although a colostomy may be protective when it is placed proximal to an anastomosis or a perforation and thus decreases the risk of complications, a colostomy only offers an advantage if it is performed correctly and is free of its own complications. For that reason, the technical performance of a colostomy must be exact and must protect the blood supply of the colon as well.

Colostomies are traditionally considered as temporary or permanent. Classically, a loop colostomy is considered temporary and an end colostomy permanent, although a loop colostomy can be permanent and an end colostomy temporary. Loop co-

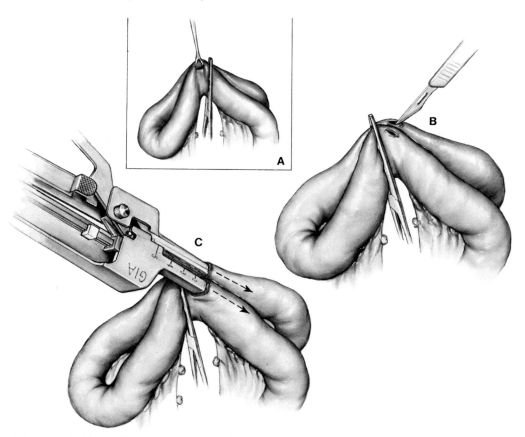

FIG. 19-7 A side-to-side anastomosis (functional end-to-end) can be constructed with the GIA and the TA 55 or TA 90. (*A*) Both segments of intestine are freed up at the appropriate locations by dividing the mesentery. Bowel to be anastomosed may be approximated with interrupted seromuscular sutures. (*B*) Small enterotomies are made on the antimesenteric border of both limbs. (*C*) The arms of the GIA are inserted into the enterotomies. The instrument is closed and the push bar is advanced. This simultaneously approximates the two limbs of intestine by parallel double rows of staples and opens the intestine between the rows.

lostomies are usually performed in areas of the colon that have a free mesentery: that is, the sigmoid colon or the right transverse colon. Although the colon can be mobilized adequately to bring it to the abdominal wall for performance of an end colostomy in almost any portion of the colon, an end colostomy is performed most commonly in the sigmoid colon, left or right transverse colon, or (rarely) the ascending colon or cecum.

LOOP COLOSTOMY. A loop colostomy is usually performed as a proximal diverting procedure for a distal obstruction or perforation. It is generally considered temporary and is closed following successful management of the distal problem. A loop colostomy is usually performed in the sigmoid colon or right transverse colon. It can be performed as a separate surgical procedure or as a complement to

a definitive surgical procedure. If done as a primary procedure, the surgical incision is typically placed over the rectus muscle in the right upper quadrant for a right transverse colostomy. The incision for a sigmoid colostomy can also be oblique, transverse, or vertical (paramedian) in the left lower quadrant. When the procedure is performed as a complement to a laparotomy, a small transverse incision can be made in either area centered over the lateral border of the rectus sheath.

The colon is freed up from any secondary attachments to the peritoneum and elevated through the incision. In the case of a sigmoid colostomy, a rod that can later fit into a specially designed appliance (Fig. 19–11A) is inserted through a small defect created in the mesentery at the mesenteric margin of the colon. A piece of rubber tubing is

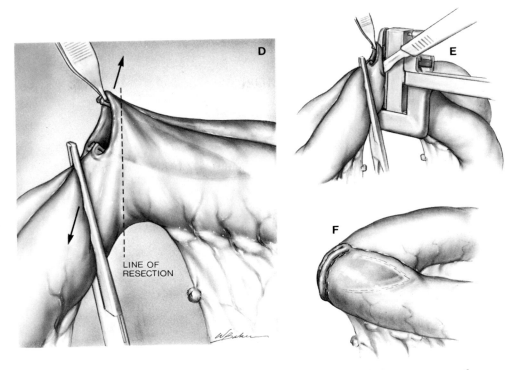

FIG. 19-7 (continued). (*D*) The line of transection of bowel is identified so as to resect the area containing the enterotomies. The lumen between the two limbs is indicated by the shaded area. The TA 55 or TA 90 is applied along this line and closed until the vernier lines on the handle line up indicating complete closure. (*E*) The resected bowel is amputated using the groove in the instrument as a guide for the knife. (*F*) The completed functional end-to-end anastomosis. The staple line can be reinforced with sutures if desired.

connected to both ends to keep it in place. A No. 20 plastic chest tube also works well. In the case of a right transverse colostomy, the omentum should be freed up from the inferior margin of the colon for a short distance. The serosa of the colon can be attached to the peritoneum and posterior fascia. Reapproximation of the fascia under the rod may help to minimize the risk of colostomy prolapse.

After the loop of colon has been brought through the fascia and secured with the rod or sutures, it can be left closed for a period of 24 to 72 hours to prevent contamination, or the colostomy can be opened immediately in the operating room by making a longitudinal incision along the tinea (Fig. 19-11B). Alternatively, after the longitudinal incision is made, the edges of the open colon can be sutured to the margin of the surgical defect (allowing the rod to protrude on either side), which results in a primarily matured colostomy (Fig. 19-11C).

END COLOSTOMY. When the sigmoid colon must be resected without preoperative bowel prepara-

tion, a primary anastomosis is inappropriate. In such a setting, an end colostomy with either a Hartmann pouch (closure of the distal rectum) or a mucous fistula (attaching the distal end of the open bowel to the abdominal wall like a colostomy) can be performed. After resection of the bowel, sigmoid colostomy is performed by excising a circular defect of skin at the appropriate point. It is helpful to have the site of an end sigmoid colostomy identified by an enterostomal therapist preoperatively to minimize the likelihood of placing the colostomy in a fold of the abdominal wall or too close to the anterior superior iliac spine or groin crease, which could cause difficulties in the fitting of the appliance. This prior identification is rarely possible, however, in an emergency setting, where an estimate of the location of the colostomy should be made. Traditionally, an end sigmoid colostomy is placed at the midpoint of a line connecting the umbilicus to the anterior superior iliac spine (Fig. 19-12A). This point is generally acceptable except in obese or elderly

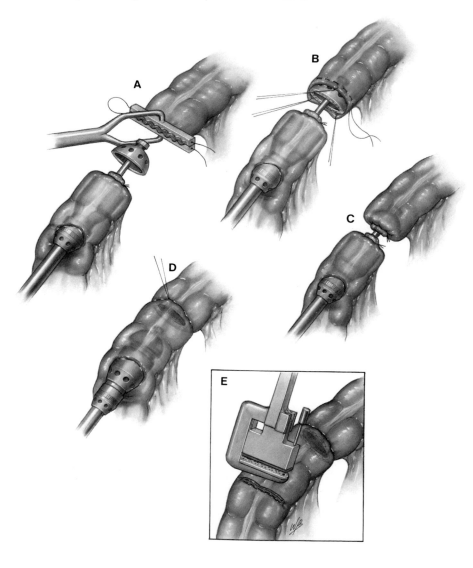

FIG. 19–8 The technique of end-to-end anastomosis is demonstrated with the EEA. (*A*) The EEA instrument is inserted through a colotomy in the antimesenteric taenia, the cone (anvil) is reattached, and the free end of the bowel is secured around the rod with a purse-string suture. (*B*) Intestine is advanced on the anvil after placement of purse-string suture near the free margin. (*C*) The purse-string suture is tied and the instrument is closed, drawing free margins of bowel together. (*D*) The instrument is fired and free margins of bowel are severed, removing a round segment of mucosa and anastomosing the two segments of bowel. (*E*) The colotomy site is closed with a single application of the TA 55 or TA 90 instrument. Staple lines are reinforced with Lembert sutures of No. 3-0 silk.

patients. In these patients, it is helpful to place the colostomy as high as possible to facilitate colostomy care.

When the site for the colostomy has been chosen and the circle of skin and underlying soft tissue has been removed, either the anterior rectus fascia along the lateral edge of the rectus muscle can be incised in a cruciate fashion or a circular defect can be excised (Fig. 19–12B). The rectus muscle is not divided, but the external and internal oblique muscles are bluntly separated. An opening that will accommodate three fingers is made in the underlying posterior sheath and transversalis fascia (Fig. 19–12C). The end of the colon is brought through the defect, taking care not to twist the colon on its mesentery.

It is frequently helpful during an emergency resection to use the GIA stapler to simultaneously divide the bowel and close the ends to prevent contamination. In patients with a fatty mesentery, it is helpful to divide the mesentery from its point of attachment to the bowel over a distance of several centimeters from the end of the cut colon. In a less fatty mesentery, this may not be necessary. The colon is attached to the posterior fascia and peritoneum with several interrupted fine sutures placed at intervals around the circumference of the bowel. The defect created between the edge of the mesentery and the lateral abdominal wall is eliminated by suturing the mesenteric margin to the peritoneum with interrupted or continuous suture. The

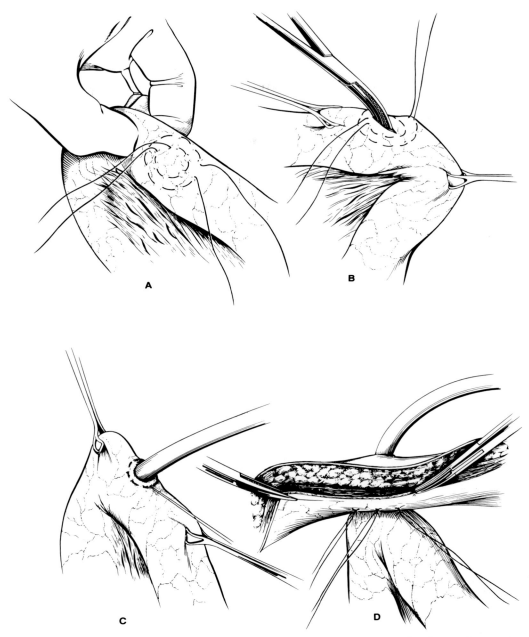

FIG. 19–9 Enterostomy. (*A*) Note the concentric purse-string sutures with the free ends opposite each other. (*B*) After a stab wound is made with a scalpel, the patency of the mucosal wound is established with a clamp. (*C*) After introducing the tube, the purse-string sutures are both tied. (*D*) The intestine is tacked to the peritoneum.

abdominal incision is closed before the colostomy is opened and matured. After the abdominal skin has been reapproximated and an occlusive dressing applied, the clamp on the end of the colon is removed or the staple line effectively closing the end

of the colon is excised. The colostomy is matured primarily by placing four quadrant delayed-absorbable No. 2-0 sutures initially (Fig. 19–13A). These sutures are placed by taking a bite of dermis, a sero-muscular bite of colon approximately 3 cm from

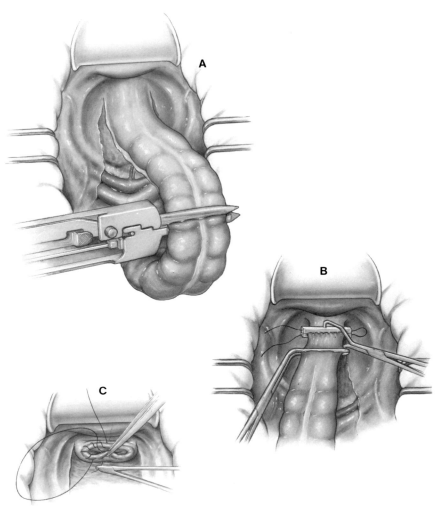

FIG. 19–10 (A) In preparation for a sigmoid colostomy, the colon can be transected to avoid spillage by using the GIA instrument. (B) Resection of the rectosigmoid colon is done with a right-angle clamp applied to the proximal side of bowel and a polypropylene suture placed around the distal end of the bowel, using a purse-string instrument and a straight needle. (C) If the terminal rectum is to be used as a site for drainage of the pelvis, a continuous suture is placed around the circumference of the open end of the bowel.

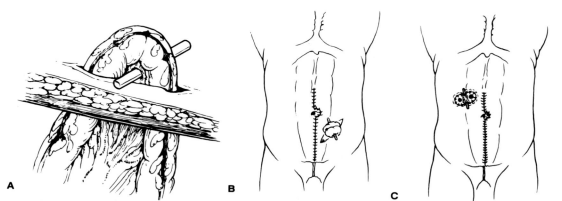

FIG. 19–11 Loop colostomy. (A) A rod or segment of vinyl tubing is inserted through an opening at the edge of the mesentery. (B) The abdominal incision is closed. The loop sigmoid colostomy is shown, with rod in place, prior to opening the colon with the electrocautery along the tinea. The rod can be secured with an appliance (Hollister), or a segment of rubber tubing attached to both ends. (C) Alternatively, as shown with this right transverse colostomy, the stoma can be matured primarily over the rod.

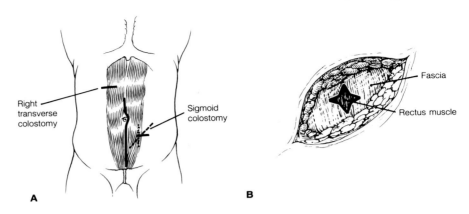

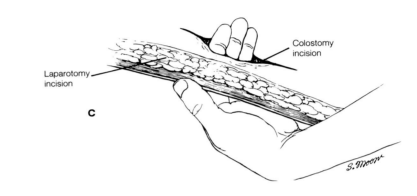

FIG. 19–12 End colostomy. (*A*) A midline abdominal incision is indicated. Sites for sigmoid colostomy (transverse, oblique, or vertical paramedian incisions) are indicated overlying the lateral border of the rectus muscle. (*B*) The incision is extended to the rectus fascia where a cruciate incision is made. (*C*) The rectus muscle is bluntly separated and the peritoneum is opened to allow passage of three fingers.

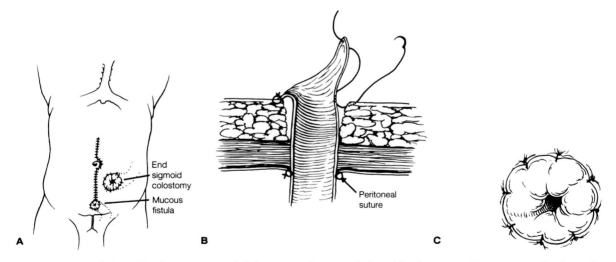

FIG. 19–13 End sigmoid colostomy. (*A*) A left lower quadrant, end sigmoid colostomy with a mucous fistula at the base of the wound. (*B*) Details of the end colostomy. Peritoneal sutures secure the colon to the abdominal wall circumferentially. A simple suture between skin edge and colon has been placed and tied. An everting suture is being placed with a bite of dermis, a seromuscular bite in the colon at skin level, and the edge of the colon. Four such sutures, one in each quadrant, will evert the stoma. (*C*) The completed end-colostomy "rosebud."

the edge of the colon, and a third bite through full thickness of the end of the colon from outside in (Fig. 19–13B). After all four sutures are placed, these are tied, which primarily everts the mucosa and matures the colostomy (Fig. 19–13C). One or two sutures can be taken between each of these quadrant sutures, again beginning with a bite of the dermis but following with a full thickness bite of the end of the colon. After all sutures have been placed, a temporary colostomy appliance is applied.

A Hartmann pouch can be created in the distal bowel segment by oversewing a previously placed staple line or by closing the end of the bowel in two layers. A mucous fistula can be created by primary attachment of the distal segment to the skin of the inferior portion of the wound, or, preferably, to a separate lower quadrant incision, after the seromuscular surface of the bowel is tacked to the surrounding fascia. Alternatively, a Stone clamp or similar crushing clamp can be left on the end of the bowel for 5 to 7 days and then removed.

A colostomy, whether temporary or permanent, will markedly alter a person's self-perception and lifestyle. Although psychological adjustment can easily be made and reinforced with the help of enterostomal therapists and ostomy clubs, one should not assume that a patient's life will not be changed materially by the addition of a colostomy. With that in mind, one can appreciate the overwhelming importance of the location of a colostomy. Modern enterostomal therapists can cope with a stoma that does not protrude adequately by using newer appliances and adhesives. Even the most ingenious enterostomal therapist, however, cannot improve on a poorly placed colostomy.

Surgery of the Anus and Rectum

Although there is no occasion requiring the gynecologic surgeon to perform major rectal surgery electively, there are many occasions when gynecologists performing vaginal plastic operations can very conveniently remove a symptomatic hemorrhoid and provide relief to the patient. However, this section deals primarily with the nonoperative management of rectal disorders.

HEMORRHOIDS

Man has paid several rather dear premiums for having assumed an upright posture; not the least of these is hemorrhoids. Few human afflictions cause more discomfort without posing any threat to life.

The story of the pathophysiology of hemorrhoids is quite simple. Increased pressure in the perianal and rectal veins causes distention with dilatation of the veins (Fig. 19–14). This may be favored by spasm in the internal sphincter and resistance to outflow. It is assumed that as the vein walls become chronically distended, varices develop. Internal hemorrhoids are covered with mucous membrane and protrude into the rectal lumen (Fig. 19–15). They are usually painless, and the primary symptom is bleeding, which may occasionally be severe enough to require transfusion. As the hemorrhoids enlarge, they may protrude through the anal opening. When this occurs, the mucocutaneous junction becomes exposed, and itching and burning may be severe. Occasionally, as a hemorrhoid prolapses through the anal opening, the external sphincter goes into spasm, and the hemorrhoid may be strangulated, with gangrene resulting. This is an excruciatingly painful process. Rupture of a perianal vessel, with hemorrhage into the perianal subcutaneous tissue, is also quite painful and is identified clinically as a thrombosed hemorrhoid.

One of the more common conditions associated with hemorrhoids in women is pregnancy. Several theories have been proposed. Possibly the increased blood volume, plus pelvic venous congestion, is a factor; arteriovenous fistulas may be of importance. If symptoms can be managed until parturition, operation may not be necessary.

Local treatment is often quite beneficial. Relief of constipation by the administration of a bulk laxative (e.g., Metamucil) is important. Sitz baths, two to four times daily, are helpful. Suppositories with local anti-inflammatory agents may be of benefit. Topical analgesic ointments should be avoided because of a high incidence of hypersensitivity with resultant burning and itching. In the case of prolapse or acute thrombosis, cold compresses of saturated magnesium sulfate solution may bring great relief. Perianal injections of local anesthetic agents may be required to relieve sphincter spasm.

Occasionally, symptomatic protruding hemorrhoids are excised at the time of vaginal surgery by the radial technique shown in Figure 19–16. Care should be exercised to avoid removing excessive anoderm, which could result in anal stenosis. Hemorrhoidectomy at this time ensures that a second operative procedure will not be needed. At the end of a week, a gentle digital examination is made. This is painful but prevents adhesion formation and constriction. It is advisable to have the patient return to the office about 2 weeks after leaving the hospital for another digital examination. If there is any tendency to stricture formation, the patient should

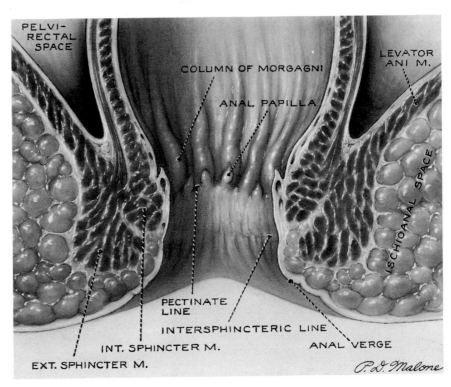

FIG. 19-14 Normal anatomy of the anus and lower rectum.

return at weekly intervals as long as necessary. Continued use of a bulk laxative allows continued regular dilatation of the anus during defecation. This prophylactic attention often prevents the formation of a troublesome stricture later.

The gynecologist may be faced with acutely thrombosed external hemorrhoids. It is important to recognize that these are, in fact, perianal hem-

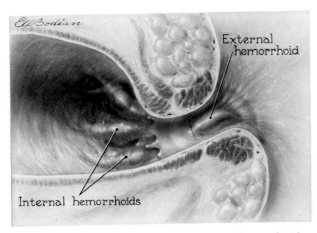

FIG. 19-15 Position of external and internal hemorrhoids.

atomas and not thrombosed blood vessels. These subcutaneous blood clots increase in size as the osmotic activity of the clot draws water into the very elastic perianal skin. If encountered during the first 3 days of onset, incision and drainage or excision with primary closure are appropriate methods of treatment. Many authorities favor excision over incision and drainage because excision precludes recurrence, postoperative bleeding, and the otherwise universal formation of skin tags. Lesions seen after 72 hours are probably best treated nonoperatively with Sitz baths, bulk-forming agents, and topical magnesium sulfate.

In 1954, Blaisdell presented a new technique for ligation of hemorrhoids using an instrument that employed a silk ligature, but premature loosening of the suture sometimes led to bleeding. In 1963, Barron modified Blaisdell's instrument, using a cone for loading the ligating drum and substituting an elastic latex rubber ring for the silk suture. Subsequently, the McGivney Hemorrhoid Ligator was developed from modifications of those of Blaisdell and Barron. Results in large series from the Cleveland Clinic, the Lahey Clinic, and others led to the conclusion that, in selected patients, elastic ligation is an acceptable form of treatment for internal hemorrhoids. Absolute contraindications are the pres-

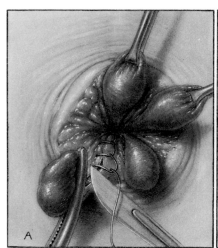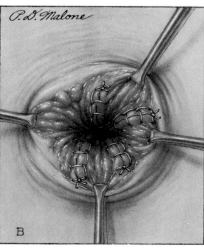

FIG. 19-16 Typical radial operation for internal hemorrhoid. (*A*) Groups of hemorrhoids are retracted with mucosa clips, and one mass of hemorrhoids is being excised. (*B*) The wounds have been sutured with continuous lock stitch of No. 0 delayed-absorbable suture.

ence of associated anorectal disease that might require operation and thrombosed hemorrhoids.

The technique of elastic ligation is quite simple (Fig. 19–17). The anoscope is inserted, and the largest hemorrhoid is selected for treatment. The cylindrical drum is placed over the hemorrhoid and the long-handled forceps is used to draw the hemorrhoid through the drum. The point at which the hemorrhoid is grasped should be at least 5 mm above the anorectal line. The handle is then closed and two rubber bands are ejected around the neck of the hemorrhoid. The patient may experience a dull ache but no significant pain. Any appreciable pain suggests the inclusion of very sensitive anoderm into the ligature. This necessitates urgent removal of the rubber band through an anoscope with a scalpel. Some patients will have a sense of fullness and the desire to defecate later in the day, and this should be discouraged for 12 to 24 hours. No more than one to two hemorrhoids should be ligated at a time; subsequent ligation should not be done for at least 3 weeks. Sloughing is usually complete in 8 days and may be associated with the passage of a small amount of red blood. Laxatives and stool softeners are usually given to avoid constipation, prevent excessive straining, and passively dilate the anal canal.

Complications are rare but include delayed hemorrhage, anal ulceration, pain, and slipping of the ligature.

ANAL FISSURE

This is a condition that rarely needs surgical treatment unless the fissure becomes chronic with scar formation. The problem is usually created by hard stool tearing the mucous membrane during defecation. Once the tear occurs, sphincter spasm follows. Each subsequent bowel movement aggravates the problem.

Management is the same as for hemorrhoids. Constipation must be alleviated and sphincter spasm relieved. A palpable abnormality, usually in the posterior midline, suggests chronicity and may require surgical intervention.

FISTULA-IN-ANO

Fistula-in-ano most often makes its presence known by the development of a perirectal abscess. The fistula usually begins in the anal crypt (Fig. 19-18). It is preceded by an inflammatory process in the crypt, which then extends through the rectal wall to contaminate the fat-containing perirectal spaces. The poor blood supply of this space makes it extremely vulnerable to infection. Fistula development is complete when the abscess drains spontaneously or is drained surgically. In the acute stage, management is aimed at the control of sepsis. Basic to the control of sepsis is the provision of adequate drainage. Since the ischiorectal space is traversed by fibrous septa, a perirectal fistula may be multiloculated. Because of the need for sigmoidoscopy through a painful anus to define the abnormality, as well as the possibility of multiloculation, perirectal abscesses are most appropriately drained in the operating room with a general anesthetic. Systemic antibiotics should be given if evidence of systemic reaction, such as leukocytosis, fever, or tachycardia is present. Special attention needs to be given to the very elderly, the debilitated, and those with associated illnesses, such as diabetes, because of the

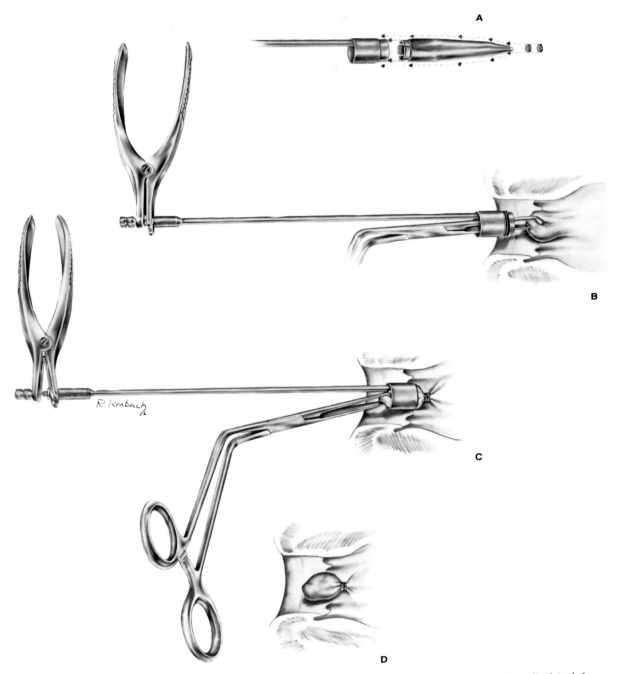

FIG. 19-17 Rubber band ligation of internal hemorrhoid. (A) Two rubber bands are loaded on the cylindrical drum. (B) The anoscope is inserted and the largest internal hemorrhoid is grasped after placing the Allis clamp *through* the cylindrical end drum. The drum is then advanced over the hemorrhoid. This must be at least 5 mm above the anorectal line. (C) The handle of the applicator is closed, ejecting the two bands at the base of the hemorrhoid. (D) Appearance of the ligated hemorrhoid with the rubber bands in place.

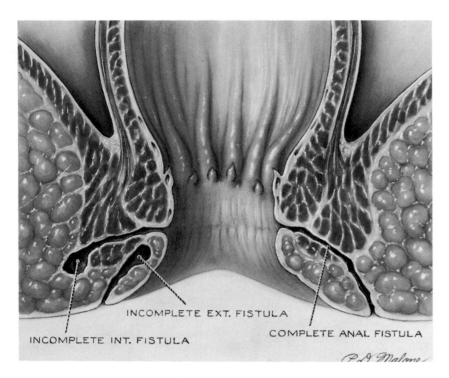

INCOMPLETE EXT. FISTULA

COMPLETE ANAL FISTULA

INCOMPLETE INT. FISTULA

FIG. 19-18 Schematic illustration of three types of fistulas.

increased likelihood of a supralevator component of the abscess. A supralevator abscess may require diversion of the fecal stream by colostomy.

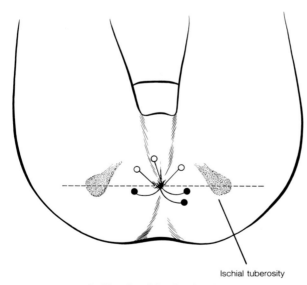

Ischial tuberosity

FIG. 19-19 Goodsall's rule of the fistula. This rule is generally valid and provides a clue to the site of the internal (mucosal) opening of a fistula-in-ano. External openings posterior to the line between ischial tuberosites enter in the posterior midline; those anterior to this line tend to have a radial course.

After a perirectal abscess is drained, a persistent fistula is common. This fistula connects the initial crypt abscess with the perianal skin. The external opening of the fistula-in-ano often gives a clue to the location of the internal opening. It is illustrated in Figure 19-19. Knowledge of this principle can be of assistance in probing a fistula, to find the internal opening. There is little need for the gynecologic surgeon to perform definitive surgery for a chronic fistula-in-ano. The need is to drain or improve spontaneous drainage of a perirectal abscess.

Bibliography

Arnold FJ, Nance RC: Volvulus of the sigmoid colon. Ann Surg 77:527, 1973

Barnett WO, Truett G, Williams R, et al: Shock in strangulation obstruction: Mechanisms and management. Ann Surg 157:747, 1963

Barron J: Office ligation of internal hemorrhoids. Am J Surg 105:563, 1963

Billig DM, Jordan PJ: Hemodynamic abnormalities in intestinal obstruction. Surg Gynecol Obstet 128:1274, 1969

Blaisdell PC: Scientific exhibit. American Medical Association, San Francisco, 1954

Bricker EA, Johnston WD: Repair of postirradiation recto-vaginal fistula and stricture. Surg Gynecol Obstet 148:499, 1979

Campbell CD, Carey LC: Shock: Differential diagnosis and immediate treatment. Postgrad Med 55:85, 1974

Classen JN, Bonardi R, O'Mara CS, et al: Surgical treatment

of acute diverticulitis by staged procedures. Ann Surg 184:582, 1976

Colcock BJ, Hume A: Radiation injury to the sigmoid and rectum. Surg Gynecol Obstet 108:306, 1959.

Corman ML, Veidenheimer MS: The new hemorrhoidectomy. Surg Clin North Am 53:417, 1973

Delancy HM: Prognostic factors in infarction of the intestine. Surg Gynecol Obstet 135:253, 1972

Dirksen PK, Matalo NM, Trelford JD: Complications following operation in the previously irradiated abdomino-pelvic cavity. Am Surgeon April 1977, p 234

Edmunds LJ, Jr, Williams GM, Welch CE: External fistulas arising from the gastrointestinal tract. Ann Surg 152:445, 1960

Fabri PJ: Intestinal ischemia in radiation enteritis. In Cooperman M (ed): Intestinal Ischemia. Mt. Kisco, New York, Futura Publishing Co, 1983

Gallagher DM, Russell TM: Surgical management of diverticular disease. Surg Clin North Am 58:563, 1978

Gehamy RA, Weakley FL: Internal hemorrhoidectomy by elastic ligation. Dis Colon Rectum 16:347, 1974

Green WW: Bowel obstruction in the aged patient. Am J Surg 118:541, 1969

Greenwald JC, Hoexter B: Repair of recto-vaginal fistulas. Surg Gynecol Obstet 146:443, 1978

Hines JR: Method of transverse loop colostomy. Surg Gynecol Obstet 141:426, 1975

Horwitz A, Smith DF, Rosensweig J: The acutely obstructed colon. Am J Surg 104:474, 1962

Kawarda Y, Brady L, Matsumoto T: Radiation injury to the large and small intestines. Am J Proctol 24:49, 1974

Leffall LO, Syphax B: Clinical aids in strangulation intestinal obstruction. Am J Surg 120:756, 1970

Lo AM, Evans WE, Carey LC: Review of small bowel obstruction at Milwaukee County General Hospital. Am J Surg 111:884, 1966

Localio SA, Stone A, Friedman M: Surgical aspects of radiation enteritis. Surg Gynecol Obstet 129:1163, 1969

McGivney JQ: The ligation treatment of internal hemorrhoids. Tex Med 63:56, 1967

Martimbeau P, Pratt JH, Gaffey TA: Small bowel obstruction secondary to endometriosis. Mayo Clin Proc 50:239, 1975

Miller TG, Abbott WO: Intestinal intubation: Practical technique. Am J Med Sci 187:595, 1934

Mortensen E, Nilsson T, Vesterhauge S: Treatment of intestinal obstruction. Dis Colon Rectum 17:638, 1974

Nadrowski LF: Pathophysiology and current treatment of intestinal obstruction. Rev Surg 31:381, 1974

Nelson SW, Christoforidis AJ, Roenigk WJ: Dangers and fallibilities of iodinated radiopaque media in obstruction of the small bowel. Am J Surg 109:546, 1965

Parks AG, Gordon PJ, Hardcastle JD: A classification of fistula in ano. Br J Surg 63:1, 1976

Plyforth RH, Holloway JB, Griffin WO: Mechanical small bowel obstruction: A plea for earlier surgical intervention. Ann Surg 1:783, 1970

Preston FW: The intestine and rectum. In Preston FW, Beal JM (eds): Basic Surgical Physiology. Chicago, Year Book Medical Publishers, 1969

Romsdahl MM, Cole WH: Diverticulitis of the colon. Arch Surg 86:751, 1963

Russell JC, Welch JP: Operative management of radiation injuries of the intestinal tract. Am J Surg 137:433, 1979

Schmitt EG, Symmonds RE: Surgical treatment of radiation-induced injuries of the small intestine. Surg Gynecol Obstet 153:896, 1981

Seyfer AE, Mologne LA, Morris RL, et al: Endometriosis causing acute small bowel obstruction: Report of a case and review of the literature. Am Surg 41:168, 1975

Smith GA, Perry JF, Jr, Yonehiro EG: Mechanical intestinal obstructions: Study of 1,252 cases. Surg Gynecol Obstet 100:651, 1955

Smith JS, Milford HE: Management of colitis caused by irradiation. Surg Gynecol Obstet 142:569, 1976

Snyder EN, McCranie D: Closed loop obstruction of the small bowel. Am J Surg 111:398, 1966

Steichern RM, Ravitch MM: History of mechanical devices and instruments for suturing. Curr Prob Surg 19:1, 1982

Steinberg DM, Liegois H, Alexander–Williams J: Long term review of the results of rubber band ligation of haemorrhoids. Br J Surg 62:144, 1975

SuFian S, Matsumoto T: Intestinal obstruction. Am J Surg 130:9, 1975

Turnbull RB, Weakley FL: Atlas of Intestinal Stomas. St Louis, CV Mosby, 1967

United States Surgical Corporation: Stapling Techniques, General Surgery, 2nd ed. 1980

Wangensteen OH, Rea CE: The distention factor in simple intestinal obstruction: An experimental study with exclusion of swallowed air by cervical esophagostomy. Surgery 5:327, 1939

Chapter 20

The Vermiform Appendix in Relation to Gynecology

The differential diagnosis between acute conditions in the pelvis and acute appendicitis is one of the most frequent that the gynecologist is called upon to make. It is also a serious one and a mistake may be fatal to the patient. The diagnosis of appendicitis may be especially difficult in the elderly and in the pregnant patient. Acute inflammation of the appendix commonly extends to the right adnexa (Fig. 20–1) and may involve the left as well when a periappendiceal abscess is located in the pelvis. When appendiceal rupture takes place, bilateral tubal involvement is common and complete or partial tubal closure may result with sterility or tubal pregnancy as sequelae. Even when the appendix is normal, the gynecologist and obstetrician must decide whether or not it should be removed during operations done for other reasons.

In 1905, Howard A. Kelly coauthored a beautifully illustrated book entitled *The Vermiform Appendix and its Diseases.* In its depiction of the pathology, clinical manifestations, and natural history of appendicitis and its complications, the book is unexcelled.

Incidental Appendectomy in Gynecologic and Obstetric Surgery

Experience and evidence in the literature support our belief and recommendation that incidental or elective or prophylactic appendectomy in gynecologic and obstetric surgery is a safe procedure and should be performed in younger women, unless the appendix is not conveniently available or the patient's condition is such that her well-being might be placed in jeopardy by the removal of the appendix. In other words, we believe that incidental appendectomy should be done unless there are contraindications.

Ever since the first recorded incidental appendectomy was performed in 1734 by Amyard, there has been much controversy concerning the routine performance of this procedure. Today, some of the most frequently done pelvic operations are hysterectomy, cesarean section, salpingectomy, oophorectomy, and tubal ligation. In these operations, the appendix is usually available for removal if the operator decides to do so and the patient agrees. That the controversy still exists is apparent from reports indicating that most gynecologic and obstetric operations are still done without incidental removal of the appendix. For example, in 1967, Loeffler and Stearn reported that only 26.5% of 555 patients had appendectomy at the time of total hysterectomy. In 1977, Hays found that most training programs recommend the performance of incidental appendectomy with uncomplicated abdominal hysterectomy. But the percentages were 66% in favor and 27% against, indicating that the controversy persists.

There are three main reasons to do incidental appendectomy:

1. To reduce future mortality and morbidity from appendicitis, including infertility following perforated appendix.
2. To eliminate undiagnosed incidental pathology in the appendix.
3. To eliminate the appendix from diagnostic consideration when the patient has abdominal or pelvic complaints in the immediate postoperative period and in future years.

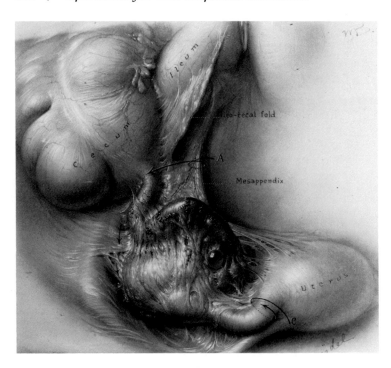

FIG. 20-1   As illustrated in this original Max Broedel drawing, inflammatory disease of the appendix may involve the fallopian tube or vice versa. Extensive adhesions may form. The tube and the appendix may be removed as a single mass.

Although the incidence of appendicitis is greater among teenagers and much less frequent in elderly women, the incidence in women over 20 and under 50 years of age is still significant. The overall lifetime risk of females developing appendicitis is about 1 in 6 at birth and 1 in 50 at 50 years of age. The risk of females developing appendicitis within the next year of life is greatest in the fifteen- to nineteen-year-old age group, in which it is about 1 in 99. Of special concern to the obstetrician is the difficulty in diagnosing appendicitis in pregnancy and the resultant increase in fetal loss. Hewitt and coworkers have estimated that for women the death rate secondary to acute appendicitis is 1 in 1100 for all ages up to 80 years of age. Of course, it is well known that although appendicitis is less common among elderly women, it is more difficult to diagnose in this group. As a result, the mortality rate is increased. Nevertheless, pointing out that 80% of cases of appendicitis in Wisconsin occur in patients between the ages of 5 and 30, with a rapid fall in subsequent years, Nockerts and coworkers feel that incidental appendectomy cannot be justified in the elderly. Unless epidemiologic data prove to the contrary, however, we will continue to offer incidental appendectomy to patients up to 50 years of age, believing that the hazards of acute appendicitis following pelvic operations without appendectomy are great enough to warrant routine removal of the appendix in these younger patients. The appendix

of an older patient should be inspected, and it should be removed if an abnormality is discovered.

Acute perforated appendicitis, especially when associated with pelvic abscess and peritonitis, has been associated with subsequent infertility. In the study by Wiig and coworkers, of 48 patients under 25 years of age who developed appendicitis with simple perforation, 19% were infertile; of 16 patients with pelvic abscess, 31% were infertile. In the control group of 58 patients, 12% could not have children. A study by Powley also found an increased incidence of infertility following appendicitis. It may be advisable, therefore, for young girls to have an incidental appendectomy performed whenever this can be done conveniently during abdominal or pelvic operations done for other reasons.

In addition to preventing appendicitis in future years, incidental appendectomy offers the advantage of removing unsuspected pathology. In the series of 532 cases reported by Taniguchi and Kilkenny, a relatively high incidence of acute inflammation was found in appendices removed incidental to pelvic laparotomies: 9.6% showed catarrhal appendicitis and 0.9% showed subacute or early acute appendicitis. In a study of 45 incidental appendectomy specimens, Melcher found only 12 to be normal. Among the pathologic findings in the abnormal appendices were acute, subacute, and chronic appendicitis, carcinoid tumors, and endometriosis. Others have confirmed that approximately 10% of incidental appendectomy specimens show significant pathology. The incidence will obviously depend on how carefully the appendix is examined by the pathologist.

Ectopic pregnancy and endometriosis have been reported in association with appendicitis. Indeed, the appendix is a frequent site of involvement in patients with pelvic endometriosis, although endometriosis will rarely be confined only to the appendix. Pittaway found endometriosis in 13% of appendices removed from patients with pelvic endometriosis at the Johns Hopkins Hospital. In 38%, the appendix was grossly normal when histologic evidence of endometriosis was found. The author concluded from the study that

1. Appendectomy is warranted in patients who are not interested in having children and are undergoing definitive surgery for endometriosis.
2. Appendectomy should be done when the appendix is abnormal even in patients with endometriosis who are undergoing surgery to restore fertility.
3. In this latter group, routine appendectomy to remove occult appendiceal endometriosis is probably unnecessary.

We agree with these recommendations.

The appendix is the most common site for carcinoid tumors, with an incidence of 0.03% of all appendices removed. Almost all appendiceal carcinoids are benign. It is rare for the carcinoid syndrome to be present. In a collected series of 1173 appendiceal carcinoid tumors, Sanders and Axtell reported that only 2.9% showed evidence of metastasis. Of two carcinoid tumors found by Melcher among 45 incidental appendectomies, one had spread into the surrounding adipose tissue. In Waters' series of 830 patients in whom elective appendectomy was performed, six appendiceal carcinoid tumors were suspected or diagnosed on gross surgical appearance.

In the final analysis, it may be admitted that the main reason to perform incidental appendectomy is to eliminate the appendix from consideration when a patient presents with perplexing pelvic or abdominal pain. In spite of medical progress in many other areas, the diagnosis of appendicitis still remains difficult in many cases. The complication of acute appendicitis in the first several weeks after pelvic laparotomy or cesarean section is undoubtedly rare but could have serious consequences because of the difficulty of interpreting physical signs and laboratory data in the postoperative patient. Howkins reported four cases in which appendicitis occurred within a week of hysterectomy. However, in many other large series of abdominal hyster-

ectomies without appendectomy there are no recognized cases of appendicitis in the postoperative recovery period. But over and over again the appendix does cause considerable confusion in the diagnosis of obscure abdominal and pelvic disease. An excellent example is the study by Isaacs and Knaus of nongenital pelvic tumors that mimicked gynecologic disease. Of 470 patients operated on for suspected tubo-ovarian pathology, 27 were found to have unsuspected nongenital pelvic tumors at the time of laparotomy. Chronic appendiceal infection was found most often. Of course, acute appendicitis is often confused with acute salpingitis, ectopic pregnancy, twisted or ruptured ovarian cyst, and other conditions within the abdomen and female pelvis. When such conditions arise, it is a significant diagnostic advantage to know that the patient has had a previous incidental appendectomy.

Incidental appendectomy could not be justified if it could not be done safely. Elective surgery must always be safe. There is ample evidence that, provided good judgement is used, no increase in morbidity or mortality occurs when incidental appendectomy is performed at the time of routine abdominal hysterectomy, salpingectomy, tubal ligation, or cesarean section. The studies of Pittaway, of Waters, of Loeffler and Stearn, of Wilson and colleagues, and of others confirm this. Of course, it cannot be denied that there are complications of incidental appendectomy just as with any operative procedure. These include bleeding and hematoma formation; adhesion formation with subsequent intestinal obstruction; blow-out of the appendiceal stump with abscess or fecal fistula or both; and others. These complications have, in fact, been reported in patients who have had an incidental appendectomy, as one might expect. One cannot have a zero complication rate with any operative procedure done in great numbers. The complication rate is not negligible, but we believe that it is low enough to justify routine incidental appendectomy under proper circumstances. These include care in performance of the procedure; satisfactory condition of the patient during the operation, including satisfactory tolerance of the anesthetic; and easy exposure of the appendix. If the patient has lost a great deal of blood or the operation has been unusually prolonged, incidental appendectomy should be performed only when significant pathology of the appendix is found. Incidental appendectomy should not be performed in the presence of bowel obstruction.

There are no data on whether or not incidental appendectomy has a deleterious effect on fertility when done at the time of an operation whose purpose is to restore or enhance fertility. In other words, should an incidental appendectomy be done in conjunction with a microsurgical tubal reconstruction operation or a myomectomy or a uterine unification operation? The fact that there is no significant difference in postoperative febrile morbidity does not preclude the possibility of a mild, subclinical, localized peritonitis that might cause pelvic and peritubal adhesions, with the possibility of affecting fertility adversely. For this reason, we usually do not remove the appendix when the operation is done for the primary purpose of restoring or enhancing fertility. The appendix is inspected at the end of the operation and is removed only if there is significant gross pathology.

Until recently, the removal of the appendix incidentally at cesarean section or at tubal ligation in the postpartum period was considered ill-advised. Larsson was one of the first to advocate incidental appendectomy with cesarean section. Since then there have been other proponents of this procedure. Sweeney compared the results for 230 cesarean section patients on whom appendectomy was performed with the results for a control group of 230 cesarean section patients without appendectomy. Except for a 16-minute increase in operative time for those with appendectomy, there were no significant differences between the groups: there was no increase in operative risk, no difference in postoperative febrile morbidity, and no increase in the duration of hospitalization among the patients in the appendectomy group. Douglas and Stromme reported no significant complications in more than 500 selected cases of cesarean section where incidental appendectomy was performed. Waters electively removed the appendix at the time of cesarean section during a personal experience of 40 years. Wilson and colleagues found no increase in morbidity when appendectomy was combined with cesarean section, cesarean tubal ligation, cesarean hysterectomy, postpartum tubal ligation, or postpartum hysterectomy. Incidental appendectomy should be done with caution when cesarean section is done for prolonged labor, prolonged rupture of the membranes, or amnionitis and is most acceptable in patients who are having an elective cesarean section.

The practice of incidental appendectomy at the time of operation for tubal ectopic gestation is more controversial. We tend to agree with Pelosi and colleagues that the prognosis for subsequent pregnancy is so dismal after operation for ectopic pregnancy that any additional possible insult should be avoided if possible.

In 1949, Bueno of Spain reported three cases of incidental appendectomy at the time of vaginal hysterectomy. Subsequently, McGowan reported the performance of 10 incidental appendectomies through the vagina without complications. Although incidental appendectomy at the time of vaginal hysterectomy is not considered acceptable practice in our clinic, it may not be absolutely contraindicated when adequate exposure and mobility of the appendix and its base is possible.

Acute Appendicitis

The diagnosis of acute appendicitis is based primarily on history and physical examination. A correlation with the pathophysiology of acute appendicitis is illustrated in Figure 20–2. The typical pain of acute appendicitis is diffuse and mild and initially located in the epigastrium and periumbilical region, subsequently to become more severe and localized in the right lower quadrant. Anorexia, nausea, and occasional vomiting are usually present. This classic sequence may be found in 50% of patients. Contrariwise, it should be emphasized that the typical presentation is absent in the remaining 50%. Atypically, pain may be localized in the right lower quadrant in the beginning or it may remain diffuse throughout the abdomen. The location and magnitude of the pain may vary with the position of the appendix and the age of the patient. Elderly patients may have less severe pain and delayed localization in the right lower quadrant. Indeed, appendicitis in the elderly presents a real challenge to early diagnosis since very few abnormal clinical findings may be present in early stages of the disease and even in the presence of advanced disease. This is the reason for the higher incidence of appendiceal perforation and consequently morbidity and mortality rates in older patients. The diagnosis is more difficult and the incidence of appendiceal perforation is also higher in infants and children. Improvement in the results for these two age groups will depend on a higher index of suspicion and a lower threshold for intervention, which will inevitably result in the removal of a larger number of normal appendices. But removal of a normal appendix in a patient who is thought to have appendicitis, a potentially lethal disease, should not be considered an unnecessary operation. More elderly patients and children die of appendicitis because of failure to operate early enough when the diagnosis is in doubt than die from removal of a normal appendix. Unfortunately, more than 30% of elderly patients will be found to have a ruptured appendix when the operation is finally done.

On physical examination, patients with appendicitis will have tenderness to direct palpation, rebound tenderness, and muscle guarding in the right

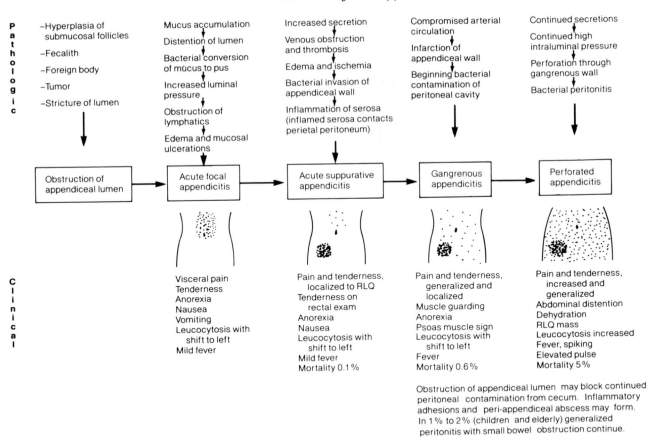

FIG. 20-2 Some pathologic and clinical correlations in appendicitis. (Modified from Condon, 1981; DeVore, 1980)

lower abdominal quadrant over the point where the inflamed appendiceal serosa is in contact with the parietal peritoneum. Rovsing's sign (pain in the right lower quadrant when pressure is applied in the left lower quadrant) as well as psoas and obturator muscle signs may be positive. Rectal and pelvic examinations should always be done and will often reveal tenderness high on the right side of the pelvis. Indeed, a pelvic mass from an inflamed appendix can sometimes be felt on pelvic examination. The appendix is located at the pelvic brim or low in the pelvis in 30% of patients. The rectovaginal-abdominal examination is also necessary to rule out gynecologic and other problems. As the disease progresses to gangrene and appendiceal rupture occurs, a mass consisting of inflammatory adhesions, omentum, indurated bowel, mesentery, and pockets of purulent exudate can usually be felt in the right lower quadrant or by pelvic examination. Tenderness and muscle rigidity are more pronounced. If the infection fails to localize, generalized peritonitis ensues with diffuse tenderness, guarding, distention, ileus, dehydration, tachycar-

dia, and spiking fever. All of these signs may be less apparent in the elderly. There is no evidence that appendicitis is more frequent in any particular phase of the menstrual cycle.

Routine laboratory determinations and special diagnostic procedures are not especially helpful except to rule out other diseases that cause a similar clinical picture. A detailed analysis of laboratory findings has been published by Andersen and associates. The white cell count is usually elevated and the differential count will show a shift to the left in most patients with appendicitis. In elderly patients, on the other hand, the white cell count may be elevated only slightly or not at all even though the differential count is abnormal. The erythrocyte sedimentation rate is elevated when the appendix is severely inflamed. Some white cells and red cells may be present in the urine with appendicitis, although with concomitant bacteriuria a urinary tract infection is a more likely diagnosis. Abdominal x-rays, barium enema, and ultrasonography are usually not helpful. It may be possible to locate an appendiceal abscess with ultrasonography or CT scan and, once located, its progress and response to therapy may be followed.

The diagnostic error for acute appendicitis in all adults is 20% to 30%, and this figure has been acceptable. The diagnostic error in adult females in the reproductive years is higher because of the frequent occurrence of nearby gynecologic diseases that confuse the clinical picture. Although appendectomy with removal of a normal appendix carries a very minimal mortality risk to the patient, there is some morbidity to be considered. Therefore, efforts should be made to improve diagnostic accuracy. Laparoscopy has been used in recent years to define more accurately the cause of pelvic pain and to eliminate an appendectomy when the appendix is normal. According to Leape and Ramenofsky, Deutsch and colleagues, approximately one-third of selected patients suspected of having appendicitis did not require appendectomy after laparoscopy was performed. A few false positive and false negative examinations were reported, however. The plan of operation (different incision, and so on) was altered in some patients who were found to have another condition. In doubtful cases of suspected early appendicitis, diagnostic accuracy will be improved by laparoscopy.

TREATMENT OF ACUTE APPENDICITIS

There is general agreement that the treatment of acute appendicitis in the nonperforated stage is immediate appendectomy. Clinical experience and numerous reports on mortality show clearly the advantage of early operation. The current operative mortality for appendicitis without perforation is essentially nil, while even following perforation, the overall mortality has been reduced to less than 5%. Obviously, antibiotics and earlier surgical intervention have contributed to the improvement in the statistics.

Thus, there is no controversy concerning the treatment of the appendicitis per se, but there is considerable difference of opinion concerning the treatment of the principal complication, namely abscess. We believe that, as a general policy, an immediate operation should be performed when the diagnosis is made, regardless of the stage of the disease.

Our general rule is to operate immediately through a McBurney incision in cases of acute appendicitis. However, when the diagnosis is uncertain and there is a possibility that other surgery may be required, either a low midline or right paramedian incision may be used. Occasionally, one may diagnose a well walled-off abscess that is palpable abdominally in a patient whose history suggests strongly that she is improving. It may be apparent from her history that she is not as ill as she was previously and that the walled-off abscess is subsiding. Such a patient should be kept under close observation, with frequent white blood counts, differential counts, and repeated radiological evaluation of the dilated bowel pattern for documented evidence of clinical improvement. Serial ultrasonography examinations or CT scans are helpful. Operation should be deferred as long as improvement continues. During the period of observation, the patient should have the advantage of intensive antibiotic therapy. If there is evidence of spread of infection, or if the patient's general condition becomes worse, surgical intervention is carried out immediately. Our reason for making this exception to the rule of immediate operation is that, in our experience with cases of this kind, patients who were treated conservatively responded better than those who were operated upon immediately. Some of the latter patients died of obstruction or peritonitis with septic shock. In retrospect, it appears that such patients probably would have continued to improve if surgical intervention had been omitted at that stage.

When appendiceal abscesses are operated upon, it is our custom to make a transverse incision directly over the abscess. The abscess cavity is entered with the greatest of care to avoid breaking up the adhesions that are responsible for the walling-off of the abscess. If the appendix can be removed readily without danger of injury to the bowel wall or of dissemination of the infection, appendectomy is done; if appendectomy is not feasible, the abscess is simply drained. Intensive antibiotic therapy is continued. When the abscess is localized in the cul-de-sac, it may be drained by colpotomy; two cigarette drains are placed in the cavity. Generally, we perform an appendectomy 6 or 8 weeks after the abscess has ceased to drain. In a few patients who have responded well, have no evidence of active infection, and have medical contraindications to operation, interval appendectomy may be postponed indefinitely as long as the patient remains well.

Perhaps the term *immediate operation* should be defined. In the usual case of unruptured appendicitis, the operation is done as soon as the operating room can be made ready. On the other hand, very ill patients with abscess or generalized peritonitis are often dehydrated, the serum electrolytes may be abnormal, gastric and intestinal distention is marked, and there may be circulatory collapse from gram-negative shock. Often intensive preoperative treatment is required for a very limited period of time until the patient's condition improves and is stable enough for her to tolerate general anesthesia. Unnecessary delay in surgery is one of the major factors in the very high mortality associated with ruptured appendix in the elderly patient. Such patients are admitted to the hospital and placed in Fowler's position. A nasogastric tube is passed and suction is started. High-dose, intravenous antibiotics are administered, including 20 to 40 million units of penicillin and 1 g to 1.5 g of the aminoglycoside kanamycin per day or other appropriate agents, such as clindamycin, that are effective against coliform bacteria, in an effort rapidly to produce adequate blood levels and tissue perfusion of the antibiotics. One of the newer cephalosporins or metronidazole may be indicated if an agent effective against *Bacteroides fragilis* is needed. The question of antibiotics for appendicitis—when they should be used, which ones to give, in what dosage, and for how long—is an area of active clinical research.

Postoperatively, supportive treatment is continued in the ill patient. All food and fluids by mouth are forbidden. Nasogastric suction is continued until distention has disappeared and there is clinical evidence of intestinal activity. Intensive antibiotic therapy is continued until the patient is well on her way to recovery. If drains are required for residual abscess material in the pelvis, we prefer a separate stab-wound incision rather than a drain placed in one end of the incision to decrease the incidence of secondary infection of the incision. Infection of the wound occurs in 5% to 10% of the reported cases of acute appendicitis, depending on the severity of the infection and the virulence of the offending organism. Incisional infection occurs in 34% to 50% of the cases where the appendix has ruptured. The important points in surgical technique to assist primary wound healing in these infected cases include minimal tissue trauma, meticulous hemostasis, and the use of the least possible amount of absorbable suture material buried in the wound. Nonabsorbable suture material should not be used in this incision closure. We are convinced, as are Ackerman and others, that the use of subcutaneous drains and subcutaneous antibiotic irrigations is important in reducing wound infection if primary closure is used in cases with a ruptured appendix.

It may be advisable, occasionally, to omit primary closure of the subcutaneous fat and skin and rely on secondary healing from the base of the incision. The open incision may be irrigated or sprayed with an antibiotic solution (Neosporin) and packed with sterile gauze. In 3 to 5 days the pack is removed and the skin margins are closed with sutures or simply drawn together with sterile adhesive strips. It has been our experience, however, that primary wound closure results in fewer postoperative incisional hernias.

Technique of Appendectomy

The appendix and the cecum are delivered. Usually this is a simple matter, but in some instances an immobile cecum, adhesions, or retrocecal position of the appendix may make it difficult. When the appendix is mobile, the mesoappendix may be conveniently grasped near the tip of the appendix with a Babcock clamp and the appendix supported with an additional Babcock clamp near its base.

The mesoappendix can then be ligated en masse with No. 3-0 delayed-absorbable suture, if it is sufficiently mobile (Fig. 20–3A). Often ligation of the mesoappendix en masse is not feasible, and, if this is the case, it is clamped with Kelly clamps in a succession of small bites; each segment of the clamped mesoappendix is ligated individually. Packs are then placed around the appendix to isolate it from the operative field.

A purse-string suture of medium silk is placed about the base of the appendix (Fig. 20–3B). The circumference of the purse string should be large enough to permit easy inversion of the stump. A half-knot is placed in the silk. A cuff of peritoneum is turned back after a circular incision is made about the base of the appendix (Fig. 20–3C) to permit complete occlusion of the appendiceal lumen when the stump is ligated. The appendix is crushed at the point of denudation with a Kelly or Halsted clamp and ligated with No. 3-0 delayed-absorbable suture (Fig. 20–3D). A Kelly clamp is placed on the appendix a short distance distal to the ligature, leaving sufficient space between the ligature and the clamp to permit the passage of the cautery or scalpel.

The appendix is amputated with the scalpel, although amputation with a cautery is an equally good technique. The appendix and the attached clamps are dropped into a small basin kept on the operating table for receiving the appendix and the instruments that might be contaminated in doing the appendectomy. The peritoneal edge of the appendix stump is grasped by the assistant with a mosquito clamp, and the ligature about the base of the appendix is cut short. The stump is inverted (Fig. 20–3E,F) and the purse string is drawn tight (Fig. 20–4). The mosquito clamp is dropped into the appendix basin, and the basin is passed from the operating table.

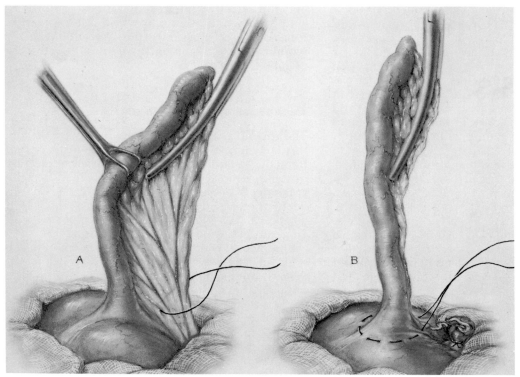

FIG. 20-3 Technique of appendectomy. (A) Appendix is delivered and supported with Kelly and Babcock clamps as the mesoappendix ligated. Often this can be done with a single ligature of No. 3-0 delayed-absorbable suture as illustrated. (B) A purse-string of medium silk has been placed about the base of the appendix.

The site of inversion of the appendiceal stump into the cecum should be covered over with the mesoappendix or any convenient flap of fat located around the terminal ileum (Fig. 20-3, G, H). If the appendiceal stump has not been inverted but has been left exposed, it is especially important that it be covered. If the appendix was retrocecal, this step may not be necessary.

We are aware that there are criticisms of a technique of appendectomy that includes burying a ligated appendiceal stump. An abscess may form in the cecal wall leading to blow-out of the cecum. A space-occupying mass in the cecum may be found on barium enema and lead to diagnostic confusion. However, these problems are rare. We still prefer to bury the appendiceal stump and have it isolated completely rather than run the risk of localized infection and adhesion formation or even intestinal obstruction from adhesions to an exposed stump. Admittedly, inversion of the stump is more applicable when a normal appendix is being removed, as in incidental appendectomy. It is less feasible when an inflamed appendix is being removed. If

the appendix is gangrenous or perforated, the stump generally should not be buried.

Appendicitis in Pregnancy

During pregnancy acute appendicitis—and especially its sequelae—present serious dangers for both mother and fetus. Brant noted an incidence of acute appendicitis of 1 in 1789 pregnancies (0.06%), while Taylor reported an increase in the frequency of this complication of pregnancy to 1 in 704 cases. Babaknia and coauthors found the incidence of appendicitis to be 1 in 1500 pregnancies (0.07%) over a 12-year period. Earlier reports by Baer, Reis, and Arens recorded the incidence to be approximately 0.17 percent. The incidence of acute appendicitis does not seem to be increased during pregnancy above that of the nonpregnant state, but the diagnosis is often delayed. In our clinics and in others, acute appendicitis occurs more frequently during the second trimester (50%) than in the first trimester (10%) or third trimester (35%). Five percent of cases

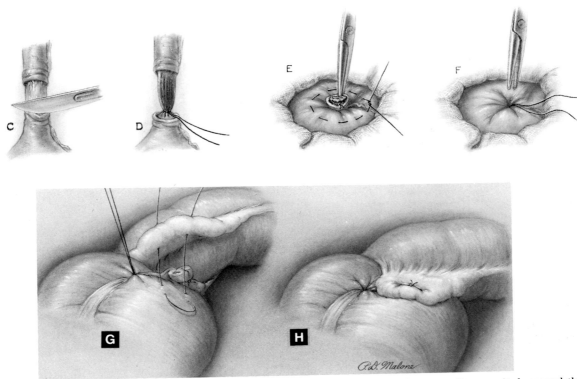

FIG. 20–3 (continued). (*C*) An incision through the serosa is made about the appendix near its base and the serosa is pushed down. (*D*) The appendix has been crushed at the point where it has been freed of serosa and ligated with No. 3-0 delayed-absorbable suture. (*E*) The stump is inverted as the purse-string is drawn tight. (*F*) The mosquito clamp is withdrawn as the purse-string suture is tied. (*G*) A simple method of peritonizing the mesoappendix stump. Fine silk is used for this. (*H*) Completed appendectomy.

occur during labor or in the puerperium. The number of patients with appendiceal rupture will be highest in the third trimester.

Appendicitis is responsible for approximately 75% of all cases of an acute abdomen during pregnancy. Errors in the clinical diagnosis of acute appendicitis are quite common during pregnancy, with a normal appendix being found in between 20% and 30% of the cases at removal, as recently reported by Mohammed and Oxorn. Although this removal rate of an uninflamed appendix may seem high, this diagnostic error is far more acceptable than a delay in surgery in the case of an acute abdomen during pregnancy, which could result in appendiceal rupture and an increased risk of maternal mortality and morbidity, as well as fetal mortality.

Delay in diagnosis is consistently the reason for gangrenous and perforated appendix with associated increased risk of maternal mortality and morbidity and perinatal mortality. The incidence of gangrenous and perforated appendix has been reported to be twice as high in pregnant patients as in women who are not pregnant and is highest

in advanced pregnancy. Patient delay or a policy of observation before operating allows the inflamed appendix time to become gangrenous and to per-

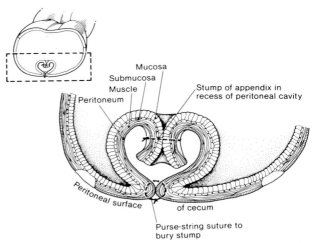

FIG. 20–4 Diagrammatic representation of inversion of the ligated appendiceal stump into the cecal wall.

forate. The incidence of perforation is only 20% in the first 24 hours of symptoms but increases to over 70% if symptoms have been present over 48 hours. In a pregnant patient, the omentum may not be able to reach the site of infection and perform its walling-off function efficiently. If rupture is followed by abscess formation, the uterus is always a part of the abscess wall because of its close proximity. Generalized peritonitis without abscess is more common in advanced pregnancy and is a serious threat to the expectant mother and her unborn child. The speed of onset and spread of peritonitis in pregnant patients may be strikingly and insidiously rapid. The patient may become seriously ill and appear moribund within 24 hours. Appendiceal perforation and involvement of the uterus in peritonitis causes uterine irritability and increases the risk of preterm labor.

DIAGNOSIS OF APPENDICITIS IN PREGNANCY

Babler's statement written in 1908 is unfortunately still pertinent today: "The mortality of appendicitis complicating pregnancy and the puerperium is the mortality of delay." Several factors cause a delay in the diagnosis of acute appendicitis in pregnant patients. Consider first that a normal pregnancy may cause some of the same symptoms as acute appendicitis and may be confusing. For example, the classic symptoms of abdominal pain, nausea, vomiting, and constipation are common to both pregnancy and appendicitis. Lower abdominal discomfort is frequently attributed to round ligament stretching, a common symptom of normal pregnancy. The evaluation of the abdomen by physical examination is more difficult in the presence of an enlarging uterus, especially since only 50% of the patients with acute appendicitis will have peritoneal irritation with rebound tenderness. Alder described a useful clinical sign to differentiate appendiceal from uterine pain. If the pain is localized in the right lower abdominal quadrant with the patient lying supine but shifts to the left when she rolls to her left side, the pain is most likely of uterine or adnexal origin. On the other hand, if the pain remains localized to the right lower quadrant after she rolls to the left, then appendicitis should be suspected.

The change in the position of the appendix during pregnancy makes the interpretation of abdominal pain and tenderness more difficult than in the nonpregnant woman. One can interpret pain and tenderness much more intelligently if one bears in mind these changes. Baer, Reis, and Arens showed by repeat roentgenographic studies throughout pregnancy and the puerperium that the appendix rotated in a counterclockwise direction, with the tip displaced near the right kidney at term. The base of the appendix underwent upward and outward displacement after the third month, caused by the enlarging uterus, reaching the level of the iliac crest at the end of the sixth month. After the seventh month of pregnancy, in 88% of their cases, the appendix was found above the iliac crest (Fig. 20–5). However, in interpreting these findings in relation to abdominal pain and tenderness, one must remember that in dealing with the abnormal appendix, in which previous attacks of appendicitis are frequent, there may be adhesions that fix it in a low position and do not permit its upward displacement. Because the appendix is embryologically a midline structure, the afferent sensory fibers to this vestigial organ register pain more frequently in the periumbilical region, as well as on both sides of the abdomen. Once local peritonitis occurs, however, the maximum tenderness is usually located in the region of the appendix.

The organ that most often leads to a mistaken diagnosis of appendicitis in pregnancy is the kidney, in which an acute urinary tract infection is frequently misdiagnosed. Since urinary tract symptoms occur in more than 50% of the cases of appendicitis in pregnancy, the patient is frequently treated initially for pyelitis of the right kidney. Acute torsion of an ovarian cyst will also mimic the clinical

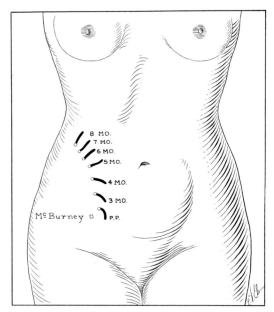

FIG. 20–5 Change of position of appendix during pregnancy (Baer JL, Reis RA, Arens RA: Appendicitis in pregnancy, with changes in position and axis of normal appendix in pregnancy. JAMA 98:1359, 1932. Copyright 1932, American Medical Association.)

signs of appendicitis in pregnancy, but in general there are fewer intestinal symptoms with this entity and the onset is more abrupt. Torsion of an ovarian cyst can be traced in many cases to strenuous physical activity such as dancing, swimming, coitus, or the like.

Although a mild leukocytosis is common in pregnancy, one should observe the white count frequently for a gradual or rapid increase and particularly for a shift in the differential leukocyte count. A white count above 16,000 per cubic millimeter and a differential count of more than 80% polymorphonuclear leukocytes suggest an acute inflammatory process but these are not specific for appendicitis. One must always be aware of the occasional case in which the white blood count remains normal throughout the acute phase of the disease. Fever is usually mild and sometimes absent.

All the above factors tend to make the diagnosis of appendicitis more difficult in pregnancy; hence a tendency to delay operation is common. The important thing for the clinician to bear in mind is the possibility of appendicitis, remembering that the symptoms of acute appendicitis are the same in a pregnant as in a nonpregnant patient. The clinician should have no concern about the possibility of removing a normal appendix during pregnancy, but should bear in mind that this additional operation is a small price to pay to avoid the increased risk to the life of the mother and fetus that accompanies a prolonged delay in the diagnosis of this disease. Although the laparoscope is beneficial in establishing the diagnosis in suspected cases, it is limited in its use by the size of the uterus.

TREATMENT OF APPENDICITIS IN PREGNANCY

Immediate operation is the treatment for acute appendicitis in pregnancy, regardless of the duration of pregnancy. Preoperative measures to improve the patient's condition should be brief and intensive. Although antibiotics may not be needed in simple acute appendicitis, antibiotic therapy should be initiated as soon as possible in all cases of suspected appendicitis so that an adequate level can be present in the tissues before the incision is made. Where a gangrenous or perforated appendix is found, antibiotics with broad-spectrum bacterial coverage should be continued or initiated immediately in both the pregnant and the nonpregnant state. One may choose to give an aminoglycoside, penicillin, and clindamycin. Second-generation cephalosporin agents, such as cefoxitin sodium (Mefoxin) may also be indicated because of their effectiveness against *Bacteroides fragilis* organisms. Ritodrine, a β-mimetic tocolytic agent, should be given prophylac-

tically to all patients beyond 16 weeks to prevent uterine contractions and premature labor. It should be continued as long as there is evidence of active infection. Although controversial, we also administer progesterone intramuscularly, especially to patients who are earlier in pregnancy than 16 weeks. Spontaneous premature termination of pregnancy is more likely when the appendix has ruptured. Delay in operating can also stem from concern about what harm the operation will do to the pregnancy, with the consequent desire to operate only when acute appendicitis is definitely present. Such a delay will result in a larger number of perforated appendices being found and a far greater harm to the pregnancy. Proper removal of a normal appendix found at operation for suspected appendicitis is rarely associated with preterm labor, especially with the prophylactic use of modern tocolytic agents.

If the pregnancy is 3 months or less in duration, the appendix may be removed through the usual gridiron incision. The more advanced the pregnancy, the higher should be the incision. If a midline incision is not used, it is important to center the incision over the point of maximum tenderness, which usually means using a high transverse muscle-cutting or a right paramedian incision. Turning the patient on her left side will minimize displacement and handling of the uterus and will relieve the compression of the vena cava by the gravid uterus. The appendectomy should be done as quickly and atraumatically as possible and the patient should be given intensive antibiotic therapy. In the case of appendiceal rupture with or without frank abscess formation, the patient should be treated immediately, in the same way as in the nonpregnant state, with the understanding that premature labor will usually occur as a result of the infection. Cesarean section should not be performed at the time of appendectomy with or without rupture in order to avoid infection in the newborn and postoperative endometritis and parametritis. Cesarean section in the third trimester patient with appendicitis is only indicated for strict obstetric reasons. When cesarean section is indicated for obstetric reasons, the fetus is near term size, and an advanced infection is present, some authors have advised that a cesarean section hysterectomy may be indicated to control the spread of the infection into the uterus and broad ligaments.

MATERNAL AND PERINATAL MORTALITY

In his 1908 collection series of 735 cases of appendicitis complicating pregnancy, labor, and the puerperium, Babler reported that the perinatal mortality was 66% and the maternal mortality was 48.5% when the appendix ruptured.

Significant progress has been made in reducing maternal and perinatal mortality from appendicitis in recent decades. The maternal mortality in the first trimester has usually been comparatively low, since diagnosis is less difficult at that stage. Black reported in 1960 that the mortality rate was 4% in the second trimester, 11% in the third trimester, and 16.7% if labor had begun. However, this high maternal mortality rate is considered to be due to the occurrence of many deaths prior to the use of antibiotics. In a 1977 review of 333 cases reported since 1963, Babaknia found only three maternal deaths (1.0%), all three of which occurred among 70 cases with a ruptured appendix (4%). In 1967, Brant reported an overall maternal mortality rate of 2% with a mortality rate of 7.3% in the last trimester. Cunningham and McCubbin reported no maternal deaths among 34 pregnant patients with documented appendicitis at Parkland Memorial Hospital between 1960 and 1975. Between 1949 and 1982, two maternal deaths from appendicitis in the antepartum period occurred at Grady Memorial Hospital. Both deaths occurred more than 26 years ago. Most reports of appendicitis complicating pregnancy since 1980 show no maternal deaths. When this is compared to the nonpregnant mortality of an unruptured acute appendicitis of 0.1%, it is evident that progress has been made in reducing maternal mortality from appendicitis.

There has also been considerable improvement in the combined fetal and neonatal (perinatal) mortality associated with appendicitis during the past two decades. Perinatal mortality is related to the duration of pregnancy and the severity of the infection. During the first trimester, spontaneous abortion may occur postoperatively in as many as 20% of cases. Midtrimester fetal loss is less common, while in the third trimester, perinatal mortality may reach as high as 15%, due primarily to prematurity. In the presence of perforation of the appendix and peritonitis, the perinatal mortality increases. McComb and Laimon recently reviewed a collected series of 171 cases of appendicitis complicating pregnancy and found that the overall perinatal mortality was 10%. The perinatal mortality was 7% when the appendix was not perforated and 30% when it was perforated. More than 20% of patients with appendicitis occurring in the third trimester will develop premature labor postoperatively. It is clear that early diagnosis and operative intervention, proper antibiotic administration, and prophylactic use of tocolytic agents to prevent preterm labor are the keys to further reduction in perinatal and maternal mortality from this disease.

Bibliography

Ackerman NB: The continuing problems of perforated appendicitis. Surg Gynecol Obstet 139:29, 1974

Adler N: A sign for differentiating uterine from extrauterine complications of pregnancy and puerperium. Br Med J 2:1194, 1951

Allen NJW, Heringer R: Coincident acute appendicitis and tubal pregnancy. Can Med Assoc J 103:531, 1970

Andersen M, Lilja T, Lundell L, Thulin A: Clinical and laboratory findings in patients subjected to laparotomy for suspected acute appendicitis. Acta Chir Scand 146:55, 1980

Arnbjornsson E: Varying frequency of acute appendicitis in different phases of the menstrual cycle. Surg Gynecol Obstet 155:709, 1982

Ashley JSA, Morris JN: Deaths from appendicitis. Lancet 1:217, 1967

Babaknia A, Parsa H, Woodruff JD: Appendicitis during pregnancy. Obstet Gynecol 50:40, 1977

Babler EA: Perforative appendicitis complicating pregnancy. JAMA 51:1310, 1908

Baer JL, Reis RA, Arens RA: Appendicitis in pregnancy, with changes in position and axis of normal appendix in pregnancy. JAMA 98:1359, 1932

Barber HRK, Graber EA: Surgical Diseases in Pregnancy. Philadelphia, WB Saunders, 1974

Bierman HR: Human appendix and neoplasia. Cancer 21:109, 1968

Black WP: Acute appendicitis in pregnancy. Br Med J 1:1938, 1960

Boyd A, Hoffmeister FJ: Cesarean section and associated surgery. Obstet Gynecol 24:533, 1964

Brant HA: Acute appendicitis in pregnancy. Obstet Gynecol 29:130, 1967

Brumer M: Appendicitis. Seasonal incidence and postoperative wound infection. Br J Surg 57:93, 1970

Bueno B: Primer caso de apendicectomia por via vaginal. Tokoginec Pract (Madrid) 8:152, 1949

Champion P, Doolittle J: Appendectomy at the time of cesarean section. Obstet Gynecol 24:533, 1964

Christhilf SM, Jr: Simplified incidental appendectomy. Surg Gynecol Obstet 122:607, 1966

Condon RE: Appendicitis. In Sabiston DC, Jr (ed): Davis-Christopher Textbook of Surgery. Philadelphia, WB Saunders, 1981

Cunningham FG, McCubbin JH: Appendicitis complicating pregnancy. Obstet Gynecol 45:415, 1975

Deutsch AA, Zelikovsky A, Reiss R: Laparoscopy in the prevention of unnecessary appendicectomies: A prospective study. Brit J Surg 69:336, 1982

DeVore GR: Acute abdominal pain in the pregnant patient due to pancreatitis, acute appendicitis, cholecystitis, or peptic ulcer disease. Clinics in Perinatology 7:349, 1980

Douglas RG, Stromme W: Operative Obstetrics, ed. 3. New York, Appleton-Century-Crofts, 1976

Editorial. Wound infection after appendectomy. Lancet 1:930, 1970

Farquharson RG: Acute appendicitis in pregnancy. Scott Med J 25:36, 1980

Finch DRA, Emanoel L: Acute appendicitis complicating pregnancy in the Oxford region. Br J Surg 61:129, 1974

Foster JH, Morgan CV, Therlkell JB, et al: Vascular malformation of the appendiceal stump. A rare cause of massive hemorrhage. JAMA 215:636, 1971

Geerdsen J, Hansen JB: Incidence of sterility in women operated on in childhood for perforated appendicitis. Acta Obstet Gynec Scand 56:523, 1977

Gilmore OJA, et al: Appendicitis and mimicking conditions. Lancet 2:421, 1975

Gomez A, Wood M: Acute appendicitis during pregnancy. Am J Surg 137:180, 1979

Greenwald JC, Fenton AN: Ovarian abscess secondary to incidental appendectomy at cesarean section. Obstet Gynecol 14:593, 1959

Grosfeld JL, Solit RWP: Prevention of wound infection in perforated appendicitis: experience with delayed primary wound closure. Am Ann Surg 168:891, 1968

Hays RJ: Incidental appendectomy: Current teaching. JAMA 238:31, 1977

Hewitt D, Milner J, LeRiche WH: Incidental appendectomy: A statistical appraisal. Can Med Assoc J 100:1075, 1969

Holtz G, Tucker E, Holtz F: Primary pure insular ovarian carcinoids. Obstet Gynecol 53:85S, 1979

Howkins J: Appendicectomy during gynaecological operations. Lancet 1:1016, 1956

Howkins J, Williams D: Total abdominal hysterectomy: 1,000 consecutive, unselected operations. Journal of Obstetrics and Gynaecology of the British Commonwealth 70:20, 1963

Isaacs JH, Knaus JV: The detection of nongenital pelvic tumors mimicking gynecologic disease. Surg Gynecol Obstet 153:74, 1981

Israel SL, Roitman HB: Cesarean section and prophylactic appendectomy: The passing of a prejudice. Obstet Gynecol 10:102, 1957

Kazarian KK, Roeder WJ, Merscheimer WL: Decreasing mortality and increasing morbidity from acute appendicitis. Am J Surg 119:681, 1970

Kelly HA, Hurdon E: The Vermiform Appendix and Its Diseases. Philadelphia, WB Saunders, 1905

Kocsard-Varo G: Physiologic role of tonsils, adenoids and the appendix in immunity. Med J Australia 2:873, 1964

Langman J, Rowland R, Vernon-Roberts B: Endometriosis of the appendix. Br J Surg 68:121, 1981

Larsson E: Elective appendectomy at time of cesarean section. JAMA 154:549, 1954

Leape LL, Ramenofsky ML: Laparoscopy for questionable appendicitis. Ann Surg 191:410, 1980

Loeffler F, Stearn R: Abdominal hysterectomy with appendectomy. Acta Obstet Gynecol Scand 46:435, 1967

MacLeod D, Howkins J: Bonney's Gynaecological Surgery, ed 7. London, Hoeber Medical Div, Harper & Row, 1964

Maier WP, Rosemond GP: A late complication of inversion of the appendiceal stump. Am J Surg 118:467, 1969

McComb P, Laimon H: Appendicitis complicating pregnancy. Can J Surg 23:92, 1980

McGowan L: Use of posterior colpotomy in the diagnosis and treatment of pelvic disease. Obstet Gynecol 21:108, 1963

McVay JR, Jr: The appendix in relation to neoplastic disease. Cancer 17:929, 1964

Melcher DH: Appendicectomy with abdominal hysterectomy. Lancet 1:810, 1971

Mohammed JA, Oxorn H: Appendicitis in pregnancy. Can Med Assoc J 112:1187, 1975

Nockerts SR, Detmer DE, Fryback DG: Incidental appendectomy in the elderly? No. Surgery 88:301, 1980

Pelosi MA, Apuzzio J, Iffy L: Ectopic pregnancy as an etiologic agent in appendicitis. Obstet Gynecol 53:45, 1979

Pittaway DE: Appendectomy in the surgical treatment of endometriosis. Obstet Gynecol 61:421, 1983

Powley PH: Infertility due to pelvic abscess and pelvic peritonitis in appendicitis. Lancet 1:27, 1965

Punnonen R, Aho AJ, Gronroos M, et al: Appendicectomy during pregnancy. Acta Chir Scand 145:555, 1979

Rubio PA, Farrell EM, Alvarez BA, et al: Endometriosis presenting as acute appendicitis. Int J Gynaecol Obstet 15:559, 1978

Sanders RJ, Axtell K: Carcinoids of the gastrointestinal tract. Surg Obstet Gynecol 119:369, 1964

Silvert MA, Meares EM, Jr: Rationale of incidental appendectomy. Urology 7:129, 1976

Sweeney WJ, III: Incidental appendectomy at the time of cesarean section. Obstet Gynecol 14:588, 1959

Taniguchi T, Kilkenny G: Prophylactic appendectomy in gynecological surgery. Am J Obstet Gynecol 60:1359, 1950

Taylor JD: Acute appendicitis in pregnancy and the puerperium. Aust NZ J Obstet Gynaecol 12:202, 1972

Thompson WT, Lynn HB: The possible relationship of appendicitis with perforation in childhood to infertility in women. J Ped Surg 6:458, 1971

Waters EG: Elective appendectomy concurrent with abdominal and pelvic surgery. Obstet Gynecol 50:511, 1977

Wiig JN, Janssen CW, Jr, Fuglesang P, et al: Infertility as a complication of perforated appendicitis. Acta Chir Scand 145:409, 1979

Wilson EA, Dilts PV, Jr, et al: Appendectomy incidental to postpartum sterilization. Am J Obstet Gynecol 116:76, 1973

Chapter 21

Dilatation of the Cervix and Curettage of the Uterus

Recamier invented the curette in 1843. Since that time, dilatation of the cervix and curettage of the endometrial cavity is the most frequent gynecologic procedure performed in the United States. It is used to diagnose uterine malignancy, to complete an incomplete or missed abortion, to evaluate the causes of infertility, to control dysfunctional uterine bleeding, and to relieve dysmenorrhea. Because medical therapy for dysfunctional uterine bleeding and dysmenorrhea has become more effective, dilatation of the cervix and curettage of the uterus is less often needed for these two problems, especially in young women. However, since it still has a major role in the diagnosis and control of abnormal uterine bleeding in older and occasionally in younger women, a proper understanding of the basic physiologic principals and clinical characteristics of normal and abnormal menstrual bleeding is essential in predicting the clinical value of a curettage.

Normal Menstrual Physiology

Normal menstrual physiology is the subject of extensive ongoing research. Excellent reviews of the subject have been written, especially by Healey and Hodgen. Menstruation is the physiologic shedding of the endometrium associated with uterine bleeding, occurring at monthly intervals from menarche to menopause. Between the menarche and the menopause, menstruation may occur 400 to 500 times. It is surprising that the physiologic process of monthly shedding and regeneration of endometrial tissue can occur so many times without producing evidence of permanent tissue damage.

In the strictest sense, the endometrium is an endocrine end-organ that contains intracellular cytoplasmic receptors that respond cyclically to the circulating blood levels of estrogen and progesterone. The endometrium sheds regularly and normally when there is proper synchronization of the hypothalamic releasing hormones that influence the release of pituitary gonadotropins that, in turn, regulate ovulation. The increasing blood levels of estrogen, principally estradiol (E_2), during the preovulatory (proliferative) phase of the cycle stimulate DNA replication and the growth of both endometrial glands and stroma by combining initially with protein receptors in the cytoplasm of the cell. Following ovulation, the increasing levels of progesterone have a suppressive effect on DNA synthesis within these cells and act as a dynamic inhibitor of cell mitosis, thereby serving as a controlling influence over endometrial cell growth. This biologic effect of progesterone is well recognized clinically and serves as the basis for its use in large doses to suppress the growth of pelvic endometriosis and well-differentiated endometrial adenocarcinoma.

Menstruation is controlled by many complex, interrelated, and incompletely understood factors. Normal menstruation results from progesterone withdrawal from an estrogen-primed endometrium. The changes in the endometrium that occur with menstruation were described by Markee by observation of endometrial tissue transplanted to the anterior chamber of the eye of the Rhesus monkey. He described the cyclic changes in the endometrial vascularity and the development of coiled vessels supplying the superficial two thirds of the endometrium. The basal one-third of the endometrium receives its blood supply from straight, short arteries. The spiral arterioles that supply the outer, functional endometrial layers are influenced by progesterone, which causes them to increase in length and also causes increased coiling and kinking. The estrogen-primed endometrium of the follicular phase is compact with relatively underdeveloped vasculature. Progesterone converts this endometrium into a thick, edematous, secretory lining that is glycogen-enriched and prepares the metabolically active stroma and glands with an increased vasculature to receive and nourish a fertilized ovum. If implantation does not occur, estrogen and progesterone levels fall and prostaglandin synthesis and lysosomal membrane rupture occur, causing constriction of the spiral arterioles, ischemic necrosis, and sloughing of the endometrium superficial to the basalis layer. This process begins in the premenstrual phase of the cycle with cessation and inspissation of glycogen secretion, depletion and disintegration of ground substance and supporting tissues, tonic contractions of spiral arterioles with reduction of blood flow to the tissues, loss of stromal edema, and kinking of the coiled spiral arterioles caused by a reduction in endometrial thickness. A generalized state of ischemia develops in the superficial layers of endometrium, bleeding into the stroma begins, acid phosphatase and prostaglandin substances released from autolized cells cause more intense vasoconstriction of spiral arterioles, and finally the devitalized tissue sloughs as small hemorrhages in the stroma coalesce. According to Bellar, coagulation factors are decreased in normal menstrual discharge. Fibrinogen is absent and plasminogen and plasmin inhibitor are decreased in amount. Menstrual blood does not clot, but as it collects in the vagina it may form red blood cell aggregates with mucoid substances, mucoproteins, and glycogen. These red cell aggregates may appear to be blood clots but contain no fibrin.

In the observations of Markee, the endometrial implants became smaller as the menstrual phase approached. The blood flow through endometrial vessels decreased and the tissue became blanched and ischemic because of contractions of the coiled vessels. After the vessels were constricted for several hours, bleeding began from breakage of the arterial walls, from diapedesis of blood cells through capillaries, and from venous channels opened by endometrial shedding. Tissue loss did not begin until several hours after the onset of bleeding. Markee felt that the degree of coiling of the spiral arterioles correlated with the amount of tissue shed.

During menstruation, the superficial compacta and the intermediate stratum spongiosum layers of the endometrium are shed, leaving the basalis layer intact. New endometrium is regenerated from the basalis. In Markee's studies, regeneration of new capillaries from the basalis could be seen. Restoration of the endometrial circulation was correlated with the cessation of menstrual bleeding. The loss of blood from the process of normal menstruation is limited by recovery of tone in the myometrium and in endometrial vasculature, cessation of cellular autolysis, eventual clotting over the endometrial surface, and finally active regeneration of glands, stroma and vessels in the basalis layer in response to rising estrogen levels in the new cycle.

In addition to estrogen and progesterone, various endometrial catabolites, enzymes, lysosomes, and prostaglandins have a role in endometrial shedding and regeneration. Cyclic changes in the synthesis of acid mucopolysaccharides influence the depolymerization of ground substance in the luteal phase, causing the release of hydrolytic enzymes and endometrial sloughing. Lysosomes in endometrial glands are released by loss of lysosomal membrane integrity from rising progesterone levels, causing destruction of endometrial cells and tissue shedding. Estrogen stimulates cyclo-oxygenase synthesis of prostaglandin $F_{2\alpha}$ and prostaglandin E from arachidonic acid, which originates in the endometrium, predominantly from linoleic acid. By contrast, progesterone inhibits this production. Receptors for prostaglandin $F_{2\alpha}$ are thought to be located in decidual spiral arterioles. Prostaglandin $F_{2\alpha}$ binding to this receptor in the late luteal phase causes vasoconstriction and controlled menstruation. Menstrual flow ceases when the basalis layer of the endometrium becomes re-epithelialized. Estrogen is the primary influence on this process but local endometrial tissue response may vary.

It is not surprising that a variety of alterations in the systems that control menstruation may occur and produce abnormal uterine bleeding, even in the absence of obvious disease. Prolonged estrogen stimulation can result in endometrium that outgrows its blood supply and has asynchronous development of endometrial glands, stroma, and blood vessels. Similarly, a failure of progesterone production may also have profound effects on endometrial glands, stroma, and blood vessels. Abnormal synthesis of acid mucopolysaccharides may result in the release of excessive amounts of hydrolytic enzymes into the stroma. Lysosome release from endometrial glands, influenced by plasma progesterone levels, may affect menstrual flow. Patients with menorrhagia produce altered types of prostaglandins from their endometrium and myometrium. Smith and associates have shown that the amount of menstrual flow is influenced by a change in the endometrial conversion of prostaglandin endoperoxide from $PGF_{2\alpha}$ to $PGE_{2\alpha}$. In their studies, women with menorrhagia synthesized mainly the vasodilator $PGE_{2\alpha}$ in the endometrium.

Menstruation has three clinical characteristics: the menstrual interval or cycle length, the duration of flow, and the amount of flow. Although the mean cycle length is 28 or 29 days, a menstrual interval of 21 to 37 days may be considered normal. A patient with a menstrual period shorter than 21 days is said to have polymenorrhea. A patient with a menstrual interval longer than 37 days is said to have oligomenorrhea. When menses have been absent for 90 days or longer, the patient is said to have amenorrhea. The menstrual interval may vary from month to month by several days. Regularity of the menstrual cycle is more important than exact approximation to the 28-day mean menstrual interval. Variation in the length of the menstrual interval in regular ovulatory cycles usually occurs in the preovulatory (proliferative) phase of the cycle, and is more frequent among the postmenarchal teenagers and in women approaching the menopause.

A duration of flow of 7 days or less is considered to be normal. Beyond 7 days, the patient is bleeding into the intermenstrual phase of the cycle, which is defined as metrorrhagia. Regardless of the length of the menstrual flow, 70% of the blood loss will usually occur by the second day and 90% by the third day. A total blood loss of 20 ml to 80 ml blood, representing 10 mg to 35 mg iron, is considered within normal limits. The mean menstrual blood loss for a normal period is approximately 40 ml. Signs of iron deficiency are present, however, in a significant proportion of women who lose more than 60 ml blood with each menstrual flow. Hallberg and associates found that iron deficiency is very common among women who lose more than 80 ml menstrual blood. Unfortunately, objective measurement of menstrual blood loss is rarely made in women complaining of heavy menstruation or women with unexplained iron deficiency anemia. The patient's history of normal or heavy menstrual blood loss is not an accurate indicator of the amount of flow. It is also difficult to estimate the amount of blood loss by counting the number of days of menstrual flow or the number of pads and tampons used, as emphasized by Grimes. Iron deficiency anemia is a late manifestation of excessive menstruation. Serum iron (ferritin) levels are more sensitive than hematocrit and hemoglobin levels in detecting depletion of iron stores before anemia develops, as shown in Guillebaud and associates' study. In our view, the availability of a convenient, standardized, objective method of measuring menstrual blood loss would improve the clinical practice of gynecology significantly, especially since 20% of women will have a problem with excessive menstrual blood loss during the reproductive years. The method of Hallberg and Nilsson is based on the simultaneous use of tampons and pads for the collection of menstrual blood. These are extracted with 5% sodium hydroxide, thus converting hemoglobin to alkaline hematin. The concentration is then determined spectrophotometrically. The method is simple and gives accurate results but is not widely used.

An alteration of the hormonal pattern at any one of the three major reproductive endocrine levels—namely, the hypothalamus, the anterior pituitary, and the ovary—will produce fluctuations in the normal levels of estrogen and progesterone, which may result in major or minor symptoms of menstrual irregularity. The more prolonged the period of endocrine imbalance, the more pronounced the menstrual abnormality, which may result in primary or secondary amenorrhea. Failure of endometrial regeneration may also result from vigorous curettage to control bleeding from either an incomplete abortion or fragments of a retained placenta. Removal of the basalis layer, originally described by Fritsch in 1894 and popularized by Asherman in 1948, results in secondary amenorrhea or oligomenorrhea with sclerosis, synechiae, or obliteration of the endometrial cavity.

The major diagnostic value of endometrial curettage is in determining the reason for abnormal uterine bleeding, whether from hormonal dysfunction, endometrial polyps, retained placental fragments, submucous leiomyomata, or uterine malignancy. All of these conditions can produce similar clinical symptoms. Continuation of abnormal menses following a dilatation and curettage may be due not only to a failure to remove all of the poorly shed endometrium, but, more commonly, to a failure to correct a coexisting endocrine dysfunction. The immediate effect of a curettage in controlling uterine bleeding is produced by the removal of endometrium that is frequently hyperplastic or has not completely shed because of steroid hormone imbalance. The bleeding arterioles and venous sinuses will usually undergo rapid thrombosis when curetted down to the basalis layer. Unfortunately, this favorable operative result may be only temporary in many patients.

Dysfunctional Uterine Bleeding

Dysfunctional uterine bleeding is a symptom complex that includes any abnormal uterine bleeding in the absence of infection, gestation, or tumor within the uterus. Such bleeding is primarily the result of altered blood levels of estrogen and progesterone, a condition in which anovulatory cycles are frequent. Abnormal stimulation and shedding of the endometrium are characteristic of this hormonal disorder, which is accompanied by increased menstrual blood loss. A similar mechanism of endocrine dysfunction causes abnormal uterine bleeding in the patient with a persistent corpus luteum, polycystic ovarian disease, or a hormone-producing tumor of the ovary. However, in the vast majority of cases of dysfunctional uterine bleeding, no gross pathologic lesion is present in the ovary. In defining the etiologic factor(s) associated with this condition, it is important that other endocrine diseases, such as hyper- or hypothyroidism, are excluded. To some extent then, the abnormal uterine bleeding called dysfunctional uterine bleeding is caused by an endocrine disorder that is exclusive of other anatomical or pathologic conditions.

PATHOPHYSIOLOGY

Using the histologic pattern of the endometrium as a guide in assessing the hormonal status of the patient, particularly at the time of curettage, has an obvious disadvantage that such information is usually after the fact. The histologic pattern of the endometrium of a woman who has been bleeding for several weeks or months sheds little light on the precise hormonal environment that precipitated the bleeding. Instead, the endometrial histology may demonstrate a mixture of the previous and the immediate endometrial response to hormonal stimulation. Therefore, retrospective studies of endometria from patients with dysfunctional uterine bleeding may have only limited clinical usefulness in determining whether the initial event was due to anovulation or to other factors. Notwithstanding this diagnostic difficulty, the endometrium of most patients with dysfunctional uterine bleeding shows only an estrogen effect in which bleeding is produced by estrogen withdrawal or estrogen breakthrough. Unopposed estrogen stimulation, in the absence of progesterone inhibition, that persists over a long period may produce progressive changes from proliferative endometrium to benign hyperplasia, adenomatous hyperplasia, and atypical adenomatous hyperplasia. Even histologic changes of low-grade adenocarcinoma have been associated with estrogen stimulation unopposed by progesterone after many years of use. In these conditions, the normal mechanisms for control of menstrual bleeding are absent. The progesterone effect on the spiral arterioles and on the biochemical composition of the stroma and glands is lacking. Shedding of the endometrium is variable, spotty, random, and disorderly. Such disorderly shedding and regeneration is associated with excessive, prolonged, and irregular menstrual flow.

Jones and associates studied the endometria from patients with dysfunctional bleeding and found hyperplasia present in 63% of the cases (Fig. 21–1). Secretory endometrium was noted in 17%, and nonsecretory endometrium of the interval, postmenstrual, or atrophic type in the remaining 20%. Thus, in at least 17% of this series, normal cyclic hormonal function and ovulation had occurred before the endometrium was examined. It is probable that many cases that showed the postmenstrual type of endometrium would have shown secretory changes had the curettage been done later.

Prospective hormonal studies using daily serum estrogen and progesterone levels are far more informative in defining anovulation than the historic studies of endometrial histology. Prospective studies provide clear evidence that the major cause of irregular shedding of the endometrium that produces clinical symptoms is failure of regular ovulation. Dysfunctional uterine bleeding must be considered to be an endocrine problem most frequently associated with an imbalance between the releasing hormones in the hypothalamus and the pituitary gonadotropins.

SYMPTOMS AND DIAGNOSIS

Dysfunctional uterine bleeding occurs most frequently at the two extremes of menstrual life, following menarche and prior to the menopause. It may also occur in the postpartum period. As it happens, these are the three times in a woman's life when anovulatory cycles are frequent. Almost any kind of abnormal bleeding may be present, including an increase in the amount of menstrual flow or an increase in the duration, or both. The usual history is of a gradual increase in amount and duration of menstrual flow, the periods becoming longer and longer until they finally merge with one another, and the bleeding is almost continuous. Intervals of several weeks of oligomenorrhea between episodes of bleeding are common. Intermenstrual spotting may be present. Menstrual bleeding in the absence of ovulation is often not associated with dysmenorrhea.

Adolescent menorrhagia is usually associated with anovulation. Of special note are those cases occurring in menarchal, teenage girls before the cyclic release of pituitary gonadotropins has become well established. When bleeding is noted before the age of normal puberty, the possibility of a feminizing

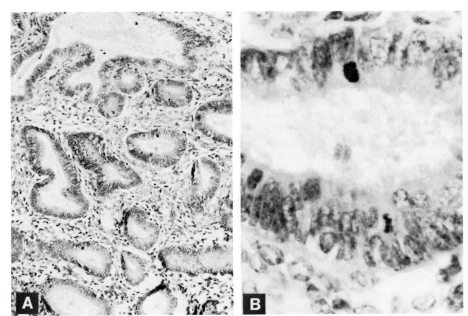

FIG. 21-1 (A) Endometrial hyperplasia before treatment showing hyperplastic cellular changes of glands. (B) Same endometrium at high-power magnification.

ovarian tumor should be considered, although this is one of the least frequent causes of precocious puberty, accounting for less than 10% of cases. However, careful general medical and endocrine examination should always be done before therapy is instituted. A dilatation and curettage is rarely needed unless there is clinical suspicion of an incomplete abortion or malignancy. In women over 35 years of age, and especially in the perimenopausal years, anovulatory cycles are also common. However, malignancy must be strongly considered as a possible cause of abnormal bleeding, and a diagnostic curettage must be done.

As mentioned, dysfunctional uterine bleeding is, to some extent, a diagnosis of exclusion. Problems of pregnancy, such as incomplete or missed abortion, subinvolution of the placental site, placental polyp, trophoblastic disease, and extrauterine pregnancy must be ruled out. All gynecologic malignancies may cause abnormal bleeding. Even common epithelial tumors of the ovary may produce estrogen and cause uterine bleeding. Submucous leiomyomata and endometrial polyps may be present in older women but are not a problem in differential diagnosis in teenagers. Excessive anovulatory bleeding is common with polycystic ovarian disease, with luteal phase defects, and with functional cysts of the ovary, especially a follicular cyst or persistent corpus luteum cyst. Blood dyscrasias that are associated with increased menstrual blood

loss include idiopathic thrombocytopenic purpura, prothrombin deficiency, and von Willebrand's disease. Menorrhagia is not uncommon in women with hypothyroidism. A forgotten IUD may be the cause of unexplained menorrhagia.

In addition to a complete history, a physical examination, and the usual laboratory investigations, other diagnostic studies that may be helpful include endometrial biopsy, thyroid function studies, hormonal assays, pregnancy test, determination of clotting factors, hysterography, hysteroscopy, and rarely, ultrasonography. A diagnostic curettage is not usually necessary in younger women, but should be done in older women. The procedure may be required for persistent bleeding in women who have recently completed a pregnancy or have had an incomplete abortion. When medical therapy is unsuccessful in young girls, a curettage may be required to stop the bleeding.

TREATMENT OF DYSFUNCTIONAL UTERINE BLEEDING

The management of patients with dysfunctional uterine bleeding differs depending on the patient's age. The most important cause of dysfunctional uterine bleeding during adolescence is an immature hypothalamic–pituitary axis. Emotional and psychogenic factors may influence this hormonal axis. Therapy should be directed toward the correction or reduction of these stressful factors. Endogenous estrogen levels are usually near normal and progesterone levels are low, resulting in an unopposed estrogen stimulation of the endometrium. This can be offset by progesterone therapy in the latter part of the cycle. One may prescribe medroxyprogesterone acetate in a dosage of 10 ml daily for the last 10 days of a planned cycle, beginning about 14 to 16 days after the onset of the previous menses if this can be determined. Combination oral contraceptive pills containing an estrogen and progestin may also be used.

In patients with dysfunctional uterine bleeding with endometrial hyperplasia, endometrial progesterone receptors are increased. Administration of progestogens to such patients will decrease DNA synthesis in the endometrium, decrease endometrial estradiol, increase endometrial estradiol inactivation by 17 β-estradiol dehydrogenase, and decrease the ratio of nuclear estradiol to estrone receptors. Through these intracellular mechanisms, the endometrial hyperplasia will usually revert to normal with progesterone therapy.

During the early reproductive years, dysfunctional uterine bleeding can usually be treated hormonally. If treatment is unsuccessful, disorders that may produce these symptoms must be ruled out. If bleeding is due to primary or secondary ovarian pathology, including polycystic ovarian disease, or physiologic cysts, the specific underlying etiology must be identified before the abnormal bleeding can be corrected. Medroxyprogesterone acetate will benefit most patients with anovulatory bleeding. If there is an episode of acute excessive bleeding, intravenous conjugated estrogens may be given to control the bleeding. Oral conjugated estrogens are then continued for three weeks. During the last week of estrogen therapy, an oral progestin is given daily. Withdrawal bleeding will occur, and the menstrual flow will usually be normal if the endometrium has been affected by the progestin.

When abnormal uterine bleeding occurs in women over 35 years of age, and especially in the perimenopausal years, a fractional uterine curettage must always be done to rule out endometrial malignancy. In this age group, organic causes of abnormal bleeding are more frequent. If adenomatous hyperplasia of the endometrium is diagnosed by the pathologist, medroxyprogesterone acetate may be indicated to decrease the endometrial responsiveness to estrogen. Follow-up endometrial biopsies will be necessary to determine the response. Endometrial curettage is often sufficient to correct minor episodes of dysfunctional uterine bleeding. However, 30% to 40% of patients in this age group will have recurrent abnormal bleeding. Curettage may need to be repeated.

Should the patient fail to respond to repeated curettage or endocrine therapy, more definitive therapy, primarily hysterectomy, should be considered in relation to the age of the patient and her desire for future childbearing. Although a hysterectomy may be considered an admission of therapeutic defeat, it is frequently an expeditious method of resolving a refractory and recurrent type of dysfunctional uterine bleeding. In general, the ovulatory type of bleeding has the poorest response to replacement hormonal therapy and the highest incidence of recurrence. When bleeding persists after repeated curettage and cyclic hormonal therapy, hysterectomy may be required. If other conditions are present that should be corrected surgically, such as a relaxed vaginal outlet, rectocele, cystocele, or uterine descensus, we recommend vaginal hysterectomy with support of the vaginal vault and repair of the vaginal wall relaxation. When hysterectomy is indicated in premenopausal women under 50 years of age, normal ovarian tissue is conserved. In a patient below 30 years of age, radical surgical treatment is to be strongly avoided, since one can almost always control the uterine bleeding by repeated curettage or by increasing amounts of cyclic hormone therapy. Today, the availability and use of estrogen and progesterone has changed the need for hysterectomy. Hysterectomy is not indicated in young women to treat dysfunctional uterine bleeding. Hysterectomy may be indicated in older women when hormonal therapy has failed and curettage has been performed at least twice.

Menorrhagia can be reduced when prostaglandin E2 and prostacyclin synthesis is decreased by flufenamic and mefenamic acid medication. Both of these drugs inhibit the cyclo-oxygenase enzyme necessary for endometrial production of prostaglandin under estrogen stimulation. These compounds are most effective when given in therapeutic dosage for 7 to 10 days before the expected onset of the next menstrual period, as shown by Fraser and Shearman.

Blood transfusions are seldom required when dysfunctional uterine bleeding is associated with anemia but may be given if the anemia is so severe that symptoms are present. Oral iron therapy should be started at the first sign of heavy menstruation to prevent depletion of iron stores, and should be given for 3 to 6 months after normal hemoglobin and hematocrit levels have been restored in patients with iron deficiency anemia. If a period of temporary amenorrhea is required to replace the depleted iron stores in the bone marrow, a pseudo-menopausal state may be produced with the continuous use of Danocrine, either 200 mg or 400 mg twice daily.

Dilatation of the Cervix

Dilatation of the cervix is carried out as a preliminary step to curettage of the uterine cavity. As a therapeutic measure, it is done for acquired or congenital cervical stenosis, for dysmenorrhea, for sterility, for introduction of intracervical and intrauterine radium or cesium, occasionally for insertion of an IUD, to allow drainage of the uterine cavity in the presence of pyometra, or as a part of other operations on the cervix.

Most indications for cervical dilatation are obvious. However, in connection with primary dysmenorrhea and sterility, there is room for controversy. It is a recognized fact that many cases of primary dysmenorrhea are not cured by cervical dilatation. Because of frequent failures, some gynecologists have almost abandoned it as a therapeutic technique. We do not subscribe totally to this pessimistic point of view. Unfortunately, in most instances it is impossible to detect those cases of dysmenorrhea that will be relieved by cervical dilatation. Often the operation must be done as a therapeutic test, but fortunately it is such a minor procedure that one is justified in performing it on that basis. In nulliparous women in whom pain is greatest just before or during the early part of the menstrual flow, there is a possibility of relief from cervical dilatation. However, this result is by no means predictable. Before proceeding with the operation, it is advisable to permit the patient to come to her own decision on whether or not her menstrual pain is sufficiently severe to justify an operation that may be of limited or no benefit.

In sterility cases, it is our custom to dilate the cervical canal thoroughly under general anesthesia after laparoscopy and tubal insufflation with a chromagen dye is completed. Among women with a long history of sterility, this combined procedure will result in a definite but small number of pregnancies.

In a postmenopausal patient with cervical stenosis, a pyometra may be discovered when the uterus is sounded. The pus should be cultured for anaerobic and aerobic organisms and the cervix should be dilated. A short, soft, rubber or plastic tube may be sutured in place to keep the cervical canal open while the uterine cavity is draining. Antibiotics are not usually indicated or necessary. A curettage of the uterine cavity should not be done until there has been adequate drainage, usually about 2 weeks later; curetting a pyometra may produce a parametritis or pelvic cellulitis in the same way as curetting an abscessed cavity. If perforation should occur, serious peritonitis might develop; therefore, antibiotic therapy is indicated. Curettage should be done after the drainage is complete because of the frequent association of pyometra with malignancy of the endometrium or endocervical canal.

TECHNIQUE OF CERVICAL DILATATION

The patient is placed on the table in the lithotomy position. A careful pelvic examination is done to locate the position of the uterine corpus. The vagina and the perineum are cleaned with the usual vaginal preparation of povidone-iodine (Betadine) and alcohol. The cervix is grasped with a 4-pronged tenaculum (Fig. 21-2, *left*) and gently drawn toward the vaginal outlet. A sound (Fig. 21-2, *right*) is passed

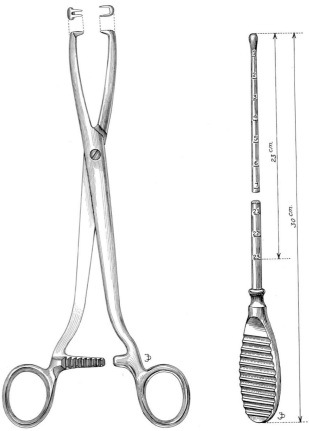

FIG. 21-2 (*Left*) Straight Jacobs clamp, used for pulling down cervix when performing curettage. (*Right*) Uterine sound.

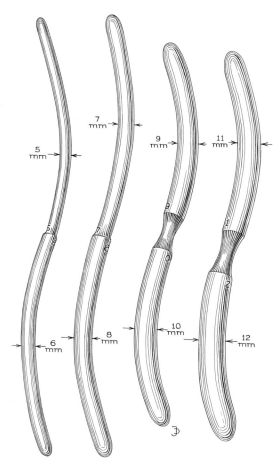

FIG. 21–3 Graduated Hegar dilators.

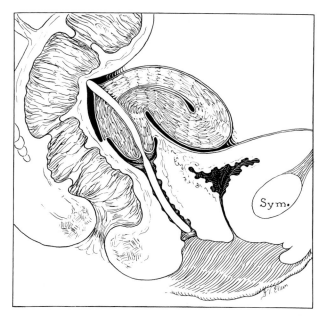

FIG. 21–4 Perforation of the acutely anteflexed uterus. The uterus was thought to be in retroposition, and the Hegar dilator was erroneously directed posteriorly.

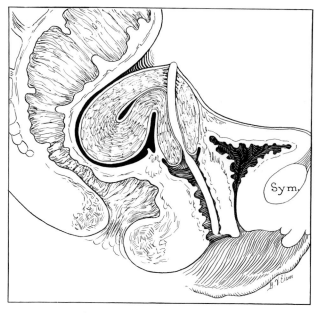

FIG. 21–5 Perforation of the retroflexed uterus. The uterus was thought to be in anteposition, and the Hegar dilator was erroneously directed anteriorly.

through the cervical canal into the uterine cavity. This must be done carefully to avoid creating a false passage. Resistance is greatest at the internal cervical os. Occasionally, a fine silver probe will be needed to find the proper passage if the canal is stenotic. Passing the uterine sound gives one confirmatory information on the position of the uterus, the length of the uterine cavity, and the angulation between the cervical canal and the uterine cavity. The degree of stenosis of the cervical canal can be detected in this manner.

The cervical canal is dilated with a small Hegar dilator (Fig. 21–3). The uterine wall may be perforated by improper passage of the dilator; usually this is due to a lack of knowledge or to disregard of the position of the uterus. When acute anteflexion is present, the dilator may perforate posteriorly (Fig. 21–4). When retrodisplacement exists, the perforation usually takes place anteriorly (Fig. 21–5). This complication may be avoided by sounding the uterine cavity before dilating the cervix and following

the direction of the endocervical canal and uterine cavity indicated by the sound. The dilator rarely perforates the fundus except when there is an atrophic postmenopausal uterus or when an invasive tumor or pregnancy has produced softening of the uterine wall. After the 3 mm or 4 mm Hegar dilator is passed, successively larger ones are used. For ordinary curettage, dilatation to 8 mm or 9 mm suffices. When dilatation is done for dysmenorrhea or sterility, we prefer to carry the dilatation up to 10 mm. There is concern that excessive dilatation may be associated with an incompetent cervix in a subsequent pregnancy.

The Hank-Bradley dilator has the same shape and contour as the Hegar dilator, but has a more tapered shank (Fig. 21–6). It also has the added advantage of a hollow center, which prevents a piston effect in which air is forced into the uterine cavity during progressive dilatation of the cervix. Because of the positive pressure created within the uterine cavity by passing a Hegar dilator, blood, endometrium, fragments of neoplastic tissue, or infected material could be forced into the fallopian tubes or peritoneal cavity. Beyth and associates have demonstrated that in a significant number of patients, endometrial tissue will be found in peritoneal fluid after curettage. Concern has been voiced about the possibility of reflux of endometrial carcinoma cells into the peritoneal cavity with forceful dilatation of a postmenopausal cervix in a patient found to harbor endometrial carcinoma. On the other hand, in the small postmenopausal uterus, it is quite easy to perforate the fundus of the uterus with the tip of the Hank's dilator while attempting to achieve the maximum dilating effect from the widest portion of the instrument. The Hank's dilator is used more commonly when curettage is being performed for an incomplete abortion since it permits the release of blood through the dilator while the cervix is being dilated. When dilatation is for removal of placental tissue, dilatation up to No. 19 or No. 20 Hank's (equivalent to a 9 mm or 10 mm Hegar) is often necessary

to permit the introduction of a large blunt curette and placental forceps.

Cervical injury is a potential problem when the cervix is forcefully dilated in preparation for removal of products of conception. The cervical tenaculum may lacerate the cervix. The internal cervical os may be damaged. The cervix is most resistant to dilatation at about 8 mm. Tapered Pratt dilators require less force than blunt Hegar dilators. The incidence of cervical incompetence may be related to the degree of cervical dilatation. Insertion of laminaria into the cervical canal several hours before cervical dilatation may make the procedure less difficult and traumatic, as suggested by Manabe and Manabe.

Curettage of the Uterus

INDICATIONS AND CONTRAINDICATIONS

It is important that dilatation and curettage be done for a proper indication, be done correctly so the most useful information is obtained, and be done safely. Like most simple procedures, it can be done correctly or incorrectly. It is not entirely devoid of danger. A curettage done properly and with aseptic technique carries with it very little risk, but if precautions are disregarded, complications and even death may result.

The chief purpose of curettage of the uterus is the removal of endometrial or endocervical tissue for histologic study in cases in which there has been abnormal uterine bleeding. Thus, a diagnosis of endometrial carcinoma may be made or excluded in women mainly over 35 years of age with abnormal bleeding or in postmenopausal women with any amount of bleeding. If a postmenopausal woman complains of vaginal bleeding of any amount and the pelvic examination does not reveal a malignancy of the cervix or vagina, a dilatation of the cervix and curettage of the uterus must be done to rule out an endometrial malignancy. Of women with postmenopausal bleeding, 10% to 25% who have a curettage will be found to have a malignancy. Generally, when the series includes a large number of private patients who report to their physician with very slight vaginal bleeding, the incidence of malignancy found will tend to be lower. One of the most important dictums to learn in gynecology is, postmenopausal bleeding requires a dilatation and curettage unless the pelvic examination reveals an obvious cervical or vaginal neoplasm. If only atrophic vaginitis, cervical polyp, or urethral caruncle are found by pelvic examination, a dilatation and curettage must still be done.

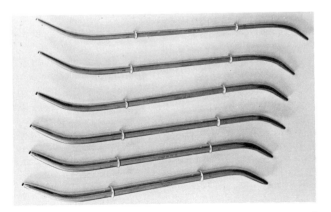

FIG. 21–6. Hank-Bradley dilators in graduated sizes. Note central canal which extends through length of dilator.

With dysfunctional bleeding in young women, a knowledge of the type of endometrium may be of value in future therapy. It is important to know if the endometrium is hyperplastic or secretory. Progesterone therapy is indicated when the endometrium is hyperplastic. When the endometrium is secretory, one must look more carefully for blood dyscrasias and uterine pathology such as submucous myomas. In sterility, a curettage done premenstrually will give information about the luteal phase of the current cycle. Evidence of inadequate progesterone effect on the endometrium may be seen histologically if the cycle is dated. Complete endometrial curettage is not recommended as a routine procedure in the work-up of patients with infertility, however. If information about endometrial histology is needed, a simple endometrial biopsy done in the office will suffice. Indeed, Taylor and Graham have suggested that endometrial curettage may be harmful as a part of the work-up of infertility patients. Laparoscopic evidence of pelvic inflammatory disease was found in a significantly higher percentage of women with infertility who had previously had an endometrial curettage. It is common practice to take infertility patients to the operating room for hysterosalpingogram, laparoscopy with retrograde dye insufflation, and dilatation and curettage. Perhaps the practice should be changed to omit the curettage and do only an endometrial biopsy.

Fractional curettage is an attempt to remove tissue samples from the endocervical canal differentially from tissue removed from the endometrial cavity. Fractional curettage of the cervical canal is indicated for patients with perimenopausal and postmenopausal bleeding who may have carcinoma of the endometrium with possible spread of the tumor to the endocervix. Curettage is also done when bleeding takes place from a cervical stump. It is frequently performed as a part of a cervical conization to rule out extension of cervical carcinoma into the endometrium. Helmkamp and associates found no evidence of endometrial abnormality in any of 114 curettage specimens removed at the time of 114 cervical conizations. These authors recommend that curettage at the time of cervical conization should not be done routinely but should be done selectively in postmenopausal and perimenopausal patients, when the cytology smear shows abnormal glandular cells and when an intrauterine abnormality is suspected. We agree with this advice.

Curettage may be combined with hysteroscopy or hysterosalpingography to look for intrauterine lesions that may be responsible for the bleeding, especially in patients with abnormal bleeding who have not responded to medical therapy. When hysterosalpingogram is done, it is helpful to have an operating room equipped with a fluoroscopy x-ray unit. The hysteroscopy or hysterosalpingogram should be done first before curettage.

The chief contraindication to curettage is infection. Acute endometritis and salpingitis constitute conditions under which curettage should be avoided. At times, however, curettage must be done for the removal of infected placental tissue, in which case it should be preceded by an adequate period of parenteral antibiotic therapy in order to achieve a therapeutic tissue level of antibiotics. Patients with endometritis associated with retained products of conception will remain unwell until the infected, necrotic material is cast off spontaneously or is removed by the curette. As stated earlier, curettage is also contraindicated when pyometra is present.

In general, we prefer to use a general anesthetic during dilatation and curettage. Not only is the procedure easier to perform with the patient fully relaxed, but it is more comfortable for the patient. Most patients, given a choice will opt for a general anesthetic for this procedure. It also provides an ideal opportunity to do a thorough examination of the pelvic organs. Prior to the examination, the bladder should be empty and an enema should have been given and expelled. If the anterior abdominal wall is relaxed from the anesthesia, a thorough pelvic examination should be done before the patient is draped. Occasionally, new and important pelvic findings will be discovered. In a study of 2666 women who required a curettage, McElin et al found an unanticipated adnexal mass in 30 patients at the time of pelvic examination under anesthesia before dilatation and curettage. Twenty-eight were benign and two were malignant. In women who are serious medical risks and require curettage for postmenopausal bleeding, we have performed the operation with no other anesthetic than hypodermic or intravenous administration of a sedative combined with paracervical nerve block.

Previously, it was common practice to do a curettage as a matter of routine before performing a hysterectomy. This practice is no longer recommended unless there are special reasons for doing so. On the other hand, if a postmenopausal patient is brought to the operating room for a gynecologic operation that does not include hysterectomy, a uterine curettage will often be done. For example, a postmenopausal woman who is having a repair of a symptomatic rectocele should usually also have a uterine curettage even if she has no symptoms related to the uterus.

It is important to understand that a single curettage will not remove all of the surface endometrium completely from the uterine cavity. Repeated studies have demonstrated the inability of a thorough curettage to remove more than 50% to 60% of the endometrium when the procedure has been done by experienced gynecologists immediately before a planned hysterectomy. Stock and Kanbour, from the McGee Hospital in Pittsburgh, have observed that in 60% of hysterectomy specimens studied, less than 50% of the endometrial surface had been curetted by a prehysterectomy curettage. They also found that in 26 cases, endometrial carcinoma had been classified as clinically normal appearing tissue on prehysterectomy curettage; 6 of these carcinomas were reported as benign on frozen section. These facts and other similar experiences have convinced us that it is difficult to be certain of the histology of the endometrium by gross examination of the curettings. If the symptoms warrant a curettage, the endometrium deserves a histologic diagnosis. It may be necessary to perform more than one curettage (usually two or three) in order to rule out polyps more convincingly and to control abnormal uterine bleeding before more definitive surgery is recommended.

TECHNIQUE OF CURETTAGE OF THE UTERUS

The perineum need not be shaved before uterine curettage. However, before the patient comes to the operating room, an enema is given and expelled so that hard stool in the rectum and sigmoid will not interfere with the accuracy of the pelvic examination under anesthesia. After the patient is anesthetized, she is placed in the lithotomy position and the bladder is emptied with a catheter. The pelvic organs are examined thoroughly before the patient is prepped and draped. The procedure includes a bimanual rectovaginal–abdominal exam. We consider the examination under anesthesia to be one of the most informative features of this operation because it can provide anatomical details of the reproductive tract that are not recognizable without anesthesia. The vagina and perineum are cleaned with the usual technique. The cervical canal is cleansed with a small cotton pledget soaked in alcohol. The uterine cavity is always sounded to determine its size and to confirm the position determined from examination under anesthesia. The cervical canal is dilated with Hegar or Hank's dilators. A dilatation to an 8 mm or 9 mm Hegar is sufficient for the usual diagnostic curettage. A gauze is placed in the posterior vaginal fornix along the posterior retractor so that the blood and the endometrium removed from the uterus may fall on it (Fig. 21–7). The uterine cavity is explored initially in search of an endometrial polyp before the curettage is performed, using a narrow stone forceps

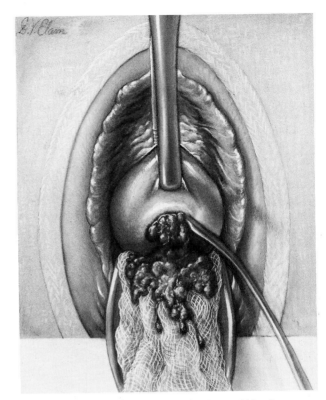

FIG. 21–7 Method of collecting curettings and blood on gauze.

(Fig. 21–8A,B). This forceps can be opened and closed as the tip of the forceps is moved systematically across the dome of the uterus and the anterior and posterior walls. This procedure is repeated several times after the uterine wall has been curetted to make certain that an area of the endometrial cavity or a polyp has not been missed.

It is important to explore the uterine cavity with a polyp forceps at each curettage. An endometrial polyp can easily be missed with an ordinary curette. As a result, unnecessary hysterectomies have been done because of supposed persistent or recurrent dysfunctional bleeding following a curettage (Fig. 21–9). If polyp forceps are routinely used, such operations may be avoided. It is easier to identify and remove an endometrial polyp if the uterine cavity is explored with the stone forceps before the uterus is curetted. In a 28-month period, during which time the forceps were used routinely at the Johns Hopkins Hospital, Josey found that the diagnosis of endometrial polyp was made 130 times. In 83 of these cases the polyp was removed by forceps. Although the sessile form of a submucous myoma is diagnosed easily by noting an irregularity of the uterine wall with the curette, the pedunculated va-

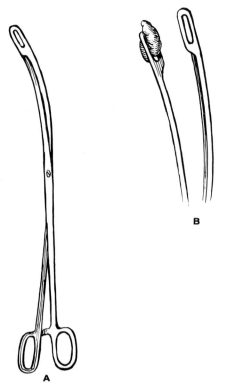

FIG. 21–8 (*A*) Ureteral stone forceps, an excellent instrument for removing endometrial polyps. (*B*) A polyp that was missed at curettage grasped in forceps.

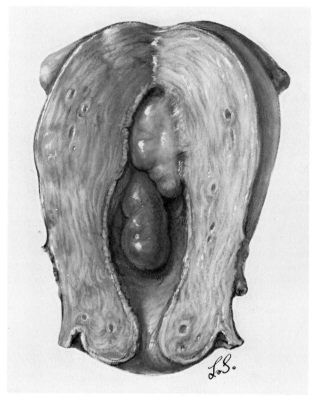

FIG. 21–9 Opened uterus, showing two separate endometrial polyps.

riety, like the endometrial polyp, may escape detection because of its narrow stalk. Often such a leiomyoma may be grasped with the polyp forceps. A uterine septum may also be detected with the forceps.

A small or medium-sized, malleable, bluntly serrated curette (Fig. 21–10) is then introduced into the uterus, and in a systematic manner the entire uterine cavity is curetted. The anterior, lateral, and posterior walls are scraped gently but firmly and finally the top of the cavity is scraped with a side-to-side movement (Fig. 21–11). The handle of the curette should never be held against the palm of the hand. Instead, it should be held gently as one would hold a pencil. The instrument is held loosely as it is inserted for the full distance. Pressure is then exerted against the uterine wall as the curette is drawn in an outward direction. Since the instrument is malleable, its curvature may be changed to conform to the contour of the uterine cavity.

The unclotted blood is absorbed quickly by the gauze sponge, leaving the relatively clean endometrium to be placed in a prepared container with

appropriate fixative. The curettings should never be mashed or scraped but should be picked carefully from the sponge with a smooth-tip forceps and placed immediately in the fixative. In so doing, the curettings are examined carefully to be certain that no fatty tissue or other unusual tissue is present. Fragments of hyperplastic endometrium may sometimes appear yellow. Teare and Rippey evaluated 1000 specimens of endometrial curettings and found that a high proportion were unsuitable for histologic assessment. The main factors contributing to the pathologist's inability to provide a useful histologic interpretation were the inadequacy of the specimen and a lack of information regarding the clinical and menstrual history.

The cervical canal should be curetted *before* dilatation of the cervical canal and curettage of the endometrial cavity if there is any suspicion of it being the site of malignancy or polyps. The Gusberg curette is a small, specially shaped instrument that is particularly useful in curetting the endocervix. A differential curettage of the endocervix, separate from the endometrium, is important in the diagnosis

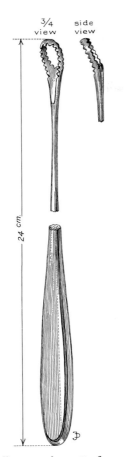

3/4 view   side view

24 cm.

FIG. 21-10   Small serrated curette for routine curettage.

of endometrial carcinoma that may have extended to the endocervix (see Chapter 33). All patients with postmenopausal bleeding should have a fractional curettage, a procedure that is frequently neglected. If the endocervical curettage is not done a second fractional curettage is required to determine the anatomical boundaries of endometrial carcinoma.

Routine blind biopsy of the cervix is usually unrewarding if a negative cytologic smear has been obtained and there is no suspicious cervical lesion. We no longer routinely do a blind biopsy of the cervix at the time of curettage unless an abnormal lesion is present. If a patient has recent negative cytology and has a profuse, recurrent, mucous discharge associated with cervicitis and Nabothian cysts, cervical cauterization will often be done at the time of curettage.

When curettage is done as a curative measure for removal of placental tissue, a large, blunt, smooth curette is used to lessen the chances of perforation and endometrial sclerosis. The larger and softer the uterus, the larger should be the curette used and the more careful should one be to avoid these complications. When large masses of placental tissue are present, the ovum forceps are most useful when used in conjunction with the curette.

COMPLICATIONS OF CERVICAL DILATATION AND UTERINE CURETTAGE

If the position and the consistency of the uterus are carefully noted on bimanual examination under

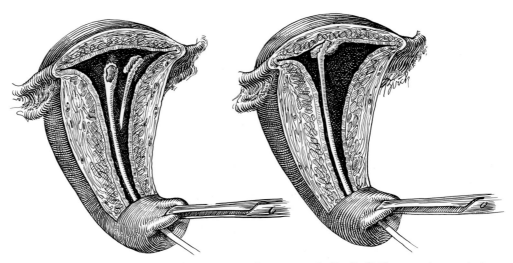

FIG. 21-11   Method of curetting the uterine cavity systematically. (*Left*) The anterior, posterior, and lateral walls of cavity are curetted systematically. (*Right*) The top of cavity is then curetted thoroughly.

anesthesia before the curettage is undertaken, perforation will rarely occur. When the position of the uterus is not known to the operator, perforation may occur with remarkable ease. Special care should be exercised in patients who have a uterus that is acutely anteflexed or retroflexed. In the presence of cervical stenosis, pregnancy, or intrauterine malignancy, perforation is more likely. The postmenopausal atrophic uterus may be perforated with only slight force applied to the uterine sound or the curette. Perforation is discovered when the sound or the curette fails to encounter resistance at the point where it normally should, as judged by the palpated size of the uterus.

Perforation by the uterine sound or cervical dilator causes less damage than perforation by the sharp curette or suction cannula. Sharp curettage for legally induced abortion has a major complication rate two to three times higher than suction curettage, according to Grimes and Cates. The two principal dangers of uterine perforation are bleeding and trauma to the abdominal viscera. Lateral perforation through the uterine vessels is especially dangerous from the standpoint of intraperitoneal hemorrhage and broad ligament hematoma formation. Damage can occur to bowel, omentum, mesentery, ureter, and fallopian tube. Perforation of the anterior or posterior wall of the uterus by a small curette in performing a diagnostic curettage is usually not a serious accident. However, it is usually necessary to discontinue the curettage. The pa-

tient should be watched carefully for signs of hemorrhage or infection. If signs of hemorrhage develop, the abdomen should be opened and the uterine wound sutured. If signs of infection occur, broad-spectrum antibiotics should be given. If a pelvic abscess develops, the abscess should be drained if possible. Serious hemorrhage or infection occur only rarely. When serious damage from perforation is suspected, laparoscopy may be done to assess the extent of the damage and the repair needed.

Fig 21–12 shows a uterus removed immediately after a perforation. The uterus was removed because of intraperitoneal bleeding. Word analyzed 70 accidental uterine perforations. Among these, an unplanned hysterectomy was done on seven unprepared patients. In none did the intraperitoneal findings indicate the need for hysterectomy. In fact, the hysterectomy only compounded the surgical error. Fifty-five patients were treated conservatively, and only one developed a complication in the form of a pelvic abscess, which was drained by colpotomy. Forty-one of the 70 perforations occurred in postmenopausal women.

When a large, boggy, postabortal, or puerperal uterus is perforated by a large curette or placental forceps in removing placental tissue, there is more danger of hemorrhage, infection, or injury to bowel. The treatment that should be given and the procedures that should be followed are discussed in Chapter 22.

According to MacKenzie and Bibby, complications

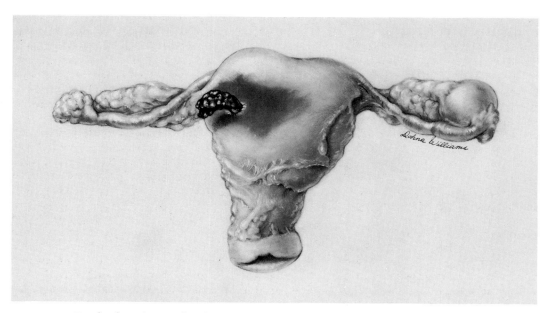

FIG. 21–12   Result of uterine perforation. Specimen removed directly after perforation.

occurred in 1.7% of patients undergoing dilatation and curettage. McElin and associates reported that 0.5% of patients had postoperative febrile morbidity following dilatation and curettage. Uterine perforation occurred in 0.63% of cases.

It should be mentioned that one should be absolutely certain that the endometrial cavity has been entered when dilatation and curettage is done for postmenopausal bleeding. A relatively stenotic internal cervical os and a fear of uterine perforation may prevent entry into the uterine cavity above the internal cervical os, resulting in a failure to curette the uterine cavity and a failure to diagnose the cause of the bleeding.

OUTPATIENT CURETTAGE

Over the years attempts have been made to lower the cost of dilatation and curettage by making it an outpatient procedure. In 1957 Vermeeren, Chamberlain, and Te Linde presented a series of 10,000 minor gynecologic operations done on an outpatient basis on the gynecology service at the Johns Hopkins Hospital. The results were quite satisfactory. These women were usually operated on under general anesthesia and were dicharged following recovery from anesthesia. Dilatation and curettage was the operation most frequently performed. The success and safety of such a program depends on careful selection of patients and a willingness to admit patients to the hospital for observation should complications occur. Today, dilatation and curettage is often done satisfactorily on an outpatient basis or in an ambulatory surgery center. Reports by Sandmire and Austin and by Martin and Rust are among many that record favorable experience with this procedure.

During the past 50 years many instruments have been devised for the sampling of endometrial tissue and evaluation of the endometrial cavity. One of the most useful instruments for outpatient use is the Novak curette. Although this curette was initially devised to obtain a sample of the endometrium by suction and aspiration, it is more commonly used as a miniature curette that contains a serrated edge surrounding its biopsy aperture. The curette is approximately 5 mm in diameter and can usually be passed through a small cervical canal, even in nulliparous women. However, the postmenopausal cervical canal is frequently stenotic and is difficult to penetrate without minimal dilatation. The Novak curette has been used for the past 50 years with increasing effectiveness in providing an adequate sample for dating the endometrium in infertility cases, as well as for the initial screening evaluation of a patient with abnormal bleeding. Its principal

value is in avoiding a formal dilatation and curettage under anesthesia if the tissue removed should contain an adenocarcinoma. However, if the cause of postmenopausal bleeding is not identified in a screening endometrial biopsy by the Novak curette, a standard curettage is obligatory. In office biopsy of the endometrium in over 20,000 patients of all ages, Hofmeister detected 273 cases of endometrial carcinoma, of which 32 (14.28%) were totally asymptomatic. The endometrial carcinoma detection rate was 1.76% of the total group of 23,202 patients. Hofmeister's routine use of the office endometrial biopsy, using a modification of the Novak and Randall curette, provides one of the largest clinical experiences to date for this instrument. Unfortunately, only patients who had continued uterine bleeding or who demonstrated an atypical endometrial pattern in the office biopsy were subjected to a complete curettage. Therefore, the true false-negative rate for the Novak-type curette in the detection of endometrial cancer has not been accurately determined. In other studies the accuracy with which endometrial cancer is detected by the Novak curette varies from 76% to 92%, as summarized by Cohen. However, a thorough endometrial curettage under anesthesia is not infallible in the detection of endometrial cancer.

More recently, the use of vacuum suction curettage has gained popularity as an office procedure not requiring general anesthesia. This technique consists of using a small metal or plastic cannula with an outside diameter of 3 mm that has a slightly curved tip and an opening on the concave surface for easy insertion through a small endocervical canal. The cannula is connected to a plastic tubular chamber containing a cylindrical plastic filter. At the opposite end of the chamber, there is a plastic spout that is connected to a negative pressure source. The apparatus is prepackaged in a sterile disposable container and the vacuum source can be either a commercial pump or a faucet in which approximately 60 cm of negative water pressure is developed for proper suction through the curette. Several improvements have been made in the technology. This instrument* has the advantage and the convenience of being completely prepared and disposable but the disadvantage of a high price, which must be borne by the patient. Several studies have compared the results of suction curettage with those of a regular curettage under anesthesia in the same patient. Cohen and associates studied 98 patients by this technique and have found that identical histologic patterns resulted from both methods. In only five patients was there no correlation between the

* Vabra Aspirator

results of the two techniques, and none of these had cancer. At the Medical University of South Carolina, Lutz and associates found the suction curettage to be 98% accurate in evaluating high-risk women with abnormal bleeding for endometrial malignant disease. We have had a similar good experience with this instrument.

Although this method may be an easy outpatient technique for evaluating the histology of the endometrium in patients with abnormal bleeding, it does not fulfill the requirements for a thorough curettage, should the cause of the uterine bleeding fail to be determined. Only if an endometrial biopsy or a suction curettage shows frank adenocarcinoma should one have total confidence in these findings. Even in the most experienced hands, endometrial carcinoma can be quite elusive. Neither the Novak curette nor the suction curettage is useful in removing an endometrial polyp. Therefore, endometrial carcinoma could be missed in a polyp, as could the source of benign bleeding. Office curettage should be used only as a screening procedure and should not be accepted as a proven substitute for a more thorough dilatation and curettage under anesthesia.

Bibliography

Akesel S, Jones GS: Etiology and treatment of dysfunctional uterine bleeding. Obstet Gynecol 44:1, 1974

Anderson ABM, Haynes PJ, Guillebaud J, et al: Reduction of menstrual blood loss by prostaglandin synthesis inhibition. Lancet 1:774, 1976

Asherman J: Amenorrhea traumatica (atretica). J Obstet Gynaecol Br Emp 55:23, 1948

Barnett JM: Suction curettage on unanesthetized outpatients. Obstet Gynecol 42:672, 1973

Beller FK: Observations on the clotting of menstrual blood and clot formation. Am J Obstet Gynecol 111:535, 1971

Beyth Y, Yaffe H, Levij I, et al: Retrograde seeding of endometrium: A sequela of tubal flushing. Fertil Steril 26:1094, 1975

Chiazze L, Jr, Brayer FT, Macisco JJ, Jr, et al: The length and variability of the human menstrual cycle. JAMA 203:377, 1968

Chimbira TH, Cope E, Anderson ABM, et al: The effects of danazol on menorrhagia, coagulation mechanisms, haematological indices and body weight. Br J Obstet Gynecol 86:46, 1979

Cohen CJ, Gusberg SB, Koffler D: Histologic screening for endometrial cancer. Gynecol Oncol 2:279, 1974

Cullen TS: Cancer of the Uterus. New York, Appleton, 1900

Davies AJ, Anderson ABM, Turnbull AC: Reduction by naproxen of excessive menstrual bleeding in women using intrauterine devices. Obstet Gynecol 57:74, 1981

Denis R, Jr, Barnett JM, Forbes SE: Diagnostic suction curettage. Obstet Gynecol 42:301, 1973

Fraser IS, Baird DT: Blood production and ovarian secretion rates of estradiol-17,3 and estrone in women with dysfunctional uterine bleeding. J Clin Endocrinol Metabol 38:727, 1974

Fraser IS, Pearse C, Shearman RP, et al: Efficacy of mefenamic acid in patients with a complaint of menorrhagia. Obstet Gynecol 58:543, 1981

Fraser IS, et al: Pituitary gonadotropins and ovarian function in adolescent dysfunctional uterine bleeding. J Clin Endocrinol Metabol 37:407, 1973

Fritsch N: Ein Fall von volligen Schwund der gebarmutter Hohle nach Auskratzung. Zentralbl Gumsrl 18:1337, 1894

Gregg RH: The praxeology of the office dilatation and curettage. Am J Obstet Gynecol 140:179, 1981

Grimes D: Estimating vaginal blood loss. J Reprod Med 22:190, 1979

Grimes D, Cates W, Jr: Complications from legally-induced abortion: A review. Obstet Gynecol Survey 34:177, 1979

Guillebaud J, Barnett MD, Gordon YB: Plasma ferritin levels as an index of iron deficiency in women using intrauterine devices. Br J Obstet Gynecol 86:51, 1979

Hallberg L, Hogdahl A, Nilsson L, et al: Menstrual blood loss and iron deficiency. Acta Med Scand 180:639, 1966

Hallberg L, Nilsson L: Constancy of individual menstrual blood loss. Acta Obstet Gynecol Scand 43:352, 1964

Hallberg L, Nilsson L: Determination of menstrual blood loss. Scand J Clin Lab Invest 16:244, 1964

Hamblen EC: Endocrinology of Woman. Springfield, Charles C Thomas, 1949

Haynes PJ, Hodgson H, Anderson ABM, et al: Measurement of menstrual blood loss in patients complaining of menorrhagia. Br J Obstet Gynecol 84:763, 1977

Healy DL, Hodgen GD: The endocrinology of human endometrium. Obstet Gynecol Survey 38:509, 1983

Helmkamp BF, Denslow BL, Boufiglio TA, et al: Cervical conization: When is dilatation and curettage indicated? Am J Obstet Gynecol 146:893, 1983

Hofmeister FJ: Endometrial biopsy: Another look. Am J Obstet Gynecol 118:773, 1974

————: Endometrial curettage. In Symmonds CM and Zuspan FT (eds): Clinical and Diagnostic Procedures in Obstetrics and Gynecology. New York, Marcel Dekker, 1984

Jensen JA, Jensen JG: Abragio mucosae uteri e aspiratione. Ugeskr Laeger 130:2121, 1968

Jensen JG: Vacuum curettage. Outpatient curettage without anesthesia: A report of 350 cases. Dan Med Bull 17:199, 1970

Josey WE: Routine intrauterine forceps exploration at curettage. Obstet Gynecol 11:108, 1958

Kelly HA: Curettage without anesthesia on the office table. Am J Obstet Gynecol 9:78, 1925

Lutz MH, Underwood PB, Jr, Kreutner A, et al: Vacuum aspiration: An efficient outpatient screening technique for endometrial disease. South Med J 70:393, 1977

MacKenzie IZ, Bibby JG: Critical assessment of dilatation and curettage in 1029 women. Lancet ii:566, 1978

Manabe Y, Manabe A: Nelaton catheter for gradual and safe cervical dilatation: An ideal substitute for laminaria. Am J Obstet Gynecol 140:465, 1981

Markee JE: Menstruation in intraocular endometrial transplants in the Rhesus monkey. Contr Embryol Carneg Justn 28:219, 1940

Martin PL, Rust JA: Surgical gynecology for the ambulatory patient. Clin Obstet Gynecol 17:205, 1974

McElin TW, Bird CC, Reeves BD, et al: Diagnostic dilatation and curettage. Obstet Gynecol 33:807, 1969

Mengert WF, Slate WG: Diagnostic dilatation and curettage

as an outpatient procedure. Am J Obstet Gynecol 79:727, 1960

Narula RK: Endometrial histopathology in dysfunctional uterine bleeding. J Obstet Gynecol India 17:614, 1967

Novak E: Relation of hyperplasia of endometrium to so-called functional uterine hemorrhage. JAMA 75:292, 1920

Novak E: A suction curette apparatus and endometrial biopsy. JAMA 104:1497, 1935

Pacheco JC, Kempers RD: Etiology of postmenopausal bleeding. Obstet Gynecol 32:40, 1968

Reyniak JV: Dysfunctional uterine bleeding. J Reprod Med 17:293, 1976

Scandmire HF, Austin SD: Curettage as an office procedure. Am J Obstet Gynecol 119:82, 1974

Smith SK, Abel MH, Kelly RW, et al: A role for prostacyclin (PG$_{I2}$) in excessive menstrual bleeding. Lancet 1:522, 1981

Smith SK, Abel MH, Kelly RW, et al: Prostaglandin synthesis in the endometrium of women with ovular dysfunctional uterine bleeding. Br J Obstet Gynecol 88:434, 1981

Southam AI, Richart RM: The prognosis for adolescents with menstrual abnormalities. Am J Obstet Gynecol 94:637, 1966

Stock RJ, Kanbour A: Pre-hysterectomy curettage: An evaluation. Obstet Gynecol 45:537, 1975

Swartz DT, Jones GES: Progesterone in anovulatory uterine bleeding: Clinical observations. Fertil Steril 8:103, 1957

Taylor PJ, Graham G: Is diagnostic curettage harmful in women with unexplained infertility? Br J Obstet Gynecol 89:296, 1982

Teare AJ, Rippey JJ: Dilatation and curettage. S Afr Med J 55:535, 1979

Tseng L, Gusberg SB, Gurpide E: Estradiol receptor and 17 B-dehydrogenase in normal and abnormal human endometrium. Ann NY Acad Sci 286:190, 1977

Vermeeren J, Chamberlain RR, Te Linde RU: Ten thousand minor gynecologic operations on an outpatient basis. Obstet Gynecol 9:139, 1957

Whitehead MI, King RJ, McQueen J, et al: Endometrial histology and biochemistry in climacteric women during estrogen and estrogen/progestogen therapy. J Roy Soc Med 72:322, 1979

Word B: Current concepts of uterine curettage. Postgrad Med 28:450, 1960

Word B, Gravlee LC, Wideman GL: The fallacy of simple uterine curettage. Obstet Gynecol 12:642, 1958

Chapter 22

Surgical Management of Abortion

David A. Grimes, M.D.

Human reproduction is an inefficient enterprise. Compared with other biologic functions, such as digestion and locomotion, reproduction is characterized by false steps. This inefficiency may relate to the complexity of the task at hand; nevertheless, if most attempts at walking resulted in stumbling, such inefficiency would cause alarm.

Inefficiency in human reproduction is manifested by pregnancy wastage. Abortion is the most frequent outcome of human conception. As determined by hormonal surveillance of early pregnancies, most human conceptions end in spontaneous abortion (Edmonds et al, 1982). Moreover, of the minority of pregnancies that do not end in spontaneous abortion, approximately one in four ends in legal abortion in the United States (Centers for Disease Control, 1983).

On a nationwide scale, the scope of the challenge posed by spontaneous and induced abortion is large. Approximately 1.5 million legal abortions are performed annually, and at least 6 million spontaneous abortions are estimated to occur each year in the United States. Thus, the surgical management of abortion is a principal focus of gynecology, and legal abortion is the gynecologic operation most frequently performed today.

This chapter provides an overview of the surgical management of abortion. It reviews the incidence, risk factors, and operative treatment of spontaneous abortion, illegal abortion, and legal abortion.

Spontaneous Abortion

INCIDENCE

The true incidence of spontaneous abortion is uncertain. This uncertainty relates to the difficulty in recognizing very early conceptions and losses. It has been estimated that 78% of conceptions fail to result in a live birth, and the pioneering histologic studies of Hertig suggested an embryonic mortality rate of 40% by the time of the expected menstrual period. However, as Shapiro put it, no method short of placing under observation a cohort of women who are subject to pregnancy tests each month can provide a satisfactory assessment of early pregnancy losses. When Edmonds and associates followed this suggestion and monitored β-hCG (human chorionic gonadotropin) in the urine of a cohort of volunteers attempting to conceive, they found that 62% of conceptions were lost before 12 weeks' gestation. Most of these losses (92%) occurred subclinically, and the woman was not aware of having been pregnant.

Most studies of spontaneous abortion deal only with pregnancies recognized by the woman. Overall spontaneous-abortion rates of 15% to 17% have been reported. These data support the clinical maxim that about one in six women who recognize they are pregnant will experience a spontaneous abortion.

RISK FACTORS

Several important risk factors for spontaneous abortion are known. The risk of spontaneous abortion increases with advancing maternal age, particularly for women over 35 years old. Likewise, the risk increases with advancing paternal age.

Race also plays an important role. At each stage of pregnancy, women of minority races have higher rates of spontaneous abortion than white women. The racial discrepancy in rates is most marked at 12 to 19 weeks' gestation (Shapiro et al, 1971).

Independent of the effect of age, the risk of spontaneous abortion increases with increasing gravidity. In addition, a history of one or more spontaneous abortions increases the risk of spontaneous abortion in subsequent pregnancies. This effect is seen at all gestational ages. On the other hand, the length of the interval between pregnancies appears to have little impact.

Both gestational age and the aging of sperm and egg appear to influence the likelihood of spontaneous abortion. In general, the probability of spontaneous abortion is inversely related to gestational age. Rates are presumably very high in the first weeks of pregnancy, though not well quantified. Assuming a total fetal loss of 22% Shapiro and associates estimated gestational age-specific rates of spontaneous abortion to be 8% at 4 to 7 weeks' gestation, 8% at 8 to 11 weeks; 5% at 12 to 19 weeks; and 2% at 20 or more weeks. Although spontaneous abortion occurs predominantly in the first 12 weeks of pregnancy (the mean is 9 weeks) (Wilcox et al, 1981), many losses occur later in pregnancy. One large study, by Guerrero and Rojas, has suggested that conceptions that do not occur near the time of the shift in basal-body temperature are more likely to be aborted than those that do.

Smoking also appears to increase the risk of spontaneous abortion significantly. Cigarette smoking is associated with a nearly doubled risk (Kline et al, 1977). Since smoking is not known to be teratogenic, its effect on spontaneous-abortion rates may be due to an increased rate of expulsion of normal conceptuses.

No seasonality of spontaneous-abortion rates has been identified. The *number* of spontaneous abortions, however, fluctuates significantly. The incidence of spontaneous abortion peaks in the spring and again in the late fall; this pattern reflects the marked seasonal variation in numbers of conceptions. However, the proportion of conceptions that end in spontaneous abortion varies little from month to month (Warren et al, 1980).

THE ROLE OF SPONTANEOUS ABORTION

Spontaneous abortion serves primarily as a quality control mechanism. Only a minority of each cohort of conceptuses survives pregnancy. Human reproduction apparently tolerates a broad diversity of conceptions; much more stringent and exacting criteria determine the probability of surviving to viability.

An extensive literature supports this teleologic role for spontaneous abortion as a screening device for abnormal pregnancies (Stein et al, 1975). The frequency of chromosomal abnormalities in aborted conceptuses is high, ranging from 30% to 61% in surveys of different populations (Hassold et al, 1980); in decreasing order of frequency, the most common abnormalities are trisomy, sex chromosome monosomy, and triploidy. The earlier the gestational age at abortion, the higher the frequency of chromosomal anomalies. Almost all anomalies, including some (such as cleft lip) that would not seem to handicap survival, increase the likelihood of spontaneous abortion.

Multiple gestations, common in other species, are atypical in humans and appear to be at high risk of fetal death. For example, in a study by Dessaive and associates of women with threatened abortion, four women with twins identified by ultrasonography at 8 weeks' gestation were followed to delivery; three delivered normal singletons, and only one delivered twins. Thus, three twins were lost without their fellow passengers in the uterus being adversely affected.

Most fetuses with abnormalities are in some way identified and rejected by the body. The incidence of chromosomal or other abnormalities in fetuses that survive this selection process is low.

PREVENTION OF SPONTANEOUS ABORTION

While an abnormal karyotype is the most important risk factor for spontaneous abortion, a variety of other risk factors have been proposed. These include endocrine defects, infections, environmental toxins, and immunologic factors.

Several surgically correctable conditions have been linked with spontaneous abortion. Uterine synechiae—that is, intrauterine adhesions—have been suggested as a cause of repeated spontaneous abortion. If synechiae are identified in this clinical setting, lysis of adhesions by hysteroscopy may be advisable.

Abnormalities of müllerian fusion have also been implicated as a cause of spontaneous abortion. Although the incidence of early abortion is probably not increased, the incidence of abortion at or after 13 weeks' gestation may be in the range of 20% to 25% (Simpson, 1981). Septate and bicornuate uteri seem to have more adverse effects than uterus bicornis bicollis. Women with müllerian anomalies who experience spontaneous abortions at or after 13 weeks' gestation may be candidates for reconstructive operations, which are described elsewhere in this text (Chapter 15).

Leiomyomas, a common condition, have also been attributed with causing spontaneous abortion. The evidence supporting this association, however, is limited. Submucous leiomyomas would be expected to have more effect than intramural or subserosal tumors. Women with leiomyomas who experience abortions at or after 13 weeks' gestation may be candidates for myomectomy, described in Chapter 11. However, current data suggest that myomectomy, if performed only because of infertility, is of minimal benefit; the effect of myomectomy on rates of spontaneous abortion has not been adequately evaluated.

MANAGEMENT

Threatened Abortion

Threatened abortion, characterized by bleeding of intrauterine origin without cervical dilation or expulsion of tissue, has traditionally been managed by watchful waiting. The likelihood of spontaneous abortion under these circumstances appears to be about 50% (Sande et al, 1980). If fetal outcome could be reliably predicted in such situations, couples might be spared substantial emotional anguish.

Fetal well-being early in pregnancy is usually determined through monitoring maternal blood or urine levels of hormones produced by the fetoplacental unit. These hormones include human chorionic gonadotropin, human placental lactogen, estriol, estradiol, and progesterone. Like hormone assays performed to determine fetal well-being late in pregnancy, such tests have two disadvantages: test results are not immediately available, and the validity of the tests varies widely. For example, for women with threatened abortion, the predictive value of an abnormally low plasma estradiol (percentage of women with an abnormal result who spontaneously abort) ranges from 53% (Eriksen and Philipsen, 1980) to 95% (Dessaive et al, 1982).

Ultrasonography has been used as a prognostic tool by a number of investigators hoping to avoid the disadvantages of hormone assays. Representative studies are listed in Table 22–1, with the validity of prediction based on ultrasonography calculated for each report. *Sensitivity* is the ability of ultrasonography to identify correctly those women who will spontaneously abort; *specificity* is the ability to identify correctly those who will not. A measure of direct interest to the clinician is the *predictive value* of an abnormal scan; that is, what percentage of women with an abnormal scan will, indeed, abort.

To be clinically useful in predicting spontaneous abortion, a test must have very high sensitivity and predictive value of an abnormal scan. Specificity and predictive value of a normal scan are of little consequence. If ultrasonography incorrectly identifies a woman as destined to have a spontaneous abortion, curettage performed on the basis of this error would abort a viable pregnancy. On the other hand, if ultrasonography incorrectly predicts a normal pregnancy outcome, no intervention ensues and no adverse effect results from the diagnostic error.

As shown in Table 22–1, the sensitivity of ultrasonography ranges from 69% to 97%, depending on the study population and diagnostic criteria used. The predictive value of an abnormal scan ranges from 74% to 100%. When morphologic criteria and evidence of fetal heart motion have been compared, the latter has been more accurate in predicting spontaneous abortion (Sakamoto and Okai, 1982). The accuracy of fetal-heartbeat determination increases with gestational age. Before 8 menstrual weeks' gestation, fetal heart motion cannot always be seen, and errors in assessing gestational age can

TABLE 22–1 *Validity of Ultrasonography in Predicting Spontaneous Abortion Among Women with Threatened Abortion*

AUTHOR	ULTRASONOGRAPHIC CRITERIA	SENSITIVITY (%)	SPECIFICITY (%)	PREDICTIVE VALUE OF ABNORMAL SCAN (%)
Duff, 1975	Morphology and fetal heart motion	92	73	86
Anderson, 1980	Fetal heart motion	97	99	98
Eriksen and Philipsen, 1980	Fetal heart motion	85	95	91
Hertz et al, 1980	Fetal heart motion	69	83	74
Sande et al, 1980	Fetal heart motion	88	84	74
Stoppelli et al, 1981	Not specified	88	93	94
Dessaive et al, 1982	Morphology and fetal heart motion	70	89	91
Sakamoto and Okai, 1982	Morphology	88	96	94
	Fetal heart motion	97	100	100

further confound interpretation of results. A woman thought to be 10 weeks pregnant and with no visible fetal heart activity could really be 6 weeks pregnant with normal, but imperceptible, cardiac activity. If fetal heart activity is absent at or after 8 weeks' gestation, and if the estimated gestational age is accurate, ultrasonography may have enough predictive value to guide intervention, if so desired. Repeating the ultrasonography exam improves the diagnostic accuracy of this procedure.

Surgical Intervention

For women with inevitable abortion (characterized by progressive cervical dilatation without expulsion of products of conception) and for those with threatened abortion in whom the pregnancy has been judged nonviable, evacuation of the uterus is appropriate management. Unless concurrent problems such as uterine infection or anemia exist, evacuation of the uterus can be handled like an elective legal abortion (described later).

Two decisions must be made: where the curettage is to take place, and by what technique. The choice between outpatient curettage in the physician's office or curettage in an emergency room may depend on the time of day and available equipment. For uncomplicated cases, hospitalization and curettage in an operating room add to the costs, inconvenience, and emotional burden occasioned by spontaneous abortion yet offer no medical benefits over outpatient curettage (Farrell et al, 1982). The choice of evacuation technique depends on the state of the cervix, gestational age, and availability of equipment. For curettage evacuations, suction curettage is preferable to sharp curettage, yet suction equipment may not be at hand. Suction curettage is both faster and safer than sharp curettage and may cause less damage to the basal layer of the endometrium. A flexible Karman cannula with syringe as a source of suction is portable, inexpensive, and convenient for outpatient use.

Distinguishing between an incomplete abortion, in which some but not all the products of conception have been expelled, and complete abortion is frequently difficult. The woman's description of tissue may not be helpful, and not all women have the presence of mind to save expelled tissue for inspection by the physician. Likewise, the aperture of the cervix, size of the uterus, and presence or absence of bleeding may not indicate whether the abortion is complete or incomplete. This distinction is important, since incomplete abortion requires evacuation of the uterus; curettage after a complete abortion is more discretionary.

In the absence of evidence that the abortion is complete, many physicians perform a curettage, which can be both diagnostic and therapeutic. Most such evacuations will yield products of conception. Unpublished data of Romero from Yale indicate that 30% of women with a recognized spontaneous abortion will not require curettage.

Alternatively, ultrasonography may provide information about the completeness of abortion. In one small series (Jeong et al, 1981), a central uterine-cavity echo was associated with absence of products of conception on curettage. This technique appears to merit further investigation.

Regardless of the completeness of abortion, the physician should know the woman's Rh type. Spontaneous abortion is a potentially sensitizing event for Rh-negative women at risk. Rates of use of Rh immunoglobulin (RhIG) after spontaneous abortion are significantly lower than after induced abortion. A 50 mcg dose should be given to RhIG candidates who abort at 12 weeks' gestation or before, and a 300 mcg dose should be administered to those who abort later in pregnancy.

Fetal Death in Utero

DEFINITIONS

Fetal death in utero (FDIU) is the cessation of fetal life before termination of pregnancy. This diagnosis is further categorized by the gestational age at fetal death and length of retention of the dead fetus. Death before the 20th week of gestation is termed *spontaneous abortion* and death thereafter, *antepartum fetal death*. If the dead fetus is retained for 8 or more weeks (or a "prolonged period"), the term *missed abortion* is used.

From both a clinical and a nosologic point of view, the proliferation of terms related to FDIU is both unnecessary and confusing; all these diagnostic categories should be viewed as variations of a single obstetric entity.

INCIDENCE

FDIU is uncommon. Approximately 200,000 women with FDIU were hospitalized in the United States from 1972 to 1978 (Dorfman et al, 1983). During this 7-year interval, approximately 22.5 million live births took place in the United States. Thus, the incidence of FDIU requiring hospitalization appears to be about 9 cases per 1000 live births. By comparison, approximately one case of FDIU and 35 legal abortions occur for every 100 live births in the United States.

MANAGEMENT

Recent data on the natural history of FDIU are scarce. Older data suggest that most dead fetuses are expelled spontaneously within 3 weeks of death (Dorfman et al, 1983). However, the gestational age at the time of death influences the probability of expulsion within a given interval: the more remote from term, the longer the time required (Foley, 1981). Only 29% of women with fetal deaths before 34 weeks' gestation delivered within 2 weeks after death, as compared with 75% of women with fetal deaths occurring later in pregnancy.

Once fetal death is confirmed, the next—and perhaps most important—step is to counsel the parents (Fig. 22–1). Helping the couple to grieve appropriately can minimize psychologic sequelae from this often devastating loss. After these two initial steps, subsequent clinical management is largely discretionary. The risk of coagulation defects within 5 weeks of fetal death is minimal, as is the risk of infection, provided the membranes are intact. However, the emotional burden of carrying a dead fetus, often for weeks, can compound the misery experienced by the parents. Thus, although either watchful waiting or uterine evacuation can be chosen, most couples opt for intervention. Since there is no compelling medical indication for one course over the other, this decision should, in general, be left to the parents after they have been fully informed about the alternatives.

If uterine evacuation is elected, the physician should confirm that the woman's coagulation system is intact before intervening. Then, two approaches to evacuation exist: surgery or labor induction. The choice between surgery and labor induction should reflect the skill and experience of the physician, the size of the fetus and uterus, the availability of equipment and drugs, and the preference of the woman (Hodgson and Ditmanson, 1980). If dilatation and evacuation (D&E) is planned, accurate determination of the size of the fetus by ultrasonography is helpful.

Suction curettage is a safe and easy way to evacuate pregnancies at or before 14 weeks' gestation; thereafter, D&E can be used by those experienced in this technique. Occasionally, hysterectomy will be appropriate treatment in this setting if there is preexisting pathology such as carcinoma *in situ* of the cervix, plus a desire for sterilization. Hysterotomy has unacceptably high morbidity, mortality, and cost; this method should not be used.

If the pregnancy is of about 15 or more weeks' gestation, and if the physician chooses not to perform a D&E procedure, labor induction can be performed by administering vaginal prostaglandin E_2 suppositories, which are both effective and safe. Their use requires little surgical skill (unlike D&E), and the suppositories simultanenously stimulate contractions and promote cervical ripening. The principal disadvantages of the suppositories are the high incidence of vomiting and diarrhea (60% and 40%, respectively) and fever from the medication itself (50%). Hence, women should be premedicated

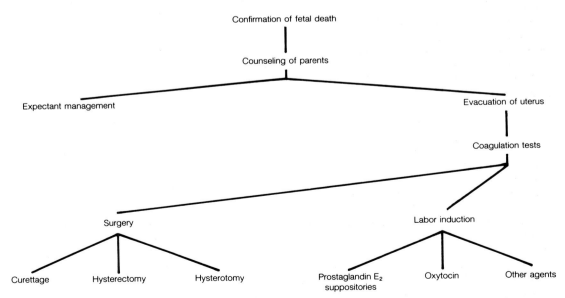

FIG. 22–1 Options for management of fetal death in utero.

with antiemetic and antidiarrheal drugs before administration of the suppositories; antipyretics and, occasionally, a cooling blanket may be required if the woman's temperature exceeds 39.4°C.

The traditional means of labor induction for cases of FDIU has been intravenous administration of oxytocin. This treatment is familiar to all gynecologists, and the medication is inexpensive. However, oxytocin lacks the efficacy of prostaglandin E_2 suppositories because the uterus is relatively insensitive to oxytocin early in pregnancy, and the cervix is frequently unfavorable for induction of labor.

Intra-amniotic abortifacients should not be used in this setting. Instillation of hypertonic saline, hyperosmolar urea, or prostaglandin F_{2a} may be hazardous because of unpredictable and potentially rapid uptake into the woman's circulation due to the altered permeability of the membranes after fetal death.

A sharp-curette check of the uterine cavity to confirm complete evacuation is probably advisable after any of these evacuation techniques. As with all pregnancy terminations, RhIG candidates should be identified and given an appropriate dose of RhIG.

COMPLICATIONS OF FETAL DEATH IN UTERO

FDIU carries risks of both morbidity and mortality for the woman. The risks of coagulation disorders and infection have received the most attention, yet recent data on their incidence are lacking. The risk of maternal death associated with FDIU is small; from 1972 to 1978, nine such deaths occurred among approximately 200,000 cases nationwide, for a death-to-case rate of 4.5 deaths per 100,000 cases (Dorfman et al, 1983).

The risk of death from FDIU increases with maternal age. The risk for women 35 years of age and older was 3.6 times that for women aged 15 to 24 years. The most frequent causes of maternal death from FDIU were uterine perforation and coagulopathy. At present, the comparative safety of available techniques for evacuating the uterus is not known.

Cervical Incompetence

INCIDENCE

Cervical incompetence is a nebulous term used to explain spontaneous abortions thought to be due to cervical factors. There is little agreement as to the definition of cervical incompetence or the appropriate diagnostic criteria; many reported cases of cervical incompetence are inconsistent with the classic picture of repetitive, acute, painless abortion in the midportion of pregnancy without associated bleeding or uterine contractions. Some physicians diagnose cervical incompetence on the basis of asymptomatic cervical dilatation observed in midpregnancy, whereas others rely on a variety of tests of unknown validity performed on nonpregnant women; for example, passage of a No. 8 (8 mm) Hegar dilator, traction on an intrauterine Foley catheter, or hysterography. A history of unexplained spontaneous abortion in the middle of pregnancy may be the most useful diagnostic criterion, yet the sensitivity and specificity of this criterion remain unknown.

This diagnostic imprecision is reflected in reported incidence rates of cervical incompetence. Rates range from 0.05 to 1 per 100 pregnancies (Cousins, 1980). Differences in diagnosis, rather than differences in populations of women, probably account for most of this variation.

RISK FACTORS

The etiology of cervical incompetence is unknown but may be multifactorial. Early theories about this problem focused on cervical trauma, such as conization, laceration, or excessive mechanical dilatation. Data are lacking, however, to confirm or refute these hypothetical risk factors. The occurrence of cervical incompetence in primigravidas suggests alternative etiologies. These may include associated uterine anomalies, prenatal exposure to diethylstilbestrol, or abnormal histology of the cervix (Cousins, 1980; Hughey and McElin, 1982). In addition, cervical incompetence may be inherited.

Cervical incompetence may be but one manifestation of a spectrum of asynchronism between the uterine corpus and cervix. In normal pregnancy and delivery, biochemical and biophysical changes in the cervix in late pregnancy allow cervical dilatation and effacement to occur synchronously with labor contractions. At one extreme of asynchronism, the corpus contracts yet cervical dilatation and effacement do not occur; this may account for the development of cervicovaginal fistulas during instillation abortions with prostaglandin F_{2a}. At the other extreme, progressive dilatation and effacement occur prematurely and in the absence of perceptible contractions (cervical incompetence). The underlying pathophysiology for many cases of cervical incompetence may be biochemical; that tying a noose around the cervix is the best available treatment suggests how limited our current understanding of this problem is.

TREATMENT

Three serious problems in published studies prohibit conclusions as to the treatment of choice for cervical incompetence. First, without a precise and reproducible definition of cervical incompetence, comparison of success rates in published reports is impossible. Second, new operations frequently are adopted into clinical practice without appropriate evidence of their efficacy. Randomized clinical trials comparing two operations are rarely done when a new operation is introduced; once the operation is accepted in clinical practice, a randomized trial is frequently judged unethical. To date, no randomized clinical trials comparing treatments for cervical incompetence have been done. Differences in rates of success in published case-series reports may be attributable in large part to differences in diagnosis, patient characteristics, and prenatal care, rather than to the treatments themselves.

Third, some of the benefit attributed to cerclage operations may not be due to the operation itself but rather to a phenomenon termed *regression to the mean* (Cole, 1982). A variable (pregnancy outcome) that is extreme or unusual when first measured (*e.g.*, fetal expulsion at 20 weeks' gestation) will tend to be nearer the mean of the population distribution at a subsequent observation (another pregnancy). Although there are methods for estimating the effect of this phenomenon in studies without comparison groups, only one study of cerclage has even considered this problem (Cole, 1982).

A variety of approaches have been used to treat cervical incompetence. Among the more innocuous, bed rest has been suggested as primary therapy as well as adjunctive therapy after cerclage. This appears to be a reasonable approach in terms of hydraulics, although data concerning efficacy are lacking.

A Smith–Hodge pessary can be used to displace the cervix posteriorly; this technique was first described by Vitsky in 1961. Although this approach has received little attention in the United States, it does have the appeal of exerting a mechanical effect without requiring an operation. Although electrocauterization of the cervix between pregnancies has been used to treat cervical incompetence in a small number of patients, this treatment has little to recommend it.

Surgery is the principal form of therapy for cervical incompetence in the United States. Two strategies have been used: primary repair of an anatomical defect and reinforcement of the cervix with a circumferential suture. The former approach, the Lash procedure, is appropriate only for women who are not pregnant and who have a demonstrable anatomical defect of the cervix. Moreover, the suggestion of diminished fertility after this operation is worrisome. Hence, the Lash procedure is infrequently used today.

Several types of cerclage procedures are currently used, with the Shirodkar and the McDonald the most common. Contraindications to cerclage include rupture of membranes, uterine bleeding, uterine contractions, chorioamnionitis, cervical dilatation greater than 4 cm, polyhydramnios, or known fetal anomaly. The Shirodkar operation places a reenforcing band around the cervix beneath the mucosa at the level of the internal os (Figs. 22–2 to 22–6). Spinal or epidural anesthesia is recommended; Trendelenburg's position and adequate retraction facilitate placement of the suture. As shown in Figures 22–4 and 22–5, the original operation used aneurysm needles to place a band of fascia lata around the cervix; then the knot was tied anteriorly. In recent years, many physicians have used a wide (*e.g.*, 5 mm) Mersilene band swedged onto large atraumatic needles, with the knot tied posteriorly to avoid erosion into the bladder. The cervical canal should remain open 3 mm to 5 mm. After the band is tied, the band and knot can be secured with several interrupted sutures of silk or other permanent material; the incisions in the mucosa are then closed with absorbable suture, thus burying the band. Opinion is divided as to whether the cerclage procedure is best performed during or between pregnancies.

Most studies (Cousins, 1980; McDonald, 1980) agree that the timing of cerclage during pregnancy influences outcome. Cerclage at around 14 weeks' gestation appears preferable. If substantial dilatation or bulging of fetal membranes has occurred, the likelihood of a successful cerclage is lessened. However, an attempt can be made to replace the protruding forewaters by means of a sterile Foley catheter (McDonald, 1980). Thereafter, the suture is placed and tied down, and the Foley balloon is deflated and withdrawn.

Postoperative care after cerclage for pregnant women has not been uniform. Although most authors advise bed rest for several days, and some advocate prophylactic antibiotics, tocolytic drugs, or progesterone, the usefulness of these measures has not been established.

The Shirodkar suture can be removed at 38 weeks' gestation or when fetal pulmonary maturity has been confirmed; it should be removed immediately if membranes rupture or labor starts. While some physicians leave a well-placed Shirodkar suture in place and deliver infants by cesarean section, the

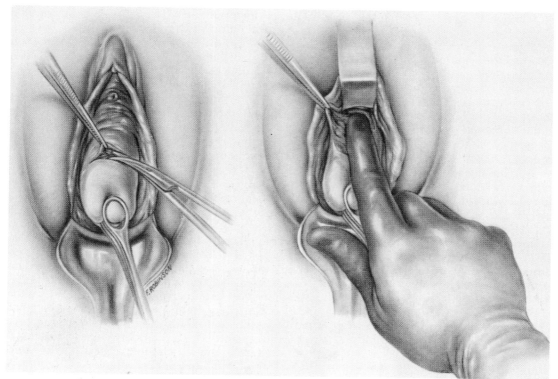

FIG. 22–2 Shirodkar cerclage operation. *(Left)* A transverse incision is made through the anterior vaginal mucosa at its junction with the cervix. *(Right)* The bladder is pushed cephalad to enable high placement of the suture.

morbidity, mortality, expense, pain, and inconvenience of cesarean delivery strongly argue against this course of action.

The McDonald procedure also places a reinforcing pulse-string suture around the proximal cervix. Unlike the Shirodkar procedure, however, the McDonald suture is not buried in its entirety (Fig. 22–7). Instead, several deep penetrations into the cervical stroma are made with a nonabsorbable suture, such as Mersilene. The advantages of this approach compared with the Shirodkar procedure are simplicity, ease of removal, and usefulness when the cervix is effaced or when fetal membranes are bulging. A notable disadvantage is the vaginal discharge associated with the exposed suture material. Since the Shirodkar and McDonald procedures have been reported to have similar efficacy, the simplicity and versatility of the McDonald operation make it preferable for most patients in need of cerclage.

Intra-abdominal cerclage may be appropriate in rare instances. Indications include traumatic cervical laceration, congenital shortening of the cervix, previous failed vaginal cerclage, and advanced cer-

vical effacement. This procedure places a band around the cervix at the level of the internal os in an avascular space between the branches of the uterine artery. Compared with the vaginal cerclage operations, this procedure has several important disadvantages: two abdominal operations are needed (one to place the suture, one for cesarean delivery); the surgery is performed in a highly vascular area adjacent to the ureters; and the complication rate is higher than with vaginal cerclage (Cousins, 1980). Hence, this approach should be used only when vaginal cerclage has failed or is not feasible (Novy, 1982).

COMPLICATIONS

Complications of cerclage range from annoying to fatal. A partial inventory of reported complications includes hemorrhage, rupture of membranes, infection (including chorioamnionitis, abscess, and death), cervical dystocia, uterine rupture, vesicovaginal fistula, and fetal death (Charles and Edwards, 1981; McDonald, 1980; Cousins, 1980). Although the

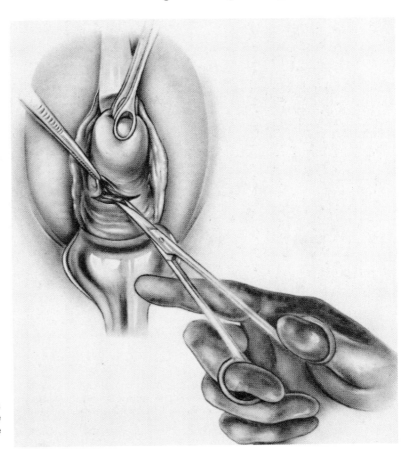

FIG. 22-3 Shirodkar cerclage operation. A transverse incision is then made through the posterior vaginal mucosa where it joins the cervix.

incidence of most of these complications is unknown, one report (Charles and Edwards, 1981) documented rates of chorioamnionitis ranging from 15 to 39 per 100 patients, depending on gestational age at the time of operation.

Illegal Abortion

INCIDENCE

Despite the widespread availability of legal abortion in the United States, small numbers of illegal procedures continue to be performed. Estimates of the incidence of illegal abortion in the United States before 1970 range from 200,000 to 1.2 million per year (Cates and Rochat, 1976); estimates for the late 1970s range from 5,000 to 23,000 per year (Binkin et al, 1982).

RISK FACTORS

Little is known about characteristics of women who obtain illegal abortions. Some inferences can be drawn, however, from the characteristics of 17 women who died from illegal abortion in the United States from 1975 to 1979 (Binkin et al, 1982). These women were older, of higher parity, and more likely to be black or Hispanic than women who died from legal abortion during these years. Slightly over half lived in the South. Thus, older black or Hispanic multiparas who live in the southern United States are more likely to die from illegal abortion than are other women.

TECHNIQUES

Although a wide variety of illegal abortion methods are used around the world, most methods in the United States can be categorized in two groups: oral abortifacients and intrauterine instrumentation. The most frequently used method reported in surveys in New York City in the 1960s (Polgar and Fried, 1976) was orally administered substances. These included turpentine, laundry bleach, and large doses of quinine. The misconception that quinine is a safe and effective oral abortifacient persists. Intrauterine

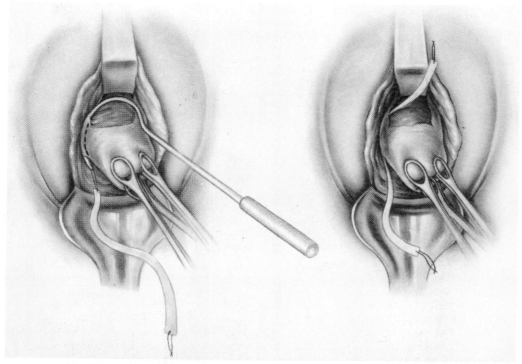

FIG. 22–4 Shirodkar cerclage operation. (*Left*) An aneurysm needle is introduced beneath the mucosa anteriorly and emerges posteriorly. (*Right*) The suture is threaded into the needle and then pulled under the mucosa on the right as the needle is withdrawn.

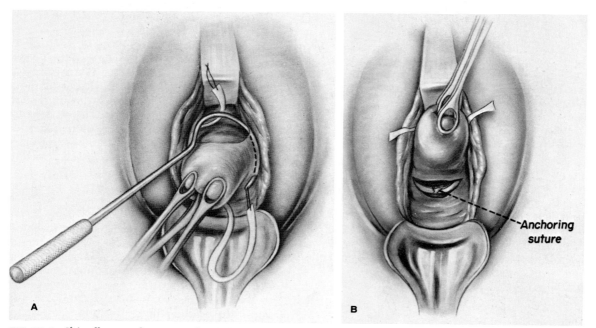

FIG. 22–5 Shirodkar cerclage operation. (*A*) A mirror image aneurysm needle is then inserted on the left side of the cervix, and the other end of the suture is brought anteriorly beneath the mucosa. (*B*) The suture is anchored posteriorly by two fine silk sutures.

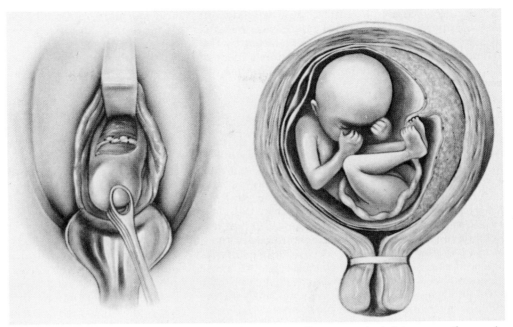

FIG. 22-6 Shirodkar cerclage operation. (*Left*) The encircling suture is tied to secure the cervix with an opening of 3 mm to 5 mm. The suture is anchored anteriorly with fine silk. (*Right*) Correct placement of the suture.

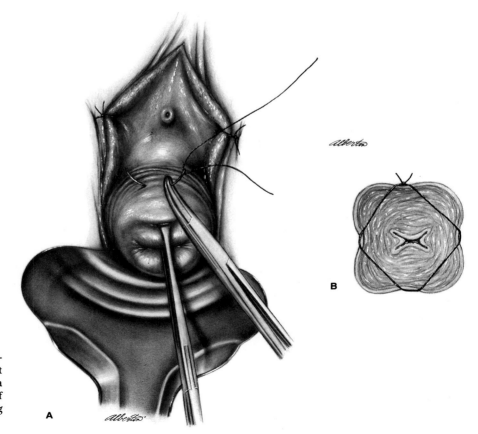

FIG. 22-7 McDonald cerclage operation. (*A*) Four bites are made at the junction of vaginal mucosa and cervix. (*B*) A cross-section of the cervix with the purse-string suture in place.

techniques were used less often; these ranged from intrauterine injection of soap or phenol disinfectants to insertion of foreign objects. As reported by the women surveyed, intrauterine techniques successfully aborted pregnancy much more often than did oral substances.

COMPLICATIONS OF ILLEGAL ABORTION

While intrauterine techniques have greater efficacy than oral abortifacients, the former also have a higher risk of complications. For example, in a 1962 study in Chile (Liskin, 1980), 42% of women who had catheter-induced abortions were hospitalized for treatment of complications, compared with 35% of those who used oral abortifacients. Other important variables influencing the likelihood of morbidity include the skill of the provider, gestational age, and availability of gynecologic care. The most frequently reported complication of illegal abortion is retained products of conception, although the incidence of this and other complications is unknown.

The number of deaths from illegal abortion in the United States declined dramatically during the 1970s. For example, the rate (illegal-abortion deaths per million women of reproductive age) decreased from 0.46 in 1972–1974 to 0.07 in 1975–1979, a reduction of 85% (Table 22–2). During the latter interval, women at both extremes of the reproductive-age span had higher death rates from illegal abortion than women of intermediate ages. However, the racial discrepancy in death rates is more striking:

the mortality rate for black and Hispanic women is more than 10 times greater than that for white women.

As with morbidity, the likelihood of mortality is strongly related to the abortion technique. Of the 17 illegal-abortion deaths from 1975 to 1979, only one followed ingestion of an abortifacient (pennyroyal oil). The other deaths were related to intrauterine techniques, ranging from injection of cleaning solutions to insertion of foreign bodies (catheters, cotton swabs, thermometers, and coat hangers). Sepsis (10 cases) and air embolism (3 cases) accounted for most of these deaths (Binkin et al, 1982).

TREATMENT

Improved management of complications of illegal abortion, in addition to the decrease in such complications, has played a major role in preventing death and permanent disability. Treatment for ingestion of toxic substances is primarily medical and will not be dealt with here. Incomplete abortion requires curettage.

Septic Abortion

The vast majority of women with septic abortion respond rapidly to uterine evacuation plus broad-spectrum antibiotics. Blood should not be given for the sole purpose of combating infection. Before beginning treatment, intrauterine and blood cultures should be obtained. An upright X-ray of the abdomen may identify a residual foreign body, gas bubbles in the uterus, or free air under the diaphragm; management is altered by these findings.

Intravenous antibiotics should be started in the emergency room. Coverage should include gram-positive, gram-negative, and anaerobic bacteria. The optimal antibiotic regimen has not been established. However, treatment guidelines (Centers for Disease Control, 1982) for pelvic inflammatory disease may be appropriate for septic abortion:

> doxycycline 100 mg, IV, twice a day
> plus
> cefoxitin 2 g, IV, four times a day
>
> or
>
> clindamycin 600 mg, IV, four times a day
> plus
> gentamicin or tobramycin 2 mg/kg, IV, followed by 1.5 mg/kg, IV, three times a day
>
> or
>
> doxycycline 100 mg, IV, twice a day
> plus
> metronidazole 1 g, IV, twice a day

TABLE 22–2 *Annual Death Rate from Illegal Abortion by Age and Race, United States, 1972–1974 and 1975–1979*

CHARACTERISTIC	RATE* 1972–1974	1975–1979
Age (yrs.)		
15–19	0.36	0.08
20–29	0.79	0.05
30–44	0.24	0.08
Race		
White	0.11	0.02
Hispanic	1.02	0.22
Black	2.36	0.31
Total	0.46	0.07

* Number of deaths per million women aged 15–44 (Binkinn, et al: Illegal-abortion deaths in the United States: Why are they still occurring? Fam Plann Perspect 14:163, 1982. Reprinted with permission from Family Planning Perspectives.)

If the woman's condition is stable, she can be taken directly from the emergency room to the operating room for curettage. Peak serum levels of antibiotics will be present within an hour of their administration. Further delay of uterine evacuation is unwarranted and may compromise recovery. Prompt elimination of the necrotic, infected tissue is critical. Tissue obtained during curettage should be transported quickly for microbiologic cultures. The yield of organisms, especially anaerobes, is often higher from a tissue specimen than from a swab inserted into the uterus.

Subsequent management is governed by the response of the woman and by microbiologic findings. All women with septic abortions should be closely observed after surgery, with special attention to vital signs and urine output, in order to detect incipient shock. Prompt, aggressive therapy (Chapter 6) is essential if septic shock develops.

Postabortal sepsis from *Clostridium perfringens* is very rare today. When this infection occurs, however, it can be catastrophic. In the absence of hemolysis, *C. perfringens* bacteremia can be managed by curettage and antibiotics. In the presence of hemolysis, hysterectomy and more aggressive medical therapy are indicated (Green and Brenner, 1978).

Legal Abortion

INCIDENCE

Legal abortion is one of the most frequently performed operations in the United States. Approximately 1.3 million procedures were reported to the Centers for Disease Control for 1980, and this figure is 15% to 20% less than the total number performed. In 1980, 362 legal abortions were performed for every 1000 live births (abortion ratio) and 25 legal abortions per 1000 women aged 15–44 years (abortion rate).

DEMOGRAPHIC CHARACTERISTICS

Women who obtain legal abortion in the United States tend to be young, white, single, and of low parity. In 1980, 29% of abortions were performed on teenagers, 36% on women 20 to 24 years old, and 35% on older women. Most women obtaining abortions were white (70%) and unmarried (77%). Most (58%) had had no previous live births.

Legal abortion in the United States is performed principally by curettage techniques early in pregnancy. In 1980, 96% of all legal abortions were performed by curettage (primarily suction curettage), 3% by intrauterine instillation, 0.1% by hysterotomy

or hysterectomy, and 1% by other methods (Centers for Disease Control, 1983). Over half (52%) of all legal abortions were performed within 8 weeks and 90% within 12 weeks of the last menstrual period; 0.9% of all abortions took place at 21 weeks' gestation or later.

TECHNIQUES

All methods of abortion can be divided into two broad categories: surgical evacuation and labor induction. Surgical evacuation includes suction curettage (vacuum aspiration), sharp curettage, D&E (defined as transcervical evacuation at or after 13 menstrual weeks' gestation), hysterotomy, and hysterectomy. Labor induction includes administration of abortifacients either systemically (vaginal or intramuscular prostaglandins) or directly into the uterus (intra-amniotic prostaglandin, hypertonic saline, hyperosmolar urea, or a combination of these). In addition, several adjuncts, such as laminaria or oxytocin, have an important role in abortion practice. This section will review the principal methods of abortion in current use; detailed descriptions of these techniques have been published elsewhere (Stubblefield, 1978; Hern, 1981).

Surgical Evacuation

Suction curettage is by far the most important method of abortion in the United States; it is the most frequently used method—and the safest. The preoperative evaluation for suction curettage should include counseling, informed consent, a brief history, and a limited physical examination. The history-taking should focus only on data of relevance to the procedure, such as gynecologic problems (e.g., leiomyomas) or medical problems (e.g., cardiac valvular disease, asthma, or drug sensitivities) that might influence the conduct of the operation. Physical examination should include the heart, lungs, abdomen, and pelvis. Although ultrasonography is not warranted on a routine basis, it is useful if the size, shape, or position of the uterus is unclear.

Few laboratory tests are required. Determination of the hematocrit (or hemoglobin) and Rh type, plus a urinalysis, are appropriate. Although screening for gonorrhea, syphilis, and cervical neoplasia is commonly done, these tests are not obligatory unless dictated by local regulations.

MENSTRUAL REGULATION. *Menstrual regulation, menstrual extraction,* or *minisuction* are euphemisms for very early suction curettage. This technique requires a flexible plastic cannula 4 mm to 6 mm in diameter, with a self-locking syringe as a source of suction (Fig. 22–8). The upper gestational-age limit for this procedure ranges from 42 to 50 days from

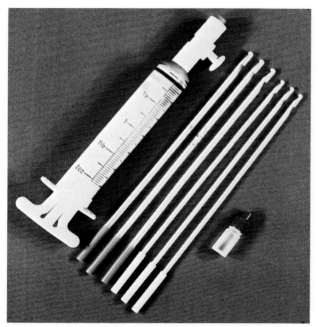

FIG. 22-8 Karman cannulas, self-locking syringe with pinch valve, and bottle of silicone lubricant. (Photograph courtesy of IPAS, Chapel Hill, North Carolina).

last menstrual period. Extensive literature in the 1970s documented the simplicity and safety of the technique (Laufe, 1977).

Menstrual regulation differs from suction curettage in several ways. First, anesthesia is not usually required, although analgesia may ease the cramping that occurs toward the end of the evacuation. Second, dilatation is often not required for menstrual regulation. If a given cannula cannot be introduced into the uterus, smaller flexible cannulas in the set can be used as dilators. After a cannula of appropriate size is inserted, the syringe is attached and the pinch valve released to begin the suctioning. Blood and tissue flow into the syringe. The abortion is performed by rotary and in-and-out movement of the cannula until the gritty feel of the endometrium is sensed and bubbles appear in the syringe. The cannula should not be removed while a vacuum exists in the syringe; likewise, the plunger of the syringe must never be advanced while the cannula is connected and is within the uterus, since air embolism can result. The syringe and cannula are disposable, although with proper care and sterilization by glutaraldehyde or ethylene oxide, the equipment can be reused many times.

Two problems occur more often with menstrual regulation than with suction curettage performed later in pregnancy: the procedure may be per- formed on women who are not pregnant, and the operation may fail to abort the pregnancy. Use of very sensitive pregnancy tests can ensure that an unnecessary procedure will not be performed; in general, the operation should not be done in the absence of a positive test. Microscopic examination of the products of conception plus careful followup with a pregnancy test and pelvic exam can reduce the likelihood of a continuing pregnancy going unnoticed.

SUCTION CURETTAGE. Suction curettage refers to dilatation of the cervix followed by vacuum aspiration of the uterine contents at 12 weeks' gestation or before. Sharp curettage, which is slower and not as safe, is analogous to diagnostic dilatation and curettage; it will not be discussed further.

Preparing the patient for surgery is simple. The woman should avoid oral intake on the day of surgery, and she should bring someone with her to the facility to take her home. The woman should empty her bladder before being placed in the dorsal lithotomy position; a catheter should not be used to drain the bladder. Shaving the perineum and washing the vulva are unnecessary; the vagina is usually washed with a povidone-iodine solution, although the benefit of this practice is not established. Likewise, routine sterile precautions (drapes, caps, masks, and gowns) are unnecessary. The physician should use a "no-touch" technique: he or she wears sterile gloves and does not touch those portions of the sterile instruments to be inserted into the uterus.

Although either local or general anesthesia can be used, use of local anesthesia predominates in the United States. While local anesthesia does not completely relieve discomfort, it is less expensive and safer than general anesthesia (Peterson et al, 1981).

To perform a paracervical block safely, the physician should use the smallest volume of the lowest concentration of local anesthetic. Local anesthetics vary in their toxicity. Chloroprocaine is substantially less toxic than lidocaine, although the latter is less expensive (Grimes and Cates, 1976). If lidocaine is used, a 0.5% concentration is safer than a 1% solution. The total dose of lidocaine should not exceed 2 mg per pound (lean weight) or 300 mg, whichever is less. Alternatively, use of local anesthesia with vasoconstrictor (e.g., epinephrine 1:200,000) slows systemic absorption of anesthetic and allows a larger total dose to be used.

The site of injection of paracervical anesthesia appears to matter little; injection at almost any site adjacent to the cervix results in excellent anesthesia. Common regimens include infiltration of the cervix at 12 o'clock (for application of the tenaculum), then injection at four sites (3, 5, 7, and 9 o'clock) or two sites (3 and 9 o'clock) at the junction of cervix and vagina. The injection should be submucosal to avoid inadvertent intravascular injection. The pain of inserting the needle can be disguised by placing the tip of a 21-gauge spinal needle against the mucosa at the chosen site and having the woman cough. The Valsalva maneuver "pops" the mucosa over the needle point—frequently without any sensation of pain. This technique works better at 3 o'clock and 9 o'clock than at 5 o'clock and 7 o'clock. Once the anesthetic has been injected, the next—and perhaps most important—step is to wait. At least 3 minutes (using a clock) should be allowed for the block to take effect; failure to wait for absorption is the usual reason for inadequate anesthesia.

Few instruments are required for suction curettage. Most physicians prefer to use a bivalve speculum. However, a speculum with standard-length blades prevents the cervix from being drawn toward the introitus during the procedure and makes the operation more difficult. The Moore modification of the Graves speculum, which has one-inch shorter blades of standard width, is well suited for this purpose and is commercially available. Two single-toothed tenaculums are helpful; one is routinely placed on the anterior cervix. If difficulty during dilatation occurs, the other can be placed on the posterior cervix to stabilize it. Although use of a uterine sound indicates the axial depth of the uterus, sounding the uterus provides no important information and carries a risk of perforation. For this reason, many experienced physicians have abandoned its use for abortion.

If the direction of the cervical canal is in question, the physician can gently probe with a small dilator. Pratt dilators are preferable to Hegar dilators for abortion, since they require less force to dilate the cervix. Other instruments required for suction curettage include: several sharp curettes of different sizes; the vacuum machine, hose, and swivel handle; and a cannula.

Traction on the cervix is important during suction curettage; it stabilizes the uterus and straightens the angle between cervix and corpus, which reduces the risk of perforation. The tenaculum should have a firm purchase on the cervix. High vertical placement at 12 o'clock, with one tooth in the canal and one on the anterior cervix, almost eliminates the risk of the tenaculum tearing through during dilatation, as can happen when less substantial horizontal application is made with the tenaculum. If the puncture site on the cervix bleeds when the tenaculum is removed, direct pressure for a brief time stops the bleeding. If the uterus is retroverted, some physicians prefer to place the tenaculum on the cervix at 6 o'clock (Fig. 22–9).

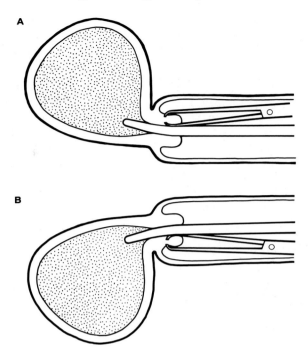

FIG. 22–9   Traction on cervix during dilatation. (*A*) The tenaculum is placed vertically on the anterior lip. (*B*) The tenaculum is placed vertically on the posterior lip for a retroverted uterus. Note the posterior direction of the dilator.

Gentleness is the key to safe cervical dilatation. The cervix should be dilated just enough to allow insertion and rotation of the desired cannula. For example, to insert an 8-mm cannula, dilatation to 25 French will allow free rotation. During dilatation, the dilator should be held between the thumb and index finger to limit the force applied; in addition, the other fingers should remain extended to prevent plunging forward in case resistance is suddenly lost. Dilatation need not start with the smallest dilator on the set; starting with a larger size (e.g., No. 15 French instead of No. 13 French) may reduce the risk of perforating the uterus or creating a false channel. If more than two fingers of force are required during dilatation, the physician should stop and reassess the situation, rather than risk injuring the cervix. One option is to use a smaller cannula than originally planned. Alternatively, the physician can pack the cervix with laminaria until snug, discontinue the procedure, then complete the operation several hours later, by which time adequate dilatation will have been achieved. Performance of the procedure in two stages is far preferable to forceful dilatation.

Laminaria are being used with increasing frequency for cervical dilatation preceding suction curettage. Laminaria are hygroscopic stalks of dried seaweed that dilate the cervix over several hours; in contrast, the process takes several minutes when mechanical dilators are used. The mode of action of laminaria is not well understood, but the principal mechanism appears to be desiccation of the cervix (Stubblefield, 1980). This desiccation may alter the ratio of collagen to ground substance, thus changing collagen cross-linkages. Alternatively, laminaria may alter the elaboration, release, or degradation of uterine prostaglandin F_{2a}. Laminaria cause the cervix to dilate away from the laminaria; whatever the mechanism, it is more complex than mere passive stretching.

Synthetic laminaria made from magnesium sulfate–impregnated polymer foam sponge appear promising in early reports. Potential advantages include uniformity of shape and size, stability, predictable dilatation, and lower costs.

Laminaria can be used conveniently in an outpatient setting. Most dilatation after laminaria insertion occurs in the first 4 to 6 hours, although dilatation will continue for about 24 hours. Placement of laminaria for 3 to 4 hours before abortion frequently dilates the cervix sufficiently for surgery. Synthetic laminaria may require only 2 hours. Laminaria use reduces fivefold the risk of both cervical injury requiring sutures and uterine perforation compared with use of metal dilators; this protective effect may be especially important for young teenagers with immature cervices who are at increased risk for cervical injury (Schulz et al, 1983).

After adequate dilatation has been obtained, a cannula is inserted into the uterus. In general, the diameter of the cannula in mm should be about one less than the weeks of gestation from last menses. For example, an 8-mm cannula is adequate for evacuating a pregnancy of 9 weeks' gestation. Some highly skilled physicians prefer to use even smaller cannulas than this guideline suggests; the advantage of needing less dilatation must be weighed against the disadvantages of longer operating time and an increased risk of incomplete abortion.

The most frequently used cannulas in the United States are clear plastic, with a slight angulation (Fig. 22–10). Rigid plastic cannulas are superior to flexible plastic cannulas. The cannula should be inserted only to the level of the lower uterine segment. The suction machine (Fig. 22–11) is turned on, and the uterine contents are then evacuated by rotation of the cannula (Fig. 22–12). In-and-out motions are not necessary and may cause perforation of the fundus and aspiration of abdominal contents. When bubbles are seen in the cannula and the interior of the cavity feels empty, a sharp curette may be used gently to confirm the completeness of evacuation.

The operation is not finished until the aspirated tissue has been examined. The physician or another trained observer must confirm in each case that

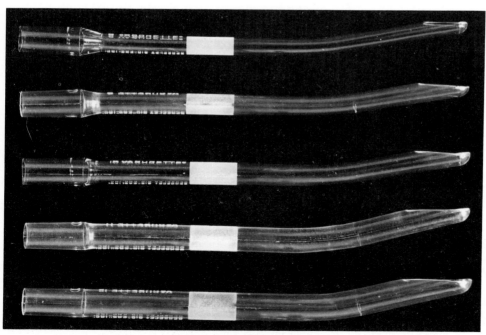

FIG. 22–10   Plastic suction cannulas 8 mm to 12 mm in diameter.

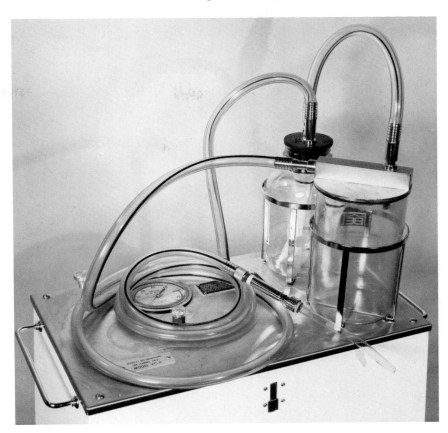

FIG. 22–11 Suction machine, tubing, swivel handle, and cannula.

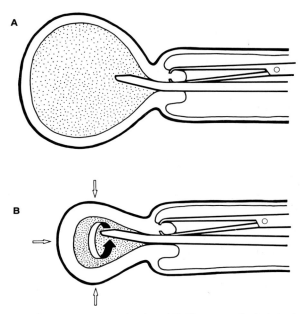

FIG. 22–12 Uterine aspiration. (*A*) The cannula is inserted just beyond the internal os. (*B*) The products of conception are evacuated by rotary motion of the cannula.

fetal tissue has been obtained, in order to exclude the possibility of an ectopic pregnancy. Since 1972, more than 10 women in the United States have died from ectopic pregnancies undetected at the time of attempted suction curettage (Rubin et al, 1980).

Pregnancies at or after 9 weeks' gestation should have recognizable fetal parts; earlier pregnancies may not. Identification of chorionic villi in these earlier pregnancies is essential. The bag of aspirated tissue should be rinsed under tap water to remove blood and clots. The tissue can then be placed in a glass baking dish and floated in water or white vinegar. The latter makes the villi appear white and facilitates their recognition. Back lighting from a horizontal X-ray viewing box is especially useful. Villi will appear soft, fluffy, and feathery, with discernible finger-like projections; in contrast, decidua appears coarse and shaggy (Figs. 22–13 and 22–14). If villi cannot be recognized with the unaided eye, a magnifying glass, dissecting microscope, colposcope, or standard microscope (×100) may enable identification of villi.

If fetal tissue is not confirmed, the woman should be reexamined, with special attention to the adnexa,

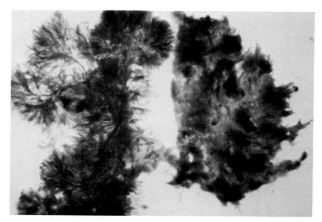

FIG. 22–13 Seen immersed in water are typical fluffy villi of placenta (*Left*) and shaggy decidua (*Right*). (Munsick RA: Clinical test for placenta in 300 consecutive menstrual aspirations. Obstet Gynecol 60:738, 1982. Reprinted with permission from The American College of Obstetricians and Gynecologists.)

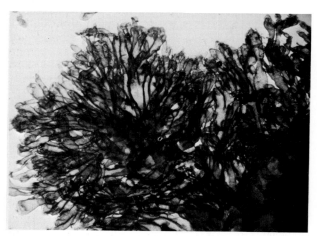

FIG. 22–14 Wet-mount microscopic appearance of placental villi. (Munsick RA: Clinical test for placenta in 300 consecutive menstrual aspirations. Obstet Gynecol 60:738, 1982. Reprinted with permission from The American College of Obstetricians and Gynecologists.)

and the uterus should be reevacuated. If no villi are recovered, a sensitive pregnancy test should be done. If positive, the woman must be presumed to have an ectopic pregnancy and should be evaluated accordingly.

ANCILLARY MEASURES.

OXYTOCICS. The usefulness of administering oxytocics during suction curettage is not established, although administering oxytocin or ergot derivatives reduces blood loss from suction curettage performed under general anesthesia. Although statis-

tically significant, the reduction in blood loss is clinically unimportant. Since blood loss is less when local rather than general anesthesia is used, oxytocics probably are not warranted on a routine basis. Although ergot derivatives are commonly given by mouth for several days after suction curettage, evidence of the benefit of this practice is lacking and the drugs cause painful uterine cramping in some women.

PROPHYLACTIC ANTIBIOTICS. As with oxytocics, the appropriate role for prophylactic antibiotics is unresolved. One large, nonrandomized cohort study (Hodgson et al, 1975) demonstrated a significant reduction in complications among the group administered prophylactic oral tetracycline. Similar results were obtained in a smaller study of oral doxycycline (London et al, 1978). In a randomized clinical trial (Sonne–Holm et al, 1981), prophylaxis with penicillin and pivampicillin reduced postabortal infections by one-half among women with a history of pelvic inflammatory disease, but no effect was observed among the other women. Yet another randomized clinical trial (Westrom et al, 1981) examined the use of a single dose of oral tinidazole; no significant differences in infection rates were observed, but the power of the study was low. Thus, the question remains unresolved. Most abortion clinics provide prophylactic antibiotics, usually tetracycline. This drug is safe, relatively inexpensive, and effective in treating both gonorrhea and chlamydial infections.

DILATATION AND EVACUATION. Dilatation and evacuation (D&E) is an extension of curettage techniques beyond the traditional (and obsolete) 12-week limit. In the United States, D&E is the method of abortion most frequently performed at or after 13 weeks' gestation. The proportion of abortions performed using D&E procedures is inversely related to gestational age: in 1980, D&E accounted for 85% of all abortions performed at 13 to 15 weeks' gestation, 44% at 16 to 20 weeks, and 30% at 21 weeks or later (Centers for Disease Control, 1983). Large studies have demonstrated that D&E has a lower morbidity rate than currently available instillation abortifacients (Grimes et al, 1977, 1980; Kafrissen et al, 1984); moreover, D&E performed at 13 to 15 weeks' gestation is associated with a lower mortality rate than instillation abortions at or after the 16th week of gestation (Cates and Grimes, 1981).

Errors in estimating gestational age, especially underestimation, can have serious consequences during a D&E procedure. Hence, confirmation of gestational age by ultrasonography is strongly advised before D&E is done.

D&E differs from suction curettage in two principal ways: D&E requires wider cervical dilatation, and forceps are needed to evacuate more advanced pregnancies. To achieve adequate dilatation, many physicians insert laminaria several hours to several days before D&E (Fig. 22–15). For example, five laminaria placed overnight result in 15-mm to 20-mm diameter dilatation with minimal or no discomfort for most women. Dilating the cervix to large diameters over several minutes may damage the cervix. Indeed, the first large study of this possibility (Hogue, unpublished data) revealed a higher incidence of low birthweight infants in subsequent desired pregnancies. Hence, in the absence of evidence to the contrary, laminaria should probably be used routinely for D&E procedures performed at or after 15 weeks' gestation.

In the 13- to 16-week interval, D&E can be done with vacuum aspiration alone; thereafter, it is accomplished primarily with forceps extraction. A cannula 14 mm in diameter will evacuate pregnancies through approximately 16 menstrual weeks' gestation. For later pregnancies, the cannula is used principally to drain amniotic fluid at the beginning of the evacuation and to draw tissue into the lower uterus for forceps extraction. Specially designed forceps for D&E are available and are far superior to standard sponge forceps. As with suction curettage, instruments should be used only in the lower uterus to minimize the risks of perforation; the only instrument to reach the fundus should be a large sharp curette to confirm that the evacuation is complete.

Complete evacuation should then be corroborated by inspection of fetal parts before the procedure is concluded. All major fetal parts must be identified. The calvarium is the component most frequently missed during the initial evacuation. Gentle explo-

ration of the fundal and cornual areas with a large curette or forceps will usually enable location and removal of the calvarium. Intraoperative ultrasonography may be helpful. If the retained tissue is not easily found and removed, the physician should discontinue the operation and administer intravenous oxytocin to the woman for 2 to 3 hours while she is under observation in the recovery room. The woman then returns to the operating room where the retained tissue will, almost invariably, be visible at the internal os, from which it can be removed in a few seconds.

In D&E abortions, the skill of the physician is of paramount importance. D&E abortion is an eclectic area of gynecology, analogous to radical cancer surgery or administration of chemotherapy, and physicians should not dabble in these activities. This is not to say that D&E is too difficult for most physicians to learn. On the contrary, residents can be taught to do D&E procedures skillfully. Facility with suction curettage is a prerequisite to learning to perform D&E abortions. The physician should study operative technique (Stubblefield, 1978; Hern, 1981). He or she should then observe and assist skilled physicians and then perform D&E procedures only under direct supervision. The gestational-age range should be advanced cautiously as skill grows. In summary, D&E is not a trivial undertaking. Attempts by an unsupervised novice to perform a D&E abortion are dangerous.

Labor Induction

Although instillation abortions have been supplanted in part by D&E, the need for labor-induction methods for abortion continues, particularly at later gestational ages. In contrast to the proportion of abortions performed using D&E, the proportion of abortions performed by instillation techniques increases with gestational age. In 1980, 3% of abortions performed at 13 to 15 weeks' gestation were done by intrauterine instillation; at 16 to 20 weeks, the percentage was 43%, and at or after 21 weeks, 61% (Centers for Disease Control, 1983).

Although prostaglandins administered intramuscularly or vaginally are available to induce abortion, intrauterine instillation of abortifacients is used much more frequently. Among the intrauterine techniques, intraamniotic instillation is customary, although some physicians prefer extraovular administration of abortifacients.

The abortifacients in current use can be divided into two groups: hypertonic solutions (*e.g.*, saline or urea) and uterotonic agents (prostaglandin F_{2a}). The mechanism of action of hypertonic solutions is unclear, but these agents usually result in fetal death from osmotic insult; labor then usually ensues.

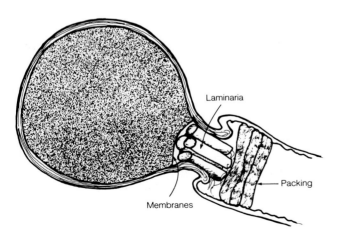

FIG. 22–15 Laminaria in place after overnight placement. (Grimes DA, Hulka JF: Midtrimester dilatation and evacuation abortion. South Med J 73:448, 1980. Reprinted by permission from the Southern Medical Journal.)

Prostaglandins appear to act directly on the myometrium to stimulate contractions.

Hypertonic solutions and uterotonic agents can be used in combination. Indeed, a combination of 80 g of urea plus 5 mg to 10 mg of prostaglandin F_{2a} injected into the amniotic sac appears superior to other instillation regimens. This urea-prostaglandin combination is significantly safer and faster than use of 200 cc of 20% saline alone as an abortifacient (Binkin et al, 1983).

Amniocentesis is required for instillation of the abortifacient. This procedure is usually performed abdominally. Some physicians prefer a "blind" insertion in the midline, several cm inferior to the level of the fundus. Others mark on the woman's abdomen the location of a pocket of amniotic fluid identified at ultrasonography. Still others use real-time ultrasonography during the needle insertion.

Preparation for the amniocentesis is similar to that for diagnostic amniocentesis. The bladder should be empty. The abdomen should be cleansed with an antiseptic, and strict aseptic technique should be used. The full thickness of the abdominal wall should be infiltrated with several ml of local anesthetic. After needle insertion, a free flow of clear amniotic fluid should be obtained. Nitrazine paper or urine dip sticks for protein can differentiate amniotic fluid from urine if necessary. Blood-tinged fluid that clears does not present a problem; grossly bloody fluid that does not clear is a contraindication to injection of hypertonic solutions. If the uterus is small, lifting the uterus anteriorly with two fingers in the vagina can facilitate amniocentesis. Alternatively, vaginal amniocentesis posterior to the cervix can be done, but the sterility of this approach is dubious.

Withdrawal of amniotic fluid is not necessary before the injection of abortifacient since withdrawing fluid apparently does not shorten the induction-to-abortion time. On the other hand, withdrawing several hundred ml fluid (and the corresponding decrease in the size of the uterus) may displace the needle tip. Hence, only enough fluid to confirm free flow need be removed.

If hypertonic solutions are used, they should be administered only by gravity drip. If correct needle placement is lost during the injection, the flow of solution stops. On the other hand, with syringe injection, hypertonic solutions can be injected forcibly into the myometrium in this situation.

Careful observation of the woman is required during instillation. No sedative or narcotic should be administered. The woman should be alert and watchful for any symptom (e.g., burning abdominal pain, severe thirst, headache, or nausea) that might indicate faulty administration or rapid systemic uptake of the abortifacient. Any such symptom dictates immediate cessation of the infusion and close observation of the woman. If the symptom persists, the instillation should be abandoned and alternative methods or agents used for the abortion.

Much of the morbidity (and mortality) associated with instillation abortion is preventable. Women in labor with instillation abortions need the same meticulous, attentive obstetric care as do women in labor with childbirth. Induction-to-abortion times of 13 to 24 hours are associated with the lowest complication rates (Binkin et al, 1983); thus, abortion within this interval should be the goal. Serious complications increase significantly with increasing induction-to-abortion times. If labor is ineffective, steps should be taken to stimulate labor. If the membranes rupture, labor must conclude within a reasonable period. Similarly, active management of a retained placenta after abortion prevents morbidity. A passive approach to desultory labor in the presence of ruptured membranes exposes the woman to unnecessary risks of complications.

ANCILLARY TECHNIQUES.   Several adjuncts can expedite instillation abortions. Administration of intravenous oxytocin shortens induction-to-abortion times with saline instillation but not with prostaglandin F_{2a} instillation. Intramuscular prostaglandin (carboprost tromethamine) or vaginal prostaglandin E_2 suppositories can be used to augment labor; these agents should be considered as the pharmacologic treatment of choice for slow or failed instillation abortions.

Direct cervical dilatation is also useful. Laminaria shorten induction-to-abortion times and protect against cervicovaginal fistulas, although this protection is not absolute. Sequential packings of laminaria may be useful if adequate dilatation is not achieved with uterotonics. Alternatively, if progress is stalled, a metreurynter can be used. A sterile Foley catheter with a 30 cc to 75 cc balloon can be inserted into the uterus, the balloon inflated with a sterile solution (not air), and the catheter tied to 0.5 kg orthopedic traction at the foot of the bed. However, this method has the obvious disadvantage of placing a foreign body in the uterus.

In many cases, the preferred means of concluding a slow induction abortion is D&E. This decision should reflect gestational age, status of the cervix, skill of the physician, and availability of equipment. Frequently, the cervix is dilated several cm and the evacuation proceeds quickly.

Hysterotomy and Hysterectomy

Neither hysterotomy nor hysterectomy should be considered a primary method of abortion. The morbidity, mortality, expense, and pain associated with these operations are greater than with alternative methods. Hysterotomy for abortion is an archaic operation with no contemporary uses. Hysterectomy for abortion should be restricted to cases in which preexisting pathology requires hysterectomy.

COMPLICATIONS OF LEGAL ABORTION

Morbidity

Legal abortion in the United States is a safe procedure. Fewer than 1 woman in 100 develops a serious complication, and fewer than 1 in 50,000 dies as a result of the operation.

Gestational age is one of two important determinants of the likelihood of morbidity. In Table 22–3, which lists serious complication rates for abortion by gestational age, the term "serious complication rates" refers to the percentage of women who had fever of 38°C or above for 3 or more days, hemorrhage requiring transfusion, or unintended surgery (excluding curettage). These data, derived from a multicenter prospective study including 84,000 abortions, relate to those women without concurrent sterilization or preexisting medical conditions and for whom followup information was available. Abortions performed at the 7- to 10-week interval were associated with the lowest incidence of serious complications. Thereafter, complications increased progressively with advancing gestational age. The finding that serious complications are more frequent at or before 6 weeks' gestation than at later gestational ages is consistent with two previous large studies in the United States; thus, this finding appears persistent and real, although the explanation is unclear.

The method of abortion is the second principal determinant of the likelihood of complications. Table 22–4, derived from the same study as Table 22–3, demonstrates that suction curettage is the safest available abortion method. The risk of serious complications associated with D&E at or after 13 weeks' gestation is higher than that associated with suction curettage and lower than that associated with instillation abortion. Of the available instillation methods, a combination of urea and prostaglandin appears to be significantly safer than either hypertonic saline or prostaglandin F_{2a}.

Abortion complications can be grouped temporally into three categories: immediate, delayed, and late complications. Immediate complications are those that develop during or within 3 hours of the operation. Delayed complications are those that occur more than 3 hours and up to 28 days after the procedure. Late complications develop thereafter.

TABLE 22–3 *Serious Complication Rates for Legal Abortion by Gestational Age, United States, 1975–1978**

GESTATIONAL AGE (WKS)	RATE[†]
≤6	0.4
7–8	0.2
9–10	0.1
11–12	0.3
13–14	0.6
15–16	1.3
17–20	1.9

* For women with follow-up and without concurrent sterilization or preexisting conditions; serious complications include fever of 38°C or higher for 3 days or more, hemorrhage requiring blood transfusion, and any complication requiring unintended surgery (excluding curettage).
† Per 100 abortions

TABLE 22–4 *Serious Complication Rates for Legal Abortion by Method, United States, 1975–1978**

METHOD	RATE[†]
Suction curettage	0.2
D&E	0.7
Saline instillation	2.1
Prostaglandin instillation	2.5
Urea/prostaglandin instillation	1.3

* For women with follow-up and without concurrent sterilization or preexisting conditions; serious complications include fever of 38°C or higher for 3 days or more, hemorrhage requiring blood transfusion, and any complication requiring unintended surgery (excluding curettage).
† Per 100 abortions

Immediate Complications

HEMORRHAGE. Reported rates of hemorrhage vary widely, reflecting both diverse definitions (100 ml to 1000 ml blood loss) and imprecision in estimating volumes of blood loss. Few studies have measured blood loss. Rates of hemorrhage ranging from 0.05 to 4.9 per 100 abortions have been reported in large case-series reports (Cates et al, 1979). However, the best index of clinically important hemorrhage is probably the rate of blood transfusion. The rate of transfusion associated with suction curettage in a large, multicenter study was 0.06 per 100 abortions (Cates et al, 1979). For abortions performed later in pregnancy, rates of 0.26 for D&E, 0.32 for urea-prostaglandin, and 1.72 for saline have been reported (Kafrissen et al, 1984; Binkin et al, 1983).

CERVICAL INJURY. Cervical injury is one of the more frequent complications of legal abortion. A broad spectrum of trauma, however, is encompassed by this term. The most common type is a superficial laceration caused by the tenaculum tearing off during dilatation. At the other extreme are the cervicovaginal fistula and the longitudinal laceration ascending to the level of the uterine vessels. Rates of cervical injury range from 0.01 to 1.6 per 100 suction curettage abortions in large case-series reports (Cates et al, 1979). The incidence of cervical injury requiring sutures has been reported to be 1 per 100 suction curettage abortions (Schulz et al, 1983).

Several risk factors for cervical injury during suction curettage have been identified. Among factors within the control of the physician, use of laminaria and performance of the abortion by an attending physician (rather than a resident) lower the risk significantly, whereas use of general anesthesia raises the risk significantly. Among factors beyond the control of the physician, a history of a prior abortion lowers the risk, while age of 17 years or less increases the risk. Use of laminaria and performance of the abortion under local anesthesia by an attending physician together yield a 27-fold protective effect.

ACUTE HEMATOMETRA. Also termed the *postabortal syndrome* or the *redo syndrome*, acute hematometra is an uncommon complication of suction curettage; its etiology is unknown. The incidence of this syndrome ranges from 0.2 to 1 per 100 suction curettage abortions according to the available literature (Sands et al, 1974).

Women with this condition develop severe cramping, usually within 2 hours of the abortion. Vaginal bleeding is less than expected. The woman may be weak and sweaty, and her uterus is enlarged and markedly tender. Treatment consists of prompt repeat suction curettage; usually neither anesthesia nor dilatation is required. Evacuation of both liquid and clotted blood leads to rapid resolution of the symptoms. An oxytocic is usually given after the repeat evacuation. Whether routine use of an oxytocic would reduce the incidence of acute hematometra is unknown.

PERFORATION. Perforation is a potentially serious but infrequent complication of abortion. According to the most recent reports, the incidence of perforation is about 0.2 per 100 suction curettage abortions (Cates et al, 1979).

Several risk factors for perforation have been identified (Grimes et al, 1984). Performance of a curettage abortion by a resident rather than by an attending physician increases the risk more than fivefold; on the other hand, cervical dilation by laminaria decreases the risk approximately fivefold. The risk of perforation increases significantly with advancing gestational age. Multiparous women have 3 times the risk of nulliparous women.

The two principal dangers of perforation are hemorrhage and damage to the abdominal contents. Lateral perforations in the cervicoisthmic region are particularly hazardous because of the proximity of the uterine vessels. Perforations of the fundus are more likely to be innocuous. Indeed, most perforations may be neither suspected nor detected.

Not all perforations require treatment. Many suspected or documented perforations require only observation. Perforation with a dilator or sound is unlikely to damage abdominal contents. On the other hand, a suction cannula or forceps in the abdominal cavity can be devastating.

If perforation is suspected, the procedure should stop immediately. If unmanageable hemorrhage, expanding hematoma, or injury to abdominal contents occurs, laparotomy should be performed promptly. Laparoscopy can be useful in documenting perforation and assessing damage; if necessary, the abortion can be completed under laparoscopic visualization.

Delayed Complications

RETAINED TISSUE. Although retained tissue after abortion may be expelled without incident, retained tissue can lead to hemorrhage, infection, or both. This complication occurs infrequently, however. Its incidence after suction curettage abortion has been reported to be less than 1 per 100 abortions.

This complication usually manifests itself within several days of the abortion. Cramping and bleeding may be accompanied by fever. When women develop pain, bleeding, and low-grade fever after abortion, retained tissue must be presumed to be present. Prompt outpatient suction curettage usually resolves the symptoms, but close followup is advisable.

INFECTION. Postabortal infection is often secondary to retained tissue. The likelihood of febrile morbidity after abortion depends upon the method used. The incidence of fever of 38°C or higher for 1 or more days is usually less than 1 per 100 abortions by suction curettage (Cates et al, 1979). Corresponding figures for D&E are 1.5 per 100 abortions; for urea-prostaglandin, 6.3; and for hypertonic saline, 5.0 (Kafrissen et al, 1984; Binkin et al, 1983).

The organisms responsible for postabortal infection are similar to those responsible for other gynecologic infections. The most frequent isolates in postabortal endometritis have been reported to be group B β-hemolytic streptococci, *Bacteroides* species, *Neisseria gonorrhoeae*, *E. coli*, and *Staphylococcus aureus* (Burkman et al, 1977). Similar organisms have been isolated from the uteri of women who have died from septic abortion in the United States.

A number of risk factors for infection are known. Women are at increased risk if they have untreated endocervical gonorrhea or if their abortion is performed late in pregnancy. Likewise, use of instillation abortion instead of D&E and use of local rather than general anesthesia for suction curettage increase the risk.

Curettage and administration of broad-spectrum antibiotics are the cornerstones of therapy. Guidelines for management have been discussed previously.

Late Complications

RH SENSITIZATION. Legal abortion is a potentially important cause of Rh sensitization for women at risk. The likelihood of sensitization increases with advancing gestational age (and, hence, larger volumes of fetal erythrocytes). One study (Simonovits et al, 1980) has quantified the risk of Rh sensitization from first trimester suction curettage without RhIG prophylaxis. A total of 3.1% of secundigravidas whose first pregnancy was terminated by suction curettage without RhIG prophylaxis were found to be sensitized in their second pregnancy. Subtracting 0.5% (the percentage of women estimated to have become sensitized primarily during the second pregnancy), the authors estimated the risk of sensitization from suction curettage to be 2.6%. Thus, on a nationwide basis, the clinical impact of failure to administer RhIG to candidates after abortion may be substantial. Candidates should receive 50 mcg of RhIG after abortions performed at or before 12 weeks' gestation or 300 mcg after abortions performed later in pregnancy.

Adverse Pregnancy Outcomes

A broad array of adverse reproductive outcomes, ranging from infertility to ectopic pregnancy, have been attributed to induced abortion. Most published reports, however, suffer from serious methodologic shortcomings that limit their usefulness. To examine the potential association between first-trimester induced abortion and subsequent reproductive performance, an exhaustive review and analysis of the

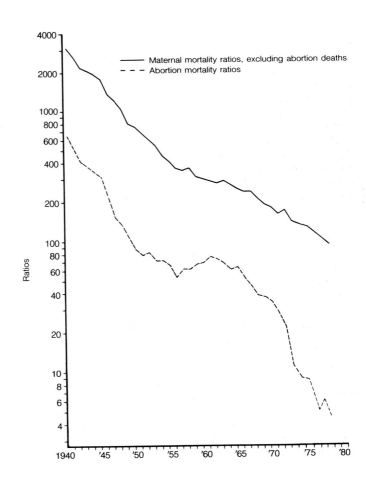

FIG. 22–16 Maternal mortality ratios (excluding abortion deaths), and abortion mortality ratios, United States, 1940–1978. Maternal mortality ratio (excluding abortion deaths) equals total maternal deaths minus abortion deaths. Mortality ratios are expressed as deaths per 1,000,000 live births. (U.S. Vital Statistics, National Center for Health Statistics)

world's literature was performed (Hogue et al, 1982). Over 150 epidemiologic studies published in 11 languages were included.

The findings of this analysis were largely reassuring. Secondary infertility and ectopic pregnancy occur so seldom that the risk of these complications is not significantly increased, even in studies with substantial power to detect differences in rates. Midtrimester spontaneous abortion is no more common among women who have had one previous abortion than among women pregnant for the first time. Similarly, the risk of premature delivery does not increase for women having undergone induced abortion.

On the other hand, low birthweight is more frequent in first births after abortion by sharp curettage performed under general anesthesia compared with first-pregnancy births. This effect is not observed after other methods of abortion, such as suction curettage. The questions of the effect of repeat induced abortion and second trimester abortion have not been adequately addressed, but sharp curettage may be associated with increased risks if it is repeated. Finally, first-born infants of women who had one induced abortion have risks of morbidity and mortality similar to those of other first-born children.

Mortality

Since 1940, the abortion mortality ratio in the United States has been declining more rapidly than the maternal mortality ratio (Fig. 22–16). The introduction of more effective contraception and increased availability of legal abortion are the most likely explanations for the accelerated decline in abortion-related deaths.

The numbers of deaths from legal, illegal, and spontaneous abortions in the United States decreased from 1972 to 1980 (Fig. 22–17). The number of deaths from illegal abortion has shown the steepest decline.

Eight women died after legal abortion in 1980, compared with 18 in 1979, 7 in 1978, and 17 in 1977 (Table 22–5). These numbers exclude deaths asso-

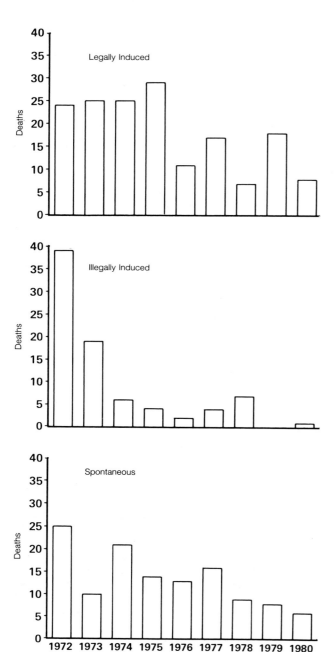

FIG. 22–17 Abortion-related deaths by category (excluding unknown category) and year, United States, 1972–1980. (Centers for Disease Control, 1983)

TABLE 22–5 *Death-to-Case Rates for Legal Abortions, by Year, United States, 1972–1980*

YEAR	DEATHS*	ABORTIONS	RATE†
1972	24	586,760	4.1
1973	25	615,831	4.1
1974	25	763,476	3.3
1975	29	854,853	3.4
1976	11	988,267	1.1
1977	17	1,079,430	1.6
1978	7	1,157,776	0.6
1979	18	1,251,921	1.4
1980	8	1,297,606	0.6

* Excludes deaths from ectopic pregnancy
† Deaths per 100,000 abortions
From Centers for Disease Control, 1983.

TABLE 22–6   Death-to-Case Rates for Legal Abortions by
Weeks of Gestation, United States, 1972–1980

WEEKS OF GESTATION	DEATHS*	ABORTIONS†	RATE‡	RELATIVE RISK§
≤8	19	4,073,472	0.5	1.0
9–10	31	2,382,516	1.3	2.6
11–12	25	1,197,915	2.1	4.2
13–15	20	419,767	4.8	9.6
16–20	55	430,907	12.8	25.6
≥21	14	91,343	15.3	30.6
Total	164	8,595,920	1.9	

* Excludes deaths from ectopic pregnancy
† Based on distribution of 6,108,658 abortions (71.1%) with weeks of gestation known
‡ Deaths per 100,000 abortions
§ Based on index rate for ≤8 menstrual weeks' gestation of 0.5 deaths per 100,000 abortions
From Centers for Disease Control, 1983.

TABLE 22–7   Death-to-Case Rates for Legal Abortions by Type of Procedure,
United States, 1972–1980

TYPE OF PROCEDURE	DEATHS*	ABORTIONS†	RATE‡	RELATIVE RISK§
Curettage	92	7,979,456	1.2	1.0
Intrauterine instillation	56	482,607	11.6	9.7
Hysterotomy/Hysterectomy	10	23,295	42.9	35.8
Other‖	6	110,562	5.4	4.5
Total	164	8,595,920	1.9	

* Excludes deaths from ectopic pregnancy
† Based on distribution of 6,408,704 abortions (74.6%) with type of procedure known
‡ Deaths per 100,000 abortions
§ Based on index rate for curettage of 1.2 deaths per 100,000 abortions
‖ Includes 2 deaths with type of procedure unknown
From Centers for Disease Control, 1983.

ciated with ectopic pregnancies occurring soon after attempted abortions. When the annual total of legal abortions was used as the denominator, the overall death-to-case rate for legal abortion was 0.6 per 100,000 abortions for 1980. This rate for legal abortion is similar to those reported during the 5 years since 1976. The aggregate death-to-case rate for legal abortion in this interval was 1.0. This figure is significantly lower than the aggregate rate of 3.7 in 1972 to 1975. Possible reasons for the decline after 1975 are: (1) the increasing percentage of abortions performed at earlier, safer gestational ages; (2) increasing experience with abortion by practicing physicians; (3) the increasing percentage of abortions performed by safer methods, such as D&E; and (4) underreporting of legal-abortion deaths after 1975. This last possibility, however, is unlikely.

The risk of death from legal abortion increases with advancing gestational age. The rate was lowest for women whose abortions were performed at or before 8 menstrual weeks' gestation, with a death-to-case rate of 0.5 per 100,000 procedures (Table 22–6). Using abortions performed at or before 8 weeks' gestation as the reference group, abortions performed at 9 to 10 weeks were 2.6 times as dangerous, and abortions performed at 13 to 15 weeks were 9.6 times as dangerous. Abortions performed at more than 20 weeks carried the greatest risk, with a death-to-case rate 30.6 times that associated with abortions performed at or before 8 weeks.

For 1972 to 1980, mortality rates were highest for hysterotomy/hysterectomy abortions and lowest for curettage, with instillation procedures intermediate (Table 22–7). Curettage was associated with a death-to-case rate of 1.2 per 100,000 abortions, compared with 11.6 for instillation and 42.9 for hysterotomy/hysterectomy. During this 9-year period, 71 women died from suction or sharp curettage procedures, 21 from D&E, 42 from saline instillation, 11 from prostaglandin instillation, 3 from use of other chemical abortifacients (*e.g.*, urea, oxytocin), 10 from hysterotomy/hysterectomy, and 6 from other or unknown methods.

Conclusion

Abortion is the most frequent outcome of human conception; thus, the surgical management of abortion and its complications is an important responsibility for physicians. Chromosomal anomalies are the single most important cause of spontaneous abortion. For women with threatened abortion, use of ultrasonography can help predict the outcome of the pregnancy. Evacuation of the uterus in cases of fetal death in utero is done primarily for psychological rather than medical indications; either curettage or labor induction can be used.

Cervical incompetence is a poorly understood cause of spontaneous abortion. Although the literature is inadequate to evaluate treatments of cervical incompetence, the McDonald cerclage operation appears preferable to the Shirodkar procedure.

Small numbers of illegal abortions continue to be done in the United States. Compared with ingestion of abortifacients, instrumentation of the uterus is both more likely to accomplish abortion and to result in complications and death.

Legally induced abortion has become one of the most frequently performed—and one of the safest—operations in the United States. Fewer than 1 per 100 of those having an abortion suffer a major complication, and fewer than 1 per 50,000 die from causes associated with the procedure. Although the rates for short-term complications of abortion are low, the potential long-term effects of abortion on subsequent fertility must be evaluated further. If the trend toward increasing percentages of women obtaining suction curettage abortions early in pregnancy persists, induced abortion should become even safer in the future.

Bibliography

Anderson SG: Management of threatened abortion with real-time sonography. Obstet Gynecol 55:259, 1980

Binkin N, Gold J, Cates W Jr: Illegal-abortion deaths in the United States: Why are they still occurring? Fam Plann Perspect 14:163, 1982

Binkin NJ, Schulz KF, Grimes DA, et al: Urea-prostaglandin versus hypertonic saline for instillation abortion. Am J Obstet Gynecol 146:947, 1983

Burkman RT, Atienza MF, King TM: Culture and treatment results in endometritis following elective abortion. Am J Obstet Gynecol 128:556, 1977

Cates W Jr, Grimes DA: Deaths from second trimester abortion by dilatation and evacuation: Causes, prevention, facilities. Obstet Gynecol 58:401, 1981

Cates W Jr, Rochat RW: Illegal abortions in the United States: 1972–1974. Fam Plann Perspect 8:86, 1976

Cates W Jr, Schulz KF, Grimes DA, et al: Short-term complications of uterine evacuation techniques for abortion at 12 weeks' gestation or earlier. In Zatuchni GI, Sciarra JJ, Speidel JJ (eds): Pregnancy Termination: Procedures, Safety, and New Developments, p 127. Hagerstown, Harper and Row, 1979

Centers for Disease Control: Abortion Surveillance 1979–1980. Issued May, 1983

Centers for Disease Control: Sexually transmitted diseases treatment guidelines 1982. Morbid Mortal Weekly Rep (Suppl) 31:35, 1982

Charles D, Edwards WR: Infectious complications of cervical cerclage. Am J Obstet Gynecol 141:1065, 1981

Cole SK: Cervical suture in Scotland: Strengths and weaknesses in the use of routine clinical summaries. Br J Obstet Gynaecol 89:528, 1982

Cousins L: Cervical incompetence, 1980: A time for reappraisal. Clin Obstet Gynecol 23:467, 1980

Dessaive R, de Hertogh R, Thomas K: Correlation between hormonal levels and ultrasound in patients with threatened abortion. Gynecol Obstet Invest 14:65, 1982

Dorfman SF, Grimes DA, Cates W Jr: Maternal deaths associated with antepartum fetal death in utero, United States, 1972–1978. South Med J 76:838, 1983

Duff GB: Prognosis in threatened abortion: a comparison between predictions made by sonar, urinary hormone assays and clinical judgement. Br J Obstet Gynaecol 82:858, 1975

Edmonds DK, Lindsay KS, Miller JF, et al: Early embryonic mortality in women. Fertil Steril 38:447, 1982

Eriksen PS, Philipsen T: Prognosis in threatened abortion evaluated by hormonal assays and ultrasound scanning. Obstet Gynecol 55:435, 1980

Farrell RG, Stonington DT, Ridgeway RA: Incomplete and inevitable abortion: Treatment by suction curettage in the emergency department. Ann Emerg Med 11:652, 1982

Foley ME: The natural history of the retained dead fetus. Ir Med J 74:237, 1981

Green SL, Brenner WE: Clostridial sepsis after abortion with PGF$_{2a}$ and intracervical laminaria tents: a case report. Int J Gynaecol Obstet 15:322, 1978

Grimes DA, Cates W Jr: Deaths from paracervical anesthesia used for first trimester abortion, 1972–1975. N Engl J Med 295:1397, 1976

Grimes DA, Hulka JF, McCutchen ME: Midtrimester abortion by dilatation and evacuation versus intra-amniotic instillation of prostaglandin F$_{2a}$: A randomized clinical trial. Am J Obstet Gynecol 137:785, 1980

Grimes DA, Schulz KF, Cates W Jr: Prevention of uterine perforation during curettage abortion. JAMA 251:2108, 1984

Grimes DA, Schulz KF, Cates W Jr, et al: Midtrimester abortion by dilatation and evacuation: A safe and practical alternative. N Engl J Med 296:1141, 1977

Guerrero V, Rojas OI: Spontaneous abortion and aging of human ova and spermatozoa. N Engl J Med 293:573, 1975

Hassold T, Chen N, Funkhouser J, et al: A cytogenetic study

of 1000 spontaneous abortions. Ann Hum Genet 44:151, 1980

Hern WM: Midtrimester abortion. Obstet Gynecol Annu 10:375, 1981

Hertz JB, Mantoni M, Svenstrup B: Threatened abortion studied by estradiol-17 beta in serum and ultrasound. Obstet Gynecol 55:324, 1980

Hodgson JE, Ditmanson GM: Unsuccessful pregnancy. Minn Med 63:134, 1980

Hodgson JE, Major B, Portmann K, et al: Prophylactic use of tetracycline for first trimester abortions. Obstet Gynecol 45:574, 1975

Hogue CJR, Cates W Jr, Tietze C: The effects of induced abortion on subsequent reproduction. Epidemiol Rev 4:66, 1982

Hughey MJ, McElin TW: The incompetent cervix. In Depp R, Eschenbach DA, Sciarra JJ (eds): Gynecology and Obstetrics, Vol 3, p 1. Philadelphia, Harper and Row, 1982

Jeong WG, Kim CH, Bernstine RL, et al: Ultrasonic sonography in the management of incomplete abortion. J Reprod Med 26:90, 1981

Kafrissen ME, Schulz KF, Grimes DA, et al: Midtrimester abortion. JAMA 251:916, 1984

Kline J, Stein ZA, Susser M, et al: Smoking: A risk factor for spontaneous abortion. N Engl J Med 297:793, 1977

Laufe LE: The menstrual regulation procedure. Stud Fam Plann 8:253, 1977

Liskin L: Complications of abortion in developing countries. Population Reports, Series F, no. 7, July 1980

London RS, London ED, Sigelbaum M, et al: Use of doxycycline in elective first trimester abortion. South Med J 71:672, 1978

McDonald IA: Cervical cerclage. Clin Obstet Gynaecol 7:461, 1980

Munsick RA: Clinical test for placenta in 300 consecutive menstrual aspirations. Obstet Gynecol 60:738, 1982

Novy MJ: Transabdominal cervicoisthmic cerclage for the management of repetitive abortion and premature delivery. Am J Obstet Gynecol 143:44, 1982

Peterson HB, Grimes DA, Cates W Jr, et al: Comparative risk of death from induced abortion at ≤12 weeks' gestation performed with local versus general anesthesia. Am J Obstet Gynecol 141:763, 1981

Polgar S, Fried ES: The bad old days: Clandestine abortions among the poor in New York City before liberalization of the abortion law. Fam Plann Perspect 8:125, 1976

Rubin GL, Cates W Jr, Gold J, et al: Fatal ectopic pregnancy after attempted legally induced abortion. JAMA 244:1705, 1980

Sakamoto S, Okai T: Ultrasonic and endocrinological aspects of first trimester miscarriage. Asia-Oceania J Obstet Gynaecol 8:105, 1982

Sande HA, Reiertsen O, Fonstelien E, et al: Evaluation of threatened abortion by human chorionic gonadotropin levels and ultrasonography. Int J Gynaecol Obstet 18:123, 1980

Sands RX, Burnhill MS, Hakim–Elahi E: Postabortal uterine atony. Obstet Gynecol 43:595, 1974

Schulz KF, Grimes DA, Cates W Jr: Measures to prevent cervical injury during suction curettage abortion. Lancet 1:1182, 1983

Shapiro S, Levine HS, Abramowicz M: Factors associated with early and late fetal loss. Adv Plann Parenth 6:45, 1971

Simonovits I, Timar I, Bajtai G: Rate of Rh immunization after induced abortion. Vox Sang 38:161, 1980

Simpson JL: Repeated suboptimal pregnancy outcome. Birth Defects 17:113, 1981

Sonne–Holm S, Heisterberg L, Hebjorn S, et al: Prophylactic antibiotics in first trimester abortions: A clinical, controlled trial. Am J Obstet Gynecol 139:693, 1981

Stein Z, Susser M, Warburton D, et al: Spontaneous abortion as a screening device. Am J Epidemiol 102:275, 1975

Stoppelli I, LoDico G, Milia S, et al: Prognostic value of hCG, progesterone, 17-beta estradiol and the echoscopic examination in threatened abortion during the first trimester. Clin Exp Obstet Gynecol 8:6, 1981

Stubblefield PG: Current technology for abortion. Current Problems in Obstetrics and Gynecology 2:1, 1978

Stubblefield PG: Present techniques for cervical dilatation. In Naftolin F, Stubblefield PG (eds): Dilatation of the uterine cervix, p 335. New York, Raven Press, 1980

Warren CW, Gold J, Tyler CW Jr, et al: Seasonal variation in spontaneous abortions. Am J Public Health 70:1297, 1980

Westrom L, Svensson L, Wolner–Hanssen P, et al: A clinical double-blind study on the effect of prophylactically administered single dose tinidazole on the occurrence of endometritis after first trimester legal abortion. Scand J Infect Dis (Suppl) 26:104, 1981

Wilcox AJ, Treloar AE, Sandler DP: Spontaneous abortion over time: Comparing occurrence in two cohorts of women a generation apart. Am J Epidemiol 114:548, 1981

Chapter 23

Malpositions of the Uterus

Retrodisplacement

ANATOMICAL CONSIDERATIONS

An understanding of the anatomical structures of the uterus and the mechanism by which it is held in its normal position of anteflexion and anteversion is important for a proper discussion of uterine displacement and appropriate surgical correction. The support system includes that of the uterus, vagina, and pelvic floor.

Typically, the portio vaginalis of the cervix points posteroinferiorly, and the uterine corpus is flexed with a wide obtuse angle on the cervix, so that when the woman is erect, the corpus lies anteriorly, resting in an anteverted position. Minor variations in the direction of the axis of both the cervix and the corpus should be considered within normal limits. Physiologic displacements also occur during pregnancy; in the third trimester the uterus becomes a practically vertical organ.

The ligamentous support system of the uterus is subject to stretching from childbearing, physical work, and aging. The fibroelastic tissue within the lower portion of the broad ligament, extending from each side of the cervix and upper vagina to the sides of the pelvis, forms the ligamenta transversalis colli (Mackenrodt's ligament), also called the cardinal ligament. Attached to the endopelvic fascia of the pelvic diaphragm, the two cardinal ligaments hold the cervix and upper vagina at that level. The softening effect of the pregnancy hormones, the weight of the pregnant uterus, the stretching of the ligaments during delivery, and the increased intra-abdominal pressure of hard work all tend to stretch the cardinal ligaments and permit the uterus to drop to a permanently lower level.

The descent of the uterus causes the corpus to fall back from its normal position. Retrodisplacement also occurs when the ligaments that normally hold the cervix in place fail to do so. Beneath the peritoneal folds, on either side of the cul-de-sac of Douglas, are the two fascial structures known as the uterosacral ligaments. These usually well developed ligaments are attached to the posterolateral surface of the cervix and proceed backward on either side of the rectum, where they are inserted into the periosteum of the sacrum, thus holding back the cervix. In the normal position, with the cervix held back, the somewhat rigid corpus lies forward so that the intra-abdominal pressure falls on the posterior surface of the corpus, maintaining it in anteposition. If the uterosacral ligaments are congenitally inadequate or have become so through childbirth, the cervix moves forward. Under such conditions the fundus of the uterus, swinging on a more or less fixed transverse axis at about the level of the internal os, moves backward, and the intra-abdominal pressure falls on the anterior surface of the corpus aggravating the retrodisplacement.

The round ligaments provide little or no support against uterine descent, but they seem to provide some support in holding the uterus in anteposition; surgical corrections of uterine malposition usually take advantage of them. Although the round ligaments do not hold the fundus forward tautly, they assist in maintaining the forward position, which is maintained by intra-abdominal pressure and by the traction of the uterosacral ligaments holding the cervix back. Once retroflexion has begun, it can be completed easily by intra-abdominal pressure on the anterior uterine surface. Most cases of retrodisplacement include both retroversion and retroflexion, although either may exist independently.

The normal nulliparous vagina is maintained in position by two structures: the cardinal ligaments and the various components of the pelvic fascia. The cardinal ligaments are firmly attached to the upper segment of the vagina and form a strong fascial sheath that inserts on the muscular pelvic wall.

Anteriorly, this pubovesicocervical fascia extends between the bladder and the vagina and stretches from its origin at the symphysis pubis beneath the bladder to where it blends with fascia that surrounds the cervix. The most lateral part of this fascia is strengthened on each side of the posterior urethra to form the important pubourethral ligaments that support the bladder neck. The upper part of this fascia is easily seen when the bladder is dissected from the anterior fornix in a total abdominal hysterectomy.

Posteriorly, similar fascia, known as the pararectal fascia, separates the vagina from the muscular wall of the rectum. The pararectal fascia gives support to the vagina and supports the anterior rectal wall from bulging into the vagina. As the levator muscles are stretched by childbirth and the levator hiatus is widened, these fascial structures become weakened and the vaginal walls lose the support of the levator ani and the urogenital diaphragm. As a result, rectocele and cystocele may develop. The weight of the uterus, especially if it is retroverted, may overwhelm the fascial support of the sagging vagina, and cause the vagina to become partially or entirely everted when uterine prolapse becomes complete.

The muscular floor of the pelvis, which is discussed in detail in Chapter 24, forms the major support on which the upper vagina rests. The middle and lower vagina is densely adherent to the muscular attachments of the puborectalis and pubococcygeus muscles, commonly called the levator crura. Tearing and separation of the medial fibers of the pubococcygeus and puborectalis muscles weaken this floor and widen the pelvic aperture through which the uterus may descend. The discussion of the mechanisms of pelvic floor relaxation in Chapter 24, together with Figures 23-1 and 23-2, provide a good understanding of uterine prolapse.

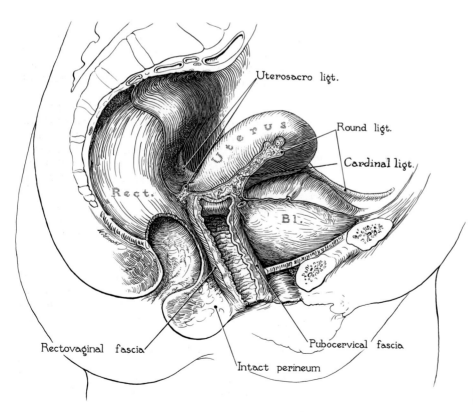

FIG. 23-1 Normal supports of uterus.

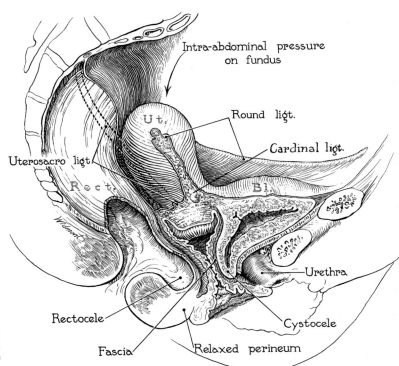

FIG. 23-2 Failure of normal supports and widening of the levator hiatus permit descent of uterus, as well as cystocele and rectocele formation.

The surgical correction of retrodisplacement of the uterus forms an interesting chapter in the development of gynecology. In 1955, Frederic Fluhmann wrote a review of the subject that is outlined in the fifth edition of this text.

SYMPTOMATOLOGY IN RELATION TO TREATMENT

The symptomatology of retrodisplacement must be appreciated before treatment is planned. It is generally estimated that one out of five women has a congenitally retrodisplaced uterus. Although retroversion occurs frequently, it generally gives rise to no symptoms at all. When symptoms do occur, they are usually slight and do not justify operative intervention. Retrodisplacement is commonly found during a routine pelvic examination in women who are completely free of symptoms. These women do not require surgery.

An uncomplicated, retroposed uterus is less apt to be responsible for symptoms than one complicated by other intrapelvic disease. Among the conditions commonly associated with and frequently a factor in the cause of retrodisplacement are: chronic salpingitis with pelvic adhesions; endometriosis; ovarian tumors; and myomata. Often these conditions are responsible for symptoms that,

in themselves, necessitate surgery. But even the complicated retrodisplaced uterus may be asymptomatic. Frequently, during surgery for some other cause, an adherent retroverted uterus is encountered with the residue of an old salpingitis, without causing the patient any discomfort.

Backache and a bearing-down type of abdominal discomfort are among the most common complaints of the erect human biped; they are the major symptoms of patients with uterine retrodisplacement. These symptoms are noticed frequently by women in whom the pelvic diaphragm is weakened and distended through repeated childbearing. Although these symptoms tend to be aggravated by the pressure of a retroverted uterus, they can occur with the uterus in a normal anteverted position as well. When the pelvic pressure and backache are relieved completely by the use of a vaginal pessary that repositions the uterus, the symptoms can be related to the altered anatomy. When there is inadequate anatomical alteration of the reproductive tract to account for these symptoms, orthopedic consultation is advisable. More frequently than not, the etiology of low back pain will be found to be positional or occupational. Surgery on the retropositioned uterus and relaxed vagina will have little benefit in relieving the symptoms of such cases.

Disturbances of Menstruation

Few menstrual symptoms can be accurately attributed to the position of the uterus. Historically, all kinds of menstrual dysfunction were commonly attributed to a retropositioned uterus; passive venous congestion was a common explanation for increased menstrual bleeding from the uterus lying in the cul-de-sac. More current understanding of the endocrinology of menstruation dispels any misconceptions about the position of the uterus and menstrual flow.

Dysmenorrhea

Primary dysmenorrhea is not related to uterine position and occurs in the anteverted as well as in the retroverted uterus. Retroplacement of the uterus may play some physiologic role in the symptoms of secondary dysmenorrhea, judging from the relief obtained, historically, by uterine suspension. It is argued that acute retroflexion of the uterus, which affords poor venous drainage of the myometrium and broad ligament, is more apt to be a factor in dysmenorrhea than *retroversion* alone. The menstrual discomfort may take the form of cramps or sacral backache. Since it frequently is difficult to evaluate the relation of uterine position to menstrual pain, the therapeutic test with the use of a vaginal pessary is helpful.

Infertility

The finding of a uterus in retroposition in a woman complaining of infertility is no indication that the position of the uterus has a direct relation to the problem. In such cases, a thorough investigation of all factors related to infertility must be made in both the man and the woman, without regard for the retroposition. Although infertility may be more common among women with retrodisplacement of the uterus, the relationship is difficult to prove except in cases with such other associated diseases as pelvic endometriosis or chronic salpingitis. With a retrodisplaced uterus, the cervix is positioned away from the posterior vaginal pool where semen is deposited. Although some investigators consider this anatomical factor to be a serious impediment to fertility, there is only limited scientific evidence to support this contention. Uterine suspension for the relief of infertility alone is seldom, if ever, justified.

Abortion

It is doubtful that uterine retroposition is ever the causative factor for abortion unless incarceration of the uterus and compromise of the blood supply have occurred. Although a chromosomal abnormality occurs in more than 50% of first trimester pregnancy losses, many early abortions have an unexplained etiology. They appear to occur no more frequently in women with retropositioned uteri than in any other group. When uterine incarceration occurs during early pregnancy, with the uterus wedged in the pelvis, the patient should be placed in the knee-chest position and an attempt should be made by digital pressure on the uterus through the rectum to displace the uterus from the cul-de-sac and put it in an anterior position. The uterus can usually be held out of the cul-de-sac by a pessary until the first trimester of pregnancy is past, at which stage the fundus will emerge from the pelvis. In the rare case in which the uterus remains incarcerated in the pelvis as pregnancy advances, careful and frequent observation of the patient is essential to prevent fixation and sacculation of the pregnant uterus. Laparotomy may be required to release the incarcerated uterus from the cul-de-sac and avoid the complication of abortion, premature delivery, fetal death in utero, fetal malformation, or uterine rupture. Uterine suspension should not be performed on the pregnant uterus.

INDICATIONS FOR UTERINE SUSPENSION

Although Fluhmann stated that suspension of the uterus is not necessary for adequate gynecologic practice, there are some young women in whom the symptoms of uterine retroversion are clear-cut and severe. Certainly, the mere presence of uterine retrodisplacement alone is not an indication for prophylactic suspension. When displacement is associated with symptomatic uterine descensus and vaginal relaxation, a vaginal hysterectomy and repair may be more appropriate. For women who desire future childbearing, there is still a place, though infrequently, for intra-abdominal suspension of the uterus when a laparotomy is done for another indication.

Uterine suspension is indicated in connection with such conservative operations as those done for endometriosis or tubal pregnancy, or in plastic operations on the tubes in the relief of infertility. To leave the uterus of an infertile patient in the cul-de-sac, where tubal adhesions may recur, while performing other conservative procedures would be to do incomplete surgery and may not completely relieve the problem.

CHOICE OF OPERATIONS

Choice of operative techniques depends to a great extent on the desirability of future pregnancies. The modified Gilliam suspension is a very good technique for suspending the uterus and preserving childbearing potential. When no future pregnancies are desired, other procedures may be more appropriate.

The modified Gilliam suspension procedure draws each round ligament through an aperature in the peritoneum near the internal inguinal ring and brings each ligament beneath the anterior rectus sheath. There, the round ligament is sutured under tension so as to hold the uterus forward. Although some patients experience transient round ligament pain with vigorous physical activity or uterine enlargement, there is no evidence that the suspension is detrimental to a subsequent pregnancy.

Many surgeons have reported satisfactory results with other types of suspensions. Some techniques have been abandoned; newer procedures give better anatomical positioning with fewer complications. In Olshausen's operation, for example, the uterus is fixed to the anterior abdominal wall. This procedure precludes the possibility of a future intrauterine pregnancy because the anchored uterus will produce severe abdominal pain as the uterus enlarges with advancing pregnancy. It also broadens the exposure of the cul-de-sac to the small intestines, which creates a serious risk of enterocele formation. In the Baldy–Webster procedure, the round ligaments are passed through the anterior and posterior leaves of the broad ligament and are sutured to the posterior surface of the uterus, leaving the support of the uterus to the hammock effect of the suspended ligaments. The extraperitoneal technique of shortening each round ligament in the inguinal canal described by Alexander and by Adams is no longer used in this country, although it is still in use in some European clinics. The operation is blind, since the uterus is not visualized unless a laparotomy is performed. The extraperitoneal approach is its only advantage.

In some cases, simple shortening of the round ligaments will not adequately hold the uterus in anteposition, regardless of the type of round ligament suspension employed. One of the more effective supplemental procedures for providing additional support is shortening the uterosacral ligaments. This is especially valuable when some descensus is present or when the cervix has been displaced anteriorly. Shortening the uterosacral ligaments helps maintain the forward position of the uterus when combined with another procedure, such as the modified Gilliam procedure. Caution should be taken to avoid excessive plication of the uterosacral ligaments, since this can result in dyspareunia and in angulation of the pelvic ureter. One or two permanent sutures that unite the uter-

osacral ligaments are sufficient when used in combination with another suspension procedure.

If future pregnancy is not desired and a vaginal plastic operation is needed, the best "suspension" operation may be vaginal hysterectomy and vaginal repair. Under these conditions, or if dysmenorrhea is a chronic problem, there is little reason for saving the uterus. Removal of the uterus will relieve the symptoms of retroposition, and at the same time insure against future trouble due to dysfunctional bleeding or uterine neoplasm.

Technique of Modified Gilliam Suspension of Uterus

The procedure begins with a modified Pfannenstiel incision, although a small midline incision could be used. Hold the uterus forward. With a Babcock clamp, grasp the middle of the round ligament, then place a traction suture around it. The suture should be placed to provide good uterine positioning when the ligaments are attached to the inside of the rectus sheath. The average distance is about 3 cm to 4 cm from the cornu, although exact positioning can only be determined by testing the uterine position with traction on the round ligaments (Fig. 23–3A).

Place an Ochsner clamp on the edge of the anterior rectus fascia at the level of the anterior superior spine of the ilium. Place a small Kelly clamp on the peritoneal edge at the same level. Then, using blunt and sharp dissection, separate the body of the rectus muscle from its fascial sheath (Fig. 23–3B). At the point of separation, insert a long Kelly clamp along the lateral margin of the rectus muscle and beneath the peritoneum as it passes along the lateral pelvic wall to the level of the internal inguinal ring. Here, elevate the peritoneum with the tip of the clamp and separate the jaws of the clamp slightly, so that an assistant can incise the peritoneum (Fig. 23–3C).

With the point of the Kelly clamp, enter the peritoneal cavity, grasp a No. 0 delayed absorbable traction suture, and draw it back out of the peritoneal cavity. By bringing the round ligament through the opening in the parietal peritoneum at the point of the internal inguinal ring, a loop is brought between the rectus muscle and its anterior sheath (Fig. 23–3D). Suture the loop of round ligament to the undersurface of the fascia, using interrupted No. 0 silk. Suture with substantial bites into the full thickness of the ligament on both sides and at the end of the loop, taking care not to encircle and strangulate the ligament (Fig. 23–3E). Repeat the procedure on the opposite round ligament. When completed, inspect inside the abdomen to be certain that no loop of bowel has been caught between the ligament and the abdominal wall. Also check to be sure that the fallopian tube was not drawn into the

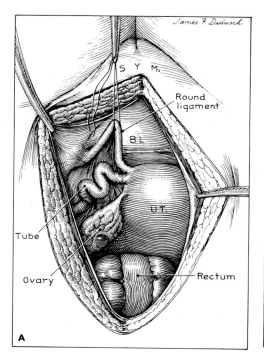

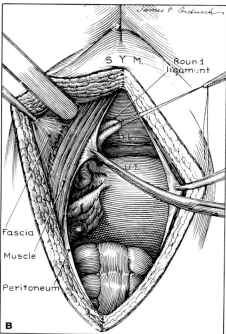

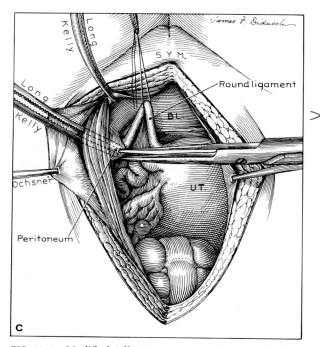

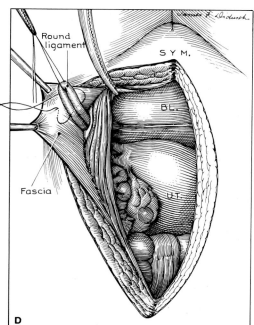

FIG. 23–3 Modified Gilliam suspension of uterus. (*A*) A traction suture of No. 0 delayed absorbable material is placed about the round ligament at an appropriate point. (*B*) The anterior rectus sheath is dissected from the body of the muscle. (*C*) A long Kelly clamp is passed around the rectus muscle, through the internal inguinal ring. The peritoneum is cut over the tip of the clamp so that it may enter the peritoneal cavity. (*D*) The traction suture is grasped by the Kelly clamp and withdrawn through the internal ring. The wound ligament is sutured to the inside of the rectus sheath with medium silk sutures.

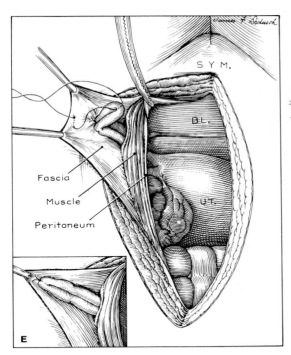

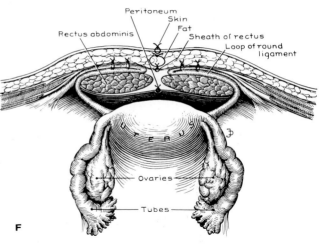

FIG. 23-3 (continued). (*E*) Another suture is anchoring the round ligament to the fascia. The inset shows the round ligament sutured to the fascia. All sutures transfix the round ligament. (*F*) Transverse section showing final result.

internal inguinal ring by excessive traction on the round ligament (Fig. 23–3F).

Technique of Shortening the Uterosacral Ligaments

Shortening of the uterosacral ligaments is easily accomplished if exposure is adequate. An assistant can hold the uterus forward by hand or with a retractor. Hold the intestines back from the pelvis with a laparotomy pack.

Grasp each uterosacral ligament with an Allis or Babcock clamp at a point just below its attachment to the uterus and bring the two ligaments together. Using No. 2-0 silk on a round needle, suture each ligament together and include a bite in the posterior surface of the cervix at the midline. Usually two or three sutures will hold the ligaments together adequately (Fig. 23–4).

The surgeon must avoid kinking or ligating the ureter, which lies in close proximity to the lateral aspect of the uterosacral ligament. Although shortening of the ligaments is necessary to hold the cervix back and to position the fundus forward, excessive tucking or folding may result in injuries to the ureter(s).

Prolapse of Uterus

The treatment of uterine prolapse and its allied conditions is a subject that has evoked considerable discussion and disagreement among many gynecologists. In many clinics, vaginal hysterectomy is done routinely and is considered to be the answer to all degrees of prolapse. In some European clinics, the Manchester operation as described by Shaw with modifications, is thought to be preferable. The Watkin's interposition operation, no longer used in North America, was originally designed for the anatomical support of a very large cystocele. This procedure used the fundus of the uterus as an obturator for the defective pelvic diaphragm. It offered a rapid method of supporting the bladder without sacrifice of coital function. Based on our current understanding of the basic anatomical defect in the levator hiatus, a common procedure used today for treating a complete uterine procidentia with a large traction enterocele is a combination of vaginoplasty with an intra-abdominal suspension of the vaginal vault.

The occurrence of progressive hydronephrosis with third-degree uterine prolapse or complete procidentia is of particular medical importance. Reports of the prevalence of this complication vary widely, from 2% in Guillemin and Cavailher's series (1948) to 92% in Franche's report (1959). These studies simply confirm the fact that the ureters are at high risk of being obstructed by the insidious process of uterine prolapse and indicate the need for an intravenous pyelogram in every patient with significant uterine prolapse.

Usually, the hydronephrosis is asymptomatic and

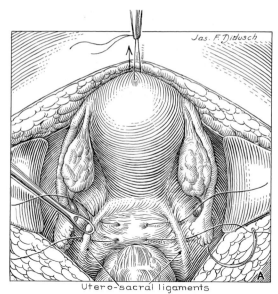

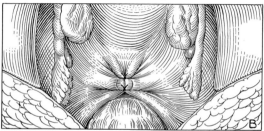

FIG. 23–4 Shortening of uterosacral ligaments. (*A*) Interrupted sutures of No. 2-0 silk or No. 0 delayed-absorbable suture are passed through the uterosacral ligaments and the posterior surface of the cervix. (*B*) Sutures have been tied, thus shortening the ligaments.

is due to downward traction of the uterine arteries against the pelvic ureters when the uterus prolapses. Frequently, repeated renal infections will draw attention to this problem, which is easily documented by an intravenous pyelogram. If obstruction has not progressed to end-stage renal parenchymal destruction, it can usually be reversed by corrective pelvic surgery.

The important factors in the evaluation of a patient with uterine prolapse are: age; general physical condition; the desirability of preserving menstruation and the childbearing function; the degree of uterine descensus; the condition of the cervix and the corpus uteri; and the presence and the degree of an associated cystocele, rectocele, or enterocele. All of these factors will be considered in discussing the various operative procedures for cure of uterine prolapse and allied conditions.

Vaginal Hysterectomy

The current technique of vaginal hysterectomy has evolved from a variety of operations as the major method of surgical treatment for symptomatic uterine prolapse in the presence of cystocele, rectocele, or enterocele. The procedure was once viewed skeptically, as revealed by Howard A. Kelly's statement in 1928: "Vaginal hysterectomy, at one time in great vogue . . . is but exceptionally resorted to in later years. . . ." Such opinions were powerful enough to prevent the use of vaginal hysterectomy at The Johns Hopkins Hospital for many years. In 1940 Te Linde, an expert vaginal surgeon, regenerated interest in vaginal surgery and began training gynecologists in the techniques.

It is interesting to note the evolution of the current indications for vaginal hysterectomy as they have developed over the past one-half of a century (Table 23–1). Still, the majority of indications throughout this period are related to pelvic relaxation and uterine bleeding, but, as a result of added indications, more than 30% of all hysterectomies performed today are by the vaginal route. For example, a recently

TABLE 23–1   Comparative Indications for Vaginal Hysterectomy*

	HEANEY 1934 (565 CASES)	DANFORTH 1938 (266 CASES)	AVERETT 1945 (2427 CASES)	KEMPERS ET AL 1959 (415 CASES)	COPENHAVER 1962 (1000 CASES)	AMIRIKIA, EVANS 1979 (1688 CASES)
Pelvic relaxation	13	57	15	61	41	13
Uterine bleeding	19	18	13	18	40	4
Uterine leiomyoma	52	11	67	2	6	56
Adenomyosis	10	—	0.3	—	—	13
Leiomyoma and adenomyosis	—	—	—	—	—	7
Carcinoma in situ of the cervix	—	—	—	16	0.2	6
Uterine retroversion	1	12	—	—	3	—
Miscellaneous	5	2	5	3	10	1

* All figures are in percentages
Adapted from Copenhaver, 1980.

added indication for vaginal surgery is the removal of a uterus with small symptomatic myomata or adenomyosis.

The liberalization of the indications of vaginal hysterectomy has often been misinterpreted to include elective sterilization, as noted by Porges and others. In view of the current instability of the family unit and the surgical mortality of 1 to 2 operative deaths per 1000 major gynecologic operations, performing a vaginal hysterectomy for elective sterilization is certainly a misuse of the procedure. Using the vaginal hysterectomy for a social indication would be comparable to performing an elective cholecystectomy or mastectomy without serious symptoms or medical indications.

Heaney Technique

In 1934, Heaney first reported the technique that, with few modifications, is probably the method that is most commonly used throughout the North American continent today. Heaney emphasized the clamping of the principal ligaments of the uterus and their immediate suture ligation. He also is credited with recommending closure of the vaginal vault, and he designed various instruments for this vaginal procedure.

The performance of a vaginal hysterectomy requires that the patient be placed in the lithotomy position with the hips located at the edge of the table so that the weighted speculum may swing free. Narrow, delicate instruments contribute to the ease in operating vaginally. Heavy, cumbersome tools may make access to the uterus impossible. In addition, a well-focused operating light is essential.

After the patient has been anesthetized and placed in the dorsolithotomy position, the vulva, perineum, and vagina are thoroughly washed with povidone-iodine (Betadine) and alcohol. The bladder is emptied with a catheter.

The labia minora when long, should be stitched back out of the way (Fig. 23–5A). If the introitus is too tight from previous perineorrhaphy, a small midline episiotomy will overcome the difficulty. A narrow vaginal fornix is a more serious obstacle to easy operating.

The cervix is grasped with a tenaculum and is pulled strongly into view. Ten ml of dilute Neo-Synephrine solution (1/200,000) or normal saline are injected into the anterior and posterior vaginal fornices (Fig. 23–5A). The judicious use of this weak vasopressor will reduce the bleeding to a minimum. However, the experience of England and associates suggests that excessive use of vasoconstricting agents has been associated with an increased incidence of postoperative cuff cellulitis and febrile morbidity. A semilunar incision is made through the mucosa

of the vaginal fornix just above the portio but below the attachment of the bladder (Fig. 23–5A). A sound or a Kelly forceps passed transurethrally into the bladder will demonstrate how low the bladder lies. Sounding the bladder can be of considerable assistance in an elderly patient with an elongated cervix who has a large, redundant cystocele and in whom tissue planes may be difficult to define because of atrophic change.

The bladder is freed from the anterior surface of the uterus by sharp dissection up to the peritoneal reflection (plica vesicouterinea) (Fig. 23–5B–D). After the loose areolar plane is entered and the fascial attachments have been excised beneath the bladder with the curved Mayo scissors, the dissection can usually be completed with the finger covered with gauze. Over-vigorous separation may create an incorrect tissue plane, which can cause a tear through the muscular wall of the bladder base.

The free peritoneal fold is identified and incised (Fig. 23–6A,B), and a narrow-bladed retractor is inserted into the peritoneal cavity to hold the bladder and the ureters forward (Fig. 23–6D,E). Occasionally, the uterus remains too high to make the vesical plica readily accessible, or a tumor low down on the cervix interferes at this point. If the bladder cannot be pushed up enough to permit easy entrance into the anterior cul-de-sac, cease work here and attempt to enter the posterior cul-de-sac.

If the bladder is torn or incised, an excessive amount of blood will appear in the operative field. Dissection should be discontinued until the source of bleeding is identified and repaired. Instill the bladder with 50 ml to 100 ml saline or sterile milk to confirm or exclude the presence of a defect in the bladder wall. If a rent has been made through the bladder wall, the rest of the bladder must be carefully loosened from its attachment to the lower uterine segment to avoid widening the opening. As soon as the bladder is completely freed from the cervix and lower uterine segment and the peritoneal cavity has been entered, the laceration in the bladder should be repaired using interrupted No. 3-0 chromic or delayed-absorbable sutures, placed through the mucosa to ensure that the bladder defect is completely closed. If the defect is small, a continuous suture may be used (see Fig. 23–6C). These sutures are followed by another interrupted row of No. 2-0 sutures passed through the muscularis and fascia of the bladder. To avoid subsequent leakage and possible fistula formation, make the bladder closure watertight and test the closure by refilling the bladder with saline or, preferably, with 100 ml sterile milk. If necessary, place additional interrupted muscle sutures to close any residual tract in the bladder wall. The free margins of the bladder

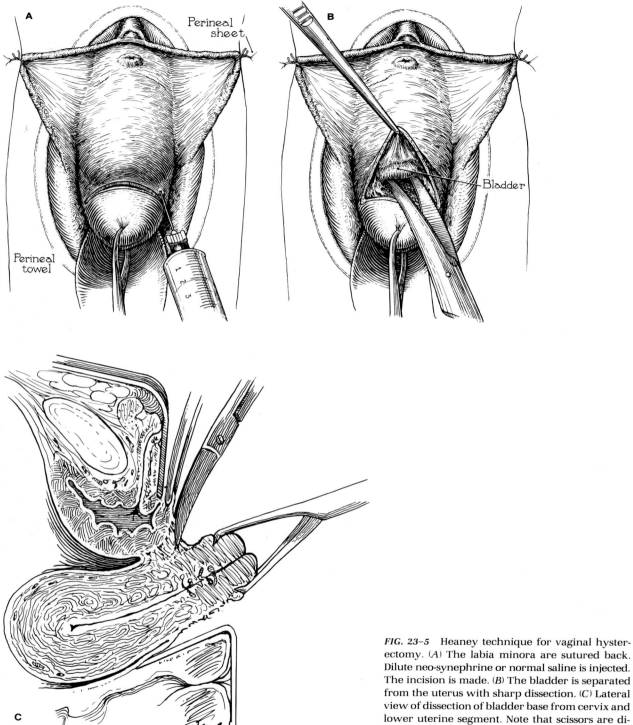

FIG. 23–5 Heaney technique for vaginal hysterectomy. (*A*) The labia minora are sutured back. Dilute neo-synephrine or normal saline is injected. The incision is made. (*B*) The bladder is separated from the uterus with sharp dissection. (*C*) Lateral view of dissection of bladder base from cervix and lower uterine segment. Note that scissors are directed toward uterus.

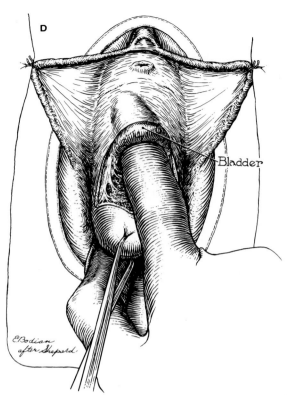

FIG. 23-5 *(continued).* (*D*) The bladder is separated to the plica of the bladder peritoneum by blunt finger dissection.

peritoneum can be advanced over the suture line and anchored to the bladder wall with fine sutures.

Following entry into the anterior cul-de-sac, the cervix is pulled strongly forward and a semilunar incision is made through the vaginal mucosa at the height of the posterior fornix, and the anterior to the posterior incisions are joined on each side of the cervix (Fig. 23-7A), taking care to avoid injury to the rectum. Occasionally, difficulty is met in entering the posterior space, and persistent attempts add to the chance of rectal injury. After cutting through the mucosa, the loose areolar plane is entered and the space is developed by sharp dissection until the peritoneum is visible (Fig. 23-7C). The peritoneum is then incised, the cul-de-sac is explored (Fig. 23-7D), and a narrow right-angle retractor is introduced. If the anterior peritoneum has not been opened, the index and middle fingers can be inserted around the uterine fundus and used to distend the peritoneum between the bladder base and the lower uterine segment. The peritoneal reflection can then be incised under direct vision (Fig. 23-7E).

Pushing back the mucosa in the attempt to see the peritoneum exposes the base of the broad (car-

dinal) ligaments. The base of the cardinal ligament is clamped separately by any narrow, curved, grooved clamp with distal teeth; the Heaney clamp is ideal for this purpose (Fig. 23-8A). The ligament is then cut on the uterine side, and the clamp is replaced by a fixation ligature using No. 0 or No. 1 delayed-absorbable suture. Next the uterosacral ligament is clamped with a Heaney clamp, excised, and transfixed with a similar suture (Fig. 23-8B–D). The ligated pedicle is held for later plication and use in the vaginal vault suspension. Excision of the uterosacral ligament usually allows the uterus to descend sufficiently so that either the anterior or the posterior cul-de-sac, if previously not accessible, may now be entered without difficulty.

A retractor placed in both the anterior and the posterior cul-de-sac allows them to be held as widely apart as possible. When the retractors are held to the left side of the patient, they provide excellent exposure of the left broad ligament, while displacing the bladder, ureter, and rectum. When the base of the broad (cardinal) ligament and the left uterosacral ligament have separately been cut and ligated, the uterine vessels can be seen. The vessels are similarly clamped, cut, and replaced by a nontransfixion suture using delayed-absorbable material (Fig. 23-8E). It is important not to transfix the uterine pedicle, because injury to the dilated vessels can result in a broad ligament hematoma.

In successive similar steps, the broad ligament on the left is disposed of as high as possible, picking up the anterior peritoneum above the uterine vessels with each successive pedicle. When further progress on the left cannot be made, the retractors are shifted to the right of the patient, and the right cardinal ligament is clamped, cut (Fig. 23-9A), and ligated. The uterosacral ligament is clamped, excised, and transfixed separately and the ligature is held in a hemostat. In similar steps the uterine vessels are ligated, and the right broad ligament is severed from the uterus as high as exposure allows.

It may happen that, after both uterine vessels are ligated, further progress in the vaginal removal of the uterus, for one reason or another, is impossible. In such an event, the cervix may be amputated, all bleeding points ligated with interrupted suture, the abdomen opened, and the operation completed from above. This impasse need cause no apprehension as long as the patient has been forewarned of this possibility.

After the broad ligaments have been excised high on each side of the uterine body, the cervix is pulled superiorly. Then the uterine body, if not too large or adherent, presents itself at the posterior opening, where it may be grasped by a tenaculum or Lahey

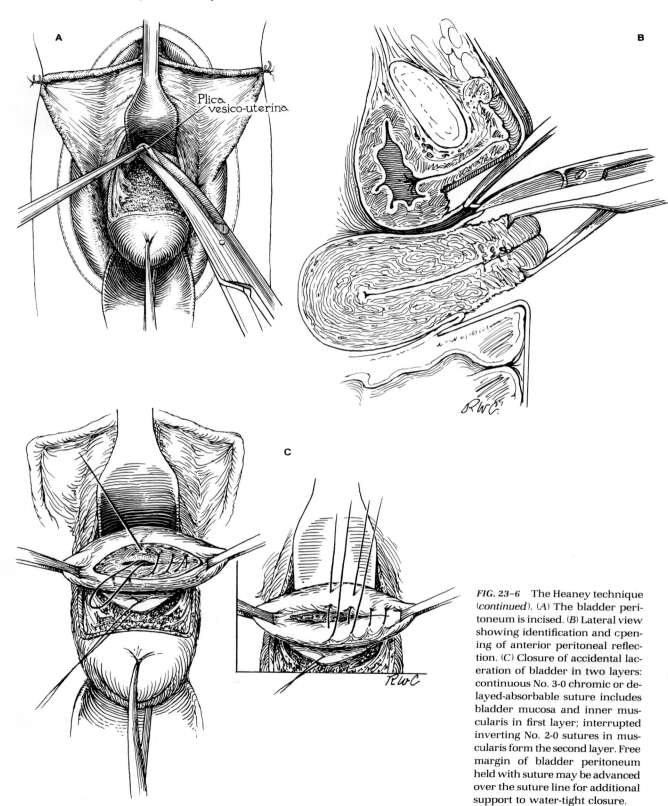

FIG. 23-6 The Heaney technique (*continued*). (*A*) The bladder peritoneum is incised. (*B*) Lateral view showing identification and opening of anterior peritoneal reflection. (*C*) Closure of accidental laceration of bladder in two layers: continuous No. 3-0 chromic or delayed-absorbable suture includes bladder mucosa and inner muscularis in first layer; interrupted inverting No. 2-0 sutures in muscularis form the second layer. Free margin of bladder peritoneum held with suture may be advanced over the suture line for additional support to water-tight closure.

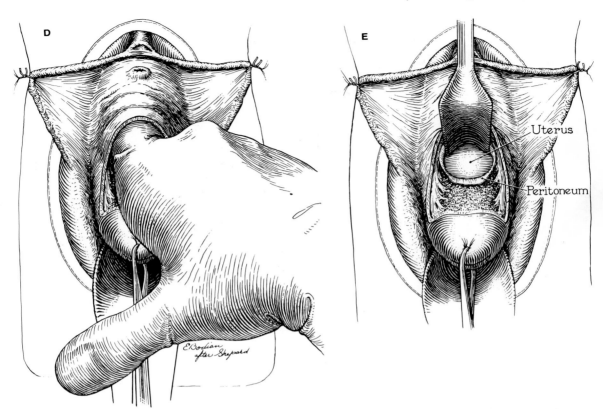

FIG. 23–6 (continued). (*D*) The pelvis is explored with the index finger. (*E*) A retractor is introduced into the peritoneal cavity.

thyroid clamp and partially pulled outside the introitus (Fig. 23–9B).

The upper portion of the broad ligament, the uterine end of the tube, the suspensory ligament of the ovary, and the round ligament on the left side can now be identified and carefully inspected. These structures are incorporated into the cornual portion of the broad ligament, which is clamped (Fig. 23–9C), cut, and doubly ligated; initially by a free tie to occlude the vascular pedicle, then by a transfixion suture placed outside the previous ligature. The clamp is replaced by a ligature for any residual portion of the upper broad ligament in the same way as was the lower part of the broad ligaments. The outer ligature on the pedicle from the tip of the broad ligament is held with a hemostat to identify this ligament at the time of peritonization and suspension of the vaginal vault (Fig. 23–10).

After the left side of the uterus is freed, the right cornual region is clamped, excised, and ligated by a similar technique. The uterus is removed and inspected to see whether any pathologic process exists that would make advisable the removal of otherwise normal adnexa.

If the body of the uterus is too large to remove intact, removal of the cervix may allow its easy delivery. If the uterus is still too large, a morcellation procedure must be done. Before morcellation, the tip of the broad ligaments should be clamped, excised, and ligated, because once the communicating branches of the ovarian vessels are securely ligated, the fear of excessive bleeding may be dismissed. The procedure is made easier by maintaining continuous traction of the uterus. The uterine size may be reduced by the removal of a series of wedge-shaped segments of the anterior wall and fundus. No piece should be cut loose from the uterine wall unless the uterus is held against possible retraction into the pelvic cavity.

When the uterus has been removed, a small laparotomy pack is introduced to hold back the intestines, and the tape from the pack is held by a hemostat. The tubes and ovaries are now inspected by drawing them into the operative field, and depending on their condition, they are retained or removed. The adnexa can almost always be inspected and examined or operated upon as easily through the vaginal incision as through the abdom-

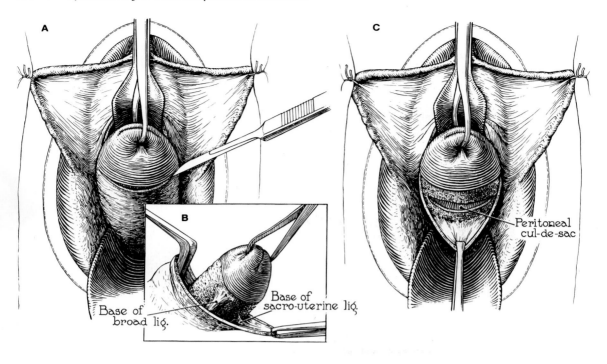

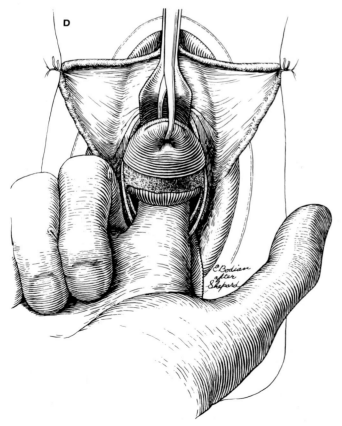

FIG. 23–7 The Heaney technique (*continued*). (*A*) Posterior transverse mucosal incision. (*B*) The uterosacral ligament and the base of the broad ligament are exposed. (*C*) The peritoneum of the cul-de-sac is exposed. (*D*) The cul-de-sac is explored.

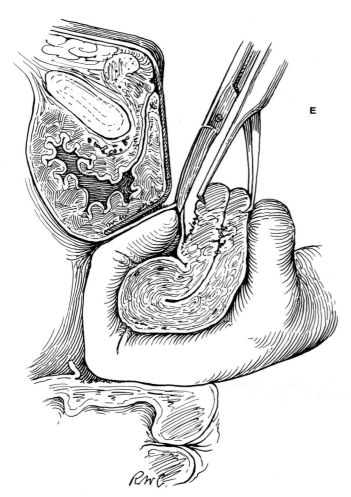

E

FIG. 23-7 *(continued).* (*E*) Lateral view of posterior cul-de-sac approach for identification and incision of bladder peritoneum between index and middle fingers.

inal route. If bleeding from the posterior vaginal mucosa or submucosa should occur, it can be controlled with a continuous No. 3-0 delayed-absorbable suture that incorporates the pelvic peritoneal margin, the submucosa, and the vaginal mucosa (Fig. 23–10, *insert*).

To remove the tube and ovary, a Babcock clamp is placed on the previously ligated pedicle and the adnexa is drawn into the operative field. When the infundibulopelvic ligament is identified, a curved Ochsner clamp is carefully placed across the entire ligament. The tube and ovary are excised and removed, leaving a good margin of the broad ligament on the pedicle (Fig. 23–11) to avoid retraction of the vessels from the clamp and subsequent bleeding. If necessary, a second clamp may be placed on the pedicle, distal to the original clamp, to make certain that the ovarian vessels are secured before the pedicle is excised and doubly ligated. A free tie is placed

snugly around the pedicle before a transfixion suture is inserted in front of the ligature. If the opposite adnexa is removed, the same technique is used.

Suspension of Vaginal Vault

Although the Heaney technique of vaginal hysterectomy was used initially in many clinics, various modifications of the original procedure have developed. Figure 23–12(1) shows the initial steps of our technique of vault suspension following removal of the uterus. The three ligamentous supports are visible on either side of the vault, including the tip of the broad ligament, the cardinal ligament in the center, and the uterosacral ligament.

The suspension is performed prior to placing the purse-string closure of the pelvic peritoneum. After the pelvis is entered through the lateral vaginal fornix, the continuous suture of No. 1 delayed-absorbable suture (Vicryl or Dexon) is placed through the

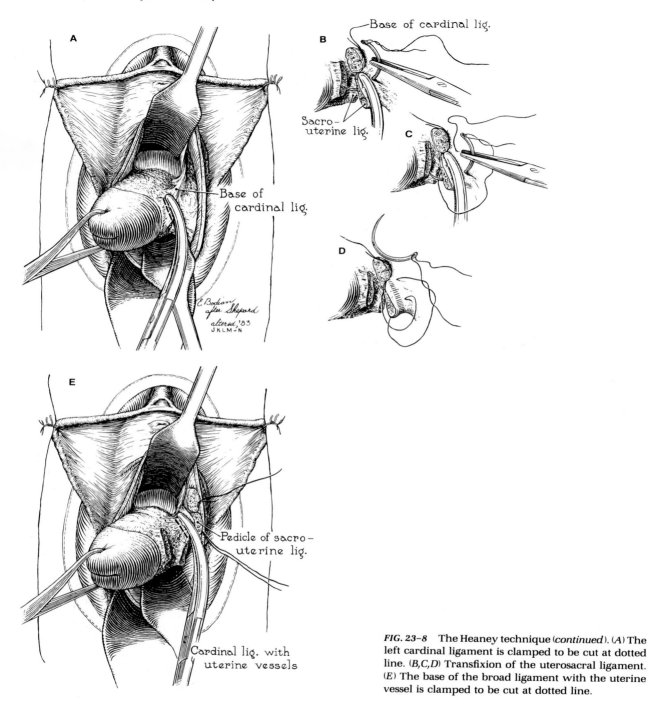

Base of cardinal lig.

A

Base of cardinal lig.

B

Sacro-
uterine lig.

C

D

E

Pedicle of sacro-
uterine lig.

Cardinal lig. with
uterine vessels

FIG. 23-8 The Heaney technique (*continued*). (*A*) The left cardinal ligament is clamped to be cut at dotted line. (*B,C,D*) Transfixion of the uterosacral ligament. (*E*) The base of the broad ligament with the uterine vessel is clamped to be cut at dotted line.

tip of the broad ligament, proximal to the tied ligature to avoid pulling the ligature off the pedicle. A deep bite is then taken in the cardinal ligament, which provides one of the main supports to the vaginal vault. The uterosacral ligament is held firmly on stretch so that a deep bite may be taken

in this structure, following which the suture is brought through the lateral vaginal mucosa to complete the suspension. The suture is held untied until the peritoneal suture is placed. The same technique is used to suspend the right side of the vaginal vault.

The practice of plicating the uterosacral ligaments

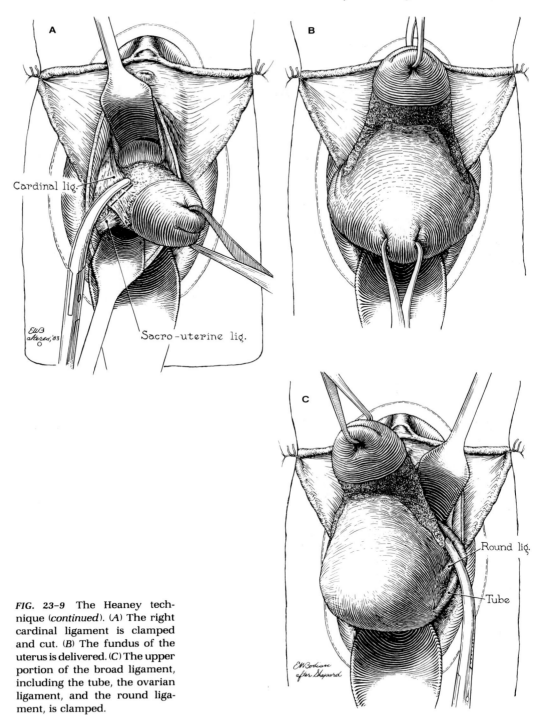

FIG. 23-9 The Heaney technique (*continued*). (*A*) The right cardinal ligament is clamped and cut. (*B*) The fundus of the uterus is delivered. (*C*) The upper portion of the broad ligament, including the tube, the ovarian ligament, and the round ligament, is clamped.

and cul-de-sac together prevents the subsequent development of an enterocele. Figure 23–12(2) illustrates one very effective technique of a posterior culdeplasty. The initial suture (2) has been placed to include the uterosacral ligaments and the cul-de-

sac peritoneum. A second suture includes the same structures but at a slightly higher level. One or more similar sutures may be placed higher in the cul-de-sac in cases in which there is marked redundancy or early enterocele formation. Figure 23–12(3) illus-

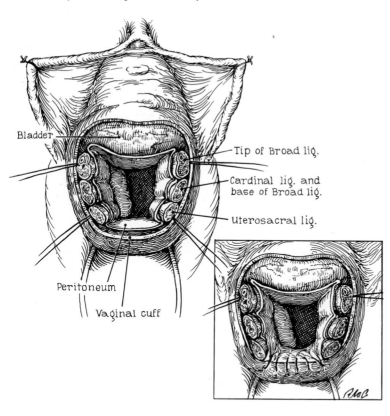

Bladder

Tip of Broad lig.

Cardinal lig. and base of Broad lig.

Uterosacral lig.

Peritoneum

Vaginal cuff

FIG. 23-10 The Heaney technique (*continued*). Cut surface of the tip of the broad ligament, the cardinal ligament, and the uterosacral ligament. (*Insert*) Posterior peritoneum is sutured to the submucosa and the posterior vaginal mucosa with No. 3-0 continuous delayed-absorbable suture to control capillary bleeding.

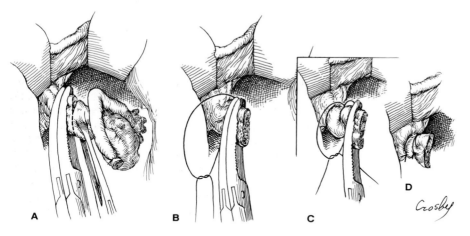

A   B   C   D

FIG. 23-11 The Heaney technique (*continued*). Adnexal removal. When removal of adnexa is indicated (*A*), the pedicle to the tip of the broad ligament is pulled into the operative field and two Heaney clamps are placed on the infundibulopelvic ligament. The ligament is excised and the tube and ovary are removed. (*B*) The ligament is ligated with a free-tie of No. 0 delayed-absorbable suture, which is placed behind the inner clamp, (*C*) transfixed to the tip of the clamp, and (*D*) tied firmly before removal of the outer clamp.

trates similar plication sutures, which originate through the posterior fornix. As shown by suture (3), the suture enters the vaginal mucosa to pass through the pelvic peritoneum. This suture picks up each uterosacral ligament, without plicating the peritoneum of the cul-de-sac, and passes back through the posterior vaginal fornix. An additional plication stitch may be placed at a slightly higher level. When tied, these latter vaginal sutures will provide additional depth to the vagina by anchoring

the posterior fornix to the uterosacral ligaments in the midline.

The procedure is completed by closing the peritoneal cavity with a continuous purse-string suture that originates in the center of the bladder peritoneum as shown in Figure 23–12(4). Note that the suture incorporates the entire circumference of the pelvic peritoneum, with particular care taken to pick up the peritoneum beyond the ligatures on the major vessels and ligaments. This will ensure

FIG. 23-12 The Heaney technique (*continued*). Suspension of vaginal vault. (*1*) A continuous suture (No. 1 delayed-absorbable) is placed through lateral vaginal wall and adjacent peritoneum; suture continues through the tip of the broad ligament, cardinal ligament, and uterosacral ligament before returning through the vaginal wall. Note that the suspension suture is placed beyond the pedicle ligatures. (*2*) After suspension completed on both sides, posterior culdeplasty sutures pass through the uterosacral ligament, cul-de-sac peritoneum, and opposite ligament (internal suture). A second suture is placed slightly higher. (*3*) External culdeplasty suture(s) are placed through the posterior fornix and passed through each uterosacral ligament before returning through cul-de-sac peritoneum and posterior fornix. (*4*) A pursestring suture encircles the peritoneal surfaces as the highest internal suture. Note that the peritoneal suture is placed above the vascular pedicles, thereby maintaining the pedicles in an extraperitoneal position to avoid intraperitoneal bleeding.

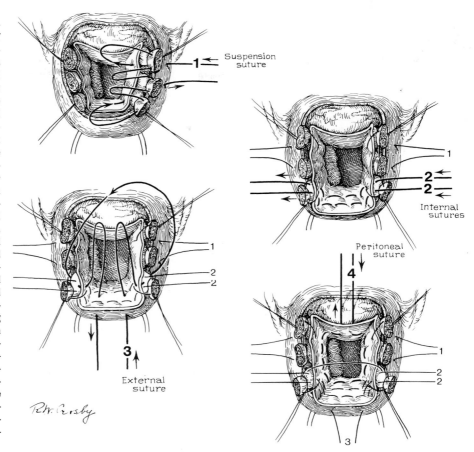

complete closure of the peritoneum, with the pedicles of the ligated vessels retained outside the peritoneal cavity. Should postoperative bleeding occur, it will remain extraperitoneal and can be drained easily through the vaginal vault.

The suspension sutures in the lateral vaginal angles are tied (Fig. 23–13[1]). The uterosacral plication sutures are now tied, both internally and in the posterior fornix (Fig. 23–13[2,3]) to insure against subsequent enterocele formation. The purse string suture in the peritoneum is now tied (Fig. 23–13[4]), which should exteriorize the pelvic pedicle. The uterosacral ligament sutures that pass through the posterior fornix will elongate the vagina by anchoring the vaginal vault to the uterosacral ligaments. The anterior vaginal repair, if needed, is initiated at this point, prior to transverse closure of the vault with figure-of-eight sutures.

Complications of Vaginal Hysterectomy

INFECTION. In recent years, there has been increasing use of the open-vault technique to reduce seroma formation in the operative site and to avoid the complication of cuff cellulitis. The prophylactic use of perioperative, broad-spectrum antibiotic agents has proven quite effective in reducing the incidence of postoperative morbidity due to infection in premenopausal women undergoing a vaginal hysterectomy, as discussed in Chapter 6 on postoperative care. The 24-hour use of a prophylactic antibiotic has reduced what was once a 20% to 30% incidence of postoperative febrile morbidity to a low rate of 5% to 10%.

A similar improvement in febrile morbidity has been noted with the use of T-tube suction drainage of the vaginal vault in the retroperitoneal space. Taking less effort and affording equally low morbidity is the use of meticulous hemostasis during the operative procedure and reefing of the margins of the vaginal cuff with a continuous locking suture. The vault is left open, and a small rubber drain may or may not be inserted beneath the closed peritoneum, depending on the presence or absence of venous oozing. This open cuff technique pre-

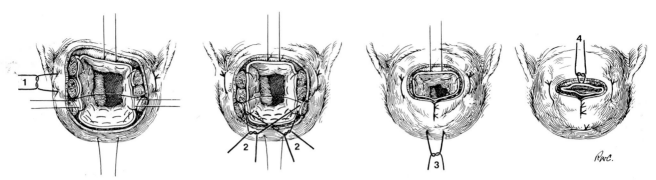

FIG. 23–13 The Heaney technique (*continued*). Suspension sutures are tied in the lateral wall of vagina (*1*). Internal culdeplasty sutures are tied next (*2*); note slight narrowing of the diameter of the vaginal vault. (*3*) External culdeplasty suture(s) are now tied. (*4*) Peritoneal suture is tied, causing pelvic pedicles to be exteriorized.

cludes the collection of serum or blood from the operative site and avoids the need for antibiotics or for drainage tubes in the vaginal vault. The vaginal cuff heals promptly, and the incidence of granulation tissue formation is no higher than when the cuff is closed tightly at the time of surgery.

BLADDER INJURY. The close anatomical relationships of the bladder, uterus, and upper vagina cause the bladder to be the most vulnerable and, understandably, the most frequently injured organ of the lower urinary tract during pelvic surgery. Bladder injury may occur during dissection of the fascial plane between the bladder base and the cervix and lower uterine segment. Although accurate data are difficult to obtain, bladder injury occurs during vaginal hysterectomy in approximately 0.5% of cases.

The incidence of bladder injury associated with vaginal hysterectomy is lower than that for abdominal hysterectomy by a ratio of approximately 1 to 6. The lower injury rate is due to the fact that when vaginal hysterectomy is selected as the operative procedure of choice, there is little deformity of the uterus, and intrapelvic pathology is usually absent. Careful dissection of the bladder base from the cervix and lower uterine segment along with identification and opening of the anterior peritoneal fold are recognized to be the most difficult technical steps of a vaginal hysterectomy. The management of bladder injury is discussed and illustrated above in the description of the operative technique for vaginal hysterectomy.

PROLAPSE OF VAGINAL VAULT. Minimal vaginal vault prolapse, too slight to make the patient conscious of it, involves the upper one-third of the vagina and is not unusual following hysterectomy. Partial prolapse, involving the upper one-half of the vagina, or complete vaginal vault prolapse is more unusual, with a reported incidence of less than 0.5% of all cases of prolapse. A prolapse occurring after total hysterectomy probably means that a deep enterocele was overlooked at the time of surgery. The routine suspension of the vaginal vault will not correct this anatomical defect or prevent future prolapse of the vault.

Vaginal prolapse resulting from a residual enterocele caused by diastasis of the levator ani muscles and separation of the attachment of the vagina to the levator crura may be symptomless immediately following hysterectomy, but the degree of prolapse and the severity of the symptoms will increase with time. Prolapse of the vaginal vault is basically caused by a significant defect in the weakened and relaxed levator plate along with a widened levator hiatus in the pelvic floor. A previously occult enterocele may become clinically manifest after a hysterectomy; residual enterocele and vault prolapse are variations of the same anatomical defect.

An occult enterocele can be missed more easily during an abdominal hysterectomy, which is usually unassociated with uterine prolapse. Since the major indication for vaginal hysterectomy is related to symptomatic uterine prolapse, an enterocele is usually evident, and surgical correction can be included in the operative procedure. A residual enterocele, which may result in vaginal vault prolapse, occurs far more frequently following vaginal hysterectomy than following an abdominal procedure.

Protrusion of a mass from the vaginal outlet is the symptom that usually brings a woman with massive prolapse of the vagina to seek relief. Walking and sitting is usually difficult for them. A cystocele and rectocele, associated with inversion of the vagina, produce severe symptoms of pelvic pressure and discomfort.

Treatment of vaginal prolapse is discussed in detail in Chapter 24 in the section on enterocele. The specific treatment of a small, medium, or large enterocele, with or without vaginal prolapse, is emphasized in that section of the text. Other important complications that can result from a vaginal hysterectomy include intra-operative and postoperative bleeding, and ureteral injury. All of these subjects are discussed in Chapters 6 and 14.

LeFORT OPERATION

The original operation, as described by Neugebauer and later by LeFort, was used for the treatment of total uterine procidentia and consisted of denuding a long narrow triangle on the anterior and posterior walls of the vagina. The base of each triangle was just below the cervix, the apex was at the outlet, and vaginal closure was brought about by approximating these denuded areas. A slightly different procedure is now used. Rectangular strips of mucosa are excised from the upper portion of the anterior and posterior vaginal walls, and the exposed submucosa and vaginal musculature are then closed.

This operation does not correct the anatomical defect associated with a complete prolapse of the uterus or vagina that is due to a large traction or pulsion enterocele. The LeFort procedure should be used only when there is a very good reason why one of the usual operations for prolapse cannot be carried out. The operation is an admission on the part of the surgeon that there is no way to cure the prolapse by a procedure that would leave a functioning vagina. Nevertheless, there are rare cases in which it is useful. Its virtue lies in the fact that it is perhaps the quickest of any of the procedures used for the cure of prolapse and that it can be done safely, under local anesthesia if necessary. The procedure is generally restricted to an elderly widow who might otherwise be condemned to the indefinite use of a pessary. Regardless of the age of the patient, the closure of the vagina should never be done without a complete understanding on the part of the patient and her spouse, if living, that the procedure will terminate her sex life.

Both stress and urge urinary incontinence may occur with the LeFort procedure because of traction of the suture line on the trigone and bladder neck. Ridley reports an incidence of urinary incontinence of 24% following the LeFort procedure. The disadvantage can be avoided by closing only the upper one-third to one-half of the anterior vaginal wall, stopping short of the area that underlies the bladder neck and the urethra. Nonetheless, part of the bladder base and the entire trigone rest on the upper one-third of the vagina, so it is difficult to close the upper vagina without placing some traction on the bladder trigone.

To avoid the risk of postoperative urinary stress incontinence, the urethra should be dissected free and a thorough plication of the vesical neck should be performed. If the patient is not sexually active, the levators are approximated very tightly, leaving only enough opening for urination. If the patient desires to retain some coital function of the vagina, the latter step is omitted although the residual depth of the outer vagina may preclude satisfactory coitus.

Obviously, this procedure is useful only for the postmenopausal female with total uterine prolapse where menses are absent. It is essential that the cervix and endometrial cavity be assessed fully by a cytologic smear and a dilatation and curettage to make certain that there is no evidence of occult uterine malignancy prior to closure of the vagina.

Technique of LeFort Operation

With the patient in the lithotomy position, the cervix is drawn out as far as possible. With total uterine procidentia, drawing out the cervix almost completely everts the vagina.

The area to be denuded anteriorly is marked out with the scalpel as indicated by the dotted line in Figure 23–14A. Sufficient mucosa should be left laterally to form a canal for drainage of cervical secretions. The area to be denuded extends to within 2 cm of the tip of the cervix and to within 5 cm of the urethral meatus, remaining away from the location of the vesical neck. In order to avoid incorporating the bladder neck and posterior urethra in the operative site, a balloon-filled urethral catheter should be used to delineate the location of the urethrovesical junction.

The mucosa is denuded from the anterior vaginal wall by a combination of sharp and blunt dissection (Fig. 23–14B). An area of mucosa of equal size and shape is denuded from the posterior vaginal wall (Fig. 23–14C).

The mucosal edges are approximated transversely below the cervix with interrupted sutures of No. 0 chromic catgut or delayed-absorbable material (Fig. 23–14D). Beginning at the top, the denuded areas are approximated with as many rows as necessary of interrupted No. 0 delayed-absorbable sutures (Fig. 23–15A,B). Finally, the outer mucosal edges are approximated with No. 0 interrupted sutures (Fig. 23–15C). Mucosa-lined tunnels left on both sides are demonstrated by the Kelly clamps (Fig. 23–15D).

HISTORICAL OPERATIONS FOR UTERINE PROLAPSE

Spalding–Richardson procedure

In 1937, Edward Richardson devised a composite operation that used and improved on the principles and techniques of various procedures already in use. Richardson's procedure included amputation

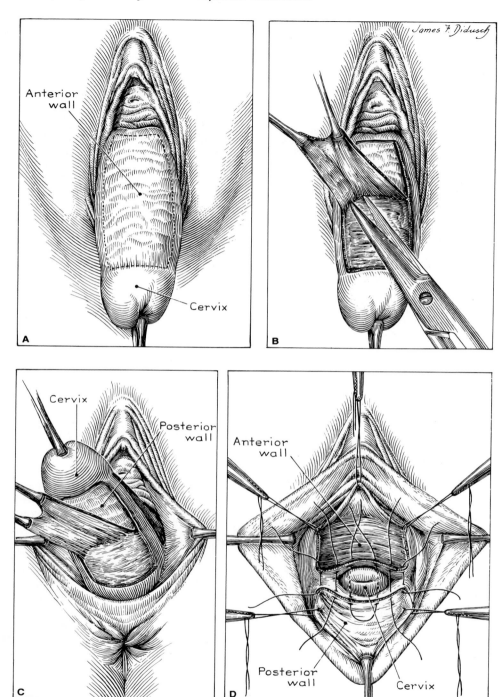

FIG. 23–14 The LeFort operation for uterine prolapse. (*A*) Dotted line indicates incision in the anterior vaginal wall. (*B*) Flap outlined is excised. (*C*) A similar flap is excised from the posterior vaginal wall. (*D*) The vaginal mucosal edge is approximated at the upper margin of the excised mucosa.

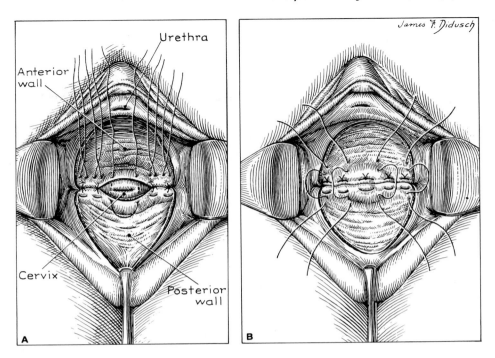

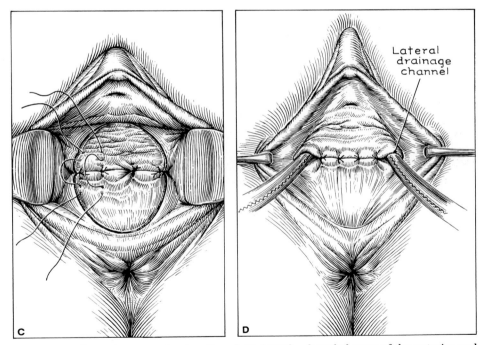

FIG. 23–15 The LeFort operation (*continued*). (*A,B,C*) The denuded areas of the anterior and the posterior wall are approximated by several horizontal layers of interrupted sutures. (*D*) The outer mucosal edges are closed. Note the tunnels that remain on either side of the vagina, which are demonstrated by Kelly clamps.

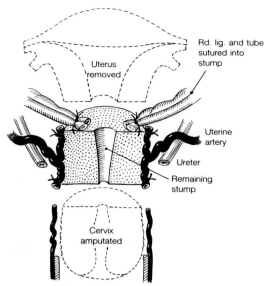

FIG. 23-16 Diagram of Spalding–Richardson composite operation indicating the portion of uterus that remains. Note that the blood supply is intact.

of the cervix; removal of the corpus at any level desired; utilization of the isthmic portion of the uterus with its broad and uterosacral ligament at-

tachments for vault support; and, finally, approximation in the midline of the pubocervical fascia beneath the urethra, the base of the bladder, and the retained portion of the isthmus of the cervix.

Richardson's plan had the following objectives: (1) to remove the hypertrophied vaginal portion of the cervix; (2) to extirpate the corpus uteri, together with the tubes and the ovaries if indicated; (3) to destroy or excise any remaining cervical canal epithelium; (4) to minimize trauma and devitalization of structures, so they could later be used for reconstruction purposes; (5) to preserve a blood supply to the cervical isthmus; (6) to ablate totally any associated enterocele through high obliteration of the cul-de-sac of Douglas; (7) to use rationally all supporting structures, namely the pubocervical fascia, the cardinal ligaments with their extraordinarily strong cervical attachments, the uterosacral and the round ligaments, the fascia of the rectovaginal septum, as well as the muscles and the fascial layers of the pelvic floor and the perineum; (8) to reestablish a vagina of normal depth and caliber; and (9) to restore normal anatomical relationships.

Richardson made no claim of originality for any of the procedures used in his operation: many of the operative steps were already in use, independently, for various conditions in gynecologic sur-

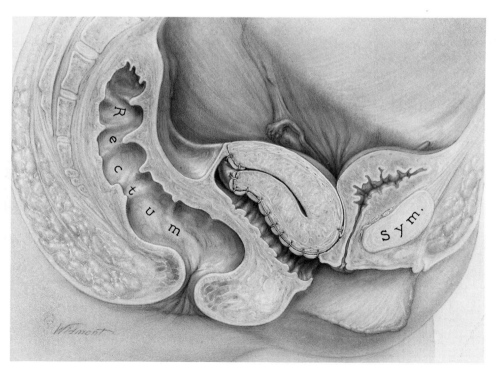

FIG. 23-17 The Watkins transposition operation. The procedure is completed with the transposed uterus fixed in its new position beneath the bladder and urethra.

gery. On reading the 1937 article, Ludwig Emge communicated with Richardson calling his attention to the description of a similar operation reported by Spalding in 1919. Spalding and Richardson each described practically identical operations; both men were motivated by the shortcomings of the other

operations for uterine prolapse in vogue at the time, and both men emphasized the same points in claiming superiority for their operations. Since the operation was described independently by the two authors, it has been called by their joint names. It is not surprising to surgeons familiar with the op-

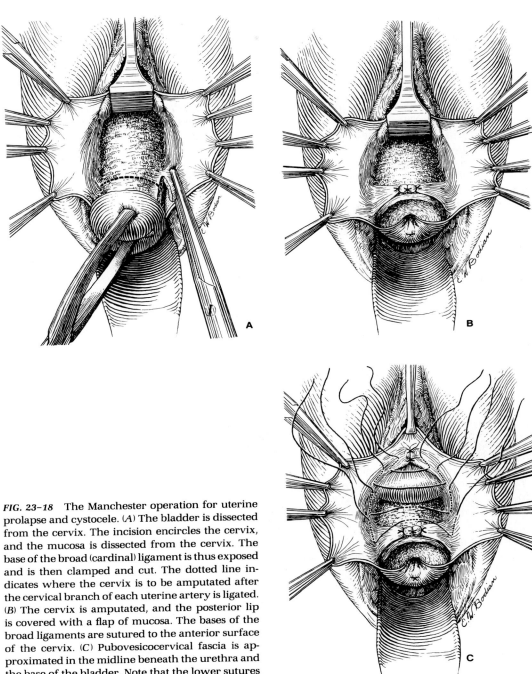

FIG. 23-18 The Manchester operation for uterine prolapse and cystocele. (*A*) The bladder is dissected from the cervix. The incision encircles the cervix, and the mucosa is dissected from the cervix. The base of the broad (cardinal) ligament is thus exposed and is then clamped and cut. The dotted line indicates where the cervix is to be amputated after the cervical branch of each uterine artery is ligated. (*B*) The cervix is amputated, and the posterior lip is covered with a flap of mucosa. The bases of the broad ligaments are sutured to the anterior surface of the cervix. (*C*) Pubovesicocervical fascia is approximated in the midline beneath the urethra and the base of the bladder. Note that the lower sutures bite into the anterior wall of the cervix.

eration that Richardson reinvented the procedure in 1937. The remarkable fact is that an operation that had such merit had escaped the general attention of gynecologists since Spalding's original article in 1919.

Although the Spalding–Richardson procedure is rarely used today in gynecologic clinics, it is recognized as one of the major surgical contributions of its time for uterine prolapse. The details of this operation are shown in Figure 23–16, and the technique is described in the original publications and in previous editions of this text.

Watkins Transposition Operation

Thomas J. Watkins first performed this operation for cystocele and uterine prolapse in 1898, and he reported it the following year. The procedure was used extensively for uterine prolapse with a very large cystocele. In most instances the results were very satisfactory. The procedure is generally known throughout this country as the interposition operation, but Watkins preferred the term transposition since the uterus was transposed beneath the bladder. Basically, the operation consisted of amputating the elongated cervix and suturing the fundus of the uterus beneath the large cystocele. The fundus was therefore used as an obturator to fill the defect in the anterior segment of the pelvic diaphragm.

Improved techniques of vaginal hysterectomy and repair of the vagina gradually led to the abandonment of the Watkins operation, and it is unlikely that recently trained gynecologists have ever seen this procedure performed. The completed procedure is shown in Figure 23–17, and the reader interested in this operation can refer to previous editions of this text for further operative details.

Manchester (Donald or Fothergill) Operation

In 1888, as related by Shaw, Donald of Manchester began treating prolapse of the uterus by the combination of anterior and posterior colporrhaphy and amputation of the cervix. This operation is still frequently performed by a number of gynecologists in Manchester and other areas of the United Kingdom. Fothergill modified the procedure slightly. The fundamental principles underlying the procedure are the same as in the operation described by Shaw in 1933, but certain details differ slightly. In Britain the operation is used for several indications, but in the United States it is usually used for the sake of expediency when a patient is unable to tolerate prolonged surgery.

Although one of the original indications for the Manchester procedure was to preserve the childbearing function of the reproductive tract, several objections have been made to the operation when future pregnancy is desired. Leonard found that, following cervical amputation, the incidence of sterility was abnormally high, premature delivery between the 6th and 8th months increased, and cervical dystocia was common. Shaw's own results would seem to condemn the operation during the childbearing period, because few of his patients subsequently had children.

As shown in Figure 23–18, the basic procedure includes excision, plication, and suturing of the cardinal ligaments to the anterior surface of the cervical stump following amputation. The operation is completed with a Sturmdorf suture placed in the anterior and posterior lips of the cervix after an anterior and posterior colporrhaphy have been completed as indicated.

Bibliography

Adams, JA: Cited by WP Graves. In Graves, WP: Gynecology. Philadelphia, W. B. Saunders. 1916

Alexander W: Quoted by Curtis. In Curtis AH (ed): Obstet Gynecol. Philadelphia, WB Saunders, 1937

Amirikia H, Evans TN: 10-year review of hysterectomies: Trends, indications, and risks. Am J Obstet Gynecol 134:431, 1979

Averett L: Vaginal hysterectomy: Indications and advantages. J Internat Coll Surg 8:53, 1945

Baldy JM: Prolapse of the uterus. Trans Am Gynecol Soc 27:25, 1912

————: Treatment of uterine retrodisplacements. Surg Gynecol Obstet 8:421, 1909

Copenhaver EH: Vaginal hysterectomy: An analysis of indications and complications among 1000 operations. Am J Obstet Gynecol 84:123, 1962

————: Vaginal hysterectomy: Past, present and future. Surg Clin North Am 60:437, 1980

Cullen TS: Use of sutures as retractors in vaginal operation for prolapse. Am J Obstet Gynecol 4:544, 1922

Danforth WC: The place of vaginal hysterectomy in present-day gynecology. Am J Obstet Gynecol 1938

Donald A: A short history of the operation of colporrhaphy with remarks on the technique. J Obstet Gynecol Br Empire 28:256, 1921

Emge LA, Durfee RB: Pelvic organ prolapse: Four thousand years of treatment. Clin Obstet Gynecol 9:997, 1966

England GT, Randall HW, Graves WL: Impairment of tissue defenses by vasoconstrictors in vaginal hysterectomies. Obstet Gynecol 61:271, 1983

Everett HS: End-result with the Watkins interposition operation. Surg Gynecol Obstet 61:403, 1935

Fluhmann CF: The rise and fall of suspension operations for uterine displacement. Bull Johns Hopkins Hosp 96:59, 1955

Fothergill WE: Anterior colporrhaphy and amputation of the cervix combined as a single operation for use in the treatment of genital prolapse. Am J Surg 29:161, 1915

Franche O, Pak-Miong-Piu, Boga-Colman C, et al: L'état des voies urinaires dans le prolapsus genital total de la femme. Urol Int 9:28, 1959

Freund HW: Uber Moderne Prolapsoperationen. Zbl Gynak 25:441, 1901

Froriep R: Chirurgische Kupfertafeln. Weimar, 1824

Gilliam DT: Round-ligament ventrosuspension of the uterus: A new method. Am J Obstet 41:299, 1900

Goodall JR, Power RMH: A modification of the LeFort operation for increasing its scope. Am J Obstet Gynecol 34:968, 1937

Graves WP: Olshauser operation for suspension of the uterus. Surg Gynecol Obstet 52:1028, 1931

Gray LA: Vaginal Hysterectomy, 3rd Ed. Springfield, Charles C Thomas, 1983

Guillemin G, Cavailher H: Les deformations vesicales et ureterales dan les prolapsus genitaux. Rev Fr Gynecol Obstet 43:93, 1948

Heaney NS: Report of 565 vaginal hysterectomies performed for benign pelvic disease. Am J Obstet Gynecol 28:751, 1934

————: Vaginal hysterectomy: Its indications and technic. Am J Surg 48:284, 1940

————: Techniques of vaginal hysterectomy. Surg Clin North Am 22:73, 1942

Hirst BC: A modification of the Alexander operation. Surg Gynecol Obstet 20:599, 1915

Kelly HA: Hysterorrhaphy. Am J Obstet 20:33, 1887

————: History of retrodisplacement of the uterus. Surg Gynecol Obstet 20:598, 1915

————: Vaginal hysterectomy. In Kelly HA (ed): Gynecology. New York, Appleton, 1928

Kempers RD, Hunter JS, Jr, Welch JS: Indications for vaginal hysterectomy. Obstet Gynecol 13:677, 1959

Kennedy JW, Campbell AD: Vaginal Hysterectomy. Philadelphia, FA Davis, 1942

Klempner E: Gynecological lesions and ureterohydronephrosis. Am J Obstet Gynecol 64:1232, 1952

Langenbeck JCM: Quoted by Senn N: The early history of vaginal hysterectomy. JAMA 25:476, 1950

Lee RA, Symmonds RE: Surgical repair of post hysterectomy vault prolapse. Am J Obstet Gynecol 112:953, 1972

LeFort L: Nouveau procede pour la Guerison, du prolapsus uterin. Bul Gen Ther 92:337, 1877

Leonard VN: The postoperative results of trachelorrhaphy in comparison with those of amputation of cervix. Surg Gynecol Obstet 18:35, 1914

Mattingly RF: Surgery in the aging female. Clin Obstet Gynecol 7:573, 1964

————: Accidental Cystotomy during vaginal hysterectomy. In Nichols DH (ed): Clinical Problems, Injuries and Complications of Gynecologic Surgery. Baltimore, Williams and Wilkins, 1983

McCall ML: Posterior culdeplasty: Surgical correction of enterocele during vaginal hysterectomy. A preliminary report. Obstet Gynecol 10:595, 1957

Neugebauer JA: Einige Worte uber die mediane Vaginalnaht, als mittel zur Beseitigung des Gebarmuttervorfalls. Zentralbl Gynaekol 5:3, 1881

Olshausen R: Uber Ventrale Operation bei Prolapsus and Retroversio Uteri. Zbl Gynak 10:698, 1886

Porges RF: Changing indications for vaginal hysterectomy. Am J Obstet Gynecol 136:153, 1980

Randall CL, Nichols DH: Surgical treatment of vaginal inversion. Obstet Gynecol 38:327, 1971

Richardson EH: An efficient composite operation for uterine prolapse and associated pathology. Am J Obstet Gynecol 34:814, 1937

Ridley JH: Evaluation of the colpocleisis operation: A report of 58 cases. Am J Obstet Gynecol 113:1114, 1972

Schauta F: Uber Prolapsoperationen. Gynak Rundschau 3:729, 1909

Senn N: The early history of vaginal hysterectomy. JAMA 25:476, 1895

Shaw WF: The treatment of prolapsus uteri, with special reference to the Manchester operation of colporrhaphy. Am J Obstet Gynecol 26:667, 1933

Sims JM: On the treatment of vesicovaginal fistula. Am J Med Sci 23:59, 1852

Spalding AB: A study of frozen sections of the pelvis with description of an operation for pelvic prolapse. Surg Gynecol Obstet 29:529, 1919

Symmonds RE, Pratt JE: Vaginal prolapse following hysterectomy. Am J Obstet Gynecol 79:899, 1960

TeLinde RW, Richardson EH, Jr: End results of the Richardson composite operation for uterine prolapse. Am J Obstet Gynecol 45:29, 1943

Watkins TJ: The treatment of cystocele and uterine prolapse after the menopause. Am J Obstet Gynecol 15:420, 1899

————: Transposition of the uterus and bladder in the treatment of extensive cystocele and uterine prolapse. Am J Obstet Gynecol 65:225, 1912

Webster JC: A satisfactory operation for certain cases of retroversion of the uterus. JAMA 37:913, 1901

Wertheim E: Zur plastischen Verwendung des Uterus bei Prolapsen. Zbl Gynak 23:369, 1899

White SC, Wartel LJ, Wade ME: Comparison of abdominal and vaginal hysterectomies. Obstet Gynecol 37:530, 1971

Chapter 24

Relaxed Vaginal Outlet, Rectocele, and Enterocele

The pelvic floor is formed chiefly by the levator ani muscles, which create a broad muscular diaphragm, aided posteriorly by the coccygeus muscles (Fig. 24–1). The levator ani consists of three distinct muscles: the iliococcygeus, the pubococcygeus, and the puborectalis. The iliococcygeal muscle arises from the posterior portion of the arcus tendineus and the ischial spine and inserts along the lateral margin of the coccyx and lower sacral vertebrae. The pubococcygeus originates from the inner aspect of the pubic bone and the proximal portion of the arcus tendineus or white fascial line. The puborectalis muscle arises from the posterior portion of the pubic bone and the inferior ramus of the pubis.

The medial portion of the levator musculature is formed by the pubococcygeus, the largest of the three muscles. The muscle passes along each side of the levator hiatus, near the urethra, vagina, and rectum. The fibers from both sides interdigitate between the rectum and the coccyx to form a median raphe, the levator plate. When this muscular portion of the pelvic diaphragm is contracted, it forms a horizontal plane supporting the rectum, vagina, and urethra.

The puborectalis lies beneath the point of origin of the pubococcygeus and the neighboring obturator fascia and deep fascia. It lies along the lateral aspect of the urethra, vagina, and rectum, inferior to the pubococcygeus. The U-shaped puborectalis muscle encircles the posterior aspect of the rectum, then returns along the opposite side of the levator hiatus to the posterior surface of the pubis. Besides providing support to the pelvic floor, vagina, and bladder neck, the puborectalis muscle also serves as a sling holding the rectum forward and providing continence control to the terminal colon.

Along with the pubococcygeus, the puborectalis muscle affixes firmly to the vagina and to the mid-portion of the urethra to provide support. Fibers from both the pubococcygeus and the puborectalis muscles send decussations to attach to the perineal body.

This pelvic diaphragm, then, is composed mainly of the pubococcygeus and coccygeus muscles, reinforced inferiorly by the puborectalis. The levator muscles contract in response to intra-abdominal pressure; the pelvic diaphragm acts as a trampoline to prevent descent of the intra-abdominal viscera. The musculature is penetrated by the urethra, vagina, and rectum, which form a central hiatus in the pelvic floor, weakening the muscular support to the pelvis.

The weakest external portion of the pelvic floor receives additional support from the urogenital diaphragm (Fig. 24–2). The musculofascial diaphragm, also known as the triangular ligament, is composed of two layers of fascia, deep and superficial. The fascial layers surround a number of supporting skeletal muscles lying within the triangular area formed by the ischial tuberosities and the inferior rami of the symphysis pubis. Within the deep fascial layer are fat, loose connective tissue, and thin, deep transverse perinei muscles. Within the superficial layer lie the superficial transverse perinei muscles, and the ischiocavernosus and bulbocavernosus muscles.

The superficial transverse perineal muscles arise from each ischial tuberosity and insert into the midline of the perineum, posterior to the vaginal introitus. The bulbocavernosus muscles arise from the midline of the perineal body, pass over the vestibular bulb and Bartholin's gland along each side of

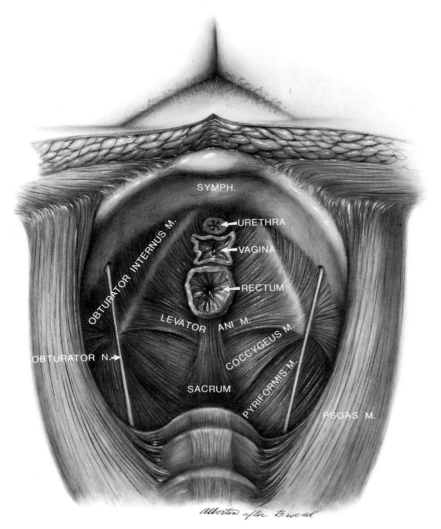

URETHRA

VAGINA

RECTUM

OBTURATOR INTERNUS M.

LEVATOR ANI M.

COCCYGEUS M.

OBTURATOR N.

SACRUM

PYRIFORMIS M.

PSOAS M.

Alberton after Broedel

FIG. 24–1 Muscular structures forming the pelvic floor in the female.

the vagina, and insert into the inferior crus of the clitoris.

The vaginal canal creates a central defect between the medial aspect of the levator muscles, and it also separates the muscles of the urogenital diaphragm into pairs. The bulbocavernosus muscles may be considered as the superficial vaginal constrictors; the levator muscles are the deep constrictors. All of the urogenital muscles are covered with fascia, which is visible during dissection in a perineal repair.

The vagina is a musculomembranous, tubal structure, extending from the cervix to the vulva. The outer orifice, the introitus, has the smallest caliber; above this, the vagina is relatively roomy. The vaginal canal, which measures approximately 8.5 cm in length in the nulliparous patient, is covered with stratified squamous epithelium. The epithelial lining is quite thin before puberty and after the menopause, and is referred to, erroneously, as a mucous membrane, because it is lubricated with mucus from the cervix and has a moist surface. During the menstrual life of a woman, the epithelial lining is much thicker and is thrown up into transverse folds or rugae.

Beneath the epithelium of the vagina are two layers of smooth muscle, an outer longitudinal and an inner circular, that are surrounded externally by the perivaginal portion of the endopelvic fascia. The fascia extends from the symphysis pubis, passes beneath the bladder, and is inserted in the anterior surface of the cervix at the level of the internal os. The endopelvic fascia is the same pubovesicocervical fascia utilized in a cystocele repair. A posterior

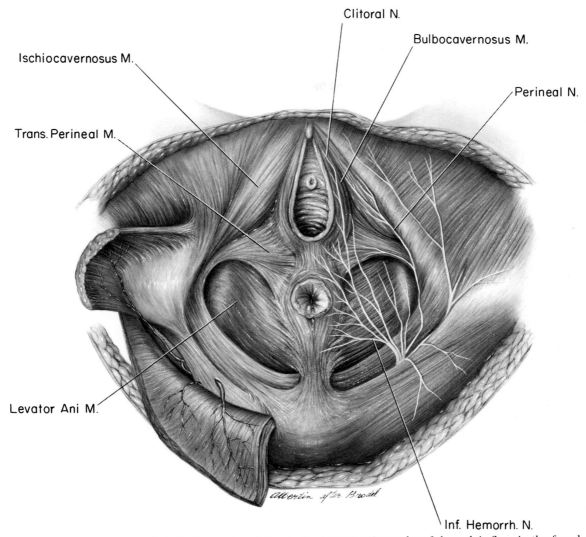

Clitoral N.

Bulbocavernosus M.

Ischiocavernosus M.

Perineal N.

Trans. Perineal M.

Levator Ani M.

Inf. Hemorrh. N.

FIG. 24–2 Urogenital diaphragm in relation to the levator ani muscles of the pelvic floor in the female.

extension of the endopelvic fascia between the rectum and vagina is utilized in a rectocele repair, although it is more attenuated and less sturdy than the anterior fascia.

The upper posterior 2 cm to 3 cm of the vagina lie in close proximity to the cul-de-sac of Douglas. Recent studies by Kuhn and Hollyock demonstrated that the base of the cul-de-sac pouch could be extended with a probe to the junction of the upper and middle third of the vagina in 93% of the patients studied. The depth of the cul-de-sac measured more than 5 cm from the lower uterine segment to the upper third of the vagina, where it separated the rectum from the vagina. If the peritoneal sac extends deeper into the rectovaginal space, it forms a peritoneal pouch, or enterocele, within which the small bowel may protrude into the vagina.

Below the level of the cul-de-sac, the vagina is separated from the rectal wall by an attenuated layer of endopelvic fascia, which forms the rectovaginal septum. At this point, weakening of the levator muscle attachment occurs, making the middle one-third of the posterior vaginal wall the most susceptible to rectocele formation should the rectum descend through the widened levator hiatus.

At the lower end of the vaginal canal, the rectum diverges due to the interdigitating muscles of the external anal sphincter and the perineal body. The perineum is formed by the union of the levator ani muscles with the bulbocavernosus and superficial transverse perinei muscles. The lowermost portion of the rectum constitutes the anal canal, which measures 2 cm to 3 cm in length. The anal canal is supported in three ways: by the external, striated sphincter muscles, including the puborectalis; by both the superficial and the deep transverse perineal muscles; and by the inferior margins of the bulbocavernosus muscles.

When the musculofascial support between the rectum and vagina weakens (including the decussating fibers of the puborectalis and pubococcygeus muscles), the cul-de-sac of Douglas deepens, and widening of the levator hiatus permits both rectocele and enterocele formation (Fig. 24–3). One of the principal mechanisms of stretching, weakening, and, often, tearing of the fascia and muscles of the pelvic floor is trauma from the descent of the infant's head through the pelvic diaphragm. Prolonged pressure of the child's head between the muscles of the pelvic floor, particularly during a prolonged second-stage of labor, weakens the rectovaginal and vesicovaginal septa. Strenuous work, straining at stool, multiple pregnancies, aging, and the orthostatic pressure of the pelvic viscera against the pelvic floor are other factors that may produce weakening of the musculofascial support, eventually causing rectocele and enterocele formation.

If an episiotomy or perineal laceration is not adequately repaired, the posterior part of the urogenital diaphragm, including the superficial transverse perinei and bulbocavernosus muscles, remains separated. Separation of the perineal attachment of the levator muscles will produce a widening of the hiatus in the pelvic diaphragm and an elongation of the puborectalis sling that holds the rectum forward at the rectal neck. Since the puborectalis also serves as one of the voluntary (striated) muscles of the anal sphincter, weakening of the puborectalis muscle may cause subsequent anal incontinence.

Trauma to the perineal body may be either complete, extending through the underlying, multi-layered anal sphincter and producing varying degrees of anal incontinence, or partial, in which case the damaged perineum may retain only a thin layer of weak connective tissue and muscle fibers. If the perineal tear extends through the rectovaginal septum, it is defined as a fourth-degree vaginal laceration.

When the levator ani muscles are seriously weakened and the levator hiatus is widened, shortening and posterior deflection of the levator plate (Fig. 24–4) may cause the cul-de-sac of Douglas to deepen and permit the development of an enterocele between the rectum and the posterior vaginal wall.

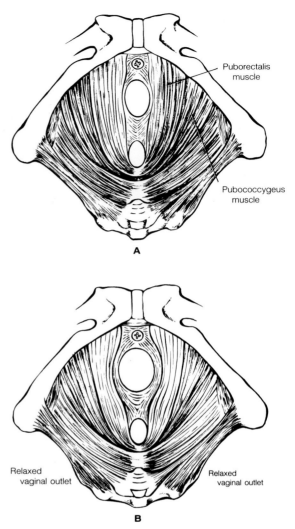

FIG. 24–3 (*A*) Perineal view of levator ani, showing the central hiatus in pelvic floor produced by penetration of urethra, vagina, and rectum. Note the decussations of levator fibers that pass between the rectum and vagina and support the hiatus. (*B*) Schematic illustration of a widened levator hiatus, showing separation of decussating fibers of the levator ani from the perineal body and the margins of the pelvic portal and shortening of the levator plate between the rectum and coccyx.

In severe cases, the enterocele may extend along the entire length of the rectovaginal septum between the vagina and the anterior rectal wall. With the passage of time, all physical activity that increases intra-abdominal pressure will contribute to the development of an enterocele by causing the peritoneal sac to dissect deeper into the area between the rectum and the vagina, where the fascia is anatomically thin and separates easily (Fig. 24–5).

Relaxed Vaginal Outlet With Rectocele

Although the terms relaxed vaginal outlet and rectocele are frequently used synonymously, each condition represents a separate anatomical entity. The conditions usually occur together in patients with significant pelvic floor relaxation, but may occur separately. Both a relaxed vaginal outlet and a rectocele may be entirely asymptomatic, requiring no treatment.

Simple relaxation of the vaginal outlet due to thinning and separation of the muscles of the perineal body is more often asymptomatic than is a rectocele. A relaxed outlet is often a contributing factor when increasing pelvic pressure is associated with uterine descensus. If either the relaxed outlet or uterine descensus requires surgical repair, both should be corrected. If a relaxed outlet exists with a symptomatic cystocele, with or without rectocele, the entire posterior vaginal wall and the perineum should be repaired along with the cystocele.

Patients often blame unsatisfactory sexual relations on the relaxed conditions of the perineum and vagina, specifically the loss of support from the bulbocavernosus, the transverse perinei, and the levator ani muscles. Complaints may originate from the patient or from her husband. Coital inadequacy may be dependent upon the degree of relaxation

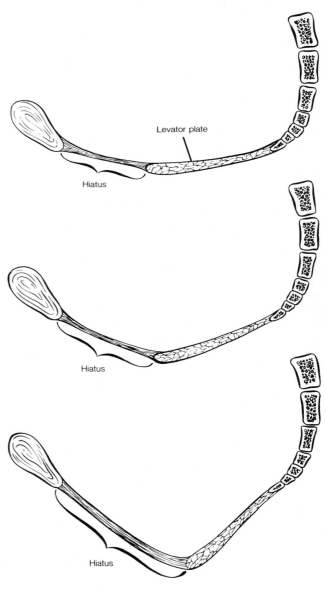

FIG. 24–4 Sagittal view of pelvic floor, showing posterior rotation of the levator plate and consequent enlargement of the levator hiatus.

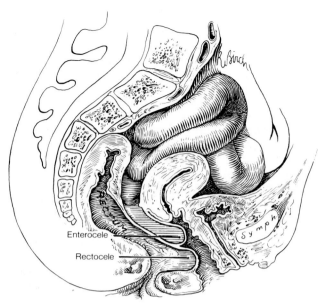

Enterocele

Rectocele

FIG. 24–5 Sagittal section of pelvis, showing relative position of rectocele and enterocele.

of the vaginal outlet and can be one of the secondary indications for perineorrhaphy, but it is rarely caused entirely by local anatomical conditions. More frequently, coital problems signal marital incompatibility, or result from increasing age and stress. The entire marital relationship should be evaluated before sexual improvement from vaginal plastic surgery is promised. As emphasized by Jeffcoate and others, dyspareunia is a frequent complication of an extensive posterior colporrhaphy and perineorrhaphy; such sexual complications could result in further deterioration of a tenuous sexual relationship.

REPAIR OF RELAXED VAGINAL OUTLET AND RECTOCELE

One of the most common complaints in women over the age of 50 is dyspareunia. This is a result of a reduction in plasma estrogen levels during the postmenopausal period that causes the vaginal epithelium to become thin and sensitive. Postmenopausal hormonal changes may lead to varying degrees of contracture of the vaginal outlet, particularly in nulliparous women and in women who have had previous perineal surgery. The eventual effects of estrogen depletion must always be considered when a vaginal repair is being planned.

The repair of a relaxed vaginal outlet and the repair of a rectocele are two distinct operative pro-

cedures. If both conditions are present they are usually repaired together. A perineal repair is often done when a rectocele is not present, whereas only occasionally does a rectocele require repair in a woman whose vaginal outlet has been well supported from a previous episiotomy.

The urogenital musculature is not visible during perineal surgery, because the muscles are ensheathed in fascia. The fascia is not dissected from the muscles because the firmest union is obtained by the healing of fascia to fascia.

Plastic surgery on the posterior vagina does not begin with a preconceived idea of the exact type of operation that will be done. Only after the vagina has been dissected, after the size and the position of the rectocele have been defined, and after the presence or the absence of an enterocele has been determined, can the surgeon make a final decision about the type and extent of operation that is required. A few standard procedures are described here, with the understanding that variations in technique must be made to fit the individual case.

Technique of Simple Perineal Repair

The ultimate size of the vaginal orifice is determined by placing Allis clamps on the inner aspect of the labia minora, along both sides of the outlet, and approximating them in the midline. The clamps should be adjusted so that the final vaginal opening will admit three fingers easily, taking into account that the levator ani and perineal muscles are completely relaxed from the general anesthesia, and that postmenopausal shrinkage may further contract the introitus.

A slightly curved, transverse incision is made posteriorly at the mucocutaneous junction connecting the two lateral Allis clamps (Fig. 24–6A). Making the incision over the perineal body toward the anus in a V-shaped fashion to a point on the perineum that is 1 cm to 2 cm from the anus provides better access to the perineal muscles by dissecting the skin overlying the posterior fourchette (Fig. 24–6B).

The mucosa of the vaginal introitus is dissected upward by blunt and sharp dissection (Fig. 24–6C). The dissection is carried only high enough to expose the fascia covering the levator muscles and to permit placing of the levator sutures, since the simple procedure does not include rectocele repair. The vaginal dissection is made vertically in the midline, placing an Allis clamp at the apex of the incision to elevate the vaginal wall (Fig. 24–6C). The vaginal mucosa is incised in an inverted V-shaped manner, with traction placed on the apex clamp. As the vaginal mucosa is dissected free from the underlying fascia, it is opened in the midline, then the excess vaginal mucosa is excised (Fig. 24–6C). Excision of a

V-shaped wedge prevents pouching of excessive tissue when the vaginal mucosa is sutured.

Interrupted stitches of No. 0 delayed-absorbable suture are placed through the pararectal fascia and levator ani muscles (Fig. 24–6D). The muscle fibers need not be exposed before placing these sutures; bold lateral stitches should include a large medial portion of the muscle mass in each bite. The number of stitches taken in the levator muscles varies, depending on the degree of relaxation and the amount of perineal support that is needed. In the average case, two or three sutures are sufficient.

Starting at the top of the incision, the vaginal mucosa is closed in the midline, using a continuous lock-stitch of No. 0 suture. When the levator region is reached, the muscles are approximated by tying the previously placed sutures (Fig. 24–6E).

The diameter of the vaginal introitus must be evaluated carefully after the levator sutures are tied. If the introitus is found to be too small, the offending suture(s) should be removed or replaced until the diameter is satisfactory. Supporting sutures are then placed in the superficial fascia. Using a small cutting needle, the mucosal suture is continued over the perineal body as a subcuticular midline stitch.

Technique of Repair of Moderate-sized Rectocele

As with a simple repair, the degree of closure of the relaxed outlet is determined before an incision is initiated at the lateral mucocutaneous border of the introitus and continued along the anterior surface of the perineal body in a V-shaped fashion to the region of the anal margin. The dissected perineal skin is excised horizontally along the vaginal outlet.

A midline vertical incision is initiated in the center of the mucosal edge by tunneling beneath the posterior mucosa with Metzenbaum scissors, incising the freed mucosa in the midline, and extending the dissection to the apex of the vagina (Fig. 24–7A). In a manner similar to an anterior repair, traction is placed on the upper margin of each segment of the mucosal dissection using an Allis clamp. The lower margins of the incision are held under tension with additional clamps while the mucosa is separated with Metzenbaum scissors from the underlying fascia. When the midline incision is completed, the vaginal mucosa is separated laterally from the pararectal fascia and muscle attachments by sharp dissection, taking care to avoid penetrating the thin mucosa (Fig. 24–7B). The lateral dissection should be extended as far as possible to mobilize the pararectal fascia and to expose the medial margins of the levator ani muscles. The terminal ends of the bulbocavernosus and transverse perinei muscles are also freed from the adherent mucosa in the lower vagina.

The pararectal fascia is then drawn over the bulging rectocele, using as many vertical mattress sutures of No. 0 delayed-absorbable suture as are necessary to reinforce and completely close the hernial space over the rectal wall (Fig. 24–7C). Interrupted stitches of No. 1 delayed-absorbable suture are placed deeply in the margins of the levator muscles, approximating the muscles and fascia sufficiently over the lower rectal wall to produce the desired support to the perineal body and posterior vaginal wall (Fig. 24–7D).

Although it is usually difficult to advance the levators over the entire posterior vagina, the plicated pararectal fascia will provide firm fascial support over the upper portion of the rectocele. By plicating the levator muscles in the midline, the levator hiatus is narrowed, providing additional support to the relaxed pelvic floor.

After any extra vaginal mucosa has been excised, the margins are closed, beginning at the apex of the vagina. This is done with a continuous lock stitch of No. 0 suture, incorporating the underlying fascia with a running suture to obliterate the dead space between vaginal wall and rectum (Fig. 24–7E). When the continuous mucosal suture reaches the levator muscles, the deep interrupted stitches are tied.

Excessive constriction of the vagina and introitus with the levator sutures must be avoided. If there is evidence that the diameter of the vagina or of the outlet is too small, the levator sutures should be removed and replaced until a satisfactory diameter is achieved (Fig. 24–8A).

After a few supporting plication sutures are placed in the fascia and underlying muscles of the perineal body, the mucosal suture is continued over the perineum as a subcuticular stitch, using a small curved cutting needle. The perineal muscle sutures, which include the lower margins of the bulbocavernosus and the transverse perinei muscles, give support to the levator hiatus and pelvic floor (Fig. 24–8B).

Technique of Repair of High Rectocele

To make certain that a rectal hernia through the relaxed levator hiatus is adequately repaired, the full length of the rectovaginal wall should be dissected out and the musculofascial repair should be performed along the entire posterior vaginal wall, whether the rectocele is of moderate size or is more extensive. The upper portion of the rectovaginal fascia is the weakest, and failure to obtain a perfect restoration of the posterior vaginal wall usually results when an inherent musculofascial weakness in the upper aspect of the wall is not recognized. Differentiation between a high rectocele and enterocele may be difficult or even impossible until

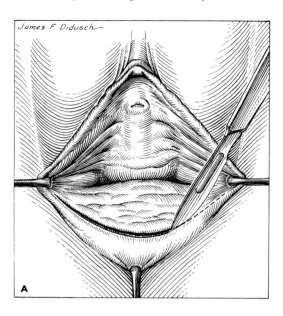

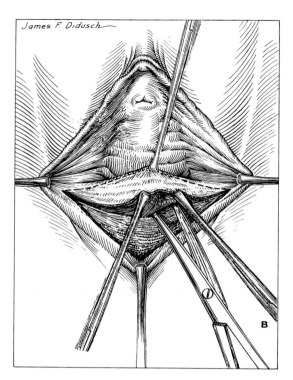

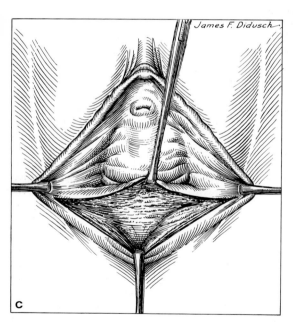

FIG. 24–6 Simple perineal repair. (*A*) An incision is made at the mucocutaneous border along the perineal body. (*B*) Alternatively, a V-shaped incision is made over the perineal body toward the anus. The dotted line indicates the line of incision of the upper flap. (*C*) The flap includes an inverted V-shaped piece of mucosa that has been excised.

the entire posterior wall is dissected to the apex of the vagina.

The repair of a high rectocele should be approached like any other posterior colporrhaphy, with the midline mucosal incision extended to the apex of the vagina. By this technique, the pararectal

fascia is identified and separated from the vaginal mucosa by sharp dissection, and mobilized as far laterally as possible, avoiding the adjacent inferior hemorrhoidal vessels. From the vaginal apex, protrusion of an additional hernial sac can be determined easily. The small bowel usually fills an en-

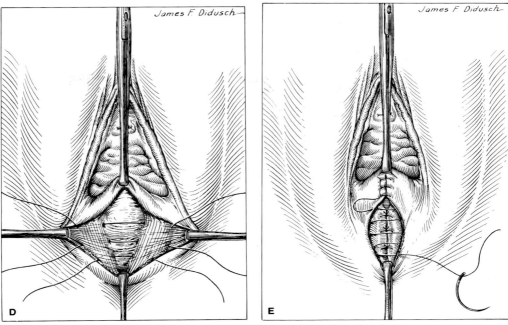

FIG. 24–6 (continued). (*D*) Three interrupted sutures have been placed in the levator ani muscles. (*E*) The levator muscles have been approximated. The mucosa has been closed with a lock stitch of No. 0 delayed-absorbable suture, and the perineal skin is being approximated with a subcuticular stitch.

terocele sac, providing a clear demarcation of the margins of the attenuated cul-de-sac peritoneum.

If no enterocele protrudes, the freed margins of the pararectal fascia are plicated with interrupted vertical mattress sutures of No. 0 delayed-absorbable suture material, making certain that the anterior rectal wall is displaced with a Kelly clamp while the sutures are tied in the midline. This series of plication sutures is best started at the apex of the vagina, where the initial suture may be anchored to the supporting tissues of the vaginal vault so that the entire hernial defect can be closed. The fascial sutures are placed in succession until the margins of the levator ani muscles can be approximated in the midline, adding further muscular support to the pelvic floor and the rectocele repair (Fig. 24–8A). The remainder of the repair follows the procedure for perineal closure.

Enterocele

Although intestinal hernias protruding through the cul-de-sac of Douglas do not occur as often as either rectal or bladder hernias (rectocele or cystocele), they must be recognized and corrected surgically for treatment to be completed successfully. An enterocele that remains unrecognized will usually appear following a hysterectomy, causing pelvic pressure and discomfort.

An enterocele that follows a hysterectomy, known as a pulsion enterocele, may appear as a result of tissue weakness caused by ischemia and necrosis at the distal ends of excised ligaments tied *en masse* during vaginal or abdominal hysterectomy. In many cases, the patient has had a previous rectocele repair. Patients complain of a mass protruding from the vaginal outlet when they stand or strain. The mass, usually bowel or omentum, will disappear when the patient lies down. The large neck of the cul-de-sac allows the bowel contents to slip in and out easily, usually without intestinal strangulation.

Like most hernias, the enterocele has an embryologic factor in its formation. During the development of the vagina, following the fusion of the müllerian ducts with the urogenital sinus, the cul-de-sac peritoneum is located deep between the rectum and the developing vagina. As the vaginal plate cannulates into the vaginal canal, the peritoneum regresses and the rectovaginal septum becomes fused. Although the cul-de-sac is commonly located in the upper one-third of the vagina, approximately 5 cm from the origin of the uterosacral ligament on the lower uterine segment, the embryologic attachment of the cul-de-sac peritoneum

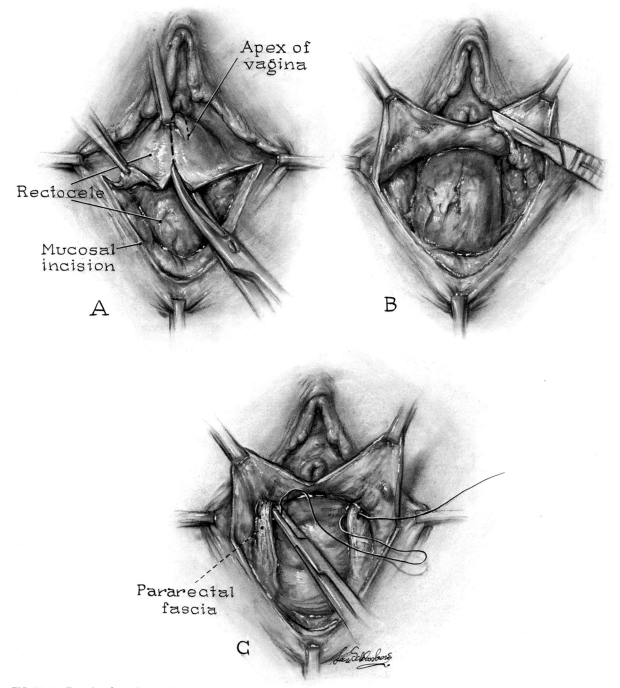

FIG. 24–7 Repair of moderate-sized rectocele. (*A*) A V-shaped incision is made from angles of introitus over perineal body; midline vertical incision extends to apex of vagina. (*B*) Pararectal fascia is separated from mucosa by sharp dissection and (*C*) plicated over anterior wall of rectum.

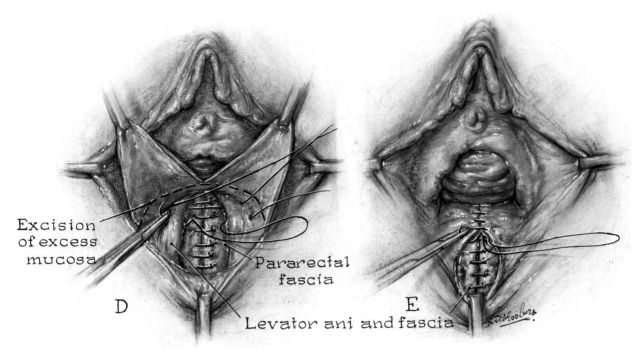

Excision of excess mucosa

Pararectal fascia

D

E

Levator ani and fascia

FIG. 24–7 (continued). (D) Levator ani muscles are approximated in the midline with deep sutures of No. 0 or 1 delayed-absorbable material. The excess vaginal mucosa is excised and the margins are closed (E) with either an interrupted or continuous suture.

to the vaginal septum can, and does, occur at a lower level, producing a deep peritoneal pouch. A congenitally deep cul-de-sac can serve as a wedge by which the small bowel dissects down into the space between the posterior vaginal wall and the anterior surface of the rectum.

The most important acquired factor promoting the formation of an enterocele is prolapse of the uterus. With progressive descent of the uterus, the cul-de-sac is pulled through the levator hiatus, deep into the vaginal canal. Intra-abdominal pressure extends the herniation, called a traction enterocele, further down.

Enteroceles are frequently misdiagnosed as high rectoceles, in spite of basic differences. The contents of an enterocele are small bowel, not rectum. Attempting a cure by performing a rectocele operation at an unusually high level without separately identifying the enterocele will not provide adequate treatment.

When an enterocele occurs, as it commonly does, in association with a rectocele, the diagnosis can be made by inspection, since the division between the two types of herniation is indicated by a transverse furrow just above the rectocele (Fig. 24–5). A finger inserted into the rectum will demonstrate the rectocele as distinct from the bulging sac that arises from a higher point. By compressing the enterocele on rectovaginal exam, it is usually possible to identify and displace small bowel in the hernial sac.

Diagnosis can be facilitated by examining the rectovaginal septum and cul-de-sac while the patient stands with one foot on a low stool, knees bent slightly, and straining by a Valsalva maneuver. Transillumination of the rectovaginal septum through the rectum does not provide enough information to warrant its use, especially since the procedure is intolerable for the patient.

REPAIR OF ENTEROCELE

After an enterocele has been diagnosed, surgical correction proceeds as for other types of hernia: isolation and complete dissection of the sac, removal of the visceral contents, excision of the sac, closure of the musculofascial defect through which the sac leaves the pelvic floor, and addition of fascial support to the closed anatomical defect. The choice of surgical technique depends upon what other conditions exist in association with the enterocele.

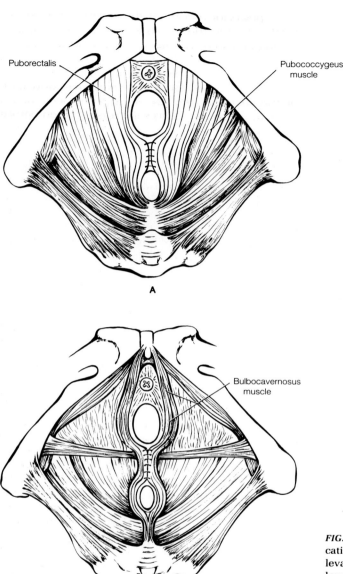

Puborectalis

Pubococcygeus muscle

A

Bulbocavernosus muscle

B

FIG. 24–8 (*A*) Schematic representation of the effect of plication of levator ani muscles in reducing the aperture of the levator hiatus, as viewed from the perineum. (*B*) Plication of lower margins of bulbocavernosus and transverse perinei muscles strengthens the support of the urogenital diaphragm and the pelvic floor.

For example, an enterocele encountered while performing a pelvic laparotomy may be closed intra-abdominally by a succession of concentric purse-string sutures, starting at the bottom of the cul-de-sac, as described by Moschcowitz for cure of rectal prolapse (Fig. 24–9). When a small pulsion enterocele occurs through the vaginal vault after a vaginal or abdominal hysterectomy, the sac is dissected and completely excised through the vagina. High ligation of the sac is accomplished by placing No. 1 delayed-absorbable or No. 0 silk sutures high along the circumference of the cul-de-sac peritoneum on the *inside* of the levator hiatus. All the available ligaments and the redundant cul-de-sac peritoneum are brought together and sutured to the vaginal vault to give it support and also to secure closure of the hernial defect.

Repair of a small or medium-sized enterocele is often part of an extensive vaginal plastic procedure for a coexisting relaxed vaginal outlet that could also include rectocele, cystocele, and uterine descensus of varying degrees. The dissection and closure procedure is described as a posterior culdeplasty in Chapter 23 (see Fig. 23–13). Usually, two or three deep bites through the uterosacral ligaments and into the cul-de-sac peritoneum will suffice to completely obliterate the site of a small or medium-sized enterocele formation. The procedure can be preventive or corrective when combined with a vaginal hysterectomy.

When a pulsion enterocele causes massive inversion of the vagina following a hysterectomy, there is insufficient ligamentous or fascial support within the levator ani diastasis to permit adequate repair by the usual vaginal approach. An abdominal colposacropexy provides a more permanent repair, using a mersilene gauze graft or an autogenous graft of rectus fascia to anchor the vault to the third or fourth sacral vertebra. Dura mater procured from autopsy sources has been used recently as an effective, lasting graft; it does not cause tissue reaction.

A very large traction enterocele accompanying total uterine procidentia requires a combined abdominoperineal procedure to place the prolapsed vagina over the levator plate and anchor the vault to the sacral vertebrae. An alternative method of repair is a sacrospinous ligament fixation of the vagina. The wide diastasis of the levator hiatus created by massive inversion of the vagina requires a surgical approach that is very different from that for the usual small enterocele.

Technique of Vaginal Repair of Small to Moderate Enterocele

A midline incision is made posteriorly as in a posterior colporrhaphy. A tunnel is made by inserting the curved Metzenbaum scissors beneath the vaginal mucosa and successively opening and closing the scissors, then incising the vagina in the midline. The process of tunneling and cutting is repeated until the apex of the vagina is reached. The vaginal wall is dissected laterally on either side to expose first a rectocele, if one is present, and then the enterocele, which appears as a peritoneal pouch.

Using blunt and sharp dissection, the enterocele sac is dissected free (Fig. 24–9A). A purse-string suture of No. 0 silk or delayed-absorbable suture material is placed on the outside of the sac at the neck. Then the sac is opened and a similar purse-string suture is placed along the inside of the sac above the levator hiatus. An additional one or two purse-string sutures placed above the initial suture and incorporating the uterosacral ligaments will provide support to the hernial repair. The purse-string sutures are tied, and the margins of the sac are trimmed.

The posterior margin of the vagina is pulled forward, placing the uterosacral ligaments under maximal tension. The ligaments are approximated in the midline with two or three interrupted sutures that bite into the stump of the ligated hernial sac (Fig. 24–9B). The tied sutures make a firm new base for the cul-de-sac (Fig. 24–9C). If a rectocele or relaxed vaginal outlet is present, it is repaired before closure.

Technique of Abdominal Repair of Enterocele (Moschcowitz Operation)

The Moschcowitz operation, which was originally devised for cure of rectal prolapse, may also be used for repairing a well-developed enterocele, specifically when this is associated with other pelvic conditions requiring a laparotomy or abdominal hysterectomy. If an unsuspected enterocele is discovered during surgery, the hernial site should be closed. Left unrepaired, the defect will enlarge with increasing age and with decreased muscular support of the pelvic diaphragm.

The patient is placed in the Trendelenburg position, and the intestines are held back in the abdominal cavity by a gauze pack. If the uterus is retained, it is held up and forward with a traction suture (Fig. 24–10). If the uterus has been removed, the posterior wall of the vaginal vault is held under traction with Allis clamps.

Beginning at the base of the sac, a purse-string suture is placed, using medium No. 0 silk to encircle the cul-de-sac of Douglas, picking up the peritoneum only, and biting very lightly into the serosa of the rectum. Successive purse-string sutures are placed, and when the region of the uterosacral ligaments is reached, good firm bites are taken through the ligaments and into the posterior surface of the vagina. The number of concentric purse-string sutures depends upon the depth of the cul-de-sac; the last, highest suture should be tied without undue tension. Usually three or four sutures will completely obliterate the anatomical defect (Fig. 24–10).

Care should be taken to avoid including the ureters in the purse-string suture. The ureters may be catheterized before the operation so that they can be identified easily by palpation, but this is not necessary if one is careful to include only the peritoneum in each stitch taken in the ureteral region.

Prevention and Repair of Enterocele in Connection with Vaginal Hysterectomy

Prevention or repair of an enterocele should be considered specifically in connection with vaginal hysterectomy, since the procedure is performed so frequently. Choice of techniques depends on

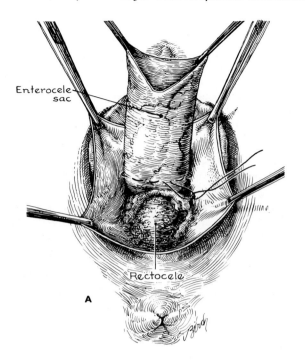

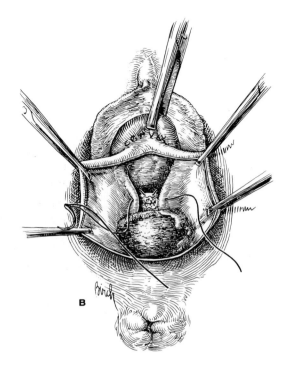

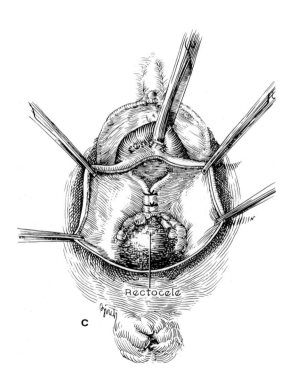

FIG. 24–9 Repair of enterocele. (*A*) A perineal incision has been made as in an operation for a rectocele. The posterior vaginal wall mucosa is divided in the midline up to the cervix. The sac of the peritoneum has been dissected out completely, then opened, and the contents pushed into the peritoneal cavity. A purse-string of No. 1 absorbable suture has been placed about the neck of the sac. Two or more such purse-string sutures are desirable. (*B*) Uterosacral ligaments that have been exposed are approximated with No. 1 delayed-absorbable sutures. The first suture bites into the posterior surface of the cervix, if present, and also the retracted neck of the sac. (*C*) The uterosacral ligaments are sutured together in the midline.

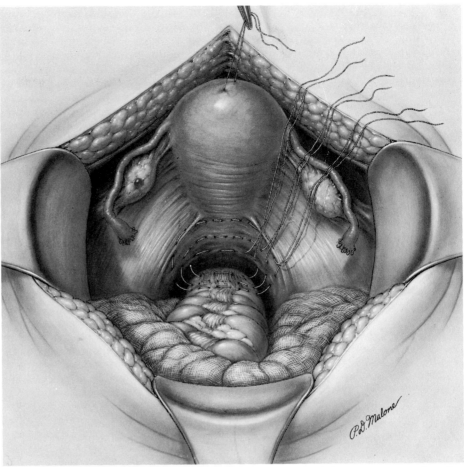

FIG. 24–10 Transabdominal method of obliteration of deep cul-de-sac or enterocele, using multiple concentric purse strings (Moschcowitz procedure).

whether the objective at the time of the hysterectomy is to prevent the development of an enterocele from a normal and from a deep cul-de-sac, or to repair a small or medium-sized enterocele associated with a well-developed rectocele.

Enteroceles that develop following a vaginal hysterectomy are usually the result of inadequate obliteration of the cul-de-sac at the time of the surgery. The space is best obliterated at the completion of the hysterectomy, when the cul-de-sac peritoneum is sutured between the uterosacral ligaments using No. 0 delayed-absorbable suture. When the sutures are tied, the space at the apex of the cul-de-sac is completely obliterated. This technique is illustrated in Chapter 23, in the section on vaginal hysterectomy. When there is a deep cul-de-sac, the redundant peritoneum is sutured to the uterosacral ligaments. The stitch is repeated two or three times

until all of the potential hernia space in the cul-de-sac is obliterated.

When either a relaxed vaginal outlet or a rectocele requires repair at the time of vaginal hysterectomy, an examination should be done to determine whether an occult enterocele is present. Frequently, this cannot be done until the posterior cul-de-sac has been opened. If an enterocele is identified, the peritoneum should be closed with a series of purse-string sutures into the uterosacral ligaments and redundant peritoneum, as described in the procedure for obliterating potential hernia space. The enterocele must be dissected free from the rectocele and closed separately. Then the rectocele and the relaxed outlet can be repaired.

In 1957, McCall described an operation for enterocele that he claimed would prevent shortening of the vagina: "a posterior culdeplasty whereby the relaxed cul-de-sac of Douglas is suspended and obliterated between the uterosacral ligaments without dissection of, or excision of, the hernia sac." Although the usual procedure for enterocele repair does shorten the vagina to some degree, few patients complain of this as a problem. McCall's technique is best applied after vaginal hysterectomy as a prophylactic measure to insure against the subsequent development of an enterocele. The procedure is particularly beneficial for a patient who has demonstrable evidence of herniation of the pelvic diaphragm with uterine descent and vaginal wall relaxation. In any enterocele repair accompanying a vaginal hysterectomy or colporrhaphy, the uterosacral ligaments and redundant cul-de-sac peritoneum should be plicated as high as possible to insure against recurrence.

Abdominal Colposacropexy for Large Enterocele and Inversion of Vaginal Vault

Inversion of the vaginal vault and vaginal prolapse is an uncommon complication of either abdominal or vaginal hysterectomy, occurring in less than 0.5% of all cases. The basic anatomical defect results from a widened levator hiatus and attenuated levator plate, which first causes uterine prolapse. Since vaginal procedures are used far more frequently than abdominal hysterectomy for uterine prolapse,

vaginal hysterectomy is the common antecedent of prolapse complications.

Normally, the upper 3 cm to 4 cm of the vagina lies in a horizontal plane when the patient is in the upright position. The horizontal portion of the vagina rests on the rectum, which in turn is supported by the pelvic diaphragm.

Berglas and Rubin (1953) were among the first to demonstrate by intramuscular injection of radiopaque contrast media into the levator plate that the rectum and upper vagina were located over the levator plate in a near-horizontal position. Their studies also confirmed radiographically that when uterine procedentia occurred, the weakened levator plate deflected posteriorly and failed to support the rectum and vagina, which then descended through a dilated levator portal. Richter, and later Nichols, demonstrated the same anatomical abnormalities in the levator plate. In more recent studies, Funt, Thompson, and Birch showed with vaginograms that the lower vagina has an oblique course and meets the upper horizontal portion of the vagina at a 130-degree angle (Fig. 24–11).

The normal axis of the upper vagina is oriented on a horizontal plane that passes over the levator plate on alignment with the third or fourth sacral vertebra. In order to restore the normal axis of the prolapsed vaginal vault, the upper vagina should

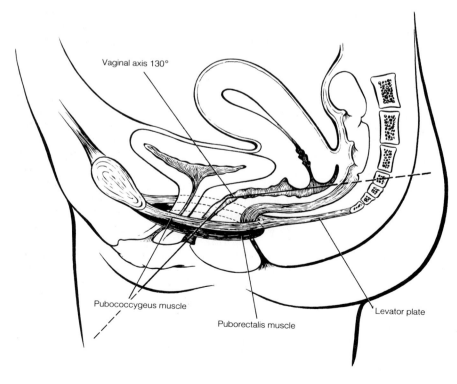

Vaginal axis 130°

Pubococcygeus muscle

Puborectalis muscle

Levator plate

FIG. 24–11 Normal axis of lower and upper vagina, which meet in a 130° angle. Upper one-third of vagina rests on the levator plate in a horizontal plane that passes through the 3rd or 4th sacral vertebra.

be repositioned over the levator plate. If the vault is held in this position, the intra-abdominal pressure will compress the vagina against the levator plate, which will assist in retaining the horizontal portion of the vagina as an intrapelvic organ.

Zacharin approaches the correction of vaginal prolapse by an abdominoperineal procedure. He closes the levator hiatus with interrupted, nonabsorbable sutures and anchors the vault to the levator plate. This combined procedure has yielded an 85% long-term success rate among patients who had multiple previous attempts at repair.

Symmonds prefers the vaginal repair of the prolapsed vault, which is resuspended to the uterosacral-cardinal ligaments after the large enterocele sac is excised and closed. His long-term cure rate approaches 87%, but the procedure has the definite disadvantage of producing significant shortening and narrowing of the vaginal canal, frequently prohibiting further coitus.

Amreich (1951) was one of the first to attach the vaginal vault to the sacrotuberous ligament by the sacral route. Since the sacrotuberous ligament was not accessible vaginally, Richter developed the technique of sacrospinous ligament suspension of the vault, which could be performed vaginally. Nichols and Randall soon adopted the sacrospinous technique as an alternative to abdominal suspension procedures.

Because the abdominal technique of colposacropexy is relatively simple, is successful, maintains vaginal depth, and restores the normal vaginal axis, the abdominal sacropexy operation is still the treatment of choice for massive inversion of the vaginal vault. Colposacropexy is always combined with a Moschcowitz closure of the deep pelvic hernia.

Usually, when vaginal prolapse occurs after either vaginal or abdominal hysterectomy, a residual cystocele, rectocele, or enterocele will also be found in various combinations. A well-preserved anterior and posterior vaginal wall may have a hernia defect at the vaginal vault through which an enterocele sac protrudes. A cystocele alone may be present with an intact poterior wall. A rectocele may be present with a well-supported bladder. In all of these cases, the restoration of the vagina to a semirigid tube greatly increases the chances for a lasting cure.

If a clear-cut enterocele develops, with or without rectocele, behind a well-supported anterior vaginal wall, the enterocele sac must be dissected and the cul-de-sac obliterated; then the rectocele can be repaired properly. This type of complication usually occurs after a vaginal hysterectomy and probably represents a potential enterocele that was neglected during surgery.

A moderate prolapse of the vaginal vault combined with enterocele, cystocele, and rectocele results from a general laxity of the urogenital musculofascial support. This combination usually can be cured by a vaginal procedure. The enterocele must be dissected with high ligation of the sac, the uterosacral ligaments must be approximated, and the uterosacral and the cardinal ligaments must be fixed to the vaginal vault as is done in a vaginal hysterectomy. Then appropriate anterior and posterior colporrhaphy should be done. If these procedures do not provide satisfactory vaginal support, an abdominal colposacropexy can be added. These vaginal procedures often result in some shortening and narrowing of the vagina.

The most difficult type of enterocele to repair is associated with complete vaginal inversion. Perhaps eversion would be a better descriptive term, for the entire vagina is everted from the introitus. These cases require an obliteration of the enterocele, a rebuilding of the anterior and the posterior vaginal walls, and a perineorrhaphy combined with an abdominal suspension of the vaginal vault (sacropexy procedure). Abdominal suspension alone may be quite satisfactory, if the tissues are adequate for support, and if the enterocele is corrected at the same time.

Several operations are useful, but the best procedure is the one appropriate for the individual case. Often a procedure must be improvised, requiring an open-minded surgeon willing to change the planned approach if necessary. Most procedures yield good immediate results; a few years of followup are required before the ultimate result can be evaluated.

Technique of Colposacropexy

The patient is initially placed in the dorsolithotomy position under anesthesia while the surgeon confirms the presence of the defect. If it is evident that the vaginal canal will require additional support after the vault has been repositioned, anterior and posterior colporrhaphy are deferred until the vaginal vault has been suspended. A posterior colporrhaphy including plication of the levator ani muscles is almost always required to provide additional support to the vagina and to the pelvic diaphragm.

Before initiating the abdominal procedure, the vaginal vault is distended with a pack, which gives form to the vault and simplifies the identification of the vaginal apex during pelvic dissection. The patient is placed in the lithotomy position, and an indwelling urethral catheter is used to drain the bladder. The abdomen is entered through a low midline abdominal incision.

An autogenous graft of rectus fascia provides an

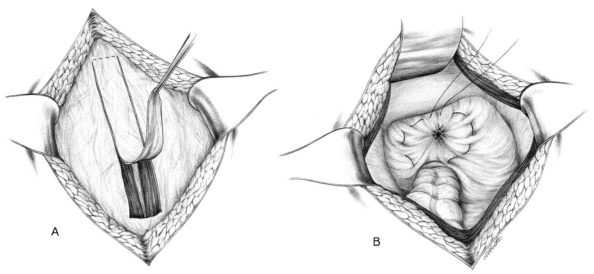

FIG. 24–12   Colposacropexy with use of autogenous fascial graft from anterior rectus sheath. Marlex mesh may also be used for the strap. (*A*) A 3 cm × 10 cm strip of fascia is excised in the midline on entering the abdomen. (*B*) Large enterocele is closed with a series of continuous purse-string sutures of No. 0 silk in the Moschcowitz procedure. Care should be taken to avoid kinking or obstructing the ureter.

excellent graft source if the anterior rectus sheath is of good quality. A strip of rectus fascia 2.5 cm to 3 cm in width is excised longitudinally for a length of 8 cm to 10 cm from the anterior surface of either rectus muscle (Fig. 24–12A). Marlex mesh is an alternative material that has proven to be permanent and nonreactive.

After the intestines have been packed into the upper abdomen, the base of the pelvis is carefully inspected, and the large hernia beneath the dilated levator hiatus is visualized. With the vagina distended by the vaginal pack, the enterocele can be identified separately from the apex of the vagina. The initial procedure is to close the pelvic hernia by the Moschcowitz procedure, using No. 0 silk suture. Three or four continuous, encircling purse-string sutures are placed from the deepest portion of the cul-de-sac to the region at the top of the vaginal vault (Fig. 24–12B). Care must be taken to avoid incorporating the ureter into the peritoneal suture.

After the hernial sac is closed, the angles of the distended vaginal vault are held with Allis clamps, and the bladder peritoneum is incised transversely across the apex of the vagina (Fig. 24–12C). The bladder base is then mobilized with sharp and blunt dissection, as is the cul-de-sac peritoneum and adjacent rectum, making certain that both the bladder base and the anterior wall of the rectum are displaced widely from the apex of the vagina (Fig. 24–12D).

The posterior parietal peritoneum overlying the sacrum is divided longitudinally, just medial to the rectosigmoid mesentery, over the region of the second, third, and fourth sacral vertebrae (Fig. 24–12E). Care must be taken to avoid trauma to the underlying middle sacral artery and veins that traverse this region. Should injury occur to these vessels, either vascular clips or direct pressure can be used to control bleeding. Pressure applied with a gauze sponge placed against the sacral vertebrae for a period of 3 to 5 minutes provides the most effective means of controlling venous bleeding in the middle sacral area. Bleeding from the middle sacral artery must be isolated and controlled by suture ligature or vascular clip.

With retraction of the sigmoid colon laterally, the third sacral vertebrae is identified, and the anterior sacral ligament is used for the placement of No. 0 Tevdek sutures. Three horizontal mattress sutures are placed through the top of the fascia graft or Mersiline mesh and the anterior sacral ligament (Fig. 24–12E,F). The graft should be trimmed to accommodate the anatomical space; any graft wider than 2.5 cm may cause compression on the medial aspect of the rectosigmoid colon. The graft is then positioned, without tension, to the apex of the vagina where three Tevdek or medium silk mattress sutures are placed in the vaginal wall and anchored to the angles and middle section of the graft (Fig. 24–12D,F).

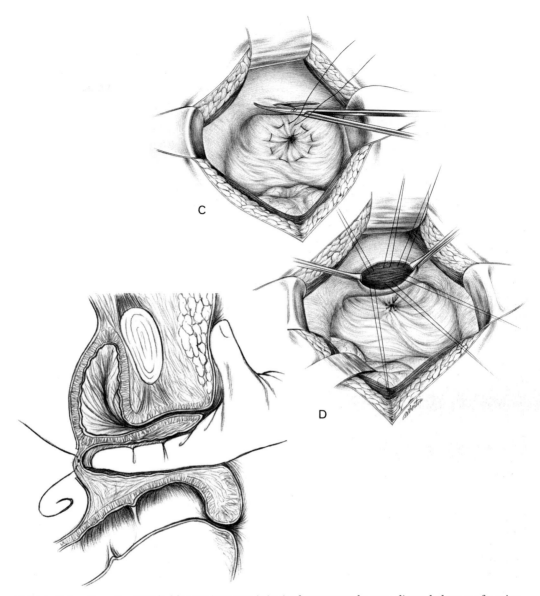

FIG. 24–12 (continued). (*C*) Bladder peritoneum is incised transversely over distended apex of vagina, after the last purse-string suture in the cul-de-sac is completed. (*D*) The surgeon's index and middle fingers are placed in the vagina to distend the vault and to guide the depth of suture placement (*insert*). Two rows of permanent suture, No. 0 Tevdek or No. 2-0 silk, are placed horizontally across the vault.

Before the sutures are placed in the vaginal vault, the vaginal pack is removed, and the right-handed surgeon places the fingers of the left hand in the vaginal vault. The surgeon's fingers serve as a guide for the proper depth of the vaginal vault sutures, making certain that the sutures do not penetrate the vaginal mucosa (Fig. 24–12D). After changing the contaminated glove and gown, if necessary the surgeon returns to the abdominal field for the remainder of the procedure.

A second row of horizontal mattress sutures may be used to strengthen the anastomosis of the graft to the vaginal vault. The sacral end of the graft should be sutured initially to the anterior sacral

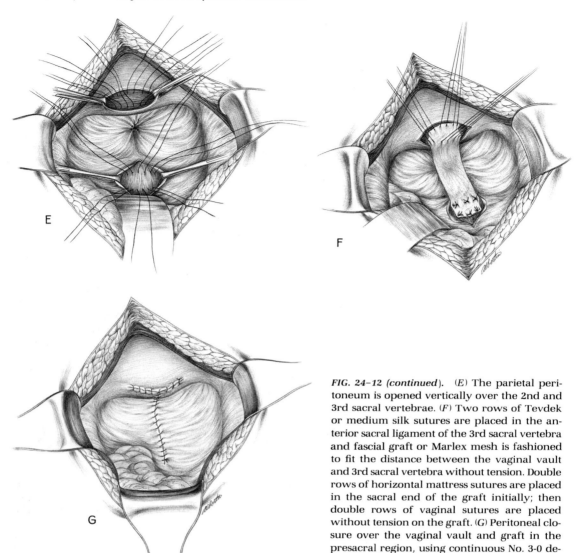

FIG. 24–12 (continued). (*E*) The parietal peritoneum is opened vertically over the 2nd and 3rd sacral vertebrae. (*F*) Two rows of Tevdek or medium silk sutures are placed in the anterior sacral ligament of the 3rd sacral vertebra and fascial graft or Marlex mesh is fashioned to fit the distance between the vaginal vault and 3rd sacral vertebra without tension. Double rows of horizontal mattress sutures are placed in the sacral end of the graft initially; then double rows of vaginal sutures are placed without tension on the graft. (*G*) Peritoneal closure over the vaginal vault and graft in the presacral region, using continuous No. 3-0 delayed-absorbable suture.

ligament, because exposure is difficult in this region. The vaginal portion of the graft can be easily attached to the vault without tension.

The bladder peritoneum is reapproximated to the cul-de-sac peritoneum with a continuous No. 3-0 delayed-absorbable suture, making certain that the graft is maintained in a retroperitoneal position. The presacral peritoneum is closed with a continuous lock-stitch of fine delayed-absorbable suture to control any residual capillary bleeding and to completely cover the entire graft (Fig. 24–12G).

Due to the loss of anatomical support to the bladder, vagina and rectum, in cases with a large diastasis of the levator muscles, the bladder neck also needs to be supported along with the pelvic floor and vaginal vault. A prophylactic Marshall–Marchetti–Krantz procedure can be performed to suspend the bladder neck and to avoid the possibility of straightening the urethrovesical junction by the sacropexy procedure. The Marshall–Marchetti–Krantz procedure is ideally suited for this type of anatomical correction and can be performed prior to closure of the abdominal wall.

At the completion of the abdominal procedure, the patient is replaced in the dorsolithotomy position and a high posterior colporrhaphy-perineorrhaphy is performed to strengthen the levator hiatus and to add considerable support to the vaginal

TABLE 24–1   *Treatment of Vault Prolapse*

STUDY (YEAR)	APPROACH	NUMBER OF PATIENTS	CURE
Symmonds (1965)	Colpocleisis/vaginectomy	16	9 (56%)
Birnbaum (1973)	Colposacropey	21	20 (95%)
Zacharin (1980)	Levator plication—vault fixation	66	56 (85%)
Symmonds (1981)	Uterosacral-cardinal ligament suspension	160	140 (87%)
Nichols (1982)	Sacrospinous fixation	163	158 (97%)
Mattingly (1982)	Moschcowitz-colposacropexy	55	53 (97%)
Richter (1982)	Sacrospinous fixation	81	50 (62%)

canal. An anterior colporrhaphy is not usually required if a Marshall–Marchetti–Krantz procedure is used, although the bladder base will need further support if a large cystocele is present.

The colposacropexy procedure has many advantages over the other methods of treatment of vaginal inversion. In the past, older patients were considered to be unsuitable medical candidates for such an extensive procedure, but with modern anesthesiology and postoperative care, older patients can now receive complete surgical repair. The colposacropexy procedure combines a repair of the anatomical defect, support to the vaginal apex, and restoration of normal depth and axis, which is necessary for continued physical activity and coital function. Several investigators have demonstrated excellent success with a variety of operative procedures (Table 24–1).

The colpocleisis (LeFort procedure) is performed infrequently in modern gynecological surgery, since the procedure causes loss of coital function and does not repair the enterocele. Only moderate success has been achieved in the past with this procedure. Total vaginectomy, a time consuming, vascular procedure, also produces only limited success and prevents future coitus.

The Zacharin procedure is one of the most effective techniques in treating vault prolapse, since it corrects the anatomical defect in the levator hiatus in patients who have sustained prolapse of the vaginal vault following hysterectomy. In this combined abdominal and vaginal surgical procedure, the cul-de-sac peritoneum is excised from the pelvis, heavy (No. 2) silk sutures are placed through the medial aspect of the levator muscles between the rectum and the bladder base, and the sutures are tied in the midline of the dilated levator hiatus, thereby approximating the margins of the levator muscles and closing the large diastasis in the pelvic diaphragm. Three or four interrupted sutures are placed in this manner to produce firm support to the pelvic floor. The abdominal surgeon then sutures the vaginal vault to the reconstituted pelvic diaphragm, using interrupted permanent sutures of No. 2-0 silk, dacron, or nylon placed in the submucosa of the vagina and anchored to the levator ani muscles. Zacharin has achieved an excellent overall success rate with this operation.

All of these procedures have greatly improved the health and well-being of aging women suffering from defects in the pelvic floor that permit massive inversion of the vagina. No longer is it necessary for women to be subjected to the discomfort and inconvenience of long-term use of the vaginal pessary for control of this anatomical defect.

Transvaginal Sacrospinous Colpopexy with Colporrhaphy*

Massive eversion of the vagina that is associated with demonstrably poor strength in the cardinal-uterosacral complex, and with coincident cystocele, rectocele, and enterocele can be corrected through a single transvaginal surgical approach. In this approach, an enterocele is identified and excised, an anterior colporrhaphy is accomplished, and the vaginal vault is firmly sewn to the surface of the coccygeus muscle–sacrospinous ligament complex. A posterior colporrhaphy, supplemented if necessary by a perineorrhaphy, completes the procedure, restoring normal vaginal depth and axis. If a prolapsed uterus is present without strong and surgically useful cardinal ligaments, a vaginal hysterectomy may precede the colpopexy and colporrhaphy.

The sacrospinous ligament is located within the substance of the coccygeus muscle, which runs from each ischial spine to the lower portion of the sacrum (Fig. 24–13). The ligament can be identified by pal-

* The section on transvaginal sacrospinous colpopexy was contributed by David H. Nichols, M.D.

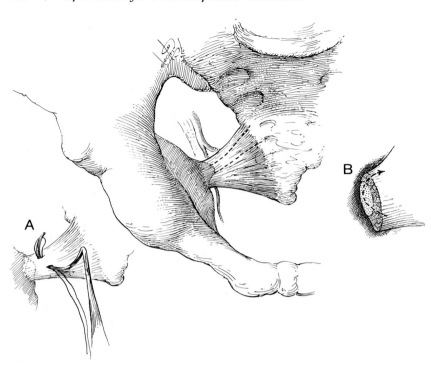

FIG. 24-13 Location of the sacrospinous ligament deep within the substance of the coccygeus muscle is shown by the dotted line. The sciatic nerve and pudendal artery are shown behind the ischial spine. To avoid them, penetration of the coccygeus muscle and sacrospinous ligament is made 1.5 fingerbreadths (2 cm–3 cm) *medial* to the ischial spine as indicated in *A*. Note that the ligature carrier has been placed *through* the muscle and ligament and not around them. The path of a ligature is shown by the dotted line in *B*; a cross-section of the sacrospinous ligament is represented by the stippled area within the coccygeus muscle. (Nichols, 1978)

pation, as the examining finger seeks first the ischial spine on either side of the pelvis and traces the finger-like thickening of the ligament that runs posteriorly from the lateral wall of the pararectal space to the hollow of the sacrum. The ischial spine and sacrospinous ligament can be palpated by transvaginal or rectal examination, or can be seen in the operative field during the surgery.

The surgical anatomy of the pararectal space includes the pudendal blood vessels and nerves posterior to the ischial spine and the sciatic nerve deeply posterior to the ligament. Trauma to these structures must be avoided. A safe procedure is best assured by placement of fixation stitches through the substance of the sacrospinous ligament 1 to 1.5 fingerbreadths (2 cm–3 cm) medial to the ischial spine. A right-handed operator may find it easier to work with the patient's right sacrospinous ligament.

Following the procedure, the vault of the vagina will deviate to the side where the attachment was made, but this deviation should not result in either dyspareunia or loss of coital function. Using both ligaments for support tends to fan out the upper portion of the vagina unnecessarily, and seems to offer no advantage.

The sacrospinous colpopexy was originally described by Paul Zweifel in Germany in 1892, then was rediscovered in 1951 by Amreich in Austria, where it was modified by Sederl and then studied

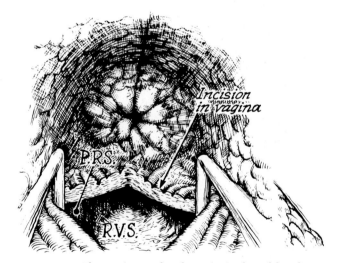

FIG. 24-14 The perineum has been incised, and by sharp dissection the vagina has been freed from the perineal body and an opening has been made into the rectovaginal space (*RVS*). The full length of the rectovaginal space is developed by blunt dissection up to the vault of the vagina. The full thickness of the posterior vaginal wall is incised to a point cranial to the rectocele. At times this will involve the full length of the posterior vaginal wall. Any enterocele present is carefully resected and the neck of the sac is closed. *PRS* = Pararectal space. (Nichols, 1981)

extensively by Richter. Preparation includes estrogen replacement therapy if necessary, administration of a broad-spectrum preventive antibiotic, and the use of full-length elastic stockings to reduce the size of the venous pool when the patient's legs are removed from the surgical stirrups.

Technique of Sacrospinous Colpopexy

Delayed-absorbable synthetic suture material is used throughout the operation. The fixation stitches are of No. 2 delayed-absorbable suture (Dexon or Vicryl)—a relatively heavy suture material, that, though absorbable, has sufficient strength that it is not likely to cut through the tissues or break while knots are being tied. The associated colporrhaphy is accomplished using the smaller sizes (No. 0 or No. 2-0) of delayed-absorbable sutures.

A V-shaped incision of an appropriate width is made through the skin overlying the perineal body. A wedge of skin and vagina is freed from the perineal body by sharp dissection, and the rectovaginal space is entered. The full length of this space is developed by blunt dissection to the vault of the vagina. The full thickness of the posterior vaginal wall is incised to a point cranial to any rectocele; at times this will involve the full length of the posterior vaginal wall (Fig. 24–14). The enterocele is carefully mobilized, the sac is opened, and digital exploration is performed to determine whether or not there are any surgically usable cardinal-uterosacral ligaments. Patients who have had a hysterectomy usually have no ligaments that could be used for further surgery.

The neck of the sac is ligated by a purse-string suture, a second purse-string is placed 1 cm distal to the first, the sac is excised, and a full length anterior colporrhaphy is usually performed. Long retractors are inserted into the rectovaginal space. An anterior retractor displaces the rectum to the patient's left, and the descending rectal septum or rectal pillar is identified. The septum separates the rectovaginal space from the pararectal space. An opening is made either bluntly or by using a sharp pointed hemostat through both layers of the descending rectal septum into the right pararectal space at the site of the ischial spine (Fig. 24–15). The opening is enlarged by spreading the points of a hemostat to permit access to the coccygeus muscle, which lies in the lateral wall of the pararectal space and contains within it the sacrospinous ligament.

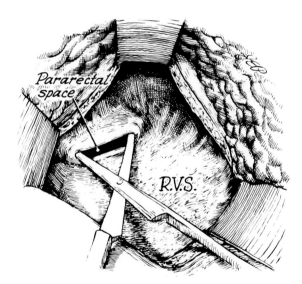

FIG. 24–15 The right cardinal ligament and the ureter have been displaced anteriorly by a Breisky–Navratil retractor in the 12 o'clock position, and the rectum has been displaced to the patient's left by a retractor in the 4 o'clock position. An opening is made either bluntly or by using a sharp-pointed hemostat through the descending rectal septum into the right pararectal space, at the site of the ischial spine. This opening is enlarged by spreading the point of the hemostat or of the Mayo scissors to permit access to the coccygeus muscle, which lies in the lateral wall of the pararectal space and contains within it the sacrospinous ligament. *RVS* = rectovaginal space. (Nichols, 1981)

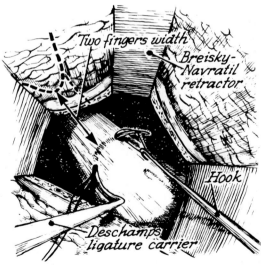

FIG. 24–16 The coccygeus muscle and the sacrospinous ligament have been penetrated by the blunt end of a long Deschamps ligature carrier at a point 1 to 2 fingerbreadths (2 cm–3 cm) medial to the ischial spine, safely away from the pudendal nerve and vessels and the sciatic nerve. The ligature carrier was previously threaded with a full uncut length of 54-inch No. 2 delayed-absorbable suture. Traction to the hook exteriorizes the suture and the Deschamps ligature carrier is removed. (Nichols, 1981)

The retractors are repositioned, exposing the depths of the pararectal space. The pelvic diaphragm is displaced laterally with a retractor. The coccygeus muscle containing the ligament is grasped with a long Babcock clamp and then penetrated, using the blunt tip of a long-handled Deschamps ligature carrier that has been threaded with a full uncut length of 54-in delayed-absorbable suture No. 2 at a point 1.5 to 2 fingerbreadths medial to the ischial spine (Fig. 24–16). The suture is made a safe distance away from the pudendal nerve and vessels and from the sciatic nerve. The Babcock clamp is then removed.

The position of the suture is carefully checked, and if the suture has been properly placed within the substance of the sacrospinous ligament, traction made to the suture will actually move the patient a small amount on the table. If the patient does not move, the suture has been inserted too superficially and it should be replaced. When passing the ligature carrier, the surgeon can feel for tissue resistance, indicating that the ligament is being penetrated. The ligature carrier *must pass through* the substance of the ligament, not around the ligament.

If it is difficult to see the ligament, because of extensive scarring from previous operative procedures, the ligature may be placed by careful palpation, making certain the rectum has been safely positioned to the opposite side. One or more sutures may be placed through the ligament, stitching *medially* from the first suture, away from the ischial spine and its underlying pudendal nerve.

One end of each suture should be threaded on a free needle that is passed through the full thickness of the fibromuscular layer of the undersurface of the vaginal wall (Figs. 24–17, 24–18). The sutures are held in separate hemostats until the redundant posterior wall has been trimmed and closure of the posterior vaginal wall has been started. The margins of the upper posterior vagina are approximated for a distance of 3 cm to 5 cm with a running submucosal stitch.

The upper portion of the posterior vaginal wall must be closed before the colpopexy stitches are tied, because once these stitches have been tied, approximation of the upper margins of the vagina is difficult. Exposure and visibility of the upper vagina are limited after the vagina has been firmly fixed in the hollow of the sacrum. When sacrospinous colpopexy stitches are tied, the undersurface of the vagina is brought into direct contact with the surface of the coccygeus muscle.

A posterior colporrhaphy completes the repair, along with a perineorrhaphy if indicated. Normal vaginal depth and a horizontally inclined axis are

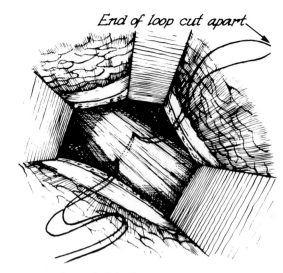

FIG. 24–17 The end of the loop is cut, resulting in two strands of suture material penetrating the ligament. The ends of these are matched into appropriate pairs of suture lengths, each held with a hemostat. (Nichols, 1981)

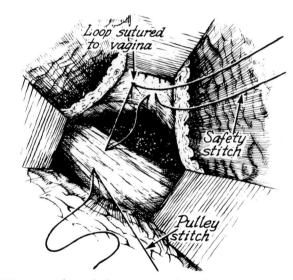

FIG. 24–18 The end of one suture is threaded on a free needle, which is then sewn to the undersurface of the vaginal wall through the full thickness of the fibromuscular layer, and fixed in this position by a single half-hitch. The end of the second piece of suture is stitched to the undersurface of the vagina 1 cm medially. These sutures are held on hemostats until the upper posterior vaginal wall is closed for 3 cm to 5 cm. After the posterior colporrhaphy has been completed and the margins of the posterior vaginal mucosa are approximated to the midportion of the vagina, the sacrospinous fixation stitches are tied, fixing the vagina to the surface of the sacrospinous ligament. (Nichols, 1981)

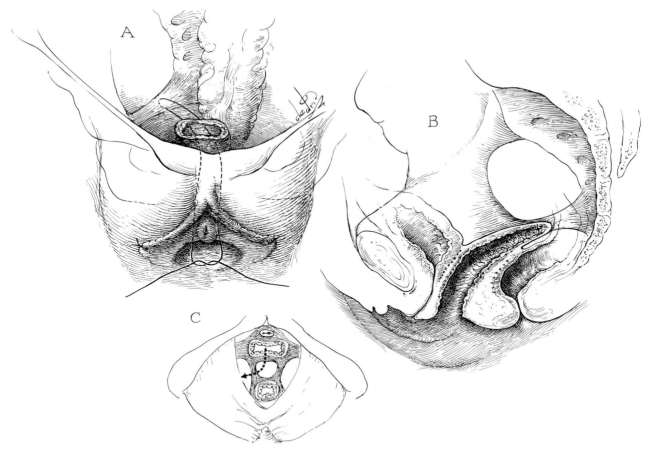

FIG. 24-19 The inverted vagina has been sewn to the right sacrospinous ligament, 1 to 2 fingerbreadths (2 cm–3 cm) medial to the ischial spine, as shown in frontal view in *A* and in sagittal view in *B*. Notice the restoration of normal vaginal depth and axis. Dotted line and arrow in *C* trace the path of the incision from the vagina into the rectovaginal space, then through the right rectal pillar to the right pararectal space, thence to the ischial spine and sacrospinous ligament. (Randall CL, Nichols DH: Surgical treatment of vaginal inversion. Obstet Gynecol 38:327, 1971. Reprinted with permission from The American College of Obstetrics and Gynecology.)

restored by the operation (Fig. 24–19). Rectal examination confirms the integrity of the rectum, and if desired, an iodoform gauze pack may be inserted for 24 hours.

Preoperative and Postoperative Care

The preoperative and postoperative care is the same as that following most vaginal reconstructive procedures. The patient begins walking the day following surgery, and normal bowel activity is stimulated then if necessary. Continuous bladder drainage is required only if anterior colporrhaphy had been performed. The average duration of hospitalization is the same as that following vaginal hysterectomy and repair.

Bibliography

Amreich J: Aetiologie und Operation des Scheidenstumpf prolapses. Wien Klin Wochenschr 63:74–77, 1951

Baden WF: Geriatric gynecology. Postgrad Med J 46:241, 1969

Beecham CT, Beecham JB: Correction of prolapsed vagina or enterocele with fascia lata. Obstet Gynecol 42:542, 1973

Berglas G, Rubin IC: Study of the supportive structures of the uterus by levator myography. Surg Gynecol Obstet 76:677, 1953

Birnbaum SJ: Rational therapy for the prolapsed vagina. Am J Obstet Gynecol 115:411, 1973

Feldman GB, Birnbaum SJ: Sacral colpopexy for vaginal vault prolapse. Obstet Gynecol 53:399, 1979

Funt MI, Thompson JD, Birch H: Normal vaginal axis. South Med J 71:1534, 1978

Goffe JR: An operation for extreme cases of procidentia with rectocele and cystocele. Med Rec 82:879, 1912

Hendee AE, Berry CM: Abdominal sacropexy for vaginal vault prolapse. Clin Obstet Gynecol 24:1217, 1982

Jeffcoate TNA: Posterior colporrhaphy. Am J Obstet Gynecol 77:490, 1959

Kuhn RJP, Hollyock VE: Observations on the anatomy of the rectovaginal pouch and septum. Obstet Gynecol 59: (No. 4) 445, 1982

McCall ML: Posterior culdeplasty: surgical correction of enterocele during vaginal hysterectomy: a preliminary report. Obstet Gynecol 10:595, 1957

Moschcowitz AV: The pathogenesis, anatomy and cure of prolapse of the rectum. Surg Gynecol Obstet 15:7, 1912

Nichols DH: Transvaginal sacrospinous fixation. The Pelvic Surgeon 1:10, 1981

Nichols DH: Effects of pelvic relaxation on gynecologic and urologic problems. Clin Obstet Gynecol 21:770, 1978

Nichols DH, Randall CL: Vaginal Surgery, 2nd ed. Baltimore, Williams and Wilkins, 1983

Nichols DH: Sacrospinous fixation for massive eversion of the vagina. Am J Obstet Gynecol 142:901–904, 1982

Nichols DH, Milley PS, Randall CL: Significance of restoration of normal vaginal depth and axis. Obstet Gynecol 36:251, 1970

Randall CL, Nichols DH: Surgical treatment of vaginal inversion. Obstet Gynecol 38:327, 1971

Richter K: Die operative Behandlung des prolabierten Scheidengrundes nach Uterusextirpation Beilrag zur Vaginalfixatio Sacrotuberalis nach Amreich. Geburtshife Frauenheilk 27:941–954, 1967

Richter K: Massive eversion of the vagina: Pathogenesis, diagnosis and therapy of the "true" prolapse of the vaginal stump. Clin Obstet Gynecol 25:897, 1982

Ridley JH: A composite vaginal vault suspension using fascia lata. Am J Obstet Gynecol 126:590, 1976

Rust JA, Botte JM, Howlett RJ: Prolapse of the vaginal vault, improved techniques for management of the abdominal approach. Am J Obstet Gynecol 125:768, 1976

Sederl J: Zur Operation des Prolapses der blind endigenden Scheide. Geburtshife Frauenheilk 18:824–828, 1958

Smout CFV, Jacoby F, Lillie EW: Gynaecological and Obstetrical Anatomy. London, Lewis Publishers, 1969

Symmonds RE, Williams TJ, Lee RA, et al: Posthysterectomy, enterocele, and vaginal vault prolapse. Obstet Gynecol 140:852, 1981

Symmonds RE, Sheldon RS: Vaginal prolapse after hysterectomy. Obstet Gynecol 25:61, 1965

TeLinde RW: Prolapse of the uterus and allied conditions. Am J Obstet Gynecol 94:444, 1966

Uhlenhuth E, Wolfe WM, Smith EM, et al: The rectogenital septum. Surg Gynecol Obstet 76:148, 1948

Ulfelder H: Enterocele. In Meigs JV, Sturgis SH (eds): Progress in Gynecology. New York, Grune and Stratton, 1970

Ward GG: Operative technique for repair of rectocele and injury to the pelvic floor. Surg Gynecol Obstet 48:399, 1929

Zacharin RF: Pulsion enterocele: Review of functional anatomy of the pelvic floor. Obstet Gynecol 55:135, 1980

Zacharin RF, Hamilton NT: Pulsion enterocele: Long-term results of an abdominoperineal technique. Obstet Gynecol 55:141, 1980

Zweifel P: Vorlesungen uber Klinische Gynakologie. Berlin, Hirschwald, 1892

Chapter 25

Stress Urinary Incontinence, Urethrocele, and Cystocele

One of the more distressing symptoms of advancing age and parity is the insidious loss of urinary control. As many as 50% of adult women are known to have some minor degree of involuntary incontinence brought on by a sudden increase in intra-abdominal pressure transmitted to the pelvic diaphragm and bladder base. Stress urinary incontinence is basically a disorder of the musculofascial support to the bladder neck and pelvic floor, involving the support mechanisms to the urethrovesical junction and posterior urethra. Trauma to the birth canal from childbirth and atrophy of the ligamentous support to the bladder base and posterior urethra are the fundamental defects associated with this disorder.

The symptoms of stress urinary incontinence are common during young adulthood but increase in severity following each successive pregnancy. Socially disabling symptoms usually appear in middle life or at the time of menopause. Stress urinary incontinence is far more common among Caucasian women than among Chinese, Eskimo, Black, or Native American women. Anatomical dissections of the pelvic fascia and urogenital diaphragm have shown the tissue quality and fascial support of the posterior urethra in oriental women to be far superior to those in Caucasian and other racial groups.

Urinary control and voiding depend upon both physiologic and anatomical elements. Four distinct factors govern normal urinary continence: (1) the urethra and bladder must maintain surface continuity; (2) intraurethral pressure must exceed intravesical pressure; (3) the detrusor muscle of the bladder must function normally; and (4) appropriate innervation must be maintained for both the smooth muscle of the urethra and the skeletal muscle that forms the external sphincter.

The anatomical factors influencing urinary incontinence are centered principally in the posterior urethral ligaments and in the levator ani muscles, which make up the pelvic diaphragm (Fig. 25–1). In Gosling's opinion, the levator ani muscles are the component most amenable to surgical correction; an important concept since frequently the symptoms of urinary incontinence are associated with anatomical defects in the levator hiatus. Herniation of the bladder base and of the posterior urethra through the levator hiatus, producing a cystourethrocele, results from stretching and relaxing of the pelvic floor—particularly the anterior portion of the urogenital diaphragm—during childbearing or from fibromuscular atrophy (Fig. 25–2).

Several other anatomical factors contribute to the high incidence of stress urinary incontinence. In the gynecoid pelvis, the wide inlet and the large diameters of the midpelvis and pelvic outlet render the posterior urethra and bladder base as sites of excessive pelvic pressure and at an increased risk for hypermobility or uncontrolled descent to a position outside the abdominal cavity. From a physiologic point of view, intra-abdominal pressure that is transmitted to the bladder should be transmitted equally to the posterior urethra (Fig. 25–3). Change of position and descent of the urethra outside the abdominal cavity would create a loss of pressure equalization, and intravesical pressure could exceed intraurethral pressure. The short length of the female urethra (4 cm) also contributes to the high incidence of this distressing disorder.

Relaxation of the musculofascial support to the bladder neck and posterior urethra can accompany advancing age, causing urinary incontinence without the development of a significant urethrocele or

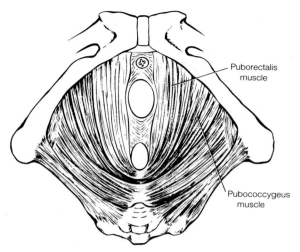

FIG. 25-1 Perineal view of the pelvic diaphragm, which is related to anatomical urinary control and support of the bladder, vagina, and rectum. The puborectalis muscle is in close approximation to the posterior urethra and sends decussating muscle fibers to support the bladder neck and urethra.

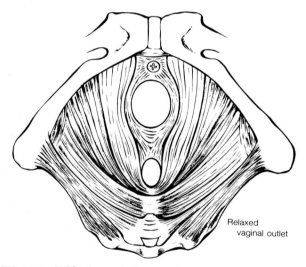

FIG. 25-2 Widening and diastasis of the levator hiatus causes relaxation of the fibromuscular support of the bladder neck and posterior urethra and usually involves herniation of the bladder base, vagina, and rectum.

cystourethrocele. Women who had previously been extremely physically active and have been subjected to prolonged periods of orthostatic pressure on the pelvic diaphragm can develop urinary incontinence. Patients usually seek medical advice and request surgical correction when the symptoms are sufficient to require the use of perineal pads for protection.

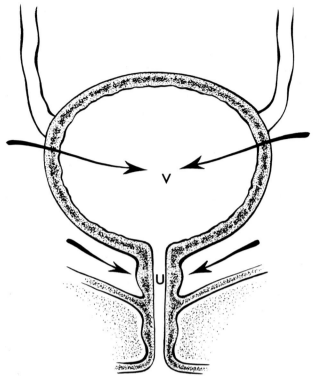

FIG. 25-3 Urinary continence is achieved by the equalization of intra-abdominal pressure to the bladder wall and posterior urethra. The intra-abdominal position of the posterior urethra ensures that intraurethral pressure (U) is higher than intravesical pressure (V). These favorable anatomical and pressure relationships assist in the maintenance of urinary continence.

Anatomy

Embryologically the bladder and urethra arise from a common mesenchymal anlage as an anterior division of the urogenital sinus, which explains why their muscular layers are similar. The urinary bladder is a hollow, muscular organ lined by transitional epithelium. The base of the bladder rests on the lower uterine segment, while the trigone is located on the upper one-third of the anterior vaginal wall. The anterior wall of the bladder lies in the space of Retzius, directly behind the symphysis pubis. The wall of the bladder is composed of three layers: an external longitudinal layer, an internal longitudinal layer, and a middle circular muscular layer. These three layers are extensively interdigitated—so much so that many anatomists describe only two layers of the bladder wall, the outer and inner layers.

The entire thickness of the bladder wall represents the detrusor muscle, which is anatomically and physiologically separate from the trigone. As the detrusor muscle converges at the internal orifice of the bladder, it arranges itself into three layers. The inner layer reaches the bladder neck and passes into the urethra to become the internal longitudinal layer of the urethra. The middle circular layer, which terminates at the level of the bladder and does not extend into the urethra, is frequently difficult to identify. The outer longitudinal layer is clearly identifiable as it converges on the bladder neck, encircling the urethrovesical junction in a horseshoe-shaped fashion, and forms a circular arrangement of smooth muscle surrounding the entire urethra. When the bladder contracts during normal voiding, it is this extension of the bladder musculature that produces funneling and shortening of the posterior urethra.

The trigone of the bladder is also composed of three layers of muscle. The deep trigonal muscle corresponds with the middle circular layer of bladder, while the inner longitudinal muscle fuses with the longitudinal muscle of the ureter and urethra. Although it is difficult to identify, an outer longitudinal muscle interdigitates with the longitudinal muscle of the bladder wall.

The urethra is approximately 3.5 cm to 4.5 cm in length. The inner longitudinal and outer circular smooth muscle layers are extensions of the smooth muscle of the bladder wall. These muscles are densely interwoven and serve as the internal urethral sphincter, which maintains a constant, tonic, intraurethral pressure. Striated sphincter muscle is concentrated in the middle third of the urethra. Some anatomists believe these striated fibers to be decussations from the deep transverse perinei muscles of the urogenital diaphragm and from the puborectalis muscle of the levator ani. Others believe that the striated muscle has no connection with the pelvic diaphragm but has a separate embryologic origin, although innervated by the same somatic nerves (S2–S4) (Fig. 25–4). As pressure profile studies demonstrate, the sphincter muscles create maximal intraurethral pressure at the mid-portion of the urethra, approximately 2 cm from the urethrovesical junction. The bulbocavernosus muscles of the urogenital diaphragm contribute little to the maintenance of urinary continence.

Physiology of Urination

The physiology of micturition involves the involuntary autonomic nervous system, both sympathetic and parasympathetic, and the voluntary somatic as well as the central nervous systems.

MOTOR FUNCTION OF THE BLADDER

Parasympathetic innervation. The detrusor muscle of the bladder is innervated by parasympathetic nerve fibers that arise from the spinal cord by way of motor axons from sacral segments S2 to S4. These fibers course through the pelvic nerve plexus, join with the hypogastric (sympathetic) nerves, and form the vesical plexus, which surrounds the urethrovesical junction and the detrusor muscle (Fig. 25–5). The parasympathetic fibers produce excitatory impulses leading to contractions of the detrusor muscle.

Sympathetic innervation. The bladder and urethra are innervated by long postganglionic sympathetic nerve fibers arising from spinal cord segments T11, T12, L1, L2. These fibers enter the pelvis primarily through the presacral (hypogastric) nerves, become incorporated in the pelvic nerve plexus and interconnect with pelvic parasympathetic ganglia that modulate the transmission of parasympathetic nerves to the detrusor. Innervation of the detrusor muscle primarily with β-adrenergic fibers results in smooth muscle relaxation, whereas innervation of the smooth muscle of the urethra by α-adrenergic nerve fibers causes depolarization and contraction (Fig. 25–5).

Somatic innervation. The striated external sphincter muscles of the urethra, the deep transverse perineal muscles of the urogenital diaphragm, and the puborectalis muscle of the levator ani receive motor fibers by way of the pudendal nerve (S2–S4). The voluntary sphincteric action of these muscles is coordinated with the smooth muscle of the bladder detrusor (Fig. 25–6).

Sensory innervation. Afferent sensory innervation from the bladder and urethra is mediated to the central nervous system by both autonomic and somatic nerve fibers. The autonomic afferent fibers sense proprioceptive (tension and volume) as well as exteroceptive (pain, temperature, touch) stimuli. Proprioceptive receptors are located between the smooth muscle fibers of the bladder wall; exteroceptive receptors have free nerve endings that are present in the mucosa and submucosa.

Most sensory nerve impulses pass from the bladder along the pelvic nerve fibers (S2–S4) to the spinal cord, where they either produce voluntary reflex activities or rise to the level of the brain stem. Depending on the specific stimulus, the urge to void travels either by way of the posterior columns (tension, volume, and sensation of touch) or by the lateral spinothalamic tracts (pain and temperature) (Fig. 25–7) to the frontal lobe of the cerebral cortex. Sensory impulses involving pain and temperature

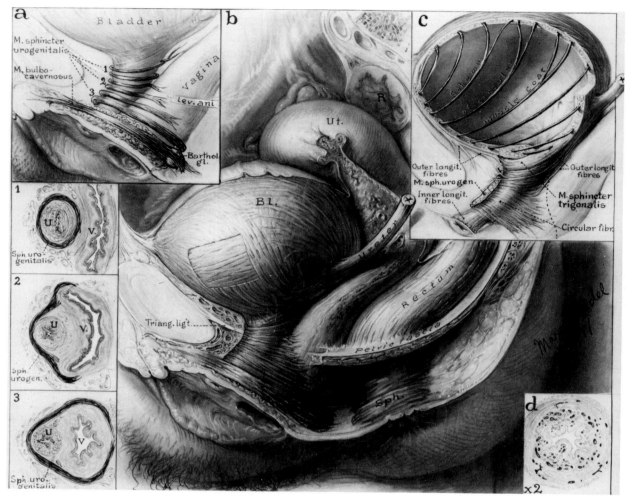

FIG. 25-4 Anatomical relationship of bladder and urethra, showing decussating fibers of the pelvic diaphragm, which encircle the urethra and provide voluntary striated muscular control. (From Kelly HA, Burnham CF: Disease of kidneys, ureters and bladder, vol 1. New York, Appleton, 1914)

sensations are transmitted from the bladder through the sympathetic pathway to the spinal cord above the level of T4, then to the brain stem and cerebral cortex.

CENTRAL NERVOUS SYSTEM CONTROL OF BLADDER FUNCTION

Four basic neurologic circuits control the act of voiding.

The cerebral motor reflex circuit includes the neural pathway between the cerebral cortex and the detrusor nuclei in the brain stem, which is integrated with the cerebellum and basal ganglia for voluntary control of voiding. (Fig. 25–8.) The specific area of the cerebral cortex concerned with voiding is located in the anteromedial portion of the frontal lobe. A specific threshold of bladder volume triggers the cortex, which releases the inhibition of the detrusor nuclei in the brain stem so voiding can occur. Voluntary control of the parasympathetic voiding reflex is a learned response, achieved during early childhood training; loss of control of this reflex pathway during senescence or following intracerebral vascular accidents results in incontinence.

The brain stem–sacral reflex circuit consists of proprioceptive sensory fibers in the bladder wall that register bladder volume and transmit it directly to the detrusor reflex center in the brain stem (Fig. 25–9). With the release of cortical suppression, afferent stimuli activate the reflex arc through motor axons descending in the spinal cord, which stimulate the sacral micturation center to produce a prolonged and complete contraction of the bladder.

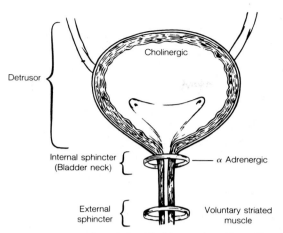

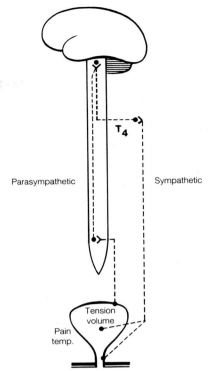

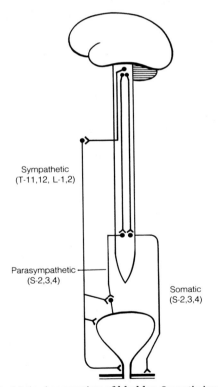

FIG. 25-5 Innervation of the bladder and urethra. The detrusor muscle of the bladder is innervated by parasympathetic cholinergic fibers (S2–S4) from the pelvis plexus whereas the smooth muscle of the entire urethra acts as an internal sphincter that is supplied principally by adrenergic (sympathetic) nerves. Maximum intraurethral pressure is exerted by striated muscular control of the pelvic diaphragm (S2–S4).

FIG. 25-7 Sensory innervation of the bladder and urethra. Bladder volume and tension impulses pass through parasympathetic fibers to spinal cord. Pain and temperature sensations pass mainly through the sympathetic nerves to a higher level of the spinal cord (T4).

FIG. 25-6 Motor innervation of bladder. Somatic innervation (S2–S4) of levator ani muscles (puborectalis) and urogenital diaphragm (deep transverse perineal) muscles, which function as the external urethral sphincter. Sympathetic innervation of the bladder and urethra is derived from T11, T12, L1, and L2. Parasympathetic innervation of the detrusor muscle arises from S2–S4, as does the somatic nerve supply.

Once the cerebral cortex inhibition has been released and a detrusor contraction has been initiated, complete emptying of the bladder is assured.

The sacrovesical–pelvic reflex coordinates detrusor muscle contraction (S2–S4) with the simultaneous relaxation of the striated muscles in the pelvic diaphragm (S2–S4) during the process of micturition (Fig. 25–10).

The cerebral–sacral reflex integrates cortical, spinal, and perineal circuits. Arising in the cerebral cortex and terminating in the pudendal nuclei of the sacral cord (Fig. 25–11), the reflex provides direct voluntary control of the striated muscles in the pelvic floor and initiates voluntary contraction and relaxation of the external urethral sphincter during the storage and voiding phases of micturition.

Mechanisms of Voiding

The cortical perception of the urge to void releases the inhibition of the detrusor center in the brain stem, then stimulates impulses through the cortical–sacral pathway to produce voluntary relaxation of the striated muscle around the urethra and in the

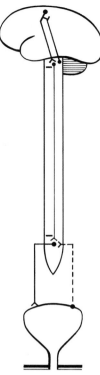

FIG. 25–8 The cerebral–brain stem reflex maintains an inhibitory suppression of the detrusor nuclei in the brain stem. Release of this inhibitory control permits voiding by detrusor stimulation.

pelvic diaphragm. The voluntary relaxation reflex stimulates involuntary sympathetic relaxation of the smooth muscle of the urethra.

The voluntary mechanisms of voiding stimulate the parasympathetic fibers in the pelvic nerve plexus (S2–S4), which cause reflex inhibition of the sympathetic, postganglionic fibers in the urethra (T11, T12, L1, L2) resulting in smooth muscle relaxation and funneling of the bladder neck and posterior urethra. Parasympathetic stimulation of the detrusor muscle initiates bladder contraction.

Voluntary contraction of the abdominal muscles causes an increase in intra-abdominal pressure that is transmitted to the bladder wall. Sensory stimuli in the bladder wall activate the parasympathetic stimulation of the detrusor muscle to initiate voiding.

The smooth muscle along the entire urethra is stimulated by α-adrenergic sympathetic fibers. The longitudinal and circular smooth muscle fibers act as an involuntary internal sphincter, creating increased smooth muscle tone and a tonic level of intraurethral pressure. Whereas the α-adrenergic fibers are concentrated mainly in the urethra with

only a few fibers in the bladder base, β-adrenergic sympathetic fibers terminate primarily in the detrusor muscle and cause relaxation of the urethral smooth muscle and bladder detrusor.

The subconscious response of the pelvic diaphragm muscles to changes in intra-abdominal pressure provides an important mechanism of bladder control for the female with normal fibromuscular support for the bladder base and pelvic diaphragm. During bladder filling, continence is maintained when intraurethral pressure exceeds intravesical pressure. A transient increase in bladder pressure must be met by a simultaneous increase in intraurethral pressure through a constriction of the striated muscle of the mid-urethra and pelvic diaphragm (Fig. 25–12). Pressure equalization augments the tone of the smooth muscle in the urethral wall, which normally keeps the urethra closed.

The concept of pressure equalization emphasizes that the equal distribution of pressure on bladder and posterior urethra is maintained by the intra-abdominal position of the posterior urethra and urethrovesical junction. Muellner proposed these pressure relationships (1958) on the basis of cineflu-

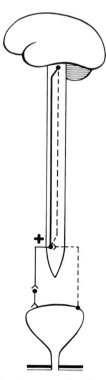

FIG. 25–9 The brain stem–sacral reflex provides activation of a prolonged and complete contraction of the detrusor muscle in response to sensory stimuli from the bladder wall.

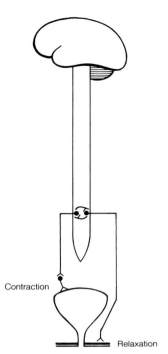

FIG. 25–10   The sacrovesical–pelvic reflex coordinates the relaxation of the striated muscle in the pelvic diaphragm with detrusor muscle contraction, permitting voiding to occur.

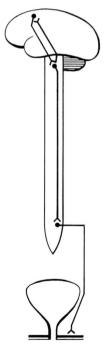

FIG. 25–11   The cerebral–sacral reflex provides direct voluntary control of the striated muscles of the pelvic diaphragm and the external urethral sphincter.

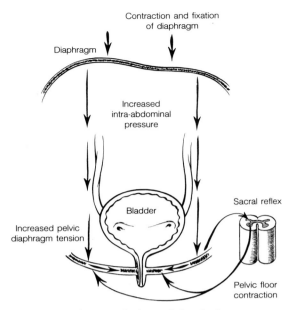

FIG. 25–12   An increase in intra-abdominal pressure causes simultaneous contraction of the pelvic diaphragm and the skeletal muscle that invests the mid-urethra. These anatomical changes maintain urethral pressure at a higher level than vesical pressure in the continent female.

roscopic voiding studies, and the theory was reinforced by the urodynamic studies of Hodgkinson (1960) and Enhorning (1961). Others, notably Turner–Warwick, have questioned this theory and contend that the reflex increase in intraurethral pressure results principally from musculofascial support of the posterior urethra and from simultaneous contraction of the smooth and skeletal muscle sphincters in response to an increase in intraurethral pressure. An insidious descent of the posterior urethra through the levator hiatus can be caused by stretching, relaxation, and elongation of the endopelvic fascia and pubourethral ligaments that attach to either side of the posterior one-third of the urethra. The gradual loss of fibromuscular support to the pelvic floor with widening of the levator hiatus is associated with an abrupt loss of urine when intra-abdominal pressure is changed by coughing, laughing, or rapid change in position.

Since fibromuscular weakening of the pelvic diaphragm causes relaxation of the anterior vaginal wall and the development of a cystocele and urethrocele, these anatomical disorders are commonly associated with stress urinary incontinence. The downward displacement and hypermobility of the posterior urethra causes a funneling of the posterior urethra and urethrovesical junction that is associated with a decrease in intraurethral pressure. These changes allow a sudden increase in intra-abdominal pressure to be transmitted directly to the bladder without a corresponding increase in intraurethral pressure. The "hydraulic wedge" in the posterior urethra, described by Hodgkinson, causes urethral incompetence and permits the immediate, involuntary escape of urine.

Preoperative Assessment of the Patient

Genuine stress urinary incontinence is defined as involuntary loss of urine immediately following an increase in intra-abdominal pressure without evidence of detrusor contraction. The preoperative evaluation of this anatomical urinary incontinence is based on an accurate history and physical examination, with the use of urodynamic studies when there is any discordance between the anatomical changes, the clinical findings, and the patient's history.

Since at least 10–15% of all primary surgical procedures fail to cure patients presumed to have an anatomical incontinence, patient selection is possibly more critical than the choice of a specific operative procedure. Patients should be asked about the use of specific medications that may interfere with normal bladder function, including both anticholinergic and α-adrenergic blocking agents. Urinary tract infections, common among patients with anatomical urinary incontinence, may provide conflicting symptoms of urinary frequency, urgency, nocturia, and urge incontinence. More important, the patient's history, derived either from written questionnaire or from direct questioning, is misleading or unreliable in 20% to 30% of cases when considered alone for a definitive diagnosis.

The poor correlation between the patient's history and urodynamic tests has been observed by Jarvis and associates (1980), Walter and Olesen (1980), McGuire and associates (1980), and by Bent and associates (1983). Therefore, only when the anatomical changes and clinical findings correlate accurately with the diagnosis of genuine stress incontinence is the patient's history considered to be reliable. When there is any variation in one or more of these clinical parameters, provocative cystometry is advisable.

Atlhough urge incontinence is commonly the result of an irritative lesion somewhere in the urinary tract, differential diagnosis of detrusor instability cannot be made on a history of urge incontinence alone. The diagnosis requires complete urodynamic investigation, including water cystoscopy, cystometry, and a study of bladder and urethral con-tractile patterns. As observed by Turner–Warwick and others, the subtle bladder dysfunction of detrusor instability may occur in conjunction with genuine stress urinary incontinence in as many as 15% of patients who report no symptoms that are typical of neurogenic disturbance. Consequently, an appropriate operative procedure can be planned only by more routine use of urodynamic studies.

To demonstrate stress incontinence anatomically, the patient is placed on the examining table with her bladder full, and she is asked to cough. If the patient has anatomical incontinence, the cough will produce an immediate spurt of urine from the urethra. Careful inspection of the anterior vaginal wall and uterine supports will define whether or not pelvic relaxation is a problem, and will show the extent of herniation of the bladder base and posterior urethra through the urogenital diaphragm.

Approximately 75% of women with urinary stress incontinence will demonstrate a moderate or large cystourethrocele on examination. If the hernia is less prominent when the patient lies supine, the Valsalva maneuver or coughing can be used to provoke the problem. If symptoms are still not apparent, test the patient in the erect position to accurately assess competence of the bladder neck and urethra.

The examiner's index and middle fingers may then be placed on either side of the urethra to elevate it slightly. This procedure, known as the Bonney–Marshall test, increases intraurethral pressure by providing paraurethral support to the anterior vaginal wall. If a strong cough does not produce leakage, the incontinence is most likely the result of an anatomical defect, not a neurologic dysfunction. Recent urethral pressure profile studies suggest that the Bonney maneuver, when applied at the time of increased intra-abdominal pressure, may create obstruction of the urethral lumen rather than augmentation of paraurethral support. Nonetheless, this test has served as a useful clinical method of documenting anatomical incontinence and has been an effective predictor of the benefit of surgically repairing a relaxed anterior vaginal wall.

A lubricated sterile Q-tip or a metal urethral catheter inserted into the urethra can be used to demonstrate posterior rotation of the bladder neck with relaxation of the pubourethral ligaments as well as hypermobility of the posterior urethra resulting from relaxation of the pelvic floor. In the continent female, the Q-tip should point in a posterior plane from the horizontal, with only mild descent of the posterior urethra when the patient is straining or when intra-abdominal pressure is increased. In the patient with anatomical urinary incontinence and progressive loss of anatomical support to the posterior urethra, the Q-tip will be elevated above the

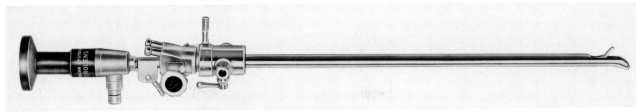

FIG. 25–13 Wappler microlens cystourethroscope. (Courtesy of American Cystoscope Makers, Inc.)

horizontal, particularly when intra-abdominal pressure is applied (see Chapter 26, Fig. 26–2).

NEUROLOGIC EXAMINATION

Examination of the sacral reflexes is important, since the sacral plexus (S2–S4) includes the important nerve fibers involved with both the parasympathetic stimulation of the bladder and the voluntary striated muscle of the pelvic diaphragm and urethra. A rectal examination or electromyographic study may be used to evaluate the tonicity of the anal sphincter, which reflects the innervation of the striated musculature of the pelvic floor and the response to increased intra-abdominal pressure. Poor external anal sphincter control due to a neurologic abnormality must be differentiated from anatomical relaxation of the perineal body. Gentle stroking of the perineal skin lateral to the anus will evoke contraction of the anal sphincter. Similarly, stimulation or squeezing of the clitoris will evoke reflex contraction of the bulbocavernosus muscle. The cough reflex will cause contraction and tension on the pelvic diaphragm through the sacral reflex, but this response can be demonstrated only by a sensitive pressure-recording catheter in the anal canal measuring anal sphincter contractility. Sensation to touch and pinprick on the perineum should be tested. Should neurologic defects be demonstrated, the patient should undergo full neurologic evaluation.

UROLOGIC STUDIES

Although urethroscopy, cystoscopy, and other urologic studies provide little additional diagnostic information about patients with primary anatomical incontinence, these procedures are essential in recurrent or complicated cases of urinary incontinence.

Water Cystoscopy

Endoscopic visualization of the bladder and urethra using a water medium allows a much better examination of the lower urinary tract than does inspection with an air cystoscope. The external ure-

thra should be cleaned by a surgical prep and protected with sterile drapes, and the patient should be put in the dorsolithotomy position. A topical anesthetic agent is then instilled into the urethra. A No. 22 French or even a No. 24 French cystoscope can be passed without dilatation of the urethra in many women, but if the urethra is tight, dilatation should be performed.

Making diagnostic cystoscopy into a routine simplifies the procedure. Each examiner should develop a specific technique, depending on the equipment available. Instruments using both foroblique and lateral viewing lens are preferable, and these can be used in the same cystoscopic sheath, such as with the Wappler microlens cystourethroscope (Figs. 25–13, 25–14, 25–15). If the Wappler microlens is not available, the McCarthy panendoscope or the Brown–Burger cystoscope is often used.

Using a cystoscope, the entire bladder can be inspected for evidence of infection, diverticuli, polyps, or foreign bodies. The ureteral orifices can be visualized and should spurt clear urine. In the rare event that a bladder tumor may have caused the clinical signs of urinary incontinence, a biopsy can be taken with the operating biopsy forceps.

When the bladder is viewed through the cystoscope, several important landmarks should be noted. The air bubble lies against the highest point of the anterior wall of the bladder and is a good point for orientation. The trigone is an inverted triangular area in the posterior bladder wall resting on the upper third of the anterior vaginal wall. The apex of this triangle is at the bladder neck, and the

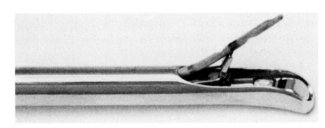

FIG. 25–14 Ureteral catheterization with lateral microlens telescope and Albarran bridge. (Courtesy of American Cystoscope Makers, Inc.)

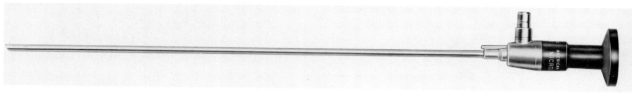

FIG. 25-15 Microlens foroblique telescope. (Courtesy of American Cystoscope Makers, Inc.)

ureteral orifices form the base of the triangle. The mucosa of the trigone is smooth, since there is no submucosa, and it is firmly attached to the bladder muscle. The mucosa of the remainder of the bladder wall has a submucosa and is loosely attached to the muscle. When the bladder is empty, it collapses into many folds, which are flattened by distention.

The bladder mucosa is composed of thin transitional epithelium, which has a pearly-white to yellowish-pink color. Through the mucosa, the submucosal vascular pattern is seen easily. When normal, the vessels are multiple, branching, delicate. Vascular inflammation may range from mild hyperemia to marked edema, mucosal hemorrhage, or ulceration. In many instances, only the trigone will be inflamed (trigonitis). Marked inflammation with multiple vesicles (bullous edema) not only indicates an inflammatory process, but also may indicate the presence of a tumor invading through the bladder wall from outside, as in carcinoma of the cervix.

After checking the bladder, carefully evaluate the urethra using the foroblique lens with the Wappler cystourethroscope or the McCarthy panendoscope. The urethra should be distended slightly by allowing the water to run freely through the urethroscope into the bladder while the total circumference of the urethra is inspected in a clockwise direction.

The female urethra is quite elastic and usually will stretch to 9 mm or 10 mm without difficulty. The mucosa at the meatus is squamous epithelium, becoming transitional within the urethra. The mucosa is pale pink, similar in appearance to the bladder mucosa but without the prominent submucosal vessels. There are longitudinal folds in the urethral mucosa, unless it is considerably stretched. With postmenopausal atrophy, the mucosa becomes smooth, pale, and less elastic.

As the cystoscope is withdrawn from the bladder, the internal sphincter (bladder neck) is seen as a circular, iris-shaped segment that closes symmetrically as the instrument passes. The sphincter mechanism is basically involuntary, but micturition can be initiated by increasing the intra-abdominal pressure and relaxing the deep transverse perineal and levator ani muscles. To stop the flow of urine,

the entire group of levator muscles and the deep transverse perineal muscles are contracted.

In addition to irregular or incomplete closure of the internal sphincter, many other signs of urethral disorders can be seen with urethroscopy: obstruction due to scarring; folds or valves, particularly in children; and inflammatory changes commonly found in the posterior urethra near the bladder neck. The mucosa may have a reddened, granular appearance, or there may be granulations or pseudopolyps. Urethral diverticula frequently are overlooked, unless purulent exudate is expressed from the orifice by pressure against the suburethral wall. Carcinoma of the urethra, although rare, can be seen and biopsied through the urethroscope.

Cystometry

Although major advances in urodynamic testing have been made during the past decade, the use of cystometry is usually reserved for patients who have symptoms of urgency, frequency, or nocturia, or episodes of urge incontinence. Elaborate electronic devices measure intravesical and intraurethral pressures, using either gas or fluid. At the same time, provocative movements, such as positional changes, coughing, and heel bouncing, can be performed to unmask the presence of bladder instability. Carbon dioxide or water can be used as a medium for cystometry, but carbon dioxide studies seem to be less accurate; carbon dioxide may be irritating to the bladder mucosa, and the test can produce false-positive results.

Hodgkinson was one of the pioneers in developing urethrocystometry with the patient in both supine and erect positions. In approximately 85% of cases, a cystometric study will detect uninhibited bladder contractions when the patient is in the supine position. In an additional 10% to 15% of cases abnormal contractions become evident when the patient is erect and making provocation movements.

Detrusor instability or dyssynergia, a condition in which the detrusor contracts spontaneously or on provocation during bladder filling, has been reported by Fischer and Gordon to be present in more than 60% of patients with at least one of the symptoms of nocturia, enuresis, urgency, frequency, or urge incontinence. If three or more of the symptoms exist, the incidence of detrusor instability increases to 80%. Because these symptoms indicate a potential neurologic dysfunction, they should be investigated with cystometry and possibly with urethral pressure profile studies.

Many reports, including the recent studies by Cardozo and associates, emphasize the difficulty in differentiating anatomical urinary incontinence from detrusor instability on the basis of history alone. Many investigators recommend that all patients with urinary incontinence should have urodynamic testing before surgery, but as only 10% to 15% of patients with stress incontinence symptoms were reported (by Turner–Warwick) to have detrusor instability, urodynamic evaluation of all of these patients probably will prove unrewarding.

When abnormal bladder symptoms are present, the gynecologist should definitely test for the presence of coexisting bladder instability. Unless the bladder is provoked by heel bounce or the standing position, as many as 30% to 40% of patients with detrusor instability may go unrecognized.

Cystometry should also be used in the evaluation of patients with recurrent urinary incontinence to exclude bladder hypertonicity, atony, or other neurologic abnormalities. The Lewis cystometer is the simplest unit to use. The bladder is distended with sterile water, using 50 ml increments or slow continuous flow, until the initial symptoms of the desire to void are demonstrated, usually when fluid volume reaches 120 ml to 200 ml.

The patient with a normal bladder volume will experience fullness at 450 ml to 600 ml and will have a stable intravesical pressure of about 15 cm to 20 cm of water. Voluntary contraction and voiding will raise the intravesical pressure to 50 cm to 80 cm of water (Fig. 25–16). There should be no uninhibited contractions, and the voiding stream should be uninterrupted.

Prior to the cystometric examination, residual urine volume should measure less than 10% of the total voided urine volume, usually less than 50 ml. Also, the bladder sensation to heat and cold can be tested by instillation of 60 ml to 90 ml of either ice water or very warm water to initiate immediate stimulation of a detrusor contraction and expulsion of the fluid within 20 to 30 seconds. The specific criteria for normal bladder function are listed below.

URODYNAMIC INDICATIONS FOR NORMAL BLADDER FUNCTION

Residual urine volume of less than 100 ml
First voiding sensation of bladder pressure at 120 ml to 200 ml

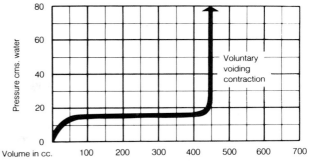

FIG. 25–16 Normal water cystometrogram and bladder function

Exteroceptive sensation
  Heat: present
  Cold: present
Proprioceptive sensation
  First desire: present at 175 ml
  Fullness: present at 450 ml
  Capacity: 500 ml
  Uninhibited contractions: none
  Voiding stream: uninterrupted
  Residual urine: 0 ml

Strong desire to void at 450 ml to 600 ml capacity
Intravesical pressure rise on bladder filling, standing, or coughing, up to 15 cm of water
Increase in intravesical pressure on voiding that does not exceed 80 cm of water
Peak voiding flow rate of 20 ml/sec for a voided volume of at least 200 ml
Ability to stop voiding on command
No loss of urine and only slight descent of bladder base on coughing

Patients who have either detrusor instability or a more serious neurologic dysfunction usually have a bladder capacity of less than 250 ml, with uninhibited contractions present (Fig. 25–17). Usually, the proprioceptive and exteroceptive sensations are absent, so patients with neurogenic bladders will not have the usual physiologic responses. A fluctuant bladder pressure, rising above the normal limits of 20 cm of water prior to involuntary contraction and voiding, usually predicts an unstable bladder. Such cases are usually at high risk for surgical failure, even when an anatomical source of urinary incontinence can be found.

Detrusor instability should be demonstrated before surgery and treated medically. More than 90% of the patients have no additional overt neuropathology. Lack of cortical inhibition of the lower sacral reflexes is considered to be the basic pathophysiologic mechanism of detrusor instability. Bladder instability is also found in patients with various demyelinating neurologic diseases, such as

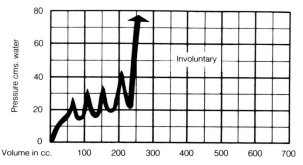

FIG. 25–17 Water cystometrogram of reflex neurogenic bladder and abnormal bladder function
Exteroceptive sensation
  Heat: absent
  Cold: absent
Proprioceptive sensation
  First desire: absent
  Fullness: specific sensation absent
  Capacity: 240 ml
  Uninhibited contractions: present
  Voiding stream: interrupted
  Residual urine: 120 ml

multiple sclerosis, and in severe forms of spina bifida.

In contrast to bladder instability, an atonic bladder may result from neurologic damage to afferent (sensory nerve) fibers. Travelling to the spinal cord mainly through the parasympathetic nerves, these fibers transmit the sensation of bladder fullness and the desire to void along the posterior spinal columns to the brain stem and sensory areas of the brain. Painful stimuli are normally transmitted along the sympathetic fibers to T4, where they enter the lateral spinothalamic tracts and continue to the brain stem.

The common spinal cord lesions—tumors, trauma, tabes dorsalis, and an advanced stage of diabetes mellitus with peripheral neuritis—are possible causes of impairment of sensory function of the bladder. Loss of bladder sensation results in the bladder becoming overdistended, which gives rise to overflow urinary incontinence and incomplete bladder emptying. Because these bladder disorders occur more commonly in the older postmenopausal patient, arteriosclerotic vascular changes are thought to be an etiologic factor contributing to urinary complications.

Urethral Pressure Profile

Demonstrating a diminished intraurethral pressure in response to an increase in intra-abdominal pressure can be particularly useful for patients with recurrent incontinence. The pressure profile is generated throughout the urethra by means of a re-

cording catheter drawn through the urethra at a predetermined rate. Normally, the mean resting pressure in the posterior urethra varies between 40 cm and 60 cm of water when evaluated by single, double, or triple lumen catheter techniques. By simultaneously measuring the resting pressure in the bladder and urethra, the urethral pressure can be compared with bladder pressure at all times, especially when abdominal and vesical pressure are increased by coughing and straining (Fig. 25–18).

Microtip transducers have now replaced fluid-filled polyethelene catheters. The transducers are placed in the bladder, urethra, and rectum. Pressure is monitored in both the supine and erect positions, with the patient making provocation movements every 30 minutes (Fig. 25–19).

A profile of intraurethral pressure can be recorded from the bladder neck to the meatus. Urethral closure pressure is the difference between resting bladder pressure and the maximum urethral pressure, usually 50 cm to 100 cm of water. The maximum urethral pressure occurs at approximately 2 cm to 2.5 cm from the urethrovesical junction and is generated by the striated muscle component of the pelvic floor and urogenital diaphragm. When any area of urethral pressure falls to less than the bladder pressure during coughing or intra-abdominal straining, urethral incontinence occurs (Fig. 25–20).

The many gradations of urethral incompetence are reflected in the varying levels of intraurethral pressure. Basic pressure profiles can be used to define the extent of the pressure deficiencies of the

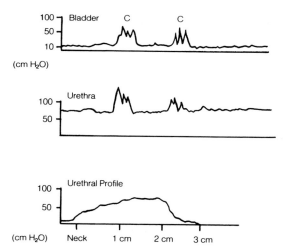

FIG. 25–18 Normal bladder and urethral pressures in a 50-year-old woman. Note that urethral pressure exceeds bladder pressure during coughing (*C*). Urethral profile shows an amplitude of 60 cm of water and an effective urethral length of 2.5 cm.

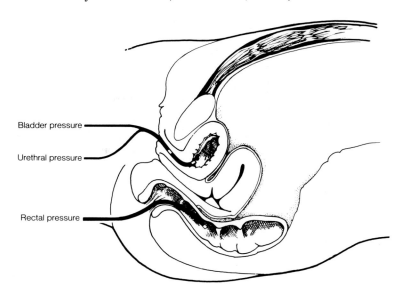

Bladder pressure

Urethral pressure

Rectal pressure

FIG. 25-19 Urodynamic monitoring of bladder function. A dual microtip transducer in the bladder and urethra and a single transducer in the rectum provide a simultaneous recording of intravesical, urethral, and abdominal pressures. (From Fantl, 1984)

urethra. The studies are also helpful in determining the benefits obtained by surgical repair of an incompetent urethra and bladder neck.

Electromyography

Electronic measurement of striated sphincter muscle contractility is of value for patients with serious neurologic dysfunction. An electromyelogram (EMG) may be obtained by inserting needle electrodes into the external urethral sphincter or by skin electrode patches to measure the contractility of the sphincter muscle. EMGs are made in conjunction with water cystometry and sometimes with urethral pressure studies. Many urodynamic instruments measure urethral, bladder, and elec-

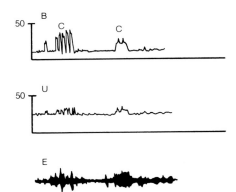

FIG. 25-20 Bladder (B) and urethral (U) pressure and anal electromyogram (E) in a patient with anatomical urinary incontinence. Bladder pressure exceeds urethral pressure with coughing (C). Electromyogram shows normal perineal muscular activity during stress.

tromyelographic pressures simultaneously while performing water cystometry for evaluation of bladder function.

Bead-Chain Cystourethrogram

Since the late 1960s, the chain cystourethrogram has become less valuable as a diagnostic tool. For many years, the cystourethrogram was used to correlate the urethrovesical anatomy with the degree of anatomical dysfunction. Since it is a static radiographic study, it offers little information concerning the urodynamic mechanisms of micturition and incontinence. Today, the cystourethrogram is used only to show the anatomical location of the urethrovesical junction preoperatively and postoperatively. As a teaching tool, the technique can provide evidence that corrective surgery has changed the posterior urethra from a dependent to a high retropubic position.

Evaluating the Patient with Urinary Incontinence

The multiplicity of techniques for assessing the urodynamic mechanisms of micturition and continence control can be perplexing to the clinician. The basic requirements for the proper evaluation of a patient with anatomical urinary incontinence can vary from clinic to clinic. Essentially, a careful history, physical examination, and neurologic evaluation will define a select group of patients with genuine anatomical urinary incontinence. When abnormal bladder symptoms are present, the gynecologist must consider the possibility of coexisting bladder instability or frank neurologic disease. Should the anatomical findings not correspond with the clinical symptoms, a more thorough urodynamic investigation should be performed before surgery. Patients with recurrent urinary incontinence following previous surgery should definitely have a complete urodynamic investigation, including water cystoscopy, urethroscopy, and cystometry.

Factors Influencing Stress Urinary Incontinence

Anatomical stress urinary incontinence is considered to result from a variety of anatomical changes, including alterations in the urethrovesical angle and urethral axis, loss of urethral length, and variations in intraurethral and intravesical pressure gradients. Hodgkinson was one of the first to suggest that patients who develop stress urinary incontinence do so as a result of the urethra and bladder base being posteriorly displaced beneath the pelvic diaphragm. These changes prevent the intra-abdominal pressure from being transmitted to the external surface of the posterior urethra. Stress urinary incontinence results because intraurethral pressure is lower than intravesical pressure. Hodgkinson's observations, along with those of Enhorning, Muellner, and others suggest that stress urinary incontinence is largely mechanical in origin and can best be corrected by restoring the urethrovesical junction to a high retropubic position above the pelvic diaphragm.

The importance of the pubourethral ligaments in the support of the bladder neck cannot be overlooked. Resuspension of the urethra to these ligaments has been the basis of surgical success for many gynecologists. Zacharin considers the key site of continence control in the female to be the paraurethral attachment of the posterior pubourethral ligaments on either side of the posterior one-third of the urethra. A variety of surgical techniques, both vaginal and abdominal, have been devised to repair the suspensory ligament defect in the posterior urethra.

Periurethral fibrosis can cause urethral rigidity, impairing the mechanisms of urethral closure. Periurethral fixation and scarring may also prevent normal funneling of the bladder neck and posterior urethra, with loss of the physiologic mobility of the posterior urethra that permits normal voiding. As a result, patients who have undergone previous surgery may have no anatomical evidence of an abnormal position of the urethra and bladder base. A history of previous surgical attempts to correct urinary incontinence is an important factor in the selection of the appropriate technique for subsequent surgical repair.

The selection of the appropriate procedure is one of the most important decisions that the surgeon must make. The type of anatomical defect is the key issue in selecting the appropriate operation.

Not all incontinent patients can be benefited by any single operative procedure. For example, both anatomical stress incontinence and herniation of the posterior urethra and bladder base through the levator hiatus (cystourethrocele) should be repaired by a primary vaginal procedure. Only by appropriately repairing the musculofascial defect of the pelvic diaphragm can there be reasonable assurance of correction of the basic problem of genuine stress urinary incontinence. When vaginal relaxation and herniation (cystourethrocele) do not exist, the urethra should be suspended by one of the various abdominal or retropubic procedures.

Restoration of normal urethral pressure depends on whether the posterior urethra and bladder neck can be elevated to a high retropubic position. In cases where the desired anatomical position cannot be achieved by the vaginal route, an abdominal or suprapubic procedure is required for adequate urethral support.

Treatment of Stress Urinary Incontinence

With widening of the levator ani hiatus due to stretching, relaxation, or atrophy of the pelvic floor musculature (Fig. 25-21), the pubourethral ligaments elongate. Alterations of the fascial ligamentous and fibromuscular support to the bladder base and posterior urethra permit hypermobility and descent of the urethrovesical junction beneath the pelvic diaphragm, the end result of pelvic floor relaxation.

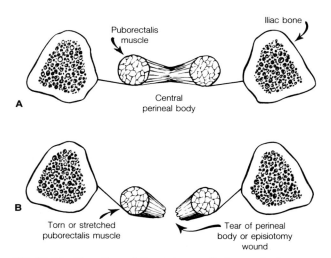

FIG. 25-21 The sling of the puborectalis is attached to the central point of the perineum (*A*). With separation or weakening of the puborectalis from childbirth or aging, support to the pelvic diaphragm is weakened and the levator hiatus is widened (*B*).

The two principal aims of surgery are to support and elevate the posterior urethra and bladder neck to a high retropubic position and to repair the anatomical defect of the pelvic diaphragm and supporting fascia. Surgical correction of urinary incontinence and repair of the pelvic diaphragm are two separate procedures; correction of one should not be done without correction of the other.

If stress incontinence is associated with a weakness of the periurethral attachments of the levator ani and pelvic fascia, any treatment that is designed to strengthen these muscles and fascial supports is appropriate. Anatomical correction requires that the levator ani muscles be relocated so that the urethral occlusive forces will be increased by the active contraction of the levator fibers. From a surgical standpoint, one of the goals of the operative procedure should be to achieve close approximation between the levator ani muscles and the urethra. Repair of a torn or stretched puborectalis portion of the levator hiatus would increase the support to the posterior urethra and bladder base.

TYPES OF ANATOMICAL DEFECTS

Stress urinary incontinence can be divided into four categories: (1) cases associated with a cystourethrocele; (2) cases following childbirth or previous surgery of the anterior vaginal wall but unassociated with demonstrable urethrocele or cystourethrocele; (3) cases occurring in nulliparous women in which no anatomical defect of the urethra or the bladder can be demonstrated; and (4) cases resulting from the improper use of the resectoscope on the vesical neck.

Most cases of stress incontinence are associated with cystourethrocele, and fortunately the operative results for this group of patients are quite successful. With loss of the tone of the urethral wall and the supporting paraurethral support from the urogenital diaphragm, the circular fibers of the vesical sphincter fail to remain closed when abdominal pressure is increased (Fig. 25–22). During surgery it is important to plicate the paraurethral and paravesical fascia carefully and to elevate the posterior urethra and urethrovesical junction to a high retropubic (intra-abdominal) position. To increase the total urethral closure pressure, the entire length of the urethra should be plicated. By approximating the relaxed paraurethral fascia along the entire urethra, the circular muscle fibers of the urethra are supported, and the total intraurethral pressure is increased.

When there is no demonstrable cystourethrocele, incontinence may result from scarring from an obstetric injury or previous surgery of the anterior vaginal wall. Scar tissue forms along the urethra, and the smooth muscle is prevented from closing normally because the surrounding tissue is fixed. When the vesical neck and urethral lumen are observed through a cystoscope, incomplete and irregular closure can be observed.

A second group of patients is made up of those in whom stress incontinence follows an unsuccessful attempt to repair a cystourethrocele. Secondary attempts at urethral plication by the vaginal

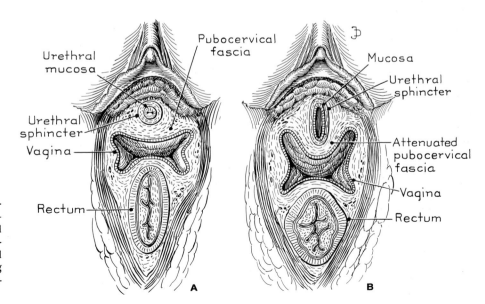

FIG. 25-22 (*A*) Schematic representation of camera-shutter–like action of normal urethral sphincter. (*B*) Schematic representation of failure of urethral sphincter to close on straining after development of urethrocele.

route are less successful in restoring continence than are primary procedures. Van Rooyen and Liebenberg have demonstrated an 89% long-term success rate with anterior colporrhaphy in a group of 150 patients, 60% of whom had documented evidence of periurethral fibrosis from previous surgery. If the recurrent incontinence is marked, treatment may be by a number of retropubic urethral suspension procedures or by a Goebell–Stoeckel strap operation.

There is a third group of women with stress incontinence who have had no children and in whom a neurologic dysfunction of the bladder cannot be demonstrated. These women are usually elderly, but on rare occasions the condition occurs in young, nulliparous women. In the older patients a loss of muscle tone of the urogenital diaphragm causes the incontinence. A plication of the sphincter and the urethra for its full length is successful in some instances, but the results are not as satisfactory as when incontinence results from childbirth. If the incontinence is severe, the Marshall–Marchetti–Krantz type of urethral suspension is the primary procedure.

A fourth group of women have stress incontinence resulting from the use of the resectoscope on the vesical neck. In 1921, Caulk reported on the treatment of contracture of the vesical neck in women by means of the cautery punch. Later, Folsom became very enthusiastic about the procedure for a condition that he referred to as female prostatism. According to Folsom's writings, he considered female "prostatism" to occur almost as frequently as the male disease. The report by Van Rooyen and Liebenberg in 1978 indicates that urologists have continued to use the resectoscope in the region of the vesical neck, even though clinical experience fails to demonstrate that specific need for the instrument. Although the instrument is aimed at relieving intraurethral obstruction, repeated resectoscopic procedures have produced scarring and rigid fixation of the urethra. The more frequently the resectoscope is used, the more women seek relief from incontinence following the procedure. In some cases, the procedure has converted mild symptoms of stress incontinence into constant and almost total incontinence, and in several cases a urethrovaginal fistula has followed an overly aggressive resectoscopic procedure.

The choice of operative procedure for the primary treatment of stress incontinence depends on an identification of those patients who are not ideal candidates for primary urethral plication and suspension by the vaginal route. Abdominal suspension procedures, which also have favorable cure rates (Table 25–1), would be more practical for patients with stress incontinence with the following characteristics:

Minimal anatomical relaxation of the urethra and urethrovesical junction

Other indications for abdominal surgery, including myomata uteri, ovarian cyst or benign intraabdominal disease

Weakening of the fascial or ligamentous support of the urethra *only*, but without loss of demonstrable anatomic support of the pelvic floor, when the patient is nulliparous and, usually, postmenopausal

Surgical trauma to the suspensory ligaments of the urethra and pelvic diaphragm including such procedures as radical vulvectomy

TABLE 25–1 *Abdominal Urethral Suspension Procedures*

AUTHOR (YEAR)	PROCEDURE	NUMBER OF PATIENTS	PERCENT CURE	MINIMAL FOLLOW-UP PERIOD
Stanton (1979)	Modified Burch	43	86	2 years*
Lee (1979)	Marshall–Marchetti–Krantz	227	91	2 years
Stamey (1980)	Stamey	203	91	6 months*
Quigley (1981)	Pereyra	40	82	1 year
Parnell (1982)	Marshall–Marchetti–Krantz	140	90	1 year
Richardson (1981)	Iliopectineal suspension	213	91	2 years*
Muzsnai (1982)	Suprapubic vaginopexy	98	95	6 months*
McDuffie (1981)	Marshall–Marchetti–Krantz	175	90	1 year*
McDuffie (1981)	Marshall–Marchetti–Krantz	70	86	5 years
Pereyra (1982)	Modified Pereyra	54	87	4 years
Kaufman (1981)	Marshall–Marchetti–Krantz	73	97	1 year

* Includes both primary and secondary procedures

A history of a sacral colpopexy procedure for suspension of a prolapsed vaginal vault with potential postoperative straightening of the urethrovesical junction

OPERATION FOR CYSTOURETHROCELE AND KELLY URETHRAL PLICATION

Surgical correction of cystourethrocele is directed toward restoring the fascial and muscular support to the bladder neck and urethra. The Kelly urethral plication, originally described in 1911, remains one of the primary methods of surgical repair of this condition. Kelly deserves much credit for identifying the precise anatomical deficits in the posterior urethral support mechanisms that result in stress urinary incontinence (Fig. 25–23). Although 20% of the patients on whom Kelly and Dumm reported in 1914 showed no improvement following the procedure, the majority of these had had previous surgery. Most abdominal procedures have a similar long-term cure rate today.

Historically, the Kelly method has been selected as the primary surgical treatment of choice in cases where there is demonstrable musculofascial relaxation of the levator hiatus as a result of childbearing. The success of the procedure is related to the thoroughness of the dissection and to the wide mobilization of the posterior urethra and the surrounding paraurethral fascia at the urethrovesical junction.

Two important reparative functions are required in addition to the Kelly plication sutures at the urethrovesical junction and along the entire urethra: (1) high, retropubic elevation of the urethrovesical junction from a dependent position to a position well above the urogenital diaphragm; and (2) restoration of the suburethral fascial support to strengthen the urethral musculature and consequently increase intraurethral pressure. For urinary continence to be achieved, the reparative procedure must increase the intraurethral pressure, but cannot completely obstruct the urethra. Plication of the outer urethra to the region of the external meatus, as emphasized by Kennedy, is also beneficial in restoring intraurethral and suburethral support, al-

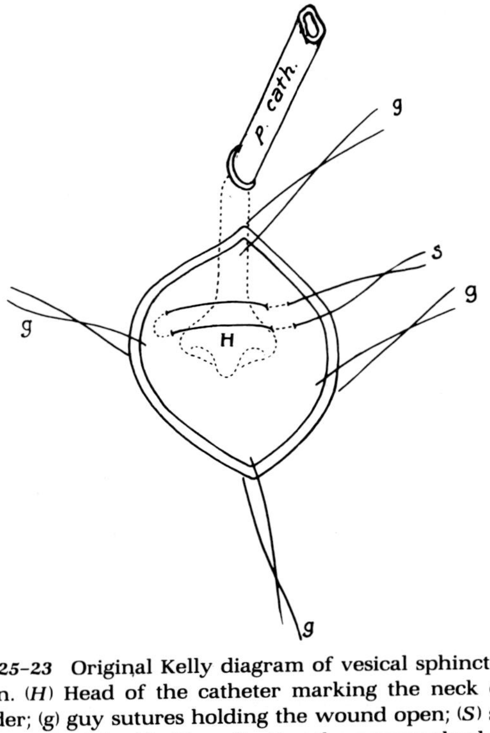

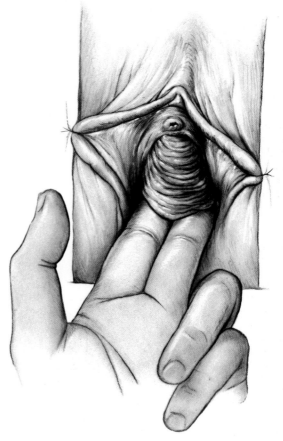

FIG. 25-23 Original Kelly diagram of vesical sphincter plication. (*H*) Head of the catheter marking the neck of the bladder; (g) guy sutures holding the wound open; (*S*) suture at the neck of the bladder plicating the paraurethral fascia.

FIG. 25-24 Anatomical relaxation of the bladder base (cystourethrocele) and fibromuscular floor of the urethra (urethrocele) with posterior rotation of the urethrovesical junction.

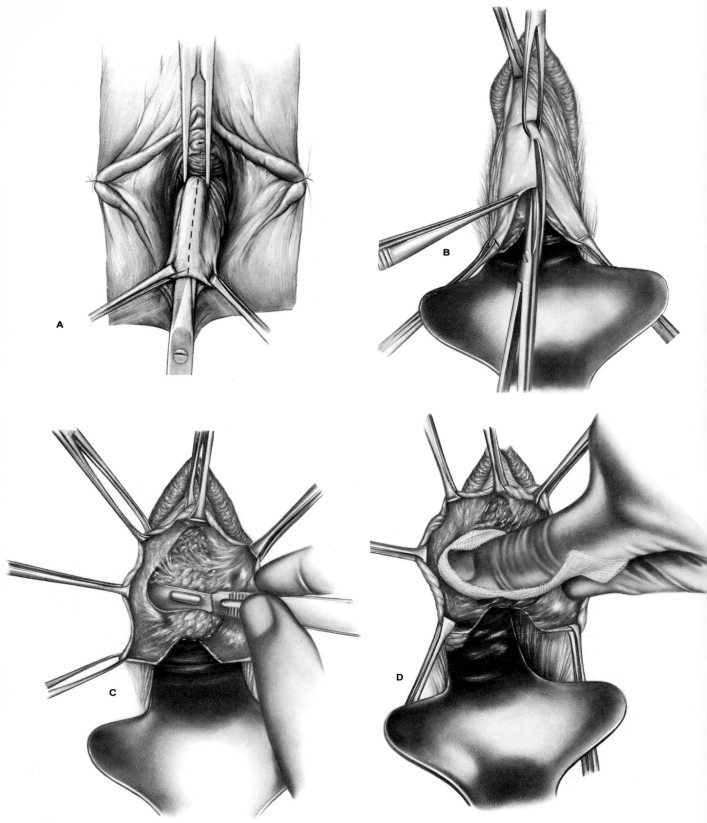

FIG. 25–25 (A,B) Technique of anterior colporrhaphy. Scissor dissection of the vaginal mucosa to the region of the external urethral meatus. Traction must be maintained on the vagina along the course of the dissection to keep the wall of the bladder separate from the vaginal mucosa in order to avoid trauma to the bladder. (C) Sharp dissection of the adherent fascia from the vaginal mucosa. The dissection should be deep enough to reach the white, relatively avascular plane just beneath the vaginal epithelium. (D) Blunt finger dissection with a single thickness of a gauze sponge to provide sufficient traction against the fascia to free it from the mucosa beneath the urethra and bladder.

FIG. 25–25 (continued). (E) Beginning at the external meatus, successive vertical mattress stitches of No. 0 delayed-absorbable suture are placed in the mobilized paraurethral fascia. A Kelly clamp depresses the floor of the urethra as the sutures are tied to avoid necrosis of the wall of the urethra. The last suture at the bladder neck is anchored to the posterior pubourethral ligament using No. 1 delayed-absorbable suture. The pubourethral ligament is grasped with a straight Ochsner clamp. The suture passes through the paraurethral fascia and is then firmly inserted through the pubourethral ligament on the posterior aspect of the symphysis pubis. A second suture is placed on the opposite side of the urethra where it incorporates the same anatomical structures. Both sutures are tied, drawing the paraurethral fascia beneath the urethra and elevating the posterior urethra to a high retropubic position.

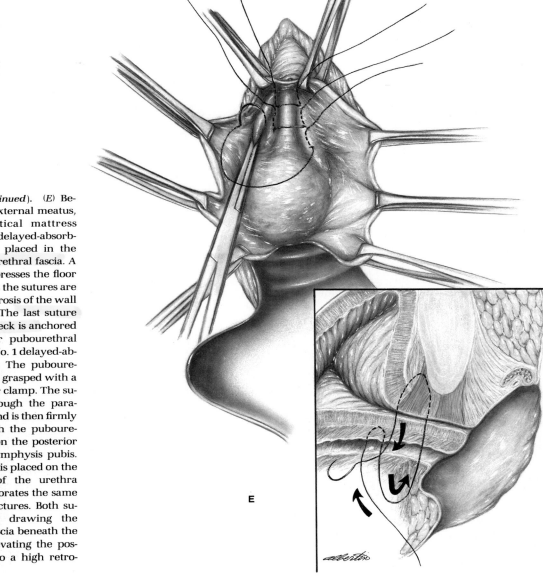

E

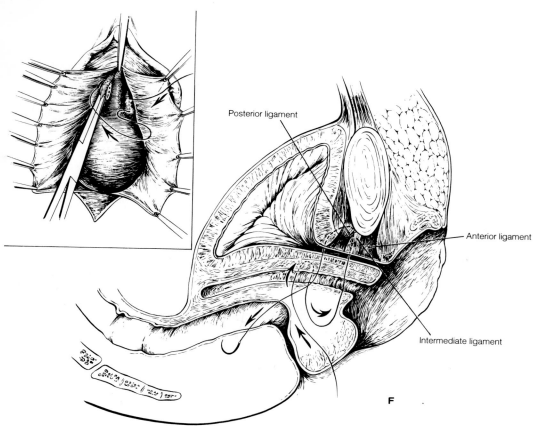

Posterior ligament

Anterior ligament

Intermediate ligament

F

FIG. 25–25 (continued). (F) Another view of the suspension of the paraurethral fascia at the urethrovesical junction to the posterior pubourethral ligament, omitting the proximal urethral plication sutures for illustrative purposes. Insert shows the placement of No. 1 delayed-absorbable suture at the urethrovesical junction, firmly anchoring the suture to the opposite posterior pubourethral ligament at the tip of the Ochsner clamp and close to the lower one-third of the posterior surface of the symphysis pubis. A similar suture is placed in the opposite paraurethral fascia and pubourethral ligament.

though the maximum surgical benefit is achieved in the region of the posterior urethra and urethrovesical junction. If mobilization of the posterior urethra is adequate, the basic plication sutures, which are strategically placed in the paraurethral fascia and anchored retropubically to the posterior pubourethral ligaments, will achieve the desired anatomical result. Excessive suturing in the region of the bladder neck should be avoided, since it does not ensure urinary continence and may instead produce excessive scarring of the urethrovesical area. Urethral scarring can result in incomplete closure, shortening of the urethra, and further disturbance in the voiding process.

Urethral plication with urethrovesical repair is performed when the defect in the pelvic diaphragm is confined to the part of the vagina beneath the urethra and the base of the bladder (Fig. 25–24).

Technique

After a midline incision is made through the vaginal mucosa extending from the apex of the vagina to the urethral meatus (Fig. 25–25A,B), the flaps of the vagina are dissected laterally with sharp knife dissection (Fig. 25–25C). The paraurethral and paravesical fascia are mobilized widely by blunt finger dissection using a single layer of a gauze sponge (Fig. 25–25D). Entry into the white-appearing avascular plane just beneath the vaginal mucosa will facilitate fascial mobilization, which should be extended to the most lateral aspects of the urethra and bladder base.

From a point less than 1 cm from the urethral meatus, successive vertical mattress sutures are made in the paraurethral fascia (Fig. 25–25E). Bites are taken parallel to, and on each side of, the urethra

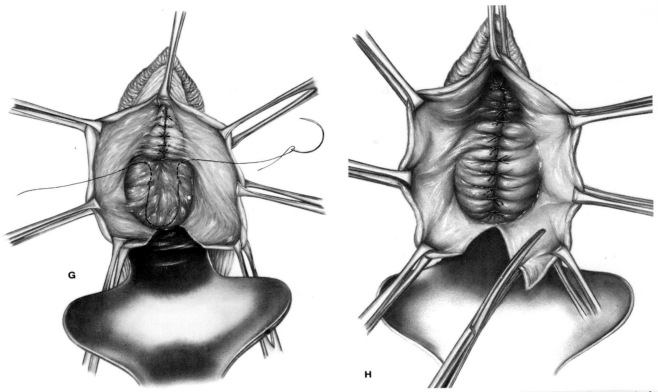

FIG. 25-25 (continued). *(G)* Repair of cystocele with a single layer of vertical mattress sutures in the mobilized paravesical fascia. *(H)* The normal urethrovesical anatomy is restored and the excess vaginal mucosa is excised. Removal of too much mucosa will cause narrowing of the caliber of the vagina.

to draw the fascia firmly beneath it. No. 0 delayed-absorbable sutures are used on a small curved needle. At the urethrovesical junction, the para-urethral fascia should be drawn carefully from its most lateral margin to add additional support to the posterior urethra.

If properly placed, the suspension suture at the urethrovesical junction should restore the posterior urethra and vesical neck to their normal retropubic (intra-abdominal) position, above the pelvic diaphragm. Most vaginal procedures for the correction of stress incontinence fail to emphasize restoration of the intra-abdominal position, which may be the explanation for unsuccessful results. The bladder neck suture must be painstakingly accurate. Placement requires the selection of strong paraurethral fascia, which is securely anchored to the reflection of the posterior pubourethral ligament along the posterior surface of the pubic bone.

The bladder neck suture begins with a firm bite in the paraurethral fascia (Fig. 25-25E,F). The suture crosses the urethra to anchor securely in the opposite pubourethral ligament high on the posterior aspect of the symphysis pubis. When tied, this suture

draws the paraurethral fascia beneath the posterior urethra and elevates it to a high retropubic position. A similar suture is placed in the opposite para-urethral fascia and pubourethral ligament, which provides additional support to the posterior urethra and reinforces the high retropubic placement of the urethra.

In most cases, the urethrovesical junction can be identified without the use of a catheter. If necessary, a Foley urethral catheter can be inserted and withdrawn, and the point where it meets obstruction noted. When the plication sutures are being placed along the course of the urethra and bladder neck, an assistant should invert the posterior floor of the urethra slightly with a Kelly clamp as each suture is tied.

The cystocele is repaired by a similar series of No. 0 delayed-absorbable plication sutures, which are placed in the mobilized paravesical fascia. The bladder base is displaced by a Kelly clamp and the sutures are tied in the midline (Fig. 25-25G). The bladder base should not be elevated too high to avoid a direct runoff-type of incontinence following surgery. Since less correction is far better than over-

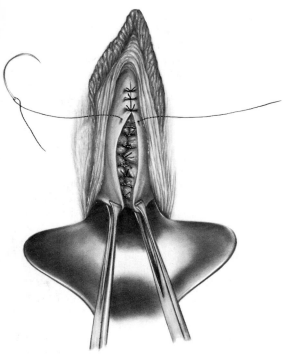

FIG. 25–25 (continued). (I) The mucosal margins are approximated in the midline with interrupted, No. 2-0 delayed-absorbable sutures which include the underlying fascia.

correction of a cystocele, second layer of plication sutures in the bladder fascia is not needed unless the cystocele is extremely large and cannot be supported by the initial suture layer.

The excess vaginal mucosa is excised (Fig. 25–25H), and the margins of the vagina are approximated in the midline using No. 2-0 delayed-absorbable suture. Including a bite of the adjacent fascia beneath the urethra and bladder with each vaginal suture will obliterate any dead space beneath the vaginal wall (Fig 25-25I). The bladder is then distended with 300 ml of saline. A suprapubic Silastic catheter (No. 12F) is then inserted percutaneously into the bladder approximately 2 cm above the pubic bone (see Chapter 6).

The Kelly plication operation and cystocele repair has been used extensively with good results (Table 25–2). More than 85% of the patients achieve long-term urinary control, 5% to 10% have improved control, while only the remaining 5% are unimproved. By doing a meticulous preoperative urologic workup of these patients, the clinician can select the most suitable candidates for this type of repair, which improves the success rate of the procedure.

Some clinics have begun to monitor intraurethral pressure during surgery to make certain that urethral pressure has been increased significantly above the intravesical pressure. Intraoperative monitoring may provide a gauge to show the amount of urethral plication needed for each procedure. If pressure is determined to be inadequate at the time of surgery, replacement sutures along the posterior urethra can be added until suspension is adequate.

For minor degrees of stress urinary incontinence, Kegel's perineal exercises should be used to strengthen the urogenital diaphragm and to increase the voluntary muscular support to the posterior urethra. As described by Kegel, this technique exercises not only the bulbocavernosus muscle, but also strengthens the superficial and deep transverse perineal and the levator ani muscles of the pelvic diaphragm. The exercise technique is beneficial for patients with minimal symptoms; Kegel was the first to emphasize the fact that herniation of the bladder and urethra through a hiatus in the pelvic diaphragm would not be corrected by this exercise.

When surgery is contraindicated or must be deferred, a patient with a cystourethrocele can be made comfortable with a vaginal pessary that provides support to the posterior urethra and bladder base. A cystocele may occur alone without anatomical stress incontinence, and it will then require separate surgical repair.

THE MARSHALL–MARCHETTI–KRANTZ OPERATION

The technique of the Marshall–Marchetti–Krantz procedure has been fundamentally unchanged

TABLE 25–2   *Vaginal Reparative Procedures (Kelly Plication)*

AUTHOR (YEAR)	PROCEDURE	NUMBER OF PATIENTS	PERCENT CURE	MINIMAL FOLLOW-UP PERIOD
Kaufman (1981)	Anterior colporrhaphy	11	100%	1 year
Beck (1982)	Anterior colporrhaphy	105	80%	2 years
Van Rooyen (1979)	Anterior colporrhaphy	102	92%	3 years*
Peters (1980)	Anterior colporrhaphy	100	90%	5 years

* Includes both primary and secondary procedures

since originally described by its authors in 1949. However, as time has passed, there have been a few changes, such as those in suture placement and types of suture material, and a few variations in the method of accomplishing the retropubic fixation of the urethra and bladder neck. Because of its low complications rate and simplicity, the procedure is the retropubic urethropexy operation of choice for many.

Technique

We have found the following modification of the Marshall–Marchetti–Krantz procedure to be satisfactory. After the pelvic examination under anesthesia, the patient is placed in a semi-frog position and a No. 24 Foley catheter with a 5-cc bulb is inserted into the bladder. Although a Pfannenstiel incision is the preferred approach to the space of Retzius, this is not always feasible if there is intra-abdominal pathology that requires a low midline approach. The intra-abdominal procedure is completed and the peritoneum is closed before dissection into the space of Retzius is begun. This is usually done by blunt dissection, which is more desirable to avoid bleeding; however, if there is distortion or obliteration by scarring of disease or previous surgery, sharp dissection must be used. Whatever oozing or bleeding is encountered can usually be controlled by pressure, individual ligature, or careful fulguration. Adequate exposure in this rather limited space may be difficult to obtain, particularly in more obese patients. The dissection is carried down toward the inferior aspect of the symphysis to within 1 cm of the external urethral meatus. The surgeon inserts two fingers into the vagina and elevates the anterior vagina and bladder neck so that the sutures may be more easily and accurately placed. The catheter demonstrates the urethra and the balloon indicates the bladder neck and trigonal area. The sutures of No. 1 delayed-absorbable material—two or three on either side—are taken. Each suture is taken (1) into the submucosa of the vaginal wall lateral to the urethra, (2) into the fascia adjacent to the wall of the urethra, and (3) into the fibrocartilage of the symphysis using a No. 4 or No. 6 Mayo round needle (Fig. 25–26A,B). This technique of the "double bite" suture placement, as described in the original procedure, gives a more secure suspension and is used whenever possible rather than a simple single suspending bite from the paraurethral tissue to the pubic fibrocartilage. In placing the pubic suture, the curvature of the needle should be followed accurately to avoid breakage of the needle or laceration of the tissue. The surgeon then changes gloves and gown, and the sutures are then tied and cut in pairs from below upward. If there is any uncertainty in identifying the proper location for the suture near the bladder neck, one should not hesitate to open the dome of the bladder transversely in order to place the suture accurately under direct vision. If this suture is placed improperly into the bladder wall, it is invariable that postoperative symptoms of recurrent urgency and frequency will develop.

We have omitted the cystopexy portion of the original procedure from the method used in our clinic in recent years, since it produced fixation and funneling of the bladder neck that resulted in increased tension on the trigone and detrusor muscle. It is usually not necessary to use any more sutures than those already placed to obliterate the space of Retzius.

A suprapubic Silastic tube (No. 12 F) is then inserted through the skin and into the bladder under direct vision for abdominal drainage prior to closure of the incision (see Chapter 6). A small Penrose drain is placed on either side of the midline in the operative area if there is residual venous bleeding, and the wound is closed per routine.

There are numerous modifications of this basic retropubic urethropexy in the manner in which the suspending sutures are placed and in the type of suture material used. The Burch technique suspends the paraurethral tissues and bladder neck to Cooper's ligament, avoiding trauma to the periosteum. This practically obviates osteitis pubis, which can be a postoperative complication, although rare, when suspension is made to the periosteum. The problem of overcorrection of the bladder neck angle is occasionally encountered in the Burch modification, leading to postoperative frequency, overflow incontinence, and chronic urinary tract infection. To avoid this problem of excessive elevation of the trigone and bladder neck, we use a nonabsorbable suture and do not attempt to draw the paraurethral fascia to Cooper's ligament, which causes the suture to be tied in a "bowstring" fashion.

Inspection of the vagina following retropubic urethropexy reveals that the entire vaginal wall, together with the urethra, is markedly elevated. Occasionally, an uncorrected cystocele remains.

POSTOPERATIVE CARE

The postoperative care of the bladder after any of these procedures may be difficult and disturbing for both patient and operator because there is practically always some derangement of bladder function and urinary tract infection. Preoperative evaluation procedures, even when meticulously and carefully done, frequently introduce infection or light up a quiescent infection in the urinary tract.

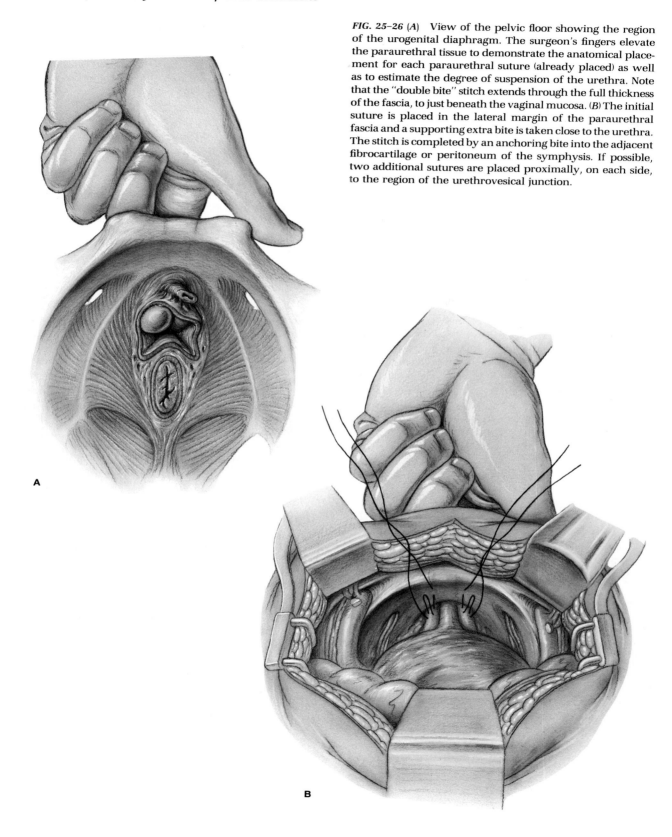

FIG. 25–26 *(A)* View of the pelvic floor showing the region of the urogenital diaphragm. The surgeon's fingers elevate the paraurethral tissue to demonstrate the anatomical placement for each paraurethral suture (already placed) as well as to estimate the degree of suspension of the urethra. Note that the "double bite" stitch extends through the full thickness of the fascia, to just beneath the vaginal mucosa. *(B)* The initial suture is placed in the lateral margin of the paraurethral fascia and a supporting extra bite is taken close to the urethra. The stitch is completed by an anchoring bite into the adjacent fibrocartilage or peritoneum of the symphysis. If possible, two additional sutures are placed proximally, on each side, to the region of the urethrovesical junction.

A

B

If obvious infection is known to be present at the time of surgery, the drug of choice, which has been previously determined by culture and sensitivity studies, is given without interruption until the bladder is emptying itself well postoperatively and the urine is free from infection.

The suprapubic Penrose drains are removed on the third postoperative day. On the fourth postoperative day, intermittent clamping of the suprapubic catheter for 3 hours is begun. The patient is then encouraged to void. If the patient cannot void spontaneously, the catheter is unclamped to allow drainage of the bladder. The cycle of clamping-unclamping is then repeated. The catheter is removed when there is consistently less than 100 ml residual urine after spontaneous voiding. The bladder should not be allowed to become distended to more than 300 ml urine. It is important to impress on the patient that at first she may be completely unable to void or may be able to void only in small amounts. If she is not reassured by this explanation, she may become apprehensive and her state of anxious tension will hamper prompt recovery. Prior to operation an explanation is given to her of just what the procedure sets out to accomplish and by what means this is done. Then she must be made to realize that a bladder weakened for such a period of time preoperatively will require some time to recover strength and function. In a few cases, the patient may have a protracted course in which voiding may be slow and difficult. This should not be too discouraging to the patient or the gynecologist. Urecholine, 10 mg to 25 mg by mouth, may be given 3 or 4 times per day for a week to help reduce bladder residual and to increase muscular tone.

Suprapubic bladder drainage by a small polyethylene or Silastic tube has made the postoperative care of the bladder much easier and reduced the incidence of urinary tract infection. It is used routinely in practically all operations of the bladder, urethra, or anterior vaginal wall.

RESULTS

When such a corrective procedure is performed as the primary effort, the degree of success is, as expected, higher than if the same procedure is done following one or more unsuccessful surgical attempts. As an example, Burch in 1968 reported a 93% success rate in 143 cases using the Cooper's ligament modification of the Marshall–Marchetti–Krantz procedure, but it is noted that 92% of the patients had had no previous surgery for correction of stress urinary incontinence.

The percentage of late failures or less than satisfactory results rises gradually for several years after the use of all procedures for the correction of stress urinary incontinence. The comparative cure rates of the Kelly plication and Marshall–Marchetti–Krantz procedures are shown in Table 25–1 and are quite similar, varying between 85% and 90%.

Even the best-conceived and best-executed procedures for correction of stress urinary incontinence will have a certain percentage of failures, and analysis of these failures can teach the operator what to be aware of in a future effort.

A most common failure is improper choice of the operative procedure. It has been pointed out in the discussion of the preoperative studies of the bladder and patient that much unnecessary trouble can be avoided if the neurologically impaired bladder is detected. This is most important because detrusor dysfunction is only aggravated by any operative procedure that causes any obstruction at the bladder neck, whether this obstruction be simply a constriction by plication, a repositioning of the bladder neck and urethra by the sling procedure, or the retropubic urethral suspension. Careful preoperative study of bladder capacity and dynamics will rule out this pitfall.

Failure of the operator to recognize urge incontinence or detrusor instability causes will result in a failure or a less than satisfactory result with the procedure. Again, proper preoperative study is emphasized.

Scarring from previous injury, surgery, or disease can be another most important factor, giving either complete or partial failure. The space of Retzius, scarred by previous surgery, requires dissection and mobilization of the urethra for proper performance of the Marshall–Marchetti–Krantz procedure.

Chronic pulmonary disease resulting an intractable cough, such as bronchiectasis, emphysema, or asthma is a frequent cause of failure of repair. It would be ideal to say that with control of the cough, one can expect improvement of the stress urinary incontinence, but too frequently this is not possible. Morbid obesity is an important contraindication to incontinence surgery. Since the pelvic floor is the target of orthostatic pressure created by the weight of the intra-abdominal viscera, obesity is one of the major high-risk factors that decreases the cure rate of all of the operative procedures.

With a basic understanding of the operative procedures discussed in this chapter, one should choose the method or improvise as the particular case demands. It is difficult to say with certainty which procedure is the best, and experience of the operator should influence the decision to some degree. Because of the simplicity, dependability, and paucity of complications, we have favored the modified Kelly plication procedure for patients requiring primary surgery in whom the urinary incontinence is associated with a demonstrable anatomical defect of the pelvic floor. In case of previous operative failure and in patients without an anatomical defect, the Marshall–Marchetti–Krantz procedure is the one most commonly used. However, the well-trained gynecologist should be comprehensively trained to deal with all the problems and vagaries of stress urinary incontinence.

Bibliography

Abrams P, Feneley R, Torrens M: Urodynamics. New York, Springer-Verlag, 1983

Asmussen M: Aspects of continence, incontinence and micturition in women based on simultaneous urethral cystometry. In Ostergard DR (ed): Gynecologic Urology and Urodynamics—Theory and Practice. Baltimore, Williams and Wilkins, 1980

Awad SA, McGinnis RH: Factors that influence the incidence of detrusor instability in women. J Urol 130:114, 1983

Ball TL, Knapp RC, Nathanson B, et al: Stress incontinence. Am J Obstet Gynecol 94:997, 1966

Ball TL, Wright KL.: Stress incontinence, complications and sequelae of the Marshall–Marchetti operation. Pacif Med Surg 73:290, 1965

Bates CP, Bradley WE, Glen ES, et al: Fourth report on the standardization of terminology of lower urinary tract function. Br J Urol 53:333, 1981

Bates CP, Bradley WE, Glen ES, et al: The standardization of terminology of lower urinary tract function. J Urol 121:551, 1979

Beck RP, McCormick S: Treatment of urinary stress incontinence with anterior colporrhaphy. Obstet Gynecol 59:269, 1982

Bent AE, Richardson DA, Ostergar DR: Diagnosis of lower urinary tract disorders in postmenopausal patients. Am J Obstet Gynecol 145:218, 1983

Blute ML, Symmonds RE, Lee RA: Repeat Marshall–Marchetti–Krantz procedure for genuine stress incontinence. Obstet Gynecol 66, 1985 (in press)

Brack CB, Guild HG: Urethral obstruction in the female child. Am J Obstet Gynecol 76:1105, 1958

Bradley WE, Scott FB: Physiology of the urinary bladder. Campbell's Urology 1:87, 1978

Brown ADG: The urodynamic management of female urinary incontinence. M.D. Thesis, Edinburgh, 1974, cited by Turner–Warwick

Burch JC: Cooper's ligament urethrovesical suspension for stress urinary incontinence Am J Obstet Gynecol 100:764, 1968

Cardozo LD, Stanton SL, Williams JE: Detrusor instability following surgery for genuine stress incontinence. Br J Urol 51:204, 1979

Caulk JR: Contractures of vesical neck in the female. J Urol 6:341, 1921

Enhorning G: Simultaneous recording of intraurethral and intravesical pressure: A study on urethral closure in stress incontinent women. Acta Chir Scand (Suppl) 276:1, 1961

Everett HS, Ridley J: Gynecological and Obstetrical Urology. Baltimore, Williams and Wilkins, 1947

———: A condemnation of resectoscopic procedures upon the female vesical neck. Urol Cutan Rev 52:80, 1948

Fantl JA: Urinary incontinence due to detrusor instability. Clin Obstet Gynecol 27:474, 1984

Fisher AM, Gordon H: The gynecologic approach to the patient with urological symptoms. Clin Obstet Gynecol 8:191, 1981

Folsom AL, O'Brien HA: The female urethra. JAMA 128:408, 1945

Ghoneim MA, Rottembourg JL, Fretin J, et al: Urethral pressure profile: Standardization of technique and study of reproducibility. Urology 5:763, 1975

Gleason DM, Reilly RJ, Bottaccini MR, et al: The urethral continence zone and its relation to stress incontinence. J Urol 112:81, 1974

Gosling JA: Why are women continent? Proc R Coll Obstet Gynecol 13 Feb, 1981

Gosling J: The structure of the bladder and urethra in relation to function. Urol Clin North Am 6:31, 1979

Green TH, Jr: Development of a plan for diagnosis and treatment of urinary stress incontinence. Am J Obstet Gynecol 83:632, 1962

———: The problem of urinary stress incontinence in the female. Obstet Gynecol Surv 23:603, 1968

———: Vaginal repair: In Stanton SL, Tanagho EA (eds): Surgery of Female Incontinence. New York, Springer-Verlag, 1980

Hodgkinson CP: Stress Urinary incontinence. Am J Obstet Gynecol 108:141, 1970

Hodgkinson CP, Cobert N: Direct urethrocystometry. Am J Obstet Gynecol 79:648, 1960

Hutch JA, Kao MS: Anatomy and Physiology of the Bladder, Trigone and Urethra. New York, Meredith, Corp, 1972

Jarvis GJ, Hall S, Stamp S, et al: An assessment of urodynamic examination in incontinent women. Br J Obstet Gynecol 87:893, 1980

Kaufman J: Operative management of stress urinary incontinence. J Urol 126:465, 1981

Kegel AH: Progressive resistance exercise in the functional restoration of the perineal muscles. Am J Obstet Gynecol 56:238, 1948

———: Exercise in the treatment of genital relaxation, urinary stress incontinence and sexual dysfunction. In Greenhill JP (ed): Office Gynecology, 9th ed. Chicago, Year Book Medical Publishers, 1971

Kelly HA: Operative Gynecology. New York, Appleton, 1909

Kelly HA, Dumm WM: Urinary incontinence in women, without manifest injury to the bladder: A report of 20 cases. Surg Gynecol Obstet 18:444, 1914

Kennedy C: Stress incontinence of urine: A survey of 34 cases treated by the Milin/Sling operation Br Med J ii:263, 1960

Kitzmiller JL, Manzer GA, Nebel WA, et al: Chain cystourethrogram for stress incontinence. Obstet Gynecol 39:333, 1972

Lee RA, Symmonds RE, Goldstein RA: Surgical complications and results of modified Marshall–Marchetti–Krantz procedure for urinary incontinence. Obstet Gynecol 53:447, 1979

Low JA, Kao MS: Intravesical and intraurethral pressure as a measure of urethral sphincter function. Obstet Gynecol 40:627, 1972

———: Patterns of urethral resistance in deficient urethral sphincter functions. Obstet Gynecol 40:634, 1972

Marchant DJ: Clinical evaluation of urinary incontinence, normal anatomy and pathophysiology. Clin Obstet Gynecol 27:434, 1984

Marshall VF, Marchetti AA, Krantz KE: The correction of stress incontinence by simple vesicourethral suspension. Surg Gynecol Obstet 88:509, 1949

Mattingly RF, Davis LE: Primary treatment of anatomic stress urinary incontinence. Clin Obstet Gynecol 27:445, 1984

McDuffie RW, Litin RB, Blundon KE: Urethrovesical suspension (Marshall–Marchetti–Krantz). Am J Surg 141:297, 1981

McGuire EJ, Lytten B, Kohorn EI, et al: Stress urinary incontinence. Obstet Gynecol 47:255, 1976

Muellner SR: The voluntary control of micturition in man. J Urol 80:473, 1958

Muzsnai D, Carrillo E, Dubin C, et al: Retropubic vaginoplasty for correction of urinary stress incontinence. Obstet Gynecol 59:113, 1982

Parnell JP, Marshall VF, Vaughn ED: Primary management of urinary stress incontinence by the Marshall–Marchetti–Krantz vesicourethropexy. J Urol 127:679, 1982

Pelosi MA, Langer A, Sama JC et al: Treatment of urinary incontinence. Obstet Gynecol 47:377, 1976

Pereyra AJ, Lebherz TB, Growdon W, et al: Pubourethral supports in perspective: Modified Pereyra procedure for urinary incontinence. Obstet Gynecol 59:643, 1982

Peters WA, Thonton WN: Selection of the primary operative procedure for stress urinary incontinence. Am J Obstet Gynecol 137:923, 1980

Quigley GJ, King SK: Transvaginal retropubic urethropexy. Am J Obstet Gynecol 139:268, 1981

Raz S, Maggio AJ, Jr, Kaufman JJ: Why the Marshall–Marchetti operation works . . . or does it. Urology 14:154, 1979

Reed T, Anderson KE, Asmussen M, et al: Factors maintaining the intraurethral pressure in women. Invest Urol 17:343, 1980

Richardson AC, Edmonds PB, Williams N: Treatment of stress urinary incontinence due to paravaginal fascial defect. Obstet Gynecol 57:357, 1981

Stamey TA: Endoscopic suspension of the vesical neck for urinary incontinence in females. Ann Surg 192(4):465, 1980

Stanton SL: Surgery of urinary incontinence. Clin in Obstet Gynaecol 5:83, 1979

Tanagho EA: Vesicourethral dynamics. In Urodynamics. Berlin, Springer-Verlag, 1973

Turner–Warwick R: Observations on the function and dysfunctions of the sphincter and detrusor mechanisms. Urol Clin North Am 6(no. 1):11, 1979

Ulmsten U, Henriksson L, Iosif S: The unstable female urethra. Am J Obstet Gynecol 144:93, 1982

Van Rooyen AJL, Liebenberg HC: A clinical approach to urinary incontinence in the female. Obstet Gynecol 53:1 1978

Walter S, Olesen KD: Urinary incontinence and genital prolapse in the female: Clinical, urodynamic and radiologic examinations. Br J Gynecol Obstet 89:393, 1982

Williams TJ: Urinary incontinence in the female. Med Clin North Am 58:729, 1974

Zacharin RF: Abdominal urethral suspension in the management of recurrent stress incontinence of urine: A 15-year experience. Obstet Gynecol 62:644, 1983

Chapter 26

The Goebell–Stoeckel Sling Operation

John H. Ridley, M.D.

Although a great majority of cases of stress incontinence of urine can be cured by a well-executed plication of the sphincter and the urethra, as described in Chapter 25, there are some failures, and one must look to another method for curing them. Failure is especially apt to result in those cases unrelated to childbirth injury in which the poor sphincter musculature has insufficient tone to control the urine when the intravesical pressure is raised. Failure with the plication operation, even in good hands, is often a consequence of previous bungling attempts in which the resulting scar tissue has made it impossible for the sphincter to contract adequately, regardless of how tightly it is plicated.

Other conditions, less frequently encountered, that are not amenable to the plication operation are congenital absence of the sphincter mechanism, which may occur as mentioned by Price in 1933. The absence of part or all of the urethra may be due to congenital deformity such as hypospadias, or be due to obstetrical or surgical accidents. In these latter cases, a urethra may be constructed, but lacking a sphincter mechanism, some procedure is required to ensure continence. In other, more common, instances, irradiation may render the urethra a virtually functionless "water-tube." Finally, there is a group in which the incontinence depends upon faulty innervation, such as may be seen in spina bifida, multiple sclerosis, and spine trauma.

One must be very careful in selecting cases for surgery that could possibly have neurologic disease. Bladder hypotonia with possible ureteral reflux contraindicates any partially obstructive procedure, which may aggravate this underlying problem. In this condition, the bladder musculature *would not* be strengthened, and the reflux *would be* aggravated, leading to an ascending chronic urinary tract infection.

Hodgkinson has made us aware of detrusor dyssynergia dysfunction, which can be a primary cause of a type of incontinence that is not correctable by surgery. Although this condition may be suspected and diagnosed in a majority of cases by accurate history and simple tests, nonetheless it requires sophisticated electronic equipment to be accurately evaluated.

Modern studies and work with highly specialized equipment have clarified some problems that heretofore have been less well understood, such as intraurethral and intravesical pressure gradients. As yet, this type of equipment is not available for general use, owing to its complexity and expense. Beck and Low have worked extensively in this field.

In all of the above groups of cases, the surgeon must seek elsewhere than the vesical neck and the urethra to create a mechanism effective in the control of the urine. Many operations have been devised, none of which has been universally successful, although some can be used to advantage in certain cases. A short summary of these attempts may be useful to the student of incontinence of urine in women. The sling technique will be presented in more detail.

Historical Development of Operative Procedures

In 1907, Giordano utilized a portion of the gracilis muscle to encircle the urethra. Deming in 1926 reported that he restored continence by this means in a woman in whom a urethral tube had been constructed previously because of epispadias.

In 1910, Goebell described an operation in which he dissected free the pyramidalis muscles, brought them down posterior to the symphysis, and encircled the urethra near its junction with the bladder. He suggested crossing the muscles if their length permitted. He reported one case in which this operation was done after constructing a urethra in a child suffering from epispadias. A second operation of this type was done on a 2-year-old child who was incontinent following an operation for meningocele. In both cases the results were reported as satisfactory. An obvious difficulty with this operation lies in the fact that the pyramidalis muscles vary greatly in their development and may be too short to encircle the urethra.

In 1914, Frangenheim used the pyramidalis muscle with an attached strap of fascia from the sheath of the rectus to encircle the male urethra. The strap was brought down retropubically around the urethra and was sutured to itself. The operation was done for incontinence following a perineal injury with stricture formation. The result was reported as perfect.

In 1917, Stoeckel combined the use of the pyramidalis muscle and the fascia strap with a plication at the sphincter region. He first dissected from the midline a strap of fascia with the pyramidalis muscles attached. The distal portion of the strap was split and brought down retropubically to the urethral region. The split ends were made to encircle the urethra and were sutured together below the urethra. He reported two cases treated successfully. In the first case, a fistula had resulted from a cesarean section. After closure of the fistula, the patient was still incontinent. By combining sphincter plication with the use of the pyramidalis muscle and the fascia strap, the patient was cured. The second case was one of a urethrocystocele associated with incontinence. The combination operation resulted in cure.

In 1932, Norman Miller modified the technique of the Goebell–Frangenheim–Stoeckel operation by bringing the pyramidalis muscle with an attached fascia strap down to and beneath the urethra anterior to the symphysis. Apparently the object of this modification was to avoid the possibility of retropubic hemorrhage, particularly from the paraurethral venous sinus frequently encountered at the bladder neck. However, it should be noted that the bleeding encountered by Miller's procedure may be most troublesome about the clitoris. In addition, the fascia strap was placed too far forward of the urethrovesical junction to be most effective.

As a result, the procedure never gained wide acceptance. As will be described, we have encountered very little difficulty from bleeding in the process of placing the fascia strap retropubically.

In 1933, Price reported the cure of urinary incontinence in a girl with congenital absence of the sacrum and the coccyx and without innervation of the sphincter. He used a sling of autogenous fascia lata, which he brought around the urethra retropubically and then attached both ends to the rectus muscle. The principles of this technique with subsequent modification have been used as a most dependable procedure and will be described in detail later in this chapter.

In 1942, Aldridge devised a modification in which he combined some of the points of the Goebell–Frangenheim–Stoeckel procedure with those of Price's procedure. Making a transverse lower abdominal incision, he developed straps of aponeurosis from the rectus sheath on both sides. He directed his incisions for the procurement of these fascia straps outward and upward, paralleling the fibers of the aponeurosis (Fig. 26–1). The fascia straps were detached laterally and the free ends were brought down through the rectus muscles, then retropubically, finally passing beneath the urethra. He depended on the elasticity of the rectus muscle to supply the proper pull on the urethra.

In 1949, Marshall, Marchetti, and Krantz reported an entirely new operation that they had carried out on 50 patients, 38 with the usual type of stress incontinence, 25 of whom had had a total of 40 standard gynecologic operations without relief. The procedure consisted of simple operative elevation and fixation of the vesical neck and the urethra by suturing them to pubic periosteum and rectus muscles by the suprapubic route with chromic catgut. A more detailed description of this procedure is given in Chapter 25.

In search for the perfect material to be used in the sling procedure, operators have used practically every conceivable type, and, as yet, no completely satisfactory agent has been found. Generally speaking, the autogenous materials, such as fascia, have functioned most dependably and with least tissue reaction. The use of foreign tissues such as ox fascia or collagen has not proved satisfactory. The use of the synthetic polyester fibers such as Dacron (Mersilene) at first seemed to be the final answer because of the availability of the material and the facility with which it could be used. However, contrary to the success reported for its use in other areas of the body, it has proved to be unsatisfactory in the experience of this operator and its use in the sling procedures is condemned. Williams and TeLinde in 1962 reported with guarded enthusiasm the use

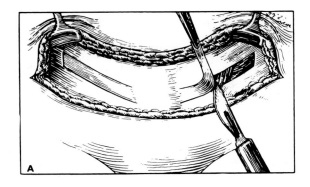

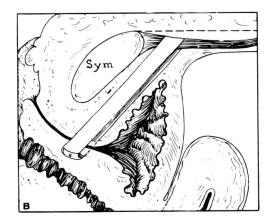

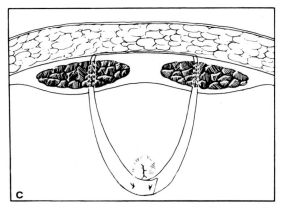

FIG. 26-1 Aldridge modification of Goebell–Frangenheim–Stoeckel operation for urinary incontinence. (*A*) The fascial strips are being separated through a Pfannenstiel incision. (*B*) The fascial strips are shown in position around the posterior portion of the urethra. Dotted line indicates position of rectus muscles when contracted. (*C*) Diagram indicating slinglike action of the fascial strips.

of Mersilene in the sling procedure, but later condemned its use as longer periods of observation were made. Ridley in 1966 reported its use in 17

cases with 4 subsequent rather serious complications. Thus, it has been concluded that this material is unsatisfactory and is condemned for further use.

The original Goebell–Frangenheim–Stoeckel procedure is now rarely performed because in many cases the abdominal fascia has been weakened by previous operative procedures. For a discussion of this technique, the reader is referred to previous editions of this text.

The literature is replete with many modifications of three basic techniques for correction of stress urinary incontinence: (1) the Kelly repair-plication procedure (described fully in the preceding chapter); (2) the sling procedure; and (3) the urethral repositioning (urethropexy) procedure (described in Chapter 25). Only time and experience will serve to evaluate them; however, the general principles of correction of stress urinary incontinence remain the same despite the passing parade of various procedures. As the understanding of stress urinary incontinence increases, the likelihood of a much more successful procedure increases, but thus far there remains an apparently irreducible number of failures resulting from any procedure. Individual surgeons will select the type of procedure in which they are most proficient and successful and will use this specific procedure in the great majority of their cases. However, surgeons should not try to fit all cases into one particular type of operation to the exclusion of the others. The surgeon must be familiar enough with all of the basic procedures to adapt the connective operation to the patient's problem.

More recent contributions have been by Green, Ball, Ingelmann–Sundberg, Pereyra, and Gunther. However, the percentage of failures and the incidence of complications remain about constant. In this chapter our recommendations will be based on our experience.

Choice of Operation

When the surgeon considers whether surgery is indicated and what is to be his choice of operation, there are many facets to be considered. In particular, and within the scope of this chapter, which is concerned primarily with cases in which stress urinary incontinence has not been cured by sphincter plication, consideration must be given to why the first efforts have failed. Although the expected percentage of success, whether it be cured or tolerably improved by the Kelly plication, is appreciably high, the failures must nevertheless be cared for by more sophisticated study and procedures. It is believed that the Kelly plication technique, with its simplicity, safety, and degree of success, should in the great majority of cases be the first effort. There is an exception to this rule, however, in cases of incontinence in women, often elderly, without anterior vaginal wall relaxation. In these cases the incontinence is apparently due to poor sphincter muscle tone and tissue weakness as a result of advancing years. Little or nothing can be expected from tightening these poor muscles. Hence, in cases of this kind that are severe enough to require correction, we have proceeded directly with the sling procedure.

The clinical experience at the Johns Hopkins Hospital through the years, and with periodic updating of the records, shows roughly 90% cure, 5% improvement, and 5% failure with the Kelly plication procedure. Other clinics with large patient loads have reported from 70% to 85% success. It seems that overall we may expect from 80% to 85% success with the properly done Kelly plication. It is felt that in the properly done Kelly plication procedure, the sutures should be placed along the entire length of the urethra. In addition, we have used a semi–purse-string suture over the ureterovesical junction for a number of years. A recent evaluation of our results shows a success rate of 85% in this plication procedure in the past 10 years. Counsellor, Brewer, and others have noted that the rate of success will gradually decline as years pass from the time of the performance of the plication, suggesting recurring tissue failure. Hence it becomes obvious that we must find muscular support elsewhere than from the damaged sphincter to give these women continence. Green and others have stressed the importance of the urethrovesical angle in relation to incontinence. More recent studies by Greenwald, Thornbury, and Dunn have cast doubt on the importance of this factor. They found the same demonstrable deformities in 12 (71%) of 17 patients who had no stress incontinence. Our own experience coincides more nearly with that of Greenwald, Thornbury, and Dunn. We have seen various types of angles in women with incontinence and with perfect control. The percentage of "normal" and "abnormal" angles in patients with and without control are such as to cause us to conclude that the angle is not the essential factor. It is true that by plication and by the sling the angle is changed, but we are convinced that this is incidental and that the factor that restores continence is the suburethral support in the region of the urethrovesical junction.

Our conclusions, however, do not mitigate the importance of and necessity for a thorough preoperative evaluation of the condition. The history is of the greatest importance in making certain that we are dealing with true stress incontinence rather than incontinence due to excessive urge. The knowledge of the type of previous surgery is important. Previous surgery often results in excessive scar tissue in the operative region, which is apt to make the contemplated surgery more difficult; but it does not rule out a further attempt, as we have cured many women with badly scarred urethras by means of a sling. It is of interest to note that a large percentage of women with stress incontinence were cured empirically years before we had the more complete understanding of the phenomenon that we have today.

In not a few instances, it is well to combine one of the strap procedures with cystocele repair and plication of the suburethral fascia. When this is done, it is well to complete the placing of the fascial strap beneath the urethra first and then to bury it beneath the suburethral fascia. In this manner the transplanted fascial strap is less liable to infection from the vagina than if it lies more superficially.

When there is a scar of previous midline abdominal incision, one should not choose an operation requiring the use of a midline fascial strap. Similarly, when the lateral fascia is scarred by a broad rectus or McBurney scar, the Aldridge lateral straps should be avoided. When a urethra has been made previously by a plastic operation and sphincter action is to be attempted, it is unwise to cut into the suburethral vaginal mucosa for fear of entering the urethral lumen. In such instances a single long strap of fascia from the midline or fascia lata may best be used in a U-shaped manner as indicated in Figure 26–1, so that a tunnel is made between the vaginal and the urethral mucosa with a small thin-bladed knife. Even this may be unsafe because of the likelihood of injuring the thin walled urethra. Two other techniques are available, as will be discussed more fully with the transected or exteriorized sling techniques.

Our experience and results with the Marshall–Marchetti–Krantz procedure have been favorable, and in many instances in which concomitant intraabdominal disease exists, it has been our first choice, since a combined abdominovaginal procedure is thereby avoided. It should be noted here that in the event of failure of the Marshall–Marchetti–Krantz procedure, our choice for the "ultimate effort," regardless of what other procedures have failed previously, is the sling procedure. This conclusion has also been put forth by Marchetti and Green and more recently by Beck. We have had a great number of successes with the sling after Marshall–Marchetti–Krantz operation failures, but we should not like to give the impression that we consider only the sling procedures after the Marshall–Marchetti–Krantz failures. Of the last 100 cases in which we used the sling procedure, 72 were failed Marshall–Marchetti–Krantz procedures. In most instances, we proceed to the sling procedure following plication failures unless intra-abdominal pathology necessitates an abdominal incision. With increasing experience and success with the fascia lata sling and with the Aldridge modification using the abdominal aponeurosis, we have favored the Goebell–Frangenheim–Stoeckel procedure more and more. Our results have been quite successful except in some neurologic cases in which the operation was done early in our experience against indications that we now more readily recognize through more careful preoperative screening.

Hodgkinson has brought to our attention the important phenomenon of detrusor dyssynergia, in which a variable amount of urine may be lost insensibly by intrinsic neuromuscular dysfunction. Although rare, this may be the primary cause of the incontinence, but it may also coexist with the aforementioned extrinsic causes and should always be suspected.

Preoperative Evaluation of the Bladder

Regardless of what method of repair is chosen, there seems to be an irreducible minimum number of cases of intractable stress urinary incontinence, that defy correction. Some of these can be identified by careful screening, and operation upon these types is obviously contraindicated. The most serious condition can indeed be aggravated by the improper choice of procedure is the atonic or otherwise neurologically impaired bladder. In all cases of stress urinary incontinence in which any procedure other than the simple Kelly plication is contemplated, it has been our routine to perform a cystometrogram to evaluate the bladder dynamics and capacity. This procedure is done without anesthesia and can be performed satisfactorily in the office. Although a Lewis Recording Cystometer is desirable, it is not absolutely necessary to have one to evaluate the bladder properly. Ridley has shown a simple technique for evaluation of the bladder as an office procedure. Again we emphasize that a careful history should be taken, particularly noting any previous surgery of the genitourinary tract and the exact subjective complaints of the patient.

The patient is allowed to void, and this specimen is saved for chemical analysis. With the patient on the examining table in dorsolithotomy position, the vulva and urethral meatus are properly prepared, using povidone-iodine, and a medium-sized straight metal catheter is carefully inserted into the urethra. By experience it can be noted what the degree of

inclination of the urethra is to the axis of the symphysis; if the catheter passes into the bladder horizontally or with the inserted tip inclined upward, the relationship of the urethra to the symphysis axis is roughly normal and the urethra is probably continent. Conversely, if the inserted tip points downward and away from the horizontal, it can be assumed that the urethra has rotated downward from the axis of the symphysis, suggesting ineffectual urethral support (Fig. 26-2). In this type of deformity we would expect improvement with proper supporting reconstruction, such as we have obtained with the sling procedure. This is only an approximation, but we find that it makes routine chain cystourethrograms unnecessary. The amount of residual urine is measured as the catheterization is completed. This amount of urine—and there is usually a sufficient amount under any circumstances—is saved for microscopic examination, cul-

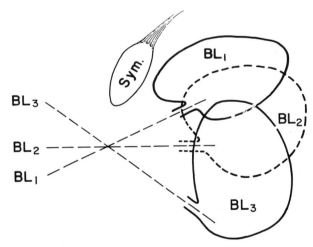

FIG. 26-2 Schematic drawing showing composite of various positions and relationships of the bladder, urethra, and symphysis pubis. BL_1, the normal position of the bladder and urethra with acute posterior urethrovesical angle and relatively close normal relationships of the axis of the urethra and symphysis pubis. This patient usually has no stress urinary incontinence. BL_2, borderline loss of urethral support with posterior rotation of the axis of the urethra and straightening of the posterior urethrovesical angle. This patient usually has moderate stress urinary incontinence. BL_3, pronounced posterior rotation of the axis of the urethra with loss of the posterior urethrovesical angle. This patient usually has a marked amount of stress urinary incontinence.

In the lithotomy examining position the gynecologist will note the position of the rigid straight catheter placed in the bladder, which gives a good indication of the inclination of the angle that the urethra has with the perpendicular axis of the symphysis pubis. (Ridley JH: Ridley's Gynecologic Surgery Errors, Safeguards and Salvage. Baltimore, Williams & Wilkins, 1974.)

ture, and sensitivity tests. Next, a Foley No. 20 catheter with a 5 cc balloon is inserted for tests of bladder capacity and dynamics. This catheter is connected to a graduated flask hanging about 90 cm (36 in) above the symphysis, and increments of 50 ml of normal saline lightly tinted with methylene blue are allowed to gravitate into the bladder. The patient is not apprehensive or uncomfortable if a detailed explanation of the planned procedure has been given to her. Allowing 10 seconds between influx of the increments of normal saline, a careful record is kept of how much saline is allowed to flow in. The end point of the test comes when the patient has a true urgency and is just beginning to have spasm for micturition. A note is made of the amount of saline used, and the bladder is now promptly allowed to begin to drain. If the patient will tolerate only 150 ml or less of the saline solution, we are dealing usually with urge incontinence or a bladder of chronic spasm (Hunner's ulcer) or of decreased capacity due to fibrosis. Any amount from 300 ml to 600 ml is classified as normal, and amounts over 600 ml suggest bladder atony or some neurologic impairment.

To test further for the amount of stress urinary incontinence, approximately 250 ml of the saline is allowed to remain in the bladder and the Foley catheter is removed. The patient is now asked to give a firm cough while the urethra is observed for evidence of leakage with the patient in the lithotomy and standing position. The Marchetti or "stress" test of evaluation of the anterior vaginal wall without compression of the urethra is done. The vaginal mucosa in the region of the urethrovesical junction is infiltrated with a wheal of local anesthetic agent just lateral to the midline on either side. This area is grasped with an Allis clamp on either side of the urethra to avoid compression, and the structures are gently thrust upward and backward to a more retropubic position. A more practical procedure is to reposition the urethrovesical junction retropubicly with the index and middle fingers without compression of the urethra to make the Marchetti test. The patient is now asked to cough firmly again. If there is no leakage with this strenuous effort, one may assume that repositioning the urethra by supporting it with a sling or by retropubic urethropexy should improve or cure the stress incontinence. All of this evaluation can be done easily and quickly at one appointment. If the patient has a history of chronic or recurring urinary tract infection or lithiasis, or if the bladder studies just completed are not within normal limits, the entire urinary tract should be further evaluated by excretory and retrograde urography and endoscopy.

There has been continuing refinement of techniques of urodynamic evaluation, with more accurate determination of flow time, differential pressure profiles of the bladder/urethra, and of myometric values.

The choice of operation for the correction of stress urinary incontinence must be even more refined if there is extraordinary scarring from previous surgery, neoplasm, or treatment thereof, or congenital deformities. Search for irregularities of sphincteric closure through the air cystoscope, water cystoscope, or by indirect air cystoscopy, described by Ridley, may be helpful in determining the presence of scarring.

Another instance in which the sling procedure is indicated is in the aged patient who has undergone previous colpocleisis for procedentia, in whom a suprapubic approach could not effectively elevate the urethra and bladder neck, but in whom the sling procedure could.

Still another example is one in which the patient has had previous surgery for construction of a congenitally or surgically absent urethra or in which there has been a successful repair of a vesicovaginal or vesicourethrovaginal fistula. The sling procedures using a split fascia lata strap, either transected and bilateral or exteriorized beneath the urethra, as described in following pages would be chosen.

Operative Procedures

THE GOEBELL–FRANGENHEIM–STOECKEL PROCEDURE USING THE FASCIA LATA STRAP

This technique has become the most dependable, the easiest, and thus the most frequently used by us as the years have gone by. Procurement of the fascia lata is quick and simple.

The patient is placed on the table in the supine position, with either thigh surgically prepared by shaving and cleaning. The site of incision is optional, depending on the patient's desire for a less noticeable scar or the gynecologist's desire for the easiest approach to and procurement of the fascia. The incision just above the lateral condyle of the femur has been used most frequently (Fig. 26–3). A 5-cm to 7-cm incision is made at right angles to the direction of the fibers of the fascia lata. The fascia is stripped of fat as well as possible with the gauzed finger, and the fascia is split by two incisions 1 cm apart in the direction parallel to the course of the fibers (Fig. 26–4). This strap is now transected 1 cm superior to its inferior attachment and this free end is threaded through the eye of the Masson fascia stripper (other equally simple fascia strippers are available) (Fig. 26–4). The fascia stripper is then thrust

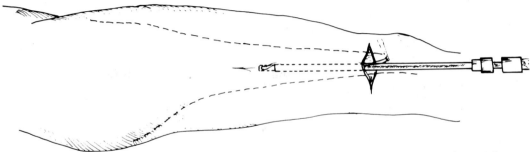

FIG. 26-3 Method of obtaining fascial strap.

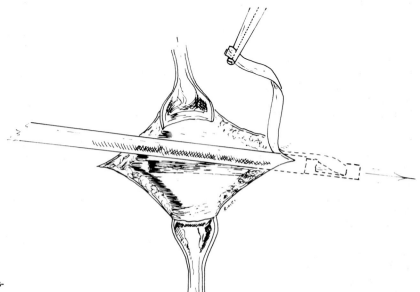

FIG. 26-4 Method of action of Masson fascial stripper.

firmly and evenly cephalad beneath the skin until it can go no further. The strap thus excised is cut by sliding the sheath over the inner tube of the stripper and the strap is removed. An additional strap of fascia lata can be taken at the same time if there is any doubt about the sufficiency of the first excision.

In some instances, if the length of the available fascia strap is insufficient, it may be lengthened by a simple plastic "turn-down" technique of hemisection (Fig. 26-5). The fascial defect within sight beneath the incision is closed with two or three interrupted sutures of No. 3-0 delayed-absorbable material and the skin closed per routine. An elastic compression bandage may be applied over the thigh if there is any evidence of bleeding, which is exceedingly rare in this procedure.

It is emphasized that the procurement of the fascia strap is easy and quick. It can be done through either the incision described above or one just in-

ferior to the greater trochanter of the femur. Because the fascia lata fibers fan out from below upward (Fig. 26-6), it is thought that the strap cut from below upward is more uniform in width and strength, thus facilitating its removal. Only rarely will the patient complain of any pain in the thigh postoperatively, and no complications have been encountered. On the contrary, however, there is a chance, although relatively infrequent in the Aldridge technique, that the patient may develop an incisional hernia at the sites where the fascia straps have been developed from the anterior abdominal aponeurosis.

The patient is now changed to a dorsolithotomy position and appropriately cleaned and draped so that a combined field of the lower abdomen and perineum is simultaneously accessible. A 7-cm to 10-cm transverse incision is made 3 cm above the symphysis down to the fibers of the anterior abdominal aponeurosis. If previous lower abdominal

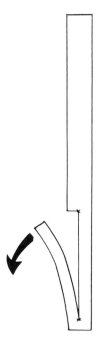

FIG. 26–5 Schematic drawing showing splicing of fascia strap to lengthen without narrowing at midpoint.

incisions have been made, the underlying fascia may be somewhat distorted or obscured by scarring, but with care it can be identified. Two small slitlike incisions about 1 cm in length are made 2 cm above the symphysis and 2 cm to either side of the midline and parallel to the direction of the aponeurotic fibers. The bladder is now completely drained and a suprapubic cystostomy is done routinely. (We use a Cystocath No. 12.) With finger dissection or blunt instrument dissection, the muscle bellies of the rectus abdominis are split or gently displaced to the midline, and the finger is thrust into the space of Retzius on either side of the midline. This dissection is gently performed and even in the presence of scarring from previous retropubic surgery, the approach can be made to the inferior aspect of the

pubic ramus. In some instances however, the scarring may be so extensive that sharp or scissors dissection must be used. It is important to "stay on the periosteum" to lessen the chance for injury to the adherent bladder. Even with this careful dissection the bladder may be entered, but this is no reason to change the operative plan. Bladder entry can be detected easily if a small amount of methylene blue has been injected into the bladder prior to this dissection. It is not feasible to attempt to repair this usually small rent in the bladder wall and with the autogenous fascia lata, healing is usually prompt. However, the patient should be closely observed postoperatively so that any retropubic extravasation or infection will be detected. These have not been a problem in our experience. After retropubic dissection has been carried out on either side and down to the inferior aspect of the pubic ramus (Fig. 26–7), the wound is lightly packed with a wet saline sponge; the operative site is shifted to the vagina.

The anterior vaginal wall is incised in the midline about 1 cm posterior to the external urethral meatus over the entire length of the urethra and to the cervix, or to the vaginal vault seam if previous hysterectomy has been performed. This allows adequate lateral dissection of the tissues of the posterior urethra and neck of the bladder as well as allowing access for repair of any concomitant cystocele. The sphincter area may be more easily determined by an indwelling balloon catheter. The subjacent vaginal fascia is dissected and developed as described in the section on colporrhaphy. Thus, one of the great advantages of the sling procedure is that any necessary vaginal surgery can be done in conjunction with the vaginal portion of the operation. In some cases, Kelly plication sutures are placed concomitantly. Again, by the use of gentle finger dissection, a shallow tunnel is developed on either side of the urethra, which is marked by an indwelling No. 16 French balloon catheter, beneath and posterior to the inferior surface of the pubic ramus. Most of the potentially troublesome bleeding that may be encountered here is avoided by blunt dis-

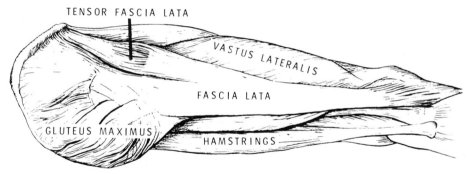

TENSOR FASCIA LATA

VASTUS LATERALIS

FASCIA LATA

GLUTEUS MAXIMUS

HAMSTRINGS

FIG. 26–6 Anatomy of fascia lata.

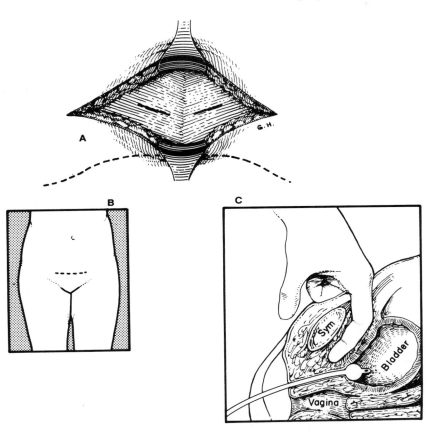

FIG. 26-7 (A) The anterior abdominal aponeurosis has been exposed and two 2-cm incisions made therein, parallel to the fibers of this fascia, 3 cm superior to level of Poupart's ligament. (B) The site of the small suprapubic incision. (C) Gentle finger dissection is done retropubically through the space of Retzius down to the level of the urogenital diaphragm and inferior aspect of the pubic ramus on either side. If space of Retzius has been scarred by previous surgery, dissection may be performed with the blunt tip of uterine dressing forceps. (Ridley JH: Ridley's Gynecologic Surgery Errors, Safeguards and Salvage. Baltimore, Williams & Wilkins, 1974.)

section reflecting the tissues from lateral to medial toward the bladder neck.

A uterine dressing forceps with a medium blunt end is of a proper curvature for gently thrusting retropubically from above downward. The tip of the clamp (Fig. 26–8) is passed through the slitlike openings of the anterior aponeurosis retropubically downward until the instrument tip can be palpated in the shallow retropubic tunnel on that side of the urethra. The tip, still closed, is gently thrust through the resistant tissue of the urogenital diaphragm into the vaginal incision. A small slit over the point of the clamp made with a scalpel may be necessary to facilitate this passage. The tip of the clamp, with the concave curve toward the symphysis, is pressed gently against the posterior surface of the bone as it is passed downward, thus minimizing the chance of injuring the bladder or of opening the venous sinuses that lie in the space of Retzius near the bladder neck. By using this technique and gentle pressure, bleeding is unlikely to occur. If it does, it is usually of venous origin and can be controlled by gentle pressure. The tip of the strap of fascia lata is grasped through the vaginal incision and drawn

retropubically. It is attached firmly with two or three sutures of No. 3-0 silk to the anterior sheath of the rectus, thus also closing securely the slitlike incision previously made.

The process of passing the uterine dressing forceps (or long Kelly clamp) retropubically into the vaginal field is repeated on the other side, and the other free end of the strap of fascia lata is drawn upward without twisting, to be attached to the anterior abdominal aponeurosis at the contralateral incision previously made. Thus, a continuous sling is formed beneath the urethra, and appropriate tension is applied before this strap of fascia lata is firmly attached to the abdominal fascia. Before final fixation of the strap is done, the operator must check to be sure that the strap has been passed *beneath* the urethra near its juncture with the bladder, and that no injury has occurred.

"Appropriate" tension of the sling beneath the urethra must be more fully described. The most frequent mistake of the less experienced operator is to suture the sling *too tight*, thus truly obstructing the urethra. It is necessary only to support the bladder neck. There can be no hard and fast rule about

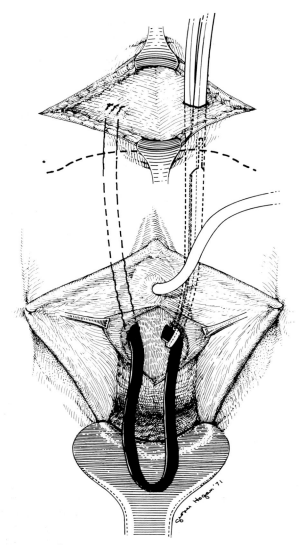

FIG. 26–8 The passage of the fascia lata strap beneath the urethra and retropubically. The strap has been anchored to the anterior abdominal fascia on the patient's right side and drawn into the vagina. It is being grasped by the uterine dressing forceps to be drawn up to the left side and anchored with proper tension at the other slitlike incision in the fascia. Thus, a sling is formed beneath the urethra at the bladder neck. The retention catheter remains in place during the entire sling procedure. (Ridley JH: Ridley's Gynecologic Surgery Errors, Safeguards and Salvage. Baltimore, Williams & Wilkins, 1974.)

what tension to apply on the strap, but it can be safely said that gentle support is desired rather than obstructing or distorting force. The tip of a curved clamp (gallbladder clamp) can be passed freely between the urethra and the fascia sling. This is one of the most important technical points in proper placement and adjustment of the tension of the sling.

With the patient in the dorsolithotomy operating position, it may be valuable to note the relative inclination of the urethra to the horizontal. As has been mentioned, a rough estimate of correct anatomical position may be demonstrated by insertion of a metal catheter into the bladder. It has been noted that proper supportive tension of the sling will bring the catheter tip to at least the horizontal with a retropubic inclination. A further test is made by filling the bladder with 300 ml or 400 ml sterile water and applying gentle suprapubic pressure. There should be no leakage. There is no obstruction to the passage of the metal catheter through the urethra after the sling is fastened. Again we say "gentle support" rather than obstructing force. This support is actually augmented and the so-called angle further corrected by gravity as the patient later assumes a sitting or an erect position.

In rare instances, because of dense scarring from previous surgical procedures, the bladder may be injured retropubically by entry into its lumen with the clamp tip. The bladder wall has become firmly adherent to the periosteal surface retropubically. One should not discontinue the operation but proceed to apply the strap regardless. This rent into the bladder heals promptly if adequate drainage is assured from the bladder itself. No foreign-body reaction results if fascia lata is used, as has been my custom since 1946. In this period, Mersilene tape was used in 17 cases but four serious complications resulted, including erosion into the urinary tract and formation of draining sinuses from foreign-body reaction. No such complications have ever been encountered using the autogenous fascia lata.

In 14 cases in which the patient was unable to void satisfactorily, in a total of 283 cases followed for 6 months or more, the fascia lata sling was completely transected transvaginally. The incision was made 1 cm to either the right or the left of the midline near where the band emerged beneath the pubic ramus. Ten of the 12 cases resulted very satisfactorily, with one failure. If the operator will wait for at least 8 weeks before transecting the sling, enough support by scar tissue will have formed to save the integrity of the original procedure.

The incision should not be made directly over the midline for fear of urethral injury. Nor should a transurethral resection be considered in those cases! In either instance the danger of causing a urethrovaginal fistula must be kept in mind.

The abdominal incision is closed and after the necessary vaginal repair work is completed, the vaginal incision is closed. The balloon retention catheter is left in the bladder and the vagina is packed with Iodoform gauze for 24 hours.

THE ALDRIDGE MODIFICATION OF THE SLING OPERATION

The Aldridge operation is similar in principle to that using the fascia lata strap. However, the fascia sling is developed bilaterally from a portion of the anterior abdominal aponeurosis, parallel to Poupart's ligament and of sufficient length laterally to accommodate any depth of the symphysis and be joined beneath the urethra.

The patient is placed on the table as described in the previous operation, except that the abdomen is draped for a transverse incision.

A semicircular transverse abdominal incision is made through the panniculus, the aponeurosis is cleared of fat over an area about 2 cm wide, and bleeding is controlled.

The strips of fascia are cut on either side of sufficient length to be carried down retropubically and encircle the urethra. The length of these strips, naturally, must be estimated and will vary, depending on the depth of the symphysis pubis; but if they are carried up to the level of the anterior superior spines of the ilia, they will be of sufficient length, even though the symphysis is quite deep. The strips will be composed of the aponeurosis of both the external and the internal oblique in the medial half, but the aponeurosis of the internal oblique laterally is replaced by muscle. Therefore the distal portion of the strap will be composed of external oblique

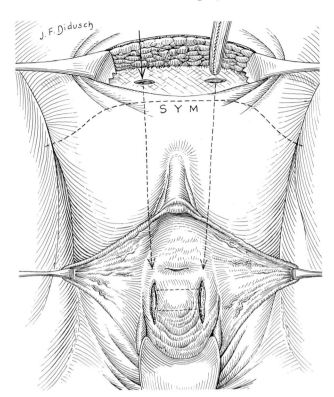

FIG. 26–10 Modified Goebell–Frangenheim–Stoeckel operation, using strap of fascia lata. Two short slits are made on either side of the urethra. A short transverse suprapubic incision has been made and the fascia has been punctured to permit the passage of a long Kelly clamp.

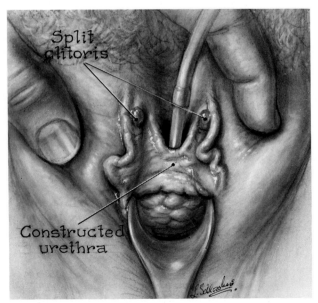

FIG. 26–9 A reconstructed urethra in a woman with hypospadias. After construction of the urethra there was no continence, but a secondary sling operation gave her continence that has persisted in spite of three vaginal deliveries.

fascia only. The straps are separated from the subjacent muscle and thus mobilized down to their bases. The medial end of each strip is left attached at about 1.5 cm from the midline (see Fig. 26–1). The incisions in the aponeuroses are then closed with continuous sutures of No. 0 polyglycolic acid; the fat is approximated with interrupted sutures of No. 3-0 polyglycolic acid, and the skin is closed with continuous fine silk, leaving a small unclosed space at the midportion of the incision. The fascia strips are placed in this space and covered with moist sponges. The closed portion of the abdominal wound is covered with sterile towels.

The operator is then seated for the vaginal portion of the operation. The labia minora may be sutured laterally for good exposure, and a posterior retractor is placed in the vagina. An Allis clip is placed near but not in the urethral meatus, and a second one is placed in the midline on the vaginal wall about 6 cm back from the first. A midline incision is then made through the vaginal mucosa, extending from about 1 cm from the urethral meatus back for about

5 cm to 8 cm. The vaginal mucosa is dissected laterally.

Any dissection made lateral to the urethra must be done cautiously and with the fingertip, as described in the previous operation. The index finger of the left hand is placed to the patient's left side of the urethra with the indwelling balloon catheter. Then, with a long uterine dressing forceps in the right hand, the space of Retzius is traversed from above downward until the tip is felt below. The handle of the clamp is kept pressed to the abdomen as the point is passed downward, thus enabling the operator more surely to keep its point gently against the periosteum of the posterior surface of the pubic bone and symphysis and so protect the bladder. If difficulty is encountered in the fascial plane of the urogenital diaphragm lateral to the urethra, a small cut with the scalpel directly over the tip of the clamp allows it to perforate. As the tip of the dressing forceps presents into the vaginal field, it is grasped by the tip of a similar clamp and pulled

upward until the lower clamp can be made to grasp the free end of the fascial straps developed from the anterior abdominal aponeurosis. Now the free end of the fascia is drawn downward retropubically into the vagina. The process is repeated on the patient's right side, the aponeurotic strips being carried downward to present into the vagina. The ends of the straps are overlapped slightly and any excess is trimmed away after these ends have been securely joined with three or four interrupted sutures of medium silk. Care is taken to get the proper amount of tension on the straps to give the patient continence, being positive that the fascia strap *supports* and *does not obstruct* the urethra. This is tested by distending the bladder through a small metal catheter and making moderate suprapubic pressure. If a cystourethrocele repair is to be done, it is completed at this point and the fascia strips are buried beneath the suburethral fascia. The excess mucosa is excised and the vaginal wound is closed with interrupted sutures of No. 0 delayed-absorbable ma-

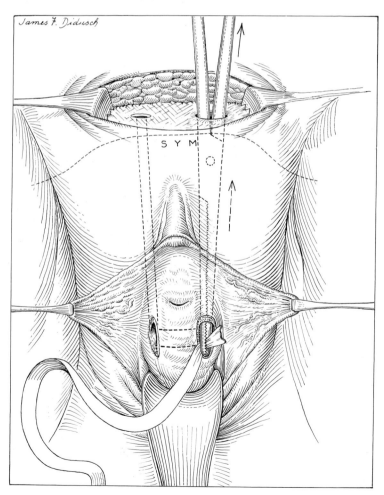

FIG. 26-11 Modified Goebell–Frangenheim–Stoeckel operation. A retropubic tunnel has been made with a uterine dressing forceps and the fascia lata has been grasped. This end is drawn upward and sutured to the fascia of the anterior abdominal wall. The dotted line shows where the *exteriorized* segment of the fascia lata sling will lie.

terial. The small midportion of the abdominal wound is then closed.

THE TRANSECTED AND THE EXTERIORIZED SLING MODIFICATIONS

Ridley has described variations of the basic technique of using the fascia lata sling that permit the creation of adequate support for the bladder neck in cases where a midvaginal incision or dissection is not feasible. For example, we are confronted at times with an ordinarily unworkable situation such as previous successful closure of a urethrovaginal or urethrovesicovaginal fistula; or with the presence of a previously constructed urethra that had been either congenitally absent or deformed by hypospadias (Fig. 26–9), or surgically absent from previous accident or slough; or with the very thin avascular vaginal membrane that follows postirradiation scarring.

The strap of fascia lata is procured as described previously, the anterior aponeurosis is exposed suprapubically and the structure slit. Careful blunt dissection is made through the space of Retzius down to the lateral aspects of the bladder neck. Vaginal incisions are made approximately 1 cm lateral to the midline of the urethra and through the subjacent fascia and scar tissue (Fig. 26–10). The point of the uterine dressing forceps is directed as described previously, lateral to the urethra with its indwelling balloon catheter, through the small vaginal slitlike incision. The strap of fascia lata is brought through the incision, fastened to the anterior abdominal aponeurosis and carried beneath the urethra into the other vaginal incision and up to the other side of the anterior abdominal aponeurosis (Fig. 26–11). Thus the sling is formed. Proper tension is applied and the ends are fastened abdominally. The vaginal portion of the sling is still exposed, but the urethra has not been exposed or injured. Alternatively, the exposed segment of fascia lata may be excised and, in a sense, transected. The intact vaginal mucous membrane overlying the urethra need not be opened. The fascia strap is now firmly fixed with medium silk sutures to the subjacent vaginal fascia and scar tissue beneath each of the small lateral vaginal incisions (Fig. 26–12). The subtending portion of the strap that is exposed is trimmed away and the vaginal incisions are closed. Three such cases have been done with excellent results, the postoperative time varying from 8 to 10 years.

In four cases in which the urethrovaginal septum was equally unworkable due to thinning or a compromised blood supply, as might be present following urethral construction or fistula repair, the strap

of the fascia lata forming the sling was brought beneath the urethra from the two small slitlike incisions just lateral to the urethra on either side (see Fig. 26–10). The fascia lata is not transected but is allowed to remain exteriorized beneath the urethra, thus forming the continuous sling (see Fig. 26–11). The two small lateral incisions through the mucosa may be partially closed, but healing has not been a problem. Within 3 or 4 weeks postoperatively, epithelialization will have taken place over the exposed or exteriorized segment of the fascia lata. This, of course, would not be possible if a foreign material is used as the sling. This technique of *exteriorization* of the fascia lata strap has virtually

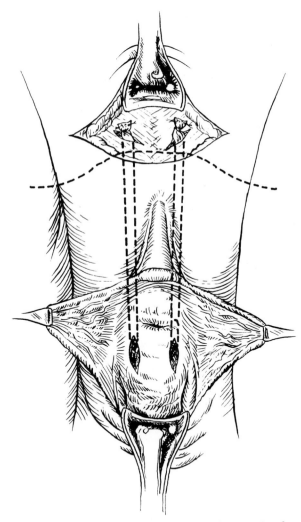

FIG. 26-12 Method of utilizing fascia straps by suturing them on either side of the urethra, a desirable method when the septum is so thin as to endanger perforation into the urethra if an attempt is made to bring the strap beneath it.

supplanted that of *transection* except in some extraordinary condition.

In some cases such as those described above in which the urethrovaginal septum is very thin due to previous surgery, Te Linde has advocated tunneling through the septum carefully, using a small-bladed knife and carrying the sling through the tunnel with an aneurysm needle. This may result in perforation or necrosis of the mucosa of the urethra or vagina. In some cases with a thin scarred suburethral area, regions of thickened and more normal mucosa can be found slightly posterior to the urethra adjacent to but not beneath the trigone. By using this area for placing the sling, continence may be obtained, although any elevation of the trigone will produce symptoms of detrusor dyssynergia that are difficult to control.

Bibliography

Aldridge AH: Transplantation of fascia for relief of urinary stress incontinence. Am J Obstet Gynecol 44:398, 1942

Ball TL, Knapp RC, Nathanson B, et al: Stress incontinence. Am J Obstet Gynecol 94:997, 1966

Ball TL, Wright KL: Stress incontinence, complication and sequelae of the Marshall–Marchetti operation. Pacif Med Surg 73:290, 1965

Beck RP, Grove D, Arnusch D, et al: Recurrent urinary stress incontinence treated by the fascia sling procedure. Am J Obstet Gynecol 120:613, 1974

Bhatia, NN and Ostergard, DR: Urodynamics in women with stress urinary incontinence. Obstet Gynecol 60:552, 1982

Burch JC: Cooper's ligament urethrovesical suspension for stress incontinence. Am J Obstet Gynecol 100:764, 1968

Christensen BC, Ostergaard E: Result of operations for stress incontinence: A study based on patients operated on during the years 1952–1960. Acta Obstet Gynecol Scand 42:367, 1964

Counsellor VS: Surgical correction of stress incontinence—methods and techniques. J Int Coll Surg 24:330, 1960

Cramer H: Fundamental and technical facts concerning Goebell's operation for urinary incontinence. Zbl Gynaek 53:342, 1929

Deming CL: Transplantation of the gracilis muscle for incontinence of urine. JAMA 86:822, 1926

Everett HS: A condemnation of resectoscopic procedures upon the female vesicle neck. Urol Cutan Rev 52:80, 1948

Frangenheim P: Zur Operativen Behandlung der Ankontinenz der Mannlichen Harnrohre. Verh Dsch Ges Chirurgie, 43rd Congress, p 149, 1914

Giordano D: Vingtieme Congress Français de Chirurgie p. 506, 1907

Goebell R: Zur Operativen Beseitigung der angeborenen Incontinentia vesicae. Z Gynäk Urol 2:187, 1910

Green TH, Jr: Development of a plan for the diagnosis and treatment of urinary stress incontinence. Am J Obstet Gynecol 83:632, 1962

Greenwald SW, Thornbury JR, Dunn LJ: Cystourethrography as a diagnostic aid in stress incontinence: an evaluation. Obstet Gynecol 29:324, 1967

Gunther RE: Letter to the Editor. Obstet Gynecol 31:295, 1968

Hodgkinson CP, Ayers MA, Drukker BH: Dyssynergic detrusor dysfunction in the apparently normal female. Am J Obstet Gynecol 86:717, 1963

Ingelman–Sundberg A: Urinary incontinence in women excluding fistulas. Acta Obstet Gynecol Scand 31:266, 1951–52

———: Partial denervation of the bladder. Acta Obstet Gynecol Scand 38:487, 1959

Jeffcoate TNA, Francis WJA: Urgency incontinence in the female. Am J Obstet Gynecol 94:604, 1966

Kelly HA: History of redisplacement of the uterus. Surg Gynecol Obset 20:598, 1915

Kennedy WT: Incontinence of urine in the female: Some functional observations of the urethra illustrated by roentgenograms. Am J Obstet Gynecol 33:19, 1937

Langmade C, Oliver J, Jr: Simplifying the management of stress urinary incontinence. Am J Obstet Gynecol 149:25, 1984

Low JA: Management of severe anatomic deficiencies of urethral sphincter function by a combined procedure with a fascia lata sling. Am J Obstet Gynecol 105:149, 1969

Marchetti AA, Marshall VF, O'Leary JF: Suprapubic vesicourethral suspension and urinary stress incontinence. Clin Obstet Gynecol 6:195, 1963

Marshall VF, Marchetti AA, Krantz KE: The correction of stress incontinence by simple vesicourethral suspension. Surg Gynecol Obstet 88:509, 1949

Miller NF: Surgical treatment of urinary incontinence in the female. JAMA 98:628, 1932

Ostergard DR: Gynecologic Urology and Urodynamics. Baltimore, Williams & Wilkins, 1980

O'Leary JA: Osteitis pubis in vesicourethral suspension. Obstet Gynecol 24:74, 1964

Parker RT, Ridley JH: Fascia lata urethrovesical suspension for stress urinary incontinence. Perspectives in Surgery, vol 1, no 4, 1978

Pereyra AJ, Lebherz TB: Combined urethrovesical suspension and vaginourethroplasty for correction of urinary stress incontinence. Obstet Gynecol 30:537, 1967

Price PB: Plastic operations for incontinence of urine and of feces. Arch Surg 26:1043, 1933

Ridley JH: Indirect air cystoscopy. South Med J 44:114, 1951

———: Appraisal of the Goebell-Frangenheim-Stoeckel sling procedure. Am J Obstet Gynecol 95:714, 1966

———: Gynecologic Surgery: Errors, Safeguards and Salvage. Baltimore, Williams & Wilkins, 1974

Robertson JR: Genitourinary Problems in Women. Springfield, Ill, Charles C Thomas, 1978

———: Endoscopic evaluation of the urethra and bladder. Clin Obstet Gynecol J 26:347, 1983

Stoeckel W: Uber die Verwendung der Muculi Pyramidales bei der operativen Behandlung der Incontinentia urinae. Zbl Gynäk 41:11, 1917

Squier JB: Postoperative urinary incontinence: Urethroplastic operation. Med Rec 79:868, 1911

Symmonds RE: Loss of urethral floor with total urinary incontinence. Am J Obstet Gynecol 103:665, 1969

Taussig FJ: A new operation for urinary incontinence in women by transposing the levator ani muscles. Am J Obstet Dis Women Child 77:881, 1918

Wharton LR, Jr, TeLinde RW: An evaluation of fascial sling operation for urinary incontinence in female patients. J Urol 82:76, 1959

Wheeless CR, Wharton LR, Dorsey JH, et al: The Goebell-Stoeckel operation for universal cases of urinary incontinence. Am J Obstet Gynecol 128:546, 1977

Williams TJ, TeLinde RW: The sling operation for urinary incontinence using Mersilene ribbon. Obstet Gynecol 19:241, 1962

Zacharin RD: Stress Incontinence of Urine. Hagerstown, Md, Harper & Row, 1972

Chapter 27

Vesicovaginal Fistulas

Before the 17th century, vesicovaginal fistula was considered a hopeless condition. The more practical-minded of those times devoted their efforts to making receptacles to catch urine, thus making the life of the victim more endurable.

The first real surgical contribution to fistula repair was made by a Dutchman, H. van Roonhuyse, whose contributions were far in advance of his time. In 1672, van Roonhuyse recommended placement of the patient in a lithotomy position, satisfactory exposure of the fistula by a retracting speculum, thorough denudation of the margins of the fistula, approximation of the denuded edges by means of quills thrust through the edges of the wound and held in place by silk threads, dressing of the wound with balsam and absorbent vaginal dressings, and keeping the patient quiet in bed until the parts had healed.

In 1839, George Hayward of Boston described the important technical point of separating the vagina from the bladder. In 1847 John Mettauer of Virginia first used twisted metal (lead) sutures. In 1845 Jobert de Lauballe described his incision for relieving tension on the suture line. In 1852, Wutzer, of Bonn, reported curing 11 of 35 patients. He was the first to use suprapubic drainage.

J. Marion Sims' first paper on vesicovaginal fistula appeared in 1852, and it is generally conceded that he is the father of surgery for vesicovaginal fistula in America. There is no doubt that he attained greater success than anyone up to his time. It is interesting to note, however, that his operation was not new. Each step had been used and described before by other surgeons. The only innovation that Sims contributed was the use of silver wire suture which was, in truth, a great step forward in fistula

repair. Sims should be given credit for enunciating clearly many principles of vesicovaginal fistula repair that are still appropriate today.

The transvesical approach was described by Trendelenburg in 1890. In 1893, von Dittel described the transperitoneal approach, dissecting the bladder from the uterus and the vagina and closing the opening in the bladder from above. Maisonneure, and later Mackenrodt, made a contribution to the technique that was of great importance. He incised the vagina in the midline across the fistula and then, with the knife and forceps, split the margins of the fistula so as to separate completely the bladder from the vaginal wall. He then closed the bladder and vaginal incisions separately. This procedure, described by Mackenrodt, approximated broad raw surfaces for healing and more nearly approached our modern methods than any technique previously described.

In 1896, Kelly described a method of closing a large bladder defect by freeing the bladder from the cervix all the way up to the peritoneum. In the same communication, Kelly mentioned using preoperative ureteral catheterization to avoid injury of the ureters, although Pawlik first recommended ureteral catheterization in vesicovaginal fistula repair in 1882. We have found this procedure to be invaluable. In 1906, Kelly described a suprapubic route of operating for vesical fistulas and could also report 12 different surgical approaches for closure of vesicovaginal fistulas.

In 1914, Latzko described a technique suited to cases of vesicovaginal fistula resulting from total hysterectomy. Later modified from the original description by Simon, it consisted of obliteration of the vaginal vault with approximation of broad areas of denuded tissue. In 1942 he reported on 31 cases of vesicovaginal fistula treated by this method, with cure in 29 cases, improvement in one case, and failure in another. Latzko's contribution has been a truly great one, and in recent years its value has been magnified because of the increased incidence of fistulas that followed the introduction of the total hysterectomy. Many others, including Garlock, Ingelman–Sundberg, Martius, Bastiaanse, and O'Connor, have contributed special techniques.

ETIOLOGY

Vesicovaginal fistulas, as seen today, fall chiefly into four groups: (1) those resulting from obstetric injury; (2) those resulting from operative accidents, chiefly during total abdominal hysterectomy; (3) those resulting from extension of carcinoma of the cervix or the radium treatment of this disease; and (4) a small group resulting from miscellaneous causes. Formerly, those following obstetric injury formed the largest group, but the improvement in obstetric methods has greatly reduced their number. However, vesicovaginal fistulas from obstetric causes are still common in developing countries, especially in Africa and Asia. The tragic social and medical circumstances of these young women have been studied by Murphy. The considerable efforts of Lawson in Ibadan (Nigeria), the Hamlins in Addis Ababa (Ethiopia) and many others toward the alleviation of this problem are indeed laudable.

The uniform use of total hysterectomy has resulted in a great increase in operative fistulas. Everett and Mattingly reviewed 149 cases of bladder fistulas operated on at the Johns Hopkins Hospital between 1933 and 1953. Of these, 44% followed gynecologic surgery, 20% resulted from obstetrical injury, 32% were related to carcinoma of the cervix and its radiation treatment and 4% were from miscellaneous causes.

Since that report, there has been a further reduction in the number of vesicovaginal fistulas caused by gynecologic cancer and its treatment with radiation or surgery, and the number caused by obstetric trauma. In the last 25 years at Grady Memorial Hospital in Atlanta, no vesicovaginal fistulas have occurred during the course of 150,000 obstetric deliveries in a predominantly black and indigent population. In the United States, about three-fourths of the cases of vesicovaginal fistulas seen are small fistulas in the vaginal vault that appear after total abdominal hysterectomy for benign disease.

ANATOMY

Fistulas may be located at any point along the anterior vaginal wall and may include any part or all of the bladder base and urethra (Fig. 27–1). They

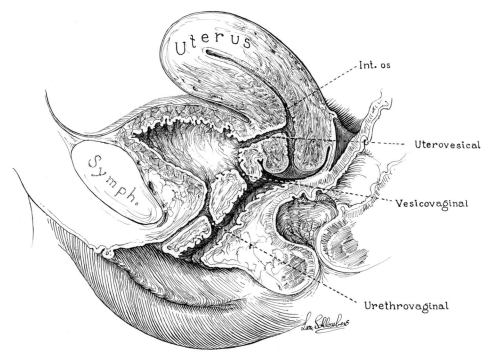

FIG. 27–1 Diagrammatic sagittal section showing locations of vesicocervical, vesicovaginal, and urethrovaginal fistula.

may be single or multiple. Although there may be a single orifice on one side and multiple orifices on the other, this is unusual.

High fistulas with the uterus *in situ* may be obstetric in etiology and may include the anterior cervical lip. High fistulas that result from radiation may also include the cervix. When a fistula follows total hysterectomy, it is high in the vaginal vault. Its posterior margin coincides with the transverse scar in the vault that results from removal of the cervix. The high fistulas are always supratrigonal in location, that is, above the interureteric ridge, although the ureteral orifices may be located near the lower edge of a high fistula. This is an important anatomical point.

Midvaginal fistulas may be located below the interureteric ridge and usually are caused by a misplaced radium applicator or anterior colporrhaphy. During prolonged obstructed labor, pressure necrosis of the bladder wall caught between the fetal head and the pubic symphysis may result in midvaginal fistulas. Difficult forceps operations may also cause midvaginal lacerations and fistulas.

The *bladder neck and upper urethra* are where obstetric fistulas are most commonly located. Fistulas in this location damage the tissue responsible for maintaining normal urinary continence. Difficult forceps operations, anterior colporrhaphies, and irradiation may cause fistulas in this location.

Massive fistulas involve loss of most or all of the vaginal wall. The anterior cervical lip, the bladder base including the trigone, and the upper urethra may be lost in extreme cases. The ureteral orifices are easily identified, spurting urine at the margins of the fistula. The dome of the bladder may prolapse through the fistula. Moir has described a circumferential vesicovaginal fistula due to extreme cases of prolonged obstructed labor. Both the anterior bladder wall behind the symphysis and the posterior bladder wall undergo pressure necrosis and slough, leaving a large area of exposed pubic bone. This obviously creates special technical problems in repair.

PREVENTION

The first and most essential step in limiting the morbidity of vesicovaginal fistulas is prevention. In the United States, major contributors to prevention have been improved obstetric management and techniques of delivery, especially the more liberal use of cesarean section for delivery with a concomitant decrease in the number of difficult forceps maneuvers and the improvements in labor management. Few American gynecologists have experience in the repair of vesicovaginal fistulas of obstetric etiology unless the experience was gained abroad.

Today, the most important measures in further reducing the incidence and morbidity of vesicovaginal fistulas must be directed toward proper techniques of gynecologic operations, especially total abdominal hysterectomy, and toward immediate recognition and repair of bladder injury at the operation of injury so that a fistula will not develop. Mattingly and Borkowf have written a complete review of this subject. Gynecologic surgery is the most common etiology of vesicovaginal fistulas in the United States and in many other developed countries in the world, and the bladder is the most common site of urinary tract injury during gynecologic surgery. The bladder is rarely injured during the course of subtotal abdominal hysterectomy. Among 75 post-hysterectomy vesicovaginal fistulas reported by Miller and George, none followed subtotal hysterectomy, 54 followed total abdominal hysterectomy, 18 followed vaginal hysterectomy, and 3 followed radical abdominal hysterectomy. Since the advent of the total abdominal hysterectomy in the late 1940s, the incidence of injury to the bladder base has increased; it occurs in approximately 0.5% to 1% of patients undergoing a total abdominal hysterectomy. The bladder is very closely related developmentally to the uterus, cervix, and vagina and is especially vulnerable to injury when a total hysterectomy is done. The base of the bladder rests on the anterior lower uterine isthmus and the cervix. The trigone of the bladder, however, is found at a level below the cervix. It is attached to the upper one-third of the anterior vaginal wall, beginning at about the anterior vaginal fornix and below, and therefore is less susceptible to injury. If the bladder is injured during its dissection away from the cervix and upper vagina, the injury will be located above the interureteric ridge in almost all cases.

Injury to the base of the bladder is three times more common with total abdominal hysterectomy than with vaginal hysterectomy. The usual cause of such injury is inadequate mobilization of the bladder or vigorous and blunt dissection in an improper plane between the bladder base and the protective pubovesicocervical fascia covering the cervix. Dissection in the proper plane to separate the bladder from the cervix and upper vagina should be done sharply and carefully with fine scissors. The use of blunt dissection, especially pushing down against the vesicocervical attachment with a sponge stick, should be discouraged, since the integrity of the bladder wall can be weakened by this technique. An intrafascial technique of removing the cervix, utilizing an inverted "T" or "V" incision in the pubovesicocervical fascia covering the cervix anteriorly, should be used whenever possible to prevent injury to the bladder and the ureters. Before clamps can be safely placed on the cardinal ligaments and before an incision is made through the anterior vaginal wall, the bladder must be thoroughly mobilized inferiorly and laterally and the vesicocervicovaginal space completely developed. Constant traction on the uterus superiorly and retraction of the bladder inferiorly with accurate placement of clamps and sutures will help prevent bladder injury. Some vesicovaginal fistulas are caused by placement of suture(s) through the bladder base when the vaginal cuff is sutured. This is usually the result of inadequate mobilization of the bladder inferiorly and laterally away from the upper vagina, or of inadequate exposure and retraction. In this instance, usually unrecognized, gradual necrosis of the bladder wall will lead to the development of a vesicovaginal fistula most commonly within the first week after surgery, when the patient will notice incontinence of urine through the vagina.

During the past three to four decades, the more frequent use of vaginal hysterectomy for the correction of anatomical pelvic relaxation and benign gynecologic disease has resulted in an increase in the number of injuries to the base of the bladder. The location of the injury is identical to that which occurs with a total abdominal hysterectomy. The vast majority of such injuries are in the supratrigonal portion of the bladder base, although in rare instances, when a cystocele repair has also been done, the injury may occur in the trigone. The correct anatomical plane between the bladder and the cervix and uterine isthmus in the midline is ordinarily easy to find and is relatively avascular. Sharp dissection in this plane with traction on the cervix inferiorly and retraction of the bladder superiorly will locate the vesicouterine fold of peritoneum promptly. After a small incision is made in the peritoneum, loops of small intestine or omentum should be identified to confirm that the peritoneal cavity rather than the bladder has been entered. Only then should the peritoneal incision be enlarged. A retractor kept beneath the bladder will protect it from harm. However, when development of the vesicocervical space is difficult or misdirected, troublesome bleeding obscures the operative field. The dissection may be too anterior and superficial and the bladder wall may be weakened or the bladder actually entered. Hopefully, the operator will not extend the incision before recognizing the error. Although most entries into the bladder are easily recognized, on occasion the operator may be misled into believing that entry into the peritoneal cavity has been made. The presence or absence of omentum or intestine seen through the entry site will distinguish between the two. Placement of an instrument (Kelly clamp or uterine sound) transurethrally into the bladder will help identify a bladder entry and can also be used to identify a proper plane of dissection between the bladder and cervix before an accidental entry is made. If the bladder mucosa is stained with methylene blue before each hysterectomy, it can be more readily identified when exposed. Leaving some urine in the bladder during vaginal surgery may also facilitate recognition of bladder injury since a spurt of urine will be seen when the bladder is entered. Vesicovaginal fistulas resulting from total vaginal hysterectomy are best prevented by finding the proper plane of dissection between the bladder base and the anterior lower uterine segment, opening the anterior peritoneum carefully, adequately mobilizing the bladder laterally, placing a retractor beneath the bladder, and properly placing clamps and ligatures on paracervical and parametrial tissue as close to the uterus as possible. Jaszczak and Evans have proposed an intrafascial technique for vaginal hysterectomy designed to avoid bladder injury among other things. Although the idea may be sound, it has not been evaluated extensively by others.

Because of the frequent use of low cervical cesarean section as a method of abdominal delivery, it can be estimated that approximately one out of every five or six women in the United States who need a hysterectomy will previously have had a cesarean section. This can cause difficulty in dissection of the vesicocervical space because of unusually dense adherence of the bladder to the lower uterine isthmus. This difficulty can be experienced with either abdominal or vaginal hysterectomy. In our experience, the dissection is less difficult with vaginal hysterectomy because the operator can use transurethral passage of an instrument to help identify a proper plane of dissection. Certainly, a history of previous cesarean section should be a warning that the dissection must be carefully performed and the bladder tested for integrity before the operation is complete. A history of prior radiation causes similar difficulties and requires similar precautions.

Repair of Bladder Injury

It has been said that to surgically injure the bladder is only a venial sin, but to fail to recognize that you have done so is a mortal one. In other words, if an injury to the bladder can be recognized at the operation of injury and can be repaired properly, a vesicovaginal fistula is not likely to occur. Since the bladder base is the most dependent portion, injuries in this location are especially likely to result in fistula formation if they are not recognized and repaired correctly. Whether the bladder wall has been weakened or the bladder has actually been entered, the extent of the injury and its proximity to the ureteral orifices should be assessed. Ordinarily, the ureteral orifices will not be involved. However, if they cannot be located, 5 ml indigo carmine given intravenously will cause blue urine to spurt from the orifices in only a few minutes, facilitating their identification. Ureteral catheters can be passed to avoid damage to or incorporation of the ureters in the repair of the bladder defect. However, this is not often necessary since the injury is almost always supratrigonal. After careful assessment of the extent of the injury, a continuous No. 3-0 delayed-absorbable suture may be used to invert and close the bladder mucosa, making certain that the entire defect is securely closed (Fig. 27-2). Formerly, a major concern was the inadvertent placement of sutures through the bladder mucosa during the repair of a bladder laceration. Today, this is no longer a matter for concern. Healing will occur provided there is accurate approximation of tissue layers. The first layer of closure should be reinforced by a second layer of continuous or interrupted No. 3-0 delayed-absorbable suture(s) placed in the musculofascial tissues imbricating and supporting the initial layer. A third layer may be used if necessary. The security of the closure must be tested by filling the bladder with at least 200 ml dilute methylene blue or sterile milk after the first layer of closure is completed.

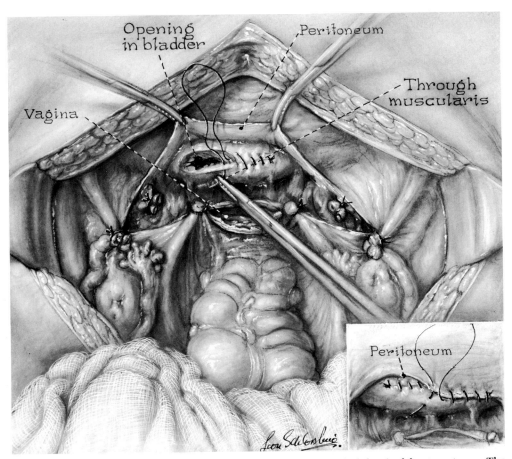

FIG. 27-2 Closure of accidental opening of bladder during total abdominal hysterectomy. The bladder is closed with a continuous No. 3-0 delayed-absorbable suture, inverting mucosa into the bladder. A second muscular layer of interrupted sutures should support the initial layer. The suture line is then reinforced by bringing the peritoneum over the operative defect and suturing it in place. Advancement of the bladder peritoneum over the suture line will protect it from postoperative pelvic cellulitis and make certain that no leakage occurs into the vagina.

Any point of leakage can be identified and reinforced. The anterior peritoneal edge behind the bladder should be sutured to the anterior vaginal cuff or to the bladder wall below the defect to interpose another layer between the site of bladder repair and the vaginal vault and to relieve tension on the suture line. This is a very useful maneuver and should be used to reinforce any suspected area of trauma to bladder muscle even if the bladder has not actually been entered. After injecting indigo carmine intravenously, cytoscopy should be performed to be certain the dye spurts from both ureteral orifices. The bladder should be kept as empty as possible for a period of 10 days following surgery. Preference should be given to a suprapubic rather than transurethral indwelling catheter, especially if the defect is low and involves the vesical neck. One should avoid placing an indwelling catheter in close proximity to the suture line inside the bladder.

Factors Influencing Vesicovaginal Fistula Formation

One of the most frequent sites of injury occurs in the bladder dome on opening the abdominal cavity. When operating abdominally, the incision in the abdominal wall must be large enough to allow adequate exposure. Performing operations for extensive pelvic disease through small incisions places the bladder and ureters and other adjacent structures at a greater risk of injury. Of course, incisions in the lower abdomen must be made carefully in order to avoid injury to the bladder dome.

One must be especially careful when making an abdominal incision in a patient who has had a previous incision. Adhesions and scarring may cause difficulty. Advancing pregnancy produces alterations in the normal relationships of the bladder to the uterus and cervix and to the abdominal wall. With growth of the uterus during pregnancy, the bladder becomes an abdominal rather than a pelvic organ. These anatomical changes account for the increased susceptibility to and frequency of injury during cesarean section, especially repeat cesarean section. In this circumstance, the bladder is more susceptible to injury not only during its dissection away from the lower uterine segment, but also when the abdominal incision is being fashioned. If the bladder neck has been chronically obstructed by a pelvic tumor, usually a leiomyomatous uterus, the bladder muscle may hypertrophy and the bladder may enlarge to the point of occupying the entire distance from the symphysis to the umbilicus. Under these circumstances, in order to avoid injury to the bladder, it may be necessary to enter the peritoneal cavity above the umbilicus. But failure to empty the bladder completely prior to surgery is one of the main errors of omission that may result in accidental bladder laceration on entering the abdomen. Insertion of an indwelling Foley catheter during the preparation of the patient for surgery is an important requirement for continued decompression of the bladder throughout the surgical procedure to avoid bladder injury.

When the bladder dome is injured, the wall of the bladder may be easily repaired in a double layered closure including an initial continuous No. 3-0 delayed-absorbable suture in the bladder mucosa reinforced by another layer of continuous or interrupted sutures in the bladder muscle. An indwelling transurethral catheter should be left in place for 7 to 10 days postoperatively depending on the extent of the injury, the security of the closure, and the location of the injury in the bladder dome (extraperitoneal or transperitoneal).

It should be understood that primary healing after intraoperative bladder injury is not dependent on placement of a large number of sutures in the bladder. Rather, tissue healing is enhanced by the accurate placement of the correct number of sutures that will approximate the bladder wall correctly and not interfere with its blood supply. It is comforting to know that the bladder has a rich collateral blood supply and will heal rapidly when closed correctly. Injury to the bladder need not be considered a dreaded and serious complication of gynecologic surgery. Indeed, the gynecologic surgeon can be encouraged to intentionally enter the bladder when it is necessary to do so to define the anatomical limits of pathology or operative procedures. In an analysis of 77 cases of recognized bladder entry, Everett and Mattingly found no case that failed to heal when repaired at the time of initial entry.

Although injuries to the bladder most commonly occur during total abdominal or vaginal hysterectomy, other gynecologic operations also place the bladder at risk of injury. In a subtotal abdominal hysterectomy, the bladder is usually drawn over the apex of the cervical stump to reperitonize the pelvis. The resultant alteration in the location of the bladder will render it more vulnerable to injury in any subsequent attempt to remove the cervix, whether done abdominally or vaginally. The exact boundary of the bladder wall is obscured by dense adhesions to the apex of the cervix.

In patients with congenital absence of the vagina, construction of a neovagina may result in bladder injury during the dissection of a space between the urethra and bladder anteriorly and the rectum posteriorly. Definition of the correct plane of dissection can be facilitated by placing a finger in the rectum and an instrument in the bladder. After a bladder injury has been properly repaired, it is essential to use a soft foam-rubber form to carry the split thickness skin graft into the new space. Total abdominal hysterectomy performed immediately after cesarean section increases the risk of bladder injury and vesicovaginal fistula formation.

A variety of operations used to correct stress urinary incontinence may result in bladder injury. Bladder injury during an anterior colporrhaphy is infrequent, but it can be avoided altogether by a careful layered dissection of the vaginal mucosa from the underlying pubovesicocervical fascia. Patients with previous bladder neck surgery are at special risk of bladder injury when a secondary abdominal retropubic procedure is done to correct recurrent stress incontinence. This type of bladder injury occurs most frequently during mobilization of the adherent bladder neck and urethra when dissecting in the space of Retzius. These injuries are particularly troublesome because their anatomical location, which limits exposure, makes them difficult to close. As a result of previous surgery, the vesical wall is frequently attentuated and friable with compromised blood supply. The surgeon should approach the scarred bladder neck with caution. Sharp, controlled dissection is less hazardous in this situation than forceful, blunt separation of the dense adhesions. An inflated catheter bulb will identify the urethrovesical junction and the location of the bladder neck. The bladder neck and the urethral margins can also be more accurately defined if the surgeon inserts the fingers into the vagina to elevate the paraurethral tissues and bladder neck into the operative field while performing the dissection and placing the sutures. When the anatomical margins of the bladder are distorted and cannot be delineated, it is preferable to open the anterior bladder wall transversely and then to perform the dissection and place the sutures with greater accuracy under direct vision. Injuries to the bladder may occur during the course of various operations to suspend the bladder neck by the retropubic placement of a fascial strap, such as in the Price or Aldridge modification of the Goebell–Frangenheim–Stoeckel operation. If cystoscopy can be a part of all these procedures, an assessment of the presence or absence and extent of bladder injury can be made and appropriate repair carried out when necessary.

In every series of vesicovaginal fistulas, there is still a significant number of patients whose fistulas are the result of treatment of gynecologic malignancies with radiation therapy or extensive pelvic surgery. Radiation has an acute effect on tissues that lasts for several months. During this acute phase, fistula formation results from destruction and sloughing of neoplastic tissue in the vesicovaginal septum, or from the acute effects of radiation on sensitive tissues. Even though most irradiated tissue may seem to recover from this acute phase, fistulas may yet appear many years later because of progressive obliterative endarteritis with resultant tissue ischemia. Evidence of this ischemia can be seen cystoscopically in patients who were irradiated for cervical cancer many years before. The bladder mucosa just above the interureteric ridge will appear pale and avascular at the point of maximum intensity of radiation. Because of this progressive ischemia over a prolonged period, vesicovaginal fistulas may appear many years after radiation. Although the dose and distribution of radiation is important, Van Nagell and associates found that the absolute dosage did not always correlate with fistula formation, nor did the patient's weight and age, suggesting that bladder tissue sensitivity to radiation varies from patient to patient and that some patients are more susceptible to fistula formation than others. They found that patients with vascular disease, as manifested by hypertension and diabetes, were particularly susceptible to fistula formation. The importance of blood supply to the area is evidence by a fourfold increase in fistula formation when simple hysterectomy was performed on patients who had previously had radiation therapy, as noted by Boronow and Rutledge. Hysterectomy further compromises the central pelvic blood supply already compromised by radiation. When extensive pelvic surgery is done after complete pelvic irradiation has been given, fistulas are especially likely to result. Although some of these are unavoidable, others could be prevented by proper irradiation dosage or distribution of rads and by use of the proper technique of extensive pelvic surgery for gynecologic malignancies. Since these fistulas are the most difficult to close, every precaution should be taken to prevent their formation.

A variety of etiologies of vesicovaginal fistulas are reported. Regrettably, a few still result from the outmoded transurethral resection of the "female prostate," thought to be the cause of bladder neck obstruction. Transurethral resections in the female should be restricted to a careful and limited resection of congenital urethral valves or folds usually found in young girls with obstruction of urinary outflow.

It is our position that the gynecologic surgeon should be technically capable of closing a bladder defect once he has created it. In this litigious era, it is important for the gynecologist to understand that the primary responsibility for the bladder injury falls on the shoulders of the surgeon who caused it and cannot be transferred to another specialist summoned to perform the repair. Injury to the urinary tract during gynecologic operations is now the second leading cause of malpractice suits against gynecologists.

SYMPTOMS AND DIAGNOSIS

The successful treatment of vesicovaginal fistula depends on an exact diagnosis. With a small fistula, the urinary leakage will be slight and, in some instances, dependent on the position of the patient. Women with such a fistula may void a good quantity of urine, whereas with larger fistulas, sufficient urine does not collect in the bladder to permit voiding. Most often, patients will be totally or almost totally incontinent of urine, will require rubber sheets to protect the mattress, and diapers or rubber pants to protect their clothing. With marked incontinence, the vulva usually becomes reddened, tender, and excoriated over time. The odor of urea may be so offensive as to be disgusting to the patient and repulsive to others. Patients often become reclusive and depressed.

Most vesicovaginal fistulas are painless. But fistulas resulting from irradiation can cause severe pain. Graham has reported 10 such cases with progressive pain, aggravated by movement or sitting. The areas of these fistulas are very tender, and often anesthesia is required for a satisfactory examination. Bacteria in the vagina split urea and produce an alkaline medium in which crystals form. The vagina and labia have greenish-gray deposits, and in many cases there are encrustations and necrotic tissue along the margins of the fistula. Since these patients have received radiation for a gynecologic malignancy, the fistula margins must be biopsied to rule out recurrent or persistent cancer. However, not all post-irradiation fistulas fall into this painful pattern.

If a fistula opening cannot be readily demonstrated by careful pelvic examination, often it may be found by filling the bladder with a dilute solution of methylene blue and then inspecting the anterior vaginal wall and vaginal vault. When the fistula is small, if the point of leakage is still not discovered with the patient in the dorsal lithotomy or knee-chest positions, the three-tampon test of Moir should be used. In this test, three cotton tampons are placed in the vagina in tandem. Methylene blue is instilled in the bladder. After having the patient walk about for 10 to 15 minutes, the tampons are removed and examined. If the lowest tampon is wet and stained blue, the patient may be presumed to have transurethral urinary incontinence. If the upper tampon is wet and blue, a vesicovaginal fistula is indicated. If the upper tampon is wet but not blue, a ureteral fistula is the likely diagnosis. Careful inspection of the tampons with regard to their position in the vagina will give some information about the location of the vaginal orifice of the fistula.

The air method of Kelly or the carbon dioxide technique of Robertson are admirably adaptive for cystoscopic examination of these patients. Although this examination is more commonly made with a water cystoscope, difficulty is experienced in filling the bladder when the opening is large unless the examination is done with the patient in the knee-chest position. However, with either water or air cystoscopy, small fistulas are often seen only with great difficulty from within the bladder. In spite of these difficulties, the cystoscopic examination should be done in order to ascertain the size and the position of the fistula and, particularly, its relation to the ureteral orifices and the vesical sphincter. It must be remembered that more than one vesicovaginal fistula may be present.

When a urinary fistula develops postoperatively, the diagnostic possibilities are a vesicovaginal fistula, a unilateral ureterovaginal fistula, bilateral ureterovaginal fistulas, or various combinations. Needless to say, an exact determination must be made before appropriate treatment can be instituted. Recalling the details of the operative procedure of injury, the surgeon may be able to suspect which kind of fistula is present. However, this suspicion should always be confirmed. If the bladder is distended with methylene blue solution, and the urine in the vagina is unstained, the communication is with the ureter. If the bladder is distended with methylene blue solution and the urine in the vagina is stained, the communication is with the bladder, but the patient might still have a ureterovaginal fistula as well. If urine in the vagina is unstained when the bladder is filled with a methylene blue solution but becomes blue when indigo carmine is injected intravenously, the communication is with the ureter, but which ureter is still not known. The findings must be confirmed by cystoscopy, which will show a failure of the ureteral orifice on the affected side to spurt urine. Attempts to pass a catheter will usually meet obstruction when the tip reaches the point of ureteral injury. Instillation of radiopaque dye through the ureteral catheter may outline the tract of a ureterovaginal fistula. Intravenous urography should be a routine part of the investigation. A hydronephrosis suggests but is not diagnostic of a ureterovaginal fistula on the same side, although these changes can also result from scarring of the edges of a vesicovaginal fistula in the region of the ureteral orifice with concomitant ureteral stenosis and dilatation above. Further discussion of the differential diagnosis of urinary fistulas can be found in Chapter 14.

MANAGEMENT PRINCIPLES

There is considerable variation among vesicovaginal fistulas in etiology, size, location, and associated features. Most vesicovaginal fistulas seen in this country are relatively small, simple fistulas in the vaginal vault that result from unrecognized bladder injury during total hysterectomy for benign gynecologic and obstetric disease. A few result from extensive surgery or pelvic irradiation for gynecologic malignancies. The major emphasis in this discussion will be given to fistulas following unrecognized bladder entry.

Complete Preoperative Investigation

As described earlier, the patient must undergo a careful evaluation of the bladder, ureters, kidney function, urethra, vagina, and other pelvic organs, tissues and disease so that the nature and extent of the fistula and associated problems can be properly assessed. This evaluation will certainly include a careful pelvic examination, cystoscopy, urethroscopy, intravenous urography, biopsy of fistula margins when indicated, and other studies. Some studies done initially to make the diagnosis may need to be repeated later as circumstances change. Repair should not be attempted in the absence of current information.

Operative Considerations

TIME OF REPAIR. Formerly, it was advised by most experienced gynecologists that, regardless of a vesicovaginal fistula's etiology or size, at least 6 months must elapse before repair is attempted, so that tissues could be completely healed. In the past 25 years, the 6-month rule has been challenged: many experts now recommend waiting only 3 to 4 months, and a few have advised repair even earlier. Fearl and Keizur found 2 or 3 months to be an adequate resolution time if the wound was a clean surgical one. Collins and Prent in 1960 reported on their experience with early repair of vesicovaginal fistulas after preoperative administration of cortisone to bring about "resolution of inflammatory reaction" around the fistula. In 15 cases, all operated on within 8 weeks and most within 4 weeks of discovery of the fistula, 13 repairs were successful on the first attempt. These acute fistulas resulted from operations for benign disease. Less favorable results were obtained when early repair was attempted in patients whose fistulas resulted from radiation or extensive surgery for gynecologic malignancy. All the

repairs were done transvaginally. Continuing to use preoperative steroids and a transvaginal approach, Collins and associates reported a 72.4% success rate in 1971 on the first attempt at even earlier repair in 29 patients without malignancy. The reparative procedures were done in the first 2 weeks after fistula discovery. In 1979, Persky and associates reported their experience with early repair (1 to 10 weeks after the initial surgery) in seven cases. All of the repairs (except one vaginal) were done by the suprapubic transvesical approach with interposition of a flap of peritoneum or omentum between the bladder and vagina at the area of closure, and all were successful. At Emory University, attempts to repair simple post-hysterectomy vesicovaginal fistulas by a Latzko operation have been successful in 14 patients when the repair was done from 2 weeks to 12 weeks following discovery of the fistula. Early in the series, five patients received preoperative steroids. Since success has been regularly achieved in recent years without steroids, we are unable to confirm that they are essential in achieving success in early repair, and we no longer recommend their use.

Those who prefer to wait 3 to 4 months to repair a vesicovaginal fistula are especially concerned that the tissues should be completely normal, and without edema and infection, so that a proper dissection, proper suturing, and proper healing will result in a successful closure. In the meantime, the patient is terribly uncomfortable. Collection devices and indwelling catheters usually do not keep her dry and may cause more perineal irritation. She is embarrassed, depressed, and restricted in her social and marital activities. She is not easily convinced that she should remain in this unpleasant state for months before anything is done. During this long period of watchful waiting, she is likely to become impatient and seek other advice. If patients with uncomplicated post-hysterectomy vesicovaginal fistulas can be offered an earlier repair with reasonable chance of success, much unpleasantness can be avoided.

When a patient develops a vesicovaginal fistula, usually in the first or second week following total hysterectomy, and evaluation shows no complicating features, a large indwelling Foley catheter should be inserted for continuous bladder drainage to facilitate spontaneous healing or eventual complete epithelialization of the fistula tract. Spontaneous healing has been reported to occur in 15% to 20% of patients. In our experience, spontaneous healing is unusual except for the very smallest fistulas only a few millimeters in diameter. Among 38 postoperative vesicovaginal fistulas, Latzko reported that 9 healed spontaneously. Greatest success was achieved when a large-caliber catheter was used and the fistula was only a few millimeters in diameter. The time required for healing varied from 17 days to 3 months.

If insertion of a urethral catheter eliminates all urine loss through the vagina, the chance of spontaneous healing is good. Some patients can tolerate a catheter connected to a leg bag for several weeks and remain relatively dry and comfortable. For those who cannot tolerate a catheter, a vaginal collecting device such as described by Wolff and Gililland can be constructed by gluing a Pezzer catheter to a fitted contraceptive diaphragm with rubber cement. The catheter is fitted to a leg bag and may be worn for the weeks or months before bladder repair is carried out. Patients who are postmenopausal, or younger patients who have had both ovaries removed, should be placed on oral estrogen. An ointment or cream containing lanolin can protect the vulva. Hot sitz baths and douches or creams containing antibacterials may help to improve tissue vascularity and reduce infection prior to surgery. Urinary antibiotics are generally not used unless there is clinical evidence of a urinary tract infection above the bladder. Acute cystitis is uncommon in conjunction with a vesicovaginal fistula.

After about a month of continuous catheter drainage, the catheter is removed. If the fistula persists, surgery can be planned. Generally, most uncomplicated post-hysterectomy vesicovaginal fistulas will be ready for repair by the eighth postsurgical week and some will be ready earlier. When edema, cellulitis, and evidence of tissue necrosis have resolved from the fistula margins, the patient's physical and mental well-being are better served by a simple surgical procedure to close the fistula rather than by wearing the catheter, prophylactically, for a longer time. It should be emphasized that complicated fistulas cannot usually be closed this soon. For example, it may take from 6 months to 2 years for the tissues around a post-irradiation fistula to be ready for surgical repair.

Very rarely a minute (<3 mm) vesicovaginal fistula may be closed by superficial bladder fulgeration. Falk and Orkin have reported success with this procedure, as have both Hyman and O'Connor. They emphasize that the tract should be free from infection and the vesicovaginal septum should not be too thin. If this rule is not observed, fulgeration may increase rather than decrease the caliber of the opening.

CHOICE OF OPERATION. The choice of the operative approach is all-important. We have come more and more to the conclusion that almost all vesicovaginal fistulas should be closed per vaginam. Simple post-hysterectomy vesicovaginal fistulas in the vaginal vault certainly should be closed with a Latzko partial colpocleisis. The operation is rapid and recovery is prompt. Extensive transperitoneal/transvesical operations are not needed to repair these simple fistulas. Even most complicated fistulas can be approached vaginally unless there are unusual circumstances. A transperitoneal or transvesical approach may be needed when the fistula margins are in close proximity to the ureteral orifices, requiring a transvesical approach to catheterize the ureters, mobilize the bladder mucosa, and close it securely without compromise of the ureters; when ureteroneocystostomy is needed; when an omental fat-flap is to be used; or when a very large fistula or contracted bladder may require bladder patching or augmentation with sigmoid colon, cecum, or ileum. We recognize that some excellent surgeons—principally urologists—such as Pfaneuf, O'Connor, Marshall, Glenn and Stevens, and others recommend and routinely use the transvesical approach to fistula repair and are successful by that method. However, we believe that it is not the preferred method of approach for the usual gynecologic vesicovaginal fistula.

PATIENT POSITIONING. When the vaginal approach is used, exposure can be accomplished best by placing the patient in the dorsal lithotomy position. The Sims lateral position and the knee–chest position are rarely used. The great majority of our fistulas are repaired in the lithotomy position. Dropping the head of the table and elevating the buttocks often facilitates exposure. On those infrequent occasions when it is necessary to approach the fistula through an abdominal incision, the patient's legs should be placed in stirrups with the knees lower than usual. In this position, the operator or the assistant, by placing the index and middle fingers in the vagina, will be able to elevate the fistula for better visualization. Also, the external urethral meatus will be available for cystoscopic examination of the bladder when the repair is completed.

SPECIAL INSTRUMENTS. It is helpful to have a cystoscope available so that the margins of the fistula in the bladder mucosa can be examined and the location of the ureteral orifices in relation to the fistula can be determined. If necessary, ureteral catheters should be inserted. The examination is best done by a surgeon who is skilled in cystoscopy, preferably by the one who is to perform the operation.

Most fistulas can be repaired correctly with a basic instrument set. It may be necessary to supplement this basic set with a few special instruments that are long and thin with fine points, such as long fine-pointed dissecting scissors, long fine-pointed tissue forceps, long, delicate needle holders, an assortment of long scalpel handles and blades, and an assortment of vaginal retractors. Technical difficulties encountered in the repair may be solved by obtaining better instruments and by innovations in their use, but are more likely to be solved by improved exposure and accessibility of the fistula itself.

FISTULA EXPOSURE. Ordinary retraction of the vaginal walls is usually sufficient for adequate exposure. However, when there is a tight vaginal outlet, scarring of the vagina, or a deep and fixed vaginal vault, an episiotomy or a Schuchardt incision (Fig. 27–3) may be needed. Such an incision should be made without hesitation if exposure and accessibility will be improved. Traction on stay sutures placed in the bladder wall on each side of the fistula can be helpful. Exposure and dissection around a small fistula can be facilitated by traction on a small urethral catheter placed through the fistula and into the bladder with the catheter bulb distended inside the bladder. The Young prostatic retractor may be used in similar fashion.

EXCISION OF THE FISTULA TRACT. The entire tract of the fistula from the vaginal orifice to the bladder orifice should be excised during the dissection. This need not necessarily be done first, but it should be accomplished at some time during the dissection. The tract is surrounded by scar tissue, and this should be removed so that normal tissue can be

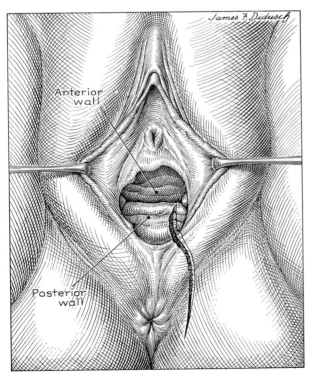

FIG. 27–3   Schuchardt's incision.

carefully approximated with sutures for better healing. Completely excising the fistula tract will inevitably result in a larger hole in the bladder, and that is as it should be. However, some surgeons are reluctant to do this, failing to understand that in order to be properly closed, the fistula must first be made larger by excising the edges of the tract completely.

WIDE MOBILIZATION OF THE VAGINAL MUCOSA AROUND THE FISTULA. So that the repair can be done in several layers, the vaginal mucosa should be mobilized widely in all directions around the fistula. The bladder muscularis should not be disturbed. At the same time, the vaginal mucosal flap should not be too thin. Any indurated tissue or scar tissue surrounding the fistula should be excised. This dissection can be facilitated by injecting sterile normal saline just beneath the vaginal mucosa to help identify the tissue planes. We prefer not to add a vasopressor to the solution because of the theoretical risk that healing might be inhibited by interference with local tissue resistance to infection. Wide dissection and mobilization of the bladder base is especially important in the closure of post-irradiation fistulas because the blood supply to the scar tissue surrounding the fistula is poor and healing is therefore at a great disadvantage. The farther away from the fistula opening one dissects, the better the blood supply becomes and the better the layered closure of the bladder wall over the fistula.

CHOICE OF SUTURES. The use of silver wire sutures for closure of a vesicovaginal fistula has been almost completely abandoned in favor of more modern suture materials. Over the years, catgut for the first two or three layers followed by a nonabsorbable synthetic suture material such as nylon, Prolene, or Dacron in the vaginal mucosa has been a favorite choice. Of course, the nonabsorbable synthetic suture in the vaginal mucosa must eventually be removed. Today, our suture preference for vesicovaginal fistula repair is for synthetic, delayed-absorbable polyglactin or polyglycolic acid sutures. These sutures retain their tensile strength longer than catgut and the tissue reaction is less than with catgut. A stronger cicatrix will have formed at the repair site by the time these sutures begin to lose their tensile strength. This is their greatest advantage when compared to catgut. Our preference is for No. 3-0 delayed-absorbable suture swaged on to a fine, small-caliber, semi-malleable, round needle. It is the most nearly ideal suture we have found for fistula repair. It can be used for all layers and does not need to be removed.

CLOSURE OF BLADDER MUCOSA. Closure of the fistula should begin by approximating the bladder mucosa with interrupted No. 3-0 delayed-absorbable sutures.

Ideally, the first row should not penetrate the bladder mucosa, but it should be taken parallel to the edge of the fistula tract so as to invert the edge within the bladder. From a practical viewpoint, this may prove to be quite difficult, and direct suture approximation of the bladder mucosa has not proven to be especially deleterious. This first row of sutures is the most important. Good bites should be taken in healthy tissue and the defect must be closed securely. The security of the closure should then be tested by instillation of 200 ml dilute methylene blue or sterile milk into the bladder. If any point of leakage is detected, it must be reinforced before proceeding. A vesicovaginal fistula repair may not be successful unless the urinary side of the fistula is securely closed.

CLOSURE OF BROAD SURFACE TO BROAD SURFACE WITH-OUT TENSION. That closure of broad surface to broad surface must be without tension is an important axiom in all types of fistula repair. Once the bladder mucosa is securely closed, it is reinforced by two or three covering layers of interrupted No. 3-0 delayed-absorbable suture placed in the bladder muscularis. If the layers do not come together without tension, a wider dissection of the bladder base is required. The excess vaginal mucosa may be trimmed away, but generous flaps should be left for approximation without tension.

All layers should be approximated in a direction that is transverse to the longitudinal axis of the vagina. There is much less tension on the suture line when layers are approximated in this direction, and there is no advantage to alternating the layers of closure with the initial layer. Unusual circumstances may dictate an exception to this rule.

URETERAL INTEGRITY. At the end of the repair, 5 ml indigo carmine should be injected intravenously with rapid infusion of parenteral fluids. The bladder should be instilled with 200 ml normal saline or distilled water, and, with a cystoscope, the dye should be observed spurting from both ureteral orifices to be certain that the ureters are not obstructed.

BLADDER DRAINAGE. It is impossible to keep the bladder completely empty and dry during the postoperative period. However, the bladder should be maintained as empty as possible and must not be allowed to become distended. Although we have always subscribed to the use of a urethral catheter for 10 days following fistula repair in order to place the operative site at rest, Falk and others have avoided the use of the postoperative catheter out of a concern over adding trauma to the bladder base. In recent years we have resolved both of these concerns by using suprapubic drainage with a No.

12 French catheter. This not only avoids trauma to the operative site, but provides bladder drainage without the need for catheterization during the time the patient initiates voiding. In using this technique, care must be taken to make certain that the suprapubic catheter does not become obstructed, for many good surgical repairs of a fistula have been ruined by overdistention of the bladder. The management of the bladder after vesicovaginal fistula repair must be an individual matter. Sometimes bladder drainage will be required for 10 to 14 days. On the other hand, if the fistula is small and the closure is undoubtedly secure, bladder drainage may be discontinued after 1 or 2 days. For this short time, a transurethral catheter may be used. It is no longer considered advisable to make a vaginal cystotomy incision for drainage.

When the fistula is large and closure is difficult, the patient should remain in bed initially for 5 to 7 days. Patients with small fistulas without much scar tissue and a secure closure may be up within 24 to 48 hours without endangering the success of the closure. We do not advise that the patient remain in a prone position with a catheter coming directly through a split mattress to a drainage bottle on the floor, nor have we used the Bradford frame or attached the catheter to suction. If adequate drainage is established so that the bladder does not become distended, the position the patient lies in postoperatively makes little difference. Bladder irrigations are not used except to clear a blocked catheter. Urinary antibiotics are unnecessary unless acute upper urinary tract infection develops. In keeping with modern theory, some surgeons have used intraoperative antibiotics to enhance tissue healing but there have been no controlled studies to support this approach. An adequate intake of fluids is required so that an adequate urine output can be maintained. The best way to keep the catheter open and avoid urinary tract infection is to ensure a high output of dilute urine, preferably as much as 75 ml/hr to 100 ml/hr.

Complicated Vesicovaginal Fistulas

Complicated fistulas are: those that are large; those that have had several unsuccessful attempts at repair; those that involve the urethra, vesical neck, or ureters; those that are associated with intestinal fistulas; and those that result from radiation for gynecologic malignancy. Although the standard principles for fistula repair still apply, and perhaps should be applied more strictly, other special techniques may be necessary to achieve continence. As mentioned earlier, a longer interval of time may be required before the tissue around the fistula is mature or healed and ready for closure. Techniques of bringing in new tissue for support and neovascularization should be considered. These include mobilization of the bulbocavernosus muscle and fat pad from the labia, the gracilis muscle from the inner thigh, or an omental fat pad. A combined transvaginal-transvesical-transperitoneal approach may be needed. The operation may need to be done in stages. For example, if a radiation vesicovaginal fistula is associated with a rectovaginal fistula and bilateral ureteral stenosis, a three-stage operation may be required. The first stage may be a ureteroileocutaneous anastomosis and colostomy. The second stage would be a closure of the fistulas. If the fistulas heal, the third stage would be a closure of the colostomy and anastomosis of the ileal conduit to the bladder.

Only when the closure of a vesicovaginal fistula is considered to be technically impossible should one consider supravesical diversion of the urinary stream. The painful post-irradiation fistulas fall into this group. In former years we transplanted the ureters into the sigmoid, but experience has taught us that transplantation into the functioning bowel may shorten the patient's life. Hydronephrosis and pyelonephritis can develop, with the attendant metabolic and electrolyte disturbance of hyperchloremic acidosis. We now rarely perform ureterosigmoid implantations. Even in patients with post-irradiation fistulas where chances for cure are not good or in whom longevity is limited by the presence of malignancy, it is preferable to anastomose the ureters to an isolated segment of ileum. When a fistula is the result of benign disease or injury but impossible to close, we believe that the implantation of the ureters into an isolated ileal loop is also the procedure of choice.

Closure of Small Vesicovaginal Fistulas

A small vesicovaginal fistula may be closed by the simple technique shown in Figure 27–4. The particular fistula pictured here resulted from too-deep fulguration of an elusive ulcer of the bladder. The patient also had stress incontinence of urine. Therefore, the operation was combined with plication of the urethrovesical angle.

Since the position of the small fistula indicated its proximity to the right ureteral orifice, the ureters were catheterized by preoperative cystoscopy. With catheters in the ureters, danger of injury to the ureters is practically eliminated.

A short midline incision is made through the vaginal mucosa from the urethral meatus to the region of the trigone (Fig. 27–4A). The vaginal mucosa is dissected free laterally and beyond the fistula. The margins of the small fistula are excised and freshened without wide dissection. A purse-string suture (No. 3-0 delayed-absorbable) is placed about the fistulous opening (Fig. 27–4B). The fistula is inverted as the purse string is tied (Fig. 27–4C). A second purse string is placed about the first, and the encircled tissue is inverted (Fig. 27–4D). Plication of the urethra and the urethrovesical angle is then carried out to relieve the urinary incontinence. A urethral or suprapubic catheter is left in the bladder for several days. This simple technique is applicable only to very small fistulas in the anterior vaginal wall.

STANDARD OPERATION FOR CLOSURE OF SIMPLE VESICOVAGINAL FISTULA. The simple technique illustrated here in Figure 27–5 may be used in closing an easily exposed fistula in which there is no excess scar tissue. It represents a more or less typical closure, if there is such a thing as a typical closure in a condition in which there is such great variation. The simple fistula for which this operation is done is shown in Figure 27–5A.

Since the fistula is close to the trigone, the ureters are first catheterized. An incision is made about the fistulous opening, and the vaginal mucosa is dissected free from the bladder for a sufficient distance in all directions to mobilize enough bladder wall for at least a double line of closure without tension. Usually a zone of about 1 cm to 2 cm is sufficient (Fig. 27–5B). The fistula tract is excised. Closure begins at one end of the fistula opening with interrupted sutures (No. 3-0 delayed-absorbable) (Fig. 27–5C). These stitches are taken either parallel to the edges of the opening, well into the bladder wall, or, alternatively, through the bladder mucosa. They should begin and end well beyond the edge of the fistula. When each suture is tied, the edges are inverted into the bladder.

At this stage of the operation, the closure is tested by introducing into the bladder about 200 ml sterilized evaporated milk (easily obtained from the hospital nursery) through a urethral catheter. The advantage of milk over methylene blue is that it does not stain the tissues if leakage occurs. A dilute solution of methylene blue also works nicely. If the suture line is not watertight, the weak point is reinforced with additional interrupted sutures, mobilizing more bladder if necessary. A second layer of No. 3-0 interrupted sutures is placed in the bladder musculature, inverting the first layer (Fig. 27–5D). A third layer of sutures may be required. A bulbocavernosus fat pad developed from the labium majus may be interposed at this point if deemed necessary.

The vaginal mucosa is trimmed and approximated with No. 3-0 interrupted sutures. This closure should

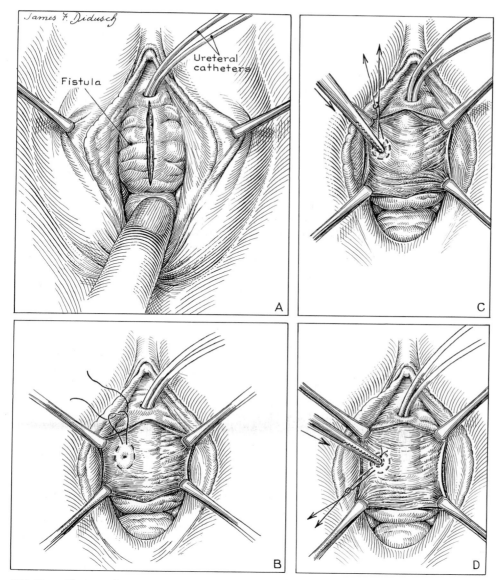

James F. Didusch

FIG. 27–4 Closure of a very small vesicovaginal fistula at the trigone. (*A*) Both ureters have been catheterized for their identification. Since in this operation the vesical sphincter was to be plicated also, a midline incision is made through the anterior vaginal wall to expose the urethral and trigonal region. (*B*) A purse string of No. 3-0 delayed-absorbable suture is placed about the opening of the fistula. (*C*) As the purse string is tied, the tissue is inverted into the bladder. (*D*) A second purse string is placed around the first. The vaginal mucosa is closed.

be made in the direction that gives the least amount of tension, which is almost always transverse to the longitudinal axis of the vagina. If ureteral catheters were previously inserted, they are now removed. A suprapubic catheter is used for bladder drainage, since a urethral catheter would almost certainly rest directly on the suture line inside the bladder.

The Modified Latzko Operation for Supratrigonal Vesicovaginal Fistula Repair

In 1913, Latzko recommended a technique of high colpocleisis, first described by Simon, as "the simplest and surest procedure for vesicovaginal fistulas following hysterectomy." In 1926, Latzko offered modification of Simon's procedure in order to eliminate the formation of bladder diverticula, and the technique now is called the Latzko operation. The principles of the operation were described in detail in 1942. Latzko reported 29 cures among 31 cases using this technique. The results are impressive since, in the majority of his patients, the fistula resulted from a radical abdominal hysterectomy for cervical cancer. Many others have reported satisfactory results since then.

The operation is basically a partial colpocleisis, an obliteration of the upper vagina for 2 cm to 3 cm around the fistula. The anterior and posterior vaginal walls with vaginal mucosa removed are then easily approximated without tension, since they naturally fall together. The upper or posterior edge of the fistula always coincides with the transverse firm scar in the vault of the vagina. A fistula that follows total abdominal or vaginal hysterectomy is usually small and supratrigonal. Therefore, the ureters are generally not in danger.

The Latzko operation is the procedure of choice when a vesicovaginal fistula develops after total hysterectomy. It cannot be done if the cervix has not been removed. Since a fistula resulting from total hysterectomy is almost always small and high in the vagina, the shortening of the vagina caused by approximation of the anterior and posterior vaginal walls is slight. In our experience, few patients have complained after operation that the vagina was too short.

Usually, the fistula may be brought into operating range by traction sutures placed in the lateral quadrants of the vaginal vault. If difficulty is encountered, greater exposure may be obtained by a mediolateral episiotomy or a true Schuchardt incision. At times, the incision may be conveniently drawn down with a Young prostatic retractor, or with a small (No. 8 Foley) urethral catheter placed through the fistula and inflated in the bladder.

Infiltration of sterile saline beneath the vaginal mucosa around the fistula will facilitate dissection. The incision should be approximately 1 cm from the fistula edge in all directions (Fig. 27–6A). The vaginal mucosa is mobilized as shown in Figure 27–6B. When the vaginal mucosa is being removed posteriorly, an effort should be made to avoid entry into the peritoneal cavity through the peritoneum of the cul de sac, although Lawson prefers to open the cul de sac directly. If an inadvertent peritoneal entry is made, it should be closed and the dissection carried out in another plane.

Latzko apparently did not feel it necessary to excise the fistulous tract. However, we strongly advise adding this step, since the margins of a scarred and epithelialized fistula may not heal well when approximated with sutures, but the margins will heal if the fibrous scarring is removed first. This should be done even if a larger hole results. This step is illustrated in Figure 27–6C. After excising the fistula tract, the bladder mucosal edges are approximated transversely with interrupted No. 3-0 delayed-absorbable sutures swaged onto a fine round needle (Fig. 27–6D). Care must be taken that the lateral margin of the bladder mucosa is closed securely by including tissue beyond the fistula margin. After placing this first line of sutures, the bladder is filled with 100 ml to 200 ml sterile evaporated milk or dilute methylene blue and tested for leakage. Points of weakness are noted and reinforced with additional mucosal sutures. This first suture line is then covered over by a second and third layer of No. 3-0 delayed absorbable sutures, each inverting the previous line of sutures and approximating the anterior and posterior vaginal walls in the process (Fig. 27–6E). Further denudation of the vaginal mucosa or dissection beneath the vaginal mucosa may ultimately be required. In fact, it is often advisable not to denude at the beginning of the operation as wide an area as may ultimately be necessary. Avoiding early complete denudation prevents blood loss that may be annoying to the operator and depleting to the patient. After the last suture is placed, the vaginal mucosa is closed with interrupted No. 3-0 delayed-absorbable sutures (Fig. 27–6F). Monofilament nylon can also be used. It is nonreactive. Nylon sutures cause less tissue maceration than silver wire, are easier to place, and permit better patient ambulation. However, both nylon and silver wire sutures must be removed later. Delayed-absorbable sutures in the vaginal mucosa are equally satisfactory in this technique, since the success or failure of the repair has already been determined by the suture layers placed in the bladder mucosa and bladder wall before the vaginal mucosa is closed.

An indwelling catheter is left in the bladder for 1 to 14 days postoperatively depending on the operator's assessment of several factors, including the size of the fistula, the health of the tissues, the security of the closure and, a history of previous unsuccessful attempts at repair.

Following an operation for fistula closure, we prefer to use a suprapubic silicone tube for bladder drainage, because the operative site can be traumatized by an indwelling transurethral catheter and voiding can be accomplished without catheterization. On the other hand, if it is anticipated that bladder drainage will be needed for only a few days, a transurethral catheter may be entirely satisfactory.

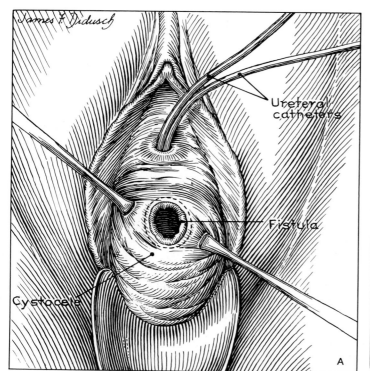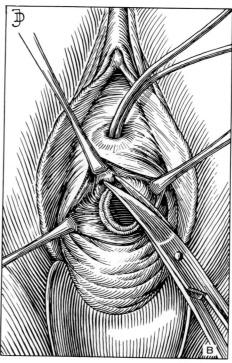

FIG. 27–5 Standard operation for closure of a simple vesicovaginal fistula. (*A*) Ureters have been catheterized to prevent encirclement of a ureter with a suture. An incision about the fistulous opening is marked by the dotted line. The scarred fistula tract should be excised. (*B*) The vaginal mucosa is dissected back from the fistulous opening for a sufficient distance to mobilize the bladder wall about the fistula.

Transabdominal Closure

In most instances, a vesicovaginal fistula can be closed by the Latzko method. However, multiple previous unsuccessful attempts at closure may produce excessive scarring and so fix the vagina that exposure from below is extremely difficult. Under these circumstances, transabdominal closure may be necessary.

With the patient in an exaggerated Trendelenburg position, the pelvis is inspected through a low midline incision. The intestines are packed back into the abdomen. The bladder is found adherent to the apex of the vagina at the site of the fistula. The peritoneum is cut at its attachment to the vagina and dissected free. It is left attached to the bladder.

When making this dissection, it should be borne in mind that a flap of peritoneum is to be brought down later between the bladder and the vagina. After freeing the peritoneal flap, a longitudinal (vertical) incision is made in the bladder dome and is extended along the posterior wall in the midline until it reaches the bladder base and the site of the

fistulous tract (Fig. 27–7A). Here, the incision encircles the fistulous tract, including the bladder and vaginal orifices (Fig. 27–7B). Then the vagina is closed with interrupted No. 3-0 delayed-absorbable sutures (Fig. 27–7C). The bladder, which has been sufficiently mobilized, is closed with two layers of sutures as shown in Figure 27–7D. If possible, the initial layer of interrupted sutures should invert the mucosal edges into the bladder cavity. The integrity of the suture line is tested by filling the bladder with sterile water through a suprapubic catheter placed in the bladder dome (Fig. 27–7E). The catheter is in a retroperitoneal position and exteriorized through the abdominal wall in a separate stab-wound incision. It is left connected to straight drainage for 12 to 14 days. The second layer, which includes the muscularis, may be closed with No. 3-0 continuous or interrupted sutures (Fig. 27–7F). After the bladder and the vagina are closed, the peritoneal flap is brought down from the bladder reflection and sutured to the anterior vaginal wall or bladder wall so that the suture line in the bladder wall is covered. An omental pedicle graft may be obtained from the

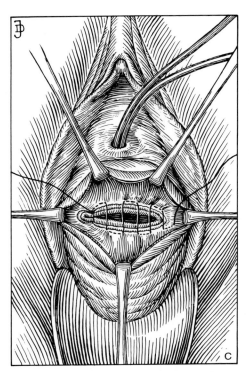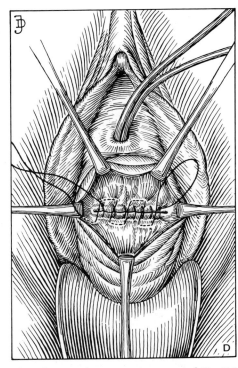

FIG. 27–5 (continued). (C) The first suture line is placed with a continuous or interrupted No. 3-0 delayed-absorbable suture, inverting tissue into the bladder. (D) A second suture line is placed, inverting the first. Excess vaginal mucosa is trimmed and approximated with interrupted No. 3-0 delayed-absorbable sutures.

transverse colon and sutured between the bladder closure and the vagina (Fig. 27–7G). A retroperitoneal drain is brought out through a separate stab-wound incision.

O'Connor described an abdominal operation for vesicovaginal fistula repair in 1951. Later, in a series of reports, O'Connor, Jr., has achieved excellent results with this operation. According to O'Connor, Jr.,

> The key to the operative procedure is bisection of the bladder with wide mobilization of the bladder and vagina, allowing for closure of the vagina and bladder in separate planes. As much dissection as possible is done to free the posterior wall of the bladder and the bladder is then opened at the dome. From this initial incision the exposure is improved by incising vertically down to the area of the fistula. Stay sutures are placed every few centimeters on either side to allow elevation of the bladder wall and the exposure is excellent as these are lifted. The fistulous tract is excised in racquet fashion, making the lateral margin wide enough to leave viable tissue for subsequent closure. Then the exposure may be helped by inserting either a balloon catheter or a Young prostatic tractor through the fistula to elevate the bladder and vagina. After generous ex-

cision of the tract, the walls of the bladder are mobilized widely away from the vagina. If there is concern regarding the ureters, catheters can be placed to visualize these structures during this part of the dissection. All non-viable or necrotic tissue is excised and the vaginal closure is done with fresh, viable tissue in 2 layers. . . . This may be further reinforced by placing fat, peritoneum, fibrous tissue or pedicled omentum over this closure. The bladder closure is then begun carefully at the apex of the incision, using a continuous suture, starting with the original knot on the outer surface of the bladder, including all muscle layers. . . . If the defect is extensive, variations of bladder flaps that are placed to cover the defect can be used but these are usually unnecessary if wide mobilization of the back wall of the bladder can be effected.

Glenn and Stevens, Wein and associates, Marshall, and others have reported good results with a similar operation. A transabdominal operation can be combined with the transvaginal approach, since it may be difficult to satisfactorily mobilize and close the vaginal side of the fistula through an abdominal incision. We have used the combined transabdominal and transvesical approach to advantage in several cases. This technique has been described by

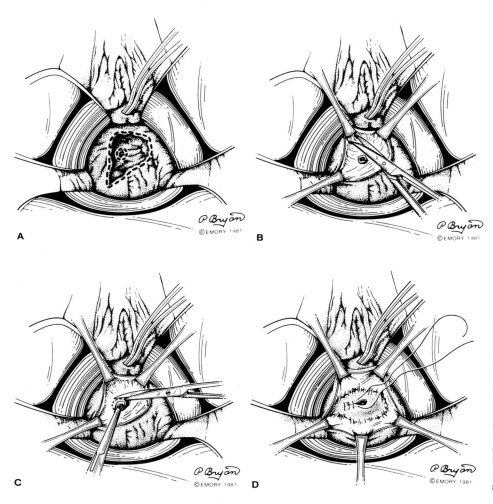

A

B

C

D

FIG. 27–6 Operation for a closure of a simple posthysterectomy vesicovaginal fistula by the Latzko technique. (*A*) Ureters have been catheterized to prevent encirclement of a ureter by a suture. Incisions about the fistula opening and about the indurated vaginal mucosa margin are marked by the dotted lines. (*B*) The vaginal mucosa is dissected back from the fistula opening for a sufficient distance to mobilize the bladder wall about the fistula. (*C*) The fistula tract is sharply and completely excised. (*D*) No. 3-0 delayed-absorbable interrupted mattress sutures taken parallel to the edge of the fistula tract are used as the initial suture line, inverting tissue into the bladder. The security of the closure should be tested by instillation of 100 ml to 200 ml dilute methylene blue or sterile milk into the bladder.

Taylor and associates, Weyrauch and Rous, and by Clarke and Holland. It should be reemphasized, however, that only in unusual circumstances is it necessary to repair a vesicovaginal fistula abdominally.

Autograft as an Aid to Fistula Closure

The tissue surrounding complicated vesicovaginal fistulas may be relatively avascular, rigid, and fibrosed. This is especially true of postirradiation fistulas where hyalinization of blood vessels and sclerotic tissue may extend for a considerable distance beyond the fistula margins. When local tissue healing is seriously impaired by irradiation, infection, diabetes, or other factors, it is usually necessary to bring fresh, normal, nonirradiated, pliable, and well-vascularized tissue into the operative field to support the repair and facilitate healing. Neovascularization from such pedicle grafts has been

proved experimentally. Small arterioles migrate from the normal into the ischemic tissues of the repair site.

Various techniques of autografting have been described. Kiricuta and Goldstein described a procedure for using pedicled omentum in the repair of difficult fistulas. According to these authors, the repair of the fistula does not even require the closure of the bladder defect. If it is technically impossible to close the bladder or vagina because of inaccessibility deep in the pelvis, the vaginal wound will eventually heal over the omental flap. Bastiaanse was also an advocate of pedicled omental grafts. Turner–Warwick has used them in a variety of ways to reconstruct the upper and lower urinary tract. A free graft of omentum cannot be used for this purpose, since the vascular supply and lymphatic drainage must be intact.

An abdominal incision must be made if an omen-

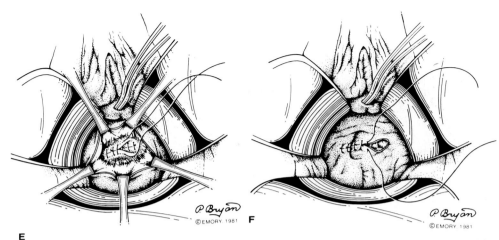

FIG. 27-6 (continued). (E) Two or three additional suture layers should approximate the bladder muscularis broad surface to broad surface without tension. No. 3-0 delayed-absorbable interrupted mattress sutures should be used. (F) The vaginal mucosa is closed transversely with interrupted No. 3-0 delayed-absorbable sutures.

tal pedicle graft is to be used, but this is rarely necessary because most fistulas can be closed by a transvaginal approach. Other grafting techniques are available in vaginal operations. Garlock described the gracilis muscle graft in 1928 and this has been modified by Ingelman–Sundberg and, more recently, by Hamlin and Nicholson. A more convenient method of pedicle grafting to provide support and neovascularization for the fistula repair was described by Martius. The graft is obtained from the labium majus on one or both sides and is composed of bulbocavernous muscle and fat. It is desirable to close the vaginal mucosa over a pedicle graft if possible. However, if it is not possible, the defect will become re-epithelialized in time. Good results with its use have been reported by Zacharin, by Patil and associates, and by Smith and Johnson. We have also found this technique extremely useful, but do not consider it necessary in routine simple fistula repairs. The Martius graft is very useful in urethral reconstruction, as discussed later.

VESICOUTERINE AND VESICOCERVICAL FISTULAS

Vesicouterine and vesicocervical fistulas are alike in etiology, symptoms, and management. Therefore, they will be considered together.

Improved obstetric practice is responsible for a reduction in the incidence of these fistulas. Although some result from instrumentation and malignancy, today almost all vesicouterine and vesicocervical fistulas are associated with injury to or necrosis of the bladder wall directly over dehiscence of a lower

uterine segment cesarean section incision. When there has been inadequate mobilization of the bladder inferiorly and laterally, the bladder may be injured with delivery of a large fetal head, or the bladder wall may be accidentally included in the sutures used to close the uterine incision. When the sutures are absorbed and a fistula forms, the patient may experience some involuntary loss of urine through the vagina or she may remain continent. However, she may complain of cyclic hematuria and amenorrhea. This symptom was called *menouria* by Youssef. In most cases, variable degrees of intermittent urinary incontinence will be present and only microscopic hematuria will be present during regular menstrual flow. Of course, vaginal examination will fail to reveal a fistula, although occasionally urine will be seen trickling through the cervical os. Cystoscopy, cystogram, and hysterogram are helpful diagnostic procedures. The vesical orifice of the fistula will always be supratrigonal in location.

Although a few fistulas have been reported to close spontaneously, most often surgery is required. The operation is fairly simple to perform and almost routinely successful. Either a transvaginal or a transabdominal approach may be used. When the fistula is high and there is no uterine descensus when traction is made on a cervical tenaculum, the repair must be performed through an abdominal incision. A dissection is carried out to separate the bladder from the cervix and lower uterine segment. Following identification of the fistula tract, the uterine and bladder defects are closed separately in lay-

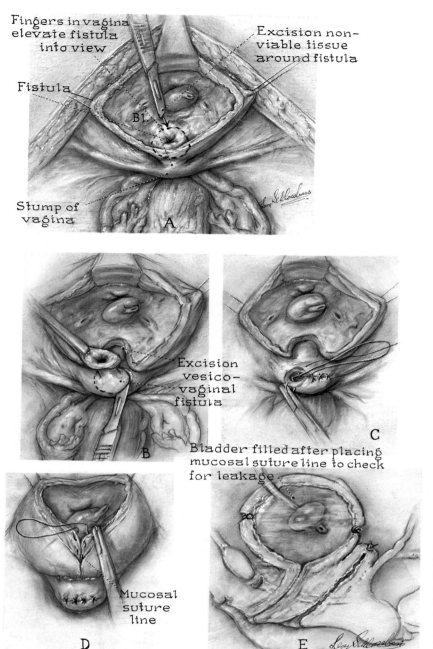

Fingers in vagina elevate fistula into view

Excision non-viable tissue around fistula

Fistula

B1

Stump of vagina

A

Excision vesico-vaginal fistula

B

C

Bladder filled after placing mucosal suture line to check for leakage

Mucosal suture line

D

E

FIG. 27-7 Transabdominal, transvesical closure of vesicovaginal fistula. (*A*) A longitudinal incision in the bladder dome illustrates the vesical opening of the fistula and its relationship to the vagina and the ureteral orifices. (*B*) The incision in the bladder wall is extended around the orifice of the fistula. The fistulous tract and its vaginal orifice are completely excised. (*C*) Interrupted No. 3-0 delayed-absorbable sutures are used to close the vaginal opening in one or two layers. (*D*) A continuous No. 3-0 delayed-absorbable suture closes the bladder mucosa longitudinally. (*E*) A suprapubic catheter is placed through the bladder dome in an extra-peritoneal location. The bladder is distended to check for security of closure.

ers. A layer of vesical peritoneum should be interposed between the two sides. Transurethral bladder drainage should be carried out for 7 to 10 days postoperatively. A hysterectomy is not required for fistula repair. If hysterectomy is done, it should be indicated for some other reason, including the presence of a large defect in the uterine wall. If the uterus is left, pregnancies can and will occur unless a tubal ligation is performed or contraception is used assiduously.

COMPLICATIONS OF FISTULA REPAIR

As soon as the last repair suture is placed, 5 ml indigo carmine should be injected intravenously, the bladder should be filled with 200 ml clear sterile

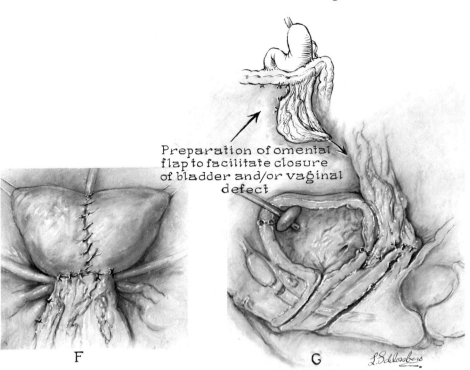

Preparation of omental flap to facilitate closure of bladder and/or vaginal defect

FIG. 27–7 (continued). (*F*) The bladder muscularis is closed with No. 3-0 delayed-absorbable continuous or interrupted sutures. (*G*) In complicated fistulas, an omental flap may be developed and sutured between the bladder closure and the vaginal closure.

F

G

saline, and a cystoscope should be gently placed into the bladder. Careful examination of the repair site for evidence of bleeding should then be carried out. The dye should be seen spurting from each ureteral orifice. By this technique, two of the most common complications of vesicovaginal fistula repair—intravesical hemorrhage and ureteral obstruction—can be diagnosed at the earliest possible moment and corrected.

When intravesical bleeding still occurs in the postoperative period and threatens the integrity of the repair by obstruction of the catheter and overdistention of the bladder, gentle attempts to evacuate the clots can be made by transurethral bladder irrigations. If these are not successful, it may be necessary to perform an immediate suprapubic cystotomy to remove the clots and suture the bleeding points in the bladder mucosa. Infection is common after such events and should be combated with antibiotics. Transfusions will be needed if significant amounts of blood are lost.

If the patient exhibits signs of ureteral obstruction (persistent fever, abdominal distention, pain, and tenderness) an intravenous pyelogram should be done immediately. Occasionally ureteral obstruction will be temporary from tissue edema caused by the fistula repair. If a complete ureteral obstruction is diagnosed, several options are available. One might consider breaking down the repair to remove the offending suture(s). This procedure may be less hazardous in a poor-risk or elderly patient than an operation to relieve the obstruction. However, it carries with it the great disappointment of failure to establish continence, since the repair will need to be redone later after a prolonged interval of waiting and may be more difficult. One also has the option of performing an abdominal operation to relieve the obstruction. After the ureter has been identified on the pelvic side wall, the choice lies between placing a T-tube in the ureter for drainage, hoping the obstruction below will be relieved spontaneously when the sutures are absorbed, or performing a ureteroneocystostomy. A percutaneous nephrostomy may be a satisfactory temporary solution attempting to preserve kidney function until a definitive repair of the ureter can be done.

The most important and dreaded complication, of course, is breakdown of the repair. This usually occurs about 7 to 10 days after operation. If the repair breaks down, large-caliber catheter drainage should be continued for several weeks to provide an adequate opportunity for the fistula to heal spontaneously. Spontaneous healing, however, will rarely occur and only under optimal conditions.

Usually only a significant reduction in the size of the fistula will result, so that the next attempt at repair will be easier and will be more likely to be successful.

Urethral Damage

Serious damage to the urethra that results in a fistula is uncommon. Formerly, obstetric injury from prolonged labor or difficult forceps delivery was the major cause of this condition. In developing countries, this is still a significant cause of urethral injury. More commonly, inadvertent urethral damage results from an unsuccessful attempt to remove an infected suburethral diverticulum. Gray reports a 25% incidence of urethrovaginal fistula in such cases, which is much higher than our own experience of 5%. Additionally, direct trauma may occur during an anterior colporrhaphy. If this is unrecognized at the time of surgery, a fistula will follow. Irradiation damage to the floor of the urethra may occur with the use of intravaginal irradiation of tumors in the lower genital tract; in most of these cases there has been extension of the tumor into the urethrovaginal septum, which subsequently breaks down with the regression of the neoplasm. We have also observed ischemia of the distal half of the urethra following repeated attempts at urethral plication for urinary incontinence that have led to a severely compromised blood supply to the urethra.

The destructive effects of lymphogranuloma venereum may cause urethral loss. Finally, some patients with congenital absence of the vagina will have loss of urethral function as a result of overzealous attempts to create a vaginal cavity by the Frank method, from frequent intercourse through the urethra, or from sloughing of the distal urethra as a complication of the Abbe–Wharton–McIndoe operation.

Loss of the distal one-third of the urethra is usually not associated with urinary incontinence, although it is often associated with loss of a well-defined urinary stream. Urine may spray from the urethra and down the insides of the thigh in an annoying fashion. The distal urethra can be sacrificed in extensive operations for the vagina and vulva without loss of continence.

Many of the principles outlined for vesicovaginal fistula repair are also applicable to repair of urethrovaginal fistulas. However, since urethrovaginal fistulas may be more difficult to repair successfully, the tissues must be as nearly normal as possible before repair is attempted. For this reason, after the diagnosis is made, a delay of several months may be necessary to allow the tissues to heal completely. Wide meticulous dissection and mobilization is essential so that tissues can be approximated exactly and without tension. Pedicle grafting is frequently necessary. Suprapubic rather than transurethral catheter drainage is always preferred. The repair must be individualized to fit the special circumstances presented by each patient.

Urethral reconstruction and restoration of continence is difficult to accomplish at the same time with a single operation. Success is generally achieved in about 50% of cases. Symmonds and Hill have pointed out that successful anatomical restoration is not synonymous with restoration of physiologic function. Little is accomplished if urethral length is restored but the patient remains incontinent. Emphasis is placed on fashioning a new urethra of small caliber using as much muscular tissue as possible, plicating the vesical neck whenever appropriate, and supporting the new repair with a pedicled bulbocavernosus muscle and fat pad if necessary. It cannot be predicted if restorative operations on the urethra will establish continence. Patients in whom continence is not established should have a retropubic cystourethropexy done after a period of at least 6 months. A Goebell–Frangenheim–Stoeckel operation has also been used in these patients but runs the risk of interfering with the urethral blood supply and causing damage to the urethral floor.

OPERATIONS FOR RESTORATION OF URETHRA AND URINARY CONTINENCE

The following operations are designed for certain cases of urinary incontinence resulting from destruction of the urethra and part of the sphincter from childbirth injury, surgery, or a diverticulum.

In the standard operation for urethral reconstruction and sphincter repair, a U-shaped flap of vaginal mucosa is dissected free and held forward, thus exposing the undersurface of the trigone and sphincter region of the bladder (Fig. 27–8A,B). Rather deep interrupted stitches of No. 3-0 delayed-absorbable suture are taken in the sphincter region. These, when tied, tighten the internal orifice (Fig. 27–8C).

The flap of mucosa is drawn downward and an area about 6 mm or 7 mm in width is denuded forward for a distance equal to the length of the flap (Fig. 27–8D).

The edge of the flap is held forward with a smooth dissecting forceps and curled under, so that the raw surface of the flap may be sutured to the anterior denuded area (Fig. 27–8E). Interrupted No. 3-0 delayed-absorbable sutures are used. This is repeated on the other side, thus forming an epithelial-lined tube to serve as a urethra. This new urethral floor is supported by a layer of paraurethral fascia that is plicated beneath the urethra with No. 3-0 delayed-absorbable sutures.

The wound is closed by approximating the mucosal edges with interrupted No. 3-0 delayed-absorbable sutures. This buries the newly constructed urethra and completely closes the wound (Fig. 27-8F,G).

To permit healing of the newly constructed urethra, a suprapubic silicone catheter is used for bladder drainage. A transurethral indwelling catheter should not be used.

We have found this procedure to be quite successful when used as the initial attempt to restore the floor of an extensively traumatized urethra. It has been less successful in cases where previous attempts to repair the urethra have failed due to the compromise of the blood supply to the long mucosal pedicle. In such cases, we prefer the following technique. This technique reestablishes the walls of the urethra along the urethral floor, as illustrated in Figure 27-9, in cases where the walls have retracted into the roof of the urethral tube. Symmonds has had excellent success in establishing urinary continence with this method. Falk and Tancer described a similar procedure and have encouraged its use. This operation emphasizes preservation of the limited blood supply to the urethral margins. By incising the vaginal mucosa at the very lateral margin of each side of the urethral remnants along the roof of the exposed urethra, leaving no more than 2 mm of vaginal mucosa attached to the urethral walls, the edges of the retracted side walls can be freed with careful sharp dissection without encroaching too far laterally on the paraurethral blood supply (Fig. 27-9A,B). The dissection should mobilize enough of the urethral walls to permit snug approximation of the edges in the posterior midline with interrupted No. 3-0 delayed-absorbable sutures over a small No. 12 French catheter (Fig. 27-9C). Although a very small urethral lumen is created by this conservative dissection, this has a distinct advantage in establishing urethral continence. The adjacent urethral fascia is then freed with sharp dissection along the side of the newly created urethral tube, avoiding deep lateral dissection and interruption of the blood supply.

Interrupted No. 3-0 delayed-absorbable sutures are placed through the fascia and musculature of the urethral tube along each side of the urethra, with each suture being held until placement has been made on both sides (Fig. 27-9C). The lower strand of each suture is then joined with the lower strand of the corresponding suture on the opposite side of the urethra and tied across the urethral floor.

The upper strand of each suture is then tied in the midline. As described by Symmonds, this produces a pulley effect that approximates broad surface of fascia and urethral muscle to broad surface (Fig. 27-9D). Alternatively, vertical mattress sutures in the fascia and adjacent urethral musculature will produce equal support to the urethral wall. The edges of the vaginal mucosa are then undermined and freed sufficiently to permit approximation in the midline without undue tension, using No. 3-0 delayed-absorbable sutures (Fig. 27-9E). It is important to remove the small urethral catheter at the completion of the procedure to avoid pressure necrosis to the suture line. It is our policy to fill the bladder with 300 ml sterile water and to insert a suprapubic silicone tube before removing the catheter because it is frequently quite difficult and hazardous to catheterize the newly constructed urethra. Should the suprapubic catheter become plugged, only the surgeon who understands the landmarks of the newly constructed urethral tube should attempt to catheterize this patient postoperatively. The bladder and urethra are left at rest for 12 to 14 days before the suprapubic catheter is clamped intermittently to initiate voiding through the reconstructed urethra.

Alternatively, before closing the vaginal mucosa, it is frequently useful to reinforce the surgical reconstruction of the urethra with a labial fat pad as shown in Figure 27-9F. This modified Martius technique adds a vascularized labial graft that will provide a new blood supply to the operative site and avoid necrosis and breakdown of the ischemic urethra. By making a U-shaped incision along the lateral and medial margins of the labium majus and minus, the fat pad overlying the bulbocavernosus muscle is dissected free, leaving a wide base of the graft at the superior aspect of the labia. The vaginal mucosa is excised along the side of the urethra adjacent to the pedicle graft to accommodate the width of the pedicle and to provide a graft site for the vulvar flap (Fig. 27-9F). The skin margins of the fat pad are then sutured to the margins of the vaginal mucosa using No. 3-0 delayed-absorbable sutures, obliterating the mucosal defect in the operative site. The vulvar skin is closed with interrupted sutures to give a flat contour to the excised labia (Fig. 27-9G). If bleeding is excessive, the labial donor site may be drained temporarily through a small lateral incision.

Repair of Urethrovesicovaginal Fistula Involving Sphincter

The operation shown in Figure 27-10 is performed for closure of vesicourethrovaginal fistula, usually one resulting from childbirth. A third of the urethra

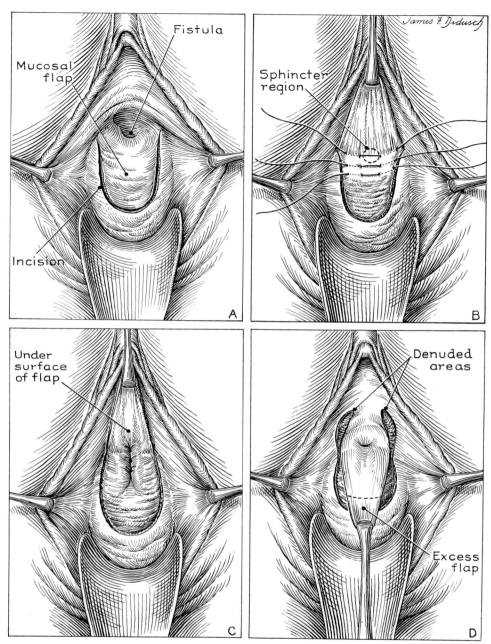

FIG. 27–8 Reconstruction of urethra and repair of sphincter. (*A*) A U-shaped incision is made through the vaginal mucosa. (*B*) The mucosal flap has been freed and pulled forward. Three interrupted sutures of No. 3-0 delayed-absorbable suture are placed to tighten the sphincter region. (*C*) The sphincter sutures have been tied, inverting the tissue. (*D*) The mucosal flap has been pulled downward, and areas have been denuded anteriorly on both sides.

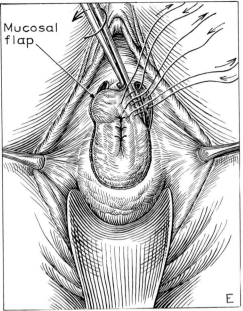

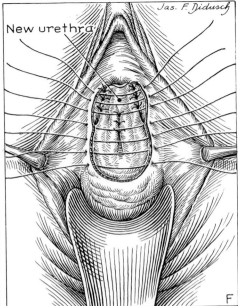

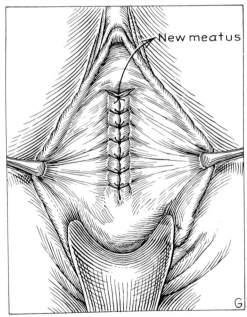

Jas. F. Didusch

FIG. 27–8 (continued). (*E*) The flap is sutured anteriorly with No. 3-0 delayed-absorbable suture, rolling the flap inward so as to approximate raw surfaces. (*F*) Mucosal edges are approximated over the newly formed urethra with interrupted sutures of No. 3-0 delayed-absorbable suture after a supporting layer of paraurethral fascia is plicated beneath the urethral floor. (*G*) Completion of reconstruction of the urethra, showing interrupted suture closure of suburethral mucosa. Urethral catheter is removed after insertion of suprapubic catheter.

may be destroyed and also a portion of the trigone. The sphincter muscles at the vesical orifice are destroyed, and the ends are retracted.

Because the bladder defect may involve the trigone in close proximity to the ureteral orifices, both ureters should be catheterized first with No. 7 French catheters. These catheters are left in place until the operation is completed.

The patient is placed on the table in the lithotomy position, and the fistula is exposed as shown in Figure 27–10A. A circular incision is made through the bladder mucosa about the edge of the opening, as indicated by the dotted line. The edges of the fistula are excised. The vaginal mucosa is dissected free from the base of the bladder and the vesical end of the urethra (Fig. 27–10B).

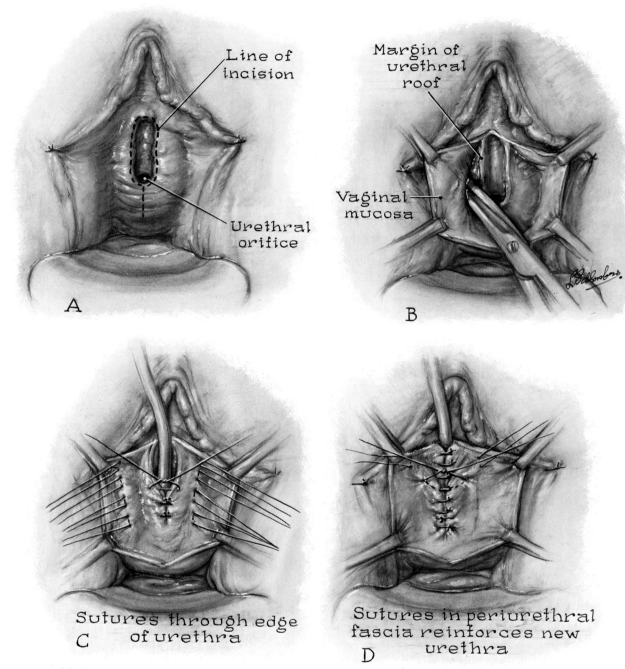

FIG. 27–9 Reconstruction of total or partial loss of urethral floor. (*A*) Line of incision along lateral margin of roof of urethra and beneath bladder base. (*B*) Enough of the urethral margins and fascia are freed from the vagina to permit approximation of the urethral mucosa in the midline. (*C*) Urethral edges are approximated in the midline over a No. 12 French catheter with interrupted No. 3-0 delayed-absorbable sutures. Mobilized urethral fascia is sutured on each side of the total length of the urethra. The lower strand of each suture is tied beneath the urethral floor (*D*) and the upper strands of the two sutures are used to pull the fascia beneath the urethra, where they are tied.

FIG. 27-9 (continued). (*E*) The vaginal mucosa is closed without tension. The bladder is filled with sterile water before the catheter is removed and a suprapubic tube is inserted. (*F*) Alternatively for additional re-inforcement, a labial fat pad is developed by a U-shaped incision along the lateral and medial aspects of the labia, leaving a broad pedicle superiorly. The lateral vaginal mucosa is resected between the urethral operative site and the labial graft (*G*). The skin margins of the labial graft are sutured to the vaginal margins with No. 3-0 interrupted delayed-absorbable suture. The labial skin margins are closed so as to produce a flat vulvar surface.

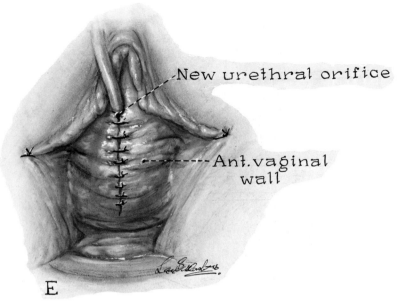

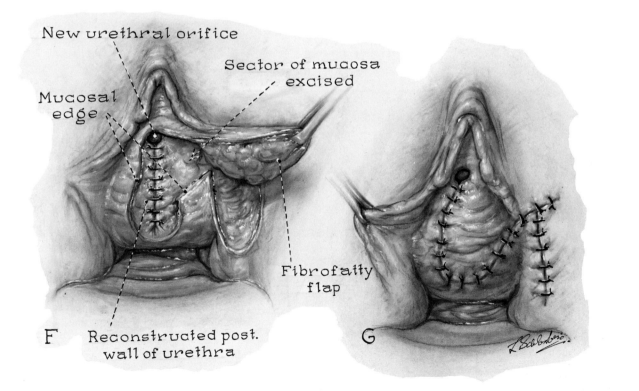

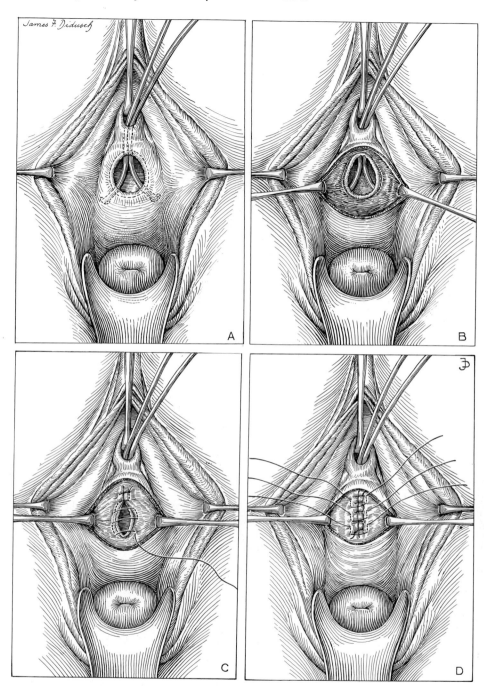

James F. Didusch

FIG. 27–10 Repair of vesico-urethrovaginal fistula, involving sphincter. (*A*) Demonstrates fistula. Both ureters have been catheterized. Dotted line indicates incision. (*B*) The vaginal mucosa has been dissected from around the fistula, exposing the base of the bladder and part of the urethra. (*C*) The fistula is closed with a continuous Cushing stitch or interrupted No. 3-0 delayed-absorbable suture. (*D*) The first suture line is reinforced with mattress sutures of No. 3-0 delayed-absorbable suture. These stitches further tighten the sphincter by drawing the subvesical fascia together.

The defect in the bladder and the urethra is closed from side to side with a continuous Cushing or interrupted No. 3-0 delayed-absorbable suture (Fig. 27-10C). The longitudinal closure is chosen in order to approximate the muscular layer of the urethrovesical junction. The suture passes into the bladder musculature and through the mucosa. When the suture is pulled taut, the margins of the fistula are brought together. The suture line is reinforced with a second layer of interrupted No. 3-0 mattress sutures as shown in Figure 27–10D. These sutures pass through the vesical fascia and musculature and thus

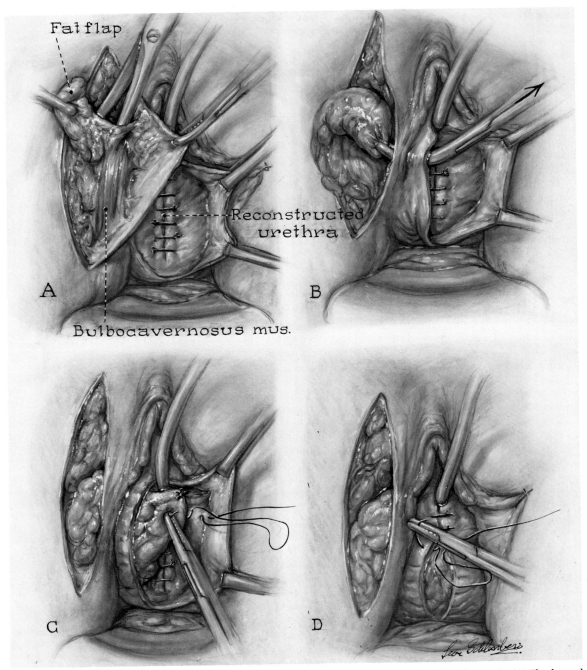

FIG. 27-11 Martius bulbocavernosus fat pad graft for urethrovaginal or vesicovaginal fistula repair. (*A*) The lateral margin of the labia majora is opened by a vertical incision and the fat pad adjacent to the bulbocavernosus muscle is mobilized, leaving a broad pedicle attached at the inferior pole. (*B,C*) The fat pad is drawn through a tunnel beneath the labia minora and vaginal mucosa and sutured with No. 3-0 delayed-absorbable sutures to the fascia of the urethra and bladder. (*D*) The vaginal mucosa is mobilized widely to permit closure in the midline. The vulvar incision is closed with interrupted No. 3-0 delayed-absorbable sutures and drained if necessary.

further approximate the retracted sphincter muscle fibers and bladder neck. A third layer can be used as indicated.

The vaginal mucosa should be closed with the least tension, preferably transversely, but vertically if necessary to avoid shortening the urethra (Fig. 27–10D). It is not necessary to avoid superimposing one suture line on the other, since tissue tension has a far greater effect on healing than overlying suture lines. The vaginal mucosa is everted as it is closed with deep vertical mattress sutures using No. 3-0 delayed-absorbable material.

The importance of suprapubic drainage to avoid trauma to the operative site cannot be stressed too strongly in a case such as this. The suprapubic catheter is removed on the 10th to 14th day when the patient is voiding normally and without an abnormal amount of residual urine.

Postirradiation Fistulas

The most intractable of all fistulas are those created by the effect of ionizing irradiation on sensitive tissues. The entire urethrovaginal or vesicovaginal septum may tolerate combined radiation doses as high as 10,000 rads before necrosis and fistula occur, but it is occasionally necessary to knowingly exceed the normal tissue tolerance in the treatment of certain malignancies of the lower genital tract. Fortunately this is uncommon, but when a radiation-induced urethrovaginal or vesicovaginal fistula does occur, every effort should be made to obtain as viable a margin of tissue around the fistula as possible before attempting a surgical closure. Therefore, it is our policy to delay repair of a radiation-induced fistula for a minimum of 6 months after its occurrence and preferably for 12 months, if possible. The key to successful closure of these fistulas is the establishment of a new blood supply to the devitalized vaginal tissues. We have found the Martius method to be very effective and to greatly reduce the previously high failure rate in attempted closure of these fistulas.

For irradiation fistulas that are located high in the vagina, we use the original Martius procedure and dissect the fat pad separately from the overlying vulvar skin, leaving one end attached to its blood supply (Fig. 27–11A). In such cases, the mobilized fatty tissue can be tunneled beneath the labia minora and vaginal mucosa to the operative site, where it can be sutured to the margins of the fistulous repair (Fig. 27–11B,C). If the fistula is large and complicated, and additional tissue is needed, the underlying bulbocavernosus muscle may be mobilized along with the fat pad. The vaginal mucosa is dissected widely and approximated over the graft of fatty tissue as the final layer of closure (Fig. 27–11D). A drain may be left beneath the labial incision. Prolonged suprapubic bladder drainage will usually be necessary.

Bibliography

Bastiaanse MA, Van Bouwdyk: The treatment of vesico-vaginal fistulas, including so-called radium fistulas. Proc R Soc Med 47:610, 1954

Boronow RC, Rutledge F: Vesico-vaginal fistula, radiation, and gynecologic cancer. Am J Obstet Gynecol 111:85, 1971

Clarke DH, Holland JB: Repair of vesicovaginal fistulas: Simultaneous transvaginal-transvesical approach. South Med J 68:1410, 1975

Collins CG, Prent D: Results of early repair of vesico-vaginal fistula with preliminary cortisone treatment. Am J Obstet Gynecol 80:1005, 1960

Collins CG, Collins JH, Harrison BR, et al: Early repair of vesicovaginal fistula. Am J Obstet Gynecol 111:524, 1971

Davis RS, Linke CA, Kraemer GK: Use of labial tissue in repair of urethrovaginal fistula and injury. Arch Surg 115:628, 1980

Everett HS, Mattingly RF: Urinary tract injuries resulting from pelvic surgery. Am J Obstet Gynecol 71:502, 1956

Everett HS, Williams TJ: Urology in the female. In Campbell MF, Harrison JB (eds): Urology, 3rd ed. Philadelphia, WB Saunders, 1970

Falk HC, Orkin LA: Nonsurgical closure of vesicovaginal fistulas. Obstet Gynecol 9:538, 1957

Falk HC, Tancer ML: Urethrovesicovaginal fistula. Obstet Gynecol 33:422, 1969

————: Loss of urethra: Report of three cases. Obstet Gynecol 9:458, 1957

Fearl CL, Keizur LW: Optimum time interval from occurrence to repair of vesicovaginal fistula. Am J Obstet Gynecol 104:205, 1968

Garlock JH: The cure of an intractable vesicovaginal fistula by the use of a pedicled muscle flap. Surg Gynecol Obstet 47:225, 1928

Glenn JF, Stevens PS: Simplified vesicovaginal fistulectomy. J Urol 110:521, 1973

Graham JB: Painful syndrome of postradiation urinary vaginal fistula. Surg Gynecol Obstet 124:1260, 1964

Gray LA: Urethrovaginal fistulas. Am J Obstet Gynecol 101:28, 1968

Hamlin RHJ, Nicholson EC: Reconstruction of the urethra totally destroyed by labour. Br Med J 2:147, 1969

Harrison KA: Obstetric fistula: one social calamity too many. Br J Obstet Gynecol 90:385, 1983

Hayward G: Case of vesicovaginal fistula, successfully treated by an operation. Am J Med Sci 24:283, 1839

Hyman RM: Coagulation therapy for small vesicovaginal fistulas. Clin Obstet Gynecol 8:465, 1968

Ingelman–Sundberg AGI: Pathogenesis and operative treatment of urinary fistulae in irradiated tissue. In Youssef AF (ed): Gynecological Urology. Springfield, Ill., Charles C Thomas Publishers, 1960

Jaszczak SE, Evans TN: Intrafascial abdominal and vaginal hysterectomy: A reappraisal. Obstet Gynecol 59:435, 1982

Kelly HA: The treatment of large vesicovaginal fistulae. Bull Johns Hopkins Hosp 7:29, 1896

————: The suprapubic route of in operating for vesical fistulae. Trans Am Gyn Soc 31:225, 1906

Kiricuta I, Goldstein AMB: The repair of extensive vesicovaginal fistulas with pedicled omentum: A review of 27 cases. J Urol 108:724, 1972

Latzko W: Behandlung Hochsitzender Blasen-und Mastdarmscheidenfisteln nach Uterusextipation mit hohem Schedienverschluss. Zentralbl Gynak 38:906, 1914

———: Post-operative vesicovaginal fistulas. Am J Surg 58:211–228, 1942

Lawson JB: Management of genitourinary fistulas. Clin Obstet Gynecol 5:209, 1975

Mackenrodt A: Die operative Heilung der Harnleiterfisteln. Ein geheilter Fall von Harnleiter-Gabarmutterfistel. 261 Gynak 18:1026, 1894

Maisónneuve JG: Clinique Chirurgicale p. 660. Paris, 1863

Martius H: Vesicovaginal therapy especially by plastic transplantation of flaps. Z Geburtsh Gynak 103:22, 1932

Marshall VF: Vesicovaginal fistulas on one urological service. J Urol 121:25, 1979

Mattingly RF, Borkowf HI: Lower urinary tract injuries in pregnancy. In Barber HR, Graber EA (eds): Surgical Diseases in Pregnancy. Philadelphia, WB Saunders, 1974

McCall ML, Bolten KA (ed and trans): Martius Gynecological Operations with Emphasis on Topographic Anatomy. Boston, Little, Brown, 1956

Mettauer JP: Vesico-vaginal fistula. Boston Med Surg J 22:154, 1840

Miller NF, George H: Lower urinary tract fistulas in women. A study based on 292 cases. Am J Obstet Gynecol 68:436, 1954

Moir JC: Vesicovaginal fistula. Proc R Soc Med 59:1019, 1966

O'Connor VJ: Suprapubic Closure of Vesicovaginal Fistula. Springfield, Ill, Charles C Thomas, 1957

O'Connor VJ, Jr: Repair of vesicovaginal fistula with associated urethral loss. Surg Gynecol Obstet 146:251, 1978

———: Review of experience with vesicovaginal fistula repair. Trans Am Assoc Genito-Urinary Surgeons 71:120, 1979

Patil V, Waterhouse K, Laungani G: Management of 18 difficult vesicovaginal and urethrovaginal fistulas with modified Ingelman–Sundberg and Martius operations. J Urol 123:653, 1980

Persky L, Herman G, Geurrier K: Non-delay in vesicovaginal fistula repair. Urology 13:273, 1979

Pfaneuf LE: Vesicovaginal fistula management—End results. Am J Obstet Gynecol 31:316, 1936

Robertson JR: Vesicovaginal fistula: The gynecologist's responsibility. Obstet Gynecol 42:611, 1973

Ridley JH: Surgery for vaginal fistulae. In Ridley JH (ed): Gynecologic Surgery: Errors, Safeguards, and Salvage. 2nd ed. Baltimore, Williams & Wilkins, 1981

Schuchardt K: Uber die paravaginale Methode der Extirpation uteri und ihre Enderfolge beim Uteruskrebs. Monatsschr Geburtsch Gynak 13:744, 1901

Simon G: Falle von Operation bei Urinfisteln am Weibe. Beobachtung einer Harnleiter Scheidenfistel. Deutsch Klin p. 311, 1856

Sims JM: On the treatment of vesico-vaginal fistula. Am J Med Sci 23:59, 1852

Smith WG, Johnson GH: Vesicovaginal fistula repair—revisited. Gyn Oncol 9:303, 1980

Symmonds RE, Hill M: Loss of the urethra: A report on 50 patients. Am J Obstet Gynecol 130:130, 1978

Tancer ML: The post total hysterectomy (vault) vesico-vaginal fistula. J Urol 123:839, 1980

Taylor JS, Hewson AD, Rachow P: Synchronous combined transvaginal transvesical repair of vesicovaginal fistulas. Aust NZ J Surg 50:23, 1980

Trendelenburg F: Operations for vesicovaginal fistula and the elevated pelvic position for operations within the abdominal cavity. Samml Vortr No. 355:3373, 1890

Turner-Warwick R: The use of the omental pedicle graft in urinary tract reconstruction. J Urol 116:341, 1976

Van Nagell JR, Jr, Parker JC, Jr, Maruyama Y, et al: Bladder or rectal injury following radiation therapy for cervical cancer. Am J Obstet Gynecol 119:727, 1974

van Roonhuyse H: Medico-chirurgical Observations. Englished out of Dutch by a Careful Hand. London, M Pitt, 1676

Von Dittel L: Abdominale Blasenscheidenfistel-Operation. Wein Klin Wchr j26:449, 1893

Wein AJ, Malloy TR, Carpinello VL, et al: Repair of vesicovaginal fistula by a suprapubic transvesical approach. Surg Gynecol Obstet 150:57, 1980

Weyrauch HM, Rous SN: Transvaginal-transvesical approach for surgical repair of vesicovaginal fistula. Surg Gynecol Obstet 123:121, 1966

Wolff HD, Jr, Gililland NA: Vaginal diaphragm catheters. J Urol 78:681, 1957

Youssef AF: "Menouria" following lower segment cesarean section: A syndrome. Am J Obstet Gynecol 73:759, 1957

Zacharin RF: Grafting as a principle in the surgical management of vesicovaginal and rectovaginal fistulae. Aust NZ J Obstet Gynaec 20:10, 1980

Chapter 28

Anal Incontinence and Rectovaginal Fistulas

Anal Incontinence

Few complications of modern gynecology and obstetrics produce so much personal discomfort and social embarrassment as the problem of fecal incontinence due to complete loss of the anal sphincter and perineal musculature (Fig. 28–1). Although gas and fecal incontinence is a relatively common problem in multiparous women, many women conceal their symptoms until the problem becomes so troublesome that they withdraw from social contacts. Loss of the anal sphincter musculature usually results from traumatic obstetric delivery, although some cases have been attributed to operations for rectal fistulas or hemorrhoids and to radical pelvic surgery, such as radical vulvectomy. A complete perineal laceration may result from a fall astride a sharp object.

The classic symptoms are present in the majority of cases: the progressive loss of control of gas and feces from the anus. The severity of symptoms generally varies with the degree of perineal laceration and sphincter loss. A few remaining external sphincter fibers left intact can provide sufficient muscular contraction to permit control of feces when the patient is constipated or when the stool is of normal consistency. When the tear extends well above the external anal sphincter, gas and feces escape at all times.

Anatomy of the Anal Canal

Modern concepts of the anatomy and physiology of defecation and anal continence are drawn primarily from the work of Shafik (1975), Parks (1975), Gaston (1948), Goligher (1955), and Milligan (1934). The complete interrelated mechanisms of defecation and anal control are more easily visualized once the principal elements of the rectoanal musculature have been delineated.

The anal canal is approximately 2.5 cm to 4 cm in length and normally remains completely collapsed due to the tonic contractions of the sphincter mechanisms (Fig. 28–2). The canal is related posteriorly to the coccyx, from which it is separated by fibrofatty tissue and by the levator ani muscles until it opens onto the perineal skin. The levator ani muscles also separate the lateral boundary of the canal from the ischiorectal fossa, through which pass the important nerves, lymphatics, and blood supply of the terminal rectum, anal canal, and perineum. The canal is fused anteriorly with the lower portion of the rectovaginal septum and the perineal body.

The anal and rectal regions of the lower colon share a common embryologic origin. During their development, the terminal end of the alimentary canal is surrounded by muscular sphincters of somatic origin. The sphincter mechanism of the anal canal (Fig. 28–2) consists of two separate anatomical structures. The internal sphincter consists of circular smooth muscle from the rectal wall, which is innervated by the autonomic nervous system and is not under voluntary control. The internal sphincter plays no voluntary role in anal continence but provides continuous tone to the anal canal from autonomic innervation. The outer sphincter is composed of four separate external skeletal muscles surrounding the anal canal. These are voluntarily controlled. The external sphincter muscles lie in close approximation with the medial margin of the strong levator ani muscles, principally the pubo-

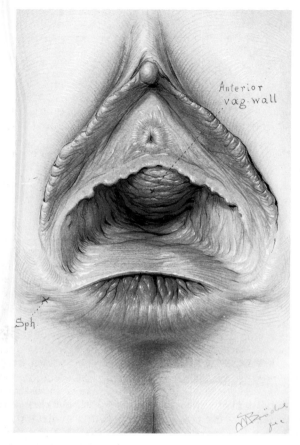

FIG. 28–1 Old third-degree laceration with complete loss of anal sphincter and perineum. Note dimples on either side due to retraction of torn sphincter.

coccygeus muscles. The tone of the levator ani is strengthened by the skeletal muscles of the anterior compartment of the urogenital diaphragm, the bulbocavernosus and transverse perinei muscles, which have a common insertion into the central perineal body between the anus and vaginal introitus.

The perineal body is an important anatomical landmark that is closely associated with the external sphincter and the anal canal. The perineal body itself includes two components of the transverse perineal muscles, a superficial and a deep muscle layer, both composed of striated muscle. The central tendon (raphe) of this transverse perineal musculature serves as a pivotal point where the external sphincter connects with the levator muscles, including the terminal end of the bulbocavernosus (see Fig. 24–2). Trauma or separation of the perineal raphe causes relaxation of the perineal body, which is attached to the base loop of the external anal sphincter. The resulting alteration of attachment generally causes loss of control of both liquid stool and gas.

Shafik's anatomical dissections and histologic sections of the anal canal show that the external anal sphincter is composed of a triple-loop system: the top, intermediate, and base. The puborectalis muscle forms the top loop of the sphincter complex at the junction of the rectum and anus (rectal neck). This U-shaped muscle encircles the rectal neck, suspends the anal canal forward toward the symphysis pubis in a near right angle, and maintains anorectal continence by closure of the rectal inlet (Fig. 28–3). The puborectalis is a striated muscle, innervated by the

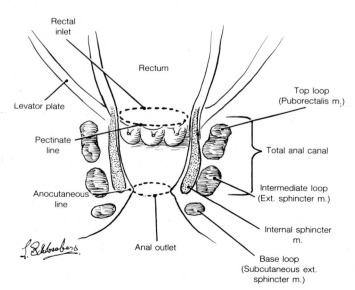

FIG. 28–2 Diagrammatic illustration of the anal canal.

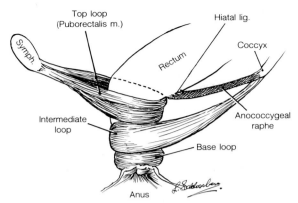

FIG. 28-3 Triple-loop external anal sphincter mechanism. The top loop represents puborectalis muscles. The intermediate loop arises and inserts in the coccyx. The base loop attaches to the perianal skin and perineal body.

inferior hemorrhoidal branch of the pudendal nerve. An extension of fibers from this muscle along the external surface of the anal canal forms the lateral external component of the longitudinal anal muscle.

The intermediate loop of the external sphincter pulls in the opposite direction from the top loop. The intermediate loop starts at the coccyx as a fibrous tendon, then evolves into a flat muscle bundle that encircles the middle segment of the anal canal and inserts into the same tendinous sheath on the coccyx (Fig. 28-3). The intermediate segment of the sphincter is innervated by the perineal branch of the fourth sacral nerve.

The base loop is the smallest component of the external anal sphincter mechanism. The base loop, which lies beneath the anal mucosa in the same plane as the internal sphincter, circles the anal orifice and attaches to the perianal skin near the midline.

This concept of the anatomy of the external anal sphincter emphasizes the role of the levator ani as an ancillary mechanism for defecation and fecal control. From a functional viewpoint, the levator ani may be divided into two components, the pubococcygeus and iliococcygeus muscles. (A detailed anatomical description of these muscles is given in Chapter 4.) The major contribution of the levator ani in anorectal control is provided by the pubococcygeal muscles and the central (anococcygeal) raphe.

The raphe extends from the coccyx to the rectal angle and incorporates the fibers of each pubococcygeal muscle as they criss-cross the center of the pelvic floor and continue to the opposite pelvic wall.

The pubococcygeus muscles include both a transverse segment (levator plate) and a longitudinal extension (anal suspensory sling) that serve specific functions in the entry and expulsion of gas and fecal content through the anal canal.

The transverse segment of the pubococcygeus (levator plate) surrounds the levator hiatus at the site of the rectal neck. Also surrounding the levator hiatus is the puborectalis muscle, located beneath the levator plate.

The levator plate is attached to the rectum by the hiatal ligament, an extension of the endopelvic fascia surrounding the levator ani. The fascia provides support by adhering the levator plate to the rectum, vagina, and urethra. The hiatal ligament permits a certain degree of mobility between the levator plate and the intrahiatal viscera during defecation and facilitates frequent changes in tonicity of the levator plate in response to such alterations of intra-abdominal pressure as coughing, laughing, or urination. The hiatal ligament provides the mechanism by which the rectal inlet is opened and closed by contraction or relaxation of the levator plate.

The musculature of the levator plate extends along the anal canal (anal suspensory ligament) and forms the intermediate layer of the longitudinal muscle of the canal wall. Ending in a central fibrous tendon, the suspensory ligament anchors to the base loop musculature and to the anal and perianal skin (Fig. 28-4). When the levator plate is voluntarily contracted, the anal canal is shortened, the rectal inlet is opened, the base loop is pulled upward and stretched open, and the anal and perianal skin is everted during the process of defecation.

The longitudinal muscle of the anal canal has three separate components: the inner smooth muscle, which blends with the wall of the anus; the intermediate striated muscular extension of the levator plate, the suspensory ligament; and the lateral striated muscular extension of the top loop of the external sphincter, the puborectalis. The major function of the striated components of the longitudinal muscle is to passively anchor the levator plate in a funnel-like fashion to the base loop of the sphincter and to the perianal skin.

In the relaxed state, the funnel-shaped levator plate releases tension on the rectal neck, which permits the rectal inlet to be pulled forward and closed by the puborectalis muscle, thereby keeping the anal canal free of feces and gas. On voluntary contraction of the levator, the levator plate is flattened, the rectal neck is retracted posteriorly by the hiatal ligament, the rectal inlet is opened, the anal canal is shortened, and the basal loop is elevated and pulled open by the attachment of the suspen-

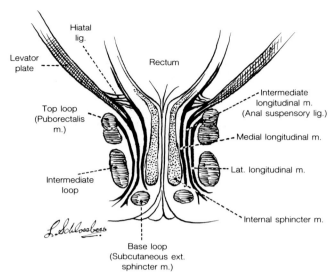

Levator plate

Hiatal lig.

Rectum

Top loop (Puborectalis m.)

Intermediate loop

Intermediate longitudinal m. (Anal suspensory lig.)

Medial longitudinal m.

Lat. longitudinal m.

Internal sphincter m.

L. Schlossberg

Base loop (Subcutaneous ext. sphincter m.)

FIG. 28–4 Coronal view of the three components of the longitudinal skeletal muscle, which is directly adjacent to the smooth muscle of the anal canal.

sory sling. By this process, feces and gas may enter the anal canal, where they are aided in their expulsion by alternate contraction and relaxation of the three separate loops of the external anal sphincter (Fig. 28–5).

During defecation or following increased intra-abdominal pressure, the pubococcygeal muscles contract and the puborectalis muscle voluntarily relaxes. This muscular interaction causes widening of the levator hiatus and widening of the rectal angle. The levator plate changes from a funneled to a flattened position on contraction, opening and elevating the rectal inlet. Contraction of the levator plate produces contraction and shortening of the anal suspensory sling (longitudinal anal muscle), which elevates the base loop of the external sphincter, shortens and widens the rectal neck, and opens the anal outlet.

Relaxation of the levator muscles causes return of the funnel shape of the levator plate, closure of the rectal inlet with relaxation of the anal suspensory sling, descent of the base loop of the external sphincter, and finally, closure of the anal outlet. The base loop located adjacent to the anal mucosa closes the anal outlet with its resting tone. Voluntary contraction of the base loop firmly seals the anal orifice and prevents passage of gas or feces. Injury to this segment of the external sphincter by obstetric trauma, such as a third-degree tear, may cause anal incontinence of gas or liquid stool.

The top loop of the external sphincter, the puborectalis muscle, closes the rectal inlet as it draws the rectal neck toward the symphysis pubis, maintaining anal continence. Relaxation of the puborectalis in conjunction with contraction of the le-

vator plate causes the rectal inlet to be elevated, opened, and drawn posteriorly, thereby allowing feces and gas to enter the anal canal during the process of defecation.

Anal continence is a function of both the external and internal sphincter. The external sphincter is responsible for voluntary continence while the internal, smooth muscle sphincter maintains involuntary continence of the anal canal.

Although the function of levator ani muscles has caused dissension among researchers, most would agree to separating the puborectalis muscle from the functioning of the classic levator ani triad. The remaining levator ani muscles, principally the pubococcygeus, serve to dilate the rectal neck during the process of defecation. The opposing action of the puborectalis muscle causes obstruction and kinking of the rectal neck by contracting and displacing the rectal inlet forward toward the symphysis pubis. Defined in this way, the levator ani plays a limited role in anal continence, and functions mainly during defecation. On contraction, the levator plate is straightened and tensed, which pulls the levator hiatal ligament laterally and posteriorly and opens the rectal neck inlet. Contraction of the anal suspensory ligament, the muscular extension of the levator plate, causes the anal canal to shorten, the rectal neck to open, and the external anal sphincter to be pulled open and the anus everted.

In contrast, the internal anal sphincter is responsible for the involuntary control of anal continence and is maintained in a continuous tonic state by autonomic innervation. The internal sphincter relaxes reflexly in response to a contraction of the smooth muscle of the rectum (detrusor) when stool

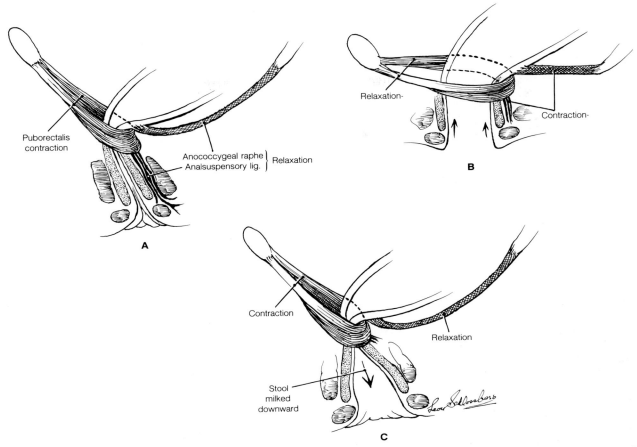

FIG. 28-5 Function of the external anal sphincter. (*A*) At rest, the rectal inlet is closed and pulled forward by contraction of puborectalis muscle. (*B*) During defecation the rectal inlet is opened and the angle is straightened by relaxation of the puborectalis muscle and contraction and flattening of the rectal plate. (*C*) Expulsion of feces from the canal is augmented by alternate contraction and relaxation of the three loops.

or flatus enters the bowel lumen above the rectal inlet. As stool enters the rectal inlet, the rectal detrusor contracts, the internal sphincter relaxes, and the rectal inlet is opened by the action of the levator plate.

For defecation to occur, the external sphincter, principally the puborectalis muscle, must voluntarily relax while the levator plate contracts and pulls the rectal inlet into an open position. The rectal inlet will not open unless the top loop of the external sphincter is voluntarily relaxed. If defecation or passage of gas is inconvenient, the external sphincter remains firmly contracted and the levator plate remains relaxed, preventing relaxation of the internal sphincter. Failure of the internal sphincter to relax will inhibit further contraction of the rectal detrusor, and the rectum will dilate above the rectal inlet to accommodate the fecal contents.

Injury to the internal sphincter can permit the involuntary passage of liquid stool and gas due to loss of tonicity of the anal canal. Such an injury is particularly noticeable when the urge to defecate is persistent from a bolus of fecal content in the terminal rectum and when the voluntary contraction of the external sphincter wanes.

The triple-loop mechanism of the external sphincter provides an explanation for the varying degrees of anal incontinence that can result when the external sphincter is partially destroyed. If the lower portion of the external anal sphincter is traumatized, the top loop of the sphincter—the puborectalis muscle—may remain intact, in which case it will obstruct the rectal neck by forward displacement and closure of the rectal inlet. In this way, a defect to the lower portion of the internal and external sphincters can be partially compensated for by voluntary sphincter control. Damage to the entire external or internal sphincter would result in total incontinence.

Reconstructive surgery should restore the right-angle configuration of the rectal neck by appropriate plication of the puborectalis muscle. The important base and intermediate loops of the sphincter should be carefully identified and repaired to ensure anatomical control of gas and liquid stool. Although it is difficult to identify the anatomy of the internal sphincter, every effort should be made to restore continuity to both the internal and external sphincter when repair of the anal canal is performed.

The major effect of a disrupted and separated perineal musculature on anal continence is mediated through the severance of the fibers of the central tendon. Perineal trauma causes a separation of the fascial septa that anchors the levator plate and the lower segments of the top loop of the external sphincter into the perineum and perianal skin. With complete loss of the perineal body by an unrepaired second-degree laceration or episiotomy breakdown, the muscular tone of the canal wall is weakened and the contractile force of the base loop of the external sphincter system is diminished. As a result, the anal canal may become incompetent for the control of gas and liquid stool. To correct a perineal defect, the separated muscles of the perineal body and the supporting muscles of the pelvic diaphragm must be reapproximated.

Treatment

A complete perineal laceration through the anal sphincter and possibly through the anal mucosa can occur during vaginal delivery and should be repaired at that time. If complete anatomical reconstruction is not achieved, symptoms will usually develop within the first 7 to 10 days following delivery. With separation of the base and intermediate loops, symptoms are usually those of incontinence of intestinal gas. Fecal incontinence occurs more commonly with complete breakdown of the perineal body, separation of the entire sphincter, and extension of the tear through the anal mucosa (a fourth-degree perineal tear).

Should repair at the time of delivery fail, a second attempt should be deferred for a minimum of 3 to 4 months, in order to provide sufficient time for return of an adequate blood supply to the margins of the defect and for return of optimum viability of the perineal tissues. A proctoscopic examination and barium enema should always precede the second attempt so that the presence of an occult rectovaginal fistula can be excluded. If anatomical findings suggest a fistula, a fistulogram should be used to demonstrate whether or not a sinus tract has formed between the vagina and the previous repair.

Three types of closure are recommended for repair of a complete perineal laceration: the layered method of repair, the Warren flap procedure, and the Noble–Mengert operation. Based on current understanding of the pathophysiology of anal incontinence, the layered method provides the optimal surgical approach for correcting a perineal laceration.

The Warren flap method was devised to avoid a mucosal incision in the anus, to provide a pedicle graft of vaginal mucosa for enlargement of the perineal skin, and to provide a more cosmetic result to the perineal body. However, the Warren technique offers no particular improvement in the results of the surgical correction of the muscular defect that produced the anal incontinence. The major advantage of the procedure is that a suture line is not created in the anal mucosa. With the Warren technique, the vaginal mucosa is turned backward and utilized as the new portion of the anterior wall of the end of the anal canal. The anal sphincter is then reapproximated over the inner portion of the vaginal flap, which is attached to the anal mucosa. The Warren flap procedure is used less frequently today than it was over a century ago when it was first described (1882).

The Noble–Mengert operation, or anal pull-through procedure as it is more commonly called, also avoids the presence of a suture line in the anal mucosa. The procedure was described originally in 1902 by Noble, but received little attention until redescribed independently by Mengert in 1955. Noble's original claims for the operation in the surgical era before the availability of antibiotics, blood banks, and modern advances in general anesthesia included: (1) elimination of the danger of infection or fecal matter from the rectum in the surgical wound; (2) avoidance of the tediousness of dissecting a vaginal flap; (3) minimal blood loss; and (4) uniformly good results.

LAYERED METHOD OF REPAIR OF COMPLETE PERINEAL LACERATION

A transverse or crescent perineal incision is used at the junction of the posterior vaginal wall and anal mucosa. The lateral margins of the incision are extended to the region of the perineal dimple created by the retracted external sphincter, and a midline incision is made along the lower one-half of the posterior vaginal wall (Fig. 28–6A).

The edges of the vaginal and rectal mucosa are grasped separately with Allis clamps, and the rectal wall is separated in the midline from the anterior vaginal mucosa with careful Metzenbaum scissor dissection. The dissection is carried laterally by sharp dissection to the region of the external anal sphincter.

The external sphincter is identified by a fibrous band that is retracted against the lateral wall of the anal canal (Fig. 28–6B). The exact anatomical margins of the external sphincter are frequently difficult to ascertain. Usually the base and intermediate loops of the external sphincter are disrupted in a complete perineal laceration; the top loop (puborectalis muscle) is attached to the inferior rami of the symphysis pubis.

To test the function of the retracted sphincter, the Allis clamps containing the muscle bundles are brought together in the midline, and the sphincter action is tested by inserting a double-gloved index finger into the rectum. If necessary, the clamps should be readjusted to incorporate more of the retracted muscle bundles, until the constricted effect of the reapproximated sphincter can be demonstrated.

Any scar tissue is excised from the margins of the rectal mucosa, and the defect in the anal mucosa is closed using a continuous suture of No. 3-0 delayed-absorbable material (Fig. 28–6C). If interrupted sutures were used as the initial layer, a small opening could be left in the mucosa through which colon bacteria and feces could enter and interfere with tissue healing. A submucosal suture would be ideal, but due to the friability of the tissue, residual tearing could occur. Complete approximation of the anal mucosa by full-thickness suturing of the mucosa is the safest method. As the mucosa are approximated, the mucosal edge is inverted by a second supporting suture that is placed into the muscle layer of the anal canal, using interrupted sutures through the submucosa and muscularis.

The sphincter ends are then united in the midline with interrupted delayed-absorbable or permanent sutures (Fig. 28–6C,D). No. 0 or No. 1 delayed-absorbable suture material has the advantage of excellent tensile strength while avoiding a permanent, foreign-body reaction should the operative site become infected with colon bacilli. Some surgeons prefer a permanent suture, preferably medium-strength silk or braided silicone-treated polyester (Tycron). Three or four sutures are used to approximate the sphincter muscle. Then the dissection is continued laterally along the anal canal and rectal wall to free the medial borders of the puborectalis muscles.

An important component of this procedure is careful identification and adequate plication of the puborectalis muscle, which serves as the top loop of the external sphincter. A series of interrupted, delayed-absorbable sutures should be placed to bring the muscle to the midline as high as possible without constricting the diameter of the vaginal canal. Extending this procedure to the midportion of the vagina can produce excellent anatomical support for the underlying anal canal and rectal neck. Because the hiatus of the puborectalis sling requires so much support, the preferred procedure is to approximate the medial margins of these muscles along the lower half of the vagina, until the sutures produce narrowing of the vaginal lumen. Delayed-absorbable sutures of No. 0 or No. 1 strength are used and provide excellent support to the underlying anorectal canal.

Further support and elevation of the perineal body is provided by plicating the transverse perineal muscles separately. Following this step, the redundant vaginal mucosa is excised, and the remaining mucosa is approximated in the midline with a continuous running No. 2-0 suture. One further effort is made to reestablish and elevate the perineal body by making a wide plication of the fascia of the perineal body followed by a subcuticular closure of the perineal skin (Fig. 28–6E). Excessive narrowing of the vaginal introitus should be avoided because it can produce a painful midline scar and troublesome dyspareunia.

PARADOXICAL RELAXING INCISION. In 1937, Miller and Brown proposed making a paradoxical incision in the inferior portion of the anal sphincter at 5 or 7 o'clock to relax the tension on the suture line. The modern method of anatomical dissection and repair of the entire external sphincter adds enough support to the sphincter muscles to make a paradoxical relaxing incision unnecessary. The procedure is fraught with physiologic risk, such as poor healing of the base loop of the sphincter with the potential for postoperative anal incontinence of gas and liquid feces.

PREOPERATIVE CARE. Preparation of the entire gastrointestinal tract with antibiotics is unnecessary. Four days prior to surgery, patients should begin using a laxative. During the 48-hour preoperative period, patients should be placed on a clear liquid diet, and stool softeners and laxatives should be continued to completely empty the colon of fecal material (Table 28–1). The bowel is then emptied prior to surgery, with enemas repeated until the return is clear. The last enema given should be a retention enema of 2% neomycin in 200 ml normal saline.

POSTOPERATIVE FEEDING. Oral feedings should not begin postoperatively for approximately 48 hours, during which time intravenous fluid replacement is maintained, and bowel function is gradually restored. Patients should begin with clear liquids for

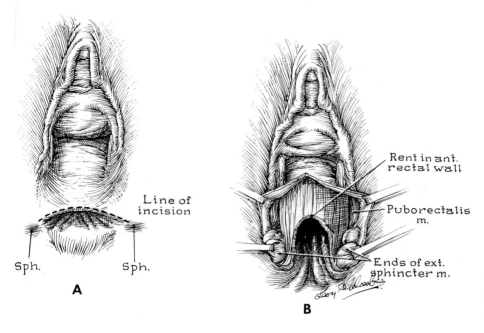

Line of incision

Sph.   Sph.

A

Rent in ant. rectal wall

Puborectalis m.

Ends of ext. sphincter m.

B

FIG. 28–6   Layered closure of a complete third-degree perineal laceration with anal extension. (*A*) A small transverse incision is made at the junction of the vaginal and rectal mucosa. A midline incision is made in the mucosa of the lower one-half of the posterior vaginal wall. (*B*) The ends of the lower portion of the anal sphincter have been identified and grasped with Allis clamps.

24 hours, with progression to a soft, low-residue diet for an additional 48 hours. A regular diet may be started when patients can intentionally pass gas or following the first soft bowel movement. To keep the terminal rectum and anal canal free of fecal material for as long as possible following surgery, the use of laxatives should be avoided for four or five days, until the mucosal suture line has healed adequately and the reparative process is well established.

WARREN-FLAP OPERATION FOR COMPLETE THIRD-DEGREE TEAR

An inverted V-shaped incision is made in the posterior vaginal mucosa, outlining the flap that is to be turned down. The lower ends of the incision should be just lateral to the dimples caused by retracted sphincter ends (Fig. 28–7A). The length of the flap should measure a minimum of 3 cm to provide sufficient vaginal mucosa to be incorporated into the anal canal and to cover the reconstructed perineal body.

Taking care to avoid injuring the bowel wall, the flap of mucosa is dissected free from the top downward (Fig. 28–7B), stopping short of the margin between the vaginal and the anal mucosa. Should this margin be perforated, the blood supply to the mucosal flap would be compromised, which would nullify the advantage of the flap technique. The properly demarcated flap will allow the areas overlying the sphincter ends to be denuded. The flap is grasped with two mucosal Allis clamps and turned down to hang over the anus.

The sphincter ends are then dissected free, using Allis clamps for traction. The ends are sutured together with 3 or 4 interrupted stitches of No. 1 delayed-absorbable or Tycron sutures (Fig. 28–7C). Sphincter tone should be tested using a double-gloved finger. If the tone is not satisfactory, a further attempt should be made to find and approximate more sphincter fibers.

The lateral aspects of the puborectalis muscle are identified, and the medial margins are brought together with a series of interrupted sutures of No. 1 delayed-absorbable material for reinforcement (Fig. 28–7D). Then the muscles are plicated in the midline as high as possible, in the manner described for the layered technique, using No. 0 or No. 1 delayed-absorbable sutures.

Closure of the vaginal mucosa is carried out as in an ordinary perineal repair. Interrupted plication stitches of No. 0 delayed-absorbable suture are used to advance the fascia and shorten the muscle fibers of the perineal body, which strengthens the external sphincter as well. The margins of the vaginal mucosa and graft are approximated in the midline by a continuous lock stitch of No. 2-0 delayed-absorbable suture. The tip end of the mucosal flap should not be trimmed too closely, even though it protrudes somewhat from the repaired perineal body; it will retract as healing is completed (Fig. 28–7E).

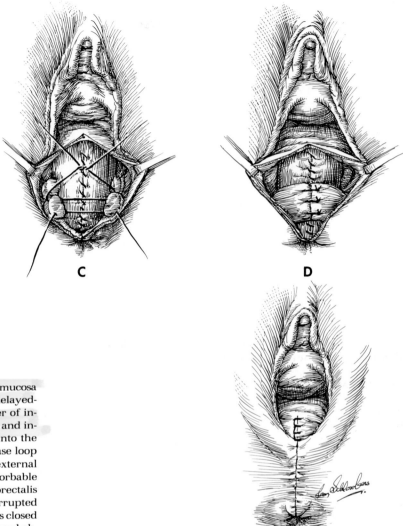

FIG. 28–6 (continued). (C) The rent in the anal mucosa has been closed with a continuous No. 3-0 delayed-absorbable suture. A second, supporting layer of interrupted sutures is placed in the submucosa and inner muscularis to invert the mucosal edges into the bowel lumen. (D) After approximating the base loop and possibly the intermediate loop of the external anal sphincter with two or three delayed-absorbable or permanent sutures as shown in C, the puborectalis muscles are brought together with deep interrupted No. 0 or No. 1 sutures. (E) The vaginal mucosa is closed with a continuous lock stitch of No. 2-0 delayed-absorbable suture, which is continued subcuticularly to approximate the perineal skin.

NOBLE–MENGERT PROCEDURE

Technique

The initial incision is initiated near the dimple in the lateral aspect of the perineum caused by the retracted external anal sphincter musculature. The incision follows the margin of the anal mucosa, along the anatomical defect in the rectovaginal septum. A small margin of vaginal mucosa is left attached to the anal wall for traction because the anal mucosa is so friable (Fig. 28–8A).

Allis clamps are placed along the margin of the anal canal, and sharp dissection with fine Metz-

enbaum scissors is used to carefully separate the anal wall from the overlying vaginal septum. Any remnants of the lower loops of the external anal sphincter, particularly the base loop, should be preserved and separated from the underlying anal wall (Fig. 28–8B). The lateral wall of the anal canal should not be extensively mobilized because doing so would cause bleeding from the inferior hemorrhoidal vessels. Using a midline incision, the vaginal mucosa is separated from the anal and lower rectal wall to the areas of the lateral vagina and underlying levator muscles. The dissection must extend into the middle or upper one-third of the vagina to permit

TABLE 28–1 *Neomycin-Erythromycin Base Colon Preparation*

Day 1:	Low-residue diet
	Bisacodyl, 1 tablet orally at 6 P.M.
Day 2:	Continue low-residue diet
	Magnesium sulfate, 30 ml 50% solution (15 g) orally at 10:00 A.M., 2:00 P.M. and 6:00 P.M.
	Saline enemas in evening until return clear
Day 3:	Clear liquid diet; supplemented intravenous fluids as needed
	Magnesium sulfate, in dose given above, at 10:00 A.M. and 2:00 P.M.
	No enemas
	Neomycin, 1 g } orally at 1:00 P.M.
	Erythromycin base, 1 g } 2:00 P.M. and 11:00 P.M.
Day 4:	Operation scheduled at 8:00 A.M

Condon RE, Nichols RL: The present position of the neomycin-erythromycin bowel prep. Surg Clin North Am 55:1332, 1975

adequate mobilization of the rectum and lower end of the anal canal without undue tension, and to prevent retraction of the reconstructed wall of the anal canal.

Mobilization of the anterior anorectal wall allows the wall to be withdrawn outside the margin of the anal orifice without difficulty (Fig. 28–8B). Then the retracted and obscured margins of the lower loops of the external anal sphincter are dissected from the lateral margins of the anal wall, with careful attention to the base loop located directly beneath the anal mucosa and perianal skin. With an Allis clamp or straight Kocher clamp placed on the attenuated muscle and its capsule, sharp dissection is continued to free both ends of the external sphincter.

Once the ends meet in the midline with traction on the anchoring clamps, the sphincter is approximated with at least three or four interrupted No. 1 delayed-absorbable or permanent sutures (Fig. 28–8C).

Although the upper loop of the sphincter is rarely traumatized by a complete perineal tear, plication of the puborectalis muscle high in the midline provides additional support to the rectal inlet and reestablishes the 90-degree angle of the rectal neck with the terminal portion of the rectal colon. The suture plication of the puborectalis is continued until there is anatomical evidence of narrowing or constriction of the vaginal canal (Fig. 28–8D). If constriction is noticed when the vagina is palpated, the uppermost suture(s) should be removed until a smooth posterior vaginal wall is reestablished.

The transverse perineal muscles and the inferior margins of the bulbocavernosus muscles are reapproximated in the midline with interrupted sutures of No. 0 or No. 1 delayed-absorbable material (Fig. 28–8E). Building a high perineal body must not cause narrowing of the vaginal introitus, which would result in introital dyspareunia.

The vaginal mucosa is trimmed, if necessary, and the margins of the posterior vaginal wall are approximated with a continuous lock stitch of No. 2-0 delayed-absorbable suture. The fascia of the perineal body is plicated with vertical mattress sutures that support the perineal repair. The continuous suture is carried over the perineal body as a subcuticular stitch, and the perianal skin is approximated at the midline.

The mobilized anterior wall of the anal canal is now drawn outside the reconstructed anal orifice and sutured without tension to the perianal skin (Fig. 28–8F). Then the excess anal mucosa is trimmed. Vertical mattress sutures of No. 0 or No. 2-0 delayed-absorbable suture are used to approximate the broad surface of the anal submucosa to the perianal skin. Any residual separation of the margins of the anal mucosa and perianal skin can be approximated with interrupted sutures.

The vagina may be packed firmly with gauze for a period of 24 hours following surgery in order to avoid the development of a hematoma in the rectovaginal septum. Other postoperative procedures are identical with those described for the layered closure and the Warren flap operations.

Although not used as frequently as the layered technique for repairing a complete perineal laceration, the Noble–Mengert operation is uniquely effective for treating a small rectovaginal fistula located inside the external sphincter. Such fistulas usually result from incomplete healing of a perineal laceration.

Rectovaginal Fistula

CAUSES AND SYMPTOMS

Rectovaginal and anovaginal fistulas result from several different causes. A fistula occurring adjacent to the external sphincter is classified as anovaginal, whereas defects more than 3 cm from the anal orifice are rectovaginal. Considered together, these fistulas occur with sufficient frequency to require a complete understanding on the part of the operating gynecologist.

Many fistulas occur after an unsuccessful attempt to repair a fourth-degree tear that extends through

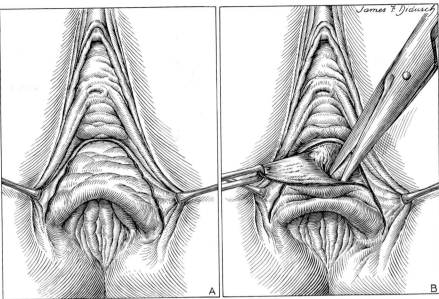

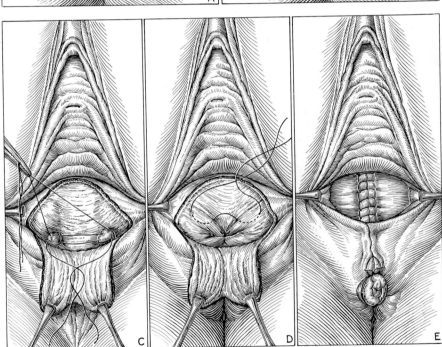

FIG. 28–7 Warren flap operation for complete third-degree tear. (*A*) Line of incision, outlining flap of vaginal mucosa. (*B*) The flap is dissected free and turned back. (*C*) The flap is retracted downward. The ends of the sphincter are delivered and are sutured with delayed-absorbable or Tycron sutures. (*D*) The sphincter ends have been united, and the puborectalis muscles are approximated in the midline with No. 0 sutures. (*E*) The vaginal incision has been closed with a continuous lock stitch that is continued subcuticularly over the perineum. The margins of the flap are included in the continuous suture, which may create a peaked appearance, temporarily, to the perineal skin. If redundant, it may be trimmed.

the anal and lower rectal mucosa. A bridge of tissue or the complete sphincter heals while the previous suture line in the anal canal above the sphincter breaks down. A low rectovaginal or anovaginal fistula of variable size results. Small and moderate-size fistulas can follow rectal injury during a posterior vaginal repair. A perirectal abscess, when opened spontaneously or surgically, may result in a fistula that opens into the vagina. The unsuccessful repair of a fistula can result in other fistulas with more scar tissue. Some uncommon causes of rectovaginal fistulas are inflammatory bowel disorders such as Crohn's disease, and systemic lupus erythematosus, a collagen-vascular disorder that produces an ulceration in the vagina and rectum with subsequent breakdown of the rectovaginal septum.

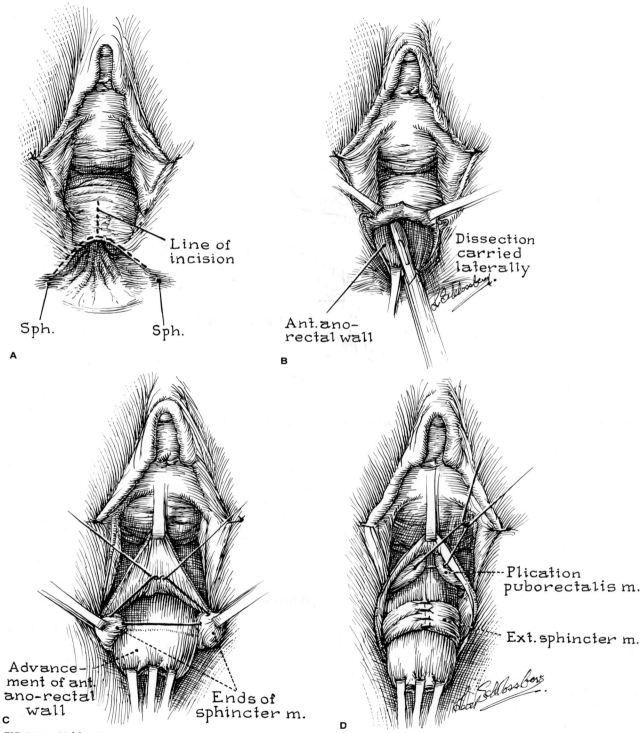

A

Line of incision

Sph. Sph.

B

Dissection carried laterally

Ant. ano-rectal wall

C

Advancement of ant. ano-rectal wall

Ends of sphincter m.

D

Plication puborectalis m.

Ext. sphincter m.

FIG. 28–8 Noble–Mengert procedure. (*A*) An initial linear incision is made in the margin of rectovaginal septum. (*B*) The anal wall is widely separated from vagina using Metzenbaum scissors or a medium-blade scalpel. (*C*) The rectal wall is withdrawn outside the site of the anal orifice and the lower loops of the external anal sphincter are dissected free and approximated with deeply placed delayed-absorbable or Tycron sutures. (*D*) Plication of puborectalis muscle is continued after ligatures are tied in external sphincter.

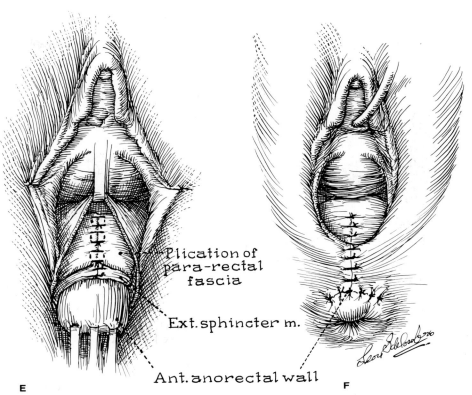

FIG. 28-8 (continued). (E) The anal wall is drawn outside the anal orifice and the pararectal fascia is plicated. (F) The vaginal mucosa and perineal skin are closed and the anal mucosa is sutured to the perianal skin.

E

Plication of para-rectal fascia

Ext. sphincter m.

Ant. anorectal wall

F

When surgery and chronic pelvic disease are combined, the risk of rectovaginal fistula is increased. For example, if the cul-de-sac has become involved in an obliterative disease process such as endometriosis, chronic inflammation, or pelvic abscess, the chances of injuring the rectum during a total hysterectomy are increased, and a fistula may form at the very top of the vagina. The risk of rectal injury is also greater when hysterectomy follows external or intracavitary irradiation in patients with uterine cancer and obliterative cul-de-sac disease. High rectovaginal fistulas also result from irradiation treatment for cervical or endometrial cancer. The fistulas are caused by radiation injury to the rectum adjacent to the posterior vaginal fornix. Rarely, destruction of carcinomatous tissue that has invaded the rectovaginal septum may result in a fistulous tract.

A small rectovaginal fistula may be entirely asymptomatic. A slight leakage of gas and seepage of feces may not be detected in the vaginal discharge. When the fistula is a bit larger, the escape of gas may be the only complaint, or there may be the complaint of fecal odor in the vaginal discharge. When the fistula is large, the entire bowel content may be evacuated through the vagina, an extremely distressing condition. As occurs with a fourth-degree

perineal laceration, voluntary constipation may reduce the amount of leakage.

DIAGNOSIS AND TREATMENT

The diagnosis of a rectovaginal fistula is usually very simple. By spreading the labia, a low fistula can be disclosed; a high fistula can be seen using a duckbill speculum. The opening in the vagina may be filled with feces, or, if the bowel has been emptied recently, the dark red rectal mucosa may be seen at the fistulous opening, contrasting with the lighter vaginal mucosa.

When the fistula is small, it may be exceedingly difficult to locate the opening between the rectum and the vagina, but the location of both orifices is essential for complete care. A small probe can be pushed through the fistula from the vaginal side, and the tip may be felt on rectal examination. If a small fistula opens into the anal canal between the anal sphincter fibers, it may be necessary to cut the fibers to lay open the fistulous tract. Injection with methylene blue may aid in proctoscopic visualization of the rectal orifice.

To enhance healing by reducing the number of bacteria in the colon and anal canal, the patient should be given a rapid bowel preparation for 72

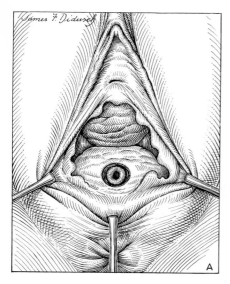
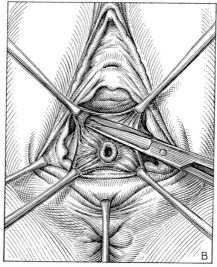
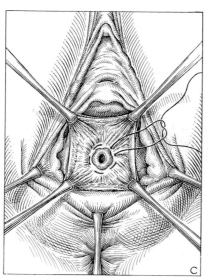
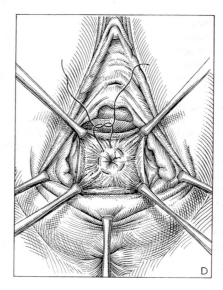

FIG. 28–9 Repair of small recto-vaginal fistula. (*A*) A circular incision through the vaginal mucosa is made about the fistulous opening. (*B*) Flaps of vaginal mucosa are dissected free for about 2 cm from the margin of the fistulous opening. (*C*) A No. 3-0 delayed-absorbable material purse-string suture is placed about the fistulous opening. (*D*) The first purse-string has been tied, inverting the fistulous opening. The second purse-string has been placed and is about to be tied.

hours preceding surgery. Bowel cleansing as described by Condon (outlined in Table 28–1) utilizes 1 g erythromycin and 1 g neomycin, given 3 times on the day preceding surgery. A few hours before the operation, the patient is given rectal irrigations with sterile saline until the fluid returns clear, and then the rectum is instilled with 200 ml 2% neomycin solution. The postoperative routine is the same as that following repair of a third-degree perineal tear.

OPERATIVE TECHNIQUE

Methodology

The surgical cure of a rectovaginal fistula may be exceedingly simply or quite complicated. Small fis-tulas may be closed by two or more purse-string sutures (Fig. 28–9). Regardless of the exact technique of closure, it is desirable to approximate broad tissue surfaces for healing. A standard technique for closure of a typical fistula is layer-for-layer closure (Fig. 28–10). When the fistula is fairly large and lies just above the sphincter or the perineal bridge, it is preferable to cut the bridge, thus converting the fistula into a complete third-degree perineal tear. The complete perineal tear is then repaired by the layered method described in Figure 28–6.

A fistula that occurs after irradiation or a fistula with scar tissue from previous surgical attempts often requires a more complicated operation. First, feces should be diverted from the field of operation

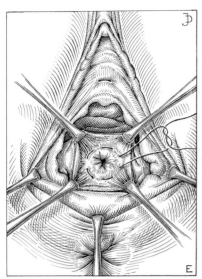
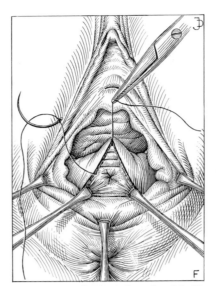
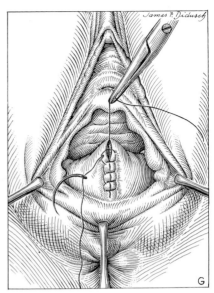

FIG. 28–9 (continued). (*E*) The second purse-string has been tied, and a third has been placed. (*F*) Submucosal–muscularis tissues are approximated with No. 2-0 continuous or interrupted delayed-absorbable sutures. (*G*) The mucosa is closed with a continuous lock stitch of No. 2-0 suture.

by performing a temporary sigmoid colostomy, such as the modified Mikulicz procedure (see Chapter 19). A transverse colostomy may also be used, utilizing essentially the same technique. The bowel is completely transected to ensure complete diversion of feces, and subsequent closure is simple.

After the colostomy, a delay of at least 8 weeks is required before the vaginal repair of the fistula should be attempted, so that the cellulitis accompanying this type of fistula will have sufficient time to heal. The process of tissue revascularization and healing cannot begin until bacterial contamination from feces passing through the fistulous tract is eliminated by a colostomy. Only when there is complete regression of the cellulitis around the fistula and when the adjacent rectovaginal septum is soft and pliable should closure of the fistula be performed.

Most high rectovaginal or sigmoidovaginal fistulas can be repaired using the Latzko technique (Fig. 28–11), but occasionally such a fistula, usually resulting from bowel injury at the time of total hysterectomy, may require transabdominal closure. Rectal fistulas induced by radiation treatment are notoriously resistant to healing after surgical repair, as a result of obliterative endarteritis and limitation of blood supply. The use of the Martius bulbocavernosus fat pad procedure as described for urethrovaginal fistula repair (Chapter 27) has improved the success rate in the closure of these difficult fistulas by transplanting a vascular graft to the operative site.

Closure of Small Rectovaginal Fistula

An incision is made in the vagina, encircling the small fistulous opening (Fig. 28–9A). With fine pointed-tip scissors, enough vaginal mucosa is dissected free to allow mobilization of the bowel wall and closure of the opening in the bowel by two or three purse-string sutures without tension (Fig. 28–9B). The first suture is placed in the submucosal opening, a few millimeters from the mucosal edge, using No. 3-0 delayed-absorbable suture (Fig. 28–9C), taking care to avoid perforating the bowel mucosa. The edges of the fistula are inverted into the lumen of the bowel as the purse-string is tied. A second purse-string suture is placed around the first in the muscularis (Fig. 28–9D). If a third purse-string can be placed without tension, it is used (Fig. 28–9E). The perirectal fascia is then approximated in the midline, using interrupted sutures of No. 0 delayed-absorbable material (Fig. 28–9F). Excess vaginal mucosa is excised, and the mucosa is closed with a continuous lock stitch of No. 2-0 suture (Fig. 28–9G).

Closure of Large Rectovaginal Fistula

An incision is made around the fistulous opening through the vaginal mucous membrane (Fig. 28–10A). The vaginal mucosa is dissected back far enough to permit mobilization of the bowel wall for closure without tension (Fig. 28–10B). Since the fistulous opening into the bowel is too large to be closed by a purse-string, a series of vertical mattress

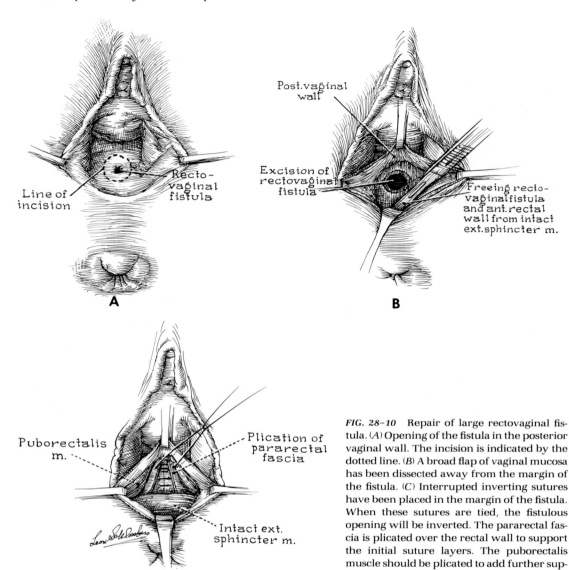

FIG. 28-10 Repair of large rectovaginal fistula. (*A*) Opening of the fistula in the posterior vaginal wall. The incision is indicated by the dotted line. (*B*) A broad flap of vaginal mucosa has been dissected away from the margin of the fistula. (*C*) Interrupted inverting sutures have been placed in the margin of the fistula. When these sutures are tied, the fistulous opening will be inverted. The pararectal fascia is plicated over the rectal wall to support the initial suture layers. The puborectalis muscle should be plicated to add further support to the anal canal and perineal body.

sutures are used (Fig. 28–10C). The bites in the tissue are taken parallel with the edges of the fistula and ideally do not enter the lumen of the bowel. Either No. 3-0 or No. 4-0 delayed-absorbable suture is most suitable for the first layer, which is reinforced by a second layer of deeper interrupted sutures into the muscular wall of the rectum. The second layer of sutures should be approximated gently, using No. 2-0 delayed-absorbable material to bring broad surface of tissue to broad surface for proper healing, and to avoid necrosis.

As an alternative to using vertical mattress sutures, the initial layer can be made with a continuous suture, inverting the edges into the bowel lumen.

The second, supporting layer is then made with interrupted mattress sutures, which invert the first layer.

After the second layer of stitches has been tied, the pararectal fascia is approximated over the fistula with No. 2-0 interrupted delayed-absorbable sutures. The puborectalis muscle may also be plicated to add further support to the closure and to correct any significant anal incontinence from damage to the external sphincter. The vaginal mucosa is closed with a continuous No. 2-0 suture. As the midline mucosal suture is placed, the subjacent fascia is picked up with each bite, thus closing all potential dead space.

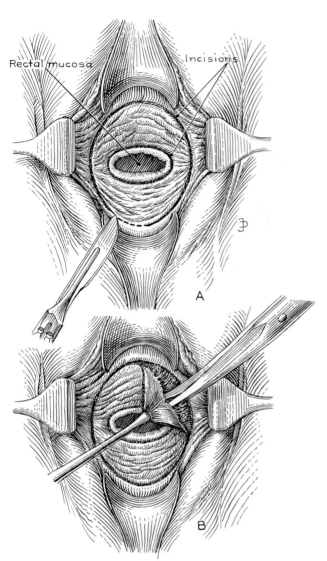

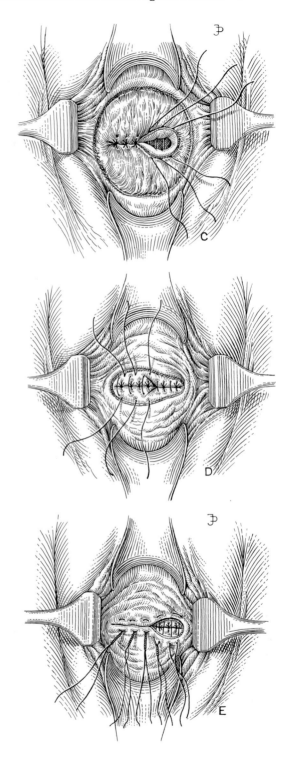

FIG. 28–11 Closure of rectovaginal fistula by Latzko technique. (*A*) Incisions around margins of fistula. (*B*) Excision of mucosa from anterior and posterior vaginal walls. (*C*) The first line of sutures is placed, inverting the edge into the rectal lumen. (*D*) The first line of sutures has been placed and tied. The second line of sutures is being placed into the rectal musculature and fascia. Note horizontal mattress sutures in the second layer. (*E*) Vertical or horizontal mattress sutures of delayed-absorbable suture form the third layer of closure.

Latzko Closure of Rectovaginal Fistula

The Latzko technique of using both the anterior and posterior vaginal walls in the closure of a vesicovaginal fistula is an effective method of closing a high rectovaginal fistula located at the apex of the vagina (Fig. 28–11).

A sufficient area around the fistula must be denuded so that broad surfaces of well-vascularized tissues can be approximated. Incisions are made around the margins of the fistula (Fig. 28–11A). Mucosa from both the anterior and the posterior vaginal walls are removed for a 2 cm to 3 cm margin (Fig. 28–11B).

With the first layer of the closure, the edges are inverted into the bowel lumen, using No. 3-0 delayed-absorbable suture (Fig. 28–11C). An alternate and frequently preferable technique for beginning closure is to use a continuous inverting suture for the first layer to assure complete closure of the rectal defect. When a colostomy has preceded the fistula repair, closure may be made by using a continuous suture and not inverting the mucosa into the bowel lumen.

In the second line, the sutures are of the horizontal mattress type; the bite of the needle is taken parallel with the suture line into the rectal musculature and fascia (Fig. 28–11D). In the last step the vaginal mucosal edges are brought together with mattress sutures of No. 0 delayed-absorbable material (Fig. 28–11E). Delayed-absorbable sutures are now used instead of silver wire. The nonreactive delayed-absorbable suture material has proven to be as effective as silver wire and produces less necrosis of the vaginal mucosa and no discomfort to the patient.

Bibliography

Ayoub SF: Anatomy of the external anal sphincter in man. Acta Anat 105:25, 1979

Berek JS, Lagasse LD, Nacker NF, et al: Levator ani transposition for anal incompetence secondary to sphincter damage. Obstet Gynecol 59:108, 1982

Birnbaum W: A method of repair for a common type of traumatic incontinence of the anal sphincter. Surg Gynecol Obstet 87:716, 1948

Blaisdell PC: A simpler yet effective repair of the incontinent sphincter ani. Surg Gynecol Obstet 112:375, 1961

Condon RE, Nichols RL: The present position of the neomycin-erythromycin bowel prep. Surg Clin North Am 55:1332, 1975

Denny–Brown D, Robertson EG: An investigation of the nervous control of defecation. Brain 58:256, 1935

Emge LA, Durfee RB: Pelvic organ prolapse—4000 years of treatment. Clin Obstet Gynecol 9:997, 1966

Gabriel WB: The Principles and Practice of Rectal Surgery, 5th ed. London, HK Lewis & Co, 1963

Garry RC: Responses to stimulation of the caudal end of the large bowel in the cat. J Physiol 78:208, 1933

Gaston EA: Physiology of faecal continence. Surg Gynaecol Obstet 87:280, 1948

Goligher JC, Leacock AG, Brossy JJ: Surgical anatomy of anal canal. Br J Surg 43:51, 1955

Howkins J (ed): Shaw's Textbook of Operative Gynecology, 3rd ed. London, E & S Livingstone, 1968

Hughes ESR, Johnson WR: Abdominoperineal levator ani repair for rectal prolapse: Technique. Aust NZ J Surg 50:117, 1980

Ingleman–Sundberg A: Transplantation of the levator muscles in the repair of complete tear and rectovaginal fistula. Acta Chir Scand 96:313, 1947

Kottmeier PK: A physiological approach to the problem of anal incontinence through use of the levator ani as a sling. Surgery 60:1262, 1966

Landeen JM, Habal MB: The rejuvenation of the anal sphincteroplasty. Surg Gynecol Obstet 149:78, 1979

Latzko W: Postoperative vesicovaginal fistulas. Am J Surg 58:211, 1942

McCall ML, Bolten KA (ed and trans): Martius Gynecological Operations with Emphasis on Topographic Anatomy. Boston, Little, Brown, 1956

Mengert WF, Fish SA: Anterior rectal wall advancement. Obstet Gynecol 5:262, 1955

Miller NF, Brown W: The surgical treatment of complete perineal tears in the female. Am J Obstet Gynecol 34:196, 1937

Milligan ETC, Morgan CN: Surgical anatomy of the anal canal, with special reference to anorectal fistulae. Lancet 2:1150, 1934

Moore FA: Anal incontinence: A reappraisal. Obstet Gynecol 41:483, 1973

Noble GH: A new technique for complete laceration of the perineum designed for the purpose of eliminating infection from the rectum. Trans Am Gynecol Soc 27:357, 1902

Parks AG: The biological basis of modern surgical practice. In: Sabiston DC Jr (ed): Davis-Christopher Textbook of Surgery, 10th ed. Philadelphia, WB Saunders, 1972

Parks AG: Anal incontinence. Proc R Soc Med 68:681, 1975

Russell TR, Gallagher DM: Low rectovaginal fistulas. Am J Surg 134:13, 1977

Shafik A: A new concept of the anatomy of the anal sphincter mechanism and the physiology of defaecation. I. The external anal sphincter: A triple-loop system. Invest Urol 12:412, 1975

———: A new concept of the anatomy of the anal sphincter mechanism and the physiology of defaecation. II. Anatomy of the levator ani muscle with special reference to puborectalis. Invest Urol 13:175, 1975

———: A new concept of the anatomy of the anal sphincter mechanism and the physiology of defaecation. III. The longitudinal anal muscle: Anatomy and role in anal sphincter mechanism. Invest Urol 13:271, 1976

———: A new concept of the anatomy of the anal sphincter mechanism and the physiology of defaecation. IV. Anatomy of the perianal spaces. Invest Urol 13:424, 1976

Warren JC: A new method of operation for the relief of rupture of the perineum through the sphincter and rectum. Trans Am Gynecol Soc 7:322, 1882

Part Four

Treatment of Pelvic Neoplasms

Chapter 29

Surgical Conditions of the Vulva

Richard F. Mattingly, M.D., and
J. Donald Woodruff, M.D.

The vulva, along with the perianal skin, is designated the anogenital area. The ectodermal tissue of the vulva must be considered separately from the vagina, the urethra, and the cervix although multifocal genital diseases often affect all of these organs.

Dermatologic Conditions of the Vulva

Dermatitis is the most common affliction of the vulva, causing major diagnostic and therapeutic problems to the dermatologist, the generalist, and the gynecologist. The dermatologist is frequently unaware of the vulvar manifestations of the common skin lesions, most of which are caused by specific irritants. The gynecologist, unfamiliar with dermatologic disease, may attempt to apply knowledge of lesions occurring in the genital canal to the neoplastic and non-neoplastic diseases of the external genitalia.

The vulvar epithelium is subject to all of the dermatologic conditions that occur elsewhere on the body. Although some of the dermatitides are seen rarely on the external genitalia (e.g., psoriasis), others, particularly those of reactive origin, are extremely common and produce major problems for the patient and the physician.

Local reactions to many otherwise simple dermatologic lesions are often exacerbated by seborrheic, eccrine, and apocrine secretions; by vaginal and cervical discharges; by menstrual blood; and by urine and fecal contamination. In addition to the normal vulvar excretions and secretions may be added the frequently irritating discharges from common vaginal infections, especially trichomonas and monilia. Other irritants are deodorants, hygiene sprays, perfumed soaps and powders, local anesthetic agents, and colored toilet tissue. Tight-fitting pants and underclothing, particularly those made of nonabsorbent synthetic fabrics, aggravate the local problems because they retain moisture and conduce to fissuring of the skin.

In the acute phase, most dermatitides do not require surgical therapy. When a dermatologic process persists, the vulvar epithelium and subcutaneous tissues become altered, with deep-seated perineural inflammation and pruritus. These may be resistant to the usual local forms of therapy, such as fluorinated hydrocortisone.

In the past, the term *leukoplakia* has been used to denote vulvar skin that has become thick and dystrophic with elongated rete pegs (acanthosis), surface hyperkeratosis, and underlying chronic inflammatory infiltrate. The term has been used vaguely to describe any type of white plaque, varying from leukoderma to cancer. Since chronic dermatitis has essentially no malignant potential, the International Society for the Study of Vulvar Disease has proposed that the condition be designated as *hyperplastic dystrophy*, which identifies more adequately its pathology. The availability of a more realistic terminology should simplify the diagnosis of vulvar disease, and, more importantly, a realistic description should prevent an unnecessary vulvectomy to remove benign white lesions.

TREATMENT OF INTRACTABLE PRURITUS

Before any therapy for vulvar lesions caused by chronic irritation is begun, an accurate tissue diagnosis must be established. The epidermis may be thickened and the skin markings accentuated (lichenification), but the extent of the epithelial proliferation cannot be assessed without biopsy. All patients should be given detailed instruction to eliminate local irritants; associated vaginitis should be treated vigorously. A thorough investigation for any systemic disease such as diabetes should be completed, and local medication for control of the symptoms must be given satisfactory trial. Vulvectomy should not be performed for chronic dermatitis or for the benign dystrophies, including lichen sclerosus.

Topical Agents

Topical agents should be tried first, although they are often ineffective because they cannot penetrate the thickened hyperkeratotic surface. Injection of the topical agent into the subepithelial dermis will circumvent the problem of thickened skin. The injection of 20 mg to 30 mg triamcinolone acetonide (Kenalog) in a localized area of approximately 12 cm has proved to be effective. The most commonly involved region is the outer surface of the labium majus. The injected solution should be rubbed thoroughly into the tissues to prevent focal irritation. Relief of symptoms occurs generally within 48 hours and remission lasts approximately 4 to 6 months (Fig. 29–1). The procedure can be repeated as the symptoms demand.

Although the subepithelial injection of steroid has almost eliminated the necessity for local alcohol injection, an occasional case is resistant to all forms of local therapy. Trauma to the vulvar skin produced by scratching with fingernails may be the most carcinogenic of a variety of agents. Vulvar pruritus is associated with fingernail trauma, which, after many years, commonly leads to malignancy. In a recalcitrant case of pruritus, the local injection of absolute alcohol produces immediate relief by affecting the nerve endings. Relief continues for at least 6 months in approximately 90% of the cases. Eliminating the itch–scratch reflex for even this short period may cure the pruritus.

TECHNIQUE OF ADMINISTRATION. Although local alcohol injection may be performed on an outpatient basis, the procedure is accomplished best under general anesthesia. The anogenital area should be shaved, cleansed, and draped. The region is marked into 1 cm squares (Fig. 29–2A) with either an autoclaved Magic Marker or a dye such as brilliant green. Then 0.2 ml absolute alcohol is injected into the subcutaneous tissues (Fig. 29–2B) at each point where the lines intersect.

The procedure should begin at the lowest level to prevent alcohol leaking from the needle point and destroying the pattern. Afer all the points have been injected, the whole area should be thoroughly massaged to prevent localization of the alcohol, and the patient should be instructed to use cold packs or hot sitz baths for 1 week.

Relief of pruritus begins immediately. The patient may feel swollen and numb for 10 days to 2 weeks, but both reactions disappear completely and relief continues for 6 months or more.

The Mering Procedure

When all forms of local treatment fail to relieve a patient's symptoms, the Mering procedure should be considered as a last resort. Although extensive surgery is required, the vulvar skin must be protected from the trauma produced by scratching.

The Mering procedure requires hospitalization for the patient and careful surgical technique from the physician (Fig. 29–3). The skin is cleansed thoroughly after being shaved, and the incision is outlined with a marking pencil. The incision is made on the outer surface of the labium majus and extends to the fascia of the urogenital diaphragm from the level of the clitoris to slightly beyond the fourchette to the level of the anal orifice, inferiorly, depending on the extent of the pruritus. The small nerves in the adjacent tissue are severed using a finger on each side, moving from the lateral aspect of the clitoris toward the midline, where the fingers meet. The procedure interrupts branches of the ilioinguinal and genitofemoral nerves (Fig. 29–4). Blunt dissection extends posteriorly to the lateral side of the rectum, outside of the external anal sphincter. If the perianal area is involved, blunt dissection should extend to the posterior limit of the anal orifice, where the two fingers meet behind the anus in the midline, breaking up the branches of the pudendal nerve.

It is important that hemostasis be meticulously

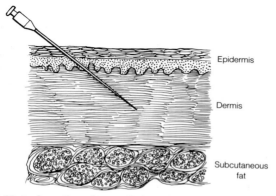

FIG. 29–1 Insertion of a needle into the subepithelial dermis for the injection of steroid for the relief of chronic pruritus.

Epidermis

Dermis

Subcutaneous fat

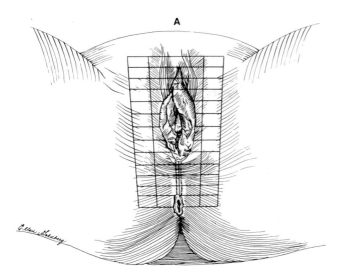

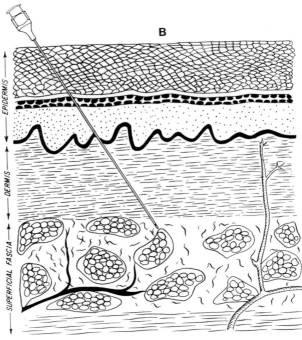

FIG. 29–2 (*A*) Marking of external genitalia into 1-cm squares in preparation for alcohol injection. (*B*) Depth of penetration of No. 25 gauge needle into the subcutaneous tissue. (Woodruff JD, Thompson B: Local alcohol injection in the treatment of vulvar pruritus. Obstet Gynecol 40:18, 1972)

controlled because the accumulation of blood and fluid may produce local cellulitis, which would delay recovery. A small drain should be placed at the dependent portion of the incision. The underlying tissue is approximated with absorbable sutures, and the skin is sutured with polyglycolic acid or polyglactin sutures. The area must be packed tightly for 48 hours, and then the patient should use ice packs or hot sitz baths until the edema has regressed.

SPECIFIC INFECTIONS

Treatment of viral infections of the vulva depends on the specific virus. Some viruses—for example, herpes and molluscum contagiosum—do not need surgical therapy. New antiherpetic medications are being introduced and should be employed instead of surgery. Recommendations to use laser beams for herpes are subject to criticism. Other viruses, such as human papillomavirus, which causes condyloma acuminatum, often require surgical intervention. Treatment of condylomata is discussed under the heading of benign solid tumors.

Although the number of diseases transmitted by sexual contact has increased, the basic group still consists of syphilis, gonorrhea, granulomatous diseases, and chancroid. In their acute phase, the lesions are treated with local or systemic therapy,

not with surgery. In the chronic stages of the granulomatous diseases, specifically lymphogranuloma venereum and granuloma inguinale, the lymphedematous distortion of the vulva does not respond to local or systemic treatment. Chronic granulomatous lesions must be inspected by biopsy, to differentiate benign lesions from malignant ones. Since chronic granulomatous lesions have often been reported to develop into cancer, a vulvectomy with wide excision of affected tissues should be performed if local and systemic therapies fail to produce satisfactory healing.

Hidradenitis

An infectious process demanding extensive local surgery is suppurative hidradenitis. This pustular disease begins as an infection in the apocrine sweat glands in the vulva. The early manifestations are frequently cyclic, since the secretory activity of the apocrine glands corresponds to the progestational phase of the menstrual cycle. Consequently, in the early stages of the disease or in the chronic pruritic phase, Fox–Fordyce disease, the use of hormonal therapy, such as oral contraceptives, may help modify the secretory activity of the glands. Once the disease infects the local tissue, local and systemic agents are generally ineffective. Often the pustules infect the entire area, so that pressure at one point may produce an exudation of purulent material

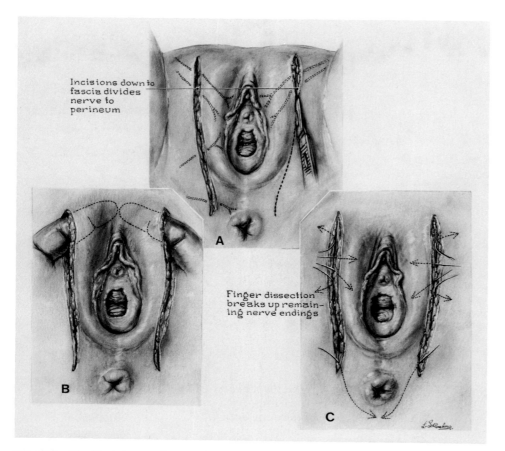

FIG. 29-3 The Mering procedure. (A) The incisions are made at the lateral margins of the labia majora, extending to the level of the clitoris superiorly and the anal orifice inferiorly. The depth of dissection is the deep fascia to incise the adipose tissue and the nerves. (B) The finger dissects the underlying tissue breaking up the fibers of the pudendal, ilioinguinal, and genitofemoral nerves. (C) The underlying tissues are approximated carefully to attain good hemostasis. A small drain should be inserted at the most dependent aspect of the incision to avoid the accumulation of blood in the operative sites.

from a distant sinus (Fig. 29-5A). Because the entire anogenital area is honeycombed by the underlying infection, simple incision into a few of the pustules is useless. Extensive debridement must be carried out to allow healing to occur from the base.

The incision extends into the underlying fat, and the involved skin is removed in segments, leaving bridges of normal skin between the excised pustules. Loose approximation of the skin edges may be carried out using polyglycolic acid or polyglactin suture material, but more commonly, the entire area is left open and treated locally to promote granulations (Fig. 29-5B). Results of therapy are rewarding in most cases, and skin grafting is usually unnecessary. The patient must be treated with antibiotics both

before and after surgery. Ampicillin is generally used, but cultures should be taken from the draining sinuses to check for organisms that are sensitive to other antibiotic agents.

Crohn's Disease

Crohn's disease, a chronic inflammatory disease of the bowel, affects the vulva and perianal area in approximately 25% to 30% of the cases in which there is the classic intestinal involvement. The draining sinuses often communicate with the vagina or the rectum and may result in fistulization. On rare occasions, the vulva may be involved even though the small and large bowel are not affected.

Before any surgical therapy is begun, diagnosis

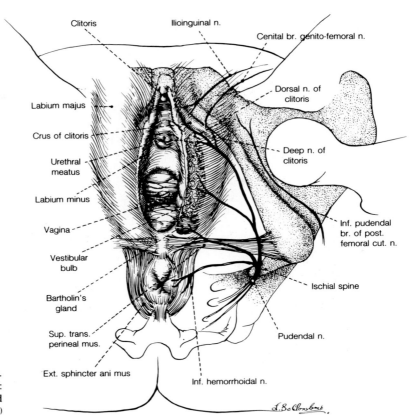

FIG. 29–4 Nerve supply to anogenital region. (Woodruff JD, Julian CG: In Ridley JH (ed): Gynecologic Surgery Errors, Safeguards and Salvage. Baltimore, Williams & Wilkins, 1974)

can be confirmed by studying the bowel or by obtaining a biopsy of the affected tissues in the perineum. The presence of noncaseating granulomas is characteristic of Crohn's disease. Further deterioration of the tissue may result from attempts to excise a draining sinus fused by Crohn's disease. Rectal incontinence may result from destruction of the anal sphincter or the development of a recto-vaginal fistula.

The currently preferred treatment is 25 mg/24 hr prednisone in addition to 750 mg/24 hr to 1000 mg/24 hr metronidazole for a minimum of 4 to 6 weeks. The treatment must be continued for a longer time if surgery is considered necessary. Although several physicians have expressed concern about using metronidazole on a long-term basis, the drug has proven to be safe and to produce excellent long-term results.

In addition to pharmacotherapy, a submucosal anal pull-through procedure may bring relief, since it brings the fistula outside the anus. A layered surgical repair of a fistula caused by Crohn's disease is usually unsuccessful, since the disease commonly recurs. Results are difficult to predict because mul-

tiple areas of the terminal colon may be affected and any affected area may involve the vagina or perineum. Antibiotic therapy should always be given during this type of surgical procedure.

Trauma

Major trauma to the vulva most often occurs when young girls experience injuries as a result of sledding or bicycling accidents. Hematomas, and occasionally lacerations, can develop from falls astride the cross-bar of a bicycle or from being thrown from a sled against an obstacle such as a tree or fence (Fig. 29–6). Trauma may also result from sexual assault.

Most traumatic injuries do not need surgical attention. Patients should be treated conservatively with bedrest, immediate application of cold packs, and, later, with hot sitz baths to reduce the edema. Antibiotics should be used to eliminate local inflammatory reactions. Should a hematoma increase in size and extend into the perineum or over the lower abdominal wall, incising the vulvar skin, evacuating the hematoma, and ligating the bleeding vessels may

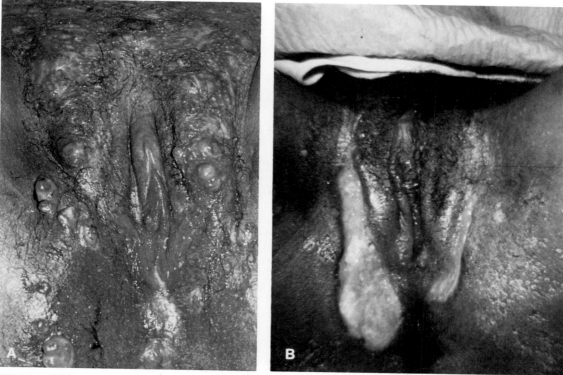

FIG. 29–5 (*A*) Extensive suppurative hidradenitis with numerous communicating sinuses. (*B*) Same vulva 4 weeks after debridement with exuberant granulations (complete healing in 2 months).

reduce the period of convalescence. When a hematoma produces urethral obstruction, evacuation may reduce the time that an indwelling urethral catheter is needed. Lacerations into the rectum or urethra should be repaired immediately.

Cysts of the Vulva

BARTHOLIN'S DUCT CYSTS

Obstruction of Bartholin's duct occurs commonly, usually near the orifice. Depending on the cause, the cyst may be mucoid or cloudy. Although such obstructions can result from gonococcal infection, other infections and trauma more commonly explain the occlusion. During a mediolateral episiotomy or a posterior colporrhaphy, for example, sutures can easily injure or even ligate the duct. The lining of the main cyst develops from transitional epithelium. The mucus-secreting glands are not affected by the obstruction, but may be distorted by the infectious process. During the acute infection, which may precede the actual cyst formation, an

abscess often develops with symptoms of tenderness, swelling, and erythema.

Incision and drainage bring almost immediate relief to the patient, and may be accomplished under local anesthesia. A small wick may be left in the cavity to maintain adequate drainage. Marsupialization can rarely be accomplished during the acute stage, but the procedure is useful for chronic or recurrent abscesses. Although injection of an antibiotic into the abscess has been tried as treatment for the acute infection, the method has proven to be no more effective than systemic antibiotic therapy.

Most small cysts of Bartholin's duct are asymptomatic, and are found during routine pelvic examinations. Patients may even be unaware of larger cysts. When symptoms do occur, patients usually complain of discomfort with coitus, or pain while sitting or walking.

Although most symptomatic Bartholin's duct cysts can be treated with a Word catheter, some will require surgery. Before deciding whether to perform marsupialization or excision of a Bartholin's duct cyst, the surgeon should consider two aspects

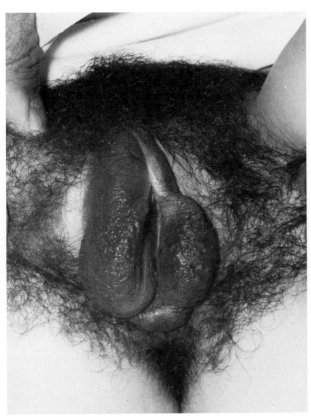

FIG. 29-6 Hematoma of the vulva. (Woodruff JD, Julian CG: In Ridley JH (ed): Gynecologic Surgery: Errors, Safeguards and Salvage. Baltimore, Williams & Wilkins, 1974)

of the problem. If the cyst recurs, a second marsupialization procedure will probably not help, since infection deep in the glandular tissue is not reached. For deep infections, excision is necessary. Another possibility is that thickening at the base of the gland could represent a neoplasm. Although uncommon, cancer must be considered, especially in the patient over the age of 40 years.

Technique of Excision of Bartholin's Duct Cyst

It is rarely necessary to excise a Bartholin's duct cyst, particularly in patients over 40 years of age, unless there is induration at the base. An elliptical incision in the vaginal mucosa is made as close as possible to the site of the gland orifice (Fig. 29-7). An incision on the mucosal side is preferable, because an incision through the vulvar skin makes it difficult to dissect the cyst wall from the very thin and delicate mucosa without incising or tearing it. If an opening is accidentally made through the mu-

cosa, a permanent fenestration may result. Usually no difficulty is encountered in dissecting the cyst from the inner surface of the vulvar skin when the incision is made on the mucosal side. Excising a small ellipse of mucosa with the cyst allows the surgeon to have a site for traction and reduces the risk of rupturing the cyst.

Since cyst formation is usually preceded by inflammation, the wall is adherent and cannot be enucleated easily with blunt dissection only. The blunt-pointed Mayo scissors serves admirably for sharp dissection of the cyst from its bed (Fig. 29-7C). The cyst can be mobilized further with the handle of the scalpel. A large cyst may develop posteriorly, and approximate the rectum. The rectal wall can easily be distinguished from the cyst by inserting a finger into the rectum during dissection.

Complete removal of the gland tissue adherent to the cyst wall is essential, for residual glandular tissue may result in the formation of a tender nodule or a recurrent cyst. The noncystic portion of the gland usually can be detected easily by palpation, because it feels quite indurated and contrasts with the surrounding soft tissues. If the margins of the cyst have become obscured, the cyst may be opened and the wall dissected from the surrounding tissue.

Directly beneath Bartholin's duct is the vestibular bulb, which is composed of anastomosing venous channels. Bleeding must be avoided when the gland is being dissected from the vascular bulb. To ensure permanent hemostasis, the entire cavity must be obliterated by approximating the walls with fine delayed-absorbable suture material after excising the cyst.

Approximation of the vaginal mucosa is accomplished best with a continuous mucosal suture of No. 1-0 delayed-absorbable material. Bleeding from the labia or vestibular bulb usually causes a postoperative hematoma of the labia, which can progress to include the mons pubis and the abdominal wall beneath Scarpa's fascia. Bedrest, ice packs, and a pressure dressing to the vulva are the methods of treatment for a hematoma; attempts to ligate the venous bleeding points will prove futile. Although the blood usually reabsorbs with time, evacuation and drainage are sometimes necessary.

If the bleeding deep in the bed of the gland seems uncontrollable, deep mattress sutures may be placed from the skin through the bleeding bed into the vagina and back. The sutures should not be tied too tightly because necrosis may result, with fenestration of the vaginal outlet. A small drain should be stitched into the bed with fine absorbable sutures to avoid the accumulation of blood and serous fluid, which could form a tender mass.

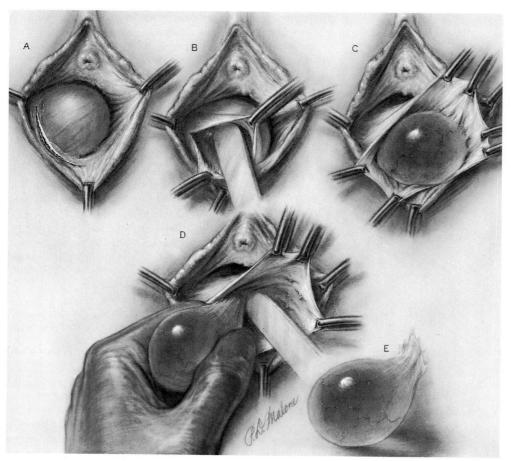

FIG. 29-7 Excision of Bartholin's gland cyst. (*A*) An incision is made in the mucosa over the cyst. (*B*) Dissection is begun, using the handle of the scalpel. (*C*) Dissection has been continued by sharp and blunt dissection. (*D*) Dissection is almost complete. (*E*) Intact cyst after removal.

Technique of Marsupialization of Bartholin's Duct Cyst

Drainage of a Bartholin's duct cyst by marsupialization is a less involved technical procedure than excision and eliminates many complications. Marsupialization is used frequently to treat a recurrent cyst. The procedure makes it possible to avoid excising the gland with the cyst and to preserve the secretory function of the gland for vaginal lubrication.

The procedure may be performed under local, regional, or general anesthesia. A wedge-shaped, vertical incision is made in the vaginal mucosa over the center of the cyst, outside the hymenal ring (Fig. 29–8A). The incision should be as wide as possible to enhance the postoperative patency of the stoma. After the cyst wall is opened and drained of its contents, the lining of the cyst is everted and sutured to the vaginal mucosa with interrupted sutures of No. 2-0 delayed-absorbable material (Fig. 29–8B). Drains and packs are not necessary, but the patient's postoperative care should include daily sitz baths beginning on the 3rd or 4th postoperative day.

As a result of closure and secondary fibrosis of the orifice following marsupialization, 10% to 15% of the cysts recur. Abscess formation is another recurring sequela of marsupialization.

Marsupialization has had limited use since the Word catheter was introduced (Fig. 29–9). The catheter accomplishes the same result as surgery with minimal or no trauma. Under local anesthesia, a small incision is made with a No. 11, pointed Bard–Parker scalpel blade at approximately the area of the normal orifice. The Word catheter is inserted through this opening, and the bulb is distended with approximately 2 cc to 3 cc saline. The nipple of the catheter is inserted into the vagina. There is essen-

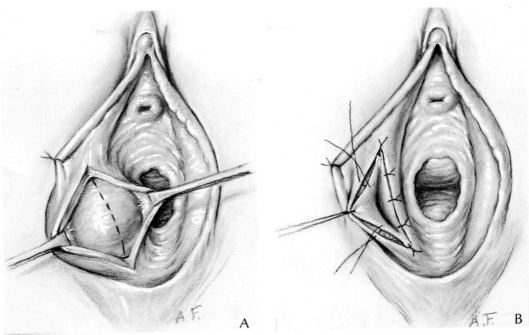

FIG. 29–8 (*A*) Incision for marsupialization. (*B*) Marsupialization. (Tancer ML, Rosenberg M, Fernandez D: Cysts of the vulvovaginal (Bartholin's) gland. Obstet Gynecol 7:609, 1956)

tially no discomfort to the procedure, and coitus may be resumed normally. In 3 to 4 weeks, the catheter can be removed by deflating the bulb. By this time, epithelialization of the orifice has taken place so that the reclosure of the duct is unlikely.

MINOR VESTIBULAR GLANDS

Numerous minor glands encircle the vaginal outlet immediately outside the hymenal ring, located superficially in comparison to the Bartholin structures (the major vestibular glands). Nonspecific infection in the small vestibular glands produces constriction of the hymen with associated dyspareunia and tenderness with motion or touch. Local procedures, antibiotics, and cortisone have been used successfully to treat the inflammatory reactions.

Excision of the hymen along with the adjacent infected glands (Fig. 29–10) has produced relief of symptoms in 90% to 95% of the cases. The incision begins just below and lateral to the urethra, includes the hymen and the 0.5 cm to 1.0 cm of tissue containing the glands, and proceeds posteriorly toward the anal orifice, where it meets the incision from the opposite side, laterally and medially to the anal outlet. As in a perineoplasty, the vaginal mucosa is undermined and approximated to the skin edges with delayed-absorbable suture. Postoperative treatment is also the same as for perineoplasty.

HYDROCELE OR CYST OF THE CANAL OF NUCK

Hydrocele is an uncommon vulvar cyst. The cyst appears as a large dilatation of the labium majus and adjacent labium minus that must be differentiated from a Bartholin's duct cyst. Figure 29–11

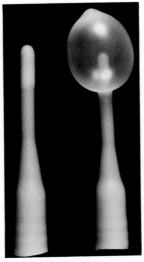

FIG. 29–9 The word catheter (*Left*) is inserted into Bartholin's duct cyst through a vaginal incision. (*Right*) The bulb is inflated with saline and the end of the catheter is placed in the vagina.

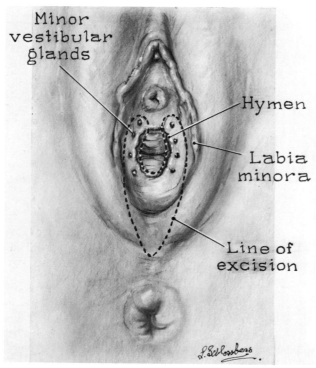

FIG. 29–10 The minor vestibular glands exit lateral to the hymenal ring. They are very superficial and thus rarely produce definable "nodules" even when chronically infected.

shows a hydrocele. The patient had received two procedures for drainage of Bartholin's duct cysts, but the mass recurred after each procedure.

The hydrocele is a dilatation of the peritoneum that accompanies the round ligament and extends from the inguinal canal into the vulva. Dilatation along the canal is known as a cyst of the canal of Nuck. Since the peritoneum may remain in the inguinal canal without close attachment to the round ligament, fluid may accumulate in this peritoneal sac. On rare occasions a loop of intestine may follow the pathway of the round ligament, forming a hernia in the vulva. When a hydrocele is treated as a Bartholin's duct cyst, peritoneal fluid reaccumulates and the hydrocele recurs.

Surgical treatment for a hydrocele begins with an incision into the mass. The external inguinal ring is identified by inserting a finger along the round ligament to the inguinal canal. The peritoneal lining is then excised from the cyst cavity, and the external inguinal ring is closed along with the subjacent tissue in the vulva. If a hernia is present, inguinal herniorrhaphy should be performed along with excision of the peritoneal covering of the round ligament.

Solid Tumors

Fibromas, fibromyomas, and lipomas rarely affect the vulva although, frequently, combinations of these elements appear as mesodermal tumors, originating in the fibromusculature of the vulvar area, in the round ligament, or in the fatty tissues of the labia majora. Hyaline degeneration usually occurs with the larger fibromyomas, and may give rise to the very rare fibrosarcoma. Lipomas are often mistaken for cystic lesions because of their consistent structure, while hernias and hydrocele of the canal of Nuck must be differentiated from tumors because they require different surgical approaches.

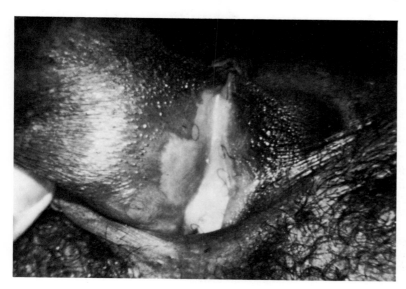

FIG. 29–11 A hydrocele is caused by the extension of a peritoneal sac with the round ligament from the inguinal canal into the vulva.

Most solid tumors should be excised, both to ascertain diagnosis and to relieve the patient's discomfort. Small pedunculated tumors can be removed by simple ligation of the stalk; the more deeply situated lesions require more extensive local dissection.

The boundaries of such mesodermal tumors are difficult to delineate, but most of the tumors are benign. Even recurrence does not signify malignant alteration; the fibromyoma tends to recur even when the original specimen had no histologic evidence of malignancy. Although a rare fibrosarcoma may rarely arise in the vulva, histological studies must be carefully made, because the lesion can be confused with the more common condition of degenerating multinucleate cells.

As in any vulvar surgery, hemostasis is important, since compression is difficult to obtain in these soft tissues. Extravasation of blood can dissect the fascial planes well out to the abdominal wall.

CONDYLOMA ACUMINATUM

Condyloma acuminatum is one of a large group of verrucous lesions caused by DNA viruses and usually transmitted by coitus. The virus associated with condyloma acuminatum is one of approximately 15 known varieties of the papilloma virus, known as HPV6. Variants of the HPV6 virus have been identified by DNA probing. Interestingly, the laryngeal papilloma is also caused by HPV6. Alterations in the vaginal milieu produced by oral contraceptives may stimulate the growth of condylomata acuminatum.

The wartlike lesions are also found in the perianal area, in the vagina, and on the cervix, and should be differentiated from other sexually transmitted diseases. Initially the lesions are reddish or reddish-brown in color owing to the surface parakeratosis. With time and exposure to local trauma, the warts become hyperkeratotic and turn gray or white in color, as any hyperkeratotic lesion will, if kept constantly moist (Fig. 29–12A).

The lesions of condyloma acuminatum are usually small, though occasionally they become massive, practically occluding the vaginal outlet. Rarely do they bleed unless evulsed by trauma, although during pregnancy, tears can occur and cause extensive bleeding of vaginal lesions. Striking vascularity between the elongated acanthotic rete pegs can be seen with a microscope (Fig. 29–12B).

The smaller lesions commonly respond to a local cauterizing agent, such as podophyllin, or a saturated solution of tri- or bichloracetic acid. Lesions more than 1 cm to 2 cm in diameter need surgical

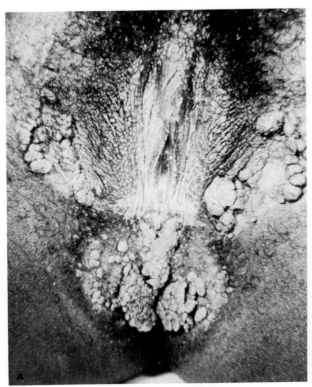
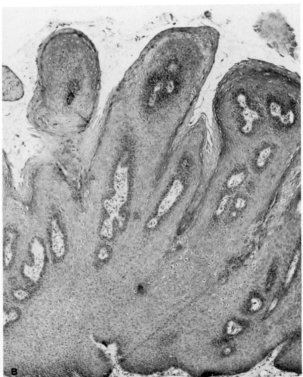

FIG. 29–12 (A) Extensive condylomatosis of anogenital area. (B) Microscopic pattern of acuminate wart.

excision, accomplished by either electrosurgery or cryosurgery. Recently, carbon dioxide laser vaporization has been employed to treat vulvar warts, using general or regional anesthesia. In experienced hands this vaporization procedure has proven to be an effective method of eradicating small lesions, but the process is much too slow for the removal of large lesions, which are preferably excised.

When electrocautery is used, the base of the small warts may be infiltrated with a local anesthetic agent; then the tumor is coagulated and removed by scraping the base with the scalpel. Regional or general anesthesia provides a better and more complete procedure for excising massive lesions. Sufficient tissue should be obtained during the procedure to prepare an autogenous vaccine to use if lesions recur. Ice packs should be used for the first 48 hours following surgery, then hot sitz baths should be used for at least 2 weeks to eliminate the local reaction to therapy.

None of the current techniques prevents recurrences, since the viral agent remains within the tissue. A connection has been made between recurrence of HPV infections and the development of neoplasia. Although the HPV6 virus can be identified in benign warts, when a malignancy occurs, the virus can no longer be identified by the peroxidase–antiperoxidase technique. Even though Koch's postulates are not fulfilled, the circumstantial evidence of a relationship is almost undeniable. Still, cellular proliferation in these papillomatous lesions may be overdiagnosed as true neoplasia, particularly in cervical lesions, but also in vulvar lesions.

HIDRADENOMA (SWEAT-GLAND TUMOR) OF THE VULVA

A rare benign tumor of the vulva, hidradenoma was first described by Schickele in 1902. The tumor is noted for its intricate proliferation pattern, which could easily be mistaken for a malignancy, resulting in unnecessary radical surgery.

Clinically, hidradenomas are small, rarely more than 1 cm in diameter (Fig. 29–13A). The tumor is sessile and covered with normal skin. Its consistency can range from firm to as soft as a sebaceous cyst, with which it is often confused. The majority of these lesions are found in the interlabial folds, in the labia majora, or in the perineum. Occasionally, a tumor may be found on the labia minora. However, since these tumors are apocrine in origin, this position is unusual. The occasional occurrence of reddish-brown pulpy material on the surface results when the tumor is evulsed through the duct of the gland.

These lesions have been studied carefully in nu-

merous laboratories, and the complex microscopic patterns have been stressed (Fig. 29–13B). The superficial papillary adenomatous pattern appears aggressive, but careful inspection shows that the glandular structures are lined by a single layer of well-organized cuboidal cells. In some parts of the tumor, the pink-staining secretory elements can be identified superficial to the basal layer. Beneath the epithelium is an indefinite layer of flattened myoepithelium cells. When the clear cell variant of the myoepithelium proliferates, an ominous picture is created, yet this clear cell hidradenoma behaves in a benign fashion. Although occasionally hidradenocarcinoma does occur, a finding of distinct adenocarcinoma in the vulva probably indicates a metastatic lesion, most commonly from the endometrium.

Hidradenomas are classically asymptomatic, and most lesions are discovered during a routine pelvic examination. Curative treatment consists of complete local excision; recurrences only result from incomplete excision.

HEMANGIOMA

Hemangiomas are common vulvar lesions that usually do not require treatment. The lesions are usually small, often multiple, and may bleed with trauma. On occasion, keratinization produces a white or gray-white appearance to the superficial surface (angiokeratoma). Hemangiomas should be differentiated from small varicosities, which are commonly seen in the postmenopausal patient.

An accurate diagnosis is imperative, because a malignant melanoma is easily misinterpreted as a hemangioma. The abrupt appearance of any hemorrhagic lesion demands differentiation including biopsy. In 2 of 11 melanomas seen in our clinic, the lesions were diagnosed as hematoma or angioma, and a correct diagnosis was provided only by a study of the biopsy tissue (Fig. 29–14).

Although carbon dioxide spray and liquid nitrogen have been used, the best treatment for congenital hemangioma is careful observation. The lesions regress spontaneously in almost all cases, and attempts at excision may be mutilating. If bleeding is a problem, the troublesome vascular channels may be ligated.

GRANULAR CELL MYOBLASTOMA (SCHWANNOMA)

Granular cell myoblastoma is an uncommon lesion that presents two major problems for the clinician and surgeon: its gross appearance is nondescript, and its diagnosis is rarely made preoperatively. Usually, during the excision process the surgeon

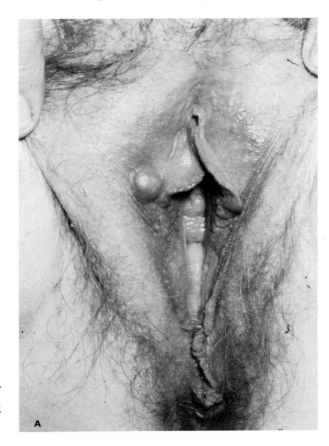

FIG. 29-13 (A) Hidradenoma of the vulva. (Novak E, Woodruff JD: Obstetric and Gynecologic Pathology, 7th ed. Philadelphia, WB Saunders, 1974) (B) Low-power magnification section of hidradenoma of the vulva.

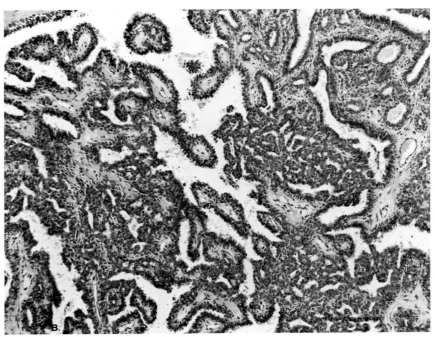

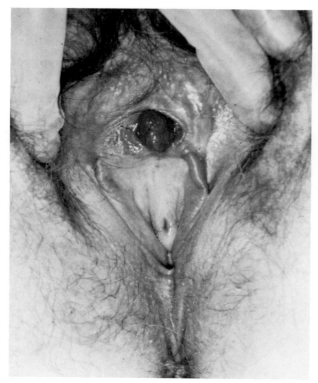

FIG. 29–14   Hemangioma of the clitoris misdiagnosed grossly as melanoma.

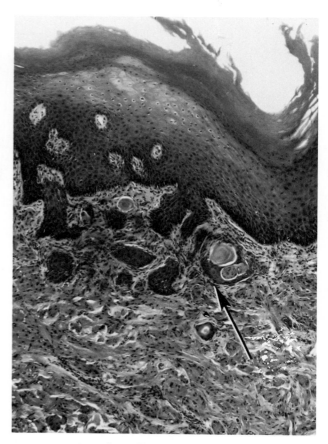

FIG. 29–15   Granular cell myoblastoma. Note the pseudo-epitheliomatous hyperplasia, nests of large pale "myoblasts" beneath the epithelium.

realizes that the tumor is not localized and that, because it has spread into the underlying tissues, total removal may not be possible. Although the tumor may recur, it is usually benign. Further excision is unnecessary unless another mass develops, suggesting increased growth.

Occasionally, the overlying pseudoepitheliomatous changes are misinterpreted as carcinoma *in situ* or early invasive cancer (Fig. 29–15). Identification is possible with recognition of the granular cells dispersed among the underlying stroma of the tumor. The epithelial atypicality results because the myoblasts are actually cells arising from the nerve sheath (thus the more correct term *schwannoma*). In a few patients, granular cell myoblastoma has been reported to be malignant, but the appearance of a second lesion at a site outside the vulva usually indicates multiple disease processes, not metastasis.

Varicocele and Varices

Varices are common on the vulva, with the larger lesions being almost routinely unilateral. As with most varicosities, treatment depends on size and symptoms. Whereas the varicocele of the scrotum arises from dilatation of the veins in the pampiniform plexus of the inguinal canal, the major lesions on the vulva are related to the pudendal veins (Fig. 29–16). Careful evaluation will usually demonstrate more extensive involvement of the tributaries of the hypogastric vein with varicosities of the gluteal vessels over the buttock.

If the patient experiences discomfort from the engorgement that follows exercise or standing for long periods, ligation is indicated, with excision of the segment of vulvar skin that contains the varices. Knowledge of the intricate vascular system supplying the external genitalia is necessary to ensure that surgery will result in long-term success and will prevent recurrences. Because drainage of the vulva is complex, ligation of vulvar varicosities is too frequently unsuccessful.

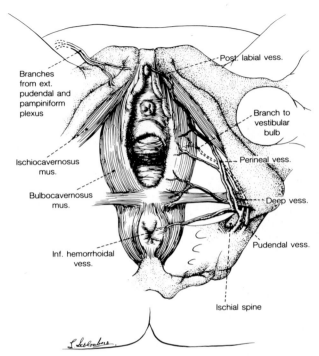

Branches from ext. pudendal and pampiniform plexus

Post. labial vess.

Branch to vestibular bulb

Ischiocavernosus mus.

Perineal vess.

Bulbocavernosus mus.

Deep vess.

Inf. hemorrhoidal vess.

Pudendal vess.

Ischial spine

FIG. 29–16 Vascular supply of the vulva.

White Lesions of the Vulva

The terms *kraurosis* and *leukoplakia* both suffer from overuse. In 1877, Schwimmer reported that leukoplakia on the buccal surfaces of the mouth was a premalignant lesion, and Beisky later described kraurosis as an atrophic lesion similar to lichen sclerosus. Since these early reports, every lesion on the vulva that appeared white and constricted the vaginal outlet was called kraurosis. And conditions as varied as leukoderma or invasive cancer have been called leukoplakia. Other terms, such as *primary senile atrophy* and *atrophic leukoplakia*, are used interchangeably and should be eliminated.

Although some physicians have suggested that they have different histopathologies, the microscopic appearance of lichen sclerosus and kraurosis is similar. A safe approach would be for surgeons to describe the anatomical appearance (*i.e.*, whether the vulva is shrunken and constricted or thickened and leathery), leaving the pathologist, familiar with both histology and anatomy, to define the cellular abnormalities.

Depigmentation Lesions

Leukoderma and **vitiligo** are terms that are used interchangeably. Treatment is not required unless the symptoms of the commonly associated chronic

CLASSIFICATION OF WHITE LESIONS OF THE VULVA

Depigmentation (leukoderma and vitiligo)
Hyperkeratosis
  Chronic infection
  Benign tumors
  Dystrophy
    Lichen sclerosus
    Hyperplasia
      Typical
      Atypical
    Mixed
Carcinoma in situ (often with parakeratosis and
      atypical pigmentation)
Invasive cancer

dermatitis cannot be controlled by local medications. The hyperkeratotic lesion, regardless of its origin, becomes whitish or grayish-white if exposed to a persistently moist atmosphere and looks like a leukoplakic plaque. Biopsies are the only reliable way to evaluate the condition accurately.

The most adequate biopsy instrument is the dermatologic, or Keyes, punch. The simple procedure can be performed under local anesthesia, can be directed at the most suspicious area, and will allow for proper histologic orientation (Fig. 29–17). The 4-mm or 6-mm instrument allows for the removal of an adequate sample that can be positioned on a filter paper or a small fragment of cucumber so that the epithelial surface will lay flat. A full-thickness section can then be prepared easily.

Hyperkeratosis

Both chronic infections and benign tumors are usually the result of dermatitides, most commonly condylomata acuminata.

In 1966, Jeffcoate first introduced the term *dystrophy* into the nomenclature of benign epithelial lesions of the vulva. Predictions about the malignant potential of vulvar dystrophy vary, but of all types of dystrophy, the one most often benign is lichen sclerosus.

Lichen sclerosus is characterized by hyperkeratosis, a thinning of the epithelium, a collagenization of the underlying tissue, and an associated inflammatory infiltrate dispersed throughout the dermis (Fig. 29–18).

Hyperplastic dystrophy is usually more dramatic than lichen sclerosus. The epithelium is thickened, the rete pegs are elongated and blunted (acanthosis), and the underlying tissue is infiltrated with chronic inflammatory cells.

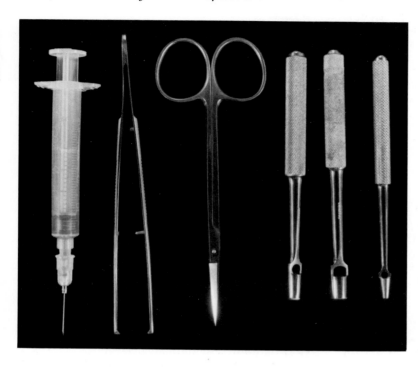

FIG. 29–17 Biopsy instruments (dermatologic punch).

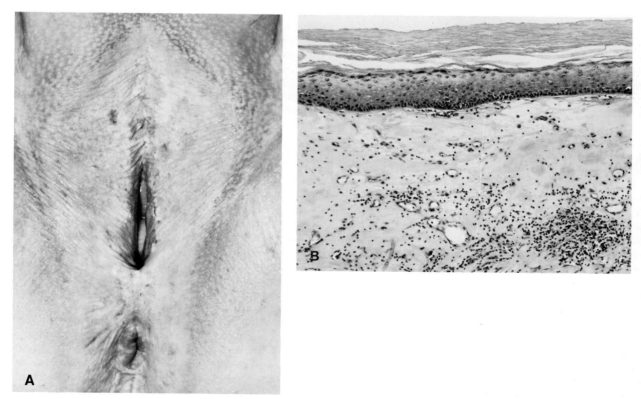

FIG. 29–18 Vulvar dystrophy. (*A*) Distorted vulva with superficial ulcerations and extensive hyperkeratosis and loss of normal architecture. (*B*) Microscopic picture of lichen sclerosus.

Hyperplastic dystrophy is a benign form of chronic dermatitis with hyperkeratosis and acanthosis. A vulvectomy should never be performed for typical hyperplastic dystrophy. The procedure is unnecessary, and may produce distortion and constriction of the outlet in addition to causing psychological trauma for the patient.

In contrast to typical hyperplasia, atypical dystrophy is related largely to chronic irritation. In addition to the features of typical hyperplasia, there is cellular atypia characterized by abnormal maturation in the acanthotic epithelium. Degrees of atypia vary from mild, with only an occasional atypical cell present, to marked, in which the abnormal cells are prevalent throughout most of the layers of the epithelium. Probably the most important feature of this condition is the very mature, abnormally keratinized cell in the basal layer of the epithelium, because the mature cells can invade the underlying tissue, even though full-thickness epithelial atypism is not demonstrated.

Dystrophic lesions are usually mixed (*i.e.*, lichen sclerosus is intermingled with the hyperplastic alterations). The diagnosis in such cases would be *mixed dystrophy*, with or without atypical hyperplasia.

Carcinoma In Situ and Invasive Cancer

The classification of white lesions includes carcinoma in situ and, occasionally, invasive cancer. In the cancerous conditions, reddish or atypically pigmented areas may coexist with the hyperkeratotic and whitish patches.

CLINICAL FEATURES, DIAGNOSIS, AND TREATMENT OF WHITE LESIONS OF THE VULVA

Lichen sclerosus may occur at any age. The disease has been noted in the prepubertal child, and it also occurs during the menstrual years. Lichen sclerosus occurs most frequently in the postmenopausal era, when the lesions are more commonly symptomatic.

During the menstrual years the lesions are usually asymptomatic. As long as the patient has no associated itching that would precipitate trauma, the malignant potential is essentially nonexistent, and treatment is unnecessary.

When lichen sclerosus is associated with hyperplastic and atypically hyperplastic epithelial changes, multiple biopsies are imperative, particularly if foci of marked hyperkeratoses are present with or without excoriation. If the biopsies reveal primarily lichen sclerosus, local testosterone ointment is the most successful agent in improving the nutrition of the dermis, thickening the epithelium,

and alleviating the symptomatology, although the treatment may not provide relief for all cases. After the presence of premalignant atypia has been ruled out by biopsy, alcohol nerve block may be used to improve the nutrition by eliminating the pruritus.

Among the vulvar hyperplasias, the most common is chronic dermatitis with hyperkeratosis. The histologic alterations of this condition are the classic symptoms of leukoplakia: hyperkeratosis, acanthosis, and inflammatory infiltrate. Except for controlling symptoms, therapy is unnecessary. Elimination of local irritants, the use of loose underclothing, and an antipruritic agent, such as hydrocortisone, are usually quite sufficient to control the symptomatology of chronic dermatitis.

Atypical epithelial alterations must be evaluated carefully, and if they persist, particularly if marked atypicality is present, either wide local excision or simple vulvectomy must be performed. Kaufman and Gardner, in a study of 100 cases of dystrophy, found that only one case was either associated with or developed carcinoma. The authors followed the lesions very carefully and made every effort to control the symptomatology. In so doing, they undoubtedly eliminated much of the carcinogenic potential for trauma resulting from scratching.

Since atypical lesions occur commonly in the postmenopausal patient, local irritation produced by associated postmenopausal vaginitis must be eliminated as a causative factor. Intravaginal estrogen thickens the epithelium and improves the nutrition of the vagina, although it has little or no effect on the postmenopausal vulvar skin, because it softens and thins the surface epithelium.

Many patients with hyperkeratosis, particularly those with lichen sclerosus, have an associated constriction of the vaginal outlet with resultant dyspareunia. Local intravaginal or vulvar applications of estrogen do not improve this condition, although every conservative effort should be made prior to any surgical approach.

Plastic surgery to the outlet (Fig. 29–19) may be helpful. By excising a triangular area of skin beneath the fourchette, the surgeon can undermine and evert the adjacent vaginal epithelium, incise the transverse perineal muscle and fascia, and cover the denuded area with the flap of vaginal mucosa. Although the suture line often lies at the anal orifice, postoperative retraction will eliminate any difficulty that might accrue from scarring near the rectal mucosa. The procedure is simple, and the use of a delayed-absorbable suture material lessens the incidence of wound breakdown, which is common when absorbable suture is used. The results of this procedure have been most satisfactory; approxi-

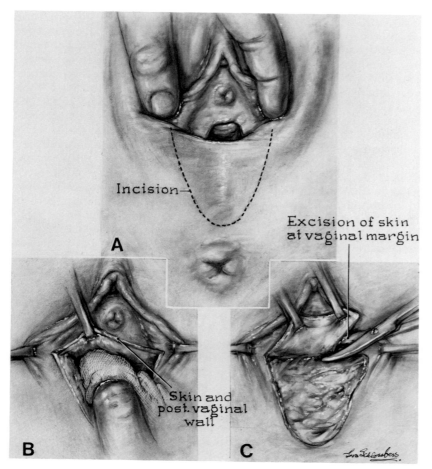

Incision

Excision of skin at vaginal margin

A

Skin and post. vaginal wall

B

C

FIG. 29-19 Perineoplasty. (*A*) The incisional line is identified. The incision must be sufficiently extensive to allow for postoperative retraction and subsequent constriction of the outlet. (*B*) The vagina is undermined to allow for exteriorization without tension. (*C*) The scarred skin of the fourchette is excised. The vaginal epithelium is preserved for exteriorization.

mately 95% of the patients are greatly relieved of dyspareunia.

Paget's Disease

The lesion originally described by Sir James Paget in 1874 has been a cause of confusion and controversy over the years, but particularly in the past few decades. The disease most commonly presents with a breast lesion that reflects an underlying malignancy in the ductile system. Most researchers have considered the alterations in the vulvar skin to represent an invasion of the epithelium by cells from the underlying malignancy in the ductile system. A possible reason why the underlying malignancy was not discovered in extramammary Paget's disease is that tissue was inadequately sectioned. Recent studies of vulvar Paget's disease indicates that there are actually two forms of the neoplasm, namely, an intraepithelial and an invasive variety.

Although undoubtedly some cases are associated with an underlying apocrine adenocarcinoma, the invasive characteristics of Paget's disease are more commonly demonstrated by foci of neoplastic cells invading directly from the basal layer, as in most skin neoplasms. The invading epithelial nests contain not only the Paget's but also the basal cells, so that locally invasive and metastatic foci contain both cellular elements.

In more than 70% of the cases, the vulvar disease is representative of in situ neoplasia and tends to remain so even though the local disease may recur frequently. One patient in our clinic had 10 local excisions of recurrences over a period of 23 years, without invasive neoplasia. Even though the appendages, particularly the hair follicles, are usually involved—as occurs when there is gland involvement with carcinoma in situ of the cervix—the lesions are still representative of in situ neoplasia, and the survival rate is unchanged. Electron microscopic studies have confirmed that Paget's tumor is of apocrine origin, substantiating the clinical picture of the lesion.

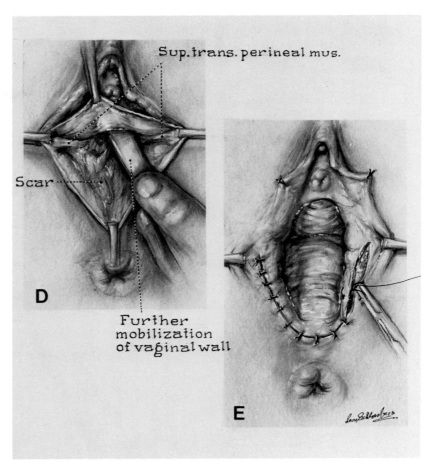

FIG. 29–19 (continued). (*D*) The vaginal epithelium is undermined sufficiently for the margins to be approximated to the skin (*E*) without tension. Occasionally, a small incision is made into the midline of the exteriorized mucosa to allow for an adequate outlet without tension.

The primary symptom of extramammary Paget's disease is itching, although some patients have discomfort and some even recognize alterations in the color of the external genitalia. The lesion is found most commonly in the early postmenopausal years.

The lesion usually appears velvety red, with dotted white epithelial islands that are grossly suggestive of carcinoma in situ (Fig. 29–20A). In some cases, the hyperkeratotic glands are the most prominent gross feature. The lesion is rarely well circumscribed and can often involve both labia without being grossly apparent. Multiple biopsies are mandatory to determine the presence of invasive disease. Since the basic treatment of Paget's disease is conservative vulvectomy, the final opinion can be made only after careful examination of many representative sections from the most grossly involved areas.

Paget's cell is identified with the use of special histochemical studies. The cell reacts positively with the mucicarmine stain, in contrast to the elements of the junction nevus. Attempts to determine histologic differences between the invasive and the in situ form of the neoplasm have regrettably not provided definite results to date.

Histologically, the vulvar Paget's cell is large, containing almost clear cytoplasm and a pale nucleus with a prominent nucleolus (Fig. 29–20B). The Paget's cell appears originally in the basal layer of the epithelium, although the basal cells themselves are intact and simply distorted by the presence of the Paget's cell. Metabolic studies have shown that the epithelium surrounding the Paget's cell is more active than is the Paget's cell. Even the most superficial layers of epithelium and the appendages, particularly the hair follicle, are involved in 75% to 90% of the cases.

Vulvectomy is justified if the lesions are multicentric or if the entire lesion cannot be evaluated by biopsy. It is necessary to rule out as thoroughly as possible the rarely found underlying carcinoma. Since the tumor is of apocrine origin, the gland-bearing areas have to be removed to eliminate the commonly involved appendages. Friedrich and others have reported instances of frequent local re-

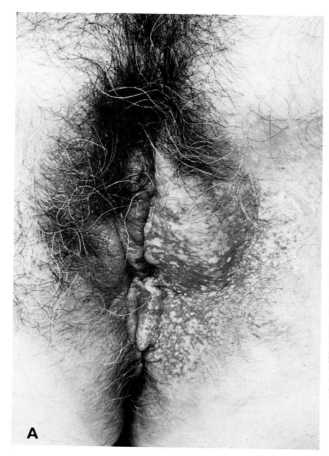

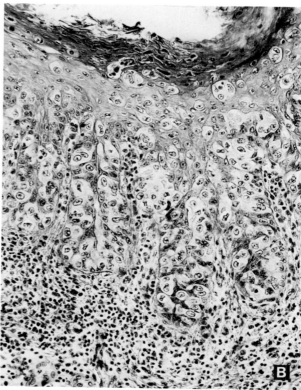

FIG. 29–20 Paget's disease of the vulva. (*A*) Gross appearance. (*B*) Microscopic appearance: note the large clear apocrine cells.

currences and associated breast neoplasia, an important relationship to watch for during follow-up of the patient with Paget's disease.

If the lesion is invasive, radical vulvectomy and groin dissection should be performed. Although the prognosis is poor for the patient with invasive disease, by adding radiation therapy, 2 of 7 patients in our clinic survived, one for more than 5 years without evidence of recurrence. In the treatment of recurrent in situ neoplasia, topical 5-fluorouracil has not been used satisfactorily in our experience, although Fetherston and Friedrich have reported some initial favorable results. Excision is still the preferred treatment; in 20 years of experience, none of the lesions that were originally in situ have returned as invasive cancer.

Carcinoma in Situ

The first two cases of carcinoma in situ of the vulvar skin were described by Bowen in 1912, when he recorded the gross and histologic features of the

disease. Bowen also stated that, although stromal invasion had not developed in patients observed over periods of 12 to 16 years, curettage and cauterization did not eliminate recurrence of the lesions. Since that time, the name *Bowen's disease* has been used to describe a clinically indolent, intraepithelial lesion that rarely if ever progresses to invasive cancer. In the past, Bowen's in situ neoplasm was considered to be extremely uncommon in the vulva. In 1943, Knight reported six patients from his experience along with another 26 he had collected from the literature. In several of the cases Knight presented, the in situ changes occurred next to invasive cancer. Other isolated examples of these uncommon malignancies have been reported by DeLima, Peterson, Robinson, and Gardner.

In 1958, Woodruff reported 13 cases of vulvar intraepithelial neoplasia and suggested that, since the histology varied from one area to another in the same section, the general term *carcinoma in situ* should be used to designate the lesion if certain microscopic criteria were fulfilled. Although the concept was not accepted wholeheartedly, clinicians are now recognizing the importance of the lesion and treating each case on an individual basis.

An increase in the incidence of carcinoma in situ was noted in a 1973 report by Woodruff and associates. Whereas only 13 cases, representing less than 20% of all vulvar neoplasia, were recorded in 1958, the current incidence of vulvar carcinoma in situ approximates that of invasive cancer. Increases could reflect: an increasing incidence of the disease; earlier diagnosis and therefore recognition of the regional nature of the lesion (cervix, vagina, or vulva); or a relationship to the increased incidence of proliferative viral lesions, specifically condylomata acuminata. Researchers have recently identified viral protein in the warty in situ lesions, although the same tests are negative when malignant alterations are present, confounding Koch's postulates. Further evaluation will show if the clinical evidence is accurate.

EPIDEMIOLOGY

AGE. Previous studies suggested that most patients with in situ vulvar neoplasia were in the early sixth decade of life. Recent investigations have uncovered a much younger age group at risk, so that the disease occasionally affects a patient in the early third decade of life.

RACE. In situ vulvar lesions seemed to have occurred in all racial groups; Charlewood even recorded cases in Bantu women. Nevertheless good epidemiologic studies have not been carried out, possibly because of a paucity of material.

PARITY. Parity does not seem to play a role in the development of carcinoma in situ of the vulva; both nulliparous and multiparous patients are susceptible to local irritants that cause the disease.

CLINICAL FEATURES

SYMPTOMS. Itching is the predominant symptom of most vulvar disease, including malignancy, yet itching was the primary symptom in only 50% of patients with in situ cancer in a series by Buscema and associates. Other presenting complaints were the presence of a lump, bleeding, or pain. In a small percentage of the cases, the lesion was discovered on routine examination, but diagnosis was made most commonly in the follow-up of cases of cervical neoplasia.

DIAGNOSIS. The best technique for early diagnosis is careful inspection of the external genitalia under a bright light, and if suspicion is aroused either by a history of pre-existing neoplasia in the lower genital canal or by the suggestion of an abnormal configuration, a magnifying glass should be used. An experienced colposcopist can describe white lesions and areas of abnormal vasculature, but as a screening procedure, colposcopy has not contributed to the early detection of vulvar neoplasia. The use of nuclear staining, specifically 1% toluidine blue and tetracycline fluorescence, has delineated foci of increased metabolic activity, but the false-negative and false-positive rates are high enough to make the results unpredictable.

Careful visual evaluation of the vulvar region should be directed at the focally white, hyperkeratotic areas, and at the more important, slightly elevated areas of skin. Atypical pigmentation, most significantly associated with gray-white areas that are even minimally ulcerated or slightly elevated above the surrounding skin, should be viewed with suspicion (Fig. 29–21A).

MICROSCOPIC FEATURES

Biopsy with a Keyes (dermatologic) punch can be performed in the office using local anesthesia. Knife biopsies often contain only the superficial layers and do not allow for the most accurate histological interpretation. Correct orientation of the tissue in the fixative is mandatory if accurate evaluation of the specimen is to be obtained. Tangential cutting may result in the erroneous diagnosis of invasive disease.

Cytology has not proven to be a satisfactory screening technique in the evaluation of the precursory cellular atypias of vulvar neoplasia. Suspicious lesions can be sampled by scraping with a saline-moistened applicator to see if any of the microscopic aberrations appear. The classic Bowenoid changes vary from one microscopic section to another, but typical sections show individual cell keratinization, corps ronds, nuclear graining, and clumping. Other microscopic variations include the erythroblastic lesion with immature cells extending from base to surface (Fig. 29–21B) and lesions that appear almost normal, being marked only by intraepithelial pearl formation at the rete tips.

MULTICENTRICITY

Multifocal areas of neoplasia involving the external genitalia and the epithelium of the lower genital canal are common; in fact, more than half the patients with intraepithelial disease in the lower genital tract have multifocal lesions between the third and fifth decades of life, which suggests an infectious origin for the neoplasia. In contrast, patients over 60 years of age with invasive or in situ cancer more commonly have unifocal disease.

When the vulva is the primary site of the lesion,

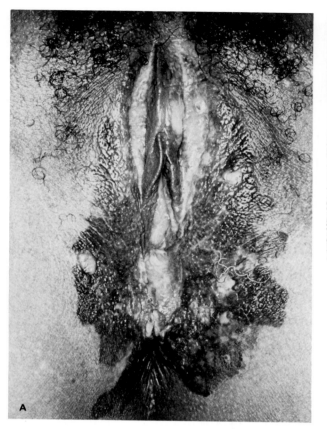

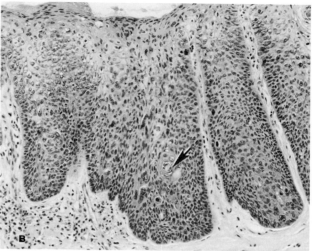

FIG. 29–21 (*A*) Carcinoma in situ of vulva showing multiple patterns, particularly atypical pigmentation. (*B*) Carcinoma *in situ* of the vulva. There is full-thickness alteration in the architecture with elongation and distortion of the rete pegs. At arrow, there is intraepithelial pearl formation. (×160)

the cervix, vagina, and perianal areas are frequent sites for associated neoplastic alterations. The combination of vulvar and cervical cancer makes up approximately 20% of all multicentric neoplasia in the lower genital tract.

The most pressing question about multifocal disease is whether invasive disease that develops from in situ lesions will arise in many foci or only in one. Only two of our cases of invasive cancer of the vulva have developed from a preceding in situ neoplasia, and both cases appeared as solitary lesions. Because the vulva and the cervix are of different embryologic origins, the tendency to correlate the histopathology of one area with that of the other can be hazardous. For example, the full-thickness changes that signal cervical intraepithelial neoplasia are not as serious when they occur on the vulva, but keratinization at the rete tips with marked atypical hyperplastic dystrophy is a most ominous feature of vulvar neoplasia.

TREATMENT AND RESULTS

Although the treatment of in situ vulvar neoplasia is basically surgical, not all patients require total vulvectomy. Except for the patient older than 50 years of age or the patient with Paget's disease, total vulvectomy is usually unnecessary in patients with in situ neoplasia. Wide local excision is usually successful following removal of enough tissue to make a careful diagnosis, provided that no other foci have been found in the area. The adjacent area can generally provide sufficient extra skin to cover minor defects. The incidence of recurrence is no greater with local excision than with total vulvectomy.

A skinning vulvectomy procedure in which the epidermis and underlying dermis are removed has been proposed for the treatment of multifocal vulvar in situ disease, but since the recurrence rate is the same as with careful local excision, there is no justification for the procedure. The skinning vulvectomy also may require taking skin from a donor site, which produces an additional scar in a patient who is usually young. Unnecessary scarring can produce constriction of the vaginal outlet and subsequent dyspareunia.

Such therapeutic measures as the use of lasers and immunotherapy have been associated with excellent results. Carbon dioxide lasers successfully vaporize diffuse areas of involvement. In spite of the success of any therapeutic approach, recurrences develop in approximately one-third of the cases.

Certain local agents have been used, with controversial results. For the young patient with multicentric foci of erythroplasia, topical 5-fluorouracil has provided a success rate of 50% to 60%. The hyperkeratotic lesion, in general, has not been responsive to 5-fluorouracil. When the treatment is successful, denudation of the epithelium is necessary, and local discomfort is unavoidable. Treatment may be continued for as long as 6 weeks, with applications two or three times daily. The advantage of using 5-fluorouracil is that the agent may seek out and destroy the foci of abnormally metabolizing tissues.

Recently an immunologic approach has been proposed for treating recurrent lesions. Once the patient has been tested to determine sensitivity, dinitrochlorobenzene is applied locally. Local application of the agent is followed by denudation of the affected skin. The agent must be used judiciously, because extensive reactions can result in the form of irritation and denudation. When local agents are used to treat recurrent in situ disease, repeat histologic study of the tissues is necessary to rule out the occurrence of invasive disease, especially in the patient over 50 years of age.

Technique of Conservative (Simple) Vulvectomy

Conservative (simple) vulvectomy is performed when premalignant lesions, such as granulomatous diseases and the more atypical hyperplasia, do not respond to medical therapy or simple surgery. Other patients who require simple vulvectomy are those with marked atypical hyperplastic dystrophy who are 60 or 70 years of age, because these women are at risk for developing invasive carcinoma. Patients over 50 years of age with extensive recurrent carcinoma in situ may need a conservative procedure, as do patients with Paget's disease of the vulva. In rare situations—for example, in an older patient with massive invasive carcinoma that is producing extreme local discomfort—a simple excision by conservative vulvectomy can be palliative. Radiation as described by Boronow may be given postoperatively.

An outline of the surgical margins is made using a coloring agent, such as brilliant green. The initial incision should be made at the vaginal outlet so that the urethral borders can be well demarcated and the vaginal epithelium undermined for a short distance (Fig. 29-22A,B). If the incision is begun at the lateral skin margins, bleeding can mask the area, making the incision at the outlet more difficult to define. When the first incision is at the outlet, a

small pack can be placed into the vagina to control the bleeding while the elliptical incision at the outer skin margins of the lesion is made.

The skin incision usually encompasses most of the labia majora, depending on the extent of the lesion. The incision through the skin is made with a knife to avoid tissue necrosis that occurs at the skin margins when an electrosurgical instrument is used. Minor vessels can be coagulated as they are clamped and cut.

The major problems develop at the clitoris, where figure-of-eight sutures must be used to control the bleeding, particularly from the dorsal vein. The second point of concern is where the pudendal vessels enter the lower one-third of the vulva, approximately at the opening of the Bartholin's duct. Branches of the pudendal vessels extend down to the anus as the external hemorrhoidals, and bleeding may be rather diffuse in this area (see Fig. 29-16).

Since the lesions for which conservative vulvectomy is performed are superficial, dissection need not extend down to the deep fascia or to the muscles of the urogenital diaphragm. Although it is unnecessary to remove the bulbocavernosus and ischiocavernosus muscles, some of these muscles may be difficult to avoid when the vulva is quite atrophic.

Removal of some of the adipose tissue, particularly in the obese patient, allows for better approximation of the skin edge to the vaginal mucosa. The incision may be carried almost to the anal orifice; however, careful dissection here is important so that the external anal sphincter is not damaged. If the disease extends onto the anal mucosa or protruding hemorrhoidal tissue, the mucosa should be dissected carefully from the underlying external sphincter, then excised beyond the tumor-free margins and sutured to the perianal skin with No. 3-0 delayed-absorbable suture. When hemostasis is achieved, the underlying tissues are approximated with No. 2-0 delayed-absorbable suture and the skin edges with No. 0 suture (Fig. 29-22C). With the use of No. 0 suture material, troublesome tissue breakdown is avoided, particularly in the area around the anal orifice, because the No. 0 suture usually resorbs slowly for a month or more. If bleeding is a problem, a small drain may be placed at the lower end of the incision, but it is better to achieve meticulous hemostasis and then use a firm pack against the area for 24 hours.

In the closure of the perineal defect around the anal orifice, it is important to evert the vaginal epithelium over the perineum in approximation to the anal orifice, rather than to suture the lateral skin edges snugly across the perineum and fourchette. Everting the vaginal skin will allow for sat-

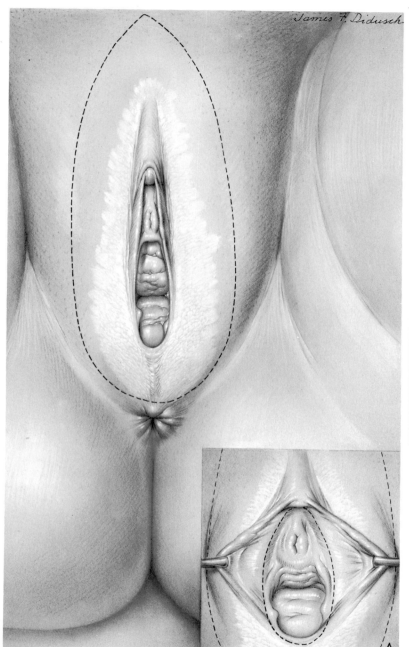

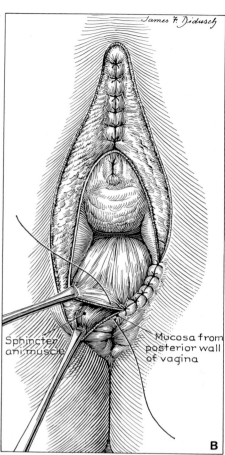

Sphincter ani muscle

Mucosa from posterior wall of vagina

FIG. 29–22   (*A,B*) Conservative vulvectomy for vulvar carcinoma in situ.

isfactory coitus, because no fissure is produced in the tightly approximated vaginal introitus.

After the tight packing has been removed in 24 hours, the entire area should be exposed. Initial application of ice packs to the operative site for 24 to 48 hours seems to provide more comfort to the patient than heat. Even better, warm air blown across the perineum is both comforting and therapeutic, because it helps keep the operative site dry, enhancing the healing process. An indwelling urethral catheter or a suprapubic catheter is used while the suture line undergoes initial healing of the skin edges. The suprapubic catheter may be maintained for 4 to 5 days, if desired. Antibiotics are not necessary for the average simple vulvectomy. On rare occasions a local cellulitis may develop, and appropriate therapy must be instituted promptly.

SKIN FLAP GRAFT. If local disease is extensive, performance of a vulvectomy can create major defects. Local epithelial flaps have been employed successfully instead of free skin grafts (Fig. 29–23), but important details of the procedure must be followed.

1. The tissues must be inspected carefully for viability
2. The incisional lines should be demarcated carefully before the operation so that the size of the flaps necessary to cover the defect is determined accurately
3. The incision must be carried down to the fascia so that the blood supply to the graft is maintained
4. The length of the flap should not exceed the width of its pedicle
5. Hemostasis must be maintained
6. The graft should be attached carefully to the underlying fascia to avoid dead space
7. Fluid accumulations beneath the skin graft must be prevented by adequate drainage and suction
8. A delayed-absorbable suture should be used to prevent early breakdown of the incision, a problem commonly noted with catgut suture
9. Pressure dressings, which may compromise the blood supply of the skin graft, should be avoided

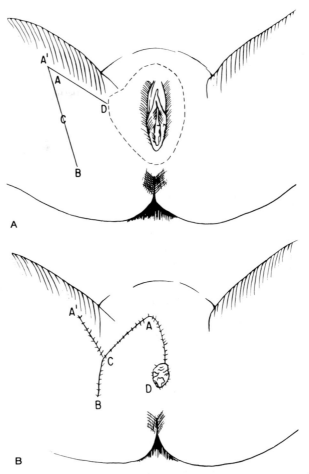

FIG. 29–23 Skin-flap graft for large defects following radical vulvectomy. (*A*) Outline of inner thigh graft site made up of triangle *ABD*. *C* represents the midpoint of the long incision. (*B*) Diagrammatic flap graft closure of vulvar defect. *A¹* to *C* represents the line of closure of the apex of the triangle.

Basal Cell Carcinoma of the Vulva

Basal cell carcinoma of the vulva differs from other forms of vulvar cancer in both treatment and prognosis. Although the tumor occurs infrequently, representing only 2% to 3% of all vulvar malignancies, the slow-growing, local in situ neoplasm presents a variety of confusing histopathologic patterns suggesting more aggressive disease. Basal cell carcinoma, previously called basal cell epithelioma, appears much like adenoid-basal (not to be confused with adenoid-cystic cancer) or like keratotic basal cell lesions. While giving the histologic appearance of invasion, the basal cells maintain continuity with the overlying epithelium and, with the exception of the squamous cell variety, rarely metastasize.

The gross lesion is characterized by a slightly elevated, rolled edge surrounding a superficial ulcer, commonly called "rodent ulcer" when appearing on other parts of the skin (Fig. 29–24A). The microscopic picture shows the deeply stained basal cells extending into the stroma from the overlying epithelium (Fig. 29–24B).

Basal cell tumors are quite radiosensitive, but the vulva is a difficult area to treat because adjacent tissues, including the vagina, urethra, and anus, will be irritated. Although simple vulvectomy has been recommended by Marcus and by others who found the origin of the lesion to be multicentric, local excision is adequate. The local recurrences of basal cell lesions can be repeatedly excised with essentially 100% cure rate. Since multifocal disease is common, recurrences in other sites are to be expected. On rare occasions, the regional lymph nodes may be involved, but more distant metastasis has not been reported.

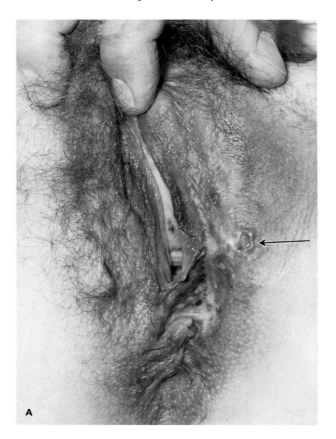

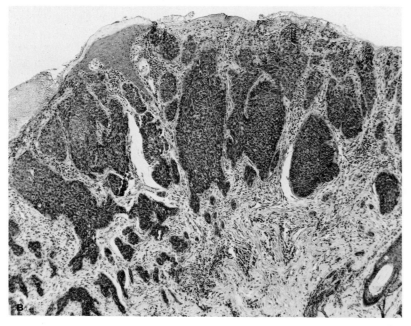

FIG. 29-24 (A) Basal cell carcinoma of the vulva. Note the elevated edge of the localized lesion. (B) Basal cell carcinoma of the vulva with deeply stained basal cells extending deep into stroma.

Invasive Carcinoma of the Vulva

Carcinoma of the vulva is one of the more uncommon malignancies of the genital tract, with a reported incidence of 3% to 4% of all gynecologic tumors. Although the vulva is the fourth most frequently affected site of female genital tract cancer—following the endometrium, cervix, and ovary—the occurrence of vulvar disease varies widely throughout the world. For example, vulvar malignancy occurs rarely in strict Muslim women who shave the pubic area frequently and who are extremely meticulous about vaginal cleansing. Vulvar disease is seen most often among women with poor vulvar hygiene and in patients who have a history of chronic vulvar irritation.

For the most part, vulvar disease affects women of advanced years; more than two-thirds of the cases occur in women between the ages of 61 and 80, with the average age being 65. Only rarely does vulvar invasive disease occur in younger patients; Hay and Cole reported a study of 52 cases of invasive cancer with an age range between 29 and 39 years. Of interest was the fact that in the Hay and Cole series, 65% of the young women (34 patients) also had tropical granulomatous disease. In general, the malignancy develops in the postmenopausal years and is associated with a prolonged period of vulvar irritation.

SYMPTOMS AND DIAGNOSIS

The most frequent symptom of vulvar malignancy is pruritus. Since vulvar dystrophy usually precedes the development of cancer, pruritus has frequently been present for months or even for years before the appearance of the carcinoma. The cancer is often painful, and when advanced, the pain may be extreme. Sometimes the appearance of a lump, an ulcer, or a bloody discharge first draws the patient's attention to the vulvar region. Another presenting symptom is burning on urination, due to irritation of the ulcerated area. When a patient complains of any or all of these symptoms, diagnosis is simple after inspection of the vulva. A nodule or raised ulceration, often on a white background, is a characteristic picture, but lymphogranuloma venereum, tuberculosis, chronic herpetic vulvitis, and other ulcerative lesions may simulate carcinoma. In all cases, a biopsy should be taken when a lesion appears on the vulva.

A question frequently asked about the diagnosis of carcinoma of the vulva is where on the diffusely abnormal vulvar skin the biopsy should be made. Because invasive carcinoma is frequently associated with dystrophic vulvar epithelial lesions, concern about missing the malignancy is valid.

Collins reported on the use of 1% solution of toluidine blue as a method of staining the abnormal epithelium. After the vulva is painted with toluidine blue, the stain is allowed to remain for 2 or 3 minutes and then removed with a decolorizing solution of 1% aqueous acetic acid. Since toluidine blue is a nuclear stain, the abnormal epithelium, particularly the areas of parakeratosis, retains the stain and identifies the suspicious areas for biopsy. False-positive results occurred in 16% of Collins' cases, but others have experienced less success in diagnosing cancer with this stain. The best method is to take multiple biopsies of the areas that appear clinically to be the most abnormal until the entire vulva has been thoroughly evaluated.

Historically, leukoplakia, a Greek word meaning *white plaque*, was considered to be a premalignant lesion. As was discussed earlier in this chapter, *leukoplakia* is a general term that is not descriptive of a specific disease process. More specific terms are now used to describe premalignant epithelial changes in the vulva. Premalignant vulvar lesions that demonstrate severe hypertrophic dystrophy have been associated with both in situ carcinoma and frank invasive carcinoma, but there is no clinical evidence to date that confirms the progression of one disease process to another.

Carcinoma of the vulva is usually relatively slow in growing, but in spite of the long time period and the fact that the growth is external, patients usually do not seek help until lesions are very advanced. Among 136 patients treated at the Medical College of Wisconsin between 1960 and 1977, 32% of the cases presented as Stage III and Stage IV disease, while 68% were diagnosed as Stage I or Stage II disease. The reasons for delay are several, but are usually related to the fact that elderly women are often unduly modest and are reluctant to consult a physician. The disease also occurs at a time in the patient's life when financial constraints are of great importance.

CLINICAL STAGING

In 1967, the International Union Against Cancer proposed a preoperative classification of the stages of vulvar cancer based on the size and location of the primary tumor (T), the spread of tumor to the regional (inguinal-femoral) nodes (N), and metastasis (M) of disease outside the regional area. This TNM classification has been in clinical use since January,

1971; the system was proposed as a more accurate method of defining the clinical status of disease prior to treatment.

TNM Classification of Vulvar Carcinoma

Classification	Description
T. PRIMARY TUMOR	
T1	Tumor confined to the vulva, 2 cm or less in largest diameter
T2	Tumor confined to the vulva, more than 2 cm in largest diameter
T3	Tumor of any size with adjacent spread to the urethra, vagina, perineum, or anus
T4	Tumor of any size infiltrating the bladder mucosa, the rectal mucosa, or both, including the upper part of the urethral mucosa, and/or fixed to the bone
N. REGIONAL LYMPH NODES	
N0	No nodes palpable
N1	Nodes palpable in one or both groins, not enlarged, mobile (not clinically suspicious of neoplasm)
N2	Nodes palpable in one or both groins, enlarged, firm, and mobile (clinically suspicious of neoplasm)
N3	Fixed or ulcerated nodes

If cytology or histology of lymph nodes reveals malignant cells, the symbol + (plus) should be added to N. If such examinations do not reveal malignant cells, the symbol − (minus) should be added to N.

Classification	Description
M. DISTANT METASTASES	
M0	No clinical metastases
M1a	Palpable deep pelvic lymph nodes
M1b	Other distant metastases

The TNM classification has proven to be too cumbersome for practical use. The Cancer Committee of the International Federation of Gynecology and Obstetrics (FIGO) adopted a revised clinical classification of vulvar carcinoma in 1976 that had actually been in use since July 1, 1974. The following clinical classification is a more useful and practical method of staging vulvar carcinoma.

FIGO Classification of Vulvar Carcinoma

Classification	Description
Stage 0	Carcinoma in situ (*e.g.*, Bowen's disease, noninvasive Paget's disease)
Stage I	Tumor confined to the vulva, 2 cm or less in largest diameter. Nodes are not palpable or are palpable in either groin, not enlarged, mobile (not clinically suspicious of neoplasm).

FIGO Classification of Vulvar Carcinoma continued

Classification	Description
Stage II	Tumor confined to the vulva, more than 2 cm in largest diameter. Nodes are not palpable or are palpable in either groin, not enlarged, mobile (not clinically suspicious of neoplasm).
Stage III	Tumor of any size with (1) adjacent spread to the urethra, all of the vagina, perineum, or anus, or (2) nodes palpable in either or both groins (enlarged, firm, and mobile, not fixed but clinically suspicious of neoplasm).
Stage IV	Tumor of any size (1) infiltrating the bladder mucosa, the rectal mucosa, or both, including the upper part of the urethral mucosa, or (2) fixed or ulcerated nodes in either or both groins, or distant metastases.

The following comparison of the two methods of staging vulvar carcinoma illustrates the complexities of the TNM classification.

Comparison of Clinical Staging

FIGO	TNM	Description
Stage 0		Carcinoma in situ, intraepithelial carcinoma.
Stage I	T1 N0 M0 T1 N1 M0	Tumor confined to the vulva, 2 cm or less in diameter. Nodes are not palpable, or are palpable in either groin, not enlarged, mobile (not clinically suspicious of neoplasm).
Stage II	T2 N0 M0	Tumor confined to the vulva, more than 2 cm in diameter.
	T2 N1 M0	Nodes are not palpable, or are palpable in either groin, not enlarged, mobile (not clinically suspicious of neoplasm).
Stage III	T3 N0 M0 T3 N1 M0 T3 N2 M0	Tumor of any size with adjacent spread to the lower urethra, vagina, perineum, and anus.
	T1 N2 M0 T2 N2 M0	Nodes palpable in either or both groins, enlarged, firm, and mobile, not fixed (but clinically suspicious of neoplasm).
Stage IV	T4 N0 M0 T4 N1 M0 T4 N2 M0	Tumor of any size that is infiltrating the bladder mucosa, the upper part of the urethral mucosa, or the rectal mucosa, and/or is

Comparison of Clinical Staging continued

FIGO	TNM	Description
Stage IV continued		
	All conditions containing N3 or M 1a or M 1b.	fixed to the bone or other distant metastases. Fixed or ulcerated nodes in either or both groins.

The clinical assessment of the status of the groin lymph nodes is used as a major indicator in individualizing treatment and in establishing a prognosis for invasive carcinoma of the vulva. The accuracy of the assessment of whether inguinal-femoral nodes are positive or negative for metastatic tumor has been summarized by Plentl and Friedman. They noted a 39% false-negative clinical error with histologically proven positive nodes and a 35% false-positive clinical error with histologically proven negative nodes. In general, clinical assessment accurately predicts positive or negative regional lymph nodes in only approximately 66% of the cases, even when performed by experienced surgeons. The experience of Way is somewhat better than that of other investigators. In comparing histological with clinical assessments, Way reports a 25% rate for false-negative and a 24% rate for false-positive clinical assessments.

The large error in clinical assessment of vulvar carcinoma means that the preoperative staging may be inaccurate in 20% to 40% of the cases that are initially classified as Stage I or Stage II lesions. The clinical error rate should be given serious consideration whenever the treatment of invasive carcinoma is planned. Friedrich has proposed a postoperative staging of vulvar cancer that is much more accurate, but it is not applicable when patients are not surgical candidates.

PROGNOSTIC FACTORS FOR INVASIVE CARCINOMA OF THE VULVA

Patterns of Lymphatic Spread

Since Mayer wrote the earliest clinicopathologic treatise on vulvar carcinoma in 1866, views have differed on the extent and type of surgical treatment advisable for the disease. The basis for recommending a lymphadenectomy of the groin originated in 1874, when the anatomist Sappey first demonstrated that the lymphatic drainage of the vulva flowed to the inguinal and femoral nodes en route to the iliac and other pelvic nodes. Groin dissection was another early treatment, based on reports from several European physicians, including Rupprecht (1893), Schauta, Kustner, and Mauclaire (1903) who advocated bilateral groin lymphadenectomy.

In his description of the treatment of malignant melanoma in 1908, Pringle was the first to recommend a monobloc excision of the vulvar tumor, including the groin lymphatics. Basset made an important contribution in his graduation thesis of 1912, recommending en bloc excision of the groin lymphatics for the primary treatment of carcinoma of the clitoris. Basset reported 147 cases of clitoral carcinoma, but an indeterminate number of these cases were obtained from autopsy studies and others were surgical cases. Interest in the en bloc surgical approach was continued by Taussig of St. Louis, who reported his initial experience in 1929 and was responsible for developing the technique in the United States. In the United Kingdom, Way achieved considerable personal experience with treatment of vulvar disease, and his description of the lymphatic drainage of the vulva (1948) was one of the important anatomical contributions influencing the treatment of vulvar carcinoma.

The use of bilateral extraperitoneal pelvic lymphadenectomy in conjunction with radical vulvectomy and groin dissection was initially suggested by Kehrer in 1918. Kehrer preferred to use two independent, low oblique groin incisions. Stoeckel, a few years before, had recommended the same surgical approach but advocated preliminary exploratory laparotomy to determine the extent of the intrapelvic and abdominal spread. Williams and Butcher revived the exploratory approach for pelvic lymphadenectomy in 1961, and the method was reported on by Byron and colleagues in 1962 and by Hacker and associates in 1981. Because spread of the disease to the para-aortic lymph nodes is uncommon in localized vulvar disease, the intraperitoneal approach is not commonly used today.

In 1963, Parry–Jones made an important contribution to our understanding of the lymphatic drainage of the vulva by extending the previous work of Way. Parry–Jones studied the pathways of lymphatic drainage by injecting patent-blue dye and colloidal iron subcutaneously into the vulva to demonstrate that the vulvar lymphatics were confined within the labiocrural folds and do not spread laterally onto the thigh. Only from the perineum were the lymphatics demonstrated to skirt the vulva onto the adjacent thigh rather than to travel exclusively along the labia majora to the inguinal-femoral nodes (Fig. 29–25). The studies also suggested that the lymphatic communication to the deep pelvic nodes occurred from channels along the urethra, outer vagina, and perineum, primarily through the internal pudendal lymphatics.

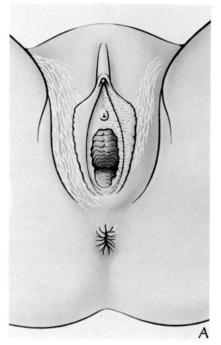
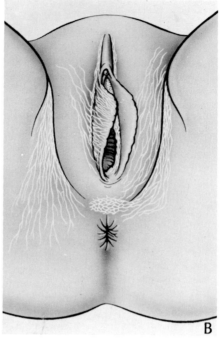

FIG. 29–25 (*A*) Lymphatic drainage of vulva demonstrating the discrete margin of lymphatic channels of the labia majora at the labiocrural fold. Periurethral and labia minora (medial surface) lymphatics may communicate with drainage of outer vagina. (*B*) Lymphatic drainage of inner aspect of thigh and perineal body of superficial inguinal and femoral nodes. (Parry–Jones E: 1963)

Studies by Iversen and Aas, using preoperative injection of radioactive technetium (^{99m}Tc colloid) into the anterior and posterior regions of the labia majora and minora and into the clitoris and perineum, showed that there are no specific differences in lymphatic drainage from any vulvar site, either to the external groin nodes or to the deep pelvic nodes. Only the clitoris and the perineum were found to have a bilateral lymph flow. Based on the understanding of the lymphatic drainage of the vulva from these studies, radical vulvectomy with groin dissection is the preferred method for treating invasive carcinoma of the vulva.

The Iversen and Aas studies showed that 28 of the 42 patients injected with ^{99m}Tc colloid showed very low, but detectable, radioactivity in the pelvic nodes removed from the side opposite their lesion, confirming the fact that a bilateral lymph flow does exist between both sides of the vulva and the deep pelvic nodes. The data also explain the occurrence of bilateral groin metastases (15%) in patients with unilateral tumors and ipsilateral groin metastasis. The work also confirms the absence of contralateral metastases in the absence of tumor spread to ipsilateral groin nodes; only 1 out of 54 studied patients had this unusual metastasis.

Depth of Stromal Invasion

The term *microinvasive* is used to describe vulvar carcinoma with tumor invasion of less than 5 mm beneath the basement epithelial membrane, but the term is misleading, and the treatment cannot be compared with that of microinvasive carcinoma of the cervix. A separate FIGO classification has not been defined for microinvasive carcinoma of the vulva. Currently, patients with these tumors are being treated more conservatively with a simple vulvectomy. Some studies suggest that simple vulvectomy is inadequate because lymph node metastasis occurs in 10% or more of such cases (Table 29–1). Although individual treatment of vulvar cancer is highly recommended, the potential for metastatic disease must be recognized. Microinvasive carcinoma, like clinically invasive vulvar carcinoma, has the potential for groin metastasis and many believe that both lesions should be treated similarly. However, some individualization of treatment for microinvasion is appropriate. If the disease is confirmed to be on one side of the vulva and does not present as a midline lesion, appropriate treatment is unilateral vulvectomy and ipsilateral groin dissection. Midline lesions have the potential for bilateral metastasis, so both groins must be dissected, as is necessary with clinically invasive carcinoma.

The histologic type and differentiation of tumor significantly influence the incidence of lymph node involvement and the 5-year survival rate. In Way's 1982 data, patients with a well-differentiated squamous carcinoma had one-third as many positive groin nodes as patients with more anaplastic tumors

TABLE 29-1   *Frequency of Lymph Node Metastasis in Microinvasive Carcinoma of the Vulva*

STUDY (YEAR)	NUMBER OF PATIENTS	NUMBER OF LYMPHADE-NECTOMIES	NODES INVOLVED	FREQUENCY (PERCENT)
Wharton et al (1974)	25	10	0	0.0
Parker et al (1975)	58	37	3	8.1
DiPaola et al (1975)	12	11	4	36.4
Kunschner et al (1978)	17	13	0	0.0
Kabulski, Franklin (1978)	23	23	5	21.7
Magrina et al (1979)	96	71	9	12.7
Buscema et al (1982)	58	40	6	15.0
Kneale et al (1982)	86	56	5	8.9
Wilkinson et al (1982)	30	27	2	6.7
Total	405	288	34	11.8

(Wilkinson EJ, Rico MJ, Pierson KK: Microinvasive carcinoma of the vulva. Int J Gynecol Pathol 1:30, 1982)

and a 30% improvement in 5-year survival. Moran and Parry–Jones found a 32% incidence of lymph node involvement among cases with well-differentiated carcinoma and a 71% incidence with poorly differentiated tumors. The experience of Podratz and associates at the Mayo Clinic was similar.

Invasive carcinoma originates primarily from the squamous epithelium (Table 29–2). Malignancies of the Bartholin's gland or the Bartholin's duct are included with carcinoma of the vulva, because the gland is located beneath the labium majus. Malignant melanoma and sarcoma are very rare in this area of the body.

Tumor Size

Tumor volume is the major criterion on which all classification systems are based. The FIGO and TNM classifications use a 2-cm diameter as the upper limit of the earliest stage of vulvar cancer because the

TABLE 29-2   *Histologic Types of Vulvar Cancer and Frequency of Occurrence*

TYPE	FREQUENCY (PERCENT)
Epidermal (squamous) lesions	90
Differentiated	75–85
Anaplastic	10–15
Basal cell	2–3
Verrucous carcinoma	2
Bartholin's carcinoma	3–5
Sarcoma	1
Malignant melanoma	3

size of the primary lesion is known to correlate with the frequency of lymph node metastases. Krupp and coworkers have recommended that the critical upper limit distinguishing Stage I from Stage II lesions be increased to 3 cm, because in their data, regional lymph node metastasis occurs infrequently in 2-cm lesions (3.8% of their cases) as compared with 3-cm lesions (9.7% of their cases). Although many clinics use a 3-cm limit between Stage I and Stage II, the international classification continues to use the 2-cm diameter of a vulvar tumor as the criterion for dividing Stage I and Stage II lesions.

TREATMENT OF INVASIVE CARCINOMA OF THE VULVA

En bloc dissection of the inguinal-femoral regions and the vulva is the time-honored treatment for frank, invasive vulvar carcinoma, and the procedure will be described in detail. The general surgical approach to the treatment of vulvar carcinoma became more individualized in the late 1960s than it had been since Basset made the initial description in 1912. Prior to 1968, all patients received a radical vulvectomy, groin dissection, and routine extraperitoneal pelvic lymphadenectomy, if surgery was feasible. Now, radical vulvectomy and groin dissection are performed without a preoperative decision to perform a deep node dissection.

During surgery a frozen-section study of suspicious groin nodes, particularly of Cloquet's sentinal nodes, is performed. If metastatic tumor is found, the deep pelvic nodes may be dissected or the dissection may be deferred. Deep node dissection is commonly omitted from the surgical treatment of vulvar cancer in order to reduce the incidence of operative and postoperative complications. Removing positive deep pelvic nodes does not offer any clear therapeutic benefit, so as an alternative, megavoltage pelvic irradiation is used as adjunctive therapy (5,500 rads, midpelvic dose). When there is no evidence of groin metastasis, deep node dissection is not recommended.

A study by Curry and associates in 1980 showed that none of their patients with three or less unilaterally positive groin nodes had positive deep pelvic nodes. The study also found that no patient had positive pelvic nodes if the ipsilateral groin nodes were negative. In a study by Hacker and associates (1983), two of three patients with three positive unilateral groin nodes had positive pelvic nodes, and five of six patients with four or more positive groin nodes had metastases to the deep pelvic nodes.

The change in treatment reflects the new understanding that deep pelvic node metastasis almost never occurs unless there is metastasis to the groin nodes. Although Krupp and Bohm found positive pelvic nodes in 4.6% of 195 patients treated with deep pelvic node dissection, only one patient in their series had pelvic lymph node metastasis in the absence of positive groin nodes. Studies from the University of California, Los Angeles (Hacker and associates, 1983), and from the Mayo Clinic (Podratz and associates, 1983) reaffirm this important therapeutic point. Whether or not postoperative irradiation is used, fewer than 10% of the patients with proven positive pelvic lymph nodes will survive for 5 years.

A still-controversial issue in treating vulvar carcinoma is whether or not a contralateral groin dissection should be performed in patients with unilateral, localized vulvar carcinoma. Morris (1977) first questioned the procedure, because few of his patients had contralateral metastasis to groin nodes where there was only ipsilateral disease. Historically, Way's findings of a 20% incidence of bilateral groin metastasis in unilateral tumors provided support for the bilateral procedure. A review of Way's total clinical experience shows that only 5% of the patients who had negative ipsilateral nodes had contralateral nodal spread. Iversen and Aas demonstrated a low incidence of flow of radioactive technetium to contralateral groin or pelvic nodes, but concluded that the main pathway for lymph node metastasis from a unilateral tumor is to the ipsilateral groin. Since the removal of deep pelvic lymph nodes with metastases does not increase the survival rate, most of the treatment protocols today concentrate on the inguinal-femoral lymph nodes and not on pelvic lymph node spread.

Feasibility of Surgery

The feasibility of surgery for patients with vulvar carcinoma is rarely limited by the extent of the lesion or the presence of metastasis to the lymph nodes of the groin. More crucial is the cardiovascular-pulmonary-renal reserve of the patient. Among 136 patients treated for invasive vulvar carcinoma at the Medical College of Wisconsin, all but one were able to receive primary surgery. Podratz at the Mayo Clinic has a comparable rate of 91%. The availability of careful postoperative cardiopulmonary and renal monitoring in intensive care units has increased the rate of operability for these older patients.

En Bloc Technique of Radical Vulvectomy with Groin Dissection

The conventional treatment for carcinoma of the vulva consists of a one-stage en bloc dissection of the inguinal and femoral lymph node regions and a total vulvectomy that includes wide surgical margins beyond the tumor. The groin incision extends in an arcuate fashion from each anterior iliac superior crest and passes 2 cm above the symphysis and inguinal ligament. The groin dissection includes the adjacent skin, underlying fat, and lymphatic channels, which lie directly over the inguinal ligament and mons pubis.

The superior and lateral incisions include the area of primary lymphatic drainage from the vulva and mons pubis to the inguinal and femoral lymphatics (Fig. 29–26). The butterfly vulvar incision of Marshall

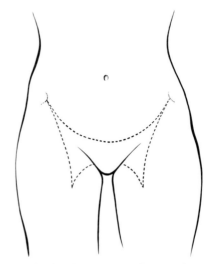

FIG. 29–26 Radical vulvectomy and groin dissection. Skin incision of Marshall and Parry–Jones, removing the area of femoral nodes without the skin of the inner thigh.

and Parry–Jones includes the skin over the region of the fossa ovalis and excludes the skin of the inner thigh. The incision extends inferiorly along the lateral aspect of the labia majora to remove all of the perineal body and the tissue around the superior aspect of the anus. The dissection avoids the necessity of undermining and skeletonizing the skin margins, which frequently undergoes necrosis due to poor blood supply. The skin and subcutaneous fat, including both Camper's and Scarpa's fascia, must be dissected to remove the superficial lymphatic channels and to avoid necrosis of skin margins.

The vulvar incision depends on the location and extent of the vulvar lesion. Parry–Jones has demonstrated that, contrary to Sappey's original description, the vulvar lymphatics drain through the labia majora and do not leave the vulva during their course to the inguinal and femoral nodes. Only from the perineum do the lymphatics extend beyond the vulva and communicate with lymphatics in the inner thigh to reach the groin nodes. The incision is confined inside the labiocrural folds and extends for 2 cm or more beyond the tumor margins; when the tumor extends laterally into or beyond the crural fold, the vulvar incision must be modified accordingly.

As shown in Figure 29–27, the gross lesion is in the region of the clitoris, whereas the extensive dystrophy is confined to the boundaries of the labium majus. All of the lesion must be removed in the dissection with a wide skin margin (at least 2 cm) from the tumor. The boundaries of the incision are marked on the skin (Fig. 29–26), with the upper incision extending 2 cm above the inguinal ligament and approximately 2 cm above the symphysis pubis. The dimensions are particularly important when vulvar lesions are in the region of the clitoris because the lymphatics of the mons are frequently involved.

The groin dissection is accomplished with two teams. This has reduced the operating time of this portion of the procedure by more than 50%. The lateral incision extends to the fascia lata, while the superior incision removes all the lymphatic and areolar tissue down to the aponeurosis of the external oblique and anterior rectus fascia. The dissection extends from the lateral aspect of inguinal ligament to the region of the mons pubis (Fig. 29–27A).

The femoral sheath is incised along the medial margin of the sartorius muscle (Fig. 29–27B) and along the lateral side of the artery, adjacent to the femoral nerve, using palpation of the femoral artery for identification. The artery is thoroughly cleaned of its sheath, the cribriform fascia. The external pudendal artery must be carefully identified and ligated because it marks the entrance of the saphenous vein into the fossa ovale, a major tributary of the femoral vein. The proximal end of the saphenous vein is transfixed and doubly ligated (Fig. 29–27C), and the femoral sheath is dissected medially as an en bloc procedure. Later, the distal segment of the saphenous vein is ligated and excised as the dissection continues toward the inner thigh.

A particular effort is made to identify and remove Cloquet's nodes (Fig. 29–28) as the deep femoral lymph chain is dissected from the surrounding artery and vein and from the tissue in the femoral canal (Fig. 29–29A). Cloquet's nodes, also called the nodes of Rosenmüller, are the sentinel nodes at the femoral ring beneath the inguinal ligament, filtering the lymphatic channels that surround the vessels in the femoral triangle. If Cloquet's nodes are found by frozen section to be negative for metastatic tumor, extraperitoneal gland dissection of the iliac, obturator, and hypogastric nodes is not necessary.

The deep inguinal chain is dissected by opening the inguinal canal from the external inguinal ring (Fig. 29–29B). The internal ring begins where the round ligament passes into the canal from the peritoneal cavity. The round ligament is excised, and the deep inguinal lymphatic tissue is removed.

If the extraperitoneal pelvic lymphadenectomy is performed at the time of the initial operation, the procedure is initiated by opening the external oblique muscle 2 cm above the inguinal ligament (Fig. 29–29C). The incision can be extended as far laterally as necessary and is continued through the internal oblique and transversalis muscles, and the iliac vessels are exposed by retracting the peritoneum medially.

Extraperitoneal lymphadenectomy includes the external iliac, common iliac, and, if accessible, the upper part of the hypogastric vessels (Fig. 29–30A). The obturator space is thoroughly cleaned. The inferior epigastric artery and vein should be ligated where they originate from the external iliac vessels, just inside the inguinal ligament, as they course upward to supply the abdominal wall. An anomalous obturator artery or vein may arise from the external iliac vessels and enter the obturator fossa along the lateral pelvic wall. The ureter is easily identified as it enters the pelvis at the bifurcation of the common iliac artery, and it should be displaced medially with the parietal perineum to avoid injury (Fig. 29–30A).

Although cleaning the deep lymphatic channels along the pelvic vessels is important, more essential is avoiding trauma to the vessel walls by excessive skeletonization. Leaving a loose layer of adventitia attached to the vessel wall can help avoid injury,

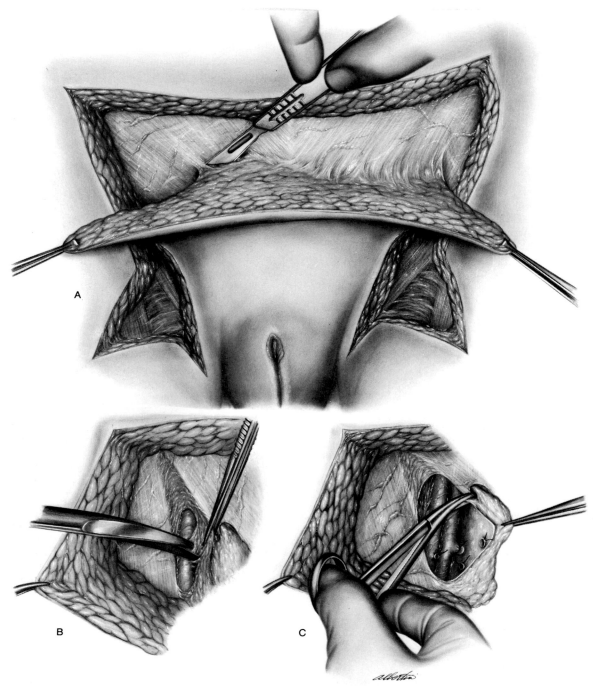

FIG. 29-27 Radical vulvectomy and groin dissection. (*A*) En bloc dissection of the groin lymphatics with attached skin and subcutaneous fat to the region of the mons pubis. (*B*) Opening of femoral sheath along medial border of sartorius muscle and the lateral side of the femoral artery. Femoral artery is cleaned of adherent fascia. Inguinal lymphatics are seen entering external inguinal ring. (*C*) Dissection of femoral sheath medially following ligation of the saphenous vein and external pudendal artery. Superficial inguinal lymph chain is seen entering inguinal canal.

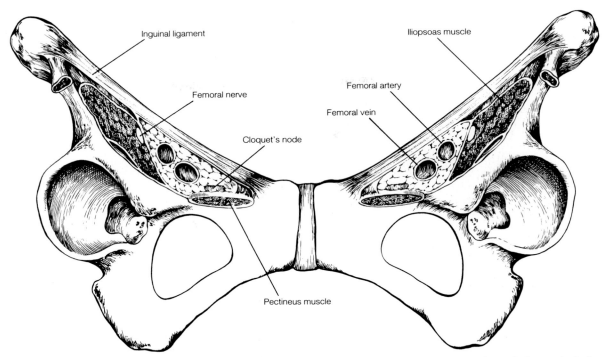

FIG. 29–28 Schematic view of Cloquet's node in the femoral triangle. The femoral triangle is bounded superiorly by the inguinal ligament, medially by the pectineus muscle, and laterally by the iliopsoas muscle.

thrombosis, and bleeding. The retroperitoneal space is routinely drained abdominally through separate stab wounds. When venous bleeding is troublesome or when there is concern for hematoma formation, mechanical suction may be applied to large-caliber polyethylene catheter drains or to Jackson-Pratt closed-suction drains to ensure adequate removal of fluid from the retroperitoneal spaces.

The external oblique, internal oblique, and transversalis muscles are closed in a two-layer fashion, with obliteration of the inguinal canal by the second suture layer. A double-layer, vest-over-pants closure of the inguinal canal may also be used. No. 1 delayed-absorbable suture is used for muscle closure.

An important step in radical vulvectomy was introduced by Baronofsky in 1948 and popularized by Way. The procedure includes transposing the sartorius muscle over the femoral neurovascular trunk to protect the femoral vessels from postoperative infection, thrombophlebitis, and possible hemorrhage, but now that prophylactic antibiotics are used, many surgeons do not perform this procedure. The origin of the sartorius muscle is excised from the anterior superior iliac spine and adjacent inguinal ligament. The muscle is freed from its fascial attachments and is sutured to the medial border of the inguinal ligament with interrupted delayed-absorbable sutures (Fig. 29–30B). The medial border of the sartorius muscle is sutured to the pectineus fascia to avoid collection of serum and exudate in the femoral space (Fig. 29–30C). Large French rubber catheters (No. 18) or Jackson–Pratt closed-suction drains are sutured in place above or below the inguinal ligament for suction drainage. The inguinal incision is then approximated by mobilizing the upper and lower skin flaps sufficiently to permit closure without tension (Fig. 29–31A). The groin specimen is wrapped in a sterile towel, and the patient is placed in the lithotomy position for the vulvectomy.

The vulvar incision is continued along the labiocrural folds or within a 2-cm margin of the vulvar tumor. The vulvar incision includes the perineal skin along the lateral side of the anus. Some conservation of uninvolved skin is acceptable, but the major portion of each side of the labia should be excised to remove the microlymphatic channels that may contain tumor emboli (Fig. 29–31A). Dissection is continued along the periosteum of the symphysis at the level of fascia of the deep musculature of the urogenital diaphragm (Fig. 29–31B). The bulbocavernosus, ischiocavernosus, and superficial transverse perinei muscles are removed in the vulvar dissection.

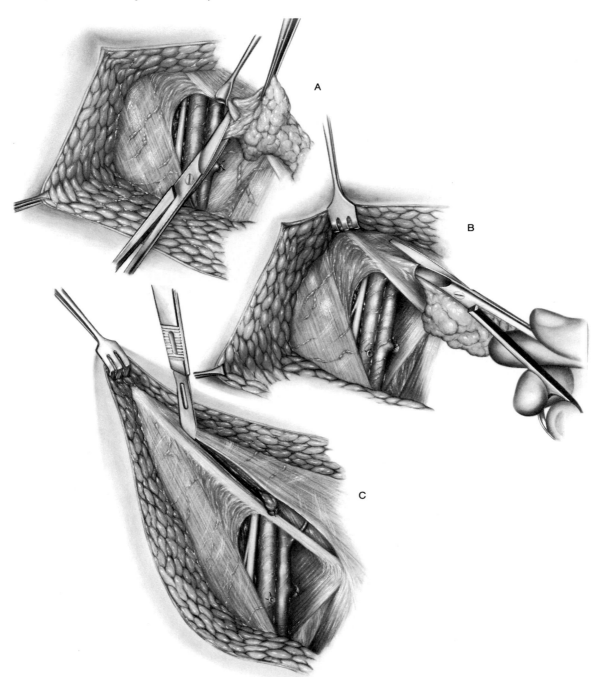

FIG. 29-29 Radical vulvectomy and groin dissection. (A) Dissection of femoral canal and Cloquet's node. The artery, vein, and nerve in the femoral triangle are completely dissected. The inguinal ligament is elevated for dissection of deep femoral lymphatics from the femoral canal. (B) Opening the inguinal canal for dissection of deep inguinal lymph chain. Scissors are placed in the external inguinal ring to open the roof of the canal. (C) Incision of external oblique muscle from inguinal canal for extraperitoneal node dissection. The round ligament protrudes from the internal inguinal ring. The inferior epigastric artery and vein (vein only shown) arise from the external iliac artery and vein above the medial border of the inguinal ligament.

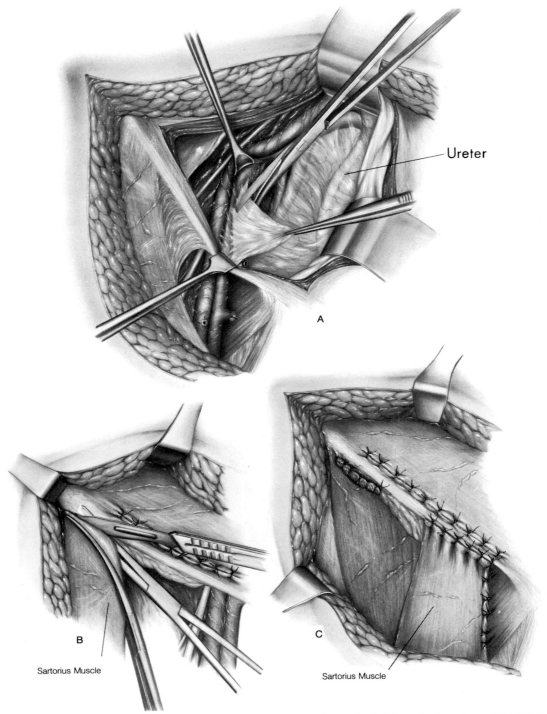

Ureter

Sartorius Muscle

Sartorius Muscle

FIG. 29–30 Radical vulvectomy and groin dissection. (*A*) Extraperitoneal pelvic lymphadenectomy. Dissection includes the external iliac, common iliac, hypogastric, and obturator lymph nodes. Ureter is reflected medially, attached to parietal peritoneum. (*B*) Excision of proximal portion of sartorius muscle at origin from anterosuperior iliac spine. (*C*) Transposed sartorius muscle over femoral vessels with suture of muscles to medial border of inguinal ligament and pectineus muscle. Abdominal musculature is closed following extraperitoneal pelvic lymphadenectomy.

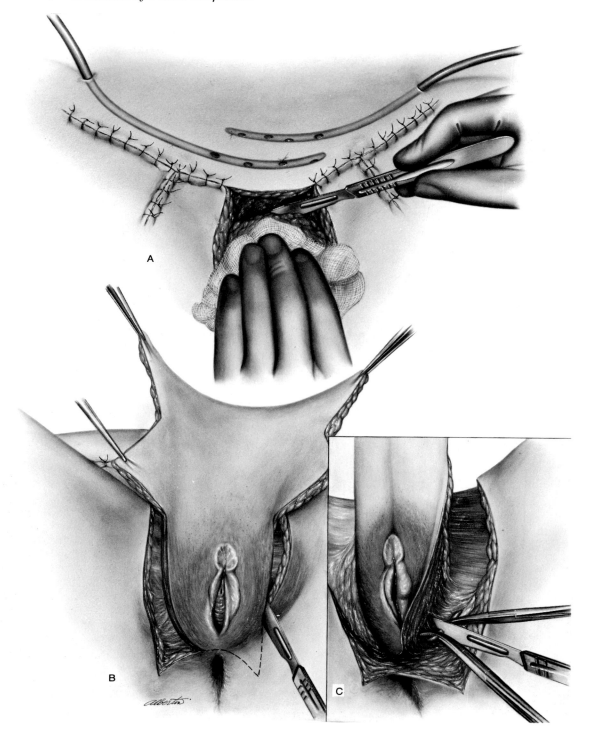

FIG. 29-31 Radical vulvectomy and groin dissection. (*A*) Closure of skin margins over groin with rubber catheter drains sutured beneath skin flap. (*B*) Vulvar incision along labiocrural fold with dissection to deep musculature of urogenital diaphragm. (*C*) Clamping and incision of internal pudendal vessels at posterior lateral margin of vulvar incision.

The internal pudendal vessels, which provide the major blood supply to the vulva, are ligated as they are identified in the dissection (Fig. 29–31C). The pudendal vessels emerge from Alcock's canal at approximately the 4 o'clock and 8 o'clock positions.

The vaginal incision is made proximal to the external urethral meatus and circumscribes the introitus just outside the carunculae hymenales (Fig. 29–32A). The mucosa of the lateral and posterior vaginal walls is undermined for 3 cm to 4 cm to form a mucosal flap for anastomosis to the perianal and vulvar skin, to avoid tension on the suture line and to avoid introital stricture. The vulva is removed after careful ligation of the blood supply to the clitoris, which can be difficult because these vessels tend to retract beneath the inferior pubic ligament. If tumor is present on the medial aspect of the labia minora near the urethra, the outer one-third of the urethra should be excised to obtain adequate tumor-free surgical margins because the lymphatics of the labia drain to the periurethral region. The outer one-third of the urethra can be removed without serious risk of urinary incontinence unless there is a prominent cystourethrocele. In such cases, plication and retropubic elevation of the urethrovesical angle is necessary.

If the outer urethra has been removed, care must be taken in approximating the skin near the excised urethra. Retraction of the urethra beneath the vulvar suture line can be avoided by anchoring the periurethral fascia to the subcutaneous fat at the lateral skin margins. The urethra should be sutured securely to the skin margins beneath the symphysis pubis to avoid retraction or formation of a hood of scar tissue over the meatus. If a hood is formed, spraying of urine may occur with voiding, which may necessitate a secondary plastic procedure to remove the hood.

Closure of the vulvar incision (Fig. 29–32B) is accomplished by slightly undermining the thigh skin flaps and the outer vaginal mucosa. The vaginal mucosa is sutured to the mobilized skin flaps of the lateral vulva or thigh with a series of vertical mattress stitches of No. 0 delayed-absorbable suture, bringing broad surface to broad surface (Fig. 29–32C). Tension on the skin margins should be avoided if at all possible. Extensive mobilization of the vaginal mucosa is occasionally required. Figure 29–33 shows the specimen after en bloc dissection.

Radical Vulvectomy with Groin Dissection Through Separate Incisions

One of the recent modifications of the en bloc dissection of the vulva and inguinal-femoral regions has been the use of a three-incision technique with separate incisions for each groin and for the vulva (Fig. 29–34). This three-incision procedure, described originally by Kehrer in 1918 and again by Byron and associates in 1962, has improved the rate of primary wound healing significantly and has also reduced the length of hospital stay. Evaluation of the technique by Hacker and colleagues showed that none of the 100 patients in their study had recurrence of tumor in the inguinal skin bridge above the symphysis pubis. Major breakdown of the groin incision occurred in only 14% of the cases, a significant improvement over the 40% to 80% incidence of wound infection and breakdown with the traditional en bloc procedure.

We have used the three-incision method with therapeutic success equal to en bloc procedure of the separate areas. Primary wound healing has also been favorable with this technique in our clinic. Lymphedema of the lower extremities has not ameliorated with the separate groin dissections, but some lymphedema is to be expected if the inguinal-femoral node dissection is complete.

TECHNIQUE. The patient is prepared for the groin and vulvar dissections in the same manner as for the en bloc procedure, using two operating teams. The lateral margin of each groin incision begins at the region of the anterior superior iliac spine, approximately 2 cm below the inguinal ligament. Each incision passes medially and obliquely along the inferior course of the inguinal ligament and terminates at a position just below the pubic tubercle, passing over the region of the fossa ovale of the femoral triangle. The inguinal and femoral regions are isolated and dissected, including Cloquet's nodes. Should an extraperitoneal pelvic lymph node dissection be warranted, the lateral margins of the incision can be extended vertically toward the head, along the lateral aspect of the lower abdominal wall.

Closure of the groin incisions is done with a two-layer technique using No. 3-0 delayed-absorbable suture to approximate the subcutaneous fat and to obliterate the underlying dead space. A large suction drain should be placed over the femoral triangle and brought out through a separate stab wound above the incision. Either a No. 18 French rubber catheter or a Jackson–Pratt closed-suction drain may be used for proper drainage of each groin. To ensure a good blood supply to the skin margins, the skin edges may be trimmed from both the medial and lateral flaps for approximately 0.5 to 1 cm each. Perioperative broad-spectrum antibiotics are given for 24 hours and may be extended for a longer period if clinically indicated. Prophylactic low-dose heparin, 5000 units, is given subcutaneously 2 hours preoperatively and every 12 hours postoperatively for approximately 7 to 10 days. Alternatively, sequential calf and thigh compression of both legs

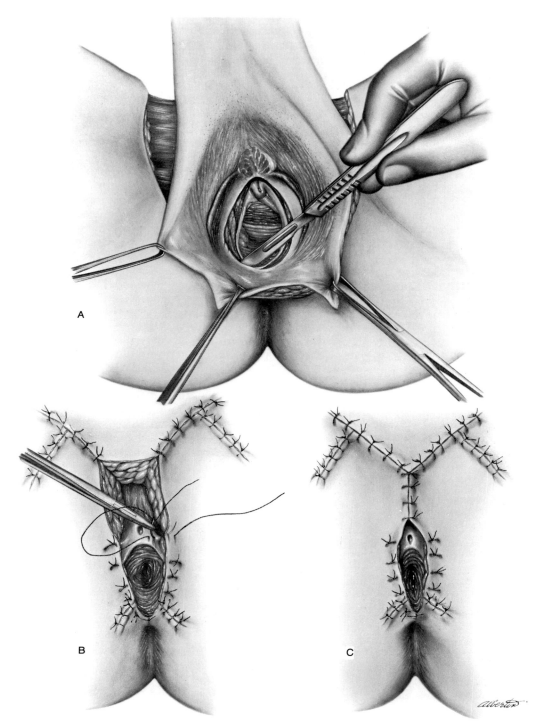

FIG. 29-32 Radical vulvectomy and groin dissection. (*A*) Vaginal incision made just above the meatus and circumscribing the introitus. (*B*) Closure of undermined vaginal mucosa to thigh skin flaps. (*C*) Complete closure of vaginal suprapubic and inguinal incision with vertical mattress sutures.

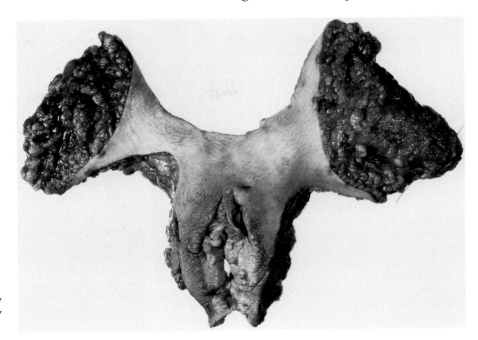

FIG. 29-33 Radical vulvectomy specimen in fresh state. (Courtesy of Eduard G. Friedrich, Jr., M.D.)

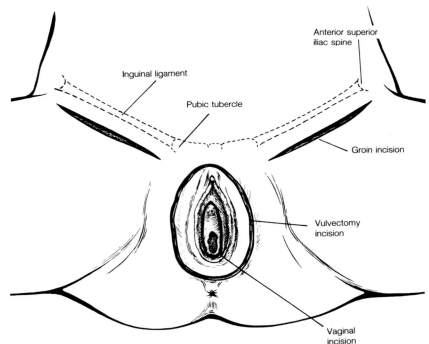

FIG. 29-34 Radical vulvectomy and groin dissection through separate incisions. The vulvectomy incision is placed along the lateral margin of the labia majora in the labiocrural folds. The vaginal incision encircles the introitus at a position that provides a tumor-free margin of 2 cm or more. The introital incision should provide a 1-cm margin from the urethral meatus unless an adjacent tumor requires the removal of the outer one-third of the urethra. Separate groin incisions are placed 2 cm below and parallel with the inguinal ligament, extending from the anterior superior iliac spine to the pubic tubercle.

may be used during and after surgery to prevent venous thrombosis.

Unilateral Radical Vulvectomy and Groin Dissection

The traditional ultraradical treatment of all stages of vulvar cancer with bilateral vulvectomy and groin dissection has been questioned for many years by serious students in this field. DiSaia and colleagues (1975) have treated patients with superficially invasive lesions (to 1 mm beneath the basement membrane) by wide local excision of the primary lesion and bilateral superficial inguinal-femoral lymphadenectomy. Only if positive superficial nodes were found by frozen section study would the cribriform fascia be opened and the deep femoral nodes be dissected. The modified procedure was used in an effort to reduce the morbidity, disfigurement, and sexual dysfunction of younger patients. None of the 60 patients treated had evidence of metastatic disease to the superficial groin nodes.

Iversen and associates and other investigators have also challenged the conventional radical treatment of patients with early, non-midline unilateral Stage I lesions. Iversen remains cautious in recommending hemivulvectomy and ipsilateral groin dissection but has used this procedure for patients with Stage I disease in whom tumor invasion is 1 cm or less with no vessel invasion. This conservative treatment is based on anatomical studies that show that the major pathway of vulvar metastasis is to ipsilateral inguinal-femoral nodes. This experience of ipsilateral groin metastasis from unilateral lesions has also been documented in 92 cases of vulvar cancer treated at the Johns Hopkins Hospital from 1970 to 1980. In all of these patients, no contralateral metastasis occurred without positive ipsilateral groin nodes.

In an effort to individualize the treatment of patients with vulvar cancer, we have carefully selected patients with mid-labial, non-midline invasive cancer of 2 cm or less for unilateral surgery. Hemivulvectomy and bilateral groin dissection are performed by a three-incision technique that separates the vulvar incision from the inguinal-femoral dissection (Fig. 29–35). It seems prudent at this time to continue to do a bilateral groin dissection despite the infrequency of a positive contralateral groin metastasis in the absence of metastasis to the ipsilateral groin nodes. Deep pelvic node dissection is no longer performed, so megavoltage irradiation is used as adjunctive treatment when there are two or more positive groin nodes. When clinical evaluation of the procedure is more complete, unilateral radical vulvectomy may become the treatment of choice for early unilateral disease.

Pelvic Exenteration for Advanced Carcinoma of the Vulva

In the infrequent case when vulvar cancer extends beyond the boundaries of the vulva to include the adjacent urinary tract or colon, ultraradical surgery, including anterior, posterior, or total pelvic exenteration, must be performed. The initial experience with advanced vulvar carcinoma was reported by Brunschwig and Daniel in 1956; from 27 cases, the operative mortality was 47%. In a survey of the literature from 1960 to 1973, Boronow found that the

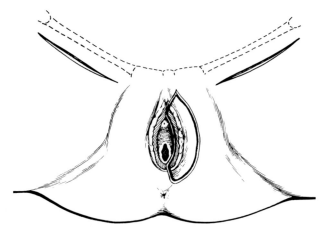

FIG. 29–35 Radical hemivulvectomy with bilateral groin dissection through separate incisions. The vulvar incision begins at the lateral side of clitoris. It continues along the labiocrural fold, laterally, and the vaginal introitus, medially, to include a 2-cm tumor-free margin, and extends to the medial aspect of the perineum. Separate groin incisions begin at the anterior superior iliac spine, 2 cm below the inguinal ligament, and extend to the pelvic tubercle.

operative mortality had declined to 10.7%, with a 5-year survival of 16%. Cavanagh and Shepherd reviewed their experience along with five other reports from the 1970s to find a collective cure rate of 47% among patients treated with exenteration and vulvectomy. In all of these cases, no one was cured who had positive node metastases.

Boronow has advocated an alternative to exenteration for advanced Stage IV lesions. The procedure includes preoperative pelvic and groin irradiation, followed 6 weeks later by a radical vulvectomy with or without groin dissection. Among 26 primary cases and 7 recurrent cases, the combined therapy resulted in 17 patients (65%) who were free of disease from 1 to 11 years after therapy. The rationale for this combination treatment seems logical because the regional lymphatic pathways of spread are treated with the megavoltage irradiation to the pelvis and groins, while the external lesion is treated by a radical vulvectomy.

In general, the cure rate from Boronow's combined therapy is similar to that from pelvic exenteration as reviewed by Phillips, Buchsbaum, and Lifshitz. Among 78 cases of pelvic exenteration for advanced vulvar cancer, including the authors' cases and those reported from the literature, there was a 48% cumulative 5-year survival rate, ranging from 20% to 66%. Since exenteration is associated with a 5% to 10% surgical mortality resulting from intraoperative or postoperative complications, and since the extensive exenteration procedure is contraindicated when there are bony or extrapelvic metastases and in debilitated patients, Boronow's combination therapy is a welcome substitute.

COMPLICATIONS OF RADICAL VULVAR SURGERY

Necrosis and Infection of Skin Flaps

The incidence of wound separation and breakdown has been improved remarkably with the use of separate groin incisions. With the three-incision technique, the incidence of significant wound breakdown has decreased from the usual 40% to 80% to less than 15% of all cases. With the reduction of tension on the skin incision and the improvement in blood supply to the skin margins, together with suction drainage beneath the incision, the problem of incision breakdown has been reduced greatly. The routine use of perioperative, broad-spectrum antibiotics has also decreased the incidence of wound infection. If after all of the advanced methods are used the incision breaks down, total healing time can be shortened using debridement and secondary closure or by making a split thickness skin graft, rather than by enforcing a long period of hospitalization to allow the wound to close slowly by secondary granulation.

Serum and Lymph Collection

Copious amounts of serum and lymph collect beneath the skin flaps in the operative site. Meticulous ligation of the margins of the lymphatic dissection will reduce the amount of this drainage significantly. Still, suction drainage collects as much as 200 ml to 300 ml a day, depending on the amount of adipose tissue in the groin and the degree of secondary infection following the operation. Large rubber or polyethylene drainage catheters are connected to low Gomco or Hemovac suction pumps and left in place as long as there is drainage beneath the skin flaps. Alternatively, a Jackson–Pratt closed-suction drain attached to the fascia of each groin with fine sutures and brought out through separate stab wounds provides excellent drainage to the groin dissection. As a rule, the drains or catheters may be advanced on the fourth or fifth day and removed within the first postoperative week.

Lymphedema

The lymphedema that usually results from vulvectomy and groin dissection is generally temporary, lasting only until secondary lymphatic drainage channels from the leg are re-established. Approximately 25% to 30% of patients have significant residual lymphedema, which is improved somewhat by the continuous use of fitted elastic stockings and by elevation of the legs to a horizontal position when sitting.

Postoperative Hemorrhage and Venous Thrombosis

Although hemorrhage from infection and necrosis of the denuded femoral vessels were formerly serious postoperative problems, they have been virtually eliminated by the procedure of transposing the sartorius muscle over the femoral vessels. The formation of a retroperitoneal hematoma from deep pelvic gland dissection remains a problem. The hematoma may localize in the cul-de-sac, where vaginal drainage can be carried out. If venous bleeding from obturator or pelvic floor veins is a problem at the time of surgery, retroperitoneal polyethylene catheter drains may be inserted and connected to low suction to avoid a pelvic hematoma.

The prophylactic use of low-dose heparin or mechanical calf and thigh compression—both during and following surgery—has reduced the incidence of venous thrombosis and thromboembolism from the lower extremities. Should thrombophlebitis or pulmonary embolism occur as a complication of hematoma formation from the pelvic veins, vigorous anticoagulation therapy is required.

Hernia

An inguinal or femoral hernia may occur postoperatively unless both canals are specifically closed at the completion of the femoral and inguinal dissection. Nonabsorbable or delayed-absorbable suture is preferable to catgut suture in approximating the inferior border of the inguinal ligament to the Cooper's ligament and the pectineus fascia. The inguinal ligament should not be transected by the deep pelvic node dissection because a postoperative hernia may result from secondary infection or from poor healing of the inguinal region.

Introital Stenosis and Dyspareunia

More than 50% of the elderly patients with carcinoma of the vulva who are sexually active at the time of radical vulvectomy confide that dyspareunia becomes a serious problem following surgery. The husbands also attest that coitus is often abandoned because of painful intercourse, while others have a general phobia of touching the genitalia where cancer had been present. Dyspareunia has been reduced greatly by advanced methods of mobilization and exteriorization of the outer vaginal mucosa. New techniques minimize the rigid circular scar at the introitus.

Even when intercourse remains possible, patients experience a marked reduction in sexual activity as a result of the negative body image that attends this type of radical surgery. Reconstruction of the vulva and perineum with the use of gracilis myocutaneous grafts after radical resection helps to improve the cosmetic appearance of the external genitalia. Although the grafting procedure increases the length of the primary surgery somewhat, the excellent functional and anatomical results are considered worthwhile for patients in whom large defects in the vulvar skin preclude primary closure. Postoperative constriction and scarring of the perineum and vulvar skin can be eliminated by using myocutaneous grafts at the time of surgery. Another procedure, a split-thickness skin graft placed over the denuded vulvar defect, is preferred by some surgeons because it takes less time than the myocutaneous flap procedure. All of these techniques have aided significantly in the attempt to preserve normal sexual function by restoring the architecture of the external genitalia following radical vulvar surgery.

HYPERCALCEMIA COMPLICATING CARCINOMA OF THE VULVA

Hypercalcemia complicating squamous cell carcinoma of the vulva was initially reported by Schatten and associates in 1958. Since that time, five additional cases have been reported in which hypercalcemia was noted without clinical evidence of osseous metastasis, renal disease, or parathyroid malfunction. The most common symptoms of this condition affect the gastrointestinal tract and include anorexia, nausea and vomiting, and constipation. Patients are frequently disoriented because of central nervous system disturbance from high calcium ion concentrations in their serum. Parathormone levels are normal, and there is no pathophysiologic evidence of primary hyperparathyroidism.

Several theories of the etiology of this uncommon paraneoplastic disorder have been advanced. A general belief ascribes the hypercalcemia to the production of a parathormone-like substance by the neoplasm. A number of tumors have been found to produce a polypeptide hormone with immunologic reactivity similar to that of parathormone, producing hypercalcemia. Epidermoid carcinoma of the lung has been the primary malignancy most frequently associated with this condition, while other less common tumors include hypernephroma, reticulum cell sarcoma, lymphoma, and epidermoid carcinoma of the head, neck, skin, and vulva.

A more uncommon finding is the occurrence of hypercalcemia in association with cancer of the endometrium and pancreas. Niebyl and associates have reported that vulvar carcinoma is the second most common gynecologic tumor to produce hypercalcemia; ovarian carcinoma is the malignancy most frequently associated with this disorder.

The hypercalcemia is abruptly resolved with removal of the parent tumor, following which the serum calcium level returns to normal, the sensorium improves, and the metabolic derangements of hypercalcemia rapidly improve. Recurrence of hypercalcemia cannot be used as a marker for recurrent disease.

OPERATIVE MORTALITY ASSOCIATED WITH INVASIVE CARCINOMA OF THE VULVA

There is still a significant mortality rate from treatment of vulvar carcinoma, mainly due to pulmonary emboli and the fact that the older patient group has a high incidence of generalized cardiovascular disease, including myocardial infarction and cerebral vascular accidents. Morley reports a surgical mortality rate of 1.8% and a hospital mortality rate of 2.1% over 40 years of experience at the University of Michigan. Since 1955, the overall operative mortality for the first 60 days following radical vulvar surgery at the Mayo Clinic was 2.2%, as reported by Podratz and colleagues. The five deaths among 223 surgical cases at the Mayo Clinic were related to pulmonary emboli, respiratory failure, myocardial infarction, and intraoperative cardiac arrest. The mortality rate at the Medical College of Wisconsin was also 2.2%, with 3 postoperative deaths among 136 operated cases within a 30-day period following surgery.

The use of low doses of heparin has decreased the incidence of postoperative pulmonary emboli and has improved the mortality rate from thromboembolism. The dosage is 5000 I.U. given 2 hours before surgery and every 12 hours following surgery for a period of 5 to 7 days. Another prophylactic method, external pneumatic calf and thigh compression, has also demonstrated a reduction of deep vein thrombosis of the lower extremities. When used during surgery and for the first 5 days postoperatively, pneumatic calf compression reduced the incidence of deep venous thrombosis from 34.6% to 12.7%, according to Clark-Pearson and associates. No postoperative deaths from pulmonary emboli occurred during the study. Venous thrombosis and pulmonary emboli have also decreased with the use of early ambulation and vigorous exercise of the lower extremities during bedrest, and with decreased cellulitis of wounds.

CURE RATE OF INVASIVE CARCINOMA OF THE VULVA

Many factors affect the possibility of curing vulvar cancer. Of the various prognostic factors, those that influence the spread of the disease beyond the vulva and the frequency of metastases to the regional lymph nodes are most important. Tumor size and location are critical. Centrally located tumors involving the urethra, vagina, perineum, anus, and rectum are known to have the highest incidence of regional lymphatic metastases. In contrast to previous reports, experience has shown that clitoral lesions do not have a preferential lymph drainage to the deep pelvic lymph nodes or a lower cure rate.

Although cure rates for vulvar carcinoma have improved, most of the favorable data are related to the treatment of patients with early disease and an absence of regional lymph node metastases. In a 20-year period at the Mayo Clinic between 1955 and 1975, Podratz and associates reported an overall absolute 5-year cure rate of 75%, compared to an expected survival of 89% based on life table analysis of control subjects matched for sex and age. When corrected for intracurrent disease, the 5-year survival rate was 90%, 81%, 68%, and 20% for stage I, II, III, and IV respectively. Local recurrences were noted in 12% of patients with stage I and 10% with stage II disease, despite the fact that the surgical margins were reportedly negative for residual tumor.

The incidence of regional node metastasis profoundly affected the Mayo Clinic statistics. Among the 175 patients who underwent inguinal-femoral lymphadenectomy, 59 (34%) demonstrated metastatic involvement in one or more nodes. The 5-year survival rate fell precipitously from 90% in patients with no node involvement to 57% for patients with a single regional node involved. A further decline in the cure rate to 37% occurred when two or more regional nodes were positive for metastatic tumor. Among the 25% of cases with bilateral groin node metastasis, the 5-year survival rate was only 29%.

Experience from 136 cases treated at the Medical College of Wisconsin shows similar cure rates. The incidence of positive groin metastases increased with the stage of the disease; 5% in Stage I, 18.5% in Stage II, 60% in Stage III, and 84% in Stage IV, for an overall incidence of 30% of positive groin nodes among the 136 cases (Table 29–3). There was a 14% incidence of deep pelvic node metastases. The corrected 5-year survival rate with negative regional and pelvic nodes was 91%, while the cure rate fell

TABLE 29-3 Incidence of Regional Node Metastases

	INCIDENCE (PERCENT)		
STAGE	UCLA* (n = 104)	OSLO† (n = 175)	MCW‡ (n = 136)
I	10.7	10	5
II	25	29.8	18.5
III	71.4	66	60
IV	100	100	84
Total	25	34	30

* University of California, Los Angeles: Hacker, et al, 1983
† Oslo: Iverson, et al, 1981
‡ The Medical College of Wisconsin: unpublished data

TABLE 29-4 Survival Rates For Vulvar Cancer

STAGE	NUMBER OF CASES	5-YEAR SURVIVAL (PERCENT)
I	1382 (30.5%)	70.0
II	1367 (30.2%)	49.1
III	1361 (30.0%)	29.8
IV	388 (8.6%)	8.2
Not Staged	33 (0.7%)	30.3
Total	4531 (100%)	46%

(FIGO Annual Report, vol 18, 1982)

to 30% in cases with positive inguinal-femoral lymph nodes. Only 2 of 19 cases with positive pelvic nodes survived 5 years (11%), and there was no case of metastasis to pelvic nodes in the absence of positive inguinal-femoral nodes.

Nearly identical data have been published by Iversen and associates from the Norwegian Radium Hospital for the period between 1956 and 1974. Among 424 patients with squamous cell carcinoma of the vulva followed for 3 to 21 years, there was an incidence of 10.5% of lymph node metastases in Stage I, 29.8% in Stage II, 66.0% in Stage III, and 100% in Stage IV lesions. Using the life table analysis, the 5-year survival rate for the entire series was 67%, with 93% in Stage I, 75% in Stage II, 50% in Stage III, and 15% in Stage IV. Only 1 of 53 patients with unilateral inguinal-femoral node metastasis was found to have contralateral lymph node spread of disease.

The survival rates of 4531 cases reported to FIGO following treatment of vulvar cancer from 120 collaborators in the 10-year period 1966 through 1975 are shown in Table 29–4.

When analyzed by the life-table method, the survival data of 3953 cases of vulvar cancer reported to FIGO during this 10-year period are similar to current cure rates from North American clinics (Fig. 29–36).

In summary, the survival of patients with carcinoma of the vulva depends on many prognostic factors, including the size of the lesion, the location of the tumor, whether the tumor is anaplastic or differentiated, and whether there is lymph node metastasis. In general, there is nearly uniform agreement that metastasis to the deep pelvic nodes does not occur in the absence of groin node metastases. Since the 5-year survival rate of 15% to 20% is not influenced by the dissection of positive pelvic nodes, there is no longer any rationale for performing this procedure. Instead, the currently preferred adjunctive treatment for the 25% to 35% of patients with positive groin nodes is megavoltage irradiation to the pelvis and groins.

RECURRENT CARCINOMA OF THE VULVA

Recurrent carcinoma of the vulva is among the most difficult of all types of genital cancer to treat. Way treated 39 patients with recurrent cancer by a variety of techniques: diathermy coagulation (10 cases), local excision (3 cases), and radical vulvectomy and node dissection (26 cases). Only 10 of the 26 patients treated by radical vulvectomy survived 5 years or more, whereas two of the three patients who had local excision of the recurrent tumor survived 5 years.

Buchler and colleagues treated 29 patients with recurrent vulvar carcinoma. Most of the tumors were confined to the perineum (18 cases) or the groin and perineum (7 cases). Recurrent perineal disease was treated mainly by wide local excision (5 patients), while three patients had radical vulvectomy with lymphadenectomy, one patient had a simple vulvectomy, and two patients required posterior exenteration. Irradiation treatment was provided by either external beam therapy or interstitial implants. Although the results were not ideal, 18 patients with perineal recurrence had an average survival of 43 months after surgery and an additional 26 months after irradiation. Two patients had no evidence of disease at 4 and 13 years.

Boronow (1982) treated seven patients with recurrent vulvar cancer with preoperative irradiation followed by vulvectomy. Five of the seven cases were alive from 1 to 3 years after therapy. Boronow's procedure is the preferred method of managing recurrent vulvar cancer, with wide local excision of perineal lesions and radiation therapy to recurrences in the groin or pelvis.

Uncommon Vulvar Malignancies

CARCINOMA OF BARTHOLIN'S GLAND

As an endodermal vestige of the urogenital sinus, Bartholin's gland is nestled beneath the bulbocavernosus muscle, inferior to the vestibular bulb. The gland lies within the fascia that separates the superficial and deep perineal compartments of the urogenital diaphragm. Composed of glandular epithelium that is arranged in an acinar fashion, the gland consists of a single layer of columnar epithelium. The duct is composed of transitional epithelium, which gradually changes to squamous epithelium at the orifice. The duct opens into the lateral wall of the vestibule just outside the hymenal ring slightly below the midplane of the vaginal introitus. Most authorities consider Bartholin's gland and its duct to be components of the vulva.

Primary carcinoma in Bartholin's gland accounts for only 3% to 5% of all vulvar malignancies. From a histologic viewpoint, the lesions may be divided into three groups: squamous carcinoma arising at the orifice, transitional cell carcinoma developing in the main duct, and adenocarcinoma or adenoid-cystic tumor arising from the glandular acini. Adenocarcinoma and adenoid-cystic carcinoma occur slightly more frequently (45%) than squamous cell carcinoma (40%), while the remaining lesions are either mixed, transitional cell, or undifferentiated tumors. Frequently, it cannot be determined whether squamous tumors originate from the vulva or from Bartholin's gland. Whenever possible, the origin of these squamous and glandular tumors should be identified, because the potential of Bartholin's gland tumors to spread to the deep pelvic

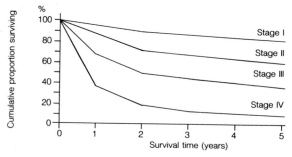

FIG. 29–36 Life-table analysis of survival rates among 3953 cases of carcinoma of the vulva by stage of disease. (FIGO Annual Report, vol 18, 1982)

nodes is greater than that of lesions that arise directly from the vulvar epithelium.

Bartholin's gland bears the name of Casper Bartholin, a Danish anatomist who described the anatomy and histology of this major vestibular gland in 1675. The first report of Bartholin's gland cancer was by Klob (1865). Since that time, several small series and individual case reports have been added to the total number of more than 200 cases.

Aquinaga collected 77 cases in 1944, Masterson and Goss added 40 additional cases to the literature in 1955, and Barclay and associates collated an additional 35 cases in 1964. Chamlian and Taylor reported one of the largest series of cases to date, which included 24 patients, and a personal series of 14 cases was reported by Leuchter and associates. Although the clinical behavior of this tumor is well documented, there are probably more unreported cases because isolated cases are rarely reported.

Diagnostic Criteria

The original criteria for diagnosing a primary cancer of Bartholin's gland were established by Homan in 1897 and included: correct anatomical position of the tumor; location deep in the labium; intact overlying skin; and presence of some elements of glandular epithelium.

Although all of these criteria may not be met by a single tumor, the anatomical site of the lesion is quite important, particularly if the remnants of the normal glandular epithelium are replaced by the tumor. It is particularly easy to misidentify an undifferentiated tumor as a lesion arising in the vulva.

Clinical Features

Patients with Bartholin's gland carcinoma are, on average, approximately 10 years younger than patients with other malignancies of the vulva. The mean age is 57 years, and the range is from 14 to 85 years. The most common symptom is the presence of a vulvar mass or the occurrence of perineal discomfort, which is frequently treated as a Bartholin's gland cyst or abscess without establishing a correct diagnosis.

The clinical diagnosis of Bartholin's gland carcinoma is frequently delayed because the tumor is located beneath the bulbocavernosus muscle; vulvar ulceration and bleeding are absent. Only when the tumor erodes through the overlying vulvar skin does bleeding occur and the symptoms become more acute. In the report by Leuchter and colleagues, 23% of their cases were incorrectly diagnosed as having a Bartholin's gland cyst or abscess and were inappropriately treated by incision and drainage or with the use of antibiotics for prolonged periods prior to the final diagnosis. The Leuchter series is typical of other reports, with a mean time of 10.8 months before the establishment of an accurate diagnosis.

Pathway of Spread

The lymphatic drainage of Bartholin's gland is similar to that of the vulva and the outer portions of the vagina. Primary lymphatic drainage is to the inguinal-femoral lymph nodes of the groin, while secondary drainage occurs by way of the internal pudendal vessels to the deep pelvic nodes. Recent studies show that approximately 37% of patients with carcinoma of Bartholin's gland will have metastases to the inguinal-femoral nodes, while approximately 18% have deep pelvic node metastases. These data resemble those for other malignancies of the vulva—in particular, squamous carcinoma—and reaffirm the fact that deep pelvic node metastases do not occur in the absence of metastatic tumor in the groin nodes. The explanation for the slight increase in deep node metastases for this disease is probably related to the late diagnosis of the lesion due to its obscured anatomical position.

Treatment

Treatment for a malignancy of Bartholin's gland or duct is similar to that for other invasive malignancies of the vulva. Although individualized treatment for this disease is important, as it is for other vulvar tumors, radical vulvectomy and groin dissection is considered to be the preferred treatment. If the disease is small and well localized to one labium, some physicians prefer to use a hemivulvectomy and bilateral groin dissection, making certain that a wide margin of tumor-free tissue is excised with the surgical specimen.

Contralateral groin node metastasis occurs infrequently with Bartholin's gland carcinoma, but bilateral node metastasis does occur when the tumor metastasizes to the ipsilateral groin nodes. Among 90 cases reviewed by Leuchter, only 1 patient of 59 who received bilateral inguinal-femoral node dissection was found to have contralateral lymph node involvement without metastasis to the ipsilateral groin. However, until a wider clinical investigation of ipsilateral inguinal-femoral lymphadenectomy has been completed, bilateral groin dissection should be performed whether the opposite labium is removed or not.

The removal of deep pelvic nodes is still controversial. Because the malignancy can spread directly to the pelvis by the internal pudendal lymph channels, Barclay and associates recommend routine pelvic lymphadenectomy as a part of the initial operation. Of the 59 cases with inguinal-femoral node dissection reviewed by Leuchter and associates, 25 included both inguinal-femoral and deep pelvic lymph node dissection. There was no case with positive pelvic lymph nodes in the absence of inguinal-femoral lymph node involvement. When metastatic tumor is found in groin nodes, an optional treatment is postoperative irradiation of the pelvis and groins. This treatment protocol is based on the fact that there is little evidence to show that resection of positive pelvic nodes has any influence on the 10% to 15% cure rate of patients with metastatic tumor to the pelvis.

The prognosis for patients with Bartholin's gland carcinoma is influenced significantly by the number of groin nodes involved with metastatic tumor. Among 90 cases reviewed by Leuchter, inguinal-femoral node metastases occurred in 37%. In the presence of negative groin nodes, a 5-year survival rate of 52% was achieved. Positive inguinal-femoral nodes reduced the 5-year survival to 36%, but five out of seven patients with only one microscopically involved node survived 5 or more years without recurrence. When two or more groin nodes were positive for tumor, only 18% of cases survived 5 years.

Although Addison and Parker consider the adenoid-cystic carcinoma to be a more favorable tumor with infrequent regional or distant metastases, a report by Wahlstrom and associates included two cases among six patients with involvement of the groin nodes. Metastases from an adenoid-cystic tumor can develop 8 to 10 years after initial treatment and may metastasize to the lung, so the tumor should be treated in the same way as all other Bartholin's gland malignancies.

Vulvar dissection for adenoid-cystic tumors should extend deeply to the level of the deep transverse perineal muscle. A tumor-free status of the deep margins of the dissection should be determined because of the close anatomical relationship of Bartholin's gland to the deep compartment of the urogenital diaphragm. When there is evidence of residual tumor in this region, postoperative irradiation is indicated.

The various treatment modalities for Bartholin's gland carcinoma have been summarized by Leuchter and associates in accordance with the 5-year survival rates (Table 29–5). Radical vulvectomy and groin dissection have clearly produced the best treatment results to date for this disease.

MELANOMA

Malignant melanoma is another of the more uncommon lesions of the external genitalia, accounting for only 3% to 5% of all vulvar malignancies, or approximately 0.1% to 0.5% of all primary neoplasms of the female genital tract. The concept that most melanomas develop from melanocytic nevi (moles) is incorrect. Although some melanomas do arise from nevi, the majority arise as de novo lesions that

TABLE 29-5 *Treatment Modalities and 5-Year Survival for Bartholin's Gland Carcinoma*

TREATMENT	PATIENTS TREATED		5-YR SURVIVORS FREE OF DISEASE	
	Number	Percent	Number	Percent
Local excision	12	13.3	1	3.8
Local excision + radiation therapy	8	8.9	2	7.7
Radical vulvectomy	4	4.5	2	7.7
Radical vulvectomy + nodes	51	56.7	20	77.0
Radical vulvectomy, nodes,* + radiation therapy	7	7.8	1	3.8
Exenteration	2	2.2	0	
Radiation therapy only	2	2.2	0	
Chemotherapy	1	1.1	0	
Biopsy only	2	2.2	0	
Unknown	1	1.1	0	
Total	90	100	26	100

* Inguinal-femoral nodes only.
(Leuchter RS, Hacker NS, Vote RL, et al: Primary carcinoma of the Bartholin's gland: A report of 14 cases and review of the literature. Obstet Gynecol 60:361, 1982)

clinically resemble nevi during certain phases of their development. An extensive discussion of the dermal pathology of melanoma is not included here; the interested reader is referred to reports by Silvers and Halperin (1978) and Balch and Milton (1985).

Melanomas may occur in any age group, most commonly in patients aged from 27 to 75 years. The lesions must be distinguished from the deep brown pattern of seborrheic keratosis and from any other chronically infected lesion. Chronically infected lesions often show pigment in the underlying tissue. Focal lesions that are hyperpigmented should be studied by excisional biopsy, not by sampling a segment of the lesion. A majority of the primary melanomas are located on the labia minora, clitoris, and introital mucosa of the vulva, whereas the majority of the epidermoid carcinomas are located on the labia majora.

An understanding of the pathogenesis of melanoma has evolved from the microanatomy of the skin. The skin of the vulva, like the skin of the body, is composed of three distinct layers: epidermis, dermis, and subcutis. Two principal epidermal cell types are related to the development of melanoma: keratinocyte, and melanocyte. The keratinocyte (squamous cell) is of ectodermal origin and gives rise to the stratified squamous epithelium and the overlying keratin layer on the vulva. The melanocyte is the pigment-producing cell in the basal layer of the vulvar epithelium and is derived from the neural crest. The melanocyte produces pigment granules in the skin and transfers them to neighboring keratinocytes. As described by Silvers and Halperin, the melanocyte is the site of pigment production, while the keratinocyte serves as a reservoir for the pigment.

The dermis lies between the epidermis and the underlying subcutis. The upper portion of the dermis contains collagen bundles and is called the *papillary dermis.* The lower two-thirds of the dermis, which contains collagen fibers that are tightly bound together, is termed *reticular dermis.*

Clark and associates and McGovern and associates have proposed a classification for primary cutaneous melanomas that is related to the microanatomy of the skin. These investigators divided primary cutaneous melanomas into three basic types: lentigo maligna melanoma, superficial spreading melanoma, and nodular melanoma. Each type has a relatively distinct clinical and histologic appearance.

Superficial spreading melanoma is the most common type, accounting for approximately 80% of melanoma cases. Nodular melanoma, unlike the other two types, does not have a clinically identifiable in situ phase. The nodular lesion apparently rises from a proliferation of melanocytes within the epidermis and rapidly extends vertically into the dermis and underlying tissues. Nodular melanoma has a poor prognosis, but fortunately it represents only 10% of all melanomas. Lentigo maligna melanoma, which accounts for the remaining 10%, and superficial spreading melanoma have a relatively long in situ phase characterized by a spread in a radial or centrifugal fashion before significant dermal invasion occurs. In situ melanomas may persist as long as 5 or more years.

The prognosis of the patient with melanoma is largely related to the histology of the lesion and the level of involvement of the underlying dermal tissues. Clark's classification of levels of involvement is as follows:

Levels of Involvement in Melanoma

Classification	Description
Level I	Intraepithelial
Level II	Extending into papillary layer of dermis
Level III	Filling dermal papillae
Level IV	Invading bundles of collagen in reticular dermis
Level V	Invading subcutaneous fat

When the subcutaneous fat has been invaded, as in the level V lesion, the potential for regional and pelvic node involvement is high, and the survival rate is low. Clark reported an 8.3% mortality rate in level II melanoma, 35.2% in level III lesions, 46.1% in level IV lesions, and 52% in level V tumors.

Treatment

The extent of treatment is tailored to the depth of invasion. In superficial lesions that extend no more than 0.5 mm in depth, wide local excision taking a 2-cm to 3-cm tumor-free margin of skin from the circumference of the tumor is considered adequate. If the disease is more invasive, a more extensive wide local excision is advocated with a tumor-free margin of approximately 5 cm.

For localized lesions, local excision is preferred to the more conventional radical vulvectomy procedure. Current experience suggests that the radical removal of regions of the vulva not involved by the melanoma is no more successful therapeutically than an extensive local resection.

Although there is controversy about the value of regional node dissection for melanoma, a safe policy is to resect the inguinal-femoral lymph nodes through separate incisions to provide some evidence of the prognosis of the disease. Although lymphadenectomy is not curative if the regional nodes

TABLE 29-6 *Vulvar Melanoma: 5-Year Survival*

STUDY	NUMBER OF CASES	NUMBER ELIGIBLE FOR 5-YEAR FOLLOW-UP	ALIVE AT 5 YEARS	
			Number	Percent
Pack and Oropeza	31*	20	7	35
Yackel et al	27	20	7	35
Morrow and Rutledge	30	14	7	50
Chung et al	44	33	10	30
Karlen et al	23	20	5	25
Total	155	107	36	(34)

* Includes 3 vaginal melanomas.
(Morrow CP: Gynecologic Oncology: Fundamental Principles and Clinical Practice, vol 2. New York, Churchill Livingstone, 1981)

are found to have metastatic tumor, the procedure allows the extent of spread of the lesion to be documented, so appropriate adjunctive therapy can be determined. Deep pelvic node dissection has no more therapeutic benefit for melanomas than for any other type of vulvar carcinoma.

Although the value of prophylactic regional node dissection for melanoma of any depth has been challenged, groin node metastasis has been documented as occurring in 20% to 45% of cases in which lymphadenectomy is performed, so there is adequate clinical indication for removal of groin nodes. Irradiation therapy has not proven to be effective in the treatment of melanoma-related groin or pelvic node metastases. The use of the chemotherapeutic agent dimethyl-triazene-imidazole-carbox-amide (DTIC) has produced tumor regression in 20% to 25% of patients with disseminated disease. Immunotherapy is also utilized in some clinics, although the treatment has been used in only a limited number of patients with only limited success as a temporary control of the disease.

Survival

Data on the survival of patients with malignant melanoma of the vulva are difficult to accumulate because the lesion occurs so infrequently. In a series reported by Morrow and Rutledge, the overall survival rate for all stages of the disease was 34% (Table 29–6).

When survival is evaluated by the level of invasion, Chung, Woodruff, and Lewis demonstrated

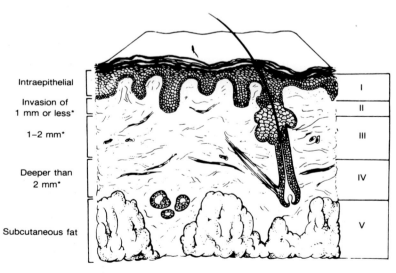

Intraepithelial

Invasion of 1 mm or less*

1–2 mm*

Deeper than 2 mm*

Subcutaneous fat

*As measured from the granular layer of surface epithelium

FIG. 29-37 Levels of invasion of vulvar melanoma. Level I (melanoma confined to the surface epithelium and pilar sheath) and level V (tumor extension into the underlying adipose tissue) are the same as Clark's levels I and V. Levels II, III, and IV are determined by measurements from the granular layer of the vulvar skin or outermost epithelial layer of the squamous mucosa. (Chung AF, Woodruff JM, Lewis JL, Jr: Malignant melanoma of the vulva: A report of 44 cases. Obstet Gynecol 45:638, 1975)

TABLE 29-7   *Vulvar Melanoma: Survival and Level of Invasion*

| LEVEL OF INVASION | NUMBER OF CASES | ALIVE AT 5 YEARS | |
		Number	Percent
II	8	7	87*
III	5	3	60
IV	15	6	40
V	5	2	40

* One patient died without recurrence.
(Adapted from Chung AF, Woodruff JM, Lewis JL: Malignant melanoma of the vulva: A report of 44 cases. Obstet Gynecol 45:638, 1975)

a very favorable result in level II lesions (Fig. 29–37) with seven of eight cases surviving 5 years or longer (87%) (Table 29–7). However, when the collagen and subcutaneous fat is invaded, only 40% of the cases survived 5 years. Among 129 cases of malignant melanoma of the vulva reported in the Annual Report of FIGO during the 10-year period 1966–1975, the 5-year cure rate was 31.8%, similar to that found by Morrow and Rutledge in 1972.

Bibliography

Addison A, Parker RT: Adenoid cystic carcinoma of Bartholin's gland: A review of the literature and report of a patient. Gynecol Oncol 5:196, 1977

Andersen BL, Hacker NF: Psychosocial adjustment following vulvectomy. Obstet Gynecol 62:457, 1983

Aquinaga A: Cancer de glandula de Bartholin. Obstet Ginecol Latinoam 2:178, 1944

Balch CM, Milton GW: Cutaneous Melanoma. Philadelphia, JB Lippincott, 1985

Ballon SC, Lagasse LD, Chang NH, et al: Primary adenocarcinoma of the vagina. Cancer 40:101, 1977

Barclay DL, Collins CR, Macey HB: Cancer of the Bartholin gland: A review and report of 8 cases. Obstet Gynecol 24:329, 1964

Baronofsky ID: Technique of inguinal node dissection. Surgery 24:555, 1948

Basset A: Traitement chirurgical operatoire de l'epithelioma primitif du clitoris. Rev Chir 46:546, 1912

Beisky A: Über kraurosis vulvae. Z Heilk (Prague), 6:69, 1885

Booher RH, McPeak CJ: Melanoma. In Nealon TF (ed): Management of the Patient With Cancer. Philadelphia, WB Saunders, 1965

Boronow RC: Therapeutic alternative to primary exenteration for advanced vulvovaginal cancer. Gynecol Oncol 1:233, 1973

———: Combined therapy as an alternative to exenteration for locally advanced vulvovaginal cancer. Cancer 49:1083, 1982

Bowen JD: Precancerous dermatoses. J Cutan Dis 30:241, 1912

Breen JL, Neubecker RD, Greenwald E, et al: Basal cell carcinoma of the vulva. Obstet Gynecol 46:122, 1975

Brunschwig A, Daniel W: Pelvic exenteration for advanced carcinoma of the vulva. Am J Obstet Gynecol 72:489, 1956

Buchler DA, Cline JC, Tunca JC, et al: Treatment of recurrent carcinoma of the vulva. Gynecol Oncol 8:180, 1979

Buscema J, Woodruff JD, Parmley TH, et al: Carcinoma in situ of the vulva. Obstet Gynecol 55:225, 1980

Byron RL, Lamb EJ, Yonemoto RH, et al: Radical inguinal node dissection in the treatment of cancer. Surg Gynecol Obstet 114:401, 1962

Calame RJ: Pelvic relaxation as a complication of radical vulvectomy. Obstet Gynecol 55:716, 1980

Cavanagh D, Shepherd JH: The place of pelvic exenteration in the primary management of advanced carcinoma of the vulva. Gynecol Oncol 13:318, 1982

Chamlian DL, Taylor HB: Primary carcinoma of Bartholin's gland: A report of 24 patients. Obstet Gynecol 39:489, 1972

Charlewood GP, Shippel S: Vulva and condylomata acuminata as a premalignant lesion in the Bantu. South African Med J 27: 149, 1953

Chung AF, Woodruff JM, Lewis JL: Malignant melanoma of the vulva: A report of 44 cases. Obstet Gynecol 45:638, 1975

Chung AF, Krumerman M: Hypercalcemia complicating vulvar carcinoma. NY State J Med 84:1763, 1977

Clark-Pearson DL, Synan IS, Hinshaw WM, et al: Prevention of postoperative venous thrombo-embolism by external pneumatic catheter compression in patients with gynecologic malignancy. Obstet Gynecol 63:92, 1984

Collins CG: Cancer of the vulva. In Marcus CC, Marcus SL (eds): Advances in Obstetrics and Gynecology. Baltimore, Williams & Wilkins, 1967

Crocker HR: Paget's disease, affecting the scrotum and penis. Trans Path Soc London 40:187, 1889

Curry SL, Wharton JT, Rutledge F: Positive lymph nodes in vulvar squamous carcinoma. Gynecol Oncol 9:63, 1980

Daly JW, Million RI: Radical vulvectomy combined with elective node irradiation for squamous carcinoma of the vulva. Cancer 34:161, 1974

Davis BL, Robinson DG: Diverticula of the female urethra: Assay of 120 cases. J Urol 104:850, 1970

DiPaola GR, Gomez-Rueda N, Arrighi L: Relevance of microinvasion in carcinoma of the vulva. Obstet Gynecol 45:647, 1975

DiSaia PJ, Creasman WT, Rich WH: An alternate approach to early cancer of the vulva. Am J Obstet Gynecol 133:825, 1979

DiSaia PJ, Morrow CP, Townsend DE (eds): Synopsis of Gynecologic Oncology. New York, John Wiley & Sons, 1975

Dodson DL, Collins CG, Macey HB: Cancer of Bartholin's gland. Obstet Gynecol 35:578, 1970

Donaldson ES, Powell DE, Hanson MB, et al: Prognostic parameters in invasive vulvar cancer. Gynecol Oncol 11:184, 1981

Dubreuilh W: Paget's disease of the vulva. Br J Dermatol 13:407, 1901

Fetherston WC, Friedrich EG, Jr: Origin and significance of vulvar Paget's disease. Obstet Gynecol 39:735, 1972

FIGO: Annual Report on the Results of Treatment in Cancer, vol 18. Stockholm, Sweden, Radiumhemmet, 1982

Franklin EW, III, Rutledge F: Prognostic factors in epidermoid carcinoma of the vulva. Obstet Gynecol 37:892, 1971

Friedrich EG, Jr, Wilkinson EJ: Mucous cyst of the vulvar vestibule. Obstet Gynecol 42:407, 1973

Friedrich EG, Jr: Vulvar Disease: Diagnosis and Management, 2nd ed. Philadelphia, WB Saunders, 1983

Gardiner J: Modified technic of inguinal lymphadenectomy. Obstet Gynecol 28:147, 1966

Green TH, Jr: Radical vulvectomy. Clin Obstet Gynecol 8:642, 1965

————: Carcinoma of the vulva: A reassessment. Obstet Gynecol 52:462, 1978

Hacker NF, Leuchter RS, Berek JS, et al: Radical vulvectomy and bilateral inguinal lymphadenectomy through separate groin incisions. Obstet Gynecol 58:574, 1981

Hacker NF, Berek JS, Lagasse LD: Management of regional lymph nodes and their prognostic influence in vulvar cancer. Obstet Gynecol 61:408, 1983

Hay DM, Cole FM: Primary invasive carcinoma of the vulva in Jamaica. J Obstet Gynaecol Brit Comm 67:821, 1961

Helwig EB. Cited by Koss LG, Ladinsky S, Brockunier A, Jr: Paget's disease of the vulva: A report of 10 cases. Obstet Gynecol 31:513, 1968

Hey W: Practical Observations in Surgery. Philadelphia, James Humphreys, 1805

Homan JH: Uber die Carcinome der gladulae Bartholini. Inaugural dissertation, Berlin, 1897

Iversen T, Aas M: Pelvic lymphoscintigraphy with ^{99m}Tc-colloid in lymph node metastases. Eur J Nucl Med 7:455, 1982

Iversen T, Abeler D, Aalders J: Individualized treatment of Stage I carcinoma of the vulva. Obstet Gynecol 57:85, 1981

Jafari K, Cartnick EN: Microinvasive squamous cell carcinoma of the vulva. Gynecol Oncol 4:158, 1976

Japaze H, Dinh T, Woodruff JD: Verrucous carcinoma of the vulva: Study of 24 cases. Obstet Gynecol 60:462, 1982

Jeffcoate TNA: Chronic vulvar dystrophies. Am J Obstet Gynecol 95:61, 1966

Julian CG, Callison J, Woodruff JD: Plastic management of extensive vulvar defects. Obstet Gynecol 38:193, 1971

Kakar VV: Prevention of fatal postoperative pulmonary embolism by low dose heparin: An international multicenter trial. Lancet ii:45, 1975

Karlen JR, Piver MS, Barlow JJ: Melanoma of the vulva. Obstet Gynecol 45:181, 1975

Kaufman RH, Gardner HL, Brown D, Jr, et al: Vulvar dystrophies: An evaluation. Am J Obstet Gynecol 120:363, 1974

Kehrer E: Soll das Vulvakarzinom operiert oder bestrahlt werden? Geburtsh & Franuenk 48:346, 1918

Knight RV: Bowen's disease. Am J Obstet Gynecol 6:514, 1943

Koss LG, Ladinsky S, Brokcunier A, Jr: Paget's disease of the vulva. Obstet Gynecol 31:513, 1968

Krupp PJ, Lee FYL, Bohm JW, et al: Prognostic parameters and clinical staging criteria in epidermoid carcinoma of the vulva. Obstet Gynecol 46:84, 1975

Krupp PJ, Bohm JW: Lymph gland metastases in invasive squamous cell cancer of the vulva. Am J Obstet Gynecol 130:943, 1978

Leuchter RS, Hacker NF, Vote RL, et al: Primary carcinoma of the Bartholin's gland: A report of 14 cases and review of the literature. Obstet Gynecol 60:361, 1982

MaGrina JF, Webb MJ, Gaffey TA, et al: Stage I squamous cell cancer of the vulva. Am J Obstet Gynecol 134:453, 1979

Marcus SL: Multiple squamous cell carcinomas involving the cervix, vagina and vulva: The theory of multicentric origin. Am J Obstet Gynecol 80:802, 1960

Masterson JG, Goss AS: Carcinoma of the Bartholin's gland: Review of the literature and report of a new case in an elderly patient treated by radical operation. Am J Obstet Gynecol 69:1323, 1955

Matthews D: Marsupialization in the treatment of Bartholin's cyst and abscesses. J Obstet Gynaecol Br Comm 73:1010, 1966

Mering JH: A surgical approach to intractable pruritis vulvae. Am J Obstet Gynecol 64:619, 1952

Moran AJ, Parry–Jones E: The surgical treatment of invasive squamous carcinoma of the vulva using a modified incision. Irish Med J 73:426, 1950

————: Cancer of the vulva: A review. Cancer (Suppl 2)48:597, 1981

Morley GW: Infiltrative carcinoma of the vulva: Results of surgical treatment. Am J Obstet Gynecol 124:874, 1976

Morris JM: A formula for selective lymphadenectomy: Its application to cancer of the vulva. Obstet Gynecol 50:152, 1977

Morrow CP, Rutledge FN: Melanoma of the vulva. Obstet Gynecol 39:745, 1972

Nakao CY, Nolan JF, DiSaia PJ, et al: "Microinvasive" epidermoid carcinoma of the vulva with an unexpected natural history. Am J Obstet Gynecol 120:1122, 1974

Niebyl JR, Genadry R, Friedrich EG, et al: Vulvar carcinoma with hypercalcemia. Obstet Gynecol 45:343, 1975

Novak ER, Woodruff JD: Gynecologic and Obstetric Pathology, 8th ed. Philadelphia, WB Saunders, 1979

Pack GT, Oropeza R: A comparative study of melanomas and epidermoid carcinomas of the vulva: A review of 44 melanomas and 58 epidermoid carcinomas (1930–1965). Rev Surg 24:305, 1967

Paget J: Disease of the mammary areola, preceding cancer of the mammary gland. St Bartholomew's Hospital Rep 10:87, 1874

Parmley T, Woodruff JD, Julian CG: Invasive vulvar Paget's disease. Obstet Gynecol 46:341, 1975

Parry–Jones E: Lymphatics of the vulva. J Obstet Gynaecol Br Comm 70:751, 1963

Phillips B, Buchsbaum HJ, Lifshitz S: Pelvic exenteration for vulvovaginal carcinoma. Am J Obstet Gynecol 141:1038, 1981

Plentl AA, Friedman EA: Lymphatic System of the Female Genitalia. Philadelphia, WB Saunders, 1971

Podratz KC, Symmonds RE, O'Brien PC, et al: Melanoma of the vulva. An update. Gynecol Oncol 16:153, 1983

Podratz KC, Symmonds RE, Taylor WF, et al: Carcinoma of the vulva: Analysis of treatment and survival. Obstet Gynecol 61:63, 1983

Pringle JH: A method of operation in cases of melanotic tumours of the skin. Edin Med J 23:496, 1908

Purola E, Widholm O: Primary carcinoma of the Bartholin's gland: Report on two cases. Acta Obstet Gynecol Scan 45:205, 1966

Rutledge FN, Boronow RC, Wharton JT: Gynecologic Oncology. New York, John Wiley and Sons, 1976

Sappy C: Traite d'Anatomie, Physiologie et Pathologie des Vaisseaux Lymphatiques, Consideres Chez l'Homme et les Vertebres. Delahaye, Paris, 1874

Schatten WE, Ship AG, Pieper WJ, et al: Syndrome resembling hyperparathyroidism associated with squamous cell carcinoma. Ann Surg 148:890, 1958

Schueller EF: Basal cell cancer of the vulva. Am J Obstet Gynecol 93:199, 1965

Schwimmer E: Die idiopathischen schlim haurt der mundhohle. Vrtljscher Dermatol Syph 9-10-510, 1877

Silvers DN, Halperin AJ: Cutaneous and vulvar melanoma: An update. Clin Obstet Gynecol 21:1117, 1978

Stoeckel W: Wie lassen sich die Dauerresultate bei der Operation des Vulvakarzinoms verbessern., Zbl Gynak 36:1102, 1912

Tancer ML: Bartholin's cysts paraurethral lesions. Clin Obstet Gynecol 8:982, 1965

Tashjian AH, Levine L, Munson PL: Immunochemical identification of parathyroid hormone in non-parathyroid neoplasms associated with hypercalcemia. J Exp Med 119:467, 1964

Taussig FJ: Leukoplakic vulvitis and cancer of the vulva (etiology, histopathology, treatment, five-year results). Trans Am Gynecol Soc 54:60, 1929

———: Diseases of the vulva. New York, Appleton–Century–Crofts, 1931

Trelford JD, Deos PH: Bartholin's gland carcinomas: Five cases. Gynecol Oncol 4:212, 1976

Tsukada Y, Lopez RG, Pickren JW: Paget's disease of the vulva. Obstet Gynecol 45:73, 1975

Wahlstrom T, Vesterinen E, Saksela E: Primary carcinoma of Bartholin's gland: A morphological and clinical study of 6 cases including a transitional cell carcinoma. Gynecol Oncol 6:354, 1978

Way S: The anatomy of the lymphatic drainage of the vulva and its influence on the radical operation for carcinoma. Ann R Coll Surg Engl 3:187, 1948

———: Carcinoma of the vulva. In Deeley TJ (ed): Modern Radiotherapy: Gynecological Cancer. London, Butterworths, 1971

———: Malignant diseases of the vulva. New York, Churchill Livingston, 1982

Way S, Benedet MD: Involvement of inguinal lymph nodes in carcinoma of the vulva. Gynecol Oncol 119:119, 1973

Wharton JT: Carcinoma of the vagina and urethra. In Rovinsky JJ (ed): Obstetrics and Gynecology, vol 2, sect 4. Hagerstown, Harper & Row, 1972

———: Carcinoma of the vagina. In Rutledge F, Boronow RC, Wharton JT (eds): Gynecologic Oncology. New York, John Wiley & Sons, 1976

Wharton JT, Gallager S, Rutledge FN: Microinvasive carcinoma of the vulva. Am J Obstet Gynecol 118:159, 1974

Wharton LR, Kearns W: Diverticulum of the female urethra. J Urol 63:1063, 1950

Wharton LR, Jr, Everett HS: Primary malignant Bartholin gland tumors. Obstet Gynecol Survey 6:1, 1951

Wheeless CR, Jr, McGibbon B, Dorsey JH, et al: Gracilis myocutaneous flap in reconstruction of the vulva and female perineum. Obstet Gynecol 54:97, 1979

Wilkinson EJ, Rico MJ, Pierson KK: Microinvasive carcinoma of the vulva. Int J Gynecol Path 1:30, 1982

Williams K, Butcher HR, Jr: A technique for inguinal and iliac lymphadenectomy. Am Surg 27:55, 1961

Woodruff JD, Julian C, Paray T, et al: The contemporary challenge of carcinoma in situ of the vulva. Am J Obstet Gynecol 115:677, 1973

Woodruff JD, Richardson EH, Jr: Malignant vulvar Paget's disease. Obstet Gynecol 10:10, 1957

Woodruff JD, Thompson B: Local alcohol injection in the treatment of vulvar pruritus. Obstet Gynecol 40:18, 1972

Woodruff JD, Hildebrandt EE: Carcinoma in situ of the vulva. Obstet Gynecol 12:414, 1958

Yackel DB, Symmonds RE, Kempers RD: Melanoma of the vulva. Obstet Gynecol 35:625, 1970

Chapter 30

Surgical Conditions of the Vagina and Urethra

THE VAGINA

Imperforate Hymen and Its Complications

Although variations in hymenal development occur, complete failure to form an orifice is rare. The hymen shown in Figure 30–1 had only a small pinhead opening, but that was sufficient to permit the entrance of sperm, and the patient was pregnant. Many cases of imperforate hymen are not reported.

SYMPTOMS OF IMPERFORATE HYMEN

If an imperforate hymen is noticed before puberty, the condition can be treated before symptoms develop. An observant mother will occasionally notice the absence of an orifice in her child's hymen before puberty, when the condition is entirely asymptomatic. When the hymen is incised, the vagina will be found to contain mucoid fluid, which results from accumulated cervical secretion.

Most patients are brought to the gynecologist at 13 to 15 years of age when their mothers begin to notice symptoms and the girls appear not to have begun menstruating. The symptoms that appear after the onset of puberty are due to the accumulation of menstrual blood. The blood of the first period or two is collected in the vagina. The vagina can hold blood from one or two cycles without undue stretching and with no other symptoms. Accumulation of menstrual blood in the vagina is termed *hematocolpos*. The patient may feel a little fatigue and have crampy discomfort suggesting menstruation, but no blood appears at the vaginal outlet.

As menstruation recurs, the vagina becomes greatly overdistended, and the cervical canal also dilates. Hematometra, which is the accumulation of menstrual blood in the uterine cavity, may form. When the intrauterine pressure reaches a certain point, there is retrograde passage of blood into the tubes, forming hematosalpinx. Adhesion formation within or at the fimbriated end of the tubes can seal them, and little or no blood may enter the peritoneal cavity. In some cases, blood passes freely into the peritoneal cavity, forming hematoperitoneum (Fig. 30–2).

The most common symptoms caused by vaginal overdistention are lower abdominal pain, discomfort in the pelvis, and pain in the lower back. Pain is often aggravated on defecation. Urination can also be difficult, because pressure of the distended vagina on the urethra may compress the urethra and prevent emptying of the bladder. Cramplike pains recur in the suprapubic region, along with the common urologic symptoms of dysuria, frequency, and urgency. Overflow incontinence may develop eventually.

When the patient is examined, a tender mass is often palpable suprapubicly, the result of uterine enlargement and upward displacement, or bladder distention, or both. If hematoperitoneum occurs, the irritation of the free blood may cause the patient to experience all the symptoms and demonstrate signs of peritonitis. Protrusion of the hymen is usually visible; in some instances the protrusion is massive and dark in color, because the occult blood shows through the stretched mucous membrane.

At the Johns Hopkins Hospital, 22 patients with an imperforate hymen were operated on between

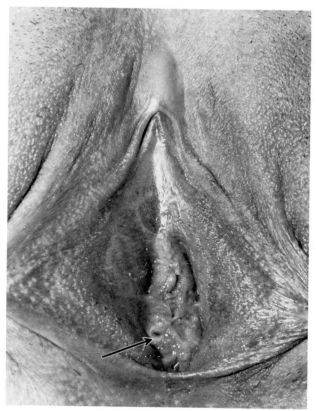

FIG. 30–1 Hymen that is almost imperforate. The pinhead-sized opening was sufficient to permit pregnancy.

1945 and 1981. The mean age at surgical correction was 14.7 years. Associated anomalies, including urinary tract anomalies, were rare. Thirteen patients subsequently conceived and 10 patients were noted to have living children at the time of the report. The greater distensibility of the vagina in adolescence probably protects patients with imperforate hymen from retrograde menstruation and subsequent development of pelvic endometriosis as long as the diagnosis is made reasonably early.

TREATMENT OF IMPERFORATE HYMEN

When an imperforate hymen is discovered before puberty, the hymenal membrane is simply incised, preferably at 2, 4, 8 and 10 o'clock. The quadrants of the hymen are then excised and the mucosal margins are approximated with fine delayed-absorbable suture (Fig. 30–3). If hematocolpos has already developed (see Fig. 30–2) all unnecessary intrauterine instrumentation should be avoided,

because of the risk of perforating the thin over-stretched uterine wall. To prevent scarring and stenosis, which could result in dyspareunia, the hymenal tissue should not be excised too close to the vaginal mucosa.

Nothing more is needed surgically unless the uterine mass does not regress within 2 to 3 weeks. Then inspection and dilatation of the cervix should be performed to make certain that drainage from the uterus is satisfactory.

Carcinoma of the Vagina

Carcinoma of the vagina is uncommon, occurring in only 2% of all patients with gynecologic cancer, and usually appearing between the ages of 55 and 65. Vaginal carcinoma results more frequently from metastases of tumors in the cervix and vulva than from conditions originating in the vagina, so differentiation is important. Lesions that encroach on the outer vagina from the vulva must also be separated from lesions originating in the vaginal canal.

FIGO has agreed on the following criteria for the classification of vaginal cancer: a vaginal growth that has extended to the portio of the cervix and has reached the area of the external os should always be considered the result of carcinoma of the cervix. A vulvar growth that has extended to the vagina should be classified as carcinoma of the vulva. A vaginal growth that is limited to the urethra should be classified separately as carcinoma of the urethra. The criteria for the definition of primary carcinoma of the vagina were established after many clinicians reported the recurrence of vaginal lesions following treatment of carcinoma in situ of the cervix. Tumors recurred in 1% to 6% of cases. Today, the extension of carcinoma in situ and invasive carcinoma of the cervix to the vaginal fornices or upper vagina can be easily excluded with the use of colposcopy. Clinicians now satisfy the staging criteria for the diagnosis of primary carcinoma of the vagina by showing a histologically negative cervix, urethra, vulva, and endometrium.

The clinical stages of carcinoma of the vagina agreed upon by FIGO are listed in Table 30–1. In 1973, Perez proposed that Stage II be divided into Stage IIa and IIb to provide a more accurate definition of the extent of the lesion. In the proposed modified FIGO classification, Stage IIa includes subvaginal infiltration not extending into the parametrial or paravaginal regions, while Stage IIb includes parametrial or paravaginal infiltration not extending to the pelvic wall.

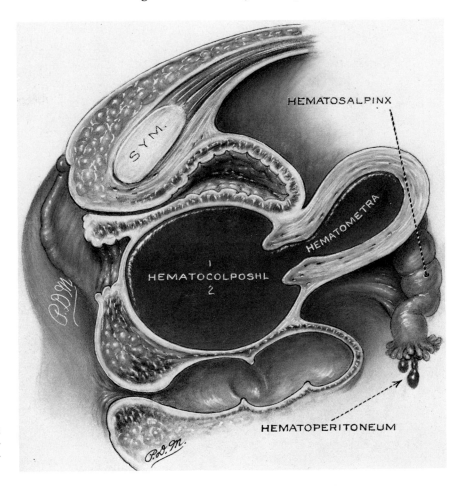

FIG. 30–2 Imperforate hymen with consequent hematocolpos, hematometra, hematosalpinx, and hematoperitoneum.

SYMPTOMS OF VAGINAL CARCINOMA

Unfortunately, the diagnosis of vaginal tumors is frequently delayed due to the lack of early symptoms. Progressive vaginal discharge and postmenopausal bleeding are the most frequent symptoms. Postcoital bleeding is not usually a common clinical feature of this tumor in the early stages, possibly because sexual activity is decreased in the population in which the tumor occurs, and bleeding does not occur until the surface epithelium has become ulcerated. The tumor will only be detected in the early stages if vaginal cytology is routinely performed for patients between the ages of 60 and 70.

The symptoms of vaginal carcinoma resemble those of cervical carcinoma except that obvious bleeding occurs later than with neoplasms on the cervix. The overt bleeding eventually forces the patient to see her physician for diagnosis. Pain is an uncommon symptom, associated only with advanced stages. Bladder symptoms occur late in the disease when the tumor has involved the anterior vaginal septum and has encroached on or invaded the base of the bladder or urethra.

HISTOPATHOLOGY OF VAGINAL CARCINOMA

Squamous carcinoma is the most common histologic type of vaginal tumor; 88% to 90% of all primary vaginal cancers are of this type. Adenocarcinoma, including DES-related cases, represents approximately 4% to 5% of vaginal cancers. Uncommon lesions such as sarcoma, including leiomyosarcoma and sarcoma botryoides, account for 2% to 3% of vaginal lesions, while melanoma is an infrequent neoplasm of the vagina (Table 30–2). Such rare tumors as endodermal sinus tumors or neoplasms originating in embryologic cloacal remnants may

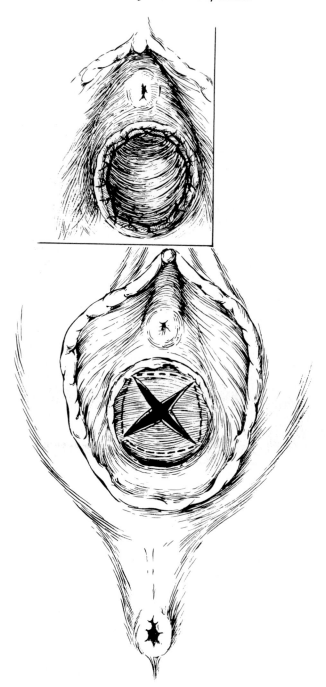

FIG. 30–3 Excision of imperforate hymen. Stellate incisions are made through the hymeneal membrane at 2, 4, 8 and 10 o'clock. The individual quadrants are excised along the lateral wall of the vagina, avoiding excision of vagina. (*Insert*) Margins of vaginal mucosa are approximated with fine delayed-absorbable suture.

TABLE 30–1   FIGO Classification of Vaginal Carcinoma

CLASSIFICATION	DESCRIPTION
	PREINVASIVE CARCINOMA
Stage 0	Carcinoma in situ, intraepithelial carcinoma
	INVASIVE CARCINOMA
Stage I	Carcinoma limited to the vaginal wall
Stage II	Carcinoma involving the subvaginal tissue, but not extending onto the pelvic wall
Stage III	Carcinoma extending onto the pelvic wall
Stage IV	Carcinoma extending beyond the true pelvis or involving the mucosa of the bladder or rectum. Bullous edema as such does not permit a case to be allotted to Stage IV.
Stage IVa	Spread of the growth to adjacent organs
Stage IVb	Spread to distant organs

TABLE 30–2   Histologic Types of Vaginal Cancer and Frequency of Occurrence

TYPE	FREQUENCY (PERCENT)
Squamous carcinoma	88–90
Adenocarcinoma (including DES-related)	4–5
Sarcoma	2–3
Leiomyosarcoma	
Sarcoma botryoides	
Melanoma	1
Other	1–2

form a transitional cell neoplasm that involves the vagina.

The fact that squamous carcinoma of the vagina occurs in 10% to 15% of cases following the finding of squamous cancer in other parts of the lower genital tract, such as the vulva or cervix, has led to the theory of multicentric origin of squamous cancer in the lower genital tract. Woodruff and others emphasize this correlation and have recommended that patients with squamous cancer in one area be categorized as high risk for the development of squamous carcinoma in other sites of the lower genital tract.

Recently, a new entity has developed in vaginal neoplasia as a result of the use of diethylstilbestrol (DES) during the first trimester of pregnancy. Women who had a history of previous spontaneous abortions or other problems with early loss of pregnancy were given DES, a nonsteroidal estrogenic hormone thought to enhance embryo implantation and placental development. DES was introduced into clinical obstetrics in 1944 in Boston and became popular and widely used during the following two decades. Only when a cluster of cases of adenocarcinoma appeared among the offspring of these patients in young women under the age of 25 in the late 1960s did Herbst, Ulfelder, and Poskanzer connect the result with the unusual coincidence.

From 1960 to 1970, from one-half to two million female offspring were exposed to DES. Fortunately, the incidence of vaginal adenocarcinoma in these young women has been quite low, ranging from 0.14 to 1.4 per 1000 exposed women. More than 400 documented cases have been reported to the DES Registry to date.

Observing the development of vaginal adenosis and adenocarcinoma in young teenage girls whose mothers were given DES before the 18th week of pregnancy started a new approach to the study of squamous tumor cells in the lower genital tract. This drug's effect provided a histologic foundation for the development of an uncommon vaginal adenocarcinoma in women under the age of 29. The strange experience also increased our understanding of the embryologic development of the vagina.

Initially, the DES-associated adenocarcinoma was thought to arise from mesonephric remnants in the vagina, and consequently the disease was mislabeled as a clear-cell carcinoma. After making an electron microscopic analysis of the ultrastructure of both the adenocarcinoma and vaginal adenosis, Richart clearly defined these lesions to be composed of columnar epithelium, similar in all respects to endocervical epithelium and of paramesonephric (müllerian) origin. The colposcopic studies of Stafl and Mattingly, as well as others, confirmed these observations.

Vaginal adenosis has been found by colposcopic examination to occur in between 34% and 90% of the exposed women, and in 50% of those with DES-associated vaginal adenocarcinoma. To date, the transition of the benign disease to frank adenocarcinoma has been observed in only one patient, reported by Blaikley in 1971. Although the hypothesis is still unproven, a strong possibility exists that the benign vaginal lesion is the cell of origin for vaginal adenocarcinoma.

ETIOLOGY OF VAGINAL CARCINOMA

During embryologic development, the vagina is formed from the columnar epithelium of the müllerian ducts and urogenital sinus. The tissue then transforms into squamous epithelium, so that the vaginal and cervical epithelia have a common embryologic origin. Squamous metaplasia has been observed with a colposcope within the vaginal adenosis; transformation of the metaplastic tissue has also been demonstrated in the development of intraepithelial neoplasia. Although many agents have been postulated as carcinogenic factors, none have been positively demonstrated. It is quite possible that squamous carcinoma arises from the effects of an oncogenic agent on the transformation zone within the foci of vaginal adenosis. The studies now being done on the effects of DES may find some interesting etiologic factors influencing vaginal carcinoma.

Carcinoma of the vagina may also share a common etiologic denominator with cervical carcinoma. Since slightly more than 50% of the cases occur in the posterior wall of the upper one-third of the vagina, which is the endpoint of vaginal coitus, vaginal carcinoma could be venereally induced. As with cervical carcinoma, primary carcinoma of the vagina usually occurs in sexually active women. Except for the cases of adenocarcinoma in young women exposed to DES, squamous carcinoma of the vagina is unquestionably associated with sexual activity.

SITE OF LESION IN VAGINAL CARCINOMA

Plentl and Friedman found that 51% of vaginal carcinoma lesions occur in the upper one-third of the vagina, 30% in the lower one-third, and 19% in the middle. In the lower one-third, lesions occur most often in the anterior wall, whereas in the upper one-third, most cases appear in the posterior vaginal wall. Although the location is noted on diagnosis, the precise site of origin is difficult to identify because the tumors have usually spread to various parts of the vagina by that time.

PATHWAYS OF SPREAD OF VAGINAL CARCINOMA

The lymphatic drainage of the vagina takes place through different pathways. The upper one-third drains by way of the cervical lymphatics, the lower one-third passes by way of the vulvar lymphatics, and the middle one-third communicates with both the upper and lower lymphatic channels. The vaginal vault and the anterior wall of the upper vagina drain to the interiliac pelvic lymph nodes, where they communicate with the external iliac, the hypogastric, and the common iliac nodes. The lymphatic drainage of the posterior vagina communicates directly with the deep pelvic nodes, including the inferior gluteal, sacral, and rectal nodes.

Because the major pathways of lymphatic drainage are to the superior and inferior gluteals and the common iliac lymph nodes, the potential for extrapelvic spread of vaginal carcinoma is great. When extrapelvic spread occurs, prognosis is generally poor. The primary site of origin of the tumor is an important indicator of lymph node metastases, whether the tumor will metastasize to the inguinal-femoral chain or to the deep pelvic lymph nodes. When the disease involves the lower one-third of the vagina, 6% to 7% of patients have metastases to the inguinal-femoral lymph nodes.

DIAGNOSIS OF VAGINAL CARCINOMA

In general, invasive carcinoma of the vagina appears as either a raised exophytic lesion or as an ulcerative, depressed lesion in the vaginal wall. Both types of lesions can be biopsied easily, and diagnosis can be established without difficulty. Vaginal cytology is usually positive if an adequate cell sample is obtained from the exfoliated lesion, although, as often happens, with cervical carcinoma, many cases of false-negative cytology occur even when an invasive lesion is present. Lugol's solution can be used to demarcate the areas for biopsy, although iodine staining is usually unnecessary if the lesion is clearly visible.

Identifying vaginal carcinoma at an early stage can be a major problem because the first lesions appear within the epithelial cells, frequently indistinguishable from the remainder of the vaginal epithelium. Only by colposcopic examination or with iodine staining can alterations in the surface epithelium of the vagina be identified. Ng and associates have achieved an accuracy of 88% to 90% in detecting dysplastic lesions in DES-exposed patients with adenosis, but their technique requires separate, four-quadrant vaginal smears from the walls of the vagina. Herbst emphasizes the advantage of iodine staining of the vagina to demonstrate occult lesions that may be associated with adenosis. Stafl and Mattingly have reported an accuracy of 96% in detecting abnormal epithelial lesions of the vagina in DES-exposed females by careful examination and colposcopy.

Since the vaginal speculum can obscure surface lesions and delay early diagnosis, the instrument should be rotated during the examination so that the entire canal can be inspected. With iodine staining, the clinician can detect multifocal lesions, but the entire vagina should also be cytologically tested. A thorough colposcopic examination can be used to detect vaginal carcinoma, if the clinician has that expertise.

TREATMENT OF VAGINAL CARCINOMA

Primary vaginal carcinoma is treated either with surgery or with radiotherapy. The choice of treatment depends on three factors: the size of the lesion, the location of the tumor in the vagina, and the clinical stage of the disease.

STAGE O LESIONS. Intraepithelial carcinoma of the vagina is by far the easiest to treat and offers the most hopeful prognosis. Either surgery or radiotherapy can be used, depending on the location of the lesion. If the disease is located in the upper vagina and the margins of the disease are distinct, a partial vaginectomy, with or without hysterectomy, is a practical and successful method of treatment.

When an epithelial lesion is multicentric, the entire vagina could require treatment, which would render the surgical approach impractical. A vaginal cylinder, such as the Bloedorn applicator, can be used for radiotherapeutic treatment to deliver 7000 rads to the vaginal surface over a period of approximately 72 hours. If the lesion is confined to the vaginal fornices, vaginal colpostats can be used to deliver a similar dosage. Lesions in the lower one-third of the vagina may be treated by partial vaginectomy or by intravaginal irradiation, using a variety of brachytherapy techniques.

Recently, the use of the carbon dioxide laser has proven to be a simple, effective method of treatment for noninvasive vaginal carcinoma. Laser therapy offers a conservative treatment for both focal and multicentric lesions without impairment of normal coital function. Because there is a risk of residual disease in 10% of laser-treated patients, careful colposcopic and cytologic follow-up is critical. Histologic study is difficult after the treated lesions are vaporized by the carbon dioxide laser.

STAGE I LESIONS. Radical surgery including hysterectomy, vaginectomy, and pelvic lymphadenectomy can be used in Stage I carcinoma of the vagina. Surgical evaluation of the para-aortic nodes should be included if lesions are bulky or extensive. Before initiating a radical procedure, the surgeon must establish that the disease is confined to the pelvis, as is done with Stage I carcinoma of the cervix.

Radical surgery is used infrequently for the treatment of invasive carcinoma of the vagina, except with very early lesions where the margins of the disease can be clearly defined and confidently re-moved. Radical surgery is difficult because the blad-der and rectum are closely attached to the vaginal walls, limiting the surgical margins. When the dis-ease occurs, as it does most commonly in the upper posterior vaginal wall, the tumor must be com-pletely freed from the underlying rectum. Radical surgery may also require the replacement of the upper vagina with a split thickness skin graft to reestablish normal vaginal length for a sexually ac-tive woman. Irradiation therapy is an alternative treatment for this stage of disease.

The radical Wertheim hysterectomy has been quite successful in treating Stage I adenocarcinoma in young women who were exposed to DES in utero. More than 75% of the patients are cured. When the disease extends beyond a Stage I lesion, the pref-erable treatment is to follow external beam mega-voltage therapy with intravaginal irradiation.

STAGE II AND STAGE III LESIONS. More extensive le-sions of the vagina pose an extremely difficult ther-apeutic problem for the gynecologist. Since the va-gina is surrounded by the levator ani muscles of the pelvic diaphragm, penetration of the lateral wall of the vagina by the invasive tumor is frequently associated with fixation of the disease to the adjacent pelvic musculature. Even radical surgery cannot effectively control the disease when it extends be-yond the confines of the vagina into the paravaginal tissues. Instead, the major method of treatment for Stage II and Stage III lesions is radiotherapy.

When Stage II lesions involve the anterior or pos-terior wall of the vaginal septum, an anterior or posterior exenteration with pelvic node dissection may be required. When the disease includes the lower one-third of the vagina, a groin dissection is necessary as well. Because surgery must be so ex-tensive, its use has been limited when the disease affects the paravaginal region (Stage IIb) or the lateral vaginal wall (Stage III).

STAGE IV LESIONS. When advanced lesions involve only the bladder or the rectum, exenteration may be required to control the disease effectively. Un-fortunately, pelvic exenteration, either anterior or posterior, can be used only when there is no other extension of the disease, and it is rare for the bladder and rectum to be involved without involvement of the adjacent paravaginal tissues. If the patient is not an acceptable surgical risk for exenteration, external beam megavoltage irradiation therapy, followed by intravaginal or interstitial irradiation, can be used to control the local disease and to offer palliation. Should the tumor not respond after 5000 rads of irradiation treatment to the whole pelvis, an ex-enteration may be required to control the disease in properly selected patients.

IRRADIATION THERAPY FOR VAGINAL CARCINOMA

Irradiation treatment of vaginal carcinoma is easily divided between lesions in the upper and middle and the lower thirds of the vagina.

UPPER AND MIDDLE THIRDS OF THE VAGINA. Because the lymphatic drainage of the upper and middle vagina extends through the hypogastric and pelvic nodes, full pelvic irradiation is necessary. Treatment usually includes a combination of techniques.

External beam megavoltage therapy using 4500 to 5000 rads focused on the midplane of the pelvis is used to treat the full pelvis and to encompass the vagina. A vaginal implant of radium, cesium, or iridium follows, delivering an additional 3000 to 4000 rads to a depth of 0.5 cm to 1.0 cm or more, de-pending on the thickness of the lesion.

At the M. D. Anderson Hospital, Brown has dem-onstrated the efficacy of using a radium needle im-plant for localized lesions. When the implant is used, high doses of radiation to the entire vagina, bladder, and rectum are avoided. Interstitial needles and ir-idium wires have been used as a primary treatment for localized vaginal lesions, and they can also be used for persistent disease.

LOWER ONE-THIRD OF THE VAGINA. Lesions in the lower one-third of the vagina frequently metastasize to the inguinal-femoral lymphatics and must be treated with full external and intravaginal irradia-tion followed by external beam irradiation treat-ment to the inguinal-femoral lymph nodes. The in-guinal-femoral regions require either a surgical groin dissection or the application of 5000 to 6000 rads of electron-beam teletherapy in addition to full pelvic irradiation. When vaginal lesions have me-tastasized to the groin lymph nodes, the cure rate is equally poor for both methods. In general, the presence of tumor in the groin nodes is a poor prog-nostic sign suggesting that the deep pelvic nodes may also be involved in approximately 6% to 7% of cases. Because the incidence of vaginal cancer is so low, the exact frequency with which the deep pel-vic nodes are involved has not been documented.

Cure Rates for Vaginal Carcinoma

In all, 561 patients with vaginal carcinoma were reported by international clinics to the FIGO Registry between 1973 and 1975. Of these, 541 patients (96.4%) received treatment, the majority by radiation. Only 37.5% of the patients were alive after 5 years.

In a retrospective analysis of 134 patients with carcinoma of the vagina treated at Washington Uni-versity, Perez and Camel report an actuarial disease-free, 5-year survival rate of 85% for Stage I lesions,

51% for Stage IIa lesions, 33% for Stage IIb lesions, 33% for Stage III lesions, and 0% for Stage IV lesions. The actuarial study demonstrates that beyond Stage I of the disease, control is poor. For Stage IIA lesions, local control of the disease was achieved in only 65% of cases at the University of Maryland because external irradiation was not used in all cases. Pelvic control was achieved in 48% of Stage IIb and Stage III lesions, but in none of the seven patients (0%) with Stage IV disease.

The results from other institutions, primarily following irradiation therapy, show that only Stage I lesions have an adequate 5-year survival rate (Table 30–3).

THE URETHRA

The female urethra develops from the caudal end of the urogenital sinus after it separates from the vaginal canal between the 8th and 12th week of embryologic life. Because they are so closely integrated, the urethra shares many common disease processes and anatomical defects with the vagina. Bacteria in the lower genital tract frequently colonize in the outer urethra, harbor in the paraurethral glands, and enter the bladder to produce acute infections. A bacterial infection in the lower genital tract may not become clinically manifest for several years, until a Skene's duct cyst or a urethral diverticulum develops.

Estrogen deficiency, which causes atrophic changes of the vaginal mucosa, can have a similar effect on the urethral mucosa. Thinning of the epithelium and irritation of the sensory nerve fibers can cause urinary frequency and dysuria. Prolapse at the external meatus may also result from atrophic changes of the urethra.

Diverticulum of the Urethra

In spite of the many documented cases of urethral diverticula, the condition has not been well recognized by the medical profession. Anderson observed a urethral diverticulum in 3% of a group of 300 women who were undergoing treatment for cervical carcinoma. The condition occurs more frequently than it is diagnosed; whenever an article about urethral diverticulum appears in the literature, there is an upsurge in the number of cases diagnosed.

ETIOLOGY OF URETHRAL DIVERTICULUM

In 1941, Parmenter suggested several congenital factors that could develop into a urethral diverticulum, including Gartner's duct, a faulty union of primal folds, cell nets, and wolffian ducts, or vaginal cysts that rupture into the urethra. Other possible causes include trauma from childbirth, instrumentation, urethral stone, urethral stricture, and infection of the urethral glands.

Of the many possible causes of urethral diverticula that have been considered, none have been proven. Two of the most probable causes are neisserian infection, although the gonococcus is seldom cultured, and infection of the suburethral tissue resulting from vaginal flora. Huffman's experiments support the concept of a suburethral infection developing into an abscess that becomes lined with epithelium. Huffman showed periurethral openings by constructing wax models of infected urethras. The usual organisms cultured are *Escherichia coli*, *Aerobacter aerogenes*, and other gram-negative bacilli; *Staphylococcus aureus*; and *Streptococcus fecalis*.

SYMPTOMATOLOGY OF URETHRAL DIVERTICULUM

Dysuria, urgency, frequency, and hematuria occurred together in 85% to 90% of 32 cases reviewed by Peters and Vaughn. Other frequently occurring symptoms are a lump in the vagina, dyspareunia, intermittent discharge from the urethra, and pain on walking. Pyuria and cystitis also occur, depending upon the location of the diverticular orifice. If the opening is sufficiently close to the outer end of the urethra, there may be no leakage of purulent exudate back into the bladder, which may explain

TABLE 30–3 *Absolute 5-Year Survival Following Irradiation Therapy for Carcinoma of the Vagina*

| FIGO STAGE | PROPORTION SURVIVING* | | |
	M.D. Anderson Hospital (1948–1967)	University of Maryland (1957–1970)	Washington University (1950–1977)
I	11/16 (69%)	5/6 (83%)	33/39 (85%)
II	13/19 (68%)	20/31 (64%)	28/60 (47%)
IIA	— —	13/20 (65%)	21/39 (51%)
IIB	— —	7/11 (63%)	7/21 (33%)
III	4/15 (27%)	8/20 (40%)	4/12 (33%)
IV	0/11 (0%)	0/7 (0%)	1/8 (19%)
I–IV	28/61 (46%)	33/64 (52%)	66/119 (53%)

* Percentage figures are in parentheses.
Adapted from Hilgers, 1978

the absence of symptoms of cystitis in 5% of cases. If the diverticulum is located in the posterior urethra near the urethrovesical junction, stress urinary incontinence may be a significant symptom. In a review of 70 cases from the Johns Hopkins Hospital, Ginsberg and Genadry found that 17% of the diverticula were located in the proximal (outer) urethra, 43% in the midurethra, and 31% in the distal (posterior) urethra; in the remaining cases, the site was not specifically identified. In our clinic, 66% or more of the diverticular orifices were located in the outer (proximal) and middle one-thirds of the urethra, while 33% were found in the posterior (distal) one-third of the urethra.

Not only are urinary tract symptoms the most common clinical expression of this urethral lesion, but a history of recurrent refractory cystitis is a clue that a diverticulum is the source of the infection.

DIAGNOSIS OF URETHRAL DIVERTICULUM

Urethral diverticula are usually small, varying from 3 mm to 3 cm in diameter. Some of the larger sacs cover the entire length of the urethra. On palpation, a suburethral mass or tenderness is commonly found. Pressure on the mass may cause the escape of urine or exudate from the urethral meatus.

An examination of the floor of the urethra through the water cystoscope while suburethral pressure is being applied will reveal an opening in 50% to 70% of cases. The pressure may force contents of the diverticulum into the urethra while it is being viewed. Some of the openings are extremely small and may be missed. Inflammatory swelling can result in edema of the orifice, which makes visualization difficult or impossible.

The diagnosis of urethral diverticulum is firmly established by means of positive pressure urethrography. A special catheter is used to block the urethra at both ends and fill it and the diverticulum under pressure with water-soluble contrast medium (Figs. 30–4, 30–5). The diverticulum then shows up clearly on a roentgenogram (Fig. 30–6). If the urethral orifice to the diverticulum is quite large, a voiding cystourethrogram together with a positive pelvic film may demonstrate the diverticulum.

Occasionally, a diverticulum occurs with no clinical evidence of inflammation. If the diverticulum is diagnosed during a careful pelvic examination, and if the patient is completely asymptomatic except for a previous history of urinary tract problems, surgery is not necessary. With a complication rate of 15% to 20%, diverticulectomy should not be considered a quick and easy procedure. Removal of an asymptomatic urethral diverticulum may create

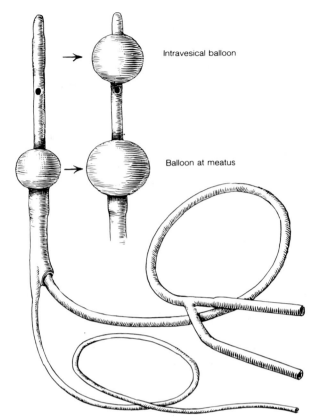

FIG. 30-4 Double ballooned catheter for positive pressure urethrography. (From Davis HJ, Cian LG: Positive pressure urethrography: A new diagnostic method. J Urol 80:34, 1958)

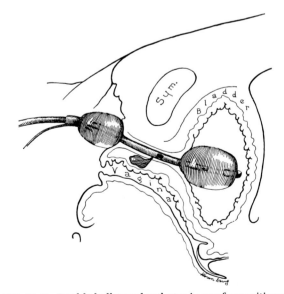

FIG. 30-5 Double ballooned catheter in use for positive pressure urethrography. (From Davis HJ, Cian LG: Positive pressure urethrography: A new diagnostic method. J Urol 80:34, 1958)

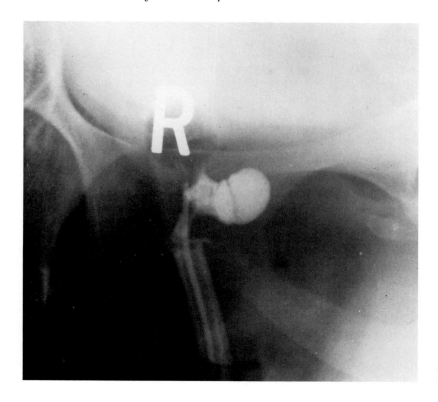

FIG. 30-6   A large urethral diverticulum filled with contrast medium.

more problems than it prevents, particularly if the sac is small or located in the floor of the posterior urethra. Only if a patient experiences acute or recurrent symptoms should urethral surgery be performed.

TREATMENT OF URETHRAL DIVERTICULUM

A diverticulum requiring treatment must be completely excised before the defect in the urethra can be closed. Failure to remove the entire diverticulum will only result in recurrence of the problem.

Many techniques have been used to identify the anatomical boundaries of the diverticulum. A method suggested by Young is to pass a sound into the diverticulum through the urethral orifice. The diverticulum can also be distended by injecting it with fibrinogen and thrombin mixed in a syringe to form a firm fibrin clot. Direct anatomical dissection of the diverticulum from the paraurethral fascia and vaginal wall offers a better success rate. The smooth covering of a diverticulum protruding into the vagina can be easily distinguished from the rugal folds of the vaginal mucosa.

If the wall of the diverticulum is left unopened until the dissection has reached the base of the sac, the neck of the diverticulum can be seen directly when it is removed. A common error is the inadvertent removal of a portion of the urethral floor along the base of the diverticulum. If the mucosa is closed with too much tension, a urethral stricture or a postoperative fistula may result.

Surgical Technique

EXCISION AND LAYERED CLOSURE.   A midline incision is made through the vaginal mucosa, which is then separated from the wall of the diverticulum (Fig. 30–7A). The wall of the diverticulum is also dissected from the paraurethral fascia in as wide a circumference as can be developed.

The diverticulum is opened and the interior of the cavity inspected. If the orifice of the diverticulum is large, the opening of the urethra can be seen easily, especially if a catheter has been placed in the urethra and bladder (Fig. 30–7B). The rest of the thin, friable mucosa of the diverticulum is separated from the vaginal mucosa and fascia, before the neck of the diverticulum is trimmed near the urethral orifice. The lining of the diverticulum becomes friable as a result of inflammatory changes, and the thin layer fragments during the dissection. Meticulous sharp dissection is required to separate the lining completely from the vagina and from the floor of the urethra. The neck of the diverticulum should be resected carefully to avoid eversion and to prevent removal of the mucosa from the urethral floor.

The urethral defect is closed with interrupted sutures of No. 3-0 chromic catgut, so that the edges can be inverted (Fig. 30–7C). After the interrupted sutures are tied, the paraurethral fascia is closed in a double layer, vest-over-pants technique. The layer of fascia from one side of the urethra is sutured beneath the opposite, overlapping fascia and fastened to the urethral wall on that opposite side. The top layer of fascia is then sutured to the underlying fascial layer. A more durable No. 2-0 delayed-absorbable suture is used to suture the fascial margins (Fig. 30–7D,E). Finally, the vaginal mucosa is trimmed and closed with interrupted No. 2-0 delayed-absorbable sutures.

The bladder is filled with 300 ml distilled water, and a suprapubic Silastic catheter is inserted and left in place until the morning of the fifth postoperative day. A suprapubic catheter is used in preference to a urethral catheter for three major reasons: to avoid trauma to the operative site; to avoid the necessity for transurethral catheterization during attempts to initiate voiding; and to avoid the discomfort of a urethral catheter. On the fifth day following surgery, the patient should attempt to void by closing the three-way stopcock of the suprapubic catheter, which allows the bladder to fill.

URETHROTOMY AND MARSUPIALIZATION. Urethrotomy has been used by Edwards and Beebe, and more recently by Kropp, to treat diverticula. By splitting the floor of the urethra from the meatus down its full length to the site of the orifice of the diverticulum, the sac can be well visualized during excision. Most cases of urethral diverticula can be repaired successfully without the added risk involved with such an extensive incision. The floor of the urethra must heal along the entire length, and healing is particularly a problem if there has been recent infection in the diverticulum.

In 1970, Spence and Duckett recommended marsupializing the diverticulum to prevent recurrence, to minimize operating time, and to reduce blood loss. This procedure has been endorsed by Lichtman and Robertson, and more recently by Ginsburg and Genadry. Although stress urinary incontinence has not been reported as a complication, the incidence would probably increase if marsupialization were used to treat lesions in the posterior urethra near the bladder base. Marsupialization is a useful procedure when diverticula occur in the outer one-third of the urethra, because a permanent opening in the outer floor of the urethra would not influence intraurethral pressure adversely.

RESULTS OF DIVERTICULECTOMY

Complications arise in about 20% of patients treated for diverticula of the urethra (Table 30–4). Urethral stricture may result when too much urethral mucosa is removed, but strictures can usually be resolved by urethral dilatations. Urethral fistula, a serious and troublesome complication of diverticulectomy, occurs in approximately 5% of treated patients.

Postoperatively, fistulas frequently result when acute or subacute infection in the walls of the diverticulum cause the urethral mucosa to become friable. The urinary incontinence that develops from a urethral fistula is far more troublesome to the patient than the initial symptoms of the diverticulum.

Closure of a urethral fistula is quite difficult because the blood supply to the floor of the urethra is delicate, and scarring and infection often result from repeated efforts to close the urethra. A fistula in the outer part of the urethra may be asymptomatic and may not need to be repaired. Patients with an outer fistula usually complain of spraying urine when voiding.

Urethral Prolapse

Although there have been few recent reports of urethral prolapse, nearly 400 cases have appeared in the English literature since 1732. More than half of the cases occurred in infants and children; the remainder occurred in elderly patients.

Urethral prolapse is characterized by a sliding outward of the urethral mucosa around the entire urethral meatus. The urethra may become cyanotic, edematous, and infarcted (Fig. 30–8). Symptoms vary greatly. Prolapse may cause no discomfort, in which case it is only detected when bloody discharge results from the breaking down of the congested tissues. Some patients complain of severe and continuous pain, with urinary frequency and tenesmus. Occasionally, in a small child, the edema and tissue reaction of the outer urethra may produce urinary retention.

Urethral prolapse is thought to result from a lack of development of or atrophic changes in the collagen and elastic tissues of the submucosa. In infants, prolapse usually follows a severe coughing or crying spell. In some older patients, too, prolapse has followed paroxysms of coughing. In older patients, the diminished tone and elasticity of tissue are considered to be etiologic factors in some cases of urethral prolapse.

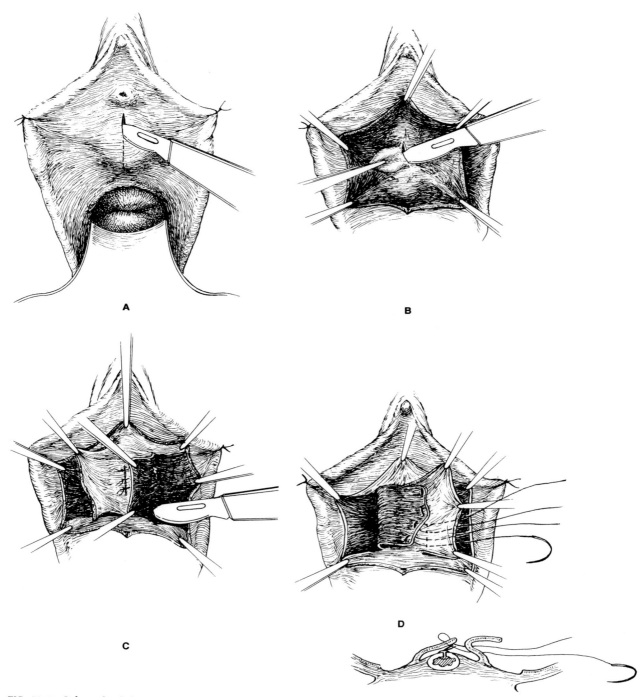

FIG. 30–7 Suburethral diverticulum. (*A*) A midline vaginal incision is made over the diverticulum. (*B*) The diverticulum is dissected from the vaginal mucosa and surrounding fascia. Freed diverticulum is excised from the floor of the urethra, avoiding removal of an excessive amount of urethral wall. (*C*)The urethra is closed with interrupted No. 3-0 delayed-absorbable sutures placed through the muscularis and mucosa to ensure mucosa-to-mucosa approximation. The paraurethral fascia is mobilized with sharp dissection from the vaginal mucosa. (*D*) The paraurethral fascia is plicated beneath urethral incision using the vest-over-pants technique. Note suture of the inner layer of fascia to the undersurface of the outer layer using horizontal mattress sutures of No. 2-0 delayed-absorbable material. Insert shows cross-sectional view of suture placement.

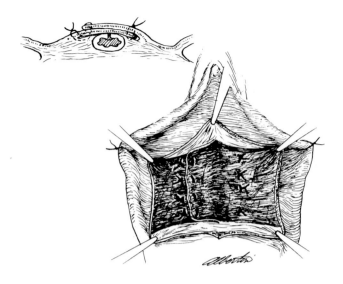

E

FIG. 30-7 (continued). (E) Completion of vest-over-pants plication of paraurethral fascia over the floor of the urethra. Note that the free margin of the outer fascia is sutured to the inner fascial layer.

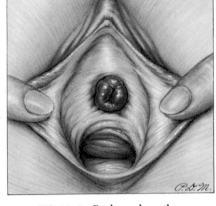

FIG. 30-8 Prolapsed urethra.

Treatment of urethral prolapse may be palliative or surgical. Hot, moist compresses provide temporary comfort. Sometimes a small mass of tissue can be reduced, but recurrence is common.

Several surgical procedures have been suggested, including the one advocated by Kelly and Burnam. The prolapsed mucosa is excised by a circular incision (Fig. 30-9A). The cut edges are then sutured with No. 3-0 chromic catgut, avoiding an excessive number of stitches, which can result in stricture of the urethral meatus (Fig. 30-9B). In most cases, circumcision has proven to be the preferable method of correction.

Cryosurgery has also been used to treat urethral prolapse. The method is extremely effective in producing complete annular necrosis and healing of the prolapsed tissue (Fig. 30-10). The cryosurgical procedure can be performed without anesthesia; for a small child, a local anesthetic is advisable. A suprapubic Silastic catheter is inserted to permit bladder drainage until complete, spontaneous voiding occurs. The catheter also helps prevent postoperative trauma to the suture line around the meatus.

TABLE 30-4 *Complications of Urethral Diverticulectomy*

OPERATIVE SERIES	NUMBER OF CASES	FISTULA	RECUR- RENCE	STRESS INCONTINENCE	STRIC- TURE	RECURRENT URINARY TRACT INFECTION	COMPLICATION RATE (PERCENT)
Wharton, TeLinde	58	4	—	1	3	5	22
Ward, et al	24	2	7	3	—	—	50
Boatwright, Moore	48	4	—	2	1	—	15
Pathak, House	42	—	—	—	—	3	7
Davis, TeLinde	84	—	10	—	—	11	26
Hoffman, Adams	60	1	—	4	1	—	10
Davis, Robinson	98	4	1	—	—	—	6
Lee	108	1	10	16	—	1	—
Ginsberg, Genadry	70	1	20	6	—	—	39
Total	592	17 (3%)	48 (8%)	32 (5%)	7 (1%)	20 (3%)	21

Adapted from Ginsberg DS, Genadry R: Suburethral diverticulum in the female. Obstet Gynecol Surv 39:1, 1984

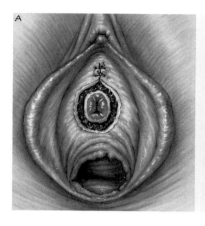
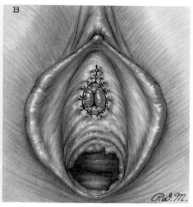

FIG. 30–9 Operation for urethral prolapse. (*A*) The prolapsed mucosa has been excised. (*B*) Completed operation; cut edges of urethral and vaginal mucosa are sutured with No. 3-0 delayed-absorbable suture material.

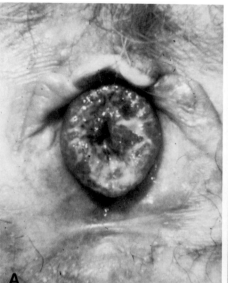
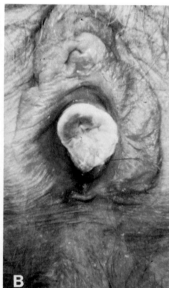
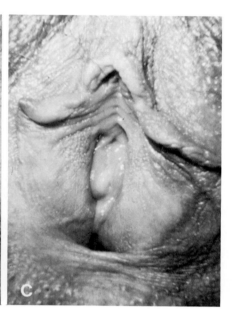

FIG. 30–10 (*A*) Urethral prolapse in an elderly female. (*B*) Regression of urethral prolapse after cryosurgery. (*C*) Repeat cryosurgery of urethral prolapse resulted in complete regression and healing of urethral meatus within 8 weeks.

Bibliography

Anderson MJF: The incidence of diverticula of the female urethra. J Urol 98:96, 1967

Annual Report on the Results of Treatment of Carcinoma of the Uterus, Vagina, and Ovary, vol 18. Stockholm, Norestedt, 1982

Benjamin J, Elliott L, Cooper JF, et al: Urethral diverticulum in adult female: Clinical aspects, operative procedure, and pathology. Urology 3:1, 1974

Blaikley JB, Dewhurst CJ, Ferreira HP, et al: Vaginal adenosis: Clinical and pathological features with special reference to malignant change. J Obstet Gynaecol Br Commonw 78:1115, 1971

Breslow A: Thickness, cross-sectional areas, and depths of invasion in the prognosis of cutaneous melanoma. Ann Surg 172:902, 1970

Brown GR, Fletcher GH, Rutledge FN: Irradiation of in situ and invasive squamous cell carcinoma of the vagina. Cancer 28:1278, 1971

Curran JW, Rendtorff RC, Chandler RW, et al: Female gonorrhea: Its relationship to abnormal uterine bleeding, urinary tract symptoms and cervicitis. Obstet Gynecol 45:195, 1975

Davis BL, Robinson DG: Diverticula of the female urethra: Assay of 120 cases. J Urol 104:850, 1970

Davis HJ, Cian LG: Positive pressure urethrography. A new diagnostic method. J Urol 80:34, 1958

Davis HJ, Te Linde RW: Urethral diverticula: An assay of 121 cases. J Urol 75:753, 1956

DiSaia PJ, Morrow CP, Townsend DE (eds): Synopsis of Gynecologic Oncology. New York, John Wiley & Sons, 1975

Edwards E, Beebe RA: Diverticula of female urethra: Review; New procedure for treatment: Report of 5 cases. Obstet Gynecol 5:729, 1955

Fenoglio C, Ferenczy A, Richard RM, et al: Scanning and transmission electron microscopic studies of vaginal adenosis and the cervical transformation zone in progeny exposed in utero to diethylstilbestrol. Am J Obstet Gynecol 126:170, 1976

Frick HC: Primary carcinoma of the vagina. Am J Obstet Gynecol 101:695, 1968

Gallup DG, Morley GW: Carcinoma in situ of the vagina: A study and review. Obstet Gynecol 46:334, 1975

Ginsberg DS, Genadry R: Suburethral diverticulum: Classification and therapeutic considerations. Obstet Gynecol 61:685, 1983

Hamilton WJ, Boyd JD, Mossman HW: Human Embryology, 3rd ed. Cambridge, W Heffer & Sons, 1962

Herbst AL, Ulfelder H, Poskanzer EC: Adenocarcinoma of the vagina: Association of maternal stilbestrol therapy with tumor appearing in young women. N Engl J Med 284:878, 1971

Herbst AL, Scully RE, Robboy SJ: The significance of adenosis and clear-cell adenocarcinoma of the genital tract in young females. J Reprod Med 14:5, 1975

Hilgers RD: Squamous cell carcinoma of the vagina. Surg Clin North Am 58:25, 1978

Hoffman MJ, Adams WE: Recognition and repair of urethral diverticula. Am J Obstet Gynecol 92:106, 1965

Huffman JW: The detailed anatomy of the paraurethral ducts in the adult human female. Am J Obstet Gynecol 55:86, 1948

Hutch JA: Anatomy and Physiology of the Bladder, Trigone and Urethra. New York, Appleton-Century-Crofts, 1972

Kamat MH, DelGaiso A, Seebode JJ: Urethral prolapse in female children. Am J Dis Child 118:691, 1969

Kanbour AE, Klionsky BK, Murphy AI: Carcinoma of the vagina following cervical cancer. Cancer 34:1838, 1974

Klaus H, Stein RT: Urethral prolapse in young girls. Pediatrics 52:645, 1973

Klobe JM: Pathologische Anatomieder Weiblichen Sexualorgane. Vien, 1864

Kropp KA: The Female Urethra. In Glenn JF (ed): Urologic Surgery. Hagerstown, Harper & Row, 1975

Lee RA: Diverticulum of the urethra: Clinical presentation, diagnosis and management. Clin Obstet Gynecol 27:490, 1984

Lichtman A, Robertson J: Suburethral diverticula treated by marsupialization. Obstet Gynecol 47:203, 1976

Lintgen C, Herbert P: Clinical-pathological study of 100 female urethras. J Urol 55:298, 1946

Livermore GR: Treatment of prolapse of the urethra. Surg Gynecol Obstet 32:557, 1921

Marcus SL: Multiple squamous cell carcinoma involving the cervix, vagina and vulva: The theory of multicentric origin. Am J Obstet Gynecol 80:802, 1960

Ng ABP, Reagan JW, Hawliczek S, et al: Cellular detection of vaginal adenosis. Obstet Gynecol 46:323, 1975

Parmenter FJ: Diverticulum of the urethra. J Urol 45:749, 1941

Pathak UN, House MJ: Diverticulum of the female urethra. Obstet Gynecol 36:789, 1970

Pempree T, Viravathana T, Slawson RG, et al: Radiation management of primary carcinoma of the vagina. Cancer 40:101, 1977

Perez AA, Camel HM: Long-term follow-up in radiation therapy of carcinoma of the vagina. Cancer 49:1308, 1982

Perez CA, Arneson AN, Galakatos A, et al: Malignant tumors of the vagina. Cancer 31:36, 1973

Perez CA, Arneson AN, Dehner LP, et al: Radiation therapy in carcinoma of the vagina. Obstet Gynecol 44:862, 1974

Peters WA, Vaughn EJ, Jr: Urethral diverticula in the female: Etiologic factors and postoperative results. Obstet Gynecol 47:549, 1976

Plentl AA, Friedman EA: Lymphatic System of the Female Genital Tract. Philadelphia, WB Saunders, 1971

Pride GL, Schultz AE, Chuprevich TW, et al: Primary invasive carcinoma of the vagina. Clinical Obstet Gynecol 53:218, 1979

Rutledge FN, Boronow RC, Wharton JT: Gynecologic Oncology. New York, John Wiley & Sons, 1976

Schubert G: Uber Scheidenbildung bei Angeborenem Vaginaldefekt. Zbl Gynak 45:1017, 1911

Sholem SL, Wechsler M, Roberts M: Management of the urethral diverticulum in women: A modified operative technique. J Urol 112, 485, 1974

Smith WG: Invasive carcinoma of the vagina. Clin Obstet Gynecol 24:503, 1981

Spence H, Duckett J: Diverticulum of the female urethra: Clinical aspects and presentation of simple operative technique for cure. J Urol 104:432, 1970

Stafl A, Mattingly RF: Vaginal adenosis: A precancerous lesion? Am J Obstet Gynecol 120:666, 1974

Stern A, Patel S: Diverticulum of the female urethra; Value of the post-void bladder film during excretory urography. Radiol 121:22, 1976

Tait L: Saccular dilatation of the urethra: Removal, cure. Lancet 2:625, 1875

Wharton JT: Carcinoma of the vagina and Urethra. In Rovinsky JJ (ed): Obstetrics and Gynecology. Hagerstown, Harper & Row, 1972

———: Carcinoma of the vagina. In Rutledge F, Boronow RC, Wharton JT (eds): Gynecologic Oncology. New York, John Wiley & Sons, 1976

Wharton JT, Kearns W: Diverticulum of the female urethra. J Urol 63:1063, 1950

Wheeles CR, Jr, McGibbon B, Dorsey JH, et al: Gracilis myocutaneous flap in reconstruction of the vulva and female perineum. Obstet Gynecol 54:97, 1979

Woodruff JD, Parmley TH: Epidermoid carcinoma of the vagina. In Hafez ECE, Evans TN (eds): The Human Vagina. New York, Elsevier North Holland, 1979

Chapter 31

Cervical Intraepithelial Neoplasia

Adolf Stafl, M.D., and Richard F. Mattingly, M.D.

Following the introduction of the Papanicolaou smear in 1943, the increased detection of preinvasive cervical cancer has been associated with a decrease in the incidence of invasive cancer and in the mortality rate from this disease. Today, 70% or more of the cervical disease is detected as in situ (Stage 0) or early invasive (Stage Ia) lesions.

The major clinical value of cervical cancer screening programs is in the detection of the disease at an earlier stage while it remains confined to the cervix and before it has spread to the regional and distant lymph nodes.

Cervical Cancer Screening

Although cytology is considered to be the most practical method for cervical cancer screening, there is some question regarding the cost-benefit ratio of this method. There is no satisfactory formula available that provides an accurate cost-benefit analysis of this or any other cancer screening technique. It is only possible to appraise the value of cytology in terms of an improvement in the morbidity and mortality of cervical cancer.

To be of value, a screening method must meet the following basic criteria: the method should be simple, inexpensive, reliable, and generally applicable. While the false-positive rate is not too critical, the false-negative rate of the screening method must be low. The disease to be screened should be of sufficient frequency in the population that early detection should produce significant decrease in morbidity and mortality. Also, appropriate and safe treatment should be available that can eradicate or alter the course of the disease. It is important to define the high-risk population for the screening of a particular disease. Cervical neoplasia is an important disease that meets most of these criteria. The uterine cervix is easily accessible for clinical evaluation, and the cytologic examination is a practical method of cervical cancer detection that has a reasonably low false-negative rate. The treatment of cervical intraepithelial neoplasia can be undertaken in most communities with a low complication rate and a good expectation of success. Invasive carcinoma of the cervix, on the other hand, is a dangerous disease which occurs in women during their productive years and will result in death if untreated.

The classic demonstration of the benefits of cytologic screening was the study by Boyes and Worth with supporting data from the British Columbia screening program. This program was started in 1949 and was designed to test the hypothesis that screening for cervical cancer was of value in reducing the incidence of invasive cervical cancer.

The main intent of the program was to test the hypothesis that screening was worthwhile in preventing the occurrence of invasive cancer. A registry was maintained in British Columbia for the prevalence and incidence of invasive cervical carcinoma as well as a registry for mortality from this disease. It was considered essential to keep the cases of preclinical invasive carcinoma separate from the cases with clinical carcinoma. The only accurate index, therefore, that can be used for evaluation of the morbidity from this disease is the incidence of clinical invasive carcinoma. As shown in Table 31–1, the incidence of invasive cancer decreased from 28.4 per 100,000 women in 1955 to 7.6 per 100,000 in 1977. The second index used in evaluating the

759

TABLE 31–1 *Incidence of Invasive Carcinoma of the Cervix in Women over 20 Years of Age in British Columbia, 1955–1977*

YEAR	POPULATION (THOUSANDS)	CLINICAL INVASIVE CARCINOMA	
		Total Cases	Incidence*
1955	422.9	120	28.4
1956	436.7	119	27.2
1957	460.9	120	26.0
1958	473.0	112	23.7
1959	478.7	108	22.6
1960	486.4	96	19.7
1961	496.0	115	23.2
1962	503.0	78	15.5
1963	513.0	98	19.1
1964	526.8	86	16.3
1965	543.2	80	14.7
1966	566.5	77	13.6
1967	592.4	85	14.3
1968	615.4	80	13.0
1969	638.2	89	13.9
1970	664.4	82	12.3
1971	687.2	73	10.6
1972	713.1	66	9.2
1973	741.4	71	9.5
1974	775.3	67	8.6
1975	805.5	70	8.7
1976	826.1	69	8.4
1977	844.6	64	7.6

* Per 100,000 women
(Boyes et al, 1981)

program was the mortality from invasive carcinoma. It was found that the refined death rate from invasive cervical cancer declined from 11.4 per 100,000 women in 1958 to 3.8 per 100,000 in 1976. The mortality from cervical carcinoma decreased by approximately 60% during the period of the study.

Because of the financial resources that are required for mass population screening, screening programs may be more appropriately aimed at populations with the highest risk for cervical cancer. There is no doubt that the highest risk group can be identified among women with certain sexual patterns. These include those women with a history of first intercourse or marriage before the age of 21, an increased number of sexual partners, and an increased rate of sexually transmitted diseases.

Concerning the optimum time for initiation of cytologic screening and for rescreening, there is agreement that a woman should have regular vaginal cytologic examinations at the time that she be-

comes sexually active. According to the report of Fidler, Boyes, and Worth, the number of cases that progress from negative to positive cytology after the age of 55 is extremely small, such that it is possible to consider decreasing the frequency of cytology screening at the age of 55 in women who have had regular cervical-vaginal cytologic smears previously. Because of the known false-negative rate of cytology of 10% to 20%, it is theoretically possible that cases of cervical cancer that were missed during the first screening will be picked up during the second. When several cytologic smears have been constantly negative during the third decade, it is considered acceptable to repeat a vaginal cytologic smear every 2 years during the fourth or fifth decade of life. However, the aim of gynecologic screening is directed not only toward the detection of cervical cancer, but also endometrial, ovarian, and breast cancer. Therefore, a yearly examination that includes a pelvic and breast examination is strongly recommended.

Epidemiology of Cervical Cancer

Many epidemiologic studies have been published concerning the environmental cofactors that are significantly correlated to the frequency of cervical cancer. These findings were supported by the retrospective study done by Nix, who reviewed hospital records and autopsy records of 100,000 Catholic nuns, among whom there was only 1 death due to cervical carcinoma. Celibacy would therefore seem to confer protection from cervical cancer.

In 1962, Rotkin and King evaluated factors that might be responsible for the development of cervical carcinoma and found that the age of first coitus was the variable of greatest clinical correlation. In this study, it was reported that among patients who began coitus between the ages of 15 and 17, twice as many had cervical cancer as in the control group. Furthermore, in contrast to rates in matched controls, comparatively few cervical cancers developed in patients who began coitus after the age of 21. There were almost none when the first coitus was as late as age 37.

The number of sexual partners is another factor that is closely related to the incidence of cervical cancer. Although it is very difficult to obtain exact data, it is well established that women with multiple sexual partners have a higher incidence of cervical cancer than matched controls.

Starreveld and associates studied the age-specific incidence of gonorrhea and cervical carcinoma. Although there is no cause-and-effect relationship between the gonococcus and cervical carcinoma, they found changes in incidence and age distribution for gonorrhea to be predictive of comparable changes in incidence and age distribution for carcinoma in situ, with a delay in presentation of approximately 5 years.

The latency period of carcinoma in situ of the cervix does not seem to vary a great deal between age groups. The results are compatible with a sexually transmitted infectious agent as an etiologic factor in cervix cancer.

Cervical cancer is more frequent in parous women than in nulliparous women, but it is not clear whether the total number of pregnancies is related to the frequency of cervical cancer. Women with a high number of pregnancies usually start sexual life early, and the early age of first intercourse might be etiologically more important than the actual number of pregnancies.

These epidemiologic data correlate well with the pathogenesis of cervical neoplasia. The period of early squamous metaplasia is the time of greatest risk for cellular transformation and for the development of cervical neoplasia. It has been shown that in this period, the young metaplastic cells near the squamocolumnar junction have phagocytic properties. If some potential mutagen is present in the vagina during this time, the epithelium may undergo some premalignant transformation. Early squamous metaplasia is most frequent in puberty, early adolescence, and the first pregnancy. Therefore, women who begin sexual activity at an early age when the metaplastic process is most active would have a greater chance of developing cervical cancer. On the basis of this hypothesis, one would predict that women who have experienced at least one pregnancy would have a higher frequency of cervical cancer than nulliparous or virginal women. A large number of sexual partners would increase the possibility of introducing a mutagen into the vagina.

A number of environmental variables are secondarily related to the frequency of cervical cancer. These variants are characteristic of the population from which women who have early intercourse and multiple sexual partners are drawn. These variables include race, socioeconomic status, occupation, education, and religion; but such factors are not independently as important in the epidemiology of the disease as those previously mentioned. Sexually transmitted diseases, such as syphilis, gonorrhea, trichomonas vaginalis, and herpes virus Type 2 infections, have also been associated with a higher frequency of cervical neoplasia. These diseases, however, are dependent upon the sexual habits of the population at risk, which classifies cervical cancer as a venereal disease.

At the present time the risk of cervical cancer is highest among the black, poor, and uneducated populations. The current trend toward changes in sexual habits, however, and specifically the lowering of the age for beginning sexual intercourse are factors that place other racial and economic groups into the high-risk population.

HERPES TYPE 2 VIRUS

Epidemiologic data concerning the pathogenesis of cervical neoplasia suggests that venereally transmitted agents may act as a possible mutagen. Viruses are obligate intracellular parasites and are likely, therefore, to interfere with DNA replication in the host. Several viruses (adenovirus, papova-viruses, SV40 virus) are unequivocally oncogenic for certain rodent species. Several other herpes viruses have been shown to induce tumors in monkeys, rabbits, chickens, and frogs. There is evidence implicating the herpes virus as oncogenic in a variety of animal species and strong, but not conclusive evidence, implicating the Epstein Barr virus as the etiologic agent of Burkitt's lymphoma in the human.

Naib has shown that women of low socioeconomic status have a high incidence of exposure to the Type 2 herpes virus as confirmed by positive serum antibody titers. The incidence of Type 2 neutralizing antibody titers was found to be significantly higher in women with preinvasive or invasive cervical carcinoma than in a control group of similar-aged gynecological patients without cervical cancer or in patients attending venereal disease clinics. While differences in incidence of positive Type 2 antibody titers have not been noted universally among women with cervical cancer (exceptions include Caucasian women in New Zealand, Mestizo women in Colombia, oriental women in Taiwan, and Jewish women in Israel, where control groups have a higher incidence of positive antibody titers), there is almost complete agreement that Caucasian and Black women in the western hemisphere who have cervical cancer have an increased incidence of positive antibody titers to herpes Type 2 infection. Royston and Aurelian reported that 31% of dyskaryotic cells from patients with invasive carcinoma showed evidence of herpes virus antigens by immunofluorescent studies. However, there was no evidence of virus antigens in frozen section biopsies from cervical tumors, which raises questions about the significance of these observations. The best evidence at present regarding the oncogenic role of the herpes Type 2 virus is indirect and does not confirm that the association of a herpes virus infection in patients with cervical cancer is one of cause and effect relationship.

HUMAN PAPILLOMAVIRUS

The role of the human papillomavirus in cervical carcinogenesis was not examined until 1976. Papillomaviruses are found in a variety of human warty lesions; condyloma acuminata, oral and laryngeal papillomas, and skin warts. For a long time, it was believed that these lesions were caused by the same virus. However, biochemical and immunologic studies have revealed that there are several serotypes of human papillomavirus (HPV). HPV 6 and 11 infections are sexually transmitted diseases that may be associated with cervical intraepithelial neoplasia. HPV 16 and 18 are two principal HPV types found in in-situ and invasive cervical carcinoma.

Warty lesions of the vulva and vagina had been recognized and described as far back as ancient times. Cervical condylomata also occur but are less readily diagnosed. They may occur in the original ectocervical squamous epithelium, and also in the metaplastic epithelium that is located in the colposcopic transformation zone. The stratified squamous epithelium covering the condyloma is characterized by parakeratosis and hyperakeratosis and also by typical cells in the outer intermediate cell layers, which show perinuclear cytoplasmic clearing or ballooning. These cells have been referred to as *koilocytotic cells*. The nuclei are usually round, rather uniform, with frequent binucleation. Meisels and associates, in a review of previously diagnosed cases of dysplasia, found that more than 70% were actually condylomata. In a correlative study of colposcopy and histology, they also demonstrated that cervical condylomata occur more frequently than previously suspected.

The prevalent pattern of condylomata on the uterine cervix is of a flat lesion (flat papilloma) that is difficult to differentiate from cervical intraepithelial neoplasia when using the colposcope. Laverty and associates introduced the term *non-condylomatous cervical wart virus infection* for these subclinical lesions. Colposcopically, these lesions produce three typical appearances: a flat acetowhite epithelium with no vessel pattern; a microvillus appearance; and a mosaic-type lesion with a large lacuna in the center of the mosaic.

The spontaneous remission of wart virus infections may explain the well-known regression of mild dysplasia. It is premature to suggest that non-condylomatous wart virus lesions are actually a precursor of cervical neoplasia. The epidemiologic behavior of the human papillomavirus lesion is similar to that of cervical neoplasia. Human papillomavirus lesions often co-exist on the cervix with dysplasia or neoplasia, can be seen in adjacent or distant areas of the squamous epithelium, or are sometimes intermingled. In terms of therapy, it does not matter if a patient has histologically proven intraepithelial cervical neoplasia alone, or has intraepithelial neoplasia along with wart virus changes, or has only wart virus lesions. The management of all of these lesions is identical.

Pathologic Features of Carcinoma in Situ

Carcinoma in situ is a term that should be applied to a microscopic picture of the surface cervical epithelium in which the individual cells have the same characteristics as invasive cancer cells have throughout the full thickness of the epithelial layer.

Figure 31–1 shows a typical section of normal stratified squamous epithelium of the cervix. In carcinoma in situ there is a complete absence of this normal stratification. The individual cells vary in size and shape and the nuclei, which are also variable in form, tend to be larger than those of the normal cells. Many of the nuclei stain heavily with hematoxylin, and mitotic figures are frequent. This microscopic picture, if seen in the depth of the cervix or in a metastatic position, would mean cancer

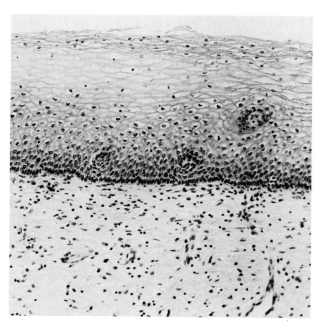

FIG. 31–1 Normal cervical epithelium. Note the stratification from deepest layer of basal cells to superficial flattened spinal cells.

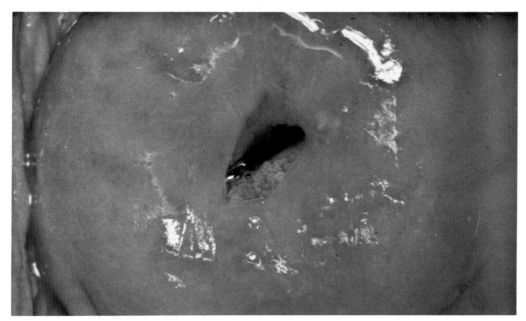

PLATE 31-1 Cervix covered with original squamous epithelium with the squamocolumnar junction near the external os. Columnar epithelium in the external os shows typical grapelike structures. The border between squamous epithelium and columnar epithelium is sharp without metaplastic changes.

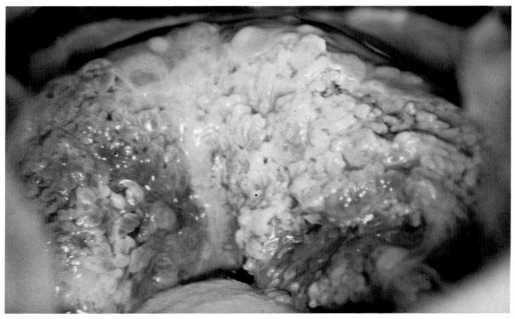

PLATE 31-2 Eversion of columnar epithelium in a pregnant (6 months) patient. Columnar epithelium is hypertrophic and produces significant amount of secretion.

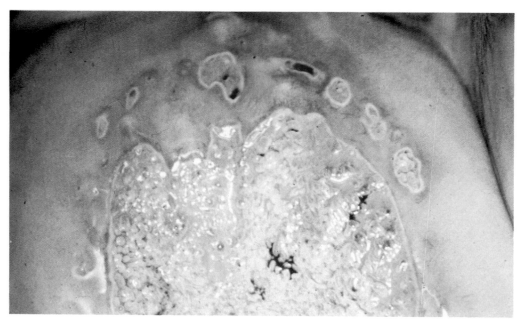

PLATE 31–3   Transformation zone. All components of the transformation zone are visible: tongues of squamous metaplasia, small islands of columnar epithelium, gland openings, and small Nabothian cysts. No abnormal colposcopic lesion is present.

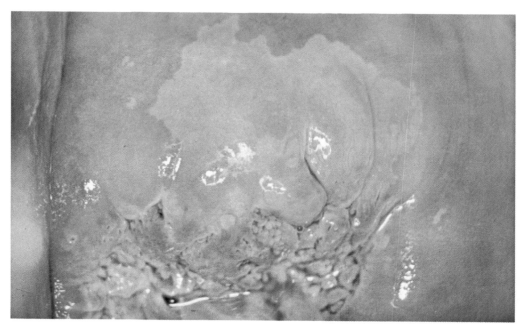

PLATE 31–4   An area of aceto-white epithelium after application of acetic acid with irregular borders. The lesion is compatible with mild dysplasia. Squamocolumnar junction is fully visible.

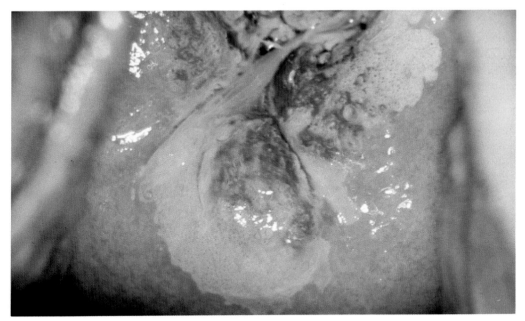

PLATE 31-5 On the posterior lip a sharp-bordered area of aceto-white epithelium with punctation. The intercapillary distance is significantly increased, and the lesion is compatible with carcinoma in situ.

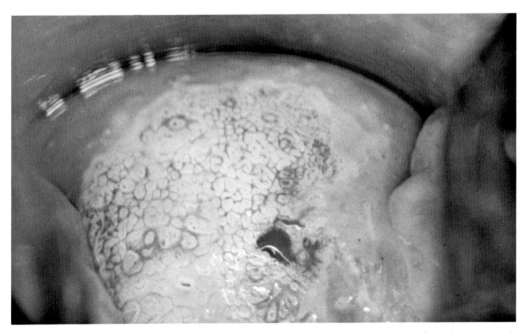

PLATE 31-6 Large area of mosaic pattern. The intercapillary distance is significantly increased, some fields of mosaic are large, some are small. The lesion is compatible with carcinoma in situ.

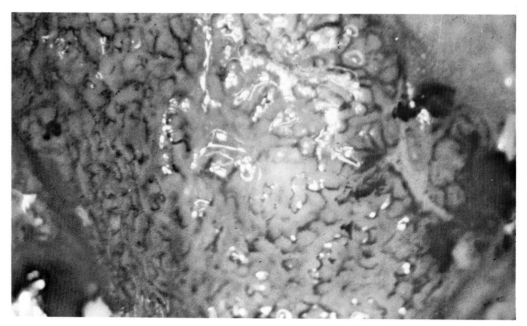

PLATE 31-7 Atypical vessels, horizontal capillaries running parallel with the surface. These vessels already are diagnostic for a microinvasive cancer.

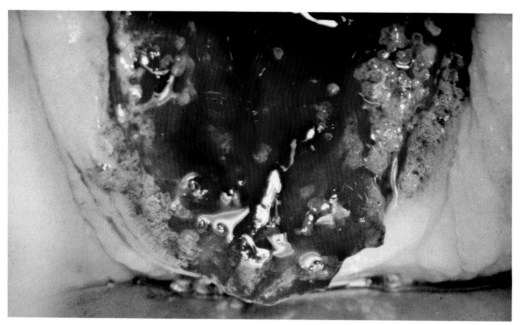

PLATE 31-8 Clinically visible invasive cervical carcinoma. The center of the lesion is necrotic with significant contact bleeding. On the periphery of the necrotic lesion, some atypical vessels are visible.

to the eye of any pathologist. Figure 31–2 illustrates a typical example.

The transition between carcinoma in situ and normal cervical epithelium is often abrupt (Fig. 31–3). On the other hand, the transition between the normal epithelial cells and the abnormal may be gradual, but when the entire thickness of the surface epithelium is composed of the cells that are abnormal, the ultimate picture is that of intraepithelial carcinoma.

Relation of Dysplasia to Carcinoma in Situ

Advances in the field of cytopathology have produced impressive correlations between the morphologic changes of the desquamated cell from the cervix and those observed by biopsy and conization. Richart followed 750 patients with abnormal smears by repeated cytologic examination and colpomicroscopy. His work suggests that approximately 30% of all patients with cervical dysplasia progress to carcinoma in situ within 2 years.

We believe that cervical dysplasia should serve as a "red flag," making the clinician acutely aware of cellular atypia. Whether due to infection, trauma, intrauterine contraceptives, or other causes, it should be investigated. The importance of follow-up studies of atypical cervical epithelium cannot be overstressed. Repeated cytologic studies with multiple cervical biopsies, utilizing the Schiller iodine stain, are essential. If the suspicious cytology persists on repeated examination and there is histologic evidence of dysplasia from cervical biopsies, more intensive studies of the cervix with colposcopy and directed biopsy or conization are required.

It would seem that there is a latent period of several years during which the intraepithelial cancer exists before becoming truly invasive. As evidence of this is the fact that the average age of women with intraepithelial cancer is about 10 years less than that of women presenting with invasive cancer.

Kurihara followed 294 patients for more than 11 years by vaginal cytology, colposcopy, and colposcopically directed biopsy of the most suspect area of the cervix without removal of the entire lesion. Using precise cytologic, histologic, and colposcopic criteria, Kurihara observed the progression of severe dysplasia to frank carcinoma in situ in 31.3% of 32 cases during the period of 1 to 7.5 years. Of 37 cases of carcinoma in situ, 54% progressed to early invasive carcinoma over a period of 1 to 7 years (Table 31–2). This study offers the unique feature of studying the *in vivo* biologic behavior of an in situ carcinoma of the cervix without the necessity of removing the

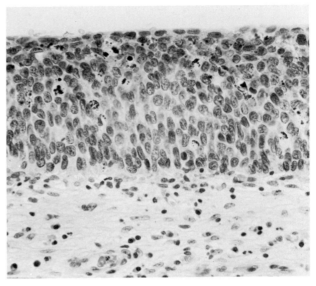

FIG. 31–2 Carcinoma in situ. Complete loss of stratification and distribution of atypical cells and mitotic figures through full thickness of epithelium. Note that there is no penetration or breakthrough of the basement membrane.

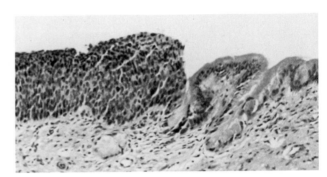

FIG. 31–3 Abrupt margin between (*left*) abnormal and (*right*) normal epithelium.

lesion by conization to determine whether there was evidence of occult invasion at the initiation of the study. It is therefore the only long-term study of its kind that provides clear evidence that carcinoma in situ will progress to invasive carcinoma if left untreated.

Another long-term study of the natural history of carcinoma in situ was performed in New Zealand by McIndoe and associates. They followed 948 patients with carcinoma in situ of the cervix for periods from 5 to 25 years. Among the 870 patients who had normal cytology follow-up, 12 (1.5%) developed invasive carcinoma. A second group of 131 continued to produce abnormal cytology consistent with cervical intraepithelial neoplasia, and 29 of

TABLE 31–2 *Long-term Follow-up Study of Untreated Cervical Intraepithelial Neoplasia, 1960–1971*

DISEASE STAGE	NUMBER OF PATIENTS	YEARS OF FOLLOW-UP	REGRESSION (PERCENT)	NO CHANGE (PERCENT)	PROGRESSION (PERCENT)
Mild-moderate dysplasia	151	1–8.0	63.6	26.5	9.9
Severe dysplasia	74	1–9.5	58.1	25.7	16.4
Severe dysplasia—borderline carcinoma in situ	32	1–7.5	25.1	43.8	31.3
Carcinoma in situ	37	1–7.0	2.7	43.2	54.0

(Kurihara et al, 1972)

them (22%) developed invasive carcinoma of the cervix or vaginal vault. This is one of the rare studies that have been conducted on the biologic behavior of carcinoma in situ without treatment.

Two histologic classifications for premalignant changes of the cervical epithelium are used. The traditional classification described mild, moderate, severe dysplasia, and carcinoma in situ. Mild dysplasia is used for lesions where abnormal cells involve the lower one-third of the epithelium (Fig. 31–4); moderate, one-half of the epithelium (Fig. 31–5); and severe dysplasia for lesions with almost full-thickness involvement, but still some differentiated cells remaining on the surface of the epithelium (Fig. 31–6A,B). Carcinoma in situ is diagnosed when complete undifferentiation of the entire thickness of the epithelium is present. Richart introduced a new concept in which dysplasia and in situ carcinoma form a biologic continuum of preinvasive neoplastic changes. The biologic behavior of any particular case of dysplasia or cervical intraepithe-

lial neoplasia cannot be accurately predicted by histologic or cytologic analysis. All significant dysplasias from mild through severe have the capacity to persist or to progress to a higher rate of abnormality or directly to invasive carcinoma (Figs. 31–7, 31–8).

Richart proposed the term *cervical intraepithelial neoplasia* (CIN), divided into three grades: CIN I corresponds to mild dysplasia, CIN II to moderate dysplasia, and CIN III to severe dysplasia or carcinoma in situ.

Cervical intraepithelial neoplasia has no clinical signs or symptoms, and therefore routine surveillance is required to detect these early lesions. Although a number of different screening techniques have been proposed over the years, the cytologic smear has proven to be the most easily applicable,

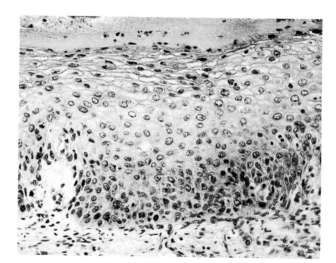

FIG. 31–4 Mild dysplasia of cervical epithelium.

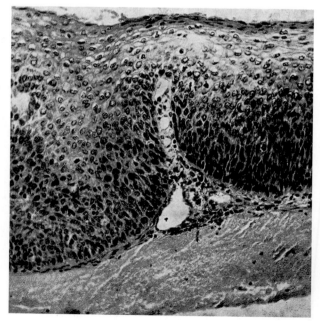

FIG. 31–5 Moderate dysplasia of cervical epithelium.

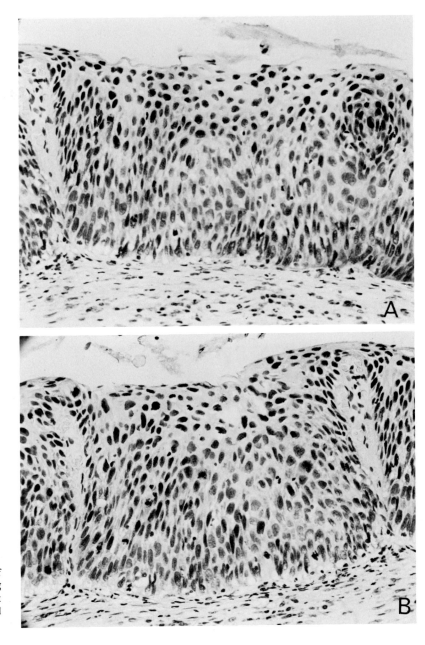

FIG. 31–6 (*A* and *B*) Severe dysplasia of cervix with epithelial changes extending through most of the surface epithelium but without the full-thickness change required for diagnosis of carcinoma in situ.

economical, and most effective tool yet devised. All women should be screened regularly when they begin sexual activity, regardless of age. Screening intervals depend on many factors but generally are 1 year. The likelihood of an abnormal Papanicolaou smear after three negative smears is very low. Some authors therefore have questioned the necessity of yearly cytologic examinations in women who have previously had three negative yearly smears. We are in favor of yearly examinations for two reasons.

First, cytologic examination is a part of a yearly gynecologic examination, which also includes a breast and pelvic examination; and second, the relatively high false-negative rate of a single smear warrants reexamination. With every subsequent cytologic smear, the false-negative rate of cytology is lower.

Richart estimated the false-negativity rate of cytology as 2.8%. In studies by Griffiths and Younge, Silbar and Woodruff, and Singleton and Rutledge,

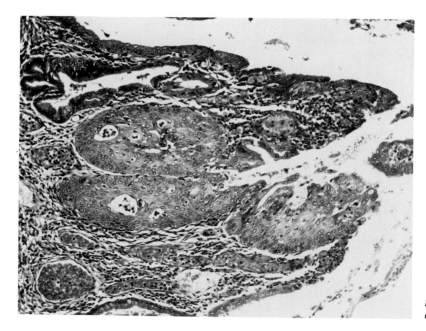

FIG. 31–7 Squamous metastasis displacing cervical glands well into cervix.

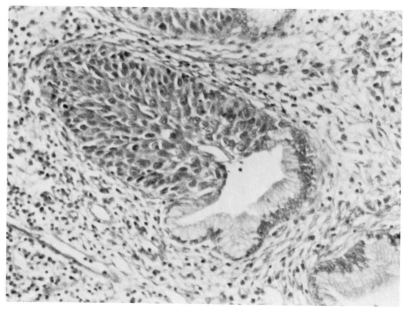

FIG. 31–8 Carcinoma in situ with involvement of endocervical clefts showing neoplastic epithelium "snowplowing" beneath glandular epithelium and filling of the gland-like lumen.

in which routine multiple cervical biopsies were obtained from Schiller negative areas (Schiller-light) in all patients with negative cytology, false-negative rates of cytology of 18.2%, 19.2%, and 20.4% were reported. Studies in which both colposcopy and cytology were used as diagnostic procedures found a false-negative rate of cytology of between 10.7% and 13.0%. Gusberg, who employed cone biopsy in the evaluation of patients with negative cytology, found the false-negativity rate to be 12.5%. In studies where

routine multiple cervical biopsies were obtained from Schiller negative areas (Schiller-light) in all patients with negative cytology, a false-negativity rate of cytology of 18.2% and 19.2% was reported. Studies in which both colposcopy and cytology have been used as diagnostic procedures demonstrate a false-negativity rate of cytology between 10.7% and 13.0%.

In cases of very early cervical neoplasia, only a few patients with abnormal cytology will have a grossly abnormal lesion on the cervix. However, if such a lesion is visible, it must be biopsied. In most patients, examination of the cervix with the unaided eye shows no difference between the cervix with a preinvasive lesion and one with benign changes. During the reproductive period of a woman's life, the squamocolumnar junction appears on the portio vaginalis of the cervix in most women. This causes the region around the cervical os to appear red and somewhat granular on direct visualization. This reddish area around the external os is described by most gynecologists as an "erosion," but a true erosion, a loss of epithelium, rarely exists in these cases. With the naked eye, it is difficult or even impossible to differentiate between the presence of columnar epithelium, early metaplasia, inflammation, or neoplasia.

A blind four-quadrant biopsy was very popular several years ago, but was associated with a significant error rate. The high error rates led other clinicians to evaluate the efficacy of taking multiple biopsies and having multiple sections examined histologically from each tissue fragment. Silbar and Woodruff performed a retrospective analysis of 185 cases in which multiple biopsies were taken and in which each tissue fragment was examined at three levels in the block. The biopsy failed to reveal the full extent of the anaplasia in 11 cases. The authors felt that this 6% error precluded the use of biopsy alone as a basis for therapy.

The largest series on this subject was reported by Sabatelle, who described the results found in 859 cases in which at least 6 to 8 biopsies were obtained from the squamocolumnar junction in cases with atypical vaginal cytology. Excluding the 189 cases in which invasive cancer was confirmed, multiple cervical biopsies in a total of 670 cases failed to show the most serious pathology in 8% of the cases.

Walter Schiller noted (1929) that glycogen was essentially absent from cervical and vaginal epithelium in cases with early squamous carcinoma. After much trial and error, he found that a weak aqueous solution of iodine would stain the glycogen contained in the normal cervical epithelium, producing a dark mahogany color, while leaving areas of carcinoma unstained. Schiller recommended that all unstained areas be carefully scraped and the tissue thus obtained be examined for the presence of neoplastic cells. It soon became apparent that not all areas of the cervix that failed to stain with iodine represented foci of carcinoma. Columnar epithelium, inflammatory areas, recent biopsy sites, and metaplastic areas also failed to take the iodine stain.

The diagnostic accuracy of office methods in detecting early cervical neoplasia is dependent on the number of cervical tissue samples obtained and the number of sections examined from each sample.

In addition, when the tissue is obtained from an area found to be suspicious by Schiller staining, the accuracy is further improved by colposcopic study and a directed biopsy. When the Schiller test is used to direct the gynecologist in obtaining multiple cervical biopsies and an endocervical curettage is performed to evaluate the tissue higher up in the canal, and when all these tissue samples are histologically examined at multiple levels in the block, a rate of accuracy is obtainable that is comparable to that of cervical conization. Unfortunately, this type of meticulous attention to detail is all too infrequent.

A patient with a Papanicolaou smear consistent with neoplasia in whom the diagnosis of invasive carcinoma has not been established by cervical biopsy should have a colposcopic examination.

Colposcopy

It should be emphasized that whereas cytology is a laboratory method of detection, colposcopy is a clinical method. Each method deals with a different aspect of neoplasia. Cytology evaluates the morphologic changes in exfoliated cells whereas colposcopy evaluates, mainly, the changes in the terminal vascular network of the cervix that reflect the biochemical and metabolic changes in the tissue.

The colposcope is basically a stereoscopic microscope by which the cervix may be visualized in bright light under 6× to 40× magnification. The examination is rapid, requiring almost the same time as the inspection of the cervix with the unaided eye. After the self-retaining speculum is inserted, the mucus is carefully removed from the cervix using a cotton swab or dry gauze. The colposcope is then focused on the cervix. During the inspection, the surface of the cervix should be moistened with normal saline. A dry epithelial surface is insufficiently transparent and allows an incomplete view of the underlying vascular pattern. In a routine colposcopic examination, a magnification of 16× is used. Optimal contrast of the vessels is achieved by the insertion of a green filter. After inspection of the cervix moistened with saline, a generous amount of 4% acetic acid is applied to the cervix. The acetic acid helps to coagulate the mucus, which can then be easily removed from the clefts and folds of columnar epithelium. Acetic acid will also temporarily remove the water from the cells, and, in areas where there is a high nuclear density (immature squamous epithelium, dysplasia, or carcinoma in situ) the epithelium will become white over a fairly well demarcated area. The effect of acetic acid is transient, lasting only a few minutes, but the acetic acid test can be repeated several times.

Colposcopy is based mainly on the stereoscopic evaluation of the transformation zone. The transformation zone is that portion of the cervix that was originally covered by columnar epithelium which, through a gradual process of squamous metaplasia, has been transformed to squamous epithelium. The transformation zone extends between the original squamocolumnar junction (border between original squamous epithelium and endocervical epithelium) and the physiological squamocolumnar junction (border between metaplastic epithelium and columnar epithelium). Colposcopically, it has been shown that cervical neoplasia develops almost exclusively within the transformation zone as a result of atypical metaplasia.

COLPOSCOPIC TERMINOLOGY

Based on the concept of the changes in the transformation zone, a revision of colposcopic terminology was adopted during the Fourth International Congress of Cervical Pathology and Colposcopy in London, England, in 1981. Colposcopic findings are divided as follows:

Normal colposcopic findings include the original squamous epithelium, normal columnar epithelium, and the transformation zone (Plates 31–1, 31–2, and 31–3).

Abnormal colposcopic findings include an atypical transformation zone in which there are colposcopic findings suggestive of cervical neoplasia, namely: mosaic, punctation, aceto-white epithelium, leukoplakia, an elevated whitened plaque of hyperkeratosis or parakeratosis, or atypical blood vessels (Plates 31–4, 31–5, 31–6, and 31–7).

Suspect frank invasive cancer includes those cases with colposcopically obvious invasive cancer which are not evident on clinical examination (Plate 31–8).

Unsatisfactory colposcopic findings are those cases in which the squamocolumnar junction cannot be visualized.

Other colposcopic findings include inflammatory changes, atropic epithelium, true erosion, and condyloma or papilloma.

DIAGNOSTIC FEATURES WITH COLPOSCOPY

Cervical neoplasia does not develop in patients with normal colposcopic findings. In patients with abnormal colposcopic findings, a colposcopic biopsy from the most suspicious lesion should be taken for histopathologic diagnosis. The histopathologic changes that are associated with mosaic, punctation, and aceto-white epithelium range from immature squamous metaplasia to carcinoma in situ. When atypical vessels are present, invasion can be expected. To predict the type of histopathologic changes that will be found in a colposcopically directed biopsy extensive clinical experience is required in the evaluation of vascular pattern, intercapillary distance, surface contour, color tone, and the clarity of demarcation of the focal lesion.

The vascular pattern is one of the most important diagnostic features. Changes in the vascular pattern correspond closely to the histologic picture. It is generally accepted that the first changes in carcinogenesis occur biochemically at the cellular level and can be detected only by very sophisticated laboratory methods, which are not clinically applicable. During the earliest stages of carcinogenesis, the morphology of the tissue proper may not be altered sufficiently for histologic diagnosis. The blood vessels, however, do react to these changes in tissue metabolism, and such vascular alterations constitute the first morphological features in the development of cervical neoplasia. These vascular changes are not detectable in 5-micron histological sections, but they are clearly visible through the colposcope. For a detailed description of the different patterns of vascular change and their diagnostic significance, the reader is referred to the colposcopic literature.

Intercapillary distance refers to the space between corresponding parts of two adjacent vessels or to the diameter delineated by a network of mosaic-like vessels. During actual colposcopy, an estimation of the intercapillary distance in abnormal areas can best be made by comparing it with that of the capillaries found in the adjacent normal epithelium. In preinvasive and invasive carcinoma of the cervix, the intercapillary distance increases as the stage of the disease advances.

Surface contour and colors. The colposcope provides stereoscopic magnification, which greatly facilitates the study of the surface contour. This may be described as smooth, uneven, granular, papillomatous, or nodular. Normal squamous epithelium has a smooth surface, whereas carcinoma in situ and early invasive cancer may both have an uneven, slightly elevated surface. Different colposcopic lesions show different colors, varying from white to deep red. The difference between the color before and the color after the acetic acid test is very important; if there is a marked change from deep red to white, a more serious histological lesion may be expected.

The border between the lesion and the adjacent normal tissue is an important feature concerned with the colposcopic diagnosis of cervical neoplasia.

The borderline between normal squamous epithelium and inflammatory lesions or mild dysplasia is quite diffuse. On the other hand, severe dysplasia and carcinoma in situ usually produce sharp bordered lesions, distinctly demarcated from the adjacent epithelium.

Unsatisfactory colposcopic findings mean that the squamocolumnar junction is not visible, a condition that occurs more often in postmenopausal women. Unsatisfactory colposcopy is present in less than 15% of patients under 45 years of age. In patients with unsatisfactory colposcopic findings, one cannot rely on colposcopy for a clinical diagnosis since the pathologic changes may be high in the endocervical canal, and other diagnostic methods (endocervical curettage or conization) are required.

At the present time, the main value of colposcopy is in the evaluation of patients with abnormal cytologic findings. With colposcopy, it is possible to localize the lesion, evaluate its extent, and obtain a directed biopsy whereby the histopathologic diagnosis can be established. Colposcopy is very accurate in differentiating between invasive and noninvasive lesions and in the differential diagnosis between inflammatory atypia and neoplasia. The limitation of colposcopy lies in its inability to detect lesions deep in the endocervical canal in cases where the squamocolumnar junction is not visible. In these cases, colposcopy is not negative but unsatisfactory, and further diagnostic steps, mainly endocervical curettage or conization, are necessary in evaluating a patient with abnormal cytology.

The term *unsatisfactory colposcopy* was not recognized in previous terminology, which explains the high false-negative rate of colposcopy reported in the German literature. When cases of unsatisfactory colposcopic findings are excluded, the true false-negative rate of colposcopy is very low.

Colposcopy is ideal for the evaluation and management of the pregnant patients with abnormal cytology. The physiologic eversion of the pregnant cervix affords good colposcopic visualization of the entire squamocolumnar junction. Such patients are excellent candidates for colposcopic evaluation of an abnormal vaginal smear. During the last 14 years, we have performed only two conizations in pregnant patients at the Milwaukee County General Hospital. A microinvasive cancer was found in both cases in directed biopsy and the conization was done to evaluate the extent of the lesion. In all other pregnant patients where a directed biopsy showed only intraepithelial cervical neoplasia, the definitive treatment was postponed until 6 weeks after delivery, at which time the surgical specimen demonstrated the identical histologic lesion as noted in

directed biopsy during pregnancy. In no case had the lesion progressed to invasive cancer.

Although colposcopy is an appropriate method for evaluation of a patient with abnormal vaginal cytology, colposcopic expertise is not available in every medical facility. Without colposcopy, the patient with abnormal cytology should have a careful speculum examination of the cervix and vagina, with the application of Lugol's solution (iodine, 3 g; potassium iodide, 6 g; water, 100 ml). Any abnormal lesion should be biopsied and endocervical curettage performed. In a case of vaginal inflammation, a wet vaginal smear should be examined and the patient should be treated according to the etiology of the vaginitis. A cytologic smear should be repeated at the time of the examination and again 2 months later. In postmenopausal women, the abnormal cytology may be caused by atrophic changes in cervicovaginal epithelium. These patients should be treated with estrogen locally and the cytologic smear should be repeated in 1 month.

When cervical biopsies show noninvasive changes, a diagnostic conization is indicated. It should be stressed that diagnostic conization is always necessary in cases where a blind cervical biopsy shows a carcinoma in situ in order to exclude the possibility of invasive carcinoma in another area of the cervix. Preferably, the patient should be referred for colposcopic study.

Conization is considered as definitive treatment of cervical carcinoma in situ when the exact limits of the lesion are defined by colposcopy, or when the histopathologic specimen has completely free margins after careful evaluation of the cone. Although conizations may be adequate treatment for in situ carcinoma in most cases, hysterectomy may still be indicated in some cases. The decision to treat a patient with carcinoma in situ by conization or hysterectomy depends on several factors: (1) age, (2) parity, (3) desire to preserve the uterus, (4) desire for permanent sterilization, (5) fear of conservative treatment, (6) reliability of the patient for continued follow-up, and (7) other gynecologic indications.

Conization of the Cervix

Cold knife conization of the cervix consists of the annular removal of a cone-shaped wedge of tissue from the cervix uteri. To be considered adequate for diagnostic purposes, the operative specimen must include uninvolved endocervical epithelium above the lesion and uninvolved ectocervix below and lateral to any lesion on the portio. Just how much tissue such a specimen should encompass must vary with the individual case. During the reproductive years, most lesions are found on the portio so that the cone will usually have a broad base and the tip will have a wide angle. In older women, where the squamocolumnar junction has shifted to a location higher in the endocervical canal, the cone specimen will be long and narrow with a sharp endocervical angle at the tip of the cone. The width of the base is best determined by including all Schiller light areas of the portio within the cone margins.

Preoperative vaginal examinations should be limited strictly, and most operators will forego the routine intravaginal prep, as both these procedures may denude the cervical epithelium, which is crucial for the histologic diagnosis. The cervix is exposed and a Lugol's stain is performed. Tenaculae or holding sutures are placed into the cervix laterally at the 3 and 9 o'clock positions beyond the margins of Schiller light epithelium. With traction on the cervix, the cervical stroma is infiltrated with 40 to 60 ml of 1:200,000 solution of Neo-Synephrine in a circumferential manner. If the injection is placed properly into the stroma, a significant amount of pressure will be required on the controlled syringe plunger. The cervix will be seen to blanch and increase somewhat in size.

The uterine canal is sounded gently and the sound is left in place to mark the course of the endocervical canal. A circular incision is then made outside the Schiller light margin beginning posteriorly with the tip of the blade directed against the metal probe in the cervical canal. The specimen should be excised in a single piece, and it is our custom to identify the 12 o'clock position on the specimen with a single suture placed into the cervical stroma. The excised tissue should not be placed in fixative at this time.

Dilatation and fractional curettage may be performed, after which the cervix may be treated in one of two ways: the cone site may be left open or Sturmdorf sutures may be used to close the raw areas. If the Sturmdorf suture is used, the suture should be placed in the posterior lip first. No. 1 delayed-absorbable sutures are used on a large cutting needle. Initially, the suture picks up the posterior flap of mucosa in the midline near the edge (Fig. 31–9). Then the suture is directed high into the endocervical canal, passing through the wall of the cervical canal and out through the portio of the posterior cervical lip near the fornix, approximately 2 cm from the site of the initial suture. As the mucosal flap is pulled forward, the other end of the suture is threaded into the cutting needle and the process of suturing through the cervical canal is repeated. The two ends of the suture should emerge on the posterior surface of the cervix about 0.5 cm

apart. Firm traction on this suture will pull the posterior mucosal flap well into the newly made cervical canal. The suture is tied and the procedure is repeated on the anterior lip.

If the cone site is left open, a superficial electrocoagulation of the bleeding points in the cervical stroma is performed, followed by application of a piece of Gelfoam sponge to the cervical defect. This is held in place with a vaginal pack that is removed in 24 hours. The cosmetic results of this method are equal to those obtained with the Sturmdorf suture technique, and there is the added theoretical advantage that one is not covering up deep residual nests of tumor that may be unable to reveal their presence by exfoliation. However, since the Sturmdorf suture is gradually released with the dissolution of the suture material, its only advantage has been in the immediate control of bleeding. Comparing these two methods of closure, Chao found no significant difference in operative blood loss or incidence of postoperative hemorrhage.

When the conization specimen is received in the laboratory, it should be opened lengthwise with a sharp knife blade at the 12 o'clock position and spread flat. The margins of the cone are pinned to a large paraffin block, care being taken not to pierce the epithelium with the holding pins. Then the entire block is placed in fixative solution. After fixation, the cone is cut lengthwise into as many sections as possible, again using a sharp thin blade. The average cone specimen can easily be divided into 15 or more tissue slices. Each slice is separately imbedded, and multiple sections are cut from each block. If five sections are obtained from each tissue slice, 75 slides will be available for histologic examination.

The number of sections examined is crucial. As reported by Burghardt, diagnostic errors will increase by 22% if only 15 histologic sections are examined from each cone instead of 80 sections. Most investigators have reported a fairly consistent diagnostic error rate for conization of 3.5%, with a range varying between 0.5% and 9.0%.

Many clinics have recommended the use of immediate frozen section interpretation of the cone specimen so that the definitive operative procedure may be performed upon receiving the report from the pathologist. Clinical experience with the conization–hysterectomy sequence has shown that the surgical morbidity rate is lowest when the hysterectomy is performed either immediately or within 48 hours after the conization. Otherwise, the hysterectomy should be deferred for 6 weeks after conization. Although the combined conization–hysterectomy technique is economically reasonable, its major drawback is the risk of missing focal areas of invasive tumor. In most instances, the patient

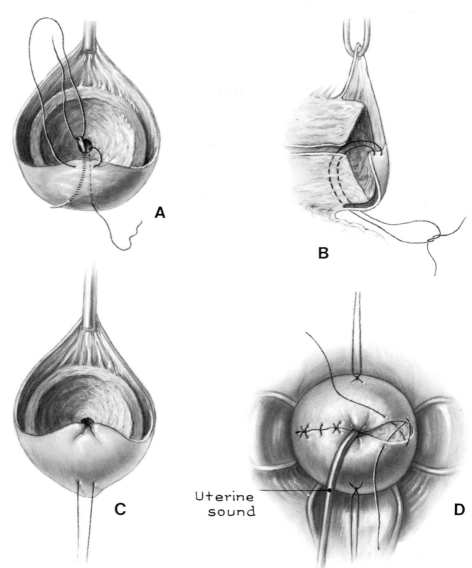

FIG. 31-9 (*A*) Mattress suture is being placed as in Sturmdorf tracheloplasty. (*B*) Method of action of suture in drawing the flap into the canal. (*C*) The lower flap has been pulled into position. (*D*) Anterior and posterior flaps have been drawn into the canal. Lateral mucosa wounds are being sutured.

Uterine sound

would be better treated by deferring the definitive treatment until the cone specimen had been studied thoroughly. This would avoid the necessity of the surgeon having to make a surgical decision with, possibly, incomplete laboratory information.

Conization is not an innocuous procedure and is associated with serious complications such as: hemorrhage, requiring transfusion in 5% to 10% of cases; stenosis; uterine perforation; pelvic cellulitis; and injury to the rectum and bladder. The bladder and rectal complications are usually seen in cases in which there is a significant atrophy with shallow vaginal fornices. Of all the complications of sharp conization of the cervix for diagnostic purposes,

none is more significant than the morbidity occurring in the pregnant patient. Following cervical conization during pregnancy, the average fetal loss is approximately 10% and the incidence of postoperative hemorrhage is 30%.

Treatment of Carcinoma in Situ

Formerly, the accepted treatment of cervical carcinoma in situ was hysterectomy with excision of a wide vaginal cuff. Although total hysterectomy remains the most common treatment in patients who have completed their childbearing, colposcopic studies have shown that foci of cervical neoplasia are often small and discrete and that such an operation may be excessive and unnecessary. In a patient with cervical intraepithelial neoplasia, there is no risk of lymphatic spread and therefore complete local excision or destruction of the pathologic lesion has become accepted in many clinics as adequate treatment. Extension of carcinoma in situ into the vaginal fornices occurs in less than 3% of patients. These cases can be identified accurately by colposcopy and only in those rare cases is removal of a wide vaginal cuff indicated. The concept that removal of a wide vaginal cuff is necessary to eliminate the "fields of neoplastic potential" is recognized now as invalid in view of the fact that the previously reported cases of recurrence of carcinoma in situ at the apex of the vagina after total hysterectomy were undoubtedly instances of inadequate excision of the entire lesion at the time of surgery. In 593 colposcopically diagnosed cases of carcinoma in situ treated by conization or hysterectomy, Coppelson has not detected a single case of recurrent carcinoma in situ in the vaginal vault. While it is well known that a patient with cervical carcinoma in situ has a higher chance of developing cancer in the lower genital tract, this lesion can develop anywhere in the vagina or on the vulva, and removal of the vaginal cuff will not protect the patient from this occurrence. Creasman and Rutledge found that 18% of 261 patients treated for cervical in situ carcinoma developed a second malignant or premalignant lesion elsewhere in the body and that half of these second cancers were found in the female genital tract. This high incidence of second primaries is significant and requires a diligent and continued search for other lesions in patients with carcinoma in situ. The same authors also agree that the recurrence of carcinoma in situ does not depend on the amount of vaginal cuff removed. The same recurrence rate (2.6%) was found if the length of removed cuff was less than 1 cm, between 1 and 3 cm, or more than 3 cm.

Cure rates with conization are higher in series in which colposcopy was used in the preoperative evaluation as reported by Ahlgren and associates. The importance of long-term follow-up is evident from a report by Kolstad and Klem. Their series of 1121 patients with carcinoma in situ represents both the largest and the longest follow-up experience available with this disease. These patients were followed from 5 to 25 years. Therapeutic conization was performed in 795 patients, of which 19 patients (2.3%) developed recurrent carcinoma in situ and 7 patients (0.9%) developed invasive cancer. Of particular interest was the finding in 238 patients with

carcinoma in situ who were treated with hysterectomy, of which 3 patients (1.2%) developed invasive cancer. This large series indicates that the recurrence rate after conization is not higher than after a conventional hysterectomy, provided that the conization is performed after colposcopic evaluation of the size and localization of the lesion. It is stressed that women having once had carcinoma in situ of the cervix will always be at some risk for recurrent disease or a second primary and therefore should be carefully followed for a much longer time than the conventional 5 years.

A hysterectomy is indicated after initial treatment of carcinoma in situ by conization when the margins of the cone specimen are not free of disease, when there is persistent abnormal cervical-vaginal cytology, or for other gynecologic indications.

In recent years, even more conservative methods than conization have been used for the treatment of cervical intraepithelial neoplasia. Chanen and Rome selected a group of 1864 nonpregnant patients in whom the margins of a noninvasive lesion were fully visible and located entirely within view of the colposcope. These patients were treated by electrocoagulation diathermy. Needle and ball electrodes were used with the standard Bovie electrosurgical unit. The needle electrodes were inserted into the cervix to a depth of 1.5 cm and multiple punctures were made over the entire abnormal transformation zone and the adjacent area of the columnar epithelium. The aim of the treatment was the destruction of the lesion and any involvement of deep glandular spaces. A ball electrode was then used to coagulate the surface of the area that had been subjected to the needle diathermy electrode. The coagulation extended into the lower endocervical canal, which had been previously dilated. The procedure was performed under general or regional anesthesia. The duration of follow-up was from 1 to 15 years. Of the 1734 patients who returned for follow-up examination after electrocoagulation diathermy treatment, 47 were found to have persistent disease. This represented an apparent primary cure rate of 97.3% for this method of treatment.

Cryosurgery has gained popularity in the treatment of cervical dysplasia and carcinoma in situ. The main advantage of cryosurgery in comparison to electrocautery is that cryosurgery is an outpatient procedure, it is done without anesthesia, and the discomfort to the patient is minimal. The refrigerants used in cryosurgery include freon ($-60°C$), carbon dioxide ($-60°C$), nitrous oxide ($-80°C$) and liquid nitrogen ($-90°C$). Townsend has treated more than 500 patients with cervical intraepithelial neoplasia by cryosurgery. Of this group, more than 200 patients had either severe dysplasia or carcinoma in situ. His method of evaluation of the patients prior to cryosurgery included repeat cytology, colposcopic examination, directed biopsies from the most suspicious areas, and endocervical curettage. He selected only those patients for cryosurgery where the entire limits of the lesion were seen and where the endocervical curettage revealed no abnormal tissue. Cryosurgery was effective in 90% of the patients treated. Of the freeze failures, about 35% occurred in patients where the lesion was so extensive that the initial freezing was inadequate. Fifteen patients have been retreated and all but one have been free of disease after the second treatment session.

In 1980, Creasman and Weed reported on 557 patients with cervical intraepithelial neoplasia who were treated by cryosurgery. Treatment failures were 9% in CIN I, 5% in CIN II, and 12% in CIN III.

The risk of recurring disease after cryosurgery was studied by Richart and associates. From nine institutions, 2839 patients were treated by cryosurgery for cervical intraepithelial neoplasia and were followed longitudinally after three negative Papanicolaou smears to ascertain the risk of recurrence. The cumulative risk of developing cervical intraepithelial neoplasia after successful cryosurgical treatment was 0.41% at year 5, 0.44% at year 10, and 0.44% at year 14. There was no significant difference in risk between patients originally treated for CIN I, CIN II, or CIN III.

In his initial report (1973), Creasman demonstrated in a group of 27 patients who received a single freeze that cervical dysplasia persisted in 48%. In 48 patients undergoing "double freeze" technique, 18% had severe dysplasia or carcinoma in situ in the surgical specimen. After this report, most authors have favored the freeze-thaw-freeze technique. Benedet and associates (1981) produced results that compared very favorably with any obtained to date by using only the standard 7-minute freeze. With new cryosurgical equipment using nitrous oxide, a double freeze is not necessary and will not produce better results.

CARBON DIOXIDE LASER THERAPY

The carbon dioxide laser is one of the new modalities of outpatient therapy for cervical intraepithelial neoplasia. The laser produces infrared energy at a wavelength of 10.6 microns. When used for the treatment of cervical intraepithelial neoplasia, the laser is attached to the colposcope and, with a micromanipulator, the laser beam is directed at the tissue that is to be destroyed. The diameter of the laser beam, at its focal point, is approximately 1.8 mm. The laser beam is totally controlled by the surgeon, so that tissue can be destroyed with precision.

The tissue, during the laser therapy, is destroyed by three mechanisms: direct tissue evaporation; necrosis caused by absorption of infrared energy (this layer of necrosis is of a uniform 50-micron thickness that is independent of the power output of the laser or duration of exposure); and necrosis resulting from the thermal burn the depth of the thermal burn (less than 1 mm) is directly related to the exposure time but is independent of the power output of the laser.

Because the amount of tissue destruction following laser treatment is less than that following cryosurgery, tissue healing is more rapid and vaginal discharge is less profuse. After cryosurgery, the entire circumference of the cervical os and squamocolumnar junction is frozen and becomes necrotic, leading to sloughing and profuse discharge. Most of the localized tissue destruction following laser therapy is by evaporation, which keeps the zone of necrosis very superficial. As a result, the amount of granulation tissue developing during the healing process is minimal.

The cure rates following laser therapy are closely related to the depth of vaporization. Jordan and Mylotte (Table 31–3) demonstrated that the depth of vaporization is more important than the severity of the cervical intraepithelial neoplasia. With a depth of destruction between 5 and 7 mm, cure rates were 92%.

One of the major disadvantages of laser therapy is the high cost of the instrument. The immobility of the instrument also limits its practical use and efficiency. So it remains questionable if the advantages of laser treatment outweigh the high cost of the instrument. Our experience suggests that laser therapy will be of most value in the management of vaginal intraepithelial lesions and that cervical neoplasia can be equally well treated by much simpler methods.

Treatment of Recurrences of Carcinoma in Situ

After the treatment of cervical carcinoma in situ, a recurrent carcinoma in situ develops in approximately 2% of patients, either in the vaginal cuff or as isolated islands in the vagina. It is our opinion that most cases of carcinoma in situ in the vaginal cuff represent residual disease that was not removed at the time of primary treatment. These cases might

TABLE 31-3 *"Cure Rate" of Cervical Intraepithelial Neoplasia Following a Single Laser Destruction to Different Depths*

DEPTH OF DESTRUCTION	CIN I		CIN II		CIN III	
	Number Treated	Percent "Cured"	Number Treated	Percent "Cured"	Number Treated	Percent "Cured"
1–2 mm	5	20	7	14	19	15
2–4 mm	18	77	18	61	56	39
4–5 mm	1	100	3	66	8	75
5–7 mm	4	75	16	100	42	92

(Jordan JA, Mylotte, MJ, Allen J: unpublished results, 1980)

have been avoided if a Schiller test or colposcopic examination of the cervix and upper vagina had been performed preoperatively to ascertain the extent of the lesion.

Controversy persists as to whether isolated islands of carcinoma in situ of the vagina found after treatment of the cervix represent a recurrent disease or a new primary lesion. It is well recognized that a woman who developed carcinoma in situ of the cervix has a higher chance of developing carcinoma of the lower genital canal, including the vagina and vulva.

In the management of recurrent carcinoma in situ of the vagina, a colposcopic evaluation is important to evaluate the extent and location of the lesions. Depending on the location and extent of the lesion and the age, and parity of the patient, one of the following modalities of treatment can be used:

Excisional biopsy
Carbon dioxide laser vaporization
Partial vaginectomy
Total vaginectomy
Topical 5-fluorouracil treatment
Irradiation therapy

Excisional biopsy can be used only in very small, isolated lesions in the vagina. When colposcopic examination 3 months after the excisional biopsy reveals that the lesion was completely removed, the patient can be followed by cytology.

Carbon dioxide laser vaporization provides an ideal modality of treatment of vaginal carcinoma in situ. After laser vaporization therapy, little granulation tissue develops and, therefore, large areas of the vagina can be treated without narrowing or scarring of the vagina. Carcinoma in situ of the vagina usually is a superficial lesion and, unlike cervical lesions, involves only squamous epithelium. A relatively superficial vaporization of the vaginal mucosa (2–3 mm depth) can completely evaporate all the pathologic tissue. The risk of injury to the

bladder or rectum is, therefore, minimal. Laser treatment of the upper one-third of the vagina can be tolerated by most patients without anesthesia. However, for treatment of the lower portion of the vagina, anesthesia is necessary. Capen and associates reported on the treatment of 15 unselected patients with vaginal intraepithelial neoplasia, primarily with carbon dioxide laser; there were two failures. However, the follow-up time was short. More failures occur after the laser treatment if there is a carcinoma in situ of the vaginal cuff after hysterectomy. In this situation, carcinoma in situ is usually buried deeper in the suture line and is not destroyed by the laser beam. Therefore, recurrences are more common in this location.

Partial vaginectomy is used for the treatment of lesions in the vaginal cuff after hysterectomy, mainly in patients in whom there was a previous failure of laser vaporization. The margins of the resection should extend at least 5 mm from a colposcopically visible lesion. The margins of the vaginal mucosa are grasped with Allis clamps and the vaginal mucosa is incised around the lesion and separated from the underlining tissue with sharp and blunt dissection. In the suture line, the vaginal mucosa must be sharply separated by scissors, carefully avoiding injury to the bladder or rectum. After the removal of the operative specimen, it is necessary for the pathologist to examine the resected margins carefully to make sure that they are free of disease. Lee and Symmonds reported 43 patients with recurrent carcinoma in situ treated by partial vaginectomy. There were no bladder or rectal injuries and no recurrence in follow-up in these cases. Our experience has been similar.

Total vaginectomy with or without skin graft is a formidable procedure and is necessary only in patients who have multicentric areas of recurrence. The technique of this procedure is described in Chapter 29. Lee and Symmonds prefer to delay the placement of the split-thickness skin graft for 3 or

4 days after the total vaginectomy in order to ensure a dry bed for the graft and a good graft take. More commonly, the vaginal canal is replaced with a split-thickness skin graft from the thigh at the time of the vaginectomy.

Topical 5-fluorouracil (5FU) treatment of in situ carcinoma of the vagina was first reported by Woodruff and associates, who treated nine patients and had only one failure. They advise frequent examination and repeat applications of the agent. Daly and Ellis treated 17 patients with 5% 5FU applied twice daily with a vaginal applicator for 14 days. Zinc oxide ointment was placed on the vulva and perineum to minimize external irritation. Of the 17 patients treated in this study, two were unable to complete the full 14-day course because of ulceration in the vaginal vestibule. The remaining 15 patients were followed for 2 to 4 years and no recurrence was detected.

Irradiation therapy is usually used in patients who have complicated medical diseases, are elderly, and are unable to tolerate any of the other modalities of treatment. Intravaginal radium or cesium is usually contained in a vaginal cylinder 3.5 cm in diameter. The radium sources are arranged so as to deliver an average dose of 7000 rads to the surface of the vagina in a single application. The depth of the effective dose is limited to the vaginal membrane and the immediate 5 mm of underlining subcutaneous tissues. Rutledge treated 31 patients with in situ vaginal cancer with irradiation therapy and no recurrence was diagnosed. The sequelae of the irradiated vagina are usually greater than those of surgical treatment of vaginal recurrences; vaginal atrophy, contracture, fibrosis, and synechiae can result unless specific efforts are taken to maintain vaginal patency with a dilator or frequent coitus. The use of estrogen vaginal suppositories or cream is also important in maintaining a functional vaginal canal following intravaginal irradiation.

Microinvasive Carcinoma

In 1961, the International Federation of Gynecology and Obstetrics (FIGO) officially subdivided Stage I cervical carcinoma into Stage Ia and Ib. The new Stage Ia classification was made to include preclinical or early stromal invasion, which is now termed *microinvasive carcinoma*. In 1971, Stage Ia was further subdivided by FIGO into early stromal invasion and occult cancer. The 1976 modification of the International Classification of carcinoma of the cervix redefined Stage Ib as either occult or clinically invasive cancer, restricting Ia to microinvasive carcinoma. Since occult invasive tumors cannot be di-

agnosed by routine clinical examination, they should be classified as *Stage Ib occult* when identified by conization of the cervix.

Diagnosis is based on microscopic examination of the tissue removed by biopsy, conization, portio amputation, or removal of the uterus. Microinvasive disease includes unambiguous cases of epithelial abnormalities with early stromal invasion (FIGO Annual Report, vol 18).

The major debate among pathologists and clinicians concerns the depth of stromal invasion that should separate Stage Ia and Ib lesions. Most clinics divide Stage Ia from Stage Ib somewhere between 3 and 5 mm of stromal invasion beneath the basement membrane, when there is no microlymphatic involvement. Other definitions include in the Stage Ib category microscopic tumors containing confluent tongues of malignant epithelium.

Since Stage Ia lesions are usually detected in asymptomatic women by vaginal cytology, and since few gross clinical features separate this microinvasive lesion from carcinoma in situ, differential diagnosis is best made by an experienced colposcopist in conjunction with a directed biopsy. If the question of microinvasion is raised from either the colposcopic findings or from the biopsy, a conization of the cervix is mandatory to rule out the possibility of frank clinical cancer. Colposcopy should be used not to make a final diagnosis, but to distinguish the most suspect areas of the cervix so they can be studied more closely. When pathologic findings include any possibility of microinvasive carcinoma, a conization is always required.

Three criteria are used to define microinvasive carcinoma: depth of stromal invasion, confluence of invading epithelial tongues, and microlymphatic or vascular involvement. Unfortunately, precise distinctions for the three factors have not been established. Depth of stromal invasion is the major criterion in making a diagnosis. Although most authorities, including the Armed Forces Institute of Pathology, agree that stromal penetration to a depth of no more than 3 mm from the basement membrane constitutes the limits of stromal extension for microinvasive disease (Fig. 31–10), the depth has not been agreed upon by the Cancer Committee of the General Assembly of FIGO, so comparisons of statistical data are difficult. Limits of the depth of invasion range from 1 to 5 mm in different studies performed at various clinics. The Armed Forces Institute of Pathology defines the depth of invasion from the surface of the epithelium rather than from the basement membrane.

Many clinics consider confluent tongues of tumor cells to represent a more advanced degree of invasion (Fig. 31–11), but this factor has not been ac-

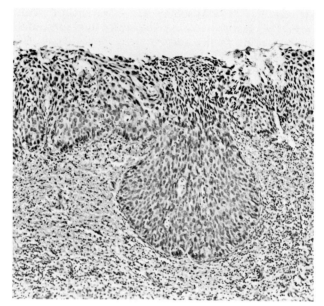

FIG. 31–10 Microinvasive carcinoma of the cervix with stromal invasion of tumor to a depth of 3 mm below the base of the epithelium in the absence of lymphatic or vascular involvement.

cepted universally as indicating frank invasive cancer. Most clinicians define Stage Ia disease (Fig. 31–12) to exclude microlymphatic or vascular involvement because of the high risk of pelvic lymph node metastases in such cases. However, the study by Roche and Norris in 1975 found no evidence of pelvic lymph node metastases following primary radical surgery and node dissection for lesions in 30 patients, 17 of whom (57%) had microlymphatic involvement.

The Committee on Nomenclature for the Society of Gynecologic Oncologists proposed a standard working definition of microinvasive disease in January, 1974:

> A microinvasive lesion should be defined as one in which neoplastic epithelium invades the stroma in one or more places to a depth of 3 mm or less below the base of the epithelium and in which lymphatic or blood vascular involvement is not demonstrated.

The committee also recommended that cases of intraepithelial carcinoma of the cervix with questionable invasion be regarded as intraepithelial carcinoma. The Society's definition of microinvasive carcinoma of the cervix is a reasonable representation of the data currently available concerning the frequency of lymph node metastases.

LYMPH NODE METASTASES

The question of occult pelvic lymph node metastases remains a major point of debate in discussions of

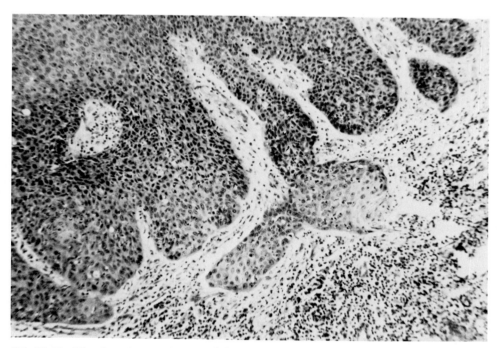

FIG. 31–11 Microinvasive carcinoma of the cervix with infiltration of confluent tongues of tumor within 5 mm from the basement membrane.

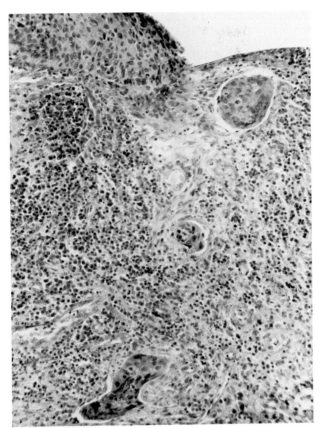

FIG. 31–12 Microlymphatic or vascular involvement of cervical carcinoma with early stromal invasion within 5 mm from basement membrane.

the treatment of microinvasive carcinoma. Averette and Nelson restricted the definition of microinvasion to penetration of less than 1 mm beneath the basement membrane with no invasion of microlymphatic or vascular spaces, and they found no lymph node metastasis among 162 patients whose treatment included pelvic lymphadenectomy.

Van Nagell and associates made detailed studies of the pelvic lymph nodes of patients with microinvasive disease. In a group of 52 patients with stromal invasion of 3 mm or less, a total of 984 lymph nodes were examined, and none had evidence of metastasis. Among 32 patients with stromal invasion of 3.1 to 5.0 mm, three (9.3%) had metastasis to the pelvic nodes.

Van Nagell's work has been supported by several other studies. Seski, Abell, and Morley reported no evidence of regional node metastasis among 37 patients with microinvasive carcinoma following pelvic lymphadenectomy when tumor invasion was 3 mm or less. In 1977, Benson and Norris reviewed reports of 57 cases with stromal invasion of 3 mm or less, with no biasing factors, and found that none

had nodal metastasis. Van Nagell more recently collected 397 cases from the literature with stromal microinvasion of 3.0 mm or less (Table 31–4). Of these, one patient (0.25%) with 1.0 mm of tumor invasion did have lymph node metastasis. More typical findings include 98 cases with stromal invasion of 3.1 to 5.0 mm in which 8 patients (8%) had positive pelvic lymph nodes. All of the data support the definition of microinvasive disease outlined by the Society of Gynecologic Oncologists: The neoplastic epithelium invades the stroma in one or more places to a depth of 3 mm or less below the basement membrane, and lymphatic or blood vascular involvement is not demonstrated.

Other studies have established clear guidelines using a three-dimensional evaluation of microinvasive carcinoma. Burghardt demonstrated the importance of tumor volume in a study of 282 patients with microinvasive disease. During the period 1958 to 1974, Burghardt showed that patients who had less than 420 cubic mm of tumor had no pelvic lymph node extension, and only one patient had pelvic recurrence of the tumor. Lohe used an upper limit of 500 cubic mm to define microcarcinoma. Although this technique of analyzing tumor volume requires the time-consuming and laborious study of a coned specimen, the three-dimensional approach provides the most accurate method of evaluation, which allows more conservative treatment for some patients.

DIAGNOSIS OF MICROINVASIVE CARCINOMA

Microinvasive carcinoma cannot be diagnosed from a random punch biopsy, nor from the colposcopic findings of superficial horizontal vessels. Conization is always required for definitive diagnosis. The accuracy of the diagnosis depends on the number of tissue blocks taken from the cone specimen and the number of histologic sections made from each block.

TREATMENT OF MICROINVASIVE CARCINOMA

Good surgical candidates who have cervical carcinoma that penetrates the stroma for 3.0 mm or less and that does not involve the capillary-like spaces should be treated with a total abdominal hysterectomy. Preferable to a vaginal approach, the abdominal procedure provides an opportunity for a complete assessment of the pelvic lymph nodes and adjacent viscera. Any unsuspected lymph node involvement can be identified during an abdominal procedure. Although some physicians restrict surgery to patients with stromal invasion of 1 mm or less, current data support a more liberal policy.

When a cone specimen demonstrates no evidence of extension of the tumor onto the portio or vaginal

TABLE 31–4 *Frequency of Lymph Node Metastasis in Microinvasive Carcinoma of the Cervix*

STUDY (YEAR)	STROMAL INVASION ≤ 3.0 MM		STROMAL INVASION 3.1 to 5.0 MM	
	Number of Cases	Cases with Positive Nodes	Number of Cases	Cases with Positive Nodes
Smith, et al (1969)	16	0	13	1
Roche, Norris (1975)	9	0	21	0
Leman, et al (1976)	32	0	3	0
Seski, et al (1977)	37	0	—	—
Taki, et al (1979)	55	0	—	—
Yajima, Noda (1979)	90	0	—	—
Hasumi, et al (1980)	106	1	29	4
van Nagell (1983)	52	0	32	3
Total	397	1 (0.25%)	98	8 (8%)

(van Nagell, et al, 1983)

fornices, an extensive vaginal cuff need not be removed, since the vaginal lymphatics are usually not involved. Recurrence in the vaginal vault is the result of failing to define the extent of the lesion prior to surgery. This can usually be prevented with a colposcopic examination before treatment.

Patients who are not good surgical risks can be treated effectively with intracavitary irradiation. One or two intracavitary applications of cesium, using the Fletcher–Suit applicator, should be used to deliver a total dose of 15,000 rads to the cervical canal and portio. Lateral pelvic wall irradiation is not given. Kottmeier has stressed the use of intracavitary irradiation therapy for microinvasive carcinoma. He has reported 5-year cure rates equal to the rates for surgery (98–99%). The only limitation on the use of intracavitary irradiation to treat microinvasive tumors is in the case where a histologic confirmation of the total tumor-bearing area cannot be obtained.

If a case is on the borderline between microinvasive and invasive cancer, the patient should be staged as a Stage Ia and treated as a Stage Ib, since the International Classification requires that the lower stage be used in any questionable lesion. Whatever the classification, it is better to overtreat than to undertreat a borderline lesion, especially one that may extend into the lymphatic drainage of the cervix.

The survival rates for microinvasive disease should reach 98% to 99% if patients are adequately studied and thoughtfully treated. Patients with stromal invasion of more than 3 mm beneath the basement membrane or with tumor invasion of the vascular or capillary-like spaces should be given a treatment plan similar to that for Stage Ib carcinoma.

Treatment for Ib lesions should include either a radical Wertheim hysterectomy with pelvic node dissection or full pelvic megavoltage irradiation.

Bibliography

Ahlgren M, Ingemarsson I, Lindberg L, et al: Conization as treatment of carcinoma in situ of the uterine cervix. Obstet Gynecol 46:135, 1975

Anderson SG, Linton EB: The diagnostic accuracy of cervical biopsy and cervical conization. Am J Obstet Gynecol 99:113, 1967

Annual Report Gynecological Cancer FIGO Vol. 18, Radiumhemmet, Stockholm, Sweden, 1975.

Benedet JL, Nickerson KG, Anderson GH: Cryotherapy in the treatment of cervical intraepithelial neoplasia. Obstet Gynecol 57:5, 1981

Benson, WL, Norris, HJ: A critical review of the frequency of lymph node metastases and death from microinvasive carcinoma of the cervix. Obstet Gynecol 49:632, 1977

Boyes DA, Worth AJ: Cytological screening for cervical cancer. In Jordan JA, Singer A (eds): The Cervix. Philadelphia, WB Saunders, 1976

Boyes DA, Worth AJ, Anderson GH: Experience with cervical screening in British Columbia. Gynecol Oncol 12:143, 1981

Burghardt E: Die diagnostische Konisation der Portio Vaginalis Uteri. Geburtsch. Frauenheilk, 23:1, 1963

Burghardt E, Holzer E: Diagnosis and treatment of microinvasive carcinoma of the cervix uteri. Obstet Gynecol 49:461, 1977

Capen CV, Masterson BJ, Magrina JF, et al: Laser therapy of vaginal intraepithelial neoplasia. Am J Obstet Gynecol 142:973, 1982

Chanen W, Rome R: Electrocoagulation diathermy for cervical dysplasia and carcinoma in situ: A 15-year survey. Am J Obstet Gynecol 61(6):673, 1983

Chao S, McCaffrey RM, Todd WD: Conization in evaluation and management of cervical neoplasm. Am J Obstet Gynecol 103:574, 1969

Coppleson M, Pixley E, Reid B: Colposcopy. Springfield, IL, Charles C Thomas, 1971

Coppleson M, Reid B: Preclinical Carcinoma of the Cervix Uteri. London, Pergamon Press, 1967

Creasman WT, Rutledge F: Carcinoma in situ of the cervix: An analysis of 861 patients. Obstet Gynecol 39:373, 1972

Creasman WT, Weed JC Jr: Conservative management of cervical intraepithelial neoplasia. Clin Obstet Gynecol 23(1):281, 1980

Crisp WE, Smith MS, Asadourian LA, et al: Cryosurgical treatment of premalignant disease of the uterine cervix. Am J Obstet Gynecol 107:737, 1970

Daly JW, Ellis GF: Treatment of vaginal dysplasia and carcinoma in situ with topical 5-fluorouracil. Obstet Gynecol 55(3):350, 1980

Fidler HK, Boyes DA, Worth AJ: Cervical cancer detection in British Columbia. J Obstet Gynaecol Br Commonw 75:392, 1968

Frenkel N, et al: A herpes simplex 2 DNA fragment and its transcription in human cervical cancer tissue. Proc Natl Acad Sci 69:3784, 1972

Green GH: The progression of pre-invasive lesions of the cervix to invasion. NZ Med J 80:279, 1974

Griffiths CT, Younge PA: The clinical diagnosis of early cervical cancer. Obstet Gynecol Surv 24:967, 1969

Gusberg SB: The relative efficiency of diagnostic techniques in the detection of early cervical cancer. A comparative study with a survey of 1,000 normal women. Am J Obstet Gynecol 65:1073, 1953

Kaufman RH, Strama T, Norton PK, et al: Cryosurgical treatment of cervical intraepithelial neoplasias. Am J Obstet Gynecol 42:881, 1973

Kivlahan C, Ingram E: Pap smear without endocervical cells. Obstet Gynecol 65:000, 1985

Kolstad P, Klem V: Long term follow-up of 1,121 cases of carcinoma in situ. Obstet Gynecol 48:125, 1976

Kottmeier HL: Erfahrungen des radiumhemmet. Stockholm, mit der behandlung des oberflachencarcinoma und des frühinvasion carcinoma der cervix. ARCH Gynäkol 207:332, 1969

Kurihara S: Study of Premalignant Lesions of the Uterine Cervix—Benign to Malignant Lesions. Keio Gijuku University School of Medicine, Tokyo, 1972

Lange P: Clinical and Histological Studies on Cervical Carcinoma; Precancerous, Early Metastasis, and Tubular Structures in the Lymph Nodes, p 40. Copenhagen, Munksgaard, 1960

Laverty C, Russel P, Hills E, et al: The significance of noncondylomatous wart virus infection of the cervical transformation zone. A review with discussion of two illustrative cases. Acta Cytol 22:195, 1978

Lee RA, Symmonds RE: Recurrent carcinoma in situ of the vagina in patients previously treated for in situ carcinoma of the cervix. Obstet Gynecol 48(1):61, 1976

Linhartova A: Comparative study of the morphology and evolution of congenital and adult ectopy of the uterine cervix. Plzen lek Shorn 37:85, 1972

Lohe KJ: Early squamous cell carcinoma of the uterine cervix. Gynecol Oncol 6:10, 1978

McIndoe WA, McLean MR, Jones RW, et al: The invasive potential of carcinoma in situ of the cervix. Am J Obstet Gynecol 61:000, 1984

Meisels A, Fortin R, Roy M: Condylomatous lesions of the cervix. II. Cytologic, colposcopic and histopathologic study. Acta Cytol 21:379, 1977

Meisels A, Fortin R: Condylomatous lesions of the cervix and vagina. I. Cytologic patterns. Acta Cytol 20:505, 1976

Naib ZM, et al: Genital herpetic infection-association with cervical dysplasia and carcinoma. Cancer 23:940, 1969

Nelson JH, Averette HE, Richart RM: Detection diagnostic evaluation and treatment of dysplasia and early carcinoma of the cervix. CA-Cancer J Clin 25:134, 1975

Peterson O: Spontaneous course of cervical precancerous conditions. Am J Obstet Gynecol 72:1063, 1956

Richart RM: Natural history of cervical intraepithelial neoplasm. Clin Obstet Gynecol 10:748, 1967

Richart RM, Townsend DE, Crisp W: An analysis of "long-term" follow-up results in patients with cervical intraepithelial neoplasia treated by cryotherapy. Am J Obstet Gynecol 137:823, 1980

Roche WD, Norris HJ: Microinvasive carcinoma of the cervix: The significance of lymphatic invasion and confluent patterns of stromal growth. Cancer 36:180, 1975

Rotkin ID: Adolescent coitus and cervical cancer: Associations of related events and increased risk. Cancer Res 27:603, 1967

Rotkin ID, King R: Environmental variables related to cervical cancer. Am J Obstet Gynecol 83:720, 1962

Royston I, Aurelian L: The association of genital herpes virus with cervical atypia and carcinoma in situ. Am J Epidemiol 91:531, 1970

Rutledge F: Cancer of the Vagina. Am J Obstet Gynecol 97:635, 1967

Sabatelle R, et al: Cervical biopsy versus conization. Cancer 23:663, 1969

Schiller W: Early diagnosis of carcinoma of the cervix. Surg Gynecol Obstet 56:210, 1933

————: Jodpinselung und Abschabung des Portioepithels. Zbl Gynak 53:1056, 1929.

————: Untersuchungen zur Entststehung der Geschwulste; Collum-carcinoma des Uterus, Virchows Arch (A) 263:279, 1927

Schottlander J, Kermauner E: Zur kenntnis des Uteruskarzinoms. Berlin, S Karger AG, 1912

Seski JC, Abell MR, Morley GW: Microinvasive squamous carcinoma of the cervix—Definition, histologic analysis, late results of treatment. Obstet Gynecol 50:410, 1977

Silbar EL, Woodruff JD: Evaluation of biopsy, cone, and hysterectomy sequence in intraepithelial carcinoma of the cervix. Obstet Gynecol 27:89, 1966

Singleton WP, Rutledge F: To cone or not to cone the cervix. Obstet Gynecol 31:430, 1968

Stafl A, Friedrich EG Jr, Mattingly RF: Detection of cervical neoplasia: Reducing the risk of error. Clin Obstet Gynecol 16:238, 1973

Stafl A, Mattingly RF: Colposcopic diagnosis of cervical neoplasia. Obstet Gynecol 41:168, 1973

Starreveld AA, Romanowski B, et al: The latency period of carcinoma-in-situ of the cervix. Obstet Gynecol 62:348, 1983

Te Linde RW: Carcinoma in situ of the cervix. Monographs on Surgery, p 5. New York, Nelson 1951

Te Linde RW, Galvin GA: The minimal histological changes in biopsies to justify a diagnosis of cervical cancer. Am J Obstet Gynecol 48:774, 1944

van Nagell JR, Greenwell N, Powell DF, et al: Microinvasive carcinoma of the cervix: Definition, histologic analysis, late results of the treatment. Obstet Gynecol 50:410, 1977

————: Microinvasive carcinoma of the cervix. Am J Obstet Gynecol 145:981, 1983

Weiner I, Burke L, Goldberger MA: Carcinoma of the cervix in Jewish women. Am J Obstet Gynecol 61:418, 1951

Woodruff JD, Parmley TH, Julian CG: Topical 5-fluorouracil in the treatment of vaginal carcinoma in situ. Gynecol Oncol 3:125, 1975

Chapter 32

Invasive Carcinoma of the Cervix

Historically, invasive cervical cancer was the most common malignancy of the female reproductive tract. Since 1950, both incidence and mortality rates have decreased so that the disease now ranks second, occurring two to three times less frequently than endometrial carcinoma. Data from the Surveillance, Epidemiology and End Results (SEER) program indicate a 50% decrease in both incidence and mortality rates of cervical cancer since 1947, or a decline of 3% to 4% per year in both white and nonwhite populations. The rates of both in situ and invasive cervical cancer have consistently been two to three times higher among black patients than among white patients, despite the significant overall reductions recorded in the epidemiologic history of the disease. For white women, the incidence rate of invasive cancer is as low as 10 per 100,000 women; but for nonwhite women, the rate is 20 to 30 per 100,000.

These improvements result from the introduction of cervical cancer screening as part of regular gynecologic examinations. Annual testing with a Papanicolaou smear has led to an increased detection of carcinoma in situ, important since in situ disease occurs 2 to 2.5 times more often than invasive disease. Also as a result of screening, from 35% to 50% of the cases of invasive cancer are now being detected when they are still at Stage I of the disease. As shown in Figure 32–1, there has been a continued increase in the number of tumors detected in Stage I (disease confined to the cervix) over the last 25 years and a decrease in more extensive disease, Stages II, III, and IV tumors. In the period from 1973 to 1975, the detection rate for Stage I tumors was approximately 15% higher than in the period from 1950 to 1954. Currently, 35% of invasive cervical cancers are detected in Stage I and 35% in Stage II.

Classification

The classification adopted in 1937 by the Health Organization of the League of Nations, which is based on gross findings of cervical cancer, is in general use abroad and in most clinics in the United States.

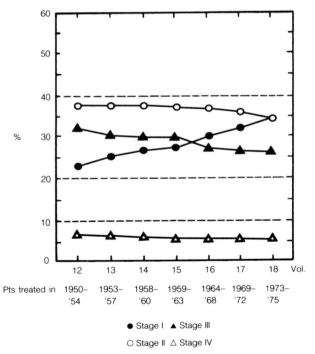

FIG. 32–1 Distribution of carcinoma of the cervix by stage, showing the incidence at each stage as a percentage of the total number treated in the 50 institutions that collaborated in volumes 12 through 18 of the FIGO Annual Report. (From FIGO Annual Report, Vol 18, 1982)

In 1950, this classification was modified to include preinvasive (in situ) cancer, which was designated Stage 0. New recommendations for the clinical classification of carcinoma of the cervix were adopted by the General Assembly of the International Federation of Gynecology and Obstetrics (FIGO) in September 1961, and changes were effected in 1971 and 1976. The following list includes all the minor modifications of the International Classification as adopted by FIGO.

FIGO Classification of Carcinoma of the Cervix

Classification	Description
STAGE 0	PREINVASIVE CARCINOMA
	Carcinoma in situ or intraepithelial carcinoma, not to be included in any statistics for invasive carcinoma
STAGE I–IV	INVASIVE CARCINOMA
I	Carcinoma strictly confined to the cervix (extension to the corpus should be disregarded)
Ia	Microinvasive carcinoma (early stromal invasion)
Ib	All other cases of Stage I. Occult cancer should be marked "occ."
II	The carcinoma extends beyond the cervix but has not extended onto the pelvic wall.
IIa	The carcinoma involves the vagina, but not the lower one-third. No obvious parametrial involvement.
IIb	Obvious parametrial involvement
III	Carcinoma extends onto the pelvic wall or lower one-third of vagina. All cases with hydronephrosis or nonfunctioning kidney should be included, unless known to be due to other causes.
IIIa	The tumor involves the lower one-third of the vagina, with no extension onto the pelvic wall.
IIIb	Extension onto the pelvic wall. Rectal examination demonstrates no cancer-free space between the tumor and the pelvic wall.
IV	Carcinoma has extended beyond the true pelvis or has involved the mucosa of the bladder or rectum. Bullous edema alone does not permit a lesion to be categorized as Stage IV.
IVa	Spread of the growth to adjacent organs
IVb	Spread to distant organs

Stages II, III, and IV are essentially unchanged from the 1971 classification; the major revision is in the redefinition of Stage I, which is discussed in detail under the section on microinvasive carcinoma, Stage Ia, in Chapter 31. The anatomical stages of cervical carcinoma are shown in Figure 32–2.

Histopathology

SQUAMOUS CARCINOMA

The principal histologic type of invasive cervical cancer, occurring in 90% of the cases, is the squamous (epidermoid) lesion. In 1923, Martzloff classified the squamous tumors into three main cell types: spinal cell (Fig. 32–3), transitional cell (Fig. 32–4), and basal cell (Fig. 32–5). Although the classification did not prove to be clinically useful, the work stimulated Broders, Reagan, and others to continue to study and categorize the clinical responses of cervical tumors to irradiation and surgery.

ADENOCARCINOMA

Although it is frequently stated that adenocarcinoma of the cervix (Fig. 32–6) makes up 3% to 5% of all cases of invasive cervical cancer, the proportion has increased in recent years. In some studies, as many as 8.5% to 10% of cases are of the adenocarcinoma type. Most investigators have found that the cellular differentiation of the glandular tumors of the endocervix can be correlated with the curability of the disease. Many classifications have been developed, including the Broders' grading of cervical adenocarcinoma from grade 1 to grade 4, from the well-differentiated to the poorly differentiated tumors. In more common use is the system similar to that for endometrial adenocarcinoma, with grade 1, 2, and 3. In general, the three grades of adenocarcinoma occur with equal frequency in the cervix.

The growth pattern of undifferentiated adenocarcinoma is most aggressive, resulting in large, bulky lesions in the cervix that may not respond to the usual dosage of irradiation. Increasing numbers of mixed adenosquamous or adenoepidermoid carcinomas of the cervix have been reported, varying in frequency from 3% to 17% of all adenocarcinomas. The biologic radiosensitivity of the mixed tumor is quite different from that of either of the pure types. The mixed lesions resemble the undifferentiated adenocarcinoma, being aggressive and responding poorly to irradiation. Studies by Glucksmann and Cherry, by Fu and associates, and Gallup and associates have shown that the mixed tumors have a lower 5-year cure rate than the more differentiated tumors.

UNUSUAL CERVICAL TUMORS

Mesonephric adenocarcinoma occurs infrequently in the cervix, and in view of its extracervical origin the lesion is usually considered separately from endocervical cancers. The generally poor prognosis for a mesonephric tumor is mainly a consequence of late diagnosis, which results in the disease being at an advanced stage when treatment is begun.

Glassy-cell carcinoma of the cervix is characterized by solid sheaths of neoplastic cells with large, hyperchromatic oval nuclei surrounded by dense, granular, acidophilic cytoplasm, giving the ground-glass appearance. Although occasionally the tumor contains clear cells and cells with vacuolated cytoplasm consisting of glycogen, it is rarely confused with a clear cell carcinoma. Glucksmann and Cherry were among the first to subclassify the mixed carcinomas into mature, signet ring, and glassy-cell types, and they recorded few 5-year cures for any of the types. Littmann and associates have reported a 5-year survival rate of 31% for patients with glassy-cell carcinoma.

Gross Pathology

In general, invasive cervical lesions are usually exophytic, infiltrative, or ulcerative. The gross lesion may often be suspected from simple palpation and inspection of the cervix. An everted carcinomatous growth may feel friable, whereas a tumor that develops beneath normal mucosa will feel stony-hard but with a smooth surface. Cervical lesions often take the form of a punched-out ulcer, but if the lesion is in the endocervical canal, even with an extensive lesion, the cervix may feel quite normal.

On inspection, the friable exophytic lesion may show a roughened, granular, bleeding surface, which may be sloughing, infected, and foul-smelling. An ulcerative lesion may look like a fairly clean punched-out ulcer, but more commonly it is crater-shaped with a necrotic base. Other types of lesions do not look particularly abnormal or carcinomatous. For example, a growth starting in the cervical canal may protrude from the external os much like a benign polyp. A stony-hard, smooth cervix that is the site of an extensive growth beneath relatively normal mucosa may look normal even when the tumor is quite advanced. The inverting, infiltrative type of growth can extend through the musculature of the cervix without changing the appearance of the cervical portio. Because cervical lesions may be deceptive, every suspicious-feeling cervix should not only be inspected through a speculum that allows good visualization, but should also be biopsied.

In a patient with a cervical lesion, a Papanicolaou vaginal smear should be obtained after inspection of the cervical lesion, and before a biopsy is taken. If a colposcope is available, an examination of the lesion should also be made before taking the biopsy. With colposcopy the exact outline of the tumor can be demarcated. The primary benefit of colposcopy, however, is in visualizing a noninvasive lesion that cannot be seen without magnification.

The biopsy specimen can be taken with any of a number of useful instruments; the Kevorkian, the Younge, and the Gaylor biopsy forceps are particularly good for taking an adequate biopsy specimen (Fig. 32–7). Conization is unnecessary when a gross lesion is present. Iodine staining should be used to outline the vaginal margins of the lesion when colposcopy is not available. Curettage of the uterine cavity is also performed as part of the diagnostic procedure, even when a tumor is obvious, in order to determine how far the lesion extends up the canal and whether or not the uterine fundus is involved. This information will be used in planning the treatment program, because extension of disease can be correlated with the prognosis for cervical carcinoma.

Prognostic Factors

The sites and pathways of spread of cervical cancer have been studied more intensively than those of any other gynecologic tumor and several specific factors related to therapeutic benefit have been defined. The factors are:

1. Tumor volume, including exophytic or endophytic (barrel-shaped) lesions
2. Vaginal or endometrial extension
3. Regional (pelvic) and distant (para-aortic) lymph-node metastases
4. Histologic grade of tumor
5. Depth of tumor invasion
6. Vascular invasion

Although the methods available for the clinical staging of cervical cancer have improved during the past 25 years, inaccuracies in defining the precise extent of the disease occur in 15% to 20% of each clinical stage. The selection of a specific method of treatment is based mainly on palpable pelvic findings from the initial examination.

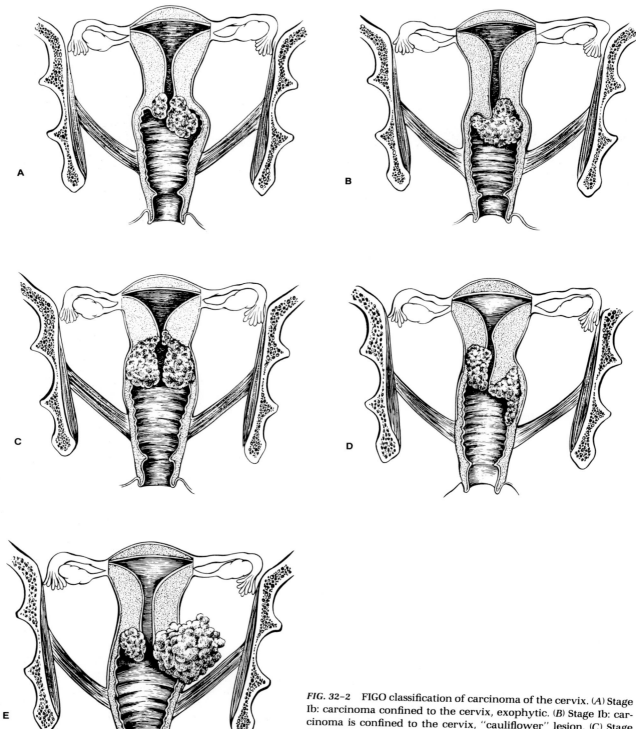

FIG. 32–2 FIGO classification of carcinoma of the cervix. (*A*) Stage Ib: carcinoma confined to the cervix, exophytic. (*B*) Stage Ib: carcinoma is confined to the cervix, "cauliflower" lesion. (*C*) Stage Ib: bulky endocervical "barrel-shaped" lesion. (*D*) Stage IIa: carcinoma extends into the upper vagina or fornix. (*E*) Stage IIb: carcinoma extends into the parametrium but does not extend to pelvic wall.

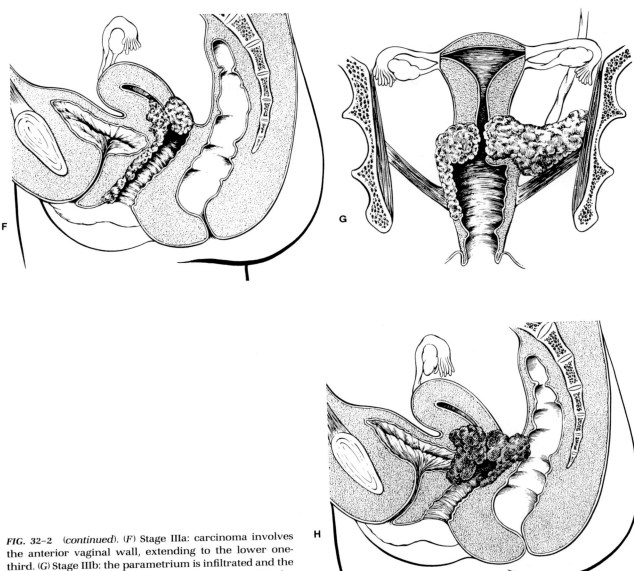

FIG. 32–2 *(continued).* (*F*) Stage IIIa: carcinoma involves the anterior vaginal wall, extending to the lower one-third. (*G*) Stage IIIb: the parametrium is infiltrated and the carcinoma extends to the pelvic wall. (*H*) Stage IVa: the bladder base and/or rectum are involved.

TUMOR VOLUME

In all stages of invasive cervical carcinoma, tumor volume is an important factor in predicting the spread of the disease and in determining the best method of treatment. Burghardt studied tumor volume as a factor in the treatment of microcarcinoma of the cervix (Stage Ia) and found that when microcarcinoma was measured accurately by serial step-sectioning, and the maximum tumor volume was less than 400 cubic mm, a variety of conser-

vative treatment programs could control the disease. When conization was the only therapy, only 1 of 44 cases was found to progress. Piver, van Nagell, Shingleton, and others found that invasive carcinoma lesions less than 2 or 3 cm in diameter were less likely to metastasize to the pelvic lymph nodes than larger lesions. The 5-year survival rate for patients with Stage Ib cervical lesions less than 3 cm in diameter ranges from 85% to 90% whereas for patients with lesions greater than 3 cm, the cure rate is 65% or less (Table 32–1).

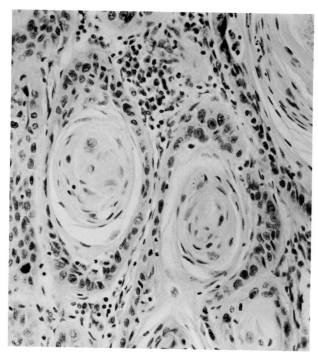

FIG. 32-3 Grade 1, well-differentiated epidermoid carcinoma of the cervix. High-power view of spinal cell type. The tumor cells contain abundant keratin that forms epithelial pearls.

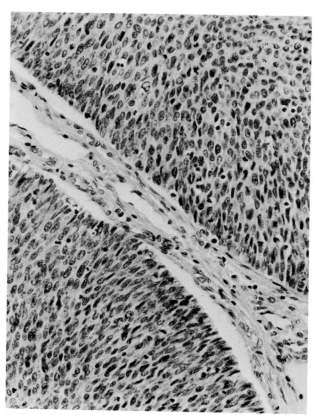

FIG. 32-5 Grade 3, poorly differentiated epidermoid carcinoma of the cervix, fat spindle or basal cell type. The tumor cells have little cytoplasm, numerous mitoses, and no keratin or epithelial pearls.

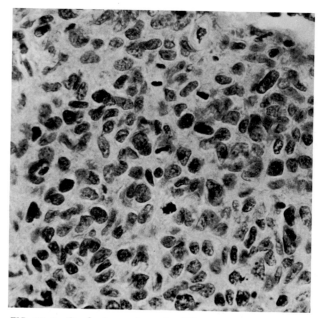

FIG. 32-4 Grade 2, moderately differentiated epidermoid carcinoma of the cervix, transitional cell type. The tumor cells are characterized by a moderate amount of cytoplasm but are without pearl formation. Extensive pleomorphism and mitosis are evident. The tumor is frequently classified as being of large-cell, non-keratinizing type.

Exophytic and bulky endophytic (barrel-shaped) lesions have a poor clinical prognosis because both have large volumes. Cells in the central portion of a large tumor mass may be well oxygenated and radiosensitive. As tumor cells extend away from the vascular source, they become more hypoxic and radioresistant. Since the effect of megavoltage irradiation on a tumor is determined mainly by blood supply, larger doses of irradiation and fractionation of the radiation are required to kill tumor cells in hypoxic, peripheral portions of a tumor mass. The ability of irradiation to cure a squamous or glandular tumor is directly related to tumor volume (Table 32-2). As the tumor volume increases to more than 2 cm in diameter, irradiation doses of more than 6000 rad are required to attain 90% control. Only by combining central brachytherapy with external beam megavoltage therapy can a dose of this magnitude be achieved.

When an exophytic tumor protrudes into the vagina from the portio of the cervix, the entire exocervix may be encompassed. The treatment pro-

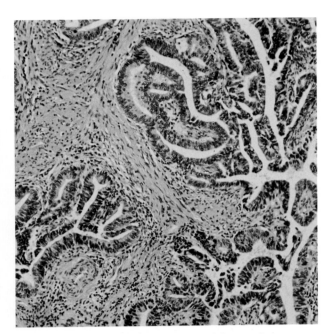

FIG. 32-6 Adenocarcinoma of the cervix.

gram can then be modified to exploit the advantages of external-beam teletherapy before using intracavitary irradiation. Because exophytic tumors have a highly vascular base, the lesions respond rapidly to external irradiation, which produces both necrobiosis from ischemia and cell death.

A tumor, particularly a Stage II tumor, that has enlarged sufficiently to produce distortion of the cervical canal or of the lower uterine segment is usually bulky and barrel-shaped (see Fig. 32-2C), and treatment with irradiation therapy alone has an unfavorable prognosis. Because of their growth pattern, bulky endophytic lesions extend beyond the therapeutic reaches of currently available intracavitary irradiation systems. The extended growth pattern is particularly evident in adeno-

carcinomas of the cervix. Consequently, these lesions require a more aggressive form of treatment, including external and intracavitary irradiation followed by surgery. Rutledge has used a simple hysterectomy following full irradiation treatment to achieve an improved 5-year survival rate of 54% for patients with Stage II lesions. When irradiation alone was used as treatment, the 5-year survival rate for patients with Stage II tumors decreased to 42%. In Rutledge's experience, patients with Stage I lesions had a satisfactory survival rate of 85% whether irradiation treatment was used alone or in combination with hysterectomy. However, in comparing the international (FIGO) statistics for bulky Stage I and II adenocarcinomas, when either surgery alone or surgery combined with irradiation therapy was used, the 5-year cure rate was 20% higher than when irradiation alone was used (Fig. 32-8).

VAGINAL OR ENDOMETRIAL EXTENSION

When invasive carcinoma of the cervix extends into the vagina, even with no parametrial involvement, the disease is associated with a much higher incidence of pelvic lymph node metastases. Piver and Chung noted a 42% incidence of pelvic node spread in Stage IIa lesions, while Averette found 2 of 9 such cases to have occult para-aortic metastases. In general, lesions extending into the vagina from the cervix are larger than 3 cm in diameter, a factor increasing the frequency of regional and distant metastases.

Extension of cervical carcinoma into the uterine fundus was initially considered to be a poor prognostic factor. The original League of Nations classification of 1937 included such lesions in the Stage II category. Over the years, classification of the disease based on fundal extension has been gradually discounted. Lesions classified as Stage Ic in 1950 were included in the broad category of Stage Ib in 1961.

Despite the change in classification, recent evidence from Washington University reported by

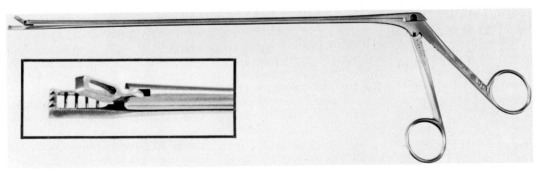

FIG. 32-7 Kevorkian square-jawed cervical biopsy forceps.

TABLE 32-1 *Correlation of Tumor Size with Incidence of Positive Nodes and Survival Rates in Cervical Cancer (Stage Ib)*

STUDY (YEAR)	NUMBER OF PATIENTS	TUMOR SIZE (CM)	POSITIVE NODES (PERCENT)	SURVIVAL (PERCENT)
Piver (1975)	96	≤3	21.2	88.5*
	52	>3	35.2	65.4
van Nagell (1977)	46	≤2	9.0	94.0†
	36	>2	31.0	40.0
Shingleton (1982)	117	≤2	12.0	91.4*
	64	>2	37.5	63.9

* 5-year survival.
† 1- to 10-year survival.

TABLE 32-2 *Relationship Between Dose and Tumor Volume in Squamous Cell Carcinoma of the Cervix**

TUMOR VOLUME	DOSE
<2 cm	5,000 rad
2 cm	6,000 rad
2-4 cm	7,000 rad
4-6 cm	7,500-8,000 rad
>6 cm	8,000-10,000 rad

* Average irradiation dose required to obtain 90% tumor control in area treated.
Modified from Fletcher GH: Clinical dose—response curves of human malignant epithelial tumors. Br J Radiol 46:1, 1973.

Perez and associates and others shows that tumor extension into the endometrial cavity lowers the 5-year survival rate of Stage Ib and IIa lesions by approximately 10% to 20%. Lesions involving the fundus also have a twofold greater incidence of distant metastases when compared to lesions without endometrial extension. Similar observations have been reported by Prempee and associates from 82 cases of Stage I and Stage II disease with endometrial extension. The absolute 5-year cure rate of 68% for Stage I and 62% for Stage II disease reflects the high risk of metastases: 20% of cases for Stage I and 24% for Stage II.

Establishing an accurate diagnosis of endometrial extension is difficult when using the microscopic study of curettings. Frequently, the curettage specimen is contaminated by the cervical tumor, so endometrial extension is not ascertained. Any historical finding indicating endometrial involvement should be given serious consideration, and the information should be used to plan the treatment. For bulky endocervical disease, a simple hysterectomy may be done in conjunction with irradiation treatment of the cervical lesion.

REGIONAL AND DISTANT METASTASES

Extension to the regional (pelvic) or to the distant (para-aortic) lymph nodes has proved to be one of the most reliable prognostic factors for patients with cervical cancer. The frequency of metastases to pelvic lymph nodes is approximately 1.5% to 2% for Stage Ia; 10% to 15% for Stage Ib; 20% to 25% for Stage IIb; greater than 35% for Stage III; and greater than 50% for Stage IV. The ability to detect positive pelvic nodes in Stage Ib disease is greatly improved when a thorough lymphadenectomy is performed, using lymphographic control before and during surgery. Kolstad has shown that when intraoperative lymphography is used, 15% to 25% more patients with Stage Ib disease will be found to have positive regional nodes.

The treatment of lymph node metastasis is a major source of controversy. Clinical evidence to date indicates that only 50% to 60% of the patients with involvement of the pelvic lymph nodes will survive 5 years, whether they receive full pelvic irradiation or no irradiation therapy.

A review of the results of postoperative irradiation for patients with Stage Ib carcinoma of the cervix and pelvic node metastasis following radical hysterectomy and lymphadenectomy was done by Morrow in 1980. The study found no statistically significant difference in the 5-year cure rates between those who received adjuvant pelvic irradiation and those who did not.

A very large individual study in Morrow's review was reported by Masterson, who operated on 600 patients with Stage Ib cervical cancer. For 103 patients (17%) with pelvic node metastases who did not receive postoperative irradiation, the 5-year cure

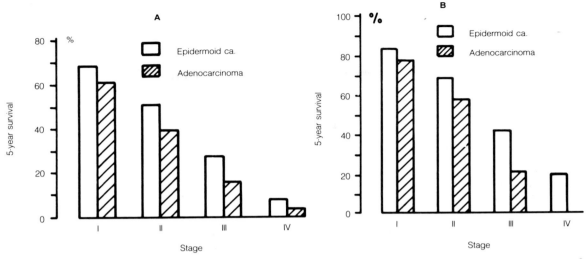

FIG. 32–8 (A) Carcinoma of the cervix uteri. Five-year survival by histologic type and stage for patients treated with irradiation alone. (B) Carcinoma of the cervix uteri. Five-year survival by histologic type and stage for patients treated with surgery either alone or in combination with radiotherapy. (From FIGO Annual Report, Vol 18, 1982)

rate was 55%. This rate was similar to that reported from other clinics for patients with comparable disease who had received irradiation. In Masterson's study, which did not include postoperative irradiation, the number of positive pelvic nodes influenced the cure rate. With one positive node, there was a 74% 5-year survival; with four or five positive nodes, there was only a 29% cure rate; and with more than five nodes, there were no 5-year cures. These studies cast some doubt on the efficacy of adjuvant pelvic irradiation therapy.

The major problem for survival is not that the regional nodes do not respond to the irradiation. Many studies have shown that current methods of irradiation will provide reasonable control of local disease less than 2 cm in diameter within the cervix, parametrium, and pelvic lymph nodes. But large, bulky cervical lesions and disease spread beyond the pelvis do not respond to current methods of treatment.

Many studies have shown that para-aortic node metastasis occurs in 10% to 15% of patients with Stage II cervical cancers, in 25% to 30% with Stage III, and in more than 40% with Stage IVa cancers. Most studies confirm that metastases to para-aortic nodes occur only when positive pelvic nodes are also present. Once a patient has been found to have pelvic node metastases, the risk of having para-aortic disease is quite high, which explains the causes of treatment failure in 148 cases of Stage III disease compiled by Fletcher and Rutledge: In only 25% of the cases was residual tumor confined to the irra-

diated pelvis; in 75%, the disease recurred outside the pelvic treatment field.

The control of metastatic tumor in lymph nodes is based on the same relationship of dose and volume as treatment of tumor in the cervix. Over the years, tumor diameter as a measure of tumor volume has been carefully correlated with the required treatment dosage (see Table 32–2). If a tumor-bearing node in the pelvic or para-aortic region is 2 cm in diameter, an irradiation dose of 6000 rad is required to control 90% of the disease. If the tumor mass is larger than 2 cm but less than 4 cm in diameter, a 7000-rad dose is needed to achieve 90% control, while a 4-cm to 6-cm lesion will require 7500 to 8000 rad.

Except for lesions confined to the cervix or immediate parametrium, it is difficult to achieve complete control of tumor masses larger than 2 cm in diameter without producing serious risk of irradiation injury to the intestinal or urinary tract. When the dose is raised to more than 6000 rad at the lateral pelvic wall, a prohibitive incidence of serious complications ensues. Because a high rate of serious bowel injury followed a para-aortic irradiation dose of 5500 rad, the total treatment dose for positive para-aortic nodes in most clinics today has been reduced to 5000 rad, given through four fields, over 5 to 5.5 weeks.

When para-aortic lymph node metastasis has progressed beyond the microscopic stage, there is little chance for control using current methods of treatment with irradiation alone. Long-term survivals have occurred only sporadically, while the mortality and serious morbidity from irradiation treatment are high.

HISTOLOGIC DIFFERENTIATION OF TUMOR

Squamous tumors are usually categorized as well differentiated, grade 1 (Fig. 32–4), moderately differentiated, grade 2 (Fig. 32–5), or poorly differentiated, grade 3 (Fig. 32–6). Since a mixture of cell types is common, cell type alone can not be used as an indicator of the outcome of treatment for most squamous tumors. Data presented by Chung and associates, Gilmore and associates, and Sedlacek, show that a higher incidence of lymph node metastasis and a lower cure rate occur among patients with poorly differentiated tumors.

Small-cell grade 3 carcinomas show a higher incidence of pelvic node metastasis (53%), of local recurrence (25%), and of distant metastases (20%) than do grade 1, Stage Ib and IIa lesions, according to studies by Chung and associates. Van Nagell presented a similar finding. Patients with small-cell grade 3 tumors had lymph-vascular space involvement in 93% of the cases, compared to 20% to 24% involvement among patients with grade 1 and grade 2 lesions.

Tumor differentiation has a greater prognostic role for adenocarcinoma of the cervix, because the cellular patterns can be correlated with the curability of the disease. As with endometrial carcinoma, well-differentiated grade 1 lesions have the best 5-year survival rate and the lowest incidence of pelvic node metastases.

Berek and associates studied 51 patients with Stage I adenocarcinoma and found a 5-year cure rate of 68.4% for those who had poorly differentiated, grade 3 tumors, whereas patients with grade 1 and grade 2 tumors had 84.2% and 77.8% cure rates. In Berek's study, patients with grade 3 tumors who had more advanced stages of cervical cancer had similar poor cure rates. In the report by Fu and associates, 67% of patients with well-differentiated tumors were alive after 5 years, whereas only 19% of patients with poorly differentiated adenocarcinoma survived that long. Shingleton considers the lower cure rate of cervical adenocarcinoma to result from the bulky tumor volume rather than from tumor grade.

Berek also studied lesion size, depth of invasion, and tumor grade in patients with adenocarcinoma to determine whether these factors influenced the status of lymph node metastases or patient survival. No positive pelvic lymph nodes were found among patients with lesions less than 2 cm in greatest diameter. Positive lymph nodes were found in 16.7% of patients with 2-cm to 4-cm lesions, and in 82.3%

of patients with lesions greater than 4 cm. Berek's study also found that pelvic lymph node metastases did not occur in patients who had a depth of tumor invasion of less than 2 mm, whereas positive nodes were found in 12.5% of patients with 2-mm to 2.5-mm invasion, in 37.5% with 5 mm to 10 mm of invasion, and in 50% in patients with greater than 10 mm of stromal invasion.

Several investigators, including Swan and Rutledge, Wheeless and Graham, and Julian and associates, have drawn attention to the fact that when there is a mixture of adenocarcinomatous and squamous elements, so-called adenosquamous tumors, the prognosis is poor and the incidence of pelvic lymph node metastases is high. Histologic combinations should be considered when comparing the prognoses of adenocarcinoma and squamous cancer of the cervix.

DEPTH OF TUMOR INVASION

Two aspects of cervical cancer that can be considered with tumor volume in making a prognosis are depth of stromal invasion and extent of cervical involvement. In a study of 139 patients with Stage I epidermoid carcinoma of the cervix, Boyce and colleagues clearly demonstrated that the depth of invasion was positively correlated with the involvement of pelvic lymph nodes and with pelvic recurrence. When the tumor had extended more than 10 mm beneath the basement membrane, 34% of the patients had positive pelvic lymph nodes, and the 5-year cure rate was only 63%. One-third of the patients had recurrences of disease in other pelvic tissue when the depth of the original tumor exceeded 10 mm.

Although the depth of cervical stromal invasion is not analyzed frequently as a prognostic factor, Abdulhayoglu and associates included stromal invasion in an analysis of prognostic factors among 35 patients with Stage Ib cervical cancer. The researchers categorized stromal invasion as involving the inner, middle, or outer one-third of the cervix. Out of 11 patients with metastases to pelvic nodes, 9 had tumor extending to the outer one-third of the cervix, while the remaining 2 cases had tumor limited to the middle one-third of the cervix. In addition to an increased risk of pelvic node metastases, advanced depth of stromal invasion was also correlated with a recurrence of pelvic disease, even when patients had negative nodes. The investigators concluded that patients who had Stage Ib cervical cancer extending to the outer one-third of the cervix with vascular invasion and little differentiation would probably benefit from adjuvant pelvic irradiation following Wertheim hysterectomy and lymphadenectomy.

VASCULAR INVASION

Although frequently overlooked, the presence of vascular invasion by tumor emboli can be used in making a prognosis for cervical cancer. Chung and associates reported that 63% of the patients with either Stage Ib or IIa carcinoma who had vascular invasion also had positive pelvic lymph nodes. Boyce and associates noted positive pelvic lymph nodes among 32% of 41 cases with vascular invasion. The incidence of vascular invasion with Stage I and Stage IIa lesions varies widely, depending on the number of sections of the cervix prepared and the depth of stromal invasion. Vascular invasion has been reported in as few as 9% and as many as 34% of Stage I lesions.

The finding of tumor in capillary-like, microlymphatic spaces is another ominous sign, portending pelvic node involvement and a generally poor prognosis. In many instances, the lymph nodes are inadequately sampled so that small microemboli associated with microlymphatic invasion are not detected. Tumor found in the capillary-like spaces within the cervix represents the earliest stage of metastatic disease and should be considered as an indication of pelvic lymph node metastases when making treatment plans.

Pretreatment Clinical Evaluation

When a diagnosis of invasive cervical cancer has been established histologically, patients require an evaluation of all pelvic organs to determine whether the tumor is confined to the cervix or has extended to the adjacent parametrium, vagina, endometrial cavity or to the bladder, ureters, or rectum. A thorough assessment requires an intravenous pyelogram, a cystoscopic examination of the bladder and urethra, a proctosigmoidoscopic study, a barium enema, and a thorough colposcopic study of the vagina and vaginal fornices. Colposcopic findings may be used for assigning a stage to the tumor, but the results must be confirmed by biopsy. When the cervical and vaginal margins of the tumor are accurately defined, a routine partial vaginectomy is not needed. Chest x-ray and cardiogram studies are used to determine cardiopulmonary disease, particularly in the older patient. Pulmonary function studies are also important, especially for evaluating patients who are candidates for radical surgery.

When pyelogram studies detect ureteral obstruc-

tion, a tumor is classified as a Stage IIIb lesion. Ureteral obstruction, either hydronephrosis or nonfunction of the kidney, has become well established as an indicator of poor prognosis and is recognized in the FIGO classification. A retrograde pyelogram may be performed after the ureteral obstruction is located for further evaluation. Kidney function studies provide important baseline information prior to treatment; serum creatinine and creatinine clearance studies are useful, as is complete urinalysis for the presence of albumin or white and red blood cells and renal tubular casts.

The bladder mucosa should also be inspected for possible bullous edema, which indicates lymphatic obstruction within the bladder wall. Evidence of disease in the bladder must be confirmed by biopsy before the lesion can be classified as Stage IV. Rectal lesions require a similar examination, because they may be related to an inflammatory process rather than to the cervical tumor.

Pretreatment pedal lymphangiography has been used by many clinics to detect pelvic and para-aortic lymph node metastases, but the procedure is associated with many false-negative and false-positive findings. When compared with lymphadenectomy, positive lymphangiograms have an accuracy rate less than 75%. Unfortunately, a lymphangiogram will only detect metastatic lesions when the parenchyma of the lymph node has become distorted, by which time the lesions are larger than 3 mm. In many clinics, including our own, a false-negative rate of 50% is not uncommon.

Lymphangiography is more appropriate for fine needle aspiration studies and for determining the completeness of lymphadenectomy during surgery than for specific diagnosis of metastatic disease. In a study of 275 patients with Stage Ib cervical carcinoma, Kolbenstvedt and Kolstad increased their surgical findings of positive pelvic lymph nodes from 15% to 25% using preoperative and intraoperative lymphangiograms. The technique is also helpful for directing lymph node dissection to suspicious lesions and for planning the extent of the radiation field at the time of irradiation therapy.

Isotope scanning of the long bones, liver, and lungs has not proven useful for evaluating the clinical extent of early cervical cancer although the technique is good for detecting distant metastases from Stage IIIb or IV lesions or from recurrent disease. Radionucleotide scans, once used preoperatively to identify metastases in liver or other viscera, have been replaced by computed tomography (CT). The CT scan also shows retroperitoneal node enlargement and other intra-abdominal masses. In experienced hands, fine needle aspiration of retroperitoneal nodes with CT-scan or sonographic direction has an accuracy rate of 75% to 85%. When the aspiration study shows cytologic evidence of neoplastic cells, a biopsy need not be performed.

When the necessary studies have been completed, a pelvic examination must be performed as part of the staging process, and the procedure should be done with the patient completely relaxed by general anesthesia. In 20% of patients, in our experience, the initial classification of the disease has proved to be incorrect on examination with general anesthesia. A careful examination usually reveals a more advanced stage of the disease than was anticipated. A fractional curettage is useful in identifying extension of the disease to the endometrium.

The pelvic examination should provide a complete evaluation of the reproductive tract, so that the location and extent of the tumor can be clearly defined. Surgical experience from pelvic lymphadenectomy has confirmed an error rate of 15% to 25% in the clinical staging of patients with Stages Ib and II lesions. In 10% to 30% of cases with Stage II or III tumors, in addition to positive findings of occult pelvic lymph nodes, other metastases occur in the para-aortic nodes.

Treatment of Invasive Cervical Carcinoma

Based on the pretreatment evaluation of the patient, including the prognostic factors of tumor size, clinical stage of the disease, and risk of pelvic node metastases, a treatment schema may be developed for invasive cervical cancer as shown.

The surgical treatment of invasive carcinoma of the cervix is limited, primarily, to those patients in whom the disease is confined to the cervix or vaginal fornix, Stage Ib or Stage IIa disease, and who are good surgical risks. Since only 35% to 40% of patients with invasive cervical cancer have a Stage Ib lesion, irradiation therapy remains the major method of treatment in most cases of this disease. Even when the disease is clinically confined to the cervix, Stage Ib lesions with a diameter greater than 2 to 3 cm are associated with a high incidence of pelvic lymph node metastasis. For example, in Piver's study, patients with a tumor size of 3 cm or less had a 21.5% incidence of pelvic node metastasis, a finding that has been confirmed by other investigators. When the lesion size was greater than 3 cm, a 35.2% incidence of positive nodes was found, and the 5-year cure rate declined from 88.5% to 65.4% (see Table 32–1). When a high risk for pelvic node metastasis exists, most clinicians in the United States prefer to treat the patient with full pelvic irradiation since the cure rates in this country for Stage Ib and IIa

Treatment Schema for Invasive Cervical Carcinoma

Disease Stage	Treatment
Stage Ia	The treatment of microinvasive cervical carcinoma is discussed in Chapter 31
Stage Ib	
Lesions ≤ 3 cm and good surgical risk	Radical Wertheim hysterectomy and pelvic node dissection or full irradiation therapy
Lesions > 3 cm or poor surgical risk	Full external and intracavitary pelvic irradiation
Large, bulky, "barrel-shaped" lesions	Full external and intracavitary pelvic irradiation followed by simple hysterectomy or modified Wertheim hysterectomy without lymphadenectomy
Stage IIa	
Lesions ≤ 3 cm and good surgical risk	Radical Wertheim hysterectomy and pelvic node dissection
Lesions > 3 cm or poor surgical risk	Full external and intracavitary pelvic irradiation
Large, bulky "barrel-shaped" lesions	Full external and intracavitary pelvic irradiation followed by simple or modified Wertheim hysterectomy
Stage IIb Stage IIIa and IIIb Stage IVa* and IVb	Full external and intracavitary pelvic irradiation

* A patient with Stage IVa lesion that extends only in the anterior or posterior direction may be a candidate for pelvic exenteration.

disease are comparable for radical surgery and irradiation therapy, despite the discrepancy in the FIGO data. Although radical surgery is much more thorough today, in terms of the extent and completeness of the pelvic node dissection, than when originally described by Wertheim at the turn of the century, tumor emboli in the pelvic microlymphatic channels are impossible to remove surgically. If adjunctive pelvic irradiation is used for patients with positive pelvic lymph nodes, it is preferable to give the irradiation treatment to the tumor-bearing area with an intact blood supply so that tissue oxygenation can be used to enhance the radiobiologic effect of the treatment.

The management of cervical cancer has gradually evolved into a team approach in which the best minds available in surgery, radiotherapy, and cellular biology are utilized.

To obtain an understanding of the present status

of the surgical treatment of cervical cancer, some historical milestones should be noted. Freund from Germany developed a technique for total hysterectomy in 1879, but the procedure resulted in an operative mortality of 50%. In 1895, Reis demonstrated two important techniques in canine experiments: lymph node removal, and excision of part of the broad ligament along with the entire uterus.

The first use of radical surgery in the United States was by J. G. Clark in 1895 while he was a resident gynecologist at the Johns Hopkins Hospital. Clark reported two cases of carcinoma of the cervix, which he treated with radical hysterectomy and pelvic lymphadenectomy. He catheterized the ureters with bougies to obtain a better dissection of the broad ligament at the lateral pelvic wall and to remove a large portion of the vagina without injuring the ureter.

In 1898, Wertheim of Vienna developed the surgical technique of removing the pelvic lymph nodes and part of the parametrium when a total hysterectomy was performed for the treatment of cervical cancer. Wertheim presented his technique in 1900 and reported his first series of 270 cases in 1905; he reported further on his experience with 500 cases in 1911.

The high mortality rate and urinary and bowel complications led surgeons to other methods. In the United States, the surgical treatment of cervical cancer was gradually replaced by radium and deep x-ray therapy from the years 1920 to 1940.

In 1939, J. V. Meigs renewed the interest in radical surgery for cervical carcinoma in the United States because he was dissatisfied with the results of irradiation therapy. Although the procedure has become known as the radical Wertheim hysterectomy, it was Meigs who routinely removed all the pelvic lymph nodes, whereas Wertheim performed a selective lymphadenectomy, removing only the enlarged and palpable nodes. Among the first 85 highly selected cases of primary invasive carcinoma of the cervix followed by Meigs (1950) for 5 years, the survival rate was 80.0% for Stage I cases and 60.7% for Stage II cases. Meigs reported that 9% of the patients developed a ureteral injury or fistula following surgery. One-third of the patients who developed a fistula had received orthovoltage irradiation before surgery.

Ureteral complications continued to plague the pelvic surgeon who performed the radical hysterectomy and pelvic lymphadenectomy. In 1962, Green reported from Meigs's clinic that a previous 12.5% ureteral complication rate, which included an 8.5% incidence of ureterovaginal fistulas and a 4% incidence of ureteral stricture, had been improved by suspending the ureters from the oblit-

erated portion of the hypogastric artery and by using continuous bladder drainage for 6 weeks following surgery. Novak, from Yugoslavia, reduced the incidence of ureteral fistulas following primary radical surgery to 2% by placing the dissected pelvic ureter on the inside (peritoneal) surface of the pelvic peritoneum and by preserving the lateral mesentery to the terminal ureter.

All of the procedures, including retroperitoneal suction-drainage of the lateral pelvis, were developed to protect the lower ureter from the pelvic cellulitis that could produce ureteral scarring and fistula formation. In general, urinary tract fistulas occur more frequently when radical surgery is performed after irradiation therapy has failed to control the central tumor. At present, in clinics with extensive experience with this procedure, an incidence of both bladder and ureter fistula following primary surgery is less than 2%.

The radical vaginal hysterectomy (Schauta–Amreich operation) has been used principally in Europe. The procedure has limited clinical application because local radical treatment of the paracervical tissue cannot reach the entire field of potential tumor spread, in particular the pelvic lymph nodes. In general, it is considered a more extensive procedure than necessary for treatment of a Stage Ia (microinvasive) disease, and an inadequate treatment for Stage Ib and IIa lesions. Therefore, it has had only limited use in this country.

IRRADIATION TREATMENT

Several different methods of intracavitary therapy were developed, including the Stockholm technique from the Radiumhemmet; the Paris technique, designed at the Curie Foundation; and the Manchester technique from England. The Stockholm radium technique consisted of high-intensity central irradiation, repeated two or three times in 3 weeks, while the Paris technique used low-intensity central irradiation continuously delivered over 1 week. The Manchester technique was derived from the Paris method and used low, hourly dosage rates requiring at least two insertions of the radiation sources. The use of radium therapy peaked in the United States between 1920 and 1940. Other radioactive elements, including cesium and iridium, are now more commonly used in central brachytherapy.

With the establishment of the roentgen as a defined unit of radiation exposure (Stockholm, 1921), irradiation dosage became a measure of the voltage of the x-ray unit. High-energy nuclear radiation sources, ranging to 25 MV for the betatron and linear accelerator, have significantly improved the cure rates following irradiation therapy. Intracavitary dose can be combined with external irradiation to best achieve the high central irradiation derived from the gamma rays of radium or cesium in addition to uniform megavoltage external irradiation with penetration of the cervix, broad ligament, and lateral pelvic walls.

To compare the survival rates of irradiation and primary surgery, Delgado analyzed the reports from patients treated for Stage I cervical cancer. The 1995 patients treated by irradiation had an average 5-year survival rate of 85.6%, which was essentially identical to the survival rate with radical surgery (Table 32–3). Patients treated with both surgery and irradiation had a very similar survival rate of 86.6%.

Einhorn reported a very favorable 5-year cure rate for Stages I and II cervical cancer treated with irradiation alone (Table 32–4). When Einhorn compared different types of tumors by volume, he found

TABLE 32–3   *5-Year Survival of Patients with Stage I Squamous Cancer of Cervix by Treatment Modality*

STUDY	NUMBER OF PATIENTS	5-YEAR SURVIVAL (PERCENT)	STUDY	NUMBER OF PATIENTS	5-YEAR SURVIVAL (PERCENT)
SURGERY			COMBINATION THERAPY		
Liu, Meigs, 1955	116	78.4	Welch et al, 1961: RT and hyst.	78	90.4
Brunschwig, Daniel, 1958	127	78.7	Currie, 1963: RT and lymph.	123	81.3
Carter et al, 1958	119	81.5	Gorton, 1964: RT and lymph.	166	86.0
Mitra, 1959	25	64.0	Kottmeier, 1964: RT and lymph.	53	79.0
Brunschwig, 1960	138	81.9	Crawford et al, 1965: RT and rad. hyst.	74	90.0
Welch et al, 1961	95	85.7	Rutledge et al., 1965: RT and lymph.	30	86.1
Green et al, 1962	315	83.0	Decker et al, 1965: RT and lymph.	44	88.6
Dobrotin, Bicheikina, 1963	349	76.2 (8 year)	Burch, Chalfant, 1970: RT and hyst.	138	85.5
Masterson, 1963	100	80.0	Nienminen, Pollanen, 1970: lymph. and RT	114	87.0
Christensen et al, 1964	168	82.7	Rampone et al, 1973: RT and lymph.	537	88.3
Brunschwig, Barber, 1966	173	81.5	Lagasse et al, 1974: RT and lymph.	60	88.3
Masterson, 1967	120	87.5	Lagasse et al, 1974: lymph. and RT	58	74.1
Masubuchi et al, 1969	296	90.5	Quigley et al, 1975: RT and lymph.	136	89.4
Crisp, 1969	98	90.0	Total	1611	86.6
Ketcham et al, 1971	28	86.0			
Park et al, 1973	126	91.0			
Newton, 1975	58	81.0			
Morley, Seski, 1976	149	91.3			
Total	2600	83.4			
RADIATION					
Makowski et al, 1962	422	81.3			
Kottmeier, 1964	611	89.5			
Crawford et al, 1965	63	46.0			
Masubuchi et al, 1969	152	88.2			
Marcial, 1970	41	87.0			
Neinminen, Pollanen, 1970	77	70.0			
Fletcher, 1971	549	91.5			
Newton, 1975	61	74.0			
Welander et al, 1975	19	89.5 (2 year)			
Total	1995	85.6			

Adapted from Delgado, 1978.

TABLE 32–4 *Cervical Cancer 5-Year Survival Rates with Irradiation Therapy Only*

CLINICAL STAGE	NUMBER OF PATIENTS	5-YEAR SURVIVAL Number	Percentage
Ia	35	35	100
Ib	60	53	88
IIa	60	39	65
IIb	53	21	40
III	38	6	16
IV	19	2	11
Total	265	156	59

Einhorn N: Frequency of severe complications after radiation therapy for cervical carcinoma. Acta Radiol Ther 14:42, 1975

the cure rate for adenocarcinoma to be comparable stage for stage with that for epidermoid cancer whether patients were treated with irradiation alone or with a combination of irradiation plus surgery. A simple total hysterectomy was used in some cases to remove the parent tumor in the endocervix if it was bulky or barrel-shaped, but lymph node dissection was not performed.

The survival rates compiled in the 1982 FIGO Annual Report (Vol. 18) from 82 collaborating institutions showed a distinctly lower cure rate for irradiation therapy than for surgery or with combination therapy, indicating that irradiation therapy techniques are not uniform internationally. There are also differences between stage-for-stage cure rates for adenocarcinoma and epidermoid carcinoma (Table 32–5). Still, data collected from 1950 to 1975 show an improvement in treatment results (Figure 32–9), due mainly to the increase in the number of cases treated in the early stages of the disease.

Complications of Irradiation Treatment

Ionizing irradiation interrupts the biochemical and metabolic processes of the human cell, causing mitotic inhibition or reproductive failure of the cell, resulting in cell death. Even cells that have received lethal doses may show no visible damage initially, but eventually they degenerate, owing to their inability to undergo continued cell division. Some cells undergo an immediate interruption of viability and rapid cellular death.

Tissue tolerance depends not only on the dose, but also on the volume of tissue irradiated and the interval between fractions of therapy. Modern irradiation therapy exploits the penetrability of the photon beams emitted by megavoltage machines. The skin is no longer a barrier; 80% of an emitted irradiation dose can be delivered to a tumor 10 cm below the surface. With this sophisticated technology, more procedures are feasible, such as whole-pelvis and whole-abdomen irradiation. Unfortunately, megavoltage rays can also produce irreversible destruction of adjacent pelvic structures.

The ideal irradiation treatment achieves the delicate balance of a dosage that can be tolerated by normal tissue while providing permanent arrest of the tumor cell. Complications occur when the ion-

TABLE 32–5 *Results of Therapy for Carcinoma of the Cervix by Histologic Type and Treatment**

STAGE	HISTOLOGY	RADIATION ALONE Number Treated	5-Year Survival Number	Percent	SURGERY, ALONE OR WITH RADIOTHERAPY Number Treated	5-Year Survival Number	Percent
I	Epidermoid ca.	2,378	1,673	70.4	3,695	3,112	84.2
	Adenocarcinoma	159	99	62.3	422	330	78.2
II	Epidermoid ca.	4,882	2,559	52.4	1,790	1,228	68.6
	Adenocarcinoma	244	98	40.2	200	116	58.0
III	Epidermoid ca.	4,452	1,258	28.3	227	96	42.3
	Adenocarcinoma	252	39	15.5	24	5	20.8
IV	Epidermoid ca.	785	64	8.2	40	8	20.0
	Adenocarcinoma	68	3	4.4	5	3	
Total	Epidermoid ca.	12,497	5,554	44.4	5,752	4,444	77.3
I–IV	Adenocarcinoma	723	239	33.1	651	454	69.7

* Combined results from 82 institutions (19,623 cases)
From FIGO Annual Report, Vol. 18, 1982

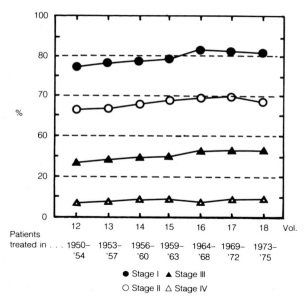

● Stage I ▲ Stage III
○ Stage II △ Stage IV

FIG. 32-9 Carcinoma of the cervix uteri. Five-year survival rates. Fifty institutions collaborated in volumes 12 through 18 of the FIGO Annual Report. (From FIGO Annual Report, Vol 18, 1982)

ization tolerance of the nonmalignant cell is exceeded. During the treatment course for cervical malignancy, the bladder and rectum are constantly at risk of receiving excessive irradiation.

One of the most frequent and most distressing complications of irradiation treatment is its effect on the vagina. The vagina may become narrowed in caliber throughout its entire length. Constriction of the upper one-third to one-half is almost inevitable and obliteration from synechiae formation is common. These changes frequently result in dyspareunia or cessation of coitus. The prophylactic use of vaginal dilators following treatment and the generous use of estrogen creams is recommended to minimize these effects.

Kottmeier reported that the complication rates for the bladder and the rectum are directly related to the dosage received. The glandular mucosa of the bowel is more radiosensitive than the transitional epithelium of the bladder. At the Radiumhemmet, rectal injuries occurred with intracavitary brachytherapy when the dosage was more than 6000 rad. When the dosage exceeded 8000 rad to the vaginal wall, serious injuries of the rectum occurred in 26.1% of the patients.

While local relief may be obtained with hydrocortisone enemas and analgesic rectal suppositories, the radiobiologic effect of the ischemic endarteritis is progressive and irreversible. Rectal-wall dosages

of greater than 6000 rad produce a high incidence of proctosigmoiditis, which frequently progresses to rectal stricture requiring a colostomy (Fig. 32–10). Even with standard treatment, a high incidence of serious rectal injuries can occur. Einhorn reported an incidence of 11% in patients treated with 5000 rad to the midplane of the pelvis.

Serious intestinal injuries from irradiation therapy should not exceed 2% to 3% of the treated cases. An increased incidence of injury to the small bowel has followed the use of high-energy megavoltage therapy, particularly in cases of fixation of the bowel in the pelvis. When adhesions cause fixation of the bowel, the total tumor dose is also delivered to the fixated segment. Piver reported 12 cases of enterovaginal and enterocutaneous fistulas following irradiation. Two-thirds of the patients had undergone a pretherapy laparotomy for surgical staging and lymph node sampling. Fixation of the small bowel into the pelvis is a frequent complication of surgical staging. The use of Schellhas's retroperitoneal approach to the para-aortic and common iliac nodes should obviate this intestinal complication.

Irradiation injuries of the bladder occur less frequently, and usually the symptoms are delayed. In Kottmeier's report, 1.4% of the patients developed serious bladder injuries following standard irradia-

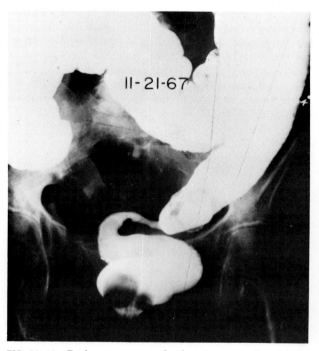

FIG. 32-10 Barium enema study showing rectosigmoid obstruction secondary to irradiation stenosis 16 years after therapy for carcinoma of the cervix.

tion therapy of 6000 rad to the outer bladder wall. When irradiation dosages exceeded 6000 rad to the internal surface of the bladder wall, injuries, including fistulas, occurred in 31.2% of the patients. The incidence of fistulas alone was only 0.8%. Ureteral damage due to irradiation treatment is uncommon. In Underwood's review, less than 0.5% of the patients who received irradiation had this rare injury, which is usually caused by displacement of intracavitary radium or cesium sources, producing ureteral fibrosis and obstruction. Monitoring with an intravenous pyelogram at yearly intervals will keep the incidence of unrecognized ureteral complications low, while providing an opportunity to examine the pelvic walls for possible neoplasia.

When intracavitary radium or cesium is combined with megavoltage external therapy, the dosage received at the lateral pelvic wall can easily exceed 6000 rad. With these high megavoltage dosages, increased incidence of pelvic cellulitis, ureteral and rectal strictures, and fistula formation can be expected. Greiss and associates found a 55% complication rate with various degrees of severity when the combined midpelvic irradiation dose exceeded 7000 rad. Meticulous monitoring of the irradiation dosage at the rectovaginal and vesicovaginal septa is crucial for maintaining the condition of the bladder and rectum. The combined irradiation dosage from external therapy and intracavitary radiation should not exceed 7000 rad throughout the entire wall of the rectum, while the outer surface of the bladder wall will tolerate 7000 to 8000 rad without serious damage.

Correlating the total dosages of intracavitary and external beam irradiation can be extremely difficult. Buchler discovered that even with the advantages of a wide clinical experience assisted by computerized dosimetry curves, a high frequency of serious bowel and bladder complications occurred, including stricture and fistula. The problems were found to result from the use of an unrestricted amount of intracavitary irradiation. The only controlling limitation in Buchler's work was the total irradiation dose to the bladder and rectum of 8000 rad, measured by scintillation probe reading.

Technique of Irradiation Treatment

The basic method of treating cervical carcinoma combines high-dosage, gamma-ray irradiation from intracavitary sources with external irradiation using high-energy megavoltage photon beams to the midplane of the pelvis, including the uterus, broad ligament, and lateral pelvic wall.

The intracavitary treatment programs have evolved from the Stockholm, Paris, or Manchester techniques. The principle involved is that a radiation dose from a central point decreases inversely as the square of the distance from the source of radiation. For example, an area that is 2 cm distant from a cesium source in the cervical canal would receive only one-fourth the dose emitted at the source. At a distance of 4 cm, the dose would be only one-sixteenth the central dose. The number of gamma rays that penetrate to the full depth of the tumor is enhanced by the use of large colpostats, which increase the distance between the radium or cesium source and the tumor surface and thus decrease the dose to the vaginal mucosa. By increasing the exposure time, a relatively larger dose can be given to the tumor while limiting the dose to the vaginal mucosa.

All methods of combined intracavitary radium or cesium (brachytherapy) and external irradiation therapy are designed to provide a dose of ionizing irradiation that is tumoricidal for both squamous cell carcinoma and adenocarcinoma of the cervix. Approximately 5500 to 6000 rad are applied to the midplane of the pelvis, the horizontal plane equidistant between the symphysis pubis and the sacrum, presumed to include the broad ligament and the lymphatics extending from the uterus to the lateral pelvic wall. Tissues adjacent to the cervical canal (Point A) receive a much higher combined irradiation dosage (approximately 8000 rad) than the 4500 to 5500 rad that are given near the lateral pelvic wall (Point B). In more precise terminology, Point A refers to the paracervical area that is located on a horizontal plane that is 2 cm lateral to the cervical canal at a level 2 cm above the external cervical os. Point B is arbitrarily located on the same horizontal plane but 5 cm from the endocervical canal. For practical purposes, many clinics consider Point B to represent the location of the lateral pelvic wall.

The 25-MV betatron unit or linear accelerator is employed for external irradiation, providing a dose-rate of 900 rad per week given in 180-rad daily fractions. The Fletcher-Suit afterloading system (Fig. 32–11) provides a convenient, safe, and efficient method of administering intracavitary irradiation. Of the many convenient isotope sources available for intracavitary irradiation (see Table 32–2), radium and cesium are used most often.

Treatment can begin with either external or intracavitary irradiation. For the more advanced lesions (Stages IIb, III, and IV) or large exophytic lesions, external irradiation is preferable initially, using opposing anterior and posterior pelvic fields (15 × 15 cm) until a midpelvic dose of 5000 to 5500 rad has been attained. Intracavitary cesium is then applied. The tissue dosages obtained by intracavitary gamma irradiation and external megavoltage x-ray

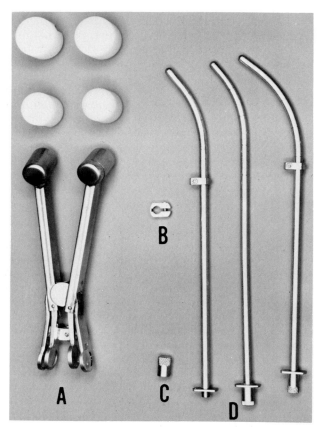

FIG. 32–11 Fletcher-Suit Afterloading System. (*A*) Afterloading colpostat (2 cm in diameter) and plastic jackets used to increase the colpostat size to medium (2.5 cm in diameter) or large (3 cm in diameter). (*B*) Keel. (*C*) Cap. (*D*) Uterine afterloading tandems (the three most useful curvatures) with metal keel to stabilize the tandem against the cervix by proper packing around it.

therapy are dissimilar on a rad-for-rad basis, varying with the geometry of the tumor and the accuracy of the application. Nonetheless, the rad (radiation absorbed dose) dosages obtained from the isodose curves of the radium or cesium implantation are combined for practical purposes with the dosage from the external beam therapy to determine the amount of total midpelvic irradiation.

The amount of cesium applied and the number of sources used depend on the volume of the tumor and the vaginal and uterine size. The duration of each application is based on the size of the uterus, the location of the lesion, the amount of external irradiation given, and the analysis of the isodose curves from a computer program. The bladder and rectum doses are calculated from computerized iso-

dose curves, so that the maximum dosage does not exceed 7000 rad to the rectum.

The biologic effectiveness of a radiation treatment program can only be determined by analyzing several factors. It is essential to know the tumor volume, the overall treatment time, the number of fractions given each week, and the amount of irradiation in each fraction in order to compare treatments given by different treatment centers. The following conclusions have been drawn from a survey of the current data on irradiation therapy.

In the treatment of Stage Ib and IIa epidermoid carcinoma of the cervix, surgery and irradiation produce similar results; the cure rate for Stage IIa lesions is somewhat lower but again is similar for both methods. Stages II, III, and IV are more effectively treated by irradiation therapy.

The incidence of serious bowel or bladder complications is slightly higher (2%–6%) with megavoltage irradiation than with surgery, and radiation injuries are far more debilitating and more difficult to correct surgically. The overall incidence of surgical fistulas is usually no more than 2%, and most injuries are correctable.

Primary radical surgery is particularly useful in the young patient with early invasive cervical cancer, because conservation of the ovaries is possible and the sclerosing effects of irradiation on the vagina and pelvis are avoided.

With either irradiation or surgery, the major emphasis in treatment is the inclusion in the plan of therapy of the pathways of tumor spread, including the cervix, vaginal fornices, parametria, and pelvic lymph nodes.

Irradiation therapy is not a panacea for gynecologic malignancies. Although some tumors are radioresistant even though a more than adequate megavoltage irradiation dosage is used, recent studies have confirmed that lateral pelvic-wall recurrence of cervical carcinoma is more often caused by inadequate irradiation dosage. Fletcher and associates showed that postirradiation recurrences are more common in extrapelvic sites than in the central or lateral pelvis.

Surgical Treatment of Invasive Cervical Carcinoma

To avoid the problems associated with irradiation therapy—particularly in young women desiring preservation of ovarian function—a radical Wertheim hysterectomy and pelvic lymphadenectomy are used for patients with Stage Ib or Stage IIa cervical carcinoma.

RADICAL WERTHEIM HYSTERECTOMY

In preparation for this procedure, patients require adequate bowel preparation, adequate hydration, and adequate blood volume.

A bowel preparation with purgatives and antibiotics is needed mainly when a radical procedure is used for radioresistant carcinoma, because in such cases the operation is usually more extensive and occasionally results in bowel injury (see Chapter 28). A liquid diet should be provided before surgery to promote complete emptying of the intestinal tract. If bowel resection is planned, a long intestinal tube (Cantor tube) is positioned in the ileum on the day before surgery.

Most of the preoperative studies require fasting or enema, so there is a tendency for the patient to become dehydrated. Dehydration is exaggerated by diarrhea produced during the extensive diagnostic studies, including intravenous pyelogram and barium enema. To provide adequate tissue hydration, 2 liters of 5% glucose in normal saline are given on the day prior to surgery, and additional intravenous fluid is given until the urinary specific gravity or plasma osmolality is within the normal range.

Blood volume studies are useful initially in evaluating red-cell mass and plasma volume but are not practical for monitoring blood replacement. Hematocrit values and plasma osmolality can be used to accurately evaluate intravascular volume and red-cell mass, both before and after surgery. Preoperative transfusion is required until a hematocrit of 40% is achieved.

The placement of a central venous catheter is considered essential for proper monitoring of the patient's intravascular compartment and cardiac reserve during and after radical surgery. Patients with cardiovascular or pulmonary disease that does not preclude radical surgery should have a Swan-Ganz catheter inserted into the pulmonary artery before surgery for accurate monitoring of cardiac and pulmonary function (see Chapters 5 and 6). The catheter should be maintained with a slow infusion, but it should not be used for intravenous fluid replacement. Baseline electrolyte studies, serum protein with albumin-globulin ratio, serum creatinine, and baseline liver function studies are also part of the normal laboratory evaluation of the patient.

Technique of the Radical Wertheim Hysterectomy

Various modifications of the radical hysterectomy and pelvic lymph node dissection have been used since Wertheim originally described the procedure. Many techniques emphasize a radical approach to one particular phase of the operation, but the management of the parametrium and the dissection of the pelvic lymph nodes constitute the important features of all versions of the procedure. The most serious complications of the operation are ureteral fistulas and stenosis, and the various modifications of the procedure were made in order to ensure an adequate blood supply to the terminal segment of the pelvic ureter. The classical Wertheim hysterectomy consists of wide resection of the parametrium, dissection of the terminal ureter from the "web" (vesicouterine ligament), wide resection of the ureterosacral ligaments, and removal of the upper 3 cm to 4 cm of the vagina and paravaginal tissues, along with a thorough pelvic lymphadenectomy.

Following proper abdominal and vaginal preparation, an indwelling catheter is placed in the bladder to keep it decompressed throughout the operative procedure. An adhesive plastic skin drape (Vi-drape) will protect the incision from bacterial contamination during prolonged surgery. A low midline incision, extending from approximately 3 cm above the umbilicus to the symphysis pubis, is required for adequate exposure. The incision is protected by a moist pack placed beneath each self-retaining retractor. As with any prolonged operative procedure, mechanical retractors should be released after 2 hours to reduce the tension from the walls of the incision and to improve the circulation through the rectus muscles.

ABDOMINAL AND PELVIC EXPLORATION. The intra-abdominal and pelvic viscera, the retroperitoneal lymph nodes, and the parietal and visceral surfaces of the peritoneal cavity must be evaluated for possible metastatic tumor. The liver surface, both hemidiaphragms, the mesentery of the large and small bowel, and the serosal surfaces of the bowel should be examined thoroughly. The kidneys should be palpated retroperitoneally to check for possible gross abnormalities.

Of paramount importance is the evaluation of the para-aortic lymph node chain. The para-aortic area must be carefully palpated from the region of the bifurcation of the aorta to the celiac plexus. Although gross metastatic disease may be easily palpable, histologic proof of the absence of metastatic disease must be provided by routine sampling of any enlarged or clinically suspicious lymph nodes from the lower portion of the aorta and vena cava. If the lower nodes below the inferior mesenteric artery and vein appear to be normal and are proven histologically by frozen-section study to be negative for metastatic tumor, the patient can be assumed with relative certainty not to have metastases higher up the lymphatic chain. Histologic proof is essential, since 15% of para-aortic node metastases are occult and occur in normal-appearing, soft lymph nodes. Patients who have undergone radical pelvic surgery and have recurrences in the upper abdomen most probably had disease in the lymphatic chain above the pelvic brim that was not recognized at the time of surgery.

The pelvic lymph node dissection can be extended routinely to include the lower 3 cm to 4 cm of the aorta and vena cava. Extrapelvic nodes are studied separately by frozen section before the hysterectomy is started. Histologic findings from extrapelvic nodes are particularly important in high-risk cases associated with one or more factors indicating a poor prognosis.

Evaluation of any extension of the pelvic tumor is carried out by examining the course of the lymphatic drainage and carefully palpating all the pelvic vessels. Clinically suspicious nodes are removed and sent for frozen section study while evaluation of the pelvis continues.

The paravesical and pararectal spaces are important anatomical landmarks because the intervening base of the broad ligament can be explored between these areas (Figure 32–12). When evidence of extracervical disease is detected in the broad ligament or at the lateral pelvic wall, the surgical procedure should be abandoned, and the patient treated with full pelvic irradiation. More than 30% of the patients with broad ligament involvement will also have pelvic lymph node metastases.

EXPLORATION OF THE PARAVESICAL SPACE. The anterior leaf of the broad ligament forms the roof of the paravesical space. Beneath the peritoneal covering, the shallow fossa is composed of loose connective tissue and fat, which is bordered medially by the lateral aspect of the bladder and laterally by the pelvic sidewall and obturator muscle. The inferior aspect of the fossa is formed by the levator ani muscles of the pelvic floor.

After completion of the abdominal and pelvic exploration, the small bowel and sigmoid colon are held out of the operative field in the upper abdomen by moist laparotomy packs, and the dissection is then initiated in the pelvis. The round ligament and infundibulopelvic ligament are clamped, excised, and ligated close to the lateral pelvic wall, and the anterior leaf of the broad ligament is opened with sharp Metzenbaum dissection, thereby allowing access to the retroperitoneal space (Fig. 32–13). The index finger can then be inserted easily into the paravesical space, which is dissected bluntly until the fascia of the levator muscles is identified (Fig. 32–14). Although there are no major blood vessels in the paravesical area, an aberrant obturator vessel may emerge from the inferior epigastric artery and course along the posterior aspect of the pubic bone to the obturator space. With gentle digital dissection, the pelvic floor can be palpated and the posterior aspect of the space can be identified, including the anterior margin of the cardinal ligament.

EXPLORATION OF THE PARARECTAL SPACE. The pararectal space lies beneath the pelvic peritoneum and extends between the uterosacral ligament and the lateral aspect of the levator muscles of the pelvic floor. The pararectal space can be opened by extending the broad ligament incision in a cephalic direction along the lateral margin of the infundibulopelvic ligament and separating the loose areolar tissue of the broad ligament (Fig. 32–15A). The pararectal space lies close to the anastomotic channels of the hypogastric vein and artery and these vessels

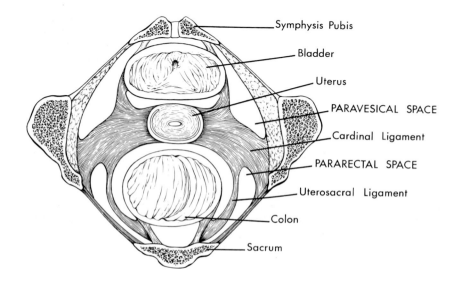

Symphysis Pubis
Bladder
Uterus
PARAVESICAL SPACE
Cardinal Ligament
PARARECTAL SPACE
Uterosacral Ligament
Colon
Sacrum

FIG. 32–12 Cross section of pelvis showing paravesical space and pararectal space. The base of the broad ligament (cardinal ligament) extends to the lateral pelvic wall and contains the major lymphatics draining the cervix.

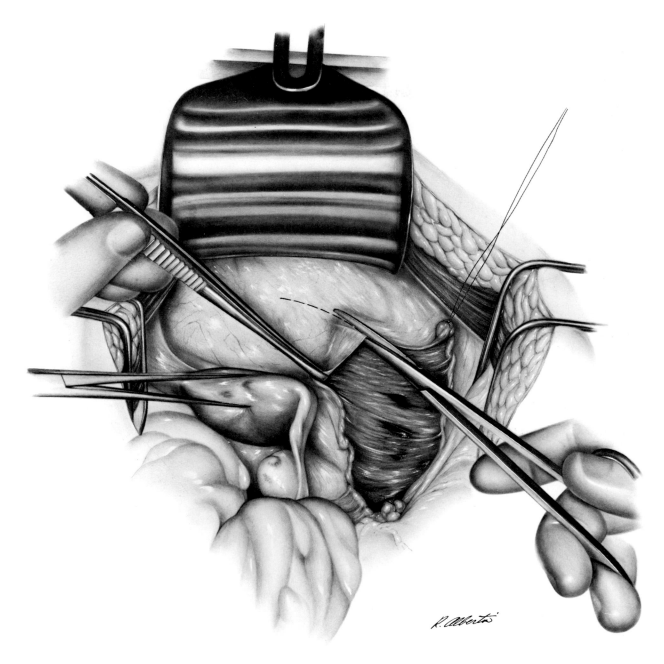

FIG. 32–13 Radical Wertheim hysterectomy. Opening the anterior leaf of the broad ligament after ligating the round ligament and infundibulopelvic ligament.

must be carefully dissected. The major branches of the hypogastric artery pass through the base of the broad ligament or along the pelvic floor, so the tissue must be carefully displaced to avoid damaging the visceral arteries and veins during blunt dissection (Fig. 32–15B). The ureter, which is medial to the paravesical and pararectal fossae, is left attached to the pelvic peritoneum.

The tissue between the paravesical and pararectal spaces constitutes the cardinal ligament, which is

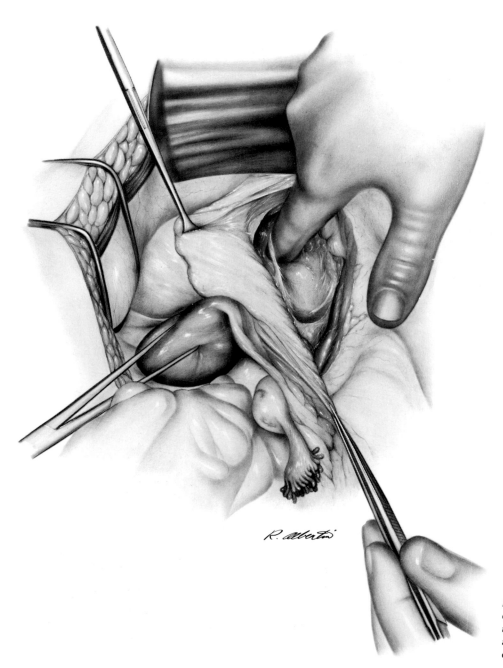

R. albertin

FIG. 32–14 Radical Wertheim hysterectomy (*continued*). Developing the paravesical space to the region of the pelvic floor.

attached to the cervix and the lateral pelvic wall (Fig. 32–15B). Care must be taken to avoid damage to the lateral sacral and hemorrhoidal vessels. If no extension of the tumor is noted during exploration of the paravesical and pararectal space, lymph node dissection may be initiated.

PELVIC LYMPHADENECTOMY. The lymphatic drainage of the pelvis is retroperitoneal and follows the course of the blood supply. Although there can be numerous variations in the lymphatic anatomy of the pelvis, the basic pattern includes lateral, superior, medial, and inferior lymph nodes and lym-

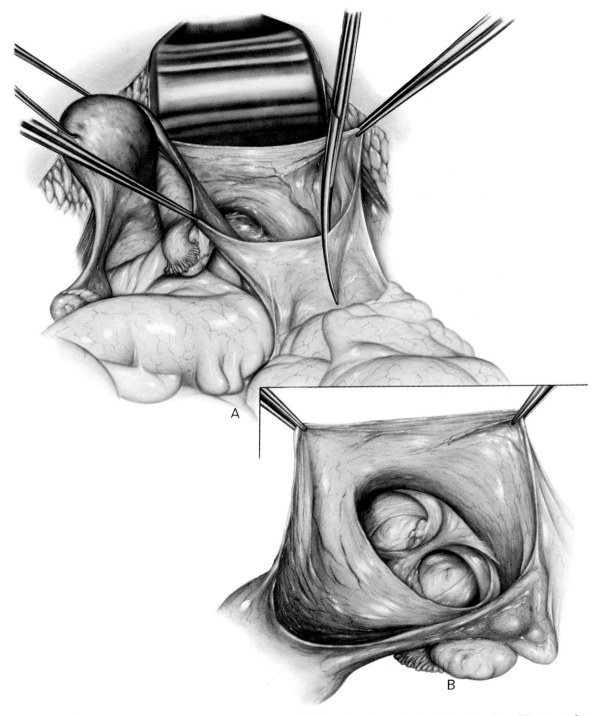

FIG. 32–15 Radical Wertheim hysterectomy (*continued*). (*A*) Opening the posterior leaf of the broad ligament for development of the pararectal fossa. (*B*) Paravesical and pararectal fossae with intervening base of broad ligament attached to the pelvic floor and lateral pelvic wall.

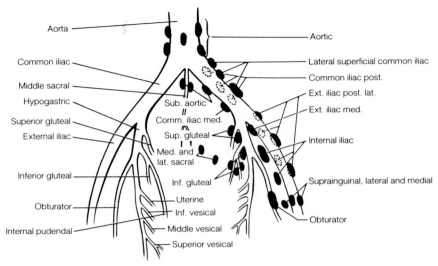

FIG. 32–16 Lymphatic drainage of the pelvis.

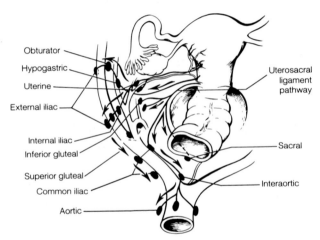

FIG. 32–17 Lymphatic drainage from the cervix through the uterosacral ligament to the lateral sacral lymph nodes.

phatic channels communicating with the common iliac, the external iliac, and the hypogastric vessels (Fig. 32–16).

An important pathway for the pelvic nodes and the thin-walled lymphatics that drain the upper vagina, cervix, and uterus courses along the posterior aspect of the endopelvic fascia (Fig. 32–17), then through the uterosacral ligament, terminating with the nodes that lie along the lateral aspect of the sacrum. The pelvic nodes communicate freely with lymphatic channels from the bifurcation of the common iliac artery near the lateral sacral and ischiosacral fossae. The deep nodes are extremely difficult to resect, because they are closely attached to the thin-walled tributaries of the hypogastric

vein. Dissection must be performed with extreme care to avoid injuring the hypogastric vein, which extends from beneath the medial side of the common iliac artery.

The most direct lymphatic drainage of the cervix and upper vagina is through the lateral parametrium (cardinal ligaments) to the hypogastric and obturator lymphatics. Due to the presence of obscured obturator veins and multiple venous tributaries from the hypogastric vein along the pelvic floor, dissection of the obturator lymphatics is difficult and is frequently associated with troublesome bleeding.

Along the iliac vessels, dissection of the lymphatic tissue begins in the region of the bifurcation of the common iliac artery and extends upward to the bifurcation of the aorta. The opening of the posterior peritoneal leaf of the broad ligament must be extended to the area of the pelvic brim, where the ureter is easily identified as it enters the pelvis at the bifurcation of the common iliac artery.

When the presacral area in the angle of the bifurcation of the aorta is being dissected, care must be taken to avoid bleeding from the middle sacral vessels and from the proximal part of the left common iliac vein, which courses through the retroperitoneal space. The middle sacral vessels should be occluded with vascular clips when they are identified. If the vessels are traumatized, bleeding can usually be controlled with positive pressure and small vascular clips.

The lymphatic tissue along the common iliac vessels is removed by sharp dissection with the points of the Metzenbaum scissors directed upward, taking care to avoid the ureter (Fig. 32–18). The ureter

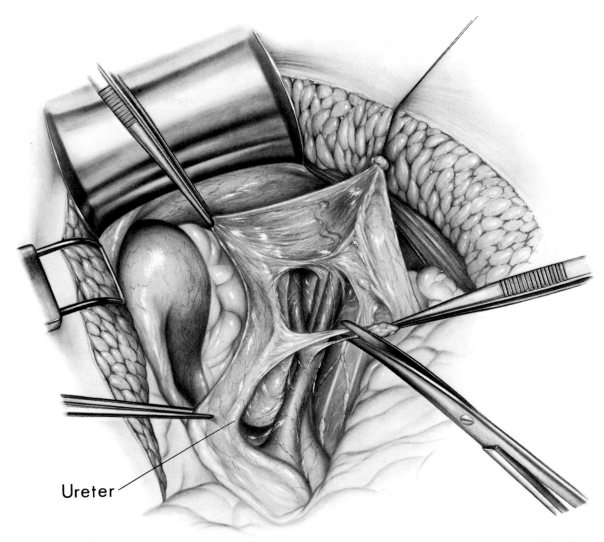

Ureter

FIG. 32–18 Radical Wertheim hysterectomy (*continued*). Pelvic lymphadenectomy with dissection of the right common iliac vessels and their branches, including the external iliac and hypogastric artery and vein. Note the attachment of the ureter to the parietal peritoneum. The genitofemoral nerve courses along the psoas muscle.

should be reflected medially during the dissection of the common iliac vessels and left attached to the parietal peritoneum in order to maintain its blood supply. The dissection is continued along the lower 2 cm to 3 cm of the aorta and vena cava, and the lymphatic tissue is clamped and excised. The pedicle is securely ligated with a No. 2-0 silk free tie to avoid lymphatic leakage and lymphocyst formation.

The loose fascial sheath should be removed from the iliac vessels, but the dissection should avoid trauma to the intima or wall of the vessels, particularly the veins. If the tumor has advanced to the adventitia of the vessel wall, skeletonizing the pelvic vessels to the point of producing a pearl-white, vas-

cular tree produces far more complications than benefits.

The common and external iliac trunks should be rotated medially and laterally with a vein retractor during the dissection to disclose the posterior lymphatic chain behind the vessels along the psoas muscle. The genitofemoral nerve, seen lateral to the external iliac vessels, should be preserved; damage to this peripheral nerve will produce postoperative discomfort in the groin and medial aspect of the thigh.

The external iliac vessels are carefully dissected to the point where they pass beneath the inguinal ligament. The inferior epigastric artery and vein arise at this point from the anterior and medial side of the external iliac vessels and then course along the anterior peritoneum into the lower abdominal wall. An anomalous obturator artery or vein may also arise from the lower portion of the external iliac or inferior epigastric vessels to course over the pelvic sidewall into the obturator space. If any of these vessels are accidentally traumatized, they should be ligated at their point of origin. To avoid bleeding in the obturator space, the vessels should be occluded with small vascular clips.

The external iliac vessels are reflected medially, and the areolar tissue directly beneath the vessels is freed from the lateral pelvic wall (Fig. 32–19A). When the obturator space has been opened, the adjacent tissue should be cleaned from the external iliac vessels. Then the artery and vein are released and are gently retracted laterally with a vein retractor to clearly expose the obturator space. Lymphatic and areolar tissue should be dissected from the obturator space to the region of the pelvic floor, avoiding trauma to the obturator nerve (Fig. 32–19B) and vessels.

Deep dissection beneath the obturator nerve is frequently complicated by bleeding from the tributaries of the hypogastric and obturator veins. Omitting this portion of the pelvic lymph node dissection provides a sanctuary for occult metastatic tumor, which can result in false assurance of the absence of tumor spread. The procedure definitely requires skill, as damage to the obturator nerve can produce motor impairment to the adductor muscles of the thigh, and can also cause sensory loss along the medial aspect of the thigh (see Fig. 4–12). The dissection should remove all of the nodes below the bifurcation of the iliac vessels, including the hypogastric nodes and the nodes in the obturator fossa. Should a node be encountered in the angle formed by the external iliac and hypogastric arteries, it must be carefully dissected, avoiding trauma to the adjacent hypogastric vein. Another step requiring particular care is the dissection of the sacroiliac plexus, just medial to the hypogastric artery and vein, near their origin. The rich collateral arterial and venous anastomoses increase the risk of bleeding from small vessels in this area. When the vessels retract into the sacral foramen, control of bleeding becomes quite difficult, although applying direct pressure over small bleeding vessels with a sponge forceps for a period of several minutes usually helps. Occasionally, hemostatic agents such as Gelfoam, thrombin solution, or microfibular collagen must be used to accelerate clot formation.

The obturator artery can be identified as it courses along the lateral pelvic wall adjacent to the easily defined obturator nerve (Fig. 32–19B). The nerve, artery, and vein advance toward the obturator foramen, where they leave the pelvis. All three structures are susceptible to trauma, particularly the obturator veins, which have a rich anastomotic network against the lateral pelvic wall where they communicate freely with the adjacent hypogastric veins. The safest procedure is to ligate or clip the obturator vessels, but should trauma occur, hemostasis is best obtained by packing the space tightly with a hot pack and allowing adequate time for a fibrin clot to form. Until clotting restores hemostatic control, dissection may continue on the opposite side.

The hypogastric artery is dissected after the visceral branches of the anterior division have been identified: the superior vesical, the uterine, middle and inferior vesical, the vaginal, and the middle hemorrhoidal arteries. The anterior division of the hypogastric artery continues along the paravesical fossa to become the obliterated umbilical ligament in the anterior abdominal wall. The superior vesical artery can be ligated without serious compromise to the blood supply of the bladder. The uterine artery should be ligated at its origin from the anterior branch of the hypogastric artery, and the uterine portion of the vessel should remain in the broad ligament as part of the roof of the paracervical web that covers the ureter. The adjacent uterine veins should be ligated in order to lessen chances of bleeding in this area.

DISSECTION OF BLADDER AND URETERS. The bladder is reflected off the lower uterine segment by incising the bladder peritoneum along its attachment to the uterus. The fascial adhesions of the base of the bladder are released from the cervix and upper vagina by sharp scissor dissection. As the bladder is gently dissected from the anterior wall of the vagina, the lower portion of the ureter is identified where it passes through the fascial fibers of the base of the broad ligament. The anterior fascial bundles are commonly called the *vesicouterine ligament* or *web*.

The fascial tunnel is carefully opened by sliding the Metzenbaum scissors, with concave surface pointed up, along the anterior and medial surface of the ureter and gently spreading the blades (Fig. 32–20A). The uterine artery and vein(s), which course along the fascial roof of the ligament, have been previously ligated. Adson clamps are used to dissect the tunnel, because their delicate tips are relatively atraumatic when placed between ureter and bladder.

Two Adson clamps are placed along the roof of the tunnel, and an incision is made between them (Fig. 32–20B), opening the tunnel and exposing the ureter attached to the posterior sheath of the broad ligament as though it were lying in a hammock (Fig.

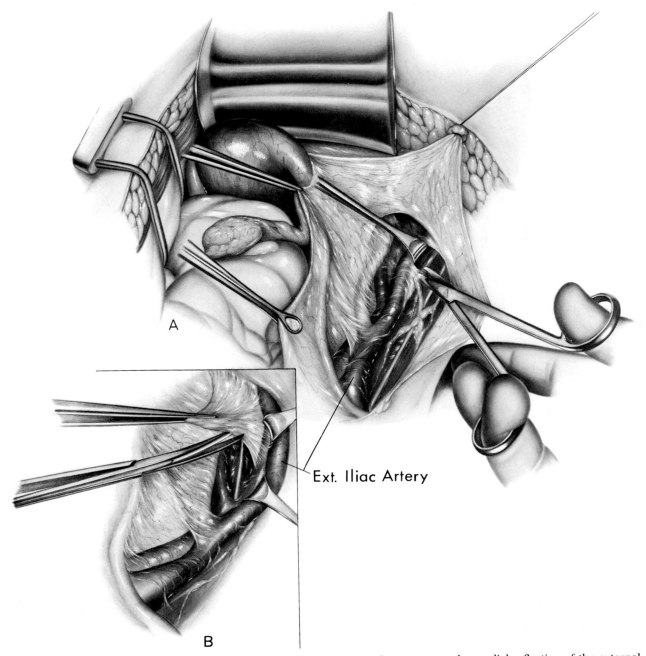

A

B

Ext. Iliac Artery

FIG. 32–19 Radical Wertheim hysterectomy (*continued*). (*A*) Entry into obturator space by medial reflection of the external iliac vessels. (*B*) Dissection of the obturator fossa showing the obturator nerve with areolar tissue attached superiorly to the external iliac vessels.

32–20C). The fascial bundles should be sutured to control bleeding, and the undersurface of the ureter should be mobilized slightly from the posterior fascial leaf of the broad ligament by gentle sharp dissection.

Every effort should be made to preserve the arteries and veins running through the web to the terminal ureter and bladder base. An excellent technique, recommended by Novak and others, is to preserve the terminal portion of the lateral mes-

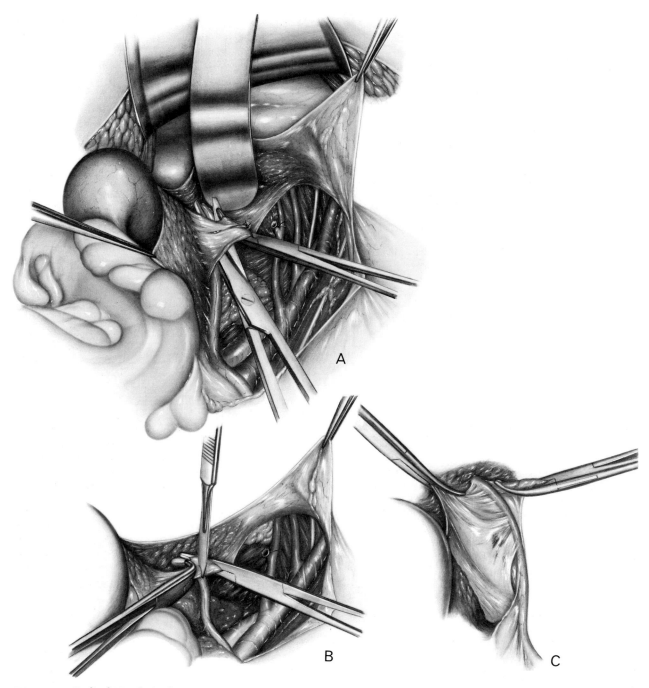

FIG. 32–20 Radical Wertheim hysterectomy (*continued*). (*A*) Metzenbaum scissors inserted above the ureter in the "web" or ureteral tunnel of the broad ligament. Note the ligated uterine artery in the anterior fascial sheath of the tunnel. (*B*) The roof of the tunnel is opened between clamps, with the ureter attached to the posterior sheath (*C*).

entery to the ureter by excising the posterior sheath along the medial aspect of the undersurface of the retracted terminal ureter to the region of the bladder base (Fig. 32–20D). Preserving the lateral segment of the terminal portion of the broad ligament not only improves the blood supply to the terminal end of the ureter, but also saves some parasympathetic and sympathetic fibers of the pelvic nerve plexus,

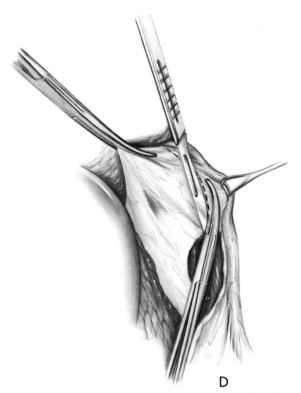

D

FIG. 32-20 (continued) (D) Excision of the posterior sheath of the vesicouterine ligament. Note the incision line along the medial border of the terminal ureter.

giving better neurogenic function to the bladder. The adventitia and muscular wall of the ureter, which contain nutrient vessels from the collateral circulation of the pelvic ureter, must also be conserved. If the blood supply to the ureter is compromised by thrombosis or trauma to the veins, fistula formation may result.

CARDINAL LIGAMENT DISSECTION. The base of the broad ligament (the cardinal ligament) may now be excised from its attachment at the lateral pelvic wall. After the ureter and hypogastric vessels have been carefully retracted from the operative field, a Wertheim clamp is placed as far lateral as possible with one jaw in the paravesical space and the other jaw in the pararectal space (Fig. 32-21A). The ligament is then excised with a scalpel, and a series of Wertheim clamps are placed along the paravaginal tissues until the dissection is completed at the pelvic floor (Fig. 32-21B). Then both margins are ligated with No. 1 delayed-absorbable suture. Should serious bleeding occur in this region because of trauma to the pelvic floor veins, hemostatic control can be obtained by firmly packing the pelvis and shifting the dissection temporarily to the opposite side.

The uterosacral ligaments, commonly called the pararectal stalks, are stretched by sharply withdrawing the uterus forward. The peritoneal reflection of the cul-de-sac of Douglas is incised, removing the peritoneal attachment to the anterior surface of the rectum (Fig. 32-22A). Care must be taken to avoid injury to the ureters, which are attached to the peritoneum just lateral to the uterosacral ligaments.

The rectovaginal septum is opened by sharp scissor dissection and deepened by blunt and sharp dissection (Fig. 32-22B). Opening the septum separates the posterior reflection of the endopelvic fascia from the lateral wall of the rectum, where the more superficial uterosacral ligaments are located. The entire fascial bundle of the uterosacral ligament is identified, clamped as far posteriorly as possible with one jaw of the Wertheim clamp in the pararectal fossa and one jaw in the rectovaginal space, and the ligament excised (Fig. 32-22C).

Dissection should be continued along the posterior endopelvic fascia to free the posterior aspect of the cervix from the pelvic floor. The paravaginal fascia, which is a continuation of the cardinal ligament, should be included in the dissection in order to incorporate all of the microlymphatic channels between the cervix and the upper vagina (Fig. 32-23A).

The bladder is then dissected free from the upper portion of the vagina. To avoid trauma to the blood supply of the bladder, sharp dissection should be used rather than blunt trauma against the base of the bladder, which could easily tear the blood vessels and musculature of the bladder wall. The fascial planes that separate the bladder and rectum from the anterior and posterior surfaces of the vagina should be dissected to free the upper 3 cm of the vagina. To remove the vaginal specimen by the open technique (Fig. 32-23B), a long straight Ochsner clamp should be applied in front of the cervix and the vagina should be opened with a scalpel. Straight Ochsner clamps are then placed along the margin of the vaginal cuff as the vagina is opened.

The vaginal vault is left open for drainage purposes, and the vaginal margins are sutured with a continuous locking stitch of No. 0 delayed-absorbable suture (Fig. 32-23C). Two soft rubber Penrose drains are placed on either side of the denuded pelvic floor and brought to the exterior surface through the open vagina. No additional support is needed for the vaginal vault, even though all of the fascial support between the uterus and the vagina has been removed. The remaining vagina, which has been shortened by approximately 3 cm, is well supported by attachments to the levator ani muscles and urogenital diaphragm. Postoperative fibrosis

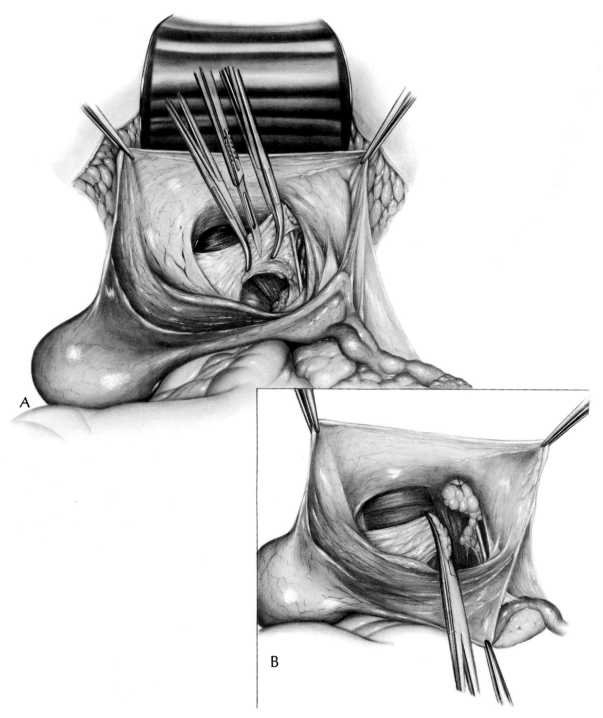

FIG. 32-21 Radical Wertheim hysterectomy (*continued*). (*A*) Clamping and incision of the lateral portion of the cardinal ligament adjacent to the lateral pelvic wall. (*B*) Excised ligament showing the pelvic floor and levator muscles. The dissected obturator nerve is seen in the obturator space.

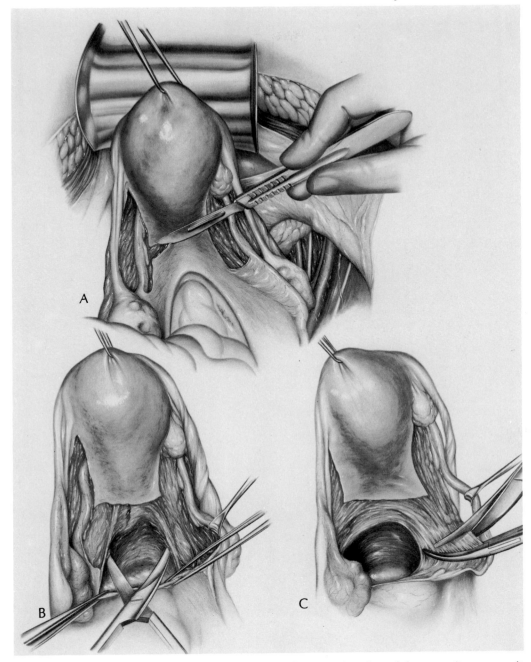

FIG. 32–22 Radical Wertheim hysterectomy (*continued*). (*A*) Cutting the cul-de-sac peritoneum as it reflects onto the rectum. Ureters course laterally devoid of peritoneum. (*B*) Dissection of the rectovaginal septum with development of the rectal stalks (uterosacral ligaments) laterally. (*C*) Clamping of the rectal stalks, including the uterosacral ligament. The ureter is gently retracted to avoid trauma.

will lend additional support to the vault. In addition, a Silastic or Jackson–Pratt catheter may be placed in each obturator fossa or along the lateral pelvic wall and brought through the abdominal wall by separate stab wounds for postoperative drainage of the pelvis. These catheters, when connected to intermittent or low-suction drainage units, are effective in preventing lymphocyst formation and in reducing the incidence of pelvic cellulitis.

The peritoneum is closed over the pelvic floor

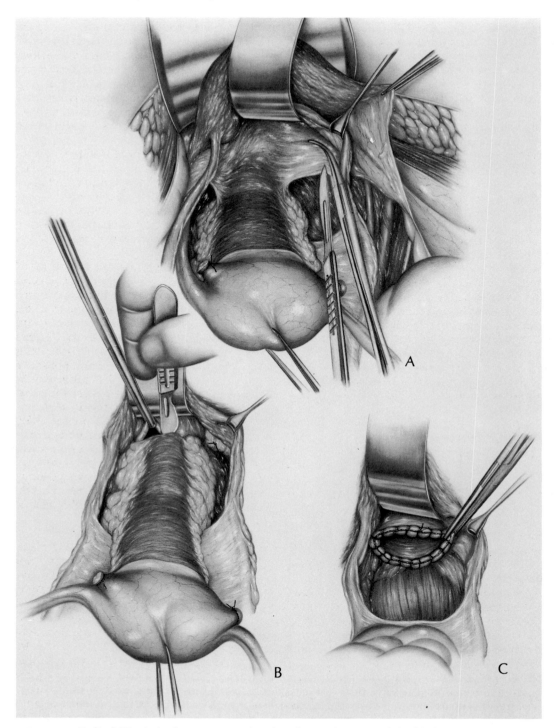

FIG. 32-23 Radical Wertheim hysterectomy (*continued*). (*A*) Dissection of the bladder from the vagina and excision of the paravaginal fascia from the lateral pelvic wall. The lower ureter is retracted from the operating field. (*B*) Opening the vagina and securing the lower vaginal cuff. The upper 2 cm to 3 cm of vagina are included with the surgical specimen. (*C*) Open vaginal cuff with continuous locking suture for hemostasis. The ureters are seen laterally and the denuded rectum posteriorly.

with a continuous locking suture, using No. 3-0 de-layed-absorbable suture material. The margins of the lateral parietal peritoneum are approximated and included with the closure of the bladder and rectal peritoneum in a continuous suture. No attempt need be made to attach the ureters to the hypogastric artery, as suggested by Green, or to place the terminal ureter on the inside of the peritoneal surface, as recommended by Novak. When the pelvis is well drained and the blood supply of the terminal ureter is preserved, fibrosis or fistula formation is not a problem.

An extra step, which has decreased the incidence of vesicovaginal and ureterovaginal fistulas, is to suture the free margin of the bladder peritoneum to the anterior vaginal cuff before closing the pelvic peritoneum. The procedure gives additional protection to the denuded bladder base by providing an extra layer of tissue between the denuded pelvis and the base of the bladder and terminal ureters.

The vaginal and abdominal drains are advanced on the third or fourth postoperative day and, if drainage has ceased, are removed on the fifth day. If drainage persists, the drains should be left in place. If all of the lymphatic channels have been ligated at the margins of the dissection, lymph drainage into the pelvis should be minimal.

POSTOPERATIVE COMPLICATIONS FOLLOWING A RADICAL WERTHEIM HYSTERECTOMY

Bladder Complications

FISTULA. Unless the patient received irradiation treatment before surgery, bladder ischemia and vesicovaginal fistula occur only infrequently. However, the posterior bladder wall may be lacerated or torn during the extensive dissection of the bladder base from the cervix and upper vagina. This injury may not be grossly visible and should routinely be checked for at the completion of the procedure by water cystoscopy or by distending the bladder with chromogen-colored saline. Suturing the bladder peritoneum to the margins of the anterior vaginal wall protects the bladder and terminal ureters from secondary infection and subsequent fistula formation. Suprapubic bladder drainage for 2 to 4 weeks postoperatively maintains the bladder and terminal ureters at rest until adequate collateral circulation has been established.

NEUROGENIC BLADDER DYSFUNCTION. Neuroanatomical studies by Smith and Ballantyne and from many clinics have demonstrated that both motor and sensory neurogenic bladder dysfunction are common complications of radical dissection of the base of

the broad ligament. Both sympathetic and para-sympathetic nerve fibers are contained in the pelvic nerve plexus, and interruption of these nerve fibers during surgery produces the problem. Green and other surgeons have shown that prolonged post-operative bladder drainage facilitates revascular-ization. Nevertheless, regeneration of both afferent and efferent autonomic nerves to the bladder base may occur slowly or not at all.

In a study at the Mayo Clinic, Webb and Sym-monds noted that sensory loss to the bladder occurred frequently among 554 patients who had undergone a radical Wertheim hysterectomy. Poor bladder sensation persisted for more than 1 year following surgery in 31.5% of the patients who required more than 14 days of catheterization following surgery.

Sasaki and associates have shown a beneficial effect on bladder function when the pars nervosa (posterior) portion of the cardinal ligament is preserved. Preservation of the lateral mesentery of the terminal ureter at the ureterovesical junction was also shown by Forney to improve both the sensory and the motor function of the bladder. Other studies by Kadar and associates and Carenza and associates have found that at least 25% of the patients who have had a radical dissection of the base of the broad ligament will have prolonged or, frequently, permanent neurogenic bladder dysfunction, including both atonic bladder and uncontrolled detrusor instability. Other problems occur more often when the entire cardinal ligament is removed: voiding dysfunction, lack of vesical sensation, and urinary incontinence. Adequate bladder retraining and the use of smooth-muscle relaxants can help patients control bladder symptoms.

Ureteral Complications

FISTULA AND STENOSIS. Devascularization and ischemic necrosis of the wall of the terminal ureter have proven to be the more serious complications of the radical Wertheim procedure: Wertheim himself had problems with this complication. Before prolonged bladder drainage was introduced along with the techniques of suspending the ureter to the obliterated portion of the hypogastric artery, Meigs's surgical patients had a 12.5% rate of significant ureteral complications, including an 8.5% incidence of ureterovaginal fistula and a 4% incidence of ureteral stricture. Novak, from Yugoslavia, reduced the incidence of ureteral fistula to 2% following primary radical surgery by placing the dissected pelvic ureter on the inside (peritoneal surface) of the pelvic peritoneum and by preserving the lateral mesentery to the terminal ureter. In our clinic, the mesentery to the terminal ureter is preserved, and the ureter is watched meticulously during the entire surgical process to prevent vascular trauma or injury to the muscularis. These techniques have reduced the incidence of ureteral fistula to less than 2%, similar to the rate reported by Webb and Symmonds at the Mayo Clinic, and by others (Table 32–6).

Pelvic Lymphocyst

The accumulation of lymph within the pelvis from retrograde lymphatic drainage was previously noted to be a common complication of the radical hysterectomy with lymphadenectomy. Historically, the complication occurred in 12.6% to 24% of cases. Prolonged drainage of the obturator space through the abdomen, as recommended by Symmonds and Pratt, together with vaginal drainage and meticulous ligation of the pelvic lymphatics, has reduced the lymphocyst to a rare event in modern surgical clinics. More commonly, the complication occurs when radical surgery is preceded by irradiation or in cases where the pelvic anatomy has been obscured.

Pelvic Cellulitis

Adequate vaginal and abdominal drainage of the operative site has greatly diminished the incidence of pelvic cellulitis following radical pelvic surgery.

In the past, patients were treated with antibiotics only if postoperative infection occurred. The current practice is to begin broad-spectrum antibiotic coverage for both aerobic (gram positive and gram negative) and anaerobic organisms immediately before surgery, and to maintain treatment for 72 hours following surgery. The use of prophylactic antibiotics has markedly reduced the incidence of pelvic cellulitis to less than 5% of all cases. If an infection does occur, the vaginal vault should be cultured and bacterial-specific, high-dose antibiotic therapy given. Only in rare cases (less than 0.5%) is it necessary to drain a pelvic abscess for secondary infection with accumulated serum and blood.

Venous Thrombosis and Pulmonary Embolus

VENOUS THROMBOSIS. The patient who undergoes radical pelvic surgery has a higher risk of developing venous thrombosis of the lower extremity than patients who have other types of gynecologic surgery. The classic triad of etiologic factors described by Virchow more than 125 years ago still applies to patients undergoing radical pelvic surgery. Postoperative alteration of blood coagulation, trauma to the vein wall, and venous stasis are all too commonly associated with radical pelvic surgery.

Pelvic lymphadenectomy invariably produces some trauma to the vein wall during the mobilization of the vessels and resection of the adherent lymphatic tissue. Tissue thromboplastin is released into the circulation during healing to accelerate the clotting mechanism, but it also produces venous thrombosis. Fibrin is likely to form at the site of injury where thromboplastin is released from the intima of the vein wall. Any area of the venous system where there is alteration in flow with stagnation of blood is susceptible to fibrin formation, particularly behind the valves of the veins in the

TABLE 32–6 *Urinary Fistulas and Operative Deaths in Nonirradiated Patients Treated by Radical Hysterectomy*

STUDY (YEAR)	NUMBER OF PATIENTS	URETERAL FISTULAS (PERCENT)	VESICAL FISTULAS (PERCENT)	OPERATIVE DEATHS (PERCENT)
Käser (1973)	717	3.3	0.6	NS
Park (1973)	156	0	0	0.64
Hoskins (1976)	224	1.3	0.45	0.89
Morley (1976)	208	4.8	0.5	1.4
Sall (1979)	349	2.0	0.8	0
Webb (1979)	423	1.4	0.7	0.3
Benedet (1980)	241	1.2	0.4	0.4
Langley (1980)	284	5.6	1.4	0
Lerner (1980)	108	0.9	0	0
Bostofte (1981)*	479	3.8	1.4	0.2
Powell (1981)	135	1.5	0	0.74
Zander (1981)	1092	1.4	0.3	1.0
Shingleton (1982)	300	1.3	0	0.3
Total	4716	2.3	0.57	0.55

* Okabayashi technique

Shingleton HM, Orr JW, Jr: Cancer of the Cervix. New York, Churchill Livingstone, 1983 lower extremities, where silent thrombosis is common.

Utilizing ^{125}I-labeled fibrinogen scanning of the lower extremities, investigators found that as many as 20% of the gynecologic patients who have had a hysterectomy develop occult venous thrombosis. Prolonged immobilization of the lower extremities during the lengthy operative procedure is a major cause of intraoperative venous stasis and clot formation. At least 50% of the patients with this complication develop it during the surgical procedure.

Heparin, in a dose of 5000 units given subcutaneously three times daily, beginning 2 hours before surgery and every 8 hours thereafter for 5 days, has decreased the incidence of thrombosis. Kakkar's study showed a decrease in postoperative cases from 24.6% in the untreated control group to 7.7% in the group treated with heparin. In Kakkar's study, 16 patients in the control group, as compared to only 2 patients in the group treated with heparin, were found on autopsy study to have died from acute, massive pulmonary embolism. Until recently, low-dose heparin was used routinely in our clinic as part of the radical Wertheim procedure as prophylaxis against venous thrombosis. However, others, notably Clarke–Pearson and associates, have found the use of low-dose heparin ineffective in preventing postoperative venous thromboses and pulmonary embolism but have found the intraoperative and postoperative use of pneumatic calf compression to be effective. The method has the added advantage that the risk of heparin-induced bleeding is eliminated. We have also found the use of sequential calf and thigh compression to be effective. The pneumatic sleeve is applied to the calf and thigh of each leg before induction of anesthesia, and pneumatic pressure is applied during surgery and throughout the first 5 postoperative days. By using calf-compression technique, Clarke–Pearson demonstrated a threefold reduction in the incidence of venous thrombosis in comparison to that associated with treatment with low-dose heparin. Use of the method has been facilitated by the development of lightweight pneumatic sleeves that permit mobility of the patient and are easily applied and removed.

PULMONARY EMBOLUS. Clinical evidence collected through ^{125}I fibrinogen scans indicates that approximately 3% to 5% of patients with occult venous thrombosis of the lower extremities will develop a pulmonary embolus. More than 50% of patients who have a fatal pulmonary embolism had "silent" venous thrombosis with no clinical evidence of the problem until the pulmonary catastrophe. Patients who have a high risk for developing thrombosis

should have routine preoperative and postoperative ^{125}I fibrinogen scanning of the lower extremities.

The day after surgery, 100 microcuries of ^{125}I-labeled fibrinogen should be injected and daily monitoring should be initiated. Should scintillation-probe scanning of the legs show a 20% or greater increase in fibrinogen uptake, bilateral venograms must be used to document the presence or absence of venous thrombosis. Kakkar's collaborative study in 1975 demonstrated by testing 4,000 surgical patients that 93% of the possible cases of venous thrombosis detected by the scanning technique could be confirmed by venography. As soon as the thrombosis is verified, full anticoagulation therapy can be started to prevent pulmonary embolism.

Only rarely does a pulmonary embolus occur after full anticoagulation has been achieved. In such cases, further migration of the venous clot must be stopped either by ligating the inferior vena cava or by using an intracaval Silastic umbrella. Although such complications are rare, even for high-risk patients, the sinister effects of thromboembolism strike suddenly and must be carefully evaluated on a daily basis.

Hemorrhage

INTRAOPERATIVE BLEEDING. Most problems with bleeding during the radical Wertheim hysterectomy occur with the dissection of the cardinal ligament and the hypogastric vessels. The many vessels of the collateral venous circulation of the hypogastric veins are particularly difficult to identify because they course among muscle bundles and fascial planes on the pelvic floor. The pararectal fossa and the cardinal ligament are also frequent sites of venous bleeding. Only meticulous dissection of the pelvic floor can prevent bleeding complications.

When venous bleeding does occur, the laceration site may be difficult to identify. Bleeding from an indefinite source can be stopped by compressing the pelvic floor veins with either a sponge stick or an abdominal pack held firmly against the entire area for no less than 7 minutes. Dissection should not proceed until full control of the bleeding has been established.

The most serious problem for hemostasis occurs when the wall of a major pelvic vein has been severely traumatized and retracts out of the operative field. Hemorrhage from a deep pelvic vein can rarely be controlled by ligating the hypogastric artery because the lower extremities and vena cava provide extensive collateral venous circulation.

Vascular clips and microfibrillar bovine collagen (Avitene) are very helpful in controlling small areas of venous oozing. Bovine collagen increases coagulation because it contains a thromboplastin-like substance. More extensive damage to the wall of the external iliac or hypogastric vein must be repaired by first placing vascular clamps above and below the area of injury and then suturing the defect.

POSTOPERATIVE HEMORRHAGE. Since all of the blood supply to the pelvis is skeletonized as part of the radical Wertheim procedure, hemorrhage can only result from bleeding that was not completely controlled during surgery. To control bleeding postoperatively, the pelvis may be packed with a multiple gauze tamponade that is extended through the open vagina and attached to an external ring (Logothetopulos pack). Pelvic packs should be advanced within 24 to 48 hours and removed shortly thereafter to prevent infection from ascending bacteria.

MODIFICATION OF THE RADICAL WERTHEIM HYSTERECTOMY

Now that the diagnosis of cervical cancer has become fairly precise in defining the tumor volume and the extent of invasion, many surgeons have begun using alternatives to the radical Wertheim hysterectomy. Since tumor is rarely found at the margins of the pelvic wall in a patient with Stage Ib cervical cancer, the rationale for removing the entire parametrium has been questioned repeatedly by surgeons and pathologists. Although tumor can traverse the microlymphatics to lymph nodes in the region of the broad ligament, metastases to the broad ligament generally do not occur when tumor is clinically confined to the cervix. Stallworthy, Kolstad, Novak, and other surgeons have maintained the attachment of the lateral mesentery to the lower ureter and have limited the parametrial dissection to the midportion of the cardinal ligament, in an effort to reduce the incidence of ureteral fistula and bladder dysfunction.

When treating patients with Stage Ib lesions, Stallworthy and Kolstad include preoperative intracavitary irradiation with surgical treatment. Irradiation therapy begins 6 weeks before surgery, delivering approximately 6000 rad to Point A in two applications of radium. Rampone, Klein, and Kolstad reported on a total of 537 patients in whom parametrial dissection was minimized, with consequent preservation of the blood supply to the lower ureter and bladder. The incidence of significant urologic complications was reduced from approximately 8% to 2.8%. The corrected 5-year survival rate of 88.3% was similar to those in many other reports that included more radical surgical treatment of the cardinal ligament. Although intracavitary irradiation is now used infrequently in conjunction with radical

Wertheim hysterectomy, we do recommend preservation of the lateral mesentery and blood supply to the terminal 2 cm of the pelvic ureter.

The modified Wertheim hysterectomy has been described in many editions of this text, because it was initially used for the treatment of carcinoma in situ, and more recently was designated for the treatment of microinvasive carcinoma. Whereas the radical Wertheim procedure removes the entire cardinal ligament and all pelvic lymph nodes, the modified Wertheim procedure, as described by Te Linde, removes the medial one-third to one-half of the cardinal ligament but does not remove the pelvic lymph nodes. As a result, the ureter is less subject to trauma, since the dissection is confined to the medial side of the widely displaced pelvic ureters and the terminal ureter is not dissected from the web. Now that colposcopy and conization are used to make a more precise diagnosis of in situ and microinvasive carcinoma, the modified Wertheim hysterectomy has a more limited use.

Rutledge uses a similar modified radical hysterectomy by displacing the ureters widely, but not dissecting them from their fascial beds, and removing the proximal one-third to one-half of the parametrium along with a wide vaginal cuff. This type of radical hysterectomy, combined with a pelvic lymphadenectomy, is the operation performed today in many clinics, since the ultraradical treatment of the cardinal ligament had done little to improve the survival rate. Removing the lateral half of the broad ligament appears to do little more than to strip the blood and nerve supply from the lower ureter and base of the bladder.

The modified Wertheim may also be used for bulky endocervical barrel-shaped tumors, both squamous and adenocarcinomatous, that require hysterectomy after full pelvic and intracavitary irradiation. In such cases, pelvic lymphadenectomy is not done. In order to remove the microlymphatics and tumor emboli that are associated with central recurrence of bulky lesions, a good margin of parametrial tissue should be removed. More radical dissection is not warranted, however, and usually results in a high incidence of fistula of the bladder, ureters, and rectum, because megavoltage irradiation must be used.

Technique of Modified Wertheim Hysterectomy

A midline incision is extended from the umbilicus to the symphysis, carrying the incision above the umbilicus for proper exposure of the pelvic organs. The intestines should be carefully held out of the operative field with moist gauze packs before the pelvis is explored manually to make certain that the tumor has not extended beyond the cervix.

The round ligament on one side is clamped, cut, and ligated at least 1 cm from the uterine cornu. The infundibulopelvic ligament is then clamped, cut, and doubly ligated well out toward the pelvic wall. The procedure is repeated on the opposite side, unless the adnexa are to be conserved, and then the clamps and the ligatures should be appropriately placed. During ligation, constant surveillance of the ureters should be maintained, to be certain they are not accidentally tied.

As is done in an ordinary hysterectomy, the incision is made so that the anterior leaf of each broad ligament is opened and the bladder peritoneum is incised where it reflects onto the anterior surface of the uterus. The bladder is then dissected from its attachment to the cervix, and the lower ureters are displaced laterally as far from the base of the broad ligament as possible, using blunt dissection with a sponge.

The peritoneum, which forms the posterior leaf of each broad ligament, is then cut downward parallel to the side of the uterus, and the structures in both bases of the broad ligaments are exposed. The ureters should then be easily palpable; they must be located to permit double ligation of the uterine vessels as far laterally as possible (Fig. 32–24A). The uterine end of the vessels should also be ligated so that the operative field may be cleared of clamps. The uterine vessels just medial to the displaced ureter should be ligated without completely freeing the ureters from their beds to avoid injuring their blood supply.

After the uterine vessels have been ligated on both sides, another bite of paracervical tissue is taken with a straight Ochsner clamp, at least 2 cm from the side of the cervix, again carefully avoiding the ureters. The clamped tissue constituting the medial one-third to one-half of the base of the broad ligament is cut and ligated with No. 0 delayed-absorbable suture placed just beyond the tip of the clamp, which is tightened as the clamp is slowly released. Sometimes a second bite of tissue has to be made parallel and lateral to the cervix below the first.

Next, the uterosacral ligaments are clamped at a point at least 1 cm to 2 cm from the cervix. The two ligaments are tied on the uterine side, and the cut is made between the clamps and the ligatures (Fig. 32–24B).

The bladder is now dissected farther down, freeing it from the pubovesicocervical fascia, which is left attached to the cervix and upper vagina. The longitudinal fibers of the fascia make it easy to recognize. Next, the lateral paravaginal tissues are clamped, cut, and ligated, approximately 2 cm lateral to either side of the vagina. Successive bites are taken with straight Ochsner clamps until a point is reached where the vagina can be cut across approximately 2 cm to 3 cm below the cervix. As the lateral clamping and ligating are continued, the bladder must be dissected further to avoid catching it or the ureter in the clamp. To prevent bleeding from either the bladder or the fascia, the vessels should be clamped and ligated as they are encountered.

When the vagina has been freed sufficiently for a 2-cm to 3-cm cuff to be amputated with the cervix, the lateral angles of the vagina, covered with the pubovesicocervical fascia, may be clamped for a short distance with curved Ochsner clamps (Fig. 32–24C). As the vagina is cut across, an assistant should grasp the anterior and the posterior vaginal walls with straight Ochsner clamps to control bleeding.

The vagina is closed with figure-of-eight No. 0 delayed-absorbable sutures. If preferred, the wound may be reefed with a continuous locking suture and left open for drainage. The vagina is suspended by suturing the cardinal, the round, and the uterosacral ligaments to its cut edge. Because the uterine vessels have been ligated so far laterally, no attempt is made to bring them into the vagina with the base of the broad ligament, as is done in conservative hysterectomy.

Carcinoma of the Cervix in Pregnancy

Invasive carcinoma of the cervix is discovered in approximately 5 per 10,000 pregnancies. The detection rate has increased since the introduction of routine cytologic smears. Still, carcinoma in situ occurs three times more frequently than invasive cancer during pregnancy: 13 cases per 10,000 pregnancies according to a study by Hacker in 1982. Figures for pregnancy-related invasive carcinoma vary somewhat. Some reports include carcinomas detected in the first 12 to 18 months postpartum, since the time interval required for the development of such cancer would probably include the period during and following the pregnancy.

To look at the statistics in another way, approximately 2.0% to 3.0% of all cases of invasive carcinoma of the cervix occur during pregnancy. Carcinoma in situ and early invasive carcinoma have approximately the same incidence in pregnant and nonpregnant women, which is not surprising since the incidence of both lesions peaks during the childbearing years.

Even though the well-known etiologic factors of cervical cancer make obstetric patients a high-risk group, Papanicolaou smears are obtained routinely in less than 60% of asymptomatic pregnant patients.

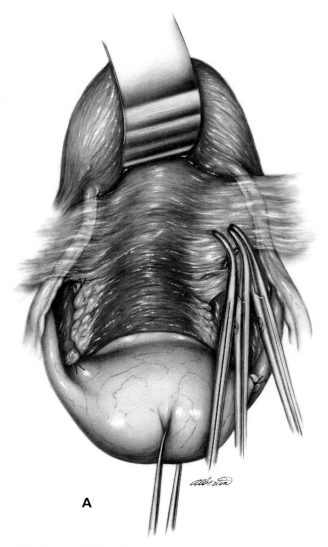

A

FIG. 32-24 Modified Wertheim hysterectomy. (*A*) Round ligaments and infundibulopelvic ligaments have been cut and ligated as in the usual hysterectomy. The broad ligament has been dissected widely by deep displacement of the bladder and terminal ureter. The right uterine vessels are clamped medial to the ureter, removing the medial one-third to one-half of the cardinal ligament with the uterus.

Once invasive carcinoma is suspected, diagnosis is often delayed by the fear of producing bleeding from the cervical scrape and biopsy.

DIAGNOSIS OF CERVICAL CARCINOMA DURING PREGNANCY

Since 75% to 80% of the pregnant patients with carcinoma of the cervix have no gross lesions, diagnosis

can only be made by a routine use of the Papanicolaou smear. Hormonal changes of the cervix that occur during pregnancy do not alter the cytologic interpretation of the Papanicolaou smear. The cytologic findings should be used to guide further evaluation of the cervix. When either a gross lesion or abnormal cytology causes a suspicion of carcinoma, the physician should not hesitate to perform a biopsy.

Modern techniques of colposcopy in conjunction with a directed biopsy from the most suspicious area of the cervix have reduced the problem of blood loss to a minimum, because the entire circumference of the cervix need not be sampled. Although the introduction of colposcopy has reduced the use of conization to only one-tenth the number of patients who previously required it, conization is still the preferred method for excluding microinvasive carcinoma, even in the pregnant patient.

Historically, conization in pregnancy has been fraught with a high incidence of residual disease, with the frequency varying from 27% to 58% (Table 32–7). Now that colposcopic localization of the lesion can be achieved, only the portion of the cervix that includes the lesion need be coned. For example, if one-half of the circumference of the cervix is devoid of any neoplastic abnormality, a cone of the total circumference is unnecessary. The depth of the cone specimen can also be planned by colposcopic examination of the neoplastic lesion. If the margin of the disease is clearly visible in the lower one-third of the cervical canal, the entire endocervix need not be removed.

The infiltration of a weak solution of Neo-Synephrine (1:200,000) into the cervix can greatly diminish the amount of blood loss from conization. A maximum of 20 ml of the solution is used throughout the procedure. Although the technique may elevate the patient's systemic blood pressure slightly and, in some patients, produce mild cardiac arrhythmia, the effect is transient and is not detrimental to placental circulation. Gelfoam, thrombin solution, microfibrillar collagen, or ligation of the descending branch of the uterine artery can also be used to control serious bleeding.

Even though the procedure is associated with an 8% to 10% incidence of postoperative bleeding, the procedure should be undertaken regardless of the duration of pregnancy if there is any question of microinvasive cancer or early invasive cancer. If a cervical lesion characteristic of invasive cancer can be observed either on gross inspection or with colposcopic studies, a directed biopsy can be used.

Colposcopic examination has been performed in our clinic on 89 pregnant patients with suspicious

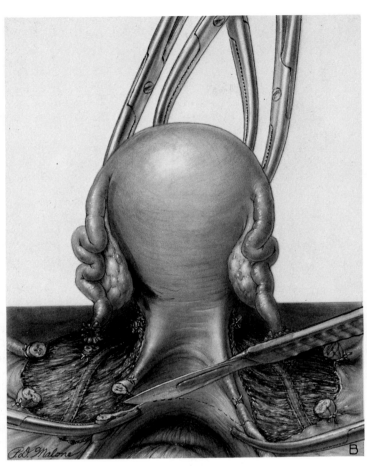

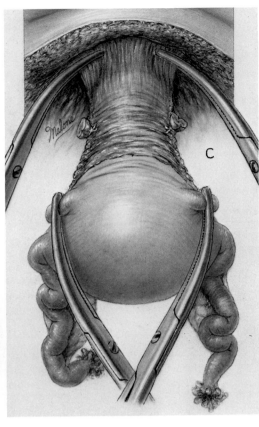

FIG. 32–24 (*continued*) (*B*) Uterosacral ligaments are clamped close to the rectum, and are being cut. The peritoneum between the two ligaments is cut as indicated by the dotted line. (*C*) The bladder is dissected down from the pubocervical fascia, well below the tip of the cervix. The pubocervical fascia is not dissected from the cervix and the vaginal wall is grasped on both sides with curved Ochsner clamps.

or positive vaginal cytology. Between 1970 and 1984, only two conization procedures had to be performed to establish a definite diagnosis of a microinvasive lesion found on colposcopy. Both patients were permitted to continue the pregnancy to term. One delivered vaginally and one delivered by cesarean section for obstetric indications.

Patients with a full-term pregnancy have an added risk of premature labor and rupture of the fetal membranes from an extensive conization procedure, but the potential for spread of invasive carcinoma poses an even greater hazard. Should labor follow a recent conization in a full-term pregnancy, the physician may prefer to perform a cesarean section rather than to risk the possibility of serious trauma or hemorrhage from a recently coned cervix.

TREATMENT OF CERVICAL CARCINOMA DURING PREGNANCY

In considering the treatment of carcinoma of the cervix during pregnancy, several factors must be taken into consideration: (1) the effect of the pregnancy on the carcinoma, (2) the effect of the carcinoma on the pregnancy, (3) the effect of the carcinoma on the method of delivery, and (4) the stage of the pregnancy when the carcinoma is detected.

Although in the past it was thought that carcinoma of the cervix was aggravated by pregnancy, current statistical evaluations of each stage of the disease show that the cure rates for pregnant women are slightly lower than those for women who are not pregnant (Table 32–8). Bosch and Marcial have shown that the survival rate for patients

TABLE 32–7 *Residual Carcinoma in Situ in Second Conization or Hysterectomy after Cervical Conization in Pregnancy*

STUDY (YEAR)	NUMBER CONIZED DURING PREGNANCY	CARCINOMA IN SITU	POSTPARTUM HYSTERECTOMY OR CONIZATION	RESIDUAL CARCINOMA IN SITU (PERCENT)
Hinde (1964)	65	65	65	18 (27.7)
Moore et al (1966)	29	19	19	7 (36.8)
Rogers, Williams (1967)	72	36	31	13 (41.9)
Smith et al (1968)	23	18	15	8 (53.3)
Mikuta et al (1968)	20	18	19	9 (47.4)
Bolognese, Corson (1969)	33	12	12	7 (58.3)
Boutselis (1972)	134	122	95	49 (51.6)
Total	376	290	256	111 (43.4)

From Hacker et al, 1982.

TABLE 32–8 *Comparison of 5-Year Survival Rates for Pregnant and Nonpregnant Women with Cervical Carcinoma*

STAGE	PREGNANT PATIENTS			NONPREGNANT PATIENTS
	Number Treated	5-Year Survival Number	Percent	5-Year Survival* (Percent)
Ib	474	348	74.5	82
II	449	214	47.8	58
III/IV	326	53	16.2	37/8
Total	1249	615	49.2	56

* Derived from FIGO Annual Report, Vol 18, 1982.
Adapted from Hacker et al, 1982.

treated during the first two trimesters of pregnancy is higher than that for women treated in the third trimester and postpartum period. Vaginal delivery is contraindicated for patients with invasive carcinoma of the cervix, since cervical dilatation and vaginal delivery can produce detrimental effects.

Prem, Makowski, and McKelvey tried a conservative approach with patients in the third trimester of pregnancy. The pregnancies were permitted to progress to 34 to 36 weeks before treatment was initiated in an effort to allow as much fetal development as possible. Stage I lesions showed the same cure rate whether or not treatment was delayed for 4 to 6 weeks. Delaying treatment is also acceptable for pregnant patients with microinvasive carcinoma of the cervix or with carcinoma in situ.

Prognosis is related primarily to the stage of the disease rather than to the stage of pregnancy.

Carcinoma in Situ

The treatment of carcinoma in situ requires no specific modification of the course of pregnancy or of the method of delivery. Once the lesion has been identified by colposcopy and a directed biopsy, the patient should be permitted to deliver vaginally. Treatment of an in situ lesion may be safely deferred until 3 to 6 months postpartum, at which time a therapeutic conization or hysterectomy is performed. If the vaginal mucosa is free of tumor on colposcopic examination, a wide vaginal cuff need not be removed routinely with a hysterectomy.

Microinvasive Carcinoma

The many reports on microinvasive disease are difficult to compare, because there is no uniform definition. According to the guidelines of the Gynecologic Oncology Society, the depth of stromal invasion is limited to 3 mm beneath the basement membrane, and the microinvasive lesion shows no evidence of involvement of the microlymphatics or capillary-like spaces. Thompson reported on 21 patients with microinvasive carcinoma in pregnancy, seven of whom had a planned delay of treatment by 5 to 28 weeks until the fetus reached term size. All of the seven patients were treated with a postpartum extended, modified Wertheim hysterectomy without lymphadenectomy, and have remained well and without recurrent disease for 3 to 10 years.

When microinvasive carcinoma occurs during pregnancy, treatment can be delayed with careful colposcopic monitoring of the cervix until a term-size fetus has been delivered vaginally or abdominally, depending on the obstetric indications. The preferred treatment, a simple hysterectomy with ovarian conservation, may be deferred until 8 to 10 weeks postpartum.

Invasive Carcinoma

FIRST TRIMESTER. When invasive cervical cancer is detected during the first trimester, treatment should be initiated immediately with complete disregard for the fetus. The choice of therapy should depend on the stage of the disease, the size of the lesion, the presence of vascular involvement, the medical condition of the patient, and the interest of the patient in retaining ovarian function. In general, the choice of therapy does not differ for the pregnant patient. Only Stage Ib and possibly early Stage IIa lesions are recommended for radical Wertheim hysterectomy with pelvic node dissection. More advanced lesions require full pelvic irradiation. When irradiation therapy is given, the external megavoltage radiation is given initially to permit the gestation to be aborted and the uterus to regress in size. The cure rates for Stage Ib disease diagnosed during the first trimester (83.3%) are no different from those for carcinoma diagnosed postpartum (81.1%), as reviewed by Hacker and coworkers. For Stage II disease, the cure rate was somewhat lower than for nonpregnant patients. Stage II patients diagnosed during the first trimester had a 5-year survival rate of 41.7%, while patients diagnosed postpartum had a 5-year survival rate of 45.1%.

SECOND TRIMESTER. When invasive cervical cancer is detected during the early part of the second trimester, definitive treatment should not be delayed. External irradiation should be used initially to produce a spontaneous abortion. Intracavitary irradiation should follow when the uterus and cervix have undergone involution and the risk of infection is decreased. For patients who are candidates for surgical treatment, primary radical surgery should be initiated as soon as the diagnosis is established. Although the operative and postoperative morbidity is somewhat higher than in cases treated primarily by irradiation, primary surgery allows a young patient to conserve ovarian function while sparing her the undesirable sequelae of pelvic irradiation.

THIRD TRIMESTER. When invasive carcinoma is detected in or near the third trimester, particularly between the 26th and 28th week of gestation, treatment may be delayed until the 34th to 36th week, so that the fetus may have a good chance for survival. In a review of the literature since 1960, Hacker and associates reported on 1657 cases of invasive carcinoma of the cervix occurring during pregnancy. Five-year data were available on 1274 cases, including 25 cases with microinvasion. The 5-year survival rates among patients treated immediately upon diagnosis in the third trimester were not statistically different from patients whose treatment was delayed for up to 8 weeks. The review stressed the importance of ensuring by ultrasound that the fetus was healthy and without congenital defects before deciding to delay treatment. When surgery is used during the third trimester, a classical cesarean section is performed initially and is followed with a radical hysterectomy and pelvic node dissection or full pelvic irradiation.

MODE OF DELIVERY. An unexpected finding of Hacker's review was that vaginal delivery did not seem to seriously jeopardize the prognosis for the control of the cervical cancer. When the mode of delivery was analyzed according to the stage of disease, vaginal delivery for patients with Stage Ib resulted in a 56% 5-year survival rate (65 of 117 cases), compared with a 30% rate for Stage II disease after abdominal delivery (9 of 30 cases). For Stages III and IV the 5-year survival rate after vaginal delivery was 31.7% (19 of 60 cases), while the rate after abdominal delivery was only 11% (2 of 28 cases). Since Hacker's review was retrospective, the data could not be analyzed for statistical significance. Although the thesis is unproven, most oncologists who have studied invasive disease during pregnancy favor an abdominal delivery and believe that tumor emboli can be spread in the highly vascular cervix during vaginal delivery. An additional risk is laceration of the cervix and severe hemorrhage as a consequence of a tear through a cervical tumor during rapid dilatation. Regardless of the method of delivery, it is clear from these data that the cure rates for patients with carcinoma of the cervix in pregnancy are significantly reduced by approximately 50% when compared, stage-for-stage, with nonpregnant patients. Only when the tumor is diagnosed in the first trimester and in Stage Ib disease are the cure rates comparable.

CHOICE OF THERAPY. The choice of therapy for a pregnant patient, just as for the nonpregnant patient, depends on the stage of the disease, the size and grade of the tumor, the presence or absence of vascular invasion, and the age and general medical health of the patient. The major advantage of primary surgery is that it allows an opportunity to conserve ovarian function and to avoid the secondary effects of irradiation on the reproductive tract of a young patient. Irradiation treatment is identical to that for the nonpregnant patient, external beam therapy of 5500 to 6000 rad to the midplane of the pelvis followed by central brachytherapy.

Pelvic Exenteration

INDICATIONS

The clinical behavior of cervical cancer, the known pathways of spread, and the protracted period of localized, central growth make this tumor suitable for en bloc treatment by pelvic exenteration. For tumors of the lower genital tract, the cervix, the vagina, and, occasionally, the vulva that have failed to respond to primary therapy and for recurrent disease confined to the central pelvis, pelvic exenteration is an important adjunctive method of treatment. On occasion, these tumors may be found to involve the urethra, bladder, or rectum and may require an exenterative procedure to encompass the disease and to effect a cure. For example, a vulvar or vaginal cancer may extend deep into the vagina, invade the adjacent organs, and require a pelvic exenteration as primary treatment.

The introduction of pelvic exenteration by Brunschwig in 1948 provided the first ultraradical surgical approach for advanced and radioresistant cervical cancer. Although the initial 10-year experience with the procedure was associated with a high morbidity and mortality rate, these early results reflected the advanced disease status of the patients selected for treatment. Later, strict guidelines regarding the indications and contraindications for exenteration were developed.

At the present time, only 40% to 50% of all patients explored for radioresistant cervical cancer are candidates for en bloc exenteration. If the dosage is accurate, most cervical cancer can be well controlled with intracavitary and megavoltage external irradiation therapy, as Jampolis documented in 1975. When irradiation therapy fails, the residual cervical cancer is usually located at the lateral pelvic wall. It may have metastasized to regional and distant sites. Both conditions limit the use of exenteration.

Following complete irradiation therapy, it is difficult to determine accurately whether or not microscopic foci of tumor are present in adjacent tissues surrounding the cervix. Perez–Mesa and Spjut have shown by pathologic study of exenteration specimens that even in cases where no clinical evidence exists, the bladder and rectum are commonly involved with tumor—the rates of occurrence being 61% and 44%, respectively. With such evidence, Brunschwig, Bricker, Schmitz, Parsons, and others

agreed that faced with an unresponsive tumor following external and intracavitary irradiation, the most radical surgical procedure may prove to be the most successful.

Even if the malignancy has not extended to the contiguous organs, such as the rectum and bladder, these organs can no longer be considered normal. Pelvic irradiation results in an obliterative endarteritis with progressive ischemia of the pelvic viscera. If a radical hysterectomy is added with skeletonization of the remaining blood supply of the pelvis, a fistula rate of at least 10% to 15% can be expected for the lower bowel and urinary tract. A total pelvic exenteration, which removes bladder, uterus, vagina, and rectum as an en bloc procedure, avoids this type of morbidity, and at the same time provides the maximum opportunity for complete eradication of the disease.

The pelvic surgeon must maintain an openminded policy about the types of radical procedure that may be utilized. Occasionally, a patient will have fascial planes and tissues that are pliable and will dissect easily, so a Wertheim operation can be used for cancer that recurs after irradiation. If a radical hysterectomy and lymphadenectomy are not feasible, either an anterior pelvic exenteration, including the bladder, uterus, and vagina, or a total pelvic exenteration should be utilized. A posterior exenteration, which would include rectum, uterus, and vagina, has been associated with an unacceptably high urinary tract fistula rate when used after full pelvic irradiation.

Indications According to Stage of Disease

Patients with radioresistant Stage Ib cervical carcinoma are the best candidates for exenteration surgery. The more advanced the tumor, the more difficult is the en bloc removal of the disease. Even with Stage II lesions, patients have a decreased survival rate, because the procedure may not completely encompass the tumor.

If tumor is found adherent to the fascia of the pelvic musculature or invading the fascial sheath of the iliac vessels, the procedure must be abandoned. When positive pelvic lymph nodes are found after complete irradiation therapy, the prognosis is poor. Parsons reported that no patients survived for 5 years when pelvic exenteration for radioresistant cervical carcinoma revealed positive pelvic lymph nodes. More recent studies found a 5-year survival rate of 5% to 15% of the patients with positive pelvic nodes found during an exenteration procedure (Table 32–9).

Exenteration has been considered as a primary procedure for a rare Stage IV cervical malignancy

TABLE 32–9   *Effect of Pelvic Lymph Node Metastasis on Survival following Pelvic Exenteration*

	NEGATIVE NODES		POSITIVE NODES	
STUDY (YEAR)	Number of Patients	5-Year Survival (Percent)	Number of Patients	5-Year Survival (Percent)
Barber, Jones (1971)	166	17.4	97	5.1
Creasman, Rutledge (1975)	29	27.0	14	14.0
Symmonds et al (1975)	139	39.0	59	13.0
Averette et al (1984)	92	–	6	0.0
Morley (1985)	73	63.0	10	0.0

that has spread anteroposteriorly, involving the bladder and rectum. The use of irradiation therapy in such cases frequently produces uncorrectable fistulas following necrosis and slough of the tumor. Even though recent experience has produced better results—Rutledge treated Stage IV lesions with irradiation therapy and showed a cure rate of 28%, without vesicovaginal fistulas—the surgical results are still superior. Ketcham reported a 5-year survival rate of 48% among 65 patients treated with a primary exenteration.

Pelvic exenteration should not be used as a palliative procedure. The morbidity, mortality, and complication rates are too high to warrant such extensive surgery, especially if treatment condemns a patient to spend the first 6 months of the remaining year of her life recovering from the surgical procedure. Even palliative urinary diversion in patients with advanced pelvic malignancy and bilateral ureteral obstruction does not improve longevity. Among 90 patients treated with urinary diversion in a study by Meyer and colleagues, only 30% lived more than 6 months, and all ultimately died as a result of the cervical malignancy.

Other types of carcinoma may or may not be suited to treatment by exenteration. Carcinoma of the endometrium has too rapid an extrapelvic spread by hematogenous and lymphatic routes to be benefited by this type of surgery. Brunschwig's early experience in 1961 with exenteration for recurrent endometrial carcinoma was very poor and there has been no success with this treatment since that report.

If a Stage IV vaginal or vulvar carcinoma destroys the urethra or extends into the bladder or rectum, it may require an anterior, posterior, or total pelvic exenteration. Our own experience has been limited with this type of primary treatment for cervical cancer. Total or partial exenteration is more commonly required for vulvar carcinoma in cases where the tumor extends into the anterior or pos-

terior wall of the vagina. A radioresistant vaginal carcinoma usually involves either the anterior or posterior vaginal wall, but may require a total pelvic exenteration to avoid a fistula forming in the uninvolved, yet heavily irradiated, organ.

CONTRAINDICATIONS

Contraindications to the exenteration procedure have been developed over time, as surgeons discovered signs and symptoms of far-advanced disease that would not respond to radical treatment.

Sciatic nerve pain, usually unilateral, is evidence of encroachment of tumor on the perineural sheath of the sciatic nerve plexus.

Progressive leg edema indicates lymphatic obstruction of the external iliac lymphatic channels. Since megavoltage irradiation may produce lymphatic obstruction, a lymphangiogram or CT scan should be used to make sure that leg edema is not the result of metastatic tumor.

Obstructive uropathy, with either unilateral or bilateral hydronephrosis, is a sensitive barometer of advancing cervical carcinoma. Cox and associates found that in only 40% of the patients with unilateral hydronephrosis was removal of the recurrent malignancy possible. Bilateral obstruction connoted nonresectability in more than 88% of the cases in their experience.

Extrapelvic metastasis to para-aortic or common iliac nodes or to abdominal viscera, as encountered at the time of exploration, is a contraindication for continuing the pelvic exenteration. Before surgery, a lymphangiogram or CT scan helps in evaluating possible extrapelvic metastatic disease, but both require histologic verification. Needle aspiration of a suspicious para-aortic node in experienced hands allows an accurate diagnosis in 75% to 80% of cases. Even an isolated occult metastasis to a single pelvic node will significantly influence the curability of the disease, although recent experience suggests that

5% to 15% of patients with such findings will survive for 5 or more years. When there are multiple unilateral or bilateral pelvic node metastases, the cure rate is lower than the mortality rate of the procedure.

Penetration of the tumor through the cervix with extension of the tumor into the peritoneal cavity generally signifies disease incurable by exenteration. Such advanced lesions will have disseminated cells into the peritoneal cavity, and patients will develop early extrapelvic recurrence. An adherent small bowel or sigmoid colon rarely protects the peritoneum from spread of tumor cells, even though segmental bowel resections have in rare instances been associated with prolonged survival. Extensive tumors of this type are rarely treated by exenteration; the risk-benefit ratio is such that surgery is unwarranted.

Obesity should be considered as a serious risk factor in the final evaluation of a patient considering surgery. Although weight is not an absolute contraindication, the complication rate from exenteration increases directly with the weight of the patient.

Age and medical complications are the physiologic barriers to this type of radical surgery, although the guidelines are not as precise as for other contraindications. In general, patients beyond the age of 65 are not ideal candidates, because their normal life expectancy is limited; the extent of any vascular, renal, cardiac, or pulmonary disease is usually already increased; and their ability to adapt to physiologic and psychological stress from a disfiguring procedure is less predictable.

Most cases of recurrent cervical cancer present earlier in life, so recurrent disease that appears after age 65 is more likely to be advanced beyond the boundaries of the central pelvic organs. Still, the final determination of surgical candidacy must include an unbiased, thorough medical assessment of the cardiopulmonary–renal–metabolic reserve of the patient, irrespective of the patient's age.

Psychological incapacity to adjust to the disfigurement produced by this type of radical surgery is a contraindication. Psychological assessment of the patient is one of the most important prerequisites for pelvic exenteration. Despite the close rapport that the gynecologic oncologist may have developed with a patient, she should also be counseled by a sex therapist and a psychiatrist or psychologist. Patients must have adequate preparation for the anatomical alterations, psychological reactions, and change in body image that result from exenterative surgery.

Some patients may not be capable of making the emotional adjustments required to accept disfig-

uring surgery, and they should not be forced to do so, even if their cancer may not be controlled by local treatment. If possible, a patient who is a candidate for a total or partial exenteration should be provided the opportunity to discuss the outcome with another patient who has satisfactorily adjusted to this type of surgery. Surgical candidates must be completely comfortable with their decision and should have a strong determination to make the changes in life-style that are necessary after a pelvic exenteration.

The eight contraindications are valuable as guidelines for selecting candidates who will benefit from radical pelvic surgery; they should not be considered as absolute criteria of inoperability. The only patients who are candidates for pelvic exenteration are those in whom the disease has recurred following irradiation in the central pelvis without extension to the parametrium or the lateral pelvic wall. Even when an evaluation of the pelvis is performed under anesthesia, it is difficult to determine whether a given case is operable. Unfortunately, the induration of the parametrial tissues that follows megavoltage irradiation is frequently indistinguishable from the induration of an invasive tumor. In the absence of extrapelvic metastases, the final decision about whether or not the procedure is feasible must be made during surgery, which begins with a meticulous evaluation of the pelvic viscera. The exploratory laparotomy is actually considered as the final portion of the diagnostic work-up.

TECHNIQUE OF PELVIC EXENTERATION

The total exenteration procedure is initiated abdominally, but it may require completion by the vaginal approach, depending on the factors of patient obesity, tumor depth, and the bony configuration of the pelvis. In an ideal procedure, two teams of surgeons could work from the vaginal and the abdominal routes to facilitate the deep pelvic and vaginal dissection and to shorten the operating time.

A generous midline incision is made and extended well above the umbilicus for adequate exposure. A transverse incision would limit the exposure of the upper abdomen and para-aortic lymph nodes. The free edges of the abdominal incision should be protected with moist abdominal gauze pads to avoid ischemia and to improve healing of the incision following prolonged retraction. The stomal sites are selected before surgery, with help from a stomatologist, and are marked on the skin with indelible ink so they will not be removed during presurgical cleansing.

The most important part of the procedure is the exploration of the abdominal viscera, particularly the liver surface, the peritoneal surfaces, and the para-aortic lymph nodes, for evidence of extrapelvic metastases. Para-aortic or common iliac lymph node involvement contraindicates an exenteration, so para-aortic node dissection (Fig. 32–25) and histologic study of the lymph nodes by frozen section must be completed before the pelvic dissection is continued.

The para-aortic node dissection begins at the bifurcation of the aorta (Fig. 32–25A) where the posterior peritoneum is opened with the Metzenbaum scissors, taking particular care to avoid injury to the left common iliac vein that courses beneath the aorta and right common iliac artery (Fig. 32–25B). The peritoneum is incised to a level above the inferior mesenteric artery and vein and a narrow retractor is placed beneath the upper peritoneal margin to expose the para-aortic and para-caval regions widely. Although many oncologists dissect only the lateral side of the aorta to avoid injury to the thin-walled vena cava, the para-caval nodes should also be removed and assessed for the presence or absence of occult lymph node metastasis. Using the Metzenbaum scissors, the dissection begins along the lateral margin of the left common iliac artery and continues along the side of the aorta to a level well above the inferior mesenteric vessels (Fig. 32–25B). The dissection is facilitated by having the assistant surgeon clamp the mesenteric base of each dissected node with a vascular clip (Fig. 32–25C) while the surgeon excises the gland and continues with the node dissection. Care must be taken to avoid injury to the lumbar arteries and veins that lie behind the aorta and vena cava. If bleeding should occur and the vessel has retracted beneath the great vessels, firm pressure for 5 to 7 minutes with a stick sponge against the vertebral bodies will usually cause a clot to form. Efforts to identify and clamp a lumbar vein that has been separated from the vena cava may produce a larger rent in the caval wall and cause profound hemorrhage. In such cases, vascular clamps must be placed above and below the caval rent and the defect clearly exposed and closed with fine vascular sutures. The surgeon must use extreme caution in retracting the vena cava while dissecting the para-caval nodes to avoid injury to the vessel. The caval dissection should begin along the lateral side of the right common iliac artery and extend on the side of the vena cava to the region above the inferior mesenteric vessels. It is important to clamp securely, excise, and ligate the superior and inferior lymphatic vessels in beginning and completing the node dissection. A No. 3-0 silk tie on the tip of an Adson clamp provides an excellent means of ligating these vessels and preventing a subsequent lymphocyst. If bleeding has been troublesome during this dissection, a retroperitoneal drain should be placed in the operative site and brought through the abdominal wall.

While the frozen section is being analyzed, the pelvic and peritoneal cavities can be assessed for involvement. Assessment of the parametrial tissues usually requires direct examination by opening the anterior and posterior leaves of the broad ligament. The paravesical and pararectal spaces must also be evaluated (see Figs. 32–14 to 32–16).

The decision to operate should be considered completely reversible throughout the initial exploration. If tumor is not identified or if advanced lesions cannot be completely encompassed, the operative procedure should be discontinued. As is done in the Wertheim procedure, the index finger is used to explore the avascular paravesical and pararectal spaces after ligating and excising the ovarian vessels at the pelvic brim and the round ligament near the lateral pelvic wall. Careful dissection with the finger along the lateral pelvic wall and the levator muscles of the pelvic floor can show whether or not the broad ligament and the paravesical and pararectal tissues can be resected without disturbing the arcade of pelvic blood vessels.

Exploration is continued gently into the obturator fossa by retracting the uterus and parametrium to the opposite side of the pelvis. Indurated and suspicious areas must be biopsied, particularly if there is a question of tumor extending to the fascia of the levator ani or obturator muscle. If tumor is confirmed by frozen section to be adherent to the fascia of the pelvic floor or vessels, the disease is too advanced for surgical cure, and the operation should be discontinued after the broad ligament is reattached.

If a complete evaluation with histologic studies shows that the disease can be contained, dissection of the pelvic contents should be continued by extending the peritoneal reflection of the broad ligament and incising the posterior peritoneum well below the pelvic brim (Fig. 32–26). If possible, the bladder peritoneum should be left attached to the bladder dome, and the lateral pelvic peritoneum should be saved to permit closure of the peritoneum at the completion of the operation.

A peritoneal flap is left attached to the ureter for preservation of its blood supply and utilization later in the urinary diversion. All of the tumor-free portion of the pelvic ureters that is not heavily irradiated should be conserved.

The pelvic peritoneum is incised along the mesosigmoid to the margin of the sigmoid musculature. Care must be taken to avoid injury to the middle sacral artery and vein, which enter the pelvis along the sacral promontory.

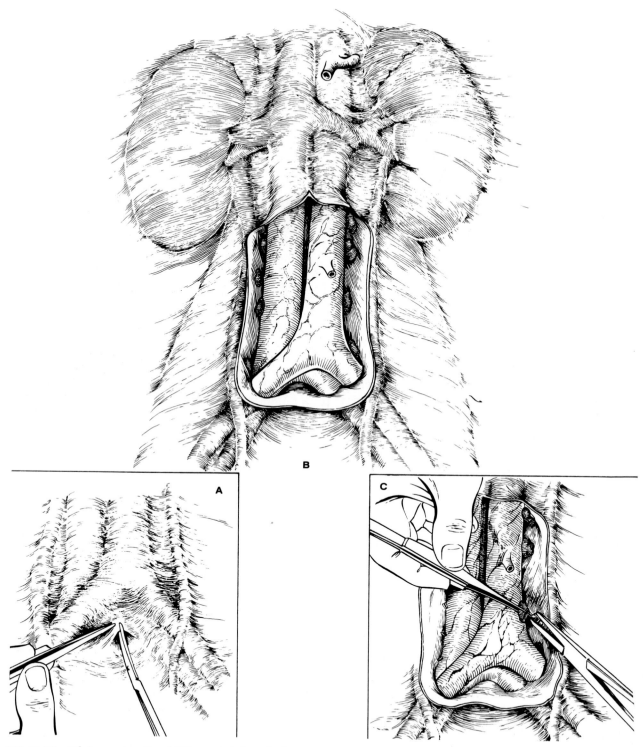

FIG. 32–25 Pelvic exenteration. (*A*) Para-aortic lymphadenectomy. The posterior peritoneum is opened below the bifurcation of the aorta, avoiding injury to the left common iliac vein. Note the close relationship of the right ureter to the vena cava. (*B*) The left common iliac vein is shown as it passes beneath the right common iliac artery. The posterior peritoneum is opened to a level well above the inferior mesenteric artery. (*C*) Nodes are removed from the lateral side of aorta. The lymphatic vessels are secured with a vascular clip to avoid lymphocyst formation. Dissection removes suspicious nodes from the lateral, anterior, and medial aspects of the aorta and vena cava.

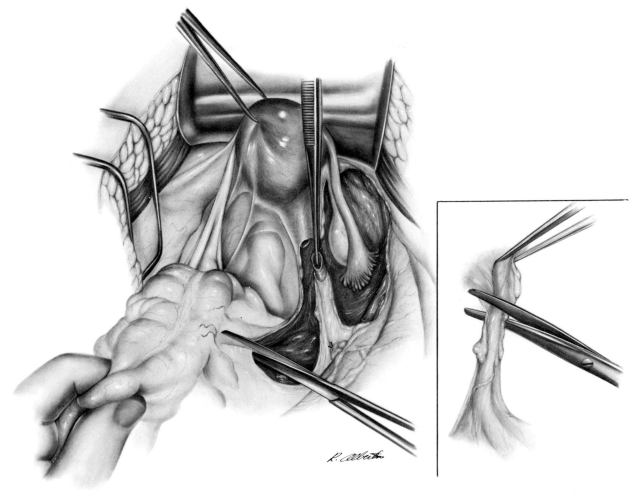

FIG. 32–26 Pelvic exenteration showing transection of the ureter and incision of the peritoneum below the pelvic brim and along the sigmoid mesentery. (*Insert*) The ureter is cut but remains attached to the pelvic peritoneum.

Urinary Diversion

Although many techniques defer the urinary diversion until the end of the operation, early diversion of the urinary tract may be beneficial if several factors are taken into consideration.

The en bloc dissection is technically easier and faster with the ureters freed from the surgical specimen and the rectum detached from the sigmoid colon. Further, the urinary diversion is the most delicate and time-consuming step in the entire procedure, and it can be accomplished more efficiently at the beginning of the operation than later, when the surgeon is fatigued. The patient could also be in a precarious condition later in the operation. In addition, early diversion provides time to evaluate the competence of the ureterointestinal anastomosis while the remainder of the pelvic dissection is completed.

If there is any concern that the disease may not be completely contained, the urinary diversion should be delayed until the pelvic tumor has been completely removed. Unnecessary trauma results when the urinary stream has been diverted to an intestinal conduit, only to find that the case is inoperable because the tumor has extended to the pelvic floor.

The procedure for using an isolated segment of the terminal ileum developed by Bricker is the most frequently used method of urinary diversion, although the sigmoid or transverse colon may also be used to construct the urinary conduit. The major advantage of the sigmoid conduit is that it does not require an end-to-end small bowel anastomosis, so the total operative time is decreased significantly. Although the transverse colon offers an unirradiated segment of bowel for the conduit, using that part of the bowel also means creating an anastomosis. The objectives are similar for all three methods: rapid urinary runoff, augmented by the peristaltic action of the large or small bowel, and the prevention of hyperchloremic acidosis. The placement of the ostia in the abdominal wall may be deferred until later in the operation in order to avoid trauma to the bowel and ureters during the remainder of the procedure.

Although used in the following procedure, the sigmoid urinary conduit has not completely replaced the conduit utilizing the more mobile terminal ileum. In fact, the ileal conduit is probably used more often than the sigmoid. In cases where intense irradiation treatment has caused fibrosis of the sigmoid colon and shortened its mesentery, the transverse colon provides a good segment of bowel and is associated with fewer complications of the ureteral anastomosis. The procedures for forming a conduit are similar whether the sigmoid colon or the distal ileum is used (see Chapter 19).

Approximately 15 cm to 18 cm of the sigmoid colon is needed for the conduit, and particular care must be used to select an area that includes a rich arcade of blood vessels from the inferior mesenteric artery (Fig. 32–27). The exact length of the bowel segment is determined by the thickness of the abdominal wall; sufficient bowel must be provided for the intra-abdominal segment without undue tension being placed on the ureteral anastomosis. In some instances, 6 cm of bowel may be used in the abdominal wall. Should additional large bowel be needed to fashion a colostomy after the construction of the urinary conduit, the descending colon can be mobilized by carefully excising its attachment from the splenic flexure to the parietal peritoneum. In preparing the conduit, care must be exercised to avoid damage to the anastomotic arcade of inferior mesenteric and superior hemorrhoidal vessels (Fig. 32–27).

After the proximal and distal ends of the sigmoid segment are divided, the proximal end of the conduit is closed with an initial layer of continuous inverting suture using No. 3-0, delayed-absorbable material (Fig. 32–27A). The next layer is made with interrupted Lembert sutures of No. 3-0 silk. The GIA autosuture surgical stapler can expedite the colon resection, important for maintaining an uncontaminated operating field (see Chapter 19). The row of staples should also be supported by an inverting layer of No. 3-0 interrupted silk sutures. The corners of the bowel must be well inverted to prevent urine leakage from the ureteral transplant. The distal pelvic colon, still attached to the pelvic tumor site, should be closed with either a continuous inverting suture or the GIA stapler to prevent soiling of the operating field during the remainder of the dissection.

The anastomosis between the ureters and the antimesenteric wall of the isolated sigmoid conduit is best created using the mucosa-to-mucosa technique of Leadbetter (Fig. 32–28). Each ureter is positioned so that the attached peritoneal flap will remain on the outer exposed surface after the ureter is attached to the mesosigmoid. Following complete mobilization, the ureter is rotated to bring the retroperitoneal portion along the inferior surface of the sigmoid pouch and mesentery, permitting the ureter to remain covered by its peritoneal flap at all times.

The adventitia of the ureter is anchored posteriorly to the serosa of the sigmoid. Three No. 4-0 silk sutures are used, beginning in the middle and followed with a suture at each edge (Fig. 32–28A,B). The sutures are placed approximately 1 cm from the end of the ureter and serve to reinforce the mucosal anastomosis.

The location for anastomosis of the left ureter is chosen to avoid encroachment on the closed end of the colon, and it should be at least 3 cm to 4 cm from the bowel suture line. The right ureter should be so implanted that it falls most naturally in line with its abdominal course, separated from the opposite ureter by at least 4 cm to 5 cm. (In Figure 32–28, the anastomoses appear close together for illustrative purposes.)

To create the openings, a small incision is made through the muscularis of the bowel, adjacent to and for the length of the ureteral orifice. In order to avoid making the opening too large, two skin hooks or empty round needles are placed as anchors, elevating the mucosa so the ureter will slide easily into the bowel lumen (Fig. 32–28C). The anchors also secure the mucosal edge until the first mucosa-to-mucosa suture is placed (Fig. 32–28D). In suturing the posterior full-thickness wall of the ureter to the mucosa of the bowel, the middle suture is placed first and followed by a suture at each end of the incision in the bowel. No. 4-0 delayed-absorbable material is used.

Silastic tubing (internal diameter 0.078 in) is used as a ureteral stent to enhance the healing process of the ureterointestinal anastomosis. As advocated by Rutledge and associates, this malleable stent is most useful for previously irradiated tissues, where anastomotic leakage is a common complication. One end of the Silastic tubing is inserted into the ureter and threaded into the renal pelvis. The opposite end is directed through the lumen of the conduit and brought out through the intestinal ostium. The

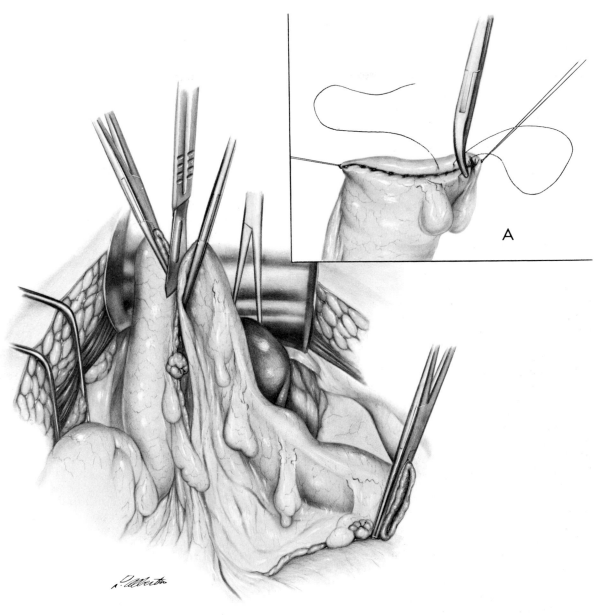

FIG. 32-27 Pelvic exenteration (*continued*). Section of the sigmoid has been excised. (*Insert A*) Two-layer closure of one end of the sigmoid segment.

catheter may be secured by sliding a small Silastic cuff (internal diameter 0.1 in) from a slightly larger piece of tubing over the stent to the region of the intestinal anastomosis. A single No. 4-0 absorbable suture placed through the bowel wall adjacent to the site of anastomosis will anchor the Silastic cuff to the wall of the conduit. The lumen of the stent should not be pierced by the suture, since it might tear or kink.

The anterior wall of the ureter is connected to the bowel mucosa in two or three locations, depending on the redundancy of the mucosal ostium. No attempt is made to produce a leak-proof anastomosis at this stage, since the second supporting layer of No. 4-0 silk serosal sutures will reinforce the anastomosis and seal the orifice. Excessive suturing of the ureter and bowel will produce tissue necrosis and possible failure of the anastomosis. No

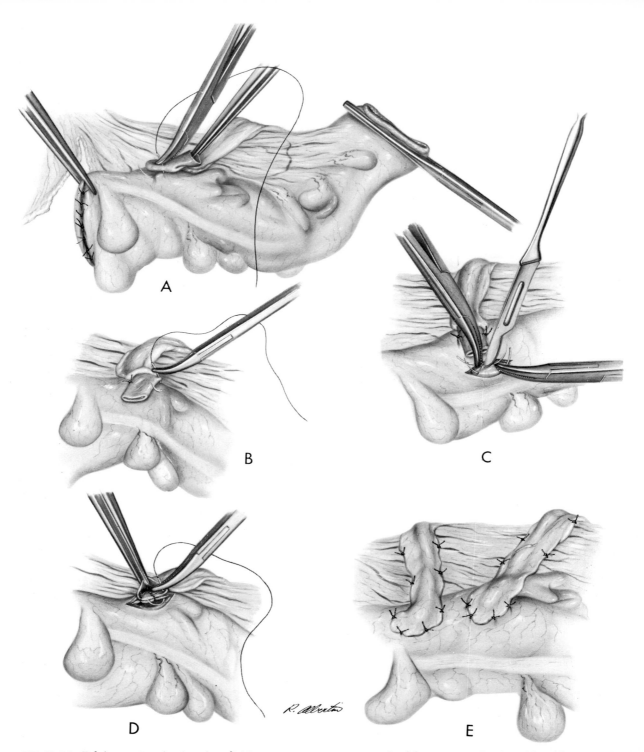

FIG. 32–28 Pelvic exenteration (*continued*). Mucosa-to-mucosa anastomosis of the ureter to the sigmoid conduit. Note that the peritoneum attached to the ureters may be used to extraperitonize the two-layer ureteral anastomosis. (*A*) The adventitia of the ureter is sutured to the serosa of the bowel with No. 4-0 silk sutures. (*B*) The lateral margin of the ureter is sutured to the serosa of the bowel. (*C*) The bowel is opened for ureteral anastomosis. The use of round needle (or skin hooks) to grasp the bowel mucosa is shown. (*D*) The ureter is anastomosed to the bowel by mucosa-to-mucosa technique, using No. 4-0 delayed-absorbable suture. (*E*) Completion of ureteral anastomosis and suture of peritoneum over anastomotic site and along the inferior surface of the bowel mesentery.

more than three additional supporting sutures should be placed in the serosa.

The peritoneal flap of the ureter is now sutured with silk to the serosa of the bowel over the anastomotic site, and then to the mesentery, so that the ureter is completely sealed inside the peritoneum (Fig. 32–28E). The peritoneal support will ensure an adequate blood supply, reinforce the anastomosis, and prevent displacement of the ureters by movement of the abdominal viscera. If the intestinal orifice has enlarged beyond the diameter of the ureteral opening, the bowel should be closed with interrupted stitches of No. 3-0 absorbable suture.

The blind end and midportion of the conduit should be securely sutured to the posterior peritoneum near the lower lumbar vertebrae. The attachment ensures that the conduit, now the bladder, remains stationary and does not fall into the pelvis. Sagging of the bladder could cause excessive tension and leakage of the ureteral anastomosis.

The ureteral Silastic catheters are removed in approximately 14 to 21 days when the suture anchoring the Silastic stent has dissolved. Irrigation with 1% neomycin solution should be used only if there is evidence of diminished drainage from either catheter. In general, the immediate outcome of the exenterative procedure is governed by the outcome of the urinary diversion. If the urinary diversion goes well, the entire operation goes well.

Pelvic Lymphadenectomy in Pelvic Exenteration

There has been much debate in recent years regarding the value of pelvic lymphadenectomy in extending the 5-year survival rate of the exenteration procedure. Although only about 5% to 15% of the patients survive 5 years or longer if the nodes are positive for metastatic tumor, even this low rate is a distinct improvement on previous experience (Table 32–9). The prognosis is very bad if more than a single isolated node is found to contain metastatic tumor; of Rutledge's patients, 77% died within 2 years following the positive pelvic node dissection.

Omitting the lymphadenectomy shortens the operating time and decreases the risk of operative hemorrhage. Performing the lymphadenectomy adds to the thoroughness of the anatomical dissection and provides anatomical guidelines for removal of the central viscera. The procedure should be accomplished quickly and cautiously. Since the tissue has usually received full irradiation treatment the lymphatic tissue is densely adherent to the blood vessels and surrounding tissues, and a meticulous lymph node dissection cannot be achieved.

The para-aortic node dissection performed during the exploratory phase of the exenteration extends to the bifurcation of the aorta and vena cava and to the proximal portion of the common iliac vessels. Dissection is continued from the common iliac artery and vein along the external iliac vessels until they pass beneath Poupart's ligament and enter the femoral canal. During the sharp dissection of the pelvic vessels, care must be taken to avoid traumatizing the vessel wall, since injury would cause a reaction in the intima of the vessel and increase the possibility of postoperative venous thrombosis and emboli. Most surgeons do not strip all the adventitia from the vessel walls, because that measure has not improved the surgical results. Leaving a filmy residue of areolar tissue is considered optimum (Fig. 32–29A). Care should also be taken to avoid injuring the inferior epigastric and anomalous obturator vessels at the lower end of the iliac vessels.

Resection of the hypogastric vessels along with the pelvic specimen was advocated in early descriptions of the procedure, but such a step is no longer considered advisable. Operative hemorrhage is far too great when the entire pelvic vascular tree is removed unless the venous system is carefully ligated. Since a case is considered inoperable if the disease has extended to the pelvic vasculature at the lateral pelvic wall, the only reason to remove the deep pelvic vessels would be to achieve a wider surgical margin, which is unnecessary.

In the current procedure, the hypogastric arteries are doubly ligated with No. 0 silk but are not excised (Fig. 32–29B). The parietal and visceral branches are occluded with hemoclips. The distal branches of the hypogastric vessels are usually included with the ligation, and may be excised with the parametrium and pararectal stalks.

Particular care must be taken with the adjacent network of communicating veins, because trauma will cause them to retract into the sacral foramina and pelvic musculature. Should retraction occur, bleeding is usually effectively stopped by packing the area firmly until a fibrin clot has formed. The use of Gelfoam moistened with thrombin solution or microfibrillar collagen (Avitene) can enhance the control of venous bleeding considerably, and these agents should be applied with pressure over the small pelvic vessels.

Continuation of the lymph node dissection into the obturator fossa (Fig. 32–30) is simplified because the blood supply to the pelvis was already ligated, and the external iliac vessels have been elevated with a vein retractor. The obturator nerve and obturator muscle should be thoroughly cleaned by sharp dissection. The distal ends of the obturator vessels are ligated or occluded with vascular clips (Fig. 32–30A) at a point before they slip through the obturator foramen. Occasionally, anomalous obturator vessels enter the distal portion of the fossa

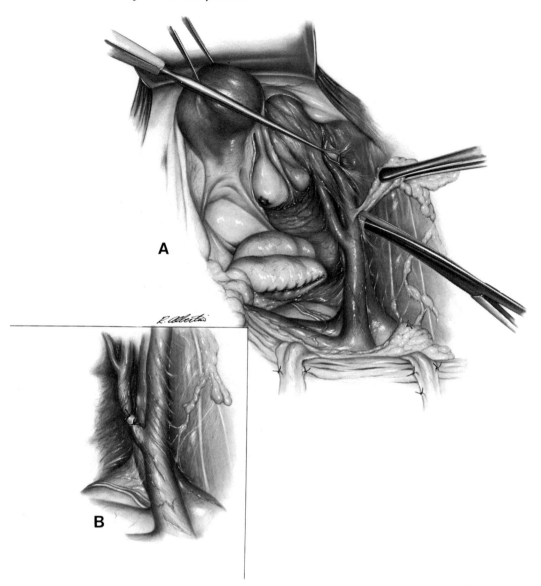

R. Alberti

FIG. 32–29 Pelvic exenteration (*continued*). Lymphatic dissection along the external iliac vessels with clamping (*A*) and ligation (*B*) of the hypogastric vessels.

from the inferior epigastric vessels. The upper portions of the sciatic nerve roots are also visible during this part of the procedure and must not be traumatized.

Deep Pelvic Dissection

The base of the broad ligament is excised at the lateral pelvic wall by placing one jaw of the Wertheim clamp in the paravesical space and the other in the pararectal space. Most of the parametrium down to the levator muscles and pelvic floor is included in the excision.

Since the major pelvic vessels were previously ligated, the rectum may be dissected bluntly from the anterior surface of the sacrum. Using strong forward traction on the rectum and uterus, one hand is inserted behind the rectum to provide support and avoid trauma to the sacral vessels (Fig. 32–31). The pararectal stalks blend with the lateral parametrial tissue and anchor the rectum and uterus to the posterolateral pelvic wall. Large Wertheim clamps are utilized to remove the parametrial tissue as close to the pelvic wall as possible (Fig. 32–31A). The distal portion of the hypogastric

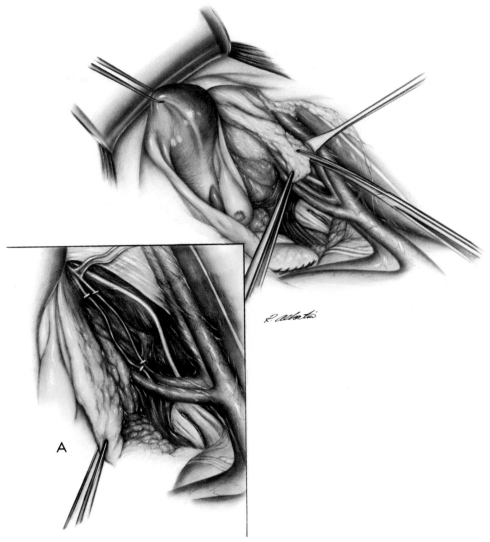

FIG. 32-30 Pelvic exenteration (*continued*). Dissection of the obturator fossa. (*Insert A*) Cleaned obturator fossa with obturator nerve retracted from the underlying obturator muscle. The obturator artery and vein are clamped and cut as they enter the obturator foramen.

vessel is included in the successive pararectal and parametrial clamps that completely free the specimen from the lateral pelvic wall.

The bladder and urethra are dissected from their subpubic attachments by both sharp and blunt dissection. Every available centimeter of bladder peritoneum is preserved, to be utilized later in the construction of a peritoneal hammock that will close the pelvic inlet from the abdominal cavity. The entire surgical specimen should be retracted cephalad to facilitate the subpubic and paravaginal dissection.

To complete the deep pelvic dissection, the rectum is retracted forward and the adherent areolar tissue is excised from the lower sacrum and coccyx (Fig. 32–32). Brisk bleeding may occur from the anterior sacral plexus of veins if each vessel is not controlled with vascular hemoclips when encountered. A pressure pack may be used for traumatized vessels.

The entire en bloc procedure can be accomplished by the abdominal route, but it is frequently easier and more expedient to use the combined abdominal-perineal approach. The separate perineal dissection is particularly useful if an effort is to be made to preserve the outer one-third of the vagina. While one surgical team is completing the deep pelvic dis-

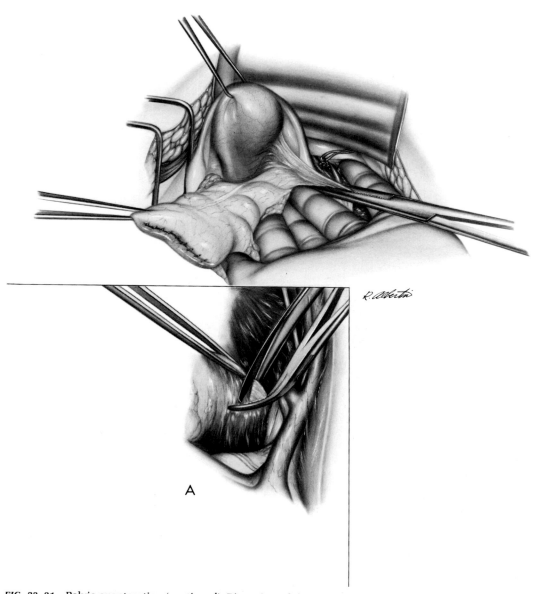

R. albertin

A

FIG. 32–31 Pelvic exenteration (*continued*). Dissection of the rectum from the anterior surface of the sacrum. (*Insert A*) Use of Wertheim clamp in excising pararectal tissue close to the pelvic wall.

section, another team incises all around the outer one-third of the vagina (Fig. 32–32A), and then the vaginal vessels on both sides are ligated.

The outer one-third of the urethra is transected, and the paraurethral vessels are secured. The paravaginal tissues are clamped and excised at the lateral pelvic wall, then the adjacent fascia and the areolar tissue are removed until the levator ani muscles are visible. At this point the vaginal dissection should communicate with the pelvic cavity, and the sur-

gical specimen is completely free except for the anal attachment.

The anus is circumscribed and closed by a continuous inverting suture so that the pelvic cavity will not be contaminated with fecal material. Next, the inferior hemorrhoidal vessels are ligated (Fig. 32–32B), and the rectum is separated from the fibers of the puborectalis portion of the levator ani muscle. Sharp-scissor dissection of the pararectal and presacral fascia completes the procedure.

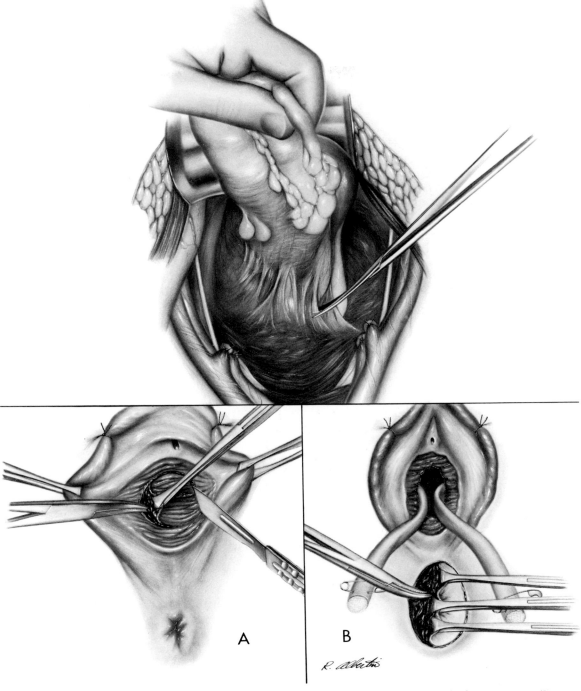

FIG. 32–32 Pelvic exenteration (*continued*). Completion of dissection of the sigmoid from the lower sacrum. (*Inserts A,B*). Vaginal and anal dissection from below done by a second team.

The entire surgical specimen is removed through the vaginal incision. The anal space is obliterated by approximation of the levator muscles in the midline, and the perineal skin is closed with a No. 3-0 delayed-absorbable subcuticular suture. A continuous locking No. 2-0 delayed-absorbable suture is placed along the excised vaginal mucosa for hemostasis, and two cigarette drains are placed in the pelvis (Fig. 32–33).

Closure of the Pelvic Peritoneum

Following a total exenteration, the pelvis is devoid of all structures except the levator ani and obturator muscles, the obturator nerve coursing across the obturator fossa, and the roots of the sciatic nerve. Vaginal drains are placed on either side of the pelvis and anchored with No. 3-0 absorbable sutures. Should there be persistent venous oozing at the time of closure, gauze packs are placed against the raw pelvis to be removed through the vagina within 48 to 72 hours. The vaginal drains remain in place until the perineal drainage has subsided, usually between the 7th and 10th days after surgery. Secondary drainage can be accomplished with large polyethylene catheters (Jackson–Pratt drains) placed through bilateral stab-wound incisions and connected to suction.

The raw pelvis should be separated from the abdominal cavity. Performing the additional step of closing the pelvic peritoneum over the operative site will decrease the incidence of postoperative intestinal obstruction significantly. Another benefit of peritoneal closure is that postoperative pelvic cellulitis is excluded from the peritoneal cavity, so the risk of peritonitis is greatly diminished. The preserved bladder peritoneum is used along with the

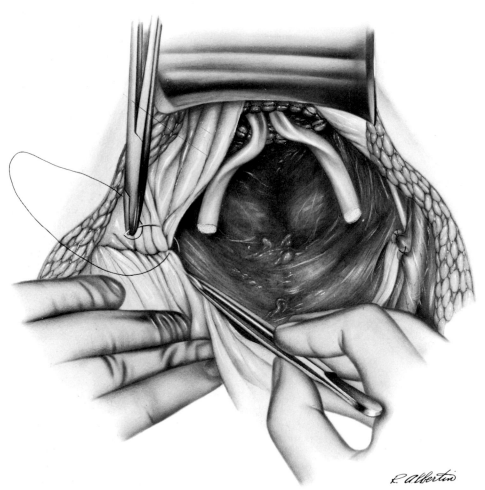

FIG. 32–33 Pelvic exenteration (*continued*). Drainage of the denuded pelvis and closure of the peritoneum.

parietal peritoneum from the anterior and lateral abdominal walls so that the pelvis can be completely closed from the abdominal cavity along the pelvic brim.

The anterior peritoneum is approximated to the residual posterior peritoneum with a continuous No. 2-0 delayed-absorbable suture. Way makes a transverse abdominal incision to conserve the peritoneum of the anterior abdominal wall, a method he calls the peritoneal "sac" procedure. Tension on the posterior peritoneum adjacent to the ureters should be avoided, because it might jeopardize the ureteral anastomosis.

The effect of this peritoneal closure is to create a peritoneal hammock across the pelvic inlet, which will gradually stretch as the small bowel settles into the pelvis. A peritoneal barrier is created between the serosa of the bowel and the raw pelvis (Fig. 32–33).

If there is insufficient peritoneum to adequately cover the entire pelvis, the omentum may be used by making a "J" pedicle graft. An adequate length of omentum is excised from the inferior margin of the transverse colon, conserving the left gastroepiploic vessels. The pedicle graft is then sutured to the free margins of the parietal and visceral peritoneum over the pelvic floor. If the omentum has been heavily irradiated and is contracted so that not enough tissue is available, the remnants of the omentum may be used as a free graft, because a parasitic blood supply will be provided from the pelvic vasculature. Recently Trelford and colleagues have used fresh human amnion with success, suturing the chorionic surface to the levator muscles and retaining the glistening amniotic surface as an extension of the pelvic peritoneum.

Construction of Neovagina

Construction of a neovagina is frequently deferred until the patient has completely healed and drainage from the pelvis through the perineum has stopped. Vaginal reconstruction is an important part of the total reconstructive procedure and should be included in the postoperative planning and completed within 6 months of the initial surgery. If the procedure has not been planned, the surgeon and the patient may disregard coital function out of concern for curing the disease.

Different methods have been used for rebuilding the vagina. One good approach is a modification of the Williams labial fusion technique, and another method, the McIndoe procedure, uses a split-thickness skin graft (see Chapter 15). Another alternative, the gracilis myocutaneous graft, requires a lengthy operative procedure that may compromise the patient's recovery from the exenterative procedure.

Although attempts have been made to use segments of colon or small bowel transplanted to the vagina at the time of the original surgery, the method has not proven to be any better than the less complicated reconstructive methods that can be performed later in the patient's recovery.

The labial reconstruction procedure designed by Williams (see Chapter 15) is very successful for young patients. When a small segment of the outer vagina can be retained, additional depth can be created for the vagina. Older patients who have atrophic labia generally have more satisfactory results from the McIndoe procedure.

Construction of Intestinal Stoma

The sites for the urinary and fecal ostia, which have been selected by the stomatologist, are marked on the abdomen with sterile methylene blue before the patient is draped. The urinary conduit is brought through the abdominal wall in the right lower quadrant, midway between the umbilicus and the anterior superior iliac spines, where a flat skin surface is available for attachment of the prosthesis. If the transverse colon is used for the urinary conduit, it can be mobilized and located in the right lower quadrant. The sigmoid colostomy site is located in the left paraumbilical area, so that the inferior pole of the fecal ostium is separated from the level of the urinary ostium.

The abdominal wall is prepared by removing an oval segment, 2 cm to 3 cm in diameter, through its entire thickness. Skin, subcutaneous fat, and external oblique fascia must all be excised so the flow of urine from the conduit will not be obstructed (Fig. 32–34A). The urinary conduit is brought through the abdominal wall, and the serosa of the bowel is sutured to the fascia of the abdominal wall. The bowel mucosa is everted, creating a raised, "rose-bud" stoma, which projects at least 1 cm from the abdominal wall. The stoma is fashioned with interrupted sutures of No. 3-0 delayed-absorbable suture, which passes initially through the skin edge, then anchors the serosa and musculature of the adjacent bowel wall, and finally passes through the free margin of the bowel mucosa (Fig. 32–34B). When the sutures are tied, the mucosa is everted over the serosa of the bowel to produce a raised stoma that directs the urine away from the skin surface (Fig. 32–34C,D), greatly reducing the chance for stricture of the ostium. Application of the urinary stoma bag is also facilitated by the raised opening.

The fecal stream is diverted to the left abdominal wall in a similar manner. The free end of the sigmoid colon is brought through the abdominal wall to the skin, just lateral to the umbilicus. Both openings cannot be placed on the same plane in the

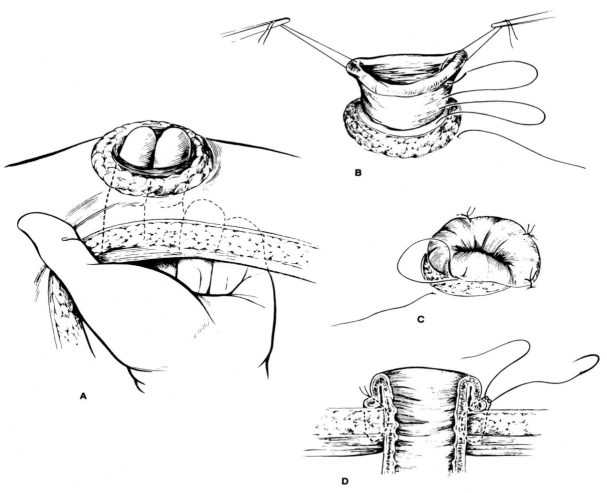

FIG. 32–34 Pelvic exenteration (*continued*). Technique for creating a bowel stoma that is elevated from the skin surface. This "rosebud" stoma is developed by (*A*) excising a wide segment of abdominal wall, (*B*) anchoring the skin margin with the adjacent wall of the exteriorized bowel, and (*C*) approximating the mucosal edge of the bowel to the skin. (*D*) The cross-sectional view demonstrates how the bowel wall is anchored to the skin margin to prevent retraction.

lower abdomen because the urinary prosthesis belt will interfere with the colostomy stoma. If anatomically feasible, the colostomy bud should be placed below the beltline for cosmetic purposes.

The serosa of both the urinary conduit and the sigmoid colostomy should be sutured to the lateral parietal peritoneum to avoid leaving peritoneal pockets for possible herniation and obstruction of bowel. Stay sutures have been omitted in recent years because they interfere with the placement of the fecal and urinary ostia. The external sutures become secondarily infected and produce necrosis of the underlying skin. In place of stay sutures, the far-near, near-far technique should be used for closing the rectus fascia and muscle. The newer method provides a stronger suture line and is based on the same surgical principles as the exterior stay sutures. If a patient is obese, a small drain should be placed at the base of the subcutaneous fat to decrease the incidence of wound infection.

ANTERIOR PELVIC EXENTERATION

When the rectum is found to be free of disease at the time of exploration and dissects easily from the vagina, an anterior pelvic exenteration is used for the treatment of radioresistant cervical carcinoma. In leaving the rectum intact in such cases and removing the remainder of the pelvic organs (uterus, vagina, and bladder), one must accept the possibility of residual tumor in small lymphatic channels in the rectal wall as well as the risk of compromising the blood supply of the rectum during the operative procedure.

The operative procedure is identical to that described for total exenteration, with the exception that the terminal ileum is used for the urinary conduit. This procedure, as introduced by Bricker, utilizes a mucosa-to-mucosa anastomosis of the ureter to the ileum following a double-layer closure of the blind end of the ileal pouch, as illustrated in Figure 32–28.

The arguments for performing a pelvic lymph node dissection are similar to those described for the total exenteration procedure. However, the hypogastric vessels are usually not sacrificed in the anterior procedure, because an effort is made to maintain the blood supply to the middle and inferior hemorrhoidal vessels while the distal portion of the anterior division of the hypogastric artery is ligated. Dissection of the parametrium is achieved by development of the paravesical and pararectal spaces including all the paracervical tissues to the lateral pelvic wall.

The uterosacral ligaments are ligated as far posteriorly as possible after mobilization of the rectum from the rectovaginal fascia by both sharp and blunt dissection. Removal of the bladder and vagina is accomplished as previously described, with preservation of as much of the bladder peritoneum as possible. The major problem at this point is the control of bleeding from the paravesical plexus of veins at the base of the bladder. If bleeding is excessive, hemoclips and firm packing usually are effective in producing hemostasis, during which time the dissection is continued on the opposite side. Peritonealization and drainage through the vagina are accomplished as previously described, and the ileal conduit is brought through the right lower abdominal wall, midway between the umbilicus and the anterior superior iliac spine. The serosa of the conduit is carefully sutured to the posterior abdominal peritoneum above the pelvic brim to avoid displacement of the conduit and tension on the ureteral anastomosis.

Although anterior pelvic exenteration is being replaced by total exenteration for recurrent cervical carcinoma, it is frequently indicated in vulvar, vaginal, or urethral carcinoma where the disease has extended to the anterior vaginal wall with involvement of the vesicovaginal septum.

COMPLICATIONS OF PELVIC EXENTERATION

The major complications following exenterative procedures are related primarily to the urinary tract and bowel. The problem of urinary tract fistulas at the site of the ureterointestinal anastomosis continues to plague the pelvic surgeon and occurs most frequently following megavoltage pelvic irradiation. Occasionally, the ureteral anastomosis fails to heal or the wall of the urinary conduit becomes involved in an area of pelvic cellulitis, with subsequent fistula formation. Rutledge has experienced a 4.5% incidence of urinary fistula among 296 patients who underwent an exenterative procedure. In the absence of ureteral obstruction, surgical correction of such fistulas should be delayed until the inflammatory reaction of the conduit and adjacent tissues has subsided, preferably in 6 to 8 weeks or longer. If stenosis of the ureter has occurred with resultant diminished renal function, as demonstrated by intravenous pyelogram and elevated serum creatinine levels, immediate repair is necessary.

Intestinal obstruction continues to be a serious problem, particularly when complete peritonization of the pelvis is not accomplished. Since the blood supply to the bowel has been impaired from previous irradiation, any additional ischemia due to adhesion formation may cause the late occurrence of either partial or complete obstruction or the development of an ileovaginal fistula. Obstruction was the most frequent serious complication (11%) in Bricker's vast experience with 207 exenterations for postirradiation carcinoma of the cervix. Of 26 patients in whom intestinal obstruction occurred, 6 (25%) died postoperatively. Bowel fistula occurred in 12.6% and obstruction in 11.6% of 198 exenterations at the Mayo Clinic, while other clinics report an incidence of 10% to 15% for similar bowel complications. Among 92 patients treated with pelvic exenteration from 1966 to 1981, Averette and colleagues experienced a 16.3% incidence of gastrointestinal fistula and a 40% operative mortality with surgical correction of the fistula. Ninety-three percent of these patients had received previous irradiation. Bowel complications have not been a major clinical problem in our own clinic, occurring in less than 5% of cases, which we feel is due to a determined effort to obtain a complete peritoneal closure of the denuded operative site. When this cannot be achieved, the remainder of the pelvis is covered by an omental graft that is brought into the pelvis along the left side of the abdominal cavity.

Way has emphasized the use of a transverse abdominal incision for pelvic exenteration in order that the anterior and posterior peritoneum can be preserved for transverse closure as an omental sac. Morley has found that a pedicle peritoneal graft of the anterior abdominal wall is useful in covering the peritoneal defect over the raw operative site and pelvic floor. We have found this technique to be useful, although closure of the abdominal incision is somewhat more difficult because of a large deficiency of peritoneum in the anterior abdominal wall.

Patients who developed an enterovaginal fistula formerly had a high mortality rate (25% to 40%) due to secondary metabolic problems. Efforts to perform an early small bowel resection along with an end-to-end and small bowel anastomosis were fraught with failure of healing of the anastomosis and recurrence of the bowel fistula. Currently, we use a bypass procedure for such cases with creation of a mucous fistula of the isolated segment of the small bowel as discussed in Chapter 19. This has reversed this potential lethal complication and eliminated the problem of nutritional deficiency as a cause of postoperative demise.

Septicemia and death resulting from resistant bacteria are serious dangers following exenteration, and intensive antibiotic therapy is frequently required. The incidence of septicemia has been reduced greatly by the prophylactic use of broad-spectrum antibiotics, which are started 24 hours prior to surgery in order to achieve an adequate tissue level at the time of surgery.

Thromboembolic disease has become a less serious problem as a result of the use of low-dose heparin, 5000 units being given subcutaneously 2 hours before surgery and at 8-hour intervals until the patient is fully ambulatory. The introduction of sequential pneumatic calf and thigh compression prior to, during, and after the surgical procedure has greatly reduced the incidence of venous thrombosis and pulmonary embolus, and it may be used in place of low-dose heparin.

The operative mortality from pelvic exenteration for recurrent carcinoma of the cervix has improved in the past decade and currently varies between 3% and 5%. In Brunschwig's original experience with total exenteration, which included 535 patients, the surgical mortality rate of 16% reflected his use of this procedure for palliative treatment in poor-risk patients. The procedure is now used only for surgical cure in carefully selected cases. An idea of the operative mortality and 5-year survival rates following pelvic exenteration in various clinics can be obtained by examining Table 32–10.

CURE RATES FOLLOWING PELVIC EXENTERATION

The total reported experience with pelvic exenteration in the English literature is less than 2500 cases. Based on the reported series to date on the treatment of radioresistant carcinoma of the cervix, the average 5-year survival rate is approximately 30% to 35% (Table 32–10).

SUMMARY

In patients with radioresistant carcinoma of the cervix, where the recurrent disease is confined to the cervix and the immediate adjacent parametrium, or has spread in an anteroposterior direction, the surgical procedure of choice is en bloc pelvic exenteration.

Because of the high incidence of urinary fistula

TABLE 32–10 *Surgical Mortality and 5-Year Survival Rates following Pelvic Exenteration*

STUDY (YEAR)	NUMBER OF PATIENTS	SURGICAL MORTALITY (PERCENT)	5-YEAR SURVIVAL (PERCENT)
Dargent (1957)	83	31.3	26.0
Smith (1963)	71	8.4	15.5
Parsons (1964)	112	14.2	21.4
Brunschwig (1965)	535	16.0	20.1
Rutledge (1965)	108	16.6	28.7
Kiselow (1967)	207* (54)†	7.8 (1.8)†	35.0
Symmonds (1968)	118	12.0	26.0
Ketcham (1970)	162‡	7.4	38.0
Brunschwig (1970)	225	8.0	19.3
Symmonds (1975)	198 (102)§	8.1 (3.0)§	33.0
Rutledge (1977)	296	13.3	48.3
Averette et al (1984)	92	24.0	37.0
Morley (1985)	100	2.0	54.7

* 1950–1965
† 1960–1965
‡ Includes 65 cases treated by primary exenteration
§ 1963–1971

formation, posterior exenteration has been largely abandoned in the treatment of patients with post-irradiation cervical carcinoma.

At the "court of last appeal," the clinical absence of gross tumor in the bladder or rectum should not deter the pelvic surgeon from a total exenteration since the surgical specimen may include residual tumor in the wall of adjacent viscera. The irradiated, ischemic bladder and rectum cannot be considered to be normal tissues and should generally be removed to ensure adequate tumor margins. However, if the rectum can be easily freed from the adjacent cervix and vagina, consideration should be given to an anterior exenteration.

Except in the most unusual circumstances, pelvic exenteration should be performed only in patients with histologically proven recurrent carcinoma. It should not be undertaken when such disease has spread beyond the pelvis. The operation has no place in palliative therapy and should be utilized only when the pelvic tumor is centrally confined and considered anatomically resectable, and where one would anticipate complete surgical control of the disease.

It is impossible to predict accurately the operability of a patient with recurrent cervical carcinoma following full irradiation therapy and resultant pelvic scarring. The inclusion of an exploratory laparotomy as a part of the tumor evaluation in patients who are candidates for a pelvic exenteration provides a definitive approach toward the use of radical surgery for an otherwise lethal disease.

The en bloc dissection is an effective, logical method of removal of radioresistant cervical carcinoma, and its acceptance by well-informed patients is excellent. Its success or failure in arresting the disease is a reflection of the proper selection of the surgical candidate by the pelvic surgeon. Consequently, the most important step in this procedure is to make certain by multiple frozen-section biopsies that the disease is confined to the pelvis and that the pelvic musculature is completely uninvolved prior to beginning the exenteration. Utilization of the avascular paravesical and pararectal anatomical spaces is helpful in the accurate evaluation of the location and extent of the neoplastic disease.

Advances in life-support mechanisms for serious physiologic and metabolic diseases have broadened the range of operative candidates for exenterative surgery and have significantly improved the operative mortality rates. Future progress will depend on continued refinements in the ability of the surgeon to detect the spread of occult tumor beyond the pelvis in order to avoid the needless effort of prolonged surgery and postoperative recovery for the majority of the cases that will ultimately succumb to the continued spread of the disease outside of the operative field.

Bibliography

CLASSIFICATION, HISTOPATHOLOGY, PROGNOSTIC FACTORS, AND TREATMENT

Abdulhayoglu G, Rich WM, Reynolds J, DiSaia PJ: Selective radiation therapy in Stage I-B uterine cervical carcinoma following radical pelvic surgery. Gynecol Oncol 10:84, 1980

Averette HE, Dudan RC, Ford JH: Exploratory celiotomy for surgical staging for cervical carcinoma. Am J Obstet Gynecol 113:1090, 1972

Averette HE, Lichtinger M, Savin M-U, et al: Pelvic exenteration: A 15-year experience in a general metropolitan hospital. Am J Obstet Gynecol 150:179, 1984

Barber HRK, Jones J: Lymphadenectomy in pelvic exenteration for recurrent cervix cancer. JAMA 215:1945, 1971

Barclay DA, Roman-Lopez JJ: Bladder dysfunction after Schauta hysterectomy. Am J Obstet Gynecol 123:519, 1975

Benson WL, Norris HJ: A critical review of the frequency of lymph node metastasis and death from microinvasive carcinoma of the cervix. Obstet Gynecol 49:632, 1977

Berek JS, Hacker NF, Fu Y-S, Sokale JR, et al: Adenocarcinoma of the uterine cervix: The influence of lesion size and grade on lymph node metastasis and prognosis. Obstet Gynecol 65:46, 1985

Berkeley C, Bonney V: The radical abdominal operation for carcinoma of the cervix uteri. Br Med J 2:445, 1916

Bohm JW, Krupp PJ, Lee FYL, et al: Lymph node metastasis in microinvasive epidermoid cancer of the cervix. Obstet Gynecol 48:65, 1976

Bonney V: Wertheim's operation in retrospect. Lancet 1:637, 1949

————: The results of 55 cases of Wertheim's operation for carcinoma of the cervix. J Obstet Gynaecol Br Comm 48:421, 1941

Boronow RC: Urologic complications secondary to radiation alone or radiation and surgery. In Delgado G, Smith NP (eds): Management of Complications in Gynecologic Oncology. New York, John Wiley & Sons, 1982

————: Stage I cervix cancer and pelvic node metastasis. Am J Obstet Gynecol 127:135, 1977

Boyce JG, Fruchter RG, Nicastri AD, et al: Vascular invasion in Stage I carcinoma of the cervix. Cancer 53:1175, 1984

————: Prognostic factors in Stage I carcinoma of the cervix. Gynecol Oncol 12:154, 1981

Bricker EM: Pelvic exenteration. In Longmire WP Jr (ed): Advances in Surgery. Chicago, Year Book Medical Publishers, 1970

————: The technique of ileal segment bladder substitution. In Meigs JV (ed): Progress in Gynecology, vol III. New York, Grune & Stratton, 1957

Bricker EM, Butcher HR Jr, Lawler WH Jr, et al: Surgical treatment of advanced and recurrent cancer of the pelvic viscera. Ann Surg 152:388, 1960

Broders AC: Grading of carcinoma. Minn Med 8:726, 1925

————: Carcinoma: Grading and practical application. Arch Pathol Lab Med 2:376, 1926

Brown RC, Buchsbaum HJ, Tewfik HH, et al: Accuracy of lymphangiography in the diagnosis of para-aortic lymph node metastases from carcinoma of the cervix. Obstet Gynecol 54:571, 1979

Brunschwig A: The surgical treatment of cancer of the cervix. Stage I & II. Am J Roentgenol 102:147, 1968

———: Radical vaginal operation (Schauta) for carcinoma of the cervix. Am J Obstet Gynecol 66:153, 1953

———: The surgical treatment of cancer of the cervix uteri. A radical operation for cancer of the cervix. Bull NY Acad Med 24:672, 1948

———: Complete excision of pelvic viscera for advanced carcinoma. Cancer 1:117, 1948

Buchler DA, Kline JC, Carr WF: Intracavitary dosimetry for carcinoma of the cervix and subsequent complications. Am J Obstet Gynecol 120:83, 1974

Buchler DA, Kline JC, Peckham BM, et al: The relationship of WSD to reactions and complications following treatment for malignant uterine cervical neoplasms. Radiology 110:687, 1974

Carenza L, Nobili F, Giacobini S: Voiding disorders after radical hysterectomy. Gynecol Oncol 13:213, 1982

Chung CK, Stryker JA, Ward SP, et al: Histologic grade and prognosis of carcinoma of the cervix. Obstet Gynecol 57:636, 1981

Clark JG: A more radical method of performing hysterectomy for cancer of the uterus. Johns Hopkins Bull, July, 1895

Clark WH Jr: The histogenesis and biologic behavior of primary human malignant melanoma of the skin. Cancer Res 29:705, 1969

Clarke-Pearson DL, Coleman RE, Synan IS, et al: Venous thromboembolism prophylaxis in gynecologic oncology: A prospective controlled trial of low dose heparin. Am J Obstet Gynecol 145:606, 1983

Clarke-Pearson DL, Jelovsek FR, Creasman WT: Thromboembolism complicating surgery for cervical and uterine malignancy: Incidence, risk factors, and prophylaxis. Obstet Gynecol 61:87, 1983

Cox EF, Ketcham AS, Villasanta U, et al: Patient evaluation for pelvic exenteration. Am Surg 30:574, 1964

Creasman WT, Rutledge F: Is positive pelvic lymphadenectomy a contraindication to radical surgery in recurrent cervical cancer? Gynecol Oncology 2:482, 1974

Davis JR, Moon LB: Increased incidence of adenocarcinoma of the uterine cervix. Obstet Gynecol 45:79, 1975

Deckers PJ, Ketcham AS, Sugerbaker EV, et al: Pelvic exenteration for primary carcinoma of the uterine cervix. Obstet Gynecol 37:647, 1971

Deckers PJ, Sugerbaker EV, Pilch YH, et al: Pelvic exenteration for late second cancers of the uterine cervix after earlier irradiation. Ann Surg 175:48, 1972

DeCosse JJ: Radiation injury to the intestinal tract. In Sabiston DC Jr (ed): Davis-Christopher Textbook of Surgery. Philadelphia, WB Saunders, 1972

———: The natural history and management of radiation into the gastrointestinal tract. Ann Surg 170:369, 1970

Delgado G: Stage I-B squamous cancer of the cervix: The choice of treatment. Obstet Gynecol Surv 31:17, 1978

Einhorn N: Frequency of severe complications after radiation therapy for cervical carcinoma. Acta Radiol Ther 14: 42, 1975

Everett HS: The effect of carcinoma of the cervix and its treatment upon the urinary tract. Am J Obstet Gynecol 38: 889, 1939

Everett HS, Brack CB, Farber GJ: Further studies on the effect of irradiation therapy for carcinoma of the cervix upon the urinary tract. Am J Obstet Gynecol 58:908, 1949

FIGO Annual Report on the Results of Treatment in Carcinoma of the Uterus, Vagina, and Ovary, vol 16. Stockholm, Radiumhemmet, 1976

———: Annual Report on the Results of Treatment in Gynecologic Cancer, vol 18. Stockholm, Radiumhemmet, 1982

Fletcher RG: Clinical dose-response curves of human malignant epithelial tumours. Br J Radiol 46:1, 1973

Forney JP: The effects of radical hysterectomy on bladder physiology. Am J Obstet Gynecol 138:374, 1980

Freund WA: Method of complete removal of the uterus. Am J Obstet Gynecol 7:200, 1879

———: Eine neue Methode der Exstirpation des ganzen Uterus. Sammlung klin Vort, No. 133 (Gynakol 41:911) Leipzig, 1878

Gallup DG, Abell MR: Invasive adenocarcinoma of the uterine cervix. Obstet Gynecol 49:596, 1977

Gallup DG, Harper RH, Stock RJ: Poor prognosis in patients with adenosquamous cell carcinoma of the cervix. Obstet Gynecol 65:1985

Glucksmann A, Cherry CP: Incidence, histology and response to radiation of mixed carcinomas (adenoacanthomas of the uterine cervix). Cancer 9:971, 1956

Green TH Jr, Meigs JV, Ulfelder H, et al: Urologic complications of radical Wertheim hysterectomy: Incidence, etiology, management and prevention. Obstet Gynecol 33:1269, 1974

———: Urologic complications of radical Wertheim hysterectomy: Incidence, etiology, management and prevention. Obstet Gynecol 20:293, 1962

Greiss FC, Blake DD, Lock FR: Complications of intensive radiation therapy for cervical carcinoma. Obstet Gynecol 18:417, 1961

Henriksen E: Distribution of metastases in Stage I carcinoma of the cervix: A study of 66 autopsied cases. Am J Obstet Gynecol 80:919, 1960

———: The lymphatic spread of carcinoma of the cervix and the body of the uterus. Am J Obstet Gynecol 58:924, 1949

Hilaris BS (ed): Afterloading: 20 Years of Experience, 1955–1975. New York, Memorial Sloan-Kettering Cancer Center, 1975

Hilgers RD: Pelvic exenteration for vaginal embryonal rhabdomyosarcoma. Obstet Gynecol 45(2):175, 1975

Hinselmann H: Zur Kenntnis der pracancerosen Veranderungen der Portio. Zbl Gynaekol 51:901, 1927

Inguilla W, Cosmi EV: Vesical, ureteral and rectal fistulas following operation for carcinoma of the cervix: Study of 1,000 consecutive cases. Am J Obstet Gynecol 99: 1078, 1967

Jampolis S, Andras EJ, Fletcher GH: Analysis of sites and causes of failures of irradiation in invasive squamous cell carcinoma of the intact uterine cervix. Radiology 115:681, 1975

Julian CG, Daikoku NH, Gillespie A: Adenoepidermoid and adenosquamous carcinoma of the uterus. Am J Obstet Gynecol 128:106, 1977

Kadar N, Saliba N, Nelson JH: The frequency, causes, and prevention of severe urinary dysfunction after radical hysterectomy. Br J Obstet Gynecol 90:858, 1983

Kakkar VV, Corrigan TP, Fossard DP: Prevention of fatal postoperative pulmonary embolism by low dose heparin. Lancet 2:45, 1975

Ketcham AS, Deckers PJ, Sugerbaker EV, et al: Pelvic exenteration for carcinoma of the uterine cervix: A 15-year experience. Cancer 26:513, 1970

Kiselow M, Butcher HR Jr, Bricker EM: Results of the radical surgical treatment of advanced pelvic cancer: A 15-year survey. Ann Surg 166:428, 1967

Kolbenstvedt A: Lymphography in the diagnosis of metastases

from carcinoma of the uterine cervix Stages I and II. Acta Radiol 16:81, 1975

Kolbenstvedt A, Kolstad P: Pelvic lymph node dissection under preoperative lymphographic control. Gynecol Oncol 2:39, 1974

Kottmeier H: Complications of radiotherapy of carcinoma of the cervix. In Marcus SL, Marcus CC (eds): Advances in Obstetrics and Gynecology, vol 1, p 633. Baltimore, Williams & Wilkins, 1967

Leman MH Jr, Benson WL, Kurman RJ, et al: Microinvasive carcinoma of the cervix. Obstet Gynecol 48:571, 1976

Littman P, Clement PB, Henrickson B, et al: Glassy cell carcinoma of the cervix. Cancer 37:2238, 1976

Liu W, Meigs JV: Radical hysterectomy and pelvic lymphadenectomy. Am J Obstet Gynecol 69:1, 1955

McGraw TA: Cases of operations for cancer of the womb. Mich Med News 2:98, 1879

Marshall CM: The newer gynecology: Some of its surgical and anatomical implications. Am J Obstet Gynecol 65:783, 1953

Martzloff KH: Epidermoid carcinoma of cervix uteri: Histologic study to determine resemblance between biopsy specimens and parent tumor obtained by radical panhysterectomy. Am J Obstet Gynecol 87:578, 1928

————: Carcinoma of the cervix uteri: A pathological and clinical study with particular reference to the relative malignancy of the neoplastic process as indicated by the predominant type of cancer cell. Bull Johns Hopkins Hosp 34:141, 1923

Masterson JG: Radical surgery in early carcinoma of cervix. Am J Obstet Gynecol 87:601, 1963

Mattingly RF: Total pelvic exenteration. Clin Obstet Gynecol 8:705, 1965

Meigs JV: Radical hysterectomy with bilateral pelvic lymph node dissections. Report of 100 cases operated on 5 years or more. Am J Obstet Gynecol 62:854, 1951

————: The Wertheim operation for carcinoma of the cervix. Am J Obstet Gynecol 49:542, 1945

————: Carcinoma of the cervix: The Wertheim operation. Surg Gynecol Obstet 78:195, 1944

Meyer JE, Green TH Jr, Yatsuhashi M: Palliative urinary diversion in carcinoma of the cervix. Obstet Gynecol 55:95, 1980

Morley GW: Pelvic exenterative therapy and treatment of recurrent carcinoma of the cervix. Semin Oncol 9:331, 1982

Morley GW, Lindenauer SM: Pelvic exenterative therapy for gynecologic malignancy: An analysis of 70 cases. Cancer 38:581, 1976

————: Pelvic exenterative therapy for gynecologic malignancy. Cancer 38:589, 1976

————: Peritoneal graft in total pelvic exenteration. Am J Obstet Gynecol 110:696, 1971

Morley GW, Seski JC: Radical pelvic surgery versus radiation therapy for Stage I carcinoma of the cervix (exclusive of microcarcinoma). Am J Obstet Gynecol 126:785, 1976

Morrow CP: Is pelvic radiation beneficial in the postoperative management of Stage Ib, squamous cell carcinoma of the cervix with pelvic node metastasis treated by radical hysterectomy and pelvic lymphadenectomy? Gynecol Oncol 10:105, 1980

Navratil E: Vaginal surgery of cervical carcinoma. Proc Am Cancer Soc, Munich, Springer-Verlag, 1968

Nelson AJ III, Fletcher GH, Wharton JT: Indications for adjunctive conservative extrafascial hysterectomy in selected cases of carcinoma of the uterine cervix. Am J Roentgenol Rad Ther Nucl Med 123:91, 1975

Nelson JH Jr, Macasaet MA: The incidence and significance of para-aortic lymph node metastases in late invasive carcinoma of the cervix. Am J Obstet Gynecol 118:749, 1974

Novak F: Gynakologische Operationstechnik. Piccin Editore-Padova, Berlin, Heidelberg, New York, Springer-Verlag, 1978

————: Procedure for the reduction of the number of utero-vaginal fistulae after Wertheim's operation. Proc Roy Soc Med 56:881, 1963

O'Quinn AG, Fletcher GH, Wharton JT: Guideline for conservative hysterectomy after irradiation. Gynecol Oncol 9:68, 1980

Orr JW Jr, Shingleton HM, Hatch KD, et al: Urinary diversion in patients undergoing pelvic exenteration. Am J Obstet Gynecol 142:883, 1982

Parry–Jones E: Lymphatics of the vulva. J Obstet Gynecol Br Comm 70:751, 1963

Parsons L: Pelvic exenteration. Clin Obstet Gynecol 2:1151, 1959

Paunier JP, Delclos L, Fletcher GH: Causes, time of death, and sites of failure in squamous cell carcinoma of the uterine cervix on intact uterus. Radiology 88:555, 1967

Peham HV, Amreich J: Operative Gynecology. Philadelphia, JB Lippincott, 1934

Perez-Mesa C, Spjut HJ: Persistent postirradiation carcinoma of cervix uteri. Arch Pathol 75:462, 1963

Piver MS, Barlow JJ: Para-aortic lymphadenectomy in staging patients with advanced local cervical cancer. Obstet Gynecol 43:544, 1974

Piver MS, Chung WS: Prognostic significance of cervical lesions size and pelvic node metastases in cervical carcinoma. Obstet Gynecol 46:507, 1975

Piver MS, Rutledge F, Smith JP: Five classes of extended hysterectomy for women with cervical cancer. Obstet Gynecol 44:265, 1974

Rampone JF, Klem V, Kolstad P: Combined treatment of Stage IB carcinoma of the cervix. Obstet Gynecol 41:163, 1973

Reagan JW, Hamonic MS, Wentz WB: Analytical study of the cells in cervical squamous-cell cancer. Lab Invest 6:241, 1957

Reis E: Eine neue Operationsmethode des Uteruscarcinoms. Z Geburtshife Gynakol 32:266, 1895

Rutledge FN, Wharton J, Fletcher GH: Clinical studies with adjunctive surgery and irradiation therapy in the treatment of carcinoma of the cervix. Cancer 38:596, 1976

Rutledge FN, Galactos AE, Wharton JT, et al: Adenocarcinoma of the uterine cervix. Am J Obstet Gynecol 122:236, 1975

Rutledge FN, Smith JP, Wharton JT, et al: Pelvic exenteration: Analysis of 296 patients. Am J Obstet Gynecol 129:881, 1977

Sasaki H, Yoshida T, Noda K, et al: Urethral pressure profiles following radical hysterectomy. Obstet Gynecol 59:101, 1982

Schauta F: Die Operation des Gebarmutterkrebses mittels des Schuchardt'schen Paravaginalschnittes. Montasschr Z Geburtschif Gynakol 15:133, 1902

Schellhas HF: Extraperitoneal para-aortic node dissection through an upper abdominal incision. Obstet Gynecol 46:444, 1975

Schmitz RL, Schmitz HE, Smith CJ, et al: Details of pelvic exenteration evolved during an experience with 75 cases. Am J Obstet Gynecol 80:43, 1960

Sedlacek TV, Mangan CE, Giuntoli RL, et al: Exploratory celiotomy for cervical carcinoma: The role of histologic grading. Gynecol Oncol 6:138, 1978

Shingleton HM, Gore H, Bradley DH, et al: Adenocarcinoma of the cervix I. Clinical evaluation and pathologic features. Am J Obstet Gynecol 139:799, 1981

Shingleton HM, Orr JW Jr: Cancer of the cervix. New York, Churchill Livingstone, 1983

Smith PH, Ballantyne B: Neuroanatomical basis for denervation of the urinary bladder following major pelvic surgery. Br J Surg 55:929, 1968

Spratt JS, Butcher HR, Bricker EM: Exenterative surgery of the pelvis, vol XII. In Dunphy JE (ed): Major Problems in Clinical Surgery. Philadelphia, WB Saunders, 1973

Stallworthy J: Pelvic cancer priorities. Am J Obstet Gynecol 126:777, 1976

Surveillance, Epidemiology and End Results: Incidence and mortality data 1973–1977. Prepared by Demographic Analysis Section, Division of Cancer Cause and Prevention, National Cancer Institute. Edited by JL Young, Jr, CL Percy, AJ Asire. Bethesda, Md, National Cancer Institute, 1981

Swan RW, Rutledge FN: Urinary conduit in pelvic cancer patients: A report of 16 years' experience. Am J Obstet Gynecol 119:6, 1974

Symmonds RE, Pratt JH, Webb MJ: Exenterative operations: Experience with 198 patients. Am J Obstet Gynecol 121:907, 1975

Symmonds RE, Webb MJ: Pelvic exenteration. In Coppleson M (ed): Gynecologic Oncology: Fundamental Principles and Clinical Practice, p 896. Edinburgh, Churchill Livingstone, 1981

Tod MC, Meredith WJ: Dosage system for use in treatment of cancer of the uterine cervix. Br J Radiol 11:809, 1938

Trelford–Sauder M, Trelford JD, Matolo NM: Replacement of the peritoneum with amnion following pelvic exenteration. Surg Gynecol Obstet 145:699, 1977

Underwood PB, Lutz MH, Smoak DL: Ureteral injury following irradiation therapy for carcinoma of the cervix. Obstet Gynecol 49:663, 1977

Van Bouwdijk-Bastiaanse MA: Vaginal hysterectomy, with special regard to use in cancer. Ned Tijdschr Geneskd 93:2132, 1949

van Nagell JR, Donaldson ES, Parker JC, et al: The prognostic significance of cell type and lesion size in patients with cervical cancer treated by radical surgery. Gynecol Oncol 5:142, 1977

van Nagell JR, Donaldson E, Wood E, et al: The significance of vascular invasion and lymphocytic infiltration in invasive cervical cancer. Cancer 41:228, 1978

van Nagell JR, Schiwietz DP: Surgical adjuncts in radical hysterectomy and pelvic lymphadenectomy. Surg Gynecol Obstet 143:735, 1976

Villasanta U: Complications of radiotherapy for carcinoma of the uterine cervix. Am J Obstet Gynecol 114:717, 1972

Watring WG, Lagasee LD, Smith ML, et al: Vaginal reconstruction following extensive treatment for pelvic cancer. Am J Obstet Gynecol 125:809, 1976

Way S: The use of the "sac" technique in pelvic exenteration. Gynecol Oncol 2:476, 1974

Webb MJ, Symmonds RE: Radical hysterectomy: A reappraisal. Obstet Gynecol 54:140, 1979

Weiner S, Wizenberg MJ: Treatment of primary adenocarcinoma of the cervix. Cancer 35:1514, 1975

Wertheim E: The extended abdominal operation for carcinoma uteri. Translated by H Grad. Am J Obstet Gynecol 66:169, 1912

———: Die erweiterte abdominale Operation bei Carcinoma Colli Uteri (Auf Grund von 500 Fallen). Berlin, Urban, 1911

———: Discussion on the diagnosis of treatment of carcinoma of the uterus. Br Med J 2:689, 1905

———: Zur Frage der Radikaloperation beim Uteruskrebs. Arch Gynakol 61:627, 1900

Wheeless CR: Small bowel bypass for complications related to pelvic malignancy. Obstet Gynecol 42:661, 1973

Wheeless CR Jr, Graham R, Graham JB: Prognosis and treatment of adenoepidermoid carcinoma of the cervix. Obstet Gynecol 35:928, 1970

CARCINOMA OF THE CERVIX IN PREGNANCY

Bosch A, Marcial VA: Carcinoma of the uterine cervix associated with pregnancy. Am J Roentgenol Rad Ther Nucl Med 96:92, 1966

Hacker NF, Berek JS, Lagasse LD: Carcinoma of the cervix associated with pregnancy. Obstet Gynecol 59(6):735, 1982

Kinch RA: Factors affecting the prognosis of cancer of the cervix in pregnancy. Am J Obstet Gynecol 82:45, 1971

Lee RB, Neglia W, Park RC: Cervical carcinoma in pregnancy. Obstet Gynecol 58:584, 1981

Mikuta JJ, Enterline HT, Braun TE Jr: Carcinoma in situ of the cervix associated with pregnancy. JAMA 204:763, 1968

Prem KA, Makowski EL, McKelvey JL: Carcinoma of the cervix with pregnancy. Am J Obstet Gynecol 95:99, 1966

Sall S, Rini S, Pineda A: Surgical management of invasive carcinoma of the cervix in pregnancy. Am J Obstet Gynecol 118:1, 1974

Thompson JD, Caputo TA, Franklin EW III, et al: The surgical management of invasive carcinoma of the cervix in pregnancy. Am J Obstet Gynecol 121:853, 1975

Chapter 33

Malignant Tumors of the Uterus

Endometrial carcinoma is the most common malignancy in the female reproductive tract, occurring in approximately 1 to 2 cases per 1000 postmenopausal women per year in the general population. This tumor is the fourth most common type of malignancy in the female, exceeded in frequency only by carcinoma of the breast, large bowel, and lung.

Although the third National Cancer Survey in the United States in 1969 and 1970 as reported by Cramer and colleagues showed no evidence of an increase in the incidence of endometrial cancer from the time of the previous survey in 1947, there was a consistent increase in the incidence between 1970 and 1975, as shown by case studies from the Connecticut Tumor Registry (Fig. 33–1), followed by a gradual decline since that time. Data collected by Walker and Jick from hospital discharge summaries in the United States show that between 1970 and 1975, the incidence of endometrial carcinoma in women aged 50 to 59 increased by 85%, from 72 to 133 cases per 100,000 women-years. From 1975 to 1979, the rates declined in this age group, returning to the starting level of 72 per 100,000 women-years in 1979. In the same period, among women aged 60 to 69 years of age, there was an 83% increase in the incidence of endometrial cancer, from 82 to 150 cases per 100,000 women-years. After the age of 70, the risk increased by 83%, from an incidence of 45 cases per 100,000 women-years in 1970 to a peak in 1978 of 83 cases per 100,000 women-years. Premenopausal women between the ages of 25 and 44 years showed no particular increased risk, and the incidence was low: 5 cases or less per 100,000 women.

The increased prominence of endometrial cancer is the result of several factors, including the decrease in the incidence of invasive cervical carcinoma, the increase in average female life expectancy, and the increase in clinical ability to detect endometrial cancer at an early stage. Women have become more aware of the risk of uterine cancer and continue to seek medical care during the postmenopausal years. There is also a strong possibility that increased estrogen use among postmenopausal women has contributed to the increased incidence of endometrial cancer.

Clinical Conditions Associated with Endometrial Cancer

OBESITY

Obesity is the risk factor most commonly associated with endometrial carcinoma. Onsrud and associates showed that the prognosis in patients with endometrial cancer who were more than 30% above ideal weight was poorer than that in patients of normal weight. Whether obesity is an associative or an etiologic factor is the subject of continued study. One theory is that circulating androgens at extraglandular sites, principally in fatty tissue, are converted to estrone, which, in turn, creates a milieu favorable to the formation of endometrial carcinoma.

MacDonald and Siiteri studied 38 premenopausal and 38 postmenopausal women whose body weights ranged from 89 to 430 pounds. They found that the metabolic rate at which androstenedione was converted to estrone increased directly with the weight of the patients. In a series of patients with endometrial cancer reported by Kottmeier, 29% weighed over 180 pounds; another 7% weighed

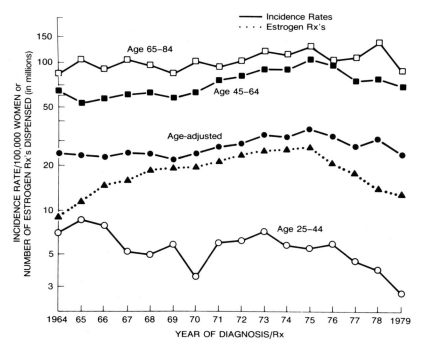

FIG. 33-1 Annual age-adjusted (1970 standard population) and age-specific incidence rates for localized cancer of the uterine corpus, corrected for hysterectomized women in Connecticut, and annual numbers of noncontraceptive oral estrogen prescriptions dispensed in the United States, 1964–1979. (Marrett LD, Meigs JW, Flannery JT: Trends in the incidence of cancer of the corpus uteri in Connecticut, 1964–1979, in relation to consumption of exogenous estrogens. Am J Epidemiol 116:62, 1982)

over 220 pounds. In Peterson's series, a total of 81% weighed over 150 pounds, while 63% of the group weighed over 200 pounds. Wynder concluded that in women 21 to 50 pounds overweight, the risk of endometrial carcinoma is increased threefold; in women 50 pounds or more over ideal weight, the risk is nine times greater than in women of normal weight. Obesity is also associated with an increase in the serum level of free, unbound estrogen because the levels of sex-hormone–binding globulin, which inactivates the estrogen molecule, are decreased.

Obese patients have a higher risk of developing other metabolic disorders, including diabetes, hypertension, and arteriosclerotic heart disease. Endometrial cancer is often associated with these metabolic derangements, which makes management all the more difficult. Obese patients with endometrial carcinoma die more often from an intercurrent disease than do patients of normal weight.

DIABETES MELLITUS

Several investigators have addressed the question of whether or not an altered carbohydrate metabolism affects or is affected by endometrial carcinoma. Most of the reports are retrospective surveys of hospital records, which provide poor data for critical evaluation. Only a few well-controlled studies have been made.

After reviewing reports linking endometrial carcinoma with altered carbohydrate metabolism and finding them inconclusive, Dunn and coworkers conducted one of the earliest controlled studies using oral glucose tolerance tests, taking the age and weight of patients into consideration. Although patients with endometrial cancer had significantly less tolerance to the glucose test than did normal women, the data did not show a relationship between altered metabolism of carbohydrates and endometrial carcinoma. Dunn estimated that 7.7% of the patients with endometrial cancer were also diabetic, an incidence similar to that for a random sample of women of the same age without cancer. Fox and Sen were also unable to show any statistically significant increase in diabetes among endometrial cancer cases.

An increased incidence of abnormal glucose tolerance has been found among women with endometrial cancer by many researchers. Kaplan and Cole reported the risk of abnormal glucose tolerance to be 2.4 times higher in the presence of this disease. Nevertheless, it has not been convincingly demonstrated that a true increase in the incidence of insulin-dependent diabetes is associated with endometrial cancer.

HYPERTENSION

It was claimed that a relationship existed between hypertension and endometrial cancer until Wynder and Dunn correlated blood pressure with body weight. Using a controlled comparison, these researchers found no statistical difference between the incidence of hypertension in patients with endometrial carcinoma and that in women without cancer.

OTHER FACTORS

Antunes and associates have provided some of the most useful information on risk factors for patients with endometrial cancer. In their study, 179 patients with endometrial cancer were compared with 155 hospitalized controls. Among all the factors studied, only excess weight, late menopause, and estrogen use were found to be associated with a statistically significant increase in the risk of this disease. Their findings showed that, compared to controls, patients with excess weight had a 2.4 times greater risk; those with a late menopause, a 2.5 times greater risk; and those using estrogen, an 8.6 times greater risk of endometrial carcinoma.

The three conditions that continue to be reported in connection with endometrial cancer also occur at approximately the same rate in women without cancer who are in the same age group. Although dubbed "the corpus cancer syndrome," the triad of obesity, diabetes mellitus, and hypertension could more appropriately be called "the postmenopausal syndrome."

Association of Estrogen with Endometrial Cancer

As early as 1936, Novak and other medical pioneers noted that women with estrogen excess or estrogen stimulation often developed endometrial adenocarcinoma. Since that time the relationship of endometrial cancer to estrogen use has been a subject of debate. Nulliparous patients treated for infertility, patients with advanced metabolic disease or delayed menopause, and patients with ovarian tumors that secrete estrogen, such as polycystic ovaries and granulosa and theca cell tumors, all have a common endocrine dysfunction, namely, anovulation and unopposed estrogen stimulation of the endometrium.

The work of several investigators supports the hypothesis that there is an association between estrogen use and the development of endometrial carcinoma. However, a direct relationship has still not been proven. There have been many epidemiologic studies designed to investigate the hypothesis of the association between endometrial cancer and estrogen use. Most were retrospective

case–control studies and one was a cohort, prospective investigation. As shown in Table 33–1, the relative risk of endometrial cancer in women using exogenous estrogen replacement was between 2.0 and 8.0 times the risk for control patients who did not use estrogen. Among the estrogen users included in these studies, the proportion using estrogens at the time of diagnosis varied between 2% and 89%. Estrogen use among controls was statistically less, as noted in the relative risk for each group of cases. As emphasized by Walker and Jick, the nationwide decline in endometrial carcinoma since 1975, when estrogen sales in the United States declined substantially, provides supportive evidence for a causal association between endometrial cancer and replacement estrogen therapy.

Patients with primary ovarian failure have been singularly devoid of endometrial carcinoma. However, Ostor and others reported that patients with gonadal dysgenesis treated with nonsteroidal estrogens were at risk to develop endometrial carcinoma. In our own experience, one patient with gonadal dysgenesis who was treated continuously for 9 years with diethylstilbestrol (DES) developed a well-differentiated endometrial adenocarcinoma. As shown in Table 33–2, the estrogen replacement most commonly given to patients with gonadal dysgenesis who developed a well-differentiated adenocarcinoma or adenosquamous carcinoma was DES. It is important to note, however, that in 7 of the 14 reported cases, the patient was given other types of estrogen, indicating that a variety of estrogen compounds can produce neoplastic changes in the endometrium. The case reported by Rosenwaks and associates is important because the patient was treated regularly with medroxyprogesterone (Provera) for 10 days of each cycle along with conjugated estrogens. This combination did not prevent the development of adenocarcinoma. Other gonadal dysgenesis patients with endometrial carcinoma reported by Ostor and by Louka were also treated with progestins. Of all of the case–control studies reported, the strongest evidence to date for an association between long-term estrogen use and endometrial carcinoma rests with the estrogen-treated cases of gonadal dysgenesis. Little endogenous estrogen is available in patients with gonadal dysgenesis other than from the adrenal gland; therefore, estrogen use is difficult to exclude as a factor related to the pathogenesis of endometrial carcinoma. Yet, there are no controls in these cases, and, therefore, the cause-and-effect relationship is not secure.

The duration of hormonal use appears to be one of the most important factors in the development of adenocarcinoma. In the cases of gonadal dys-

TABLE 33-1 Risk of Endometrial Cancer with Estrogen Replacement Therapy

STUDY (YEAR)	PERIOD OF ESTROGEN USE	WOMEN WITH CANCER		CONTROLS WITHOUT CANCER	ODDS RATIO OR CALCULATED RELATIVE RISK
		Cases of cancer	Percent using estrogens	Percent using estrogens	
Jensen et al (1954)	1.5–15 yr	105	33	21	1.9
Wynder et al (1966)	Any use	112	2	4	0.6
Dunn, Bradley (1967)	Any use	56	29	28	1.0
Smith et al (1975)	>6 mo	317	48	17	7.5
Ziel, Finkel (1975)	>1 yr	94	57	15	7.6
Mack et al (1976)	Any use	63	89	50	8.0
McDonald et al (1976)	>6 mo	145	17	8	2.3
Gray et al (1977)	>3 mo	205	27	15	2.2
Horwitz, Feinstein (1978)	>6 mo	149	30	15	2.3

(Drill VA: Relationship of estrogens and oral contraceptives to endometrial cancer in animals and women. J. Reprod Med 24: 5, 1980)

genesis, adenocarcinoma developed after periods of estrogen use ranging from 4 to 20 years. Less than 5 years is required in women who are given regular estrogen replacement therapy in the menopausal or postmenopausal period.

There are many prospective clinical studies in which progestins were administered sequentially with the estrogen and where there was no evidence of an associated endometrial adenocarcinoma. In a study of the use of estrogen–progestin as a sequential oral contraceptive for periods of 10 to 14 years reported by Leis, no cases of endometrial carcinoma were found. In a 10-year prospective study by Nachtigall and associates, 84 institutionalized

TABLE 33-2 Endometrial Carcinoma in Patients with Gonadal Dysgenesis and Estrogen Replacement

STUDY (YEAR)	NUMBER OF PATIENTS	AGE AT DETECTION (YEARS)	KARYOTYPE	DURATION OF ESTROGEN USE (YEARS)		TOTAL DOSE (g)	TYPE OF CARCINOMA
				DES	Other		
Lewis et al (1963)	1	45	45, X/46, XY	—	—	—	Adeno
Dowsett (1963)	2	28	45, X	6	—	5	Adenosquamous
Scott (1963)	3	31	45, X	4	2	9	Adenosquamous
Canlorbe et al (1967)	4	32	45, X	6	3	3	Adeno
Cutler et al (1972)	5*	29	45, X	9	1	2.8	? Adenosquamous
	6	35	45, X/46, XY	20	0	5	Adenosquamous
	7†	35	46, XXqi§	17	1	6.2	? Adeno
Wilkinson et al (1963)	8	26	45, X	9	0	2.6	Adeno
Roberts and Wells (1975)	9*	28	45, X	4	0	1.5	? Adenosquamous
McCarroll et al (1975)	10‡	35	45, X	13	0	3.7	Adeno
Sirota et al (1975)	11	27	45, X	8	—	15	Adeno
Ostor et al (1978)	12	34	45, X/47, XXX	—	—	—	Adenosquamous
	13‡	27	45, X/46, XX	—	3	15 mg	Adeno
Louka et al (1978)	14	36	45, X	0	—	0.2	Adenosquamous
Rosenwaks et al (1979)	15‡	24	45, X	—	4.2	2.5	Adeno

* Uncertain if squamous component is malignant
† Uncertain about presence of true carcinoma
‡ Patient also treated with progesterone
§ Isochromosome for the long arm of X
(Ostor AG, Fortune DW, Evans JH, et al: Endometrial carcinoma in gonadal dysgenesis with and without estrogen therapy. Gynecol Oncol 6:316, 1978)

women were given high doses of conjugated estrogen plus medroxyprogesterone acetate while 84 control cases were treated with a placebo. The groups were matched carefully for age and associated disease after 10 years of hormone use. Among the postmenopausal women receiving the estrogen-progestin replacement therapy, there were no cases of endometrial carcinoma, although an estimated 3.8 cases of endometrial carcinoma should have developed. In these cases, the use of a progestin, as recommended by Gambrell and others, showed a definite protective benefit.

Since 1922, when Schroeder first described it, the association of endometrial cancer with estrogen-producing ovarian neoplasms has become more clinically evident. Estrogen-secreting granulosa cell and theca cell tumors of the ovary have been associated with endometrial carcinoma in incidences ranging from 3.5% to 27%. Most commonly, the association is found to be present in less than 5% of cases. If endometrial cancer is associated with these functioning ovarian tumors in approximately 3.5% of the cases—that is, if there are 35 cases of endometrial cancer per 1000 women with such ovarian tumors—the risk of endometrial cancer is 10 to 50 times greater for women with estrogen-producing ovarian neoplasms than for women with normal ovaries.

In 1971, Herbst and associates showed that there was an association between the use of nonsteroidal estrogens during the first trimester of pregnancy and the occurrence of adenocarcinoma in the vagina and cervix of female offspring (see Chapter 30). Studies by Silverberg and Makowski demonstrated that 11 of 21 young women with endometrial carcinoma had used sequential estrogen-progestin combinations as birth control pills. Because of these and similar studies by Lyon and others, this contraceptive agent was removed from the marketplace.

Knab summarized the reports on prolonged postmenopausal use of estrogen and emphasized that it was associated with an increased incidence of endometrial cancer. These studies, which are retrospective and not randomized, show that women taking estrogens for 1 to 5 years have a four to five times greater risk of developing endometrial cancer than untreated women. Women who take the hormones for 7 or more years have a 13 times greater risk. Silverberg estimates that a 55-year-old woman with a life expectancy of 20 years who receives estrogen therapy for all 20 years has a 3% chance of developing endometrial carcinoma, which is nearly 40 times the normal risk of this disease for a 75-year-old woman.

The risk of endometrial cancer is reduced if the lowest dosage of estrogen is used in an interrupted pattern. Most of the studies relate to the use of conjugated estrogens, but an increased risk occurs with any type of estrogen. In most reports, the endometrial cancer is well-differentiated, with many cases diagnosed as carcinoma in situ. In fact, part of the controversy occurs because some clinicians consider many of the lesions in question to be atypical endometrial hyperplasia, not invasive carcinoma. This potential detection bias was studied by Gordon and associates, who found that three pathologist reviewers agreed on the diagnosis of endometrial cancer in 66 (74%) of the original 89 cases reported by Ziel and Finkel while at least two reviewers agreed on 82 of the cases (92%).

In a 1981 study of 28 cases of endometrial carcinoma, Horowitz and associates found that three pathology reviewers concurred with the original diagnosis of adenocarcinoma in 82% of the cases reviewed. Most of the disagreements were about whether particular lesions should be designated as markedly atypical adenomatous hyperplasia or as grade 1 endometrial cancer. Therefore, there appears to be a relatively accurate diagnosis in these lesions in some 75% to 80% of the cases.

Although the evidence is not conclusive, the data suggest that prolonged use of estrogen can have a neoplastic effect on DNA metabolism in sensitive endometrial tissue. Even without conclusive evidence, the data provide a strong warning against high-dose and continuous estrogen therapy in high-risk patients. Low doses of estrogen should be given for the shortest time needed to provide symptomatic relief in patients who have an increased risk for the development of carcinoma of the endometrium. Although routine estrogen replacement therapy is practiced more commonly in recent years because of an increasing concern about the dangers of debilitating osteoporosis, an endometrial biopsy should always be obtained *before* therapy is begun to ensure that there is no existing occult atypia or adenocarcinoma.

Despite the many reports suggesting that the risk of endometrial carcinoma is significantly increased in postmenopausal women who are given replacement estrogen therapy, there are those who contend that this strong association is the result of detection bias. It is well known that estrogen replacement therapy can induce endometrial proliferation and that endometrial bleeding frequently results from proliferation. It is suggested that estrogen-induced proliferation and bleeding lead to the discovery of preexisting endometrial carcinomas, which may then erroneously be described as estrogen-related. Horowitz and Feinstein, two noted biostatisticians who are the major protagonists of this opposing theory, remain firm in their conviction that the estrogen genesis of endometrial carcinoma is, as yet, unproven.

In a prospective screening program of 2586 asymptomatic women aged 45 years or older, Koss and associates have attempted to answer the question of whether estrogen-induced proliferative bleeding leads to the early detection of endometrial carcinoma Endometrial biopsy failed to confirm that endometrial hyperplasia preceded adenocarcinoma. Furthermore, no significant association between estrogen medication and endometrial adenocarcinoma could be shown. These investigators conclude that endometrial cancer in postmenopausal women may develop as a focal event rather than from existing diffuse endometrial hyperplasia.

Clinical Staging of Endometrial Carcinoma

Since Kelly first discussed endometrial carcinoma in 1900, many attempts have been made to define and categorize the clinical stages of the lesions. The depth of myometrial involvement and the extension of the disease were considered, but additional criteria were needed for patients who could not undergo surgery.

The four-stage clinical classification used today was developed in 1958, revised by the FIGO Cancer Committee in 1961 and 1970, and adopted officially by the FIGO General Assembly in 1976.

The FIGO classification of the stage of the disease is based on a standard of uterine cavity length and the extension of the disease beyond the uterus and pelvis. Lesions that do not enlarge the size of the uterus (8 cm or less) are considered Stage Ia while lesions that result in enlargement of the uterine cavity to more than 8 cm are categorized as Stage Ib disease. It is presumed that the increase in uterine size to more than 8 cm is related to myometrial extension of tumor. Despite the FIGO classification, an accurate assessment of myometrial involvement should be made only by histologic study of the surgical specimen.

Factors Influencing Prognosis

Among malignancies of the female reproductive tract, endometrial carcinoma has one of the more favorable prognoses, mainly because approximately 75% of the cases are diagnosed as an early Stage I, and 75% of tumors are either well-differentiated (grade 1) or moderately differentiated (grade 2) le-

FIGO Classification of Endometrial Carcinoma

Classification	Description
Stage 0	Carcinoma in situ. Histologic findings suspicious of malignancy. (Cases of Stage 0 should not be included in statistics on invasive disease.)
Stage I	Carcinoma confined to the corpus including the isthmus
Ia	The length of the uterine cavity is 8 cm or less
Ib	The length of the uterine cavity is more than 8 cm
	Stage I cases should be subgrouped with regard to the histologic type of adenocarcinoma as follows:
	Grade 1 highly differentiated adenomatous carcinoma
	Grade 2 differentiated adenomatous carcinoma with partly solid areas
	Grade 3 predominantly solid or entirely undifferentiated carcinoma
Stage II	Carcinoma involving the corpus and cervix, but not extending outside the uterus
Stage III	Carcinoma extending outside the uterus, but not outside the true pelvis
Stage IV	Carcinoma extending outside the true pelvis or obviously involving the mucosa of the bladder or rectum. (Bullous edema alone does not permit a lesion to be considered Stage IV.)
IVa	Spread of the growth to adjacent organs
IVb	Spread to distant organs

sions. The important factors related to the prognosis of carcinoma of the uterine corpus have been confined to the following: age at the time of diagnosis; histologic grade of the tumor; tumor volume, including uterine size and depth of myometrial penetration; and the extent of the disease at the time of diagnosis, including involvement of the cervix or metastasis to pelvic and para-aortic lymph nodes.

AGE

Most patients with endometrial cancer are diagnosed between the ages of 55 and 60. As few as 2% to 5% of the cases occur in women under 40. As Speert, Dockerty and associates, Fechner and Kaufman, and others have documented, younger patients usually have a steroid-producing ovarian tumor or polycystic ovarian disease.

As many as 20% to 25% of the patients with endometrial cancer are diagnosed before menopause, and these patients have a more favorable prognosis than do postmenopausal patients. Bonham collected a 24-year follow-up study of 535 patients with endometrial carcinoma in New Zealand and found that of the survivors, 27.7% had been diagnosed before menopause. The group diagnosed before menopause had an 88.8% survival rate for more than 5 years. The postmenopausal patients had a lower survival rate, which continued to decline until it stabilized after 15 years at 58.3%. Jones suggests that the improved survival rates in younger patients is related to the early diagnosis of well-differentiated tumors without myometrial invasion.

Late menopause is a recognized risk factor among women who develop endometrial carcinoma. In an epidemiologic study by Kaplan and Cole, the relative risk was 2.4 times greater among women with a menopause delayed until after the age of 52 than among women in whom menopause occurred before the age of 49. Patients in the perimenopausal age group frequently assume that irregular bleeding is physiologic, which delays the diagnosis and treatment of this disease.

HISTOLOGIC TYPE

Although adenocarcinoma with or without benign squamous components represents approximately 80% to 90% of all endometrial carcinomas, there are other less common epithelial malignancies involving the endometrium. As shown in Table 33–3, *adenosquamous carcinoma* has been noted more commonly as a part of this disease in recent years. In our experience, this type comprises less than 10% of all cases of endometrial carcinoma and represents a mixed tumor of glandular and squamous carcinoma. Originally, this tumor was considered to be a highly virulent tumor that metastasized rapidly. Salazar and associates conducted a clinicopathologic study of this tumor by comparing the clinical behavior and cure rates of 87 patients with mixed adenosquamous carcinoma with those of 260 patients with pure adenocarcinoma and 29 patients with *adenoacanthoma*. As shown by this study, the prognosis is now considered to be similar on a stage-for-stage basis to that of a pure adenocarcinoma. Historically, many gynecologists and pathologists have considered the degree of malignancy of adenosquamous carcinoma to be comparable to that of a poorly differentiated (grade 3) adenocarcinoma. Adenosquamous carcinoma occurs in an older age group than adenocarcinoma and is more frequently associated with a poorly differentiated glandular component. Based on these characteristics, it has historically been considered to carry a poorer prognosis. These beliefs have been challenged by the Salazar group. In their study, they found that there was no basic difference in incidence, clinical history, response to irradiation therapy, or prognosis between adenosquamous carcinoma, adenoacanthoma, and pure adenocarcinoma. These findings are not shared by Boronow and his colleagues in the Gynecologic Oncology Group, who had a different experience among 21 patients with adenosquamous carcinoma. Among this group, three patients (14%) had pelvic node metastases, and five patients (23.8%) had aortic node metastases. The clinical behavior of this tumor was similar to a grade 3 lesion or a tumor with deep myometrial invasion. In general, the FIGO grading system is used for tumors in which the differentiation of the glandular component is the criterion upon which the grading system is based.

Papillary adenocarcinoma has also been subclassified from the epithelial tumors of the endometrium in recent years. Christopherson and associates reported 46 patients with papillary carcinoma and described this lesion as a more aggressive type of papillary lesion. They found it to have a more anaplastic cellular pattern, to be associated with a more advanced stage of disease, and to have a 5-year cure rate of 51%, which is typical for extrauterine spread of tumor. This tumor, like *clear cell adenocarcinoma*, is extremely uncommon, and only limited clinical information regarding prognosis is available.

TABLE 33–3   *Relative Frequency of Endometrial Cancer Cell Subtypes*

STUDY (YEAR)	FREQUENCY (PERCENT)					
	Adenocarcinoma	Adenoacanthoma	Adenosquamous	Clear Cell	Papillary	Secretory
Christopherson et al (1982)	59.6	21.7	6.9	5.7	4.7	1.5
Underwood et al (1977)	70.0	14.0	7.0	1.0	8.0	—
Wentz (1982)	56.3	18.9	24.8	—	—	—
Salazar et al (1977)	69.0	8.0	23.0	—	—	—
Boronow et al (1984)	82.9	6.7	10.4	—	—	—

(Adapted from Boronow, 1983)

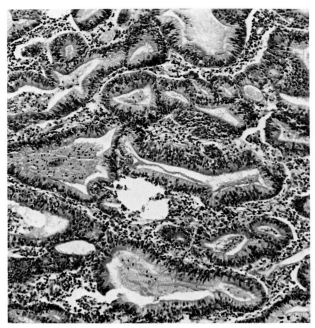

FIG. 33-2   Well-differentiated adenocarcinoma (grade 1).

HISTOLOGIC GRADE

The degree of histologic differentiation of endometrial carcinoma has become a reliable indicator of the prognosis of the disease. The rating system introduced by Broders in 1941 included four categories that have correlated well with patient survival rates over many years of analysis. Mahle used the system to categorize cellular differentiation in the endometrial cancer of 186 patients at the Mayo Clinic and demonstrated a direct relationship between histologic pattern and clinical results.

The current FIGO system of clinical staging includes only three gradations of histopathologic differentiation of endometrial carcinoma, including well-differentiated, grade 1 (Fig. 33-2); moderately differentiated, grade 2 (Fig. 33-3); and poorly differentiated, grade 3 (Fig. 33-4) tumors.

The FIGO classification is a modification in which Broders' grades 3 and 4 are combined into the FIGO grade 3. The FIGO classification was correlated with patient survival rates in a comprehensive review by Jones (Table 33-4), which showed a decrease in survival with decrease in tumor differentiation. Histologic differentiation is also related to lymph node metastasis, as Lewis, Cowdell, and Stallworthy found in a series of 107 patients who were treated by radical hysterectomy and lymph node dissection. Only 5% of the patients with well-differentiated tumors had positive pelvic lymph nodes, while 26% of the patients with poorly differentiated tumor had

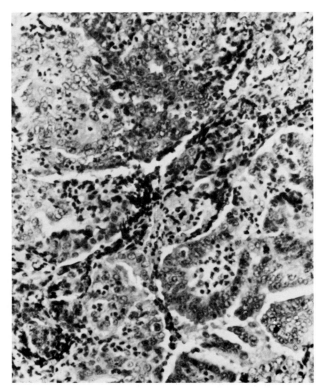

FIG.   33-3   Moderately   differentiated   adenocarcinoma (grade 2).

lymph node metastases. This early observation is supported by the data collated from the FIGO Annual Report, Volume 18, in which 69 institutional collaborators provided information on age, histol-

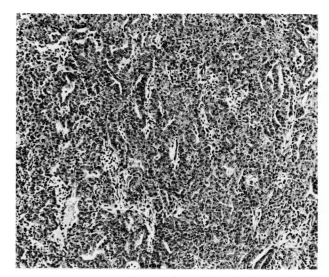

FIG. 33-4   Poorly differentiated or undifferentiated adenocarcinoma (grade 3).

TABLE 33-4 Correlation of Tumor Differentiation and 5-Year Survival Rates

TUMOR TYPE	NUMBER OF PATIENTS	5-YEAR SURVIVAL	
		Number	Percent
Grade 1	1558	1267	81
Grade 2	1515	1124	74
Grade 3	917	462	50

(Adapted from Jones HW, III: Treatment of adenocarcinoma of the endometrium. Obstet Gynecol Surv 30:147, 1975)

ogy, stage of disease, type of treatment, and 5-year survival in 11,501 cases of endometrial carcinoma (see Table 33-8). In this report, the mean age and the clinical stage were higher among patients with a grade 3 tumor than among those with grade 1 and grade 2 lesions.

TUMOR VOLUME AND EXTENSION

The extent of tumor invasion in the myometrium has been studied for correlations with the size of the uterine cavity, the frequency of pelvic node metastases, and the 5-year survival rate. Lewis, Cowdell, and Stallworthy reported that no pelvic nodes were found to be positive when the tumor involved only the endometrium or when tumor extended only to the superficial layer of the myometrium. The 5-year survival rate was 93.7% among patients with no myometrial involvement and 88.1% among those with superficial myometrial involve-

ment. Among patients who had tumors that extended within 2 mm or less from the serosal surface, 36.2% were found to have positive pelvic nodes and only 33% survived for 5 years even though they received irradiation therapy following surgery. These early data correlate well with current findings of the Gynecologic Oncology Group study as reported by Boronow and associates. In this multiinstitutional study involving 222 patients with Stage I endometrial carcinoma, there was an overall 10% incidence of positive pelvic lymph nodes (Table 33-5), which is similar to the 12% finding in the Oxford study. Deep myometrial tumor invasion of grade 3 tumors was associated with a 43.7% incidence of pelvic lymph node metastasis among the 222 cases where pelvic lymph nodes were resected. In all degrees of myometrial invasion, including superficial, intermediate, and deep myometrial extension, pelvic node metastasis was more common in patients with grade 3 tumors.

The three grades of Stage I lesions have been correlated with the extent of tumor invasion. Homesly observed 539 patients with carcinoma confined to the corpus (Stage I), and found that only one of 93 patients with deep myometrial invasion had a grade 1 lesion. Of the other 92 patients with deep myometrial extension, 48 had grade 2 lesions, 32 had grade 3 lesions and 12 were not recorded. Deep myometrial invasion resulted in a 5-year survival of only 61%.

Many investigators have analyzed Stage I adenocarcinoma for correlations between myometrial involvement and pelvic node metastasis. By col-

TABLE 33-5 Node Metastasis in Patients with Stage I Endometrial Carcinoma by Invasion and Grade

INVASION AND GRADE	NUMBER OF PATIENTS	PELVIC NODE METASTASIS		AORTIC NODE METASTASIS IN SAMPLED PATIENTS		AORTIC NODE METASTASIS OVERALL	
		Number	Percent	Number	Percent	Number	Percent
Endometrium G1	58	1	1.7	1/47	2.1	1/58	1.7
Endometrium G2	27	1	3.7	0/15	0.0	0/27	0.0
Endometrium G3	7	0	0.0	0/06	0.0	0/07	0.0
Superficial G1	27	0	0.0	0/18	0.0	0/27	0.0
Superficial G2	40	1	2.5	0/26	0.0	0/40	0.0
Superficial G3	13	3	23.1	5/11	45.5	5/13	38.5
Intermediate G1	4	0	0.0	0/02	0.0	0/04	0.0
Intermediate G2	8	2	25.0	1/04	25.0	1/08	12.5
Intermediate G3	5	1	20.0	0/03	0.0	0/05	0.0
Deep G1	4	1	25.0	0/03	0.0	0/04	0.0
Deep G2	13	6	46.2	5/09	55.5	5/13	38.5
Deep G3	16	7	43.7	5/14	35.7	5/16	31.3
Total	222	23	10.3	17/158	10.8	17/222	7.7

(Boronow et al, 1984)

lecting data from many reports, Morrow and associates reviewed 193 patients who were treated with radical hysterectomy and pelvic lymphadenectomy. They found metastases in only 3.4% of the patients with no myometrial invasion, whereas in the patients with deep myometrial involvement, 14.4% had positive pelvic nodes. The data confirmed the earlier report of Lewis and associates.

In the Gynecologic Oncology Group collaborative study, Boronow and colleagues made a clinicopathologic study of the uterus, tubes, ovaries, and pelvic lymph nodes of 222 patients and the aortic nodes of 158 patients with Stage I endometrial carcinoma. As shown in Table 33–5, among 222 patients operated on for Stage I endometrial cancer, both the grade of the tumor and the extent of myometrial invasion were important determinants of the frequency of pelvic node metastases. Pelvic nodes were involved in 10.3% of the patients, with a 2.2% incidence for grade 1, 11.4% for grade 2, and 26.8% for grade 3 tumors. Pathologic examination of surgical specimens showed that the risk of pelvic lymph node metastasis was negligible when the cancer was confined to the endometrium, regardless of the grade of the tumor. When superficial invasion to the inner one-third of the myometrium had occurred, only grade 3 lesions showed a significant incidence of pelvic node metastasis (23.1%). However, when the middle (intermediate) one-third of the myometrium had been invaded by tumor, the incidence of pelvic node metastasis for grade 2 and grade 3 tumors was 25% and 20% respectively. When deep myometrial invasion had occurred with extension of tumor to the outer one-third of the uterine wall, all grades of tumor showed a high incidence of pelvic node metastases: 25.0%, 46.2%, and 43.7% respectively for grade 1, 2, and 3 lesions.

Para-aortic node metastases were detected in 10% of the 158 patients in the Gynecologic Oncology Group study in whom lymph nodes were sampled and in 7.7% of the entire 222 cases. It is estimated that the true risk for lymph node metastasis for Stage I endometrial cancer varies between 7.7% and 10.8%. The pelvic nodes provide a valid indicator of the risk of para-aortic node metastasis. In the Gynecologic Oncology Group study, when pelvic nodes were negative only 1.5% of para-aortic nodes were found to be positive for metastatic tumor. When pelvic node metastases occurred, the para-aortic nodes were also involved in 60% of the cases. Further, this study found that 80% of Stage I tumors were grade 1 and grade 2 lesions (40% each), while 20% were poorly differentiated, grade 3 lesions. Approximately 40% of the tumors were confined to the endometrium, and 20% showed deep myome-

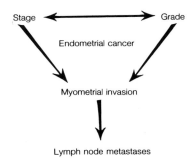

FIG. 33–5 Factors that increase the frequency of tumor metastases to pelvic and extrapelvic lymph nodes. Deep myometrial invasion is one of the most important factors associated with lymph node metastasis.

trial invasion. As noted in Table 33–5, when deep myometrial invasion occurs, between 25% and 46% of cases will have pelvic lymph node metastases. Also, when deep myometrial invasion occurs, more than 30% of the cases with grade 2 or grade 3 lesions will have para-aortic lymph node metastases.

Metastasis to the pelvic lymph nodes is also related to tumor extension into the cervical canal (Stage II). Because of the rich concentration of lymphatics in the paracervical tissues (cardinal ligaments), cervical involvement increases the potential for dissemination of tumor cells to pelvic lymph nodes. The frequency of extension of endometrial carcinoma to the isthmus and cervical canal increases with the extent of myometrial invasion. As reported by Lewis and Bundy, endocervical involvement (occult Stage II) increases from 7.3% of cases with tumor in the endometrium only, to 9.3% with superficial myometrial invasion, to 10.8% with intermediate invasion, and to 25% with deep myometrial invasion. Approximately 15% of all cases of endometrial cancer will have either occult or clinical extension of tumor to the cervix. The incidence of pelvic node metastases in Stage II disease approximates 30% and increases to nearly 45% with grade 3 lesions.

The classic triad of *stage of disease, grade of tumor,* and *myometrial extension* are independent variables that influence the frequency of tumor metastases and the curability of the disease (Fig. 33–5). In turn, each of these clinical features of the disease is related to the frequency of pelvic and extrapelvic lymph node metastases and the hematogenous spread of the tumor. Tumor permeation of lymphatic channels that drain the uterus and cervix is interrelated with the extent and location of the disease. Regardless of the stage of the disease, the overall 5-year cure rate is reduced to 50% to 55% when pelvic lymph nodes are found to contain metastatic tumor.

Pathways of Tumor Spread

Endometrial carcinoma spreads through three separate lymphatic pathways: paracervical and parametrial lymphatics, ovarian lymphatics, and round ligament lymphatics (Fig. 33–6). Although the lymphatic drainage of the uterine fundus and cervix directs most of the metastases to the pelvic lymph nodes, the para-aortic nodes are also within the pathway of metastatic spread through the ovarian (infundibulopelvic ligament) lymphatic vessels. Since the left ovarian vein drains into the left renal vein, it is understandable that distant metastases may occur directly into the upper abdomen. Although an infrequent site of lymph node metastasis, the lymphatic vessels adjacent to the round ligament provide an anatomical explanation for the uncommon occurrence of tumor involvement of the external iliac and femoral lymph nodes. The liver may be involved in tumor metastases, either from the interchange from para-aortic and portal vein lymphatics or more directly by hematogenous spread. Bone and lung metastases are more commonly the result of blood stream dissemination of tumor cells.

Diagnosis of Endometrial Carcinoma

Since abnormal uterine bleeding is common during the years just before and after the menopause, the symptom is easily overlooked, and the diagnosis of endometrial cancer may be delayed. Any patient with abnormal bleeding should have a thorough endometrial evaluation. Even if a patient is not of the typical age for endometrial cancer (55 to 65 years of age) an endometrial evaluation should be performed, since 5% of all cases occur in women under 40 years old.

The Papanicolaou smear generally detects only 50% to 60% of endometrial carcinomas. Aspiration or scraping of the endocervical canal is usually 70% to 85% effective. Reagan and Ng reported 85% accuracy for all types of endometrial cancer using both endocervical aspiration and vaginal cytology, but vaginal cytology alone detected abnormal cells in only 50% of the patients with known endometrial carcinoma.

Frost obtains better results using the cytologic material in the posterior fornix in combination with an endocervical scraping with a spatula. The problem with Frost's method is that the postmenopausal cervix does not always allow insertion of the tip of the spatula, so an endocervical specimen may not always be obtained.

The two most definitive methods that provide an adequate histopathologic study of the endometrial

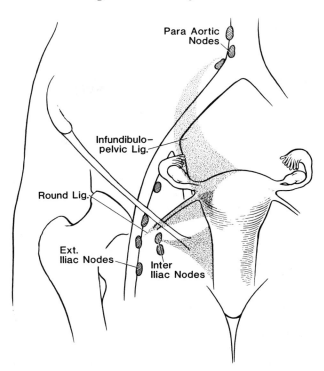

FIG. 33–6 Lymphatic pathways of tumor spread of endometrial carcinoma to pelvic and extrapelvic nodes.

tissue are, first, a cervical dilatation and fractional curettage and, second, a four-quadrant endometrial biopsy. A dilatation and fractional curettage can provide definitive results, even though a thorough curettage may fail to encompass the entire intrauterine cavity in 50% to 60% of patients. Patients of perimenopausal age should be evaluated with a fractional curettage so that the cervical canal can be assessed for possible extension or metastases of adenocarcinoma. If the endometrial specimen is positive for tumor, the separate endocervical curettings can show if there has been extension of the disease to the cervix so that appropriate treatment can be planned.

Hofmeister has used the endometrial biopsy in over 30,000 patients since 1949. Of all the patients, 187 cases (0.9%) of endometrial cancer were diagnosed. Of the women found to have endometrial cancer, 17% had no symptoms but had the biopsy as part of a routine examination during the perimenopausal years. Vaginal smears taken at the time of the biopsy were positive in only 26% of the cancer cases.

Many attempts have been made to brush, wash, or aspirate the endometrial cavity. The endometrial lavage technique introduced by Gravlee has been used with both good and bad results. Twiggs and colleagues found that endometrial lavage failed to demonstrate carcinoma in 14 of 25 proven cases of endometrial cancer. Even with adequate samples, the investigators had a 27% false-negative rate. Other clinics, however, have reported a 90% accuracy rate using endometrial lavage.

Among 93 patients referred to the Duke Medical Center with a histologic diagnosis of endometrial cancer, Creasman found a poor correlation with clinical diagnostic techniques. Among this group of patients with endometrial cancer, only 67% were identified by a Papanicolaou smear, 76% by an endometrial brush, 81% by a jet wash, and 62% by an endometrial biopsy. When the brush technique was combined with any other method, including jet wash, vabra aspirator, or endometrial biopsy, the accuracy rate improved to 91%. If any of these screening techniques is negative or obtains an inadequate sample, a complete dilatation and fractional curettage is required to properly evaluate the patient.

Patients who are using estrogen to control vasomotor symptoms of menopause require careful monitoring for signs of endometrial cancer. Any abnormal bleeding should be thoroughly evaluated, preferably by dilatation and curettage or endometrial biopsy. If a patient has abnormal bleeding, and the endometrial biopsy is negative, a full dilatation and curettage is required to study the entire endometrial surface. A Papanicolaou smear does not provide an adequate means of evaluating abnormal uterine bleeding.

Patients should not be scheduled to have a diagnostic dilatation and curettage immediately before definitive surgery unless histologic study of a frozen section specimen is done. Analyzing the curettage specimen by gross observation results in a 50% or higher rate of error in diagnosis. The tissue specimen needs to be thoroughly examined by a histopathologist if endometrial carcinoma is to be excluded.

Hysterography has been used to provide additional information once a diagnosis of endometrial cancer is made. Using a water-soluble medium, the extent, size, and precise location of the tumor can be defined. Long-term follow-up studies conducted in Sweden dispelled the initial concern that hysterography could cause retrograde dissemination of tumor cells. Devore, Schwartz, and Morris noted abnormal hysterogram findings in 40% of the patients they studied. Information about the size and contour of the uterine cavity, uterine perforation, and the location of the endometrial cancer helped in planning treatment for the patients. Tak and associates reported that pretreatment hysterography

provided enough new information to cause them to alter their treatment plans for 28% of the patients tested. Hysteroscopy has proven to be useful in visualizing the endometrial cavity and the endocervix. It can be used to document precisely any extension of the disease into the lower uterine segment and endocervical canal. Both hysteroscopy and hysterography are useful tools for planning treatment.

Treatment of Endometrial Carcinoma

Three basic methods of treatment—surgery, irradiation, and a combination of the two—are used for patients with endometrial carcinoma, based on the extent of the tumor at the time of diagnosis. In addition to histologic type, factors that determine the treatment plan include whether or not the tumor is confined to the uterus, whether or not the tumor has extended into the cervical canal, and whether or not myometrial invasion has occurred with expansion of the uterine cavity.

Although hysterectomy is considered the definitive method of therapy for endometrial carcinoma, problems involved with removing the affected uterus are of primary concern. As long ago as 1900, Cullen raised the possibility that during the hysterectomy, tumor implants could be disseminated to the remaining genital organs. In 1916, Howard Kelly suggested using intrauterine radium before surgery to sterilize the endometrium. Kelly, a pioneer in the use of radium, had noticed that treatment with intrauterine radium before a dilatation and curettage had resulted in sterilization of the endometrium in several cases.

Today, the gynecologist and radiotherapist plan treatment with advanced intracavitary techniques and high-energy megavoltage equipment for external irradiation. To completely irradiate endometrial carcinoma, treatment must encompass the entire affected area. Any extension of the tumor to the cervix or pelvic lymph nodes must also be controlled.

When surgery and irradiation are indicated, patients are usually treated first with irradiation to deter tumor dissemination and implantation on a cellular level. Before surgery, the blood supply is intact, so the oxygenated tumor bed can receive maximum effects of the irradiation.

Although the benefits of preoperative irradiation treatment are still argued, one positive effect has been well documented. A definite decrease in the incidence of vaginal recurrence results when either intracavitary or external irradiation is used in addition to surgery. In a collective review of 2264 patients, Jones showed that when surgery was used without prior irradiation, the vaginal recurrence rate was 10.3%. When postoperative vaginal radium or cesium was used, the rate of vaginal recurrence decreased to 5.2%, and the rate decreased further, to 4.6%, when preoperative radium or cesium was given. The experience in our clinic conforms with the data in Table 33–6 which show a decrease in vaginal vault recurrence varying from 4.4% to 1.5% when either external or intracavitary irradiation is used before or after surgery.

Vaginal recurrences are controlled almost equally well whether irradiation is applied to the upper vagina before or after surgery, and statistics show little difference in the effectiveness of intracavitary or external irradiation therapy. Unless a patient is at high risk for node metastases and requires full pelvic irradiation, intracavitary cesium used with vaginal colpostats effectively controls vaginal recurrence and results in fewer complications. When irradiation is used before surgery, there is no need to suture the cervix at the beginning of the hysterectomy, nor is it necessary to remove an excessively wide vaginal cuff with the hysterectomy specimen provided that the paravaginal tissues have received a tumoricidal level of irradiation.

With modern irradiation techniques, the vesicovaginal and the rectovaginal septa can be monitored while irradiation is applied. Intracavitary doses can be programmed with computerized isodose curves so that the precise irradiation dose to the bladder base, the rectum, and the entire broad ligament can be recorded. These improved techniques have increased the effectiveness of irradiation therapy while decreasing the incidence of injury to the bowel and bladder.

In many cases, surgery is performed 48 to 72 hours after central irradiation treatment. Immediate surgery has several advantages for both physician and patient. The patient can be treated completely during one hospital admission. The surgeon benefits because the pelvic tissues will not show the irradiation effects, so that the surgical specimen can be studied to determine both histologic grade and extent of myometrial invasion.

An important advance in the treatment of recurrent endometrial carcinoma is the use of progesterone in recurrent tumors that have high levels of progesterone receptors. Information about progesterone receptor levels obtained from tumor tissue in surgical specimens at the time of initial treatment may prove to be useful in the treatment of any recurrence.

Every case of endometrial carcinoma should be assessed individually. Treatment should be planned to obtain the best advantage from any method or combination of methods while also decreasing as much as possible the risks or complications. A general treatment plan based on these priorities is summarized in Table 33–7.

STAGE Ia

When the uterine cavity measures 8 cm or less and the tumor tissue is well-differentiated (grade 1), a total abdominal hysterectomy with bilateral salpingo-oophorectomy is performed and any suspicious pelvic or para-aortic nodes are removed. Preoperative irradiation is not required. Stage Ia, grade 1 lesions must be confirmed by fractional dilatation and curettage to ensure that there is no involvement of the endocervix.

If the removed uterus shows that the tumor has involved either the middle third or the outer third of the myometrium, postoperative irradiation should be given. A midpelvic dose of 5400 rad is given to the upper vagina and entire pelvis using

TABLE 33–6   *Vaginal Vault Recurrence in Stage I Endometrial Carcinoma According to Treatment Method*

STUDY (YEAR)	SURGERY ONLY		SURGERY PLUS IRRADIATION	
	Number	Percent	Number	Percent
Homesley (1976)	12/369	3.2	1/61	1.6
Lewis (1977)	7/194	3.6	4/380	1.0
Bean (1978)	1/107	0.9	0/130	0.0
Prem (1979)	7/131	5.3	1/63	1.6
Piver (1979)	4/53	7.5	4/136	2.9
Alders (1980)	19/277	6.9	5/263	1.9
Overall	50/1131	4.4	15/1033	1.5

(Adapted from Lifshitz S, Bernstein SG, 1983)

TABLE 33-7   Treatment Plan for Adenocarcinoma of the Endometrium

STAGE	EXTERNAL IRRADIATION (XRT)*	INTRACAVITARY IRRADIATION (BRACHYTHERAPY)†	SURGERY‡
Stage Ia Small uterus ≤ 8 cm G1 tumor	Postop—only if moderate or deep myometrial invasion: 5400 r over 5.5 weeks	None	TAH, bilat. SO Sample enlarged pelvic and para-aortic nodes
Small uterus ≤ 8 cm G2 tumor	Postop—only if moderate or deep myometrial invasion: 5400 r over 5.5 weeks or Preop—5000 r over 5 weeks	Preop—single application, Fletcher–Suit (F–S) afterloading technique Colpostats—7000 r surface dose (4000 r if following XRT)	TAH, bilat. SO (48 hr post-brachytherapy or 4 weeks post-XRT) Sample enlarged pelvic and para-aortic nodes
Small uterus ≤ 8 cm G3 tumor	Preop—5400 r over 5.5 weeks	Preop—single application, F–S afterloading technique Colpostats—4000 r surface dose following XRT	TAH, bilat. SO (4 weeks post-XRT) Sample enlarged pelvic and para-aortic nodes
Stage Ib Slightly enlarged uterus ≤10 cm, G1, G2 tumor§	Postop (a) if moderate or deep myometrial invasion (b) if positive pelvic nodes or Preop—5400 r over 5.5 weeks	Preop—single application, F–S afterloading technique Colpostats—7000 r surface dose (4000 r if following XRT)	TAH, bilat. SO (48 hr post-brachytherapy or 4 weeks post XRT) Sample enlarged pelvic and para-aortic nodes
Moderately enlarged uterus, 10 to 12 cm, G2 or G3 tumor	Preop—5400 r over 5.5 weeks	Preop—single application, following XRT (as below)	TAH, bilat. SO (4 weeks post-brachytherapy) Sample enlarged pelvic and para-aortic nodes
Greatly enlarged uterus, >12 cm, G2 or G3 tumor	Preop—5400 r over 5.5 weeks	Preop—single application, F–S afterloading technique following XRT Colpostats—4000 r surface dose	TAH, bilat. SO (4 weeks post-brachytherapy) Sample enlarged pelvic and para-aortic nodes
Stage II Extension to cervix, G1, G2, or G3 tumor	Preop—5400 r over 5.5 weeks	Preop—single application, F–S afterloading technique following XRT Colpostats—4000 r surface dose	TAH, Bilat. SO (4 weeks post-brachytherapy) Sample enlarged pelvic and para-aortic nodes.
Stage III Usually enlarged uterus, G1, G2, or G3 tumor	Preop—5400 r over 5.5 weeks	Preop—single application, F–S afterloading technique following XRT Colpostats—4000 r surface dose, possible second application	TAH, Bilat. SO if possible (4 weeks post-brachytherapy) Sample enlarged pelvic and para-aortic nodes
Stage IVa Usually enlarged uterus, G1, G2, or G3 tumor, extension to bladder and/or rectum	5000–6000 r midpelvic dose	Individualized Rx (a) interstitial needles (b) vaginal cylinder	Rarely a surgical candidate —may require colostomy for symptomatic control —urinary diversion rarely indicated - exenteration contraindicated

TABLE 33–7 *Treatment Plan for Adenocarcinoma of the Endometrium (continued)*

STAGE	EXTERNAL IRRADIATION (XRT)*	INTRACAVITARY IRRADIATION (BRACHYTHERAPY)†	SURGERY‡
Stage IVb Extrapelvic spread to distant organs (extrapelvic nodes, abdomen, lung, bone, etc.)	Individualized Rx, irradiation used for local control of symptomatic disease	Individualized Rx	TAH, bilat. SO for tumor debulking, if possible Irradiation or hormonal or chemotherapy treatment

* 25-megavolt teletherapy, delivering total midpelvic dose of 5000–5400 r in daily fractions of 180–200 r over 5–6 week period.
† Fletcher–Suit tandem colpostats afterloading applicator using cesium, giving average depth dose of 6000 r to 1 cm beneath endometrial surface within 48–72 hours and 7000 r to the vaginal surface (4000 r if prior XRT).
‡ Total abdominal hysterectomy, bilateral salpingo-oophorectomy with 2-cm vaginal cuff.
§ All Stage Ib grade 3 lesions should receive preoperative external and intracavitary irradiation.

the 25 megavolt teletherapy unit to deliver daily fractions of 180 to 200 rad for 5 to 5.5 weeks.

If deep myometrial invasion has occurred, the patient with a grade 1 tumor has a 25% chance of having metastases in the pelvic lymph nodes according to the study by Boronow and associates. In these cases, the treatment field must include the pelvis and lateral pelvic walls.

Preoperative irradiation should be used for patients with grade 2 or 3 tumors, to prevent dissemination of tumor cells during surgery. Grade 2 tumors may be treated with a single intracavitary application of cesium by the afterloading technique to deliver 6000 gamma rad to a depth of 1 cm beneath the endometrial surface. Vaginal colpostats should also be used to deliver 7000 rad to the vaginal surface, and both intrauterine and vaginal treatment (brachytherapy) should be completed within 48 to 72 hours. Immediately after the brachytherapy delivery systems are removed, a total abdominal hysterectomy with bilateral salpingo-oophorectomy can be performed. Any suspicious pelvic or para-aortic lymph nodes should be removed and undergo histologic study.

Alternatively, some oncologists prefer to give 5000 rad preoperatively because of the risk of pelvic lymph node metastases with grade 2 lesions. A single central application of cesium, using the Fletcher–Suit applicator, would also be used in such cases. In cases of Stage Ia, grade 3 tumors that show no evidence of endocervical involvement, preoperative external irradiation should be delivered over the course of 5.5 weeks. Approximately 5400 rad of external irradiation should be given to the pelvic midplane with the 25-megavolt teletherapy or similar unit in an attempt to treat the lateral pelvis and any pelvic node metastases. A single intracavitary application of cesium along with the insertion of vaginal colpostats giving 4000 rad vaginal surface dose will provide maximum tumoricidal effect to both the uterine lesion and adjacent lymphatic channels. Surgery may be performed 4 weeks after the irradiation is completed. If the patient has tolerated the irradiation therapy with no evidence of bowel injury, the surgeon will usually have no difficulty during the operation.

STAGE Ib

When the uterine cavity is enlarged to more than 8 cm, treatment should include preoperative irradiation, regardless of the histologic grade of the tumor. The ideal brachytherapy dose is 6000 gamma rad given by Fletcher–Suit applicator to a depth of 1.0 cm to 1.5 cm beneath the endometrial surface, while 7000 gamma rad are applied to the vaginal surface with colpostats. The dosage should be delivered over 48 to 72 hours, and the rectum and bladder should be displaced carefully from the vaginal sources to avoid irradiation damage. Computer programming of the isodose curves can be used to check the dosage at the wall of the uterus and of contiguous organs.

Alternatively, the patient may be treated with external irradiation, with 5400 rad being delivered to the midplane of the pelvis over 5.5 weeks. This treatment should be followed by a single application of cesium, by either the Fletcher–Suit applicator or a similar intracavitary device along with vaginal colpostats. The intracavitary irradiation should deliver an additional 6000 gamma rad to the endometrium and to a myometrial depth of 1 cm. The vaginal colpostat should give a 4000-rad surface dose. Four weeks following completion of external and intracavitary irradiation, or 48 to 72 hours following intracavitary irradiation alone, total abdominal hysterectomy, bilateral salpingo-oophorectomy, and evaluation of the pelvic and para-aortic lymph nodes are done. Any suspicious lymph nodes should be removed during surgery and evaluated. Positive nodes, along with moderate (middle third) or deep (outer third) myometrial invasion in the surgical specimen, are indications for full external beam irradiation following surgery, if not given preoperatively.

Although grade 2 tumors in a moderately enlarged uterus (< 12 cm) can be treated preoperatively in a similar manner, the addition of preoperative external irradiation is preferable because of the increased incidence of pelvic node metastases from this moderately undifferentiated malignancy. Applying a midpelvic dose of 5400 rad of external irradiation over 5.5 weeks to the patients with a Stage Ib tumor who are at high risk for lymph node metastases is much better than giving external irradiation therapy postoperatively, when indicated, after intracavitary therapy has been given prior to surgery, since such treatment requires midline shielding that may result in undertreatment of some areas in the pelvis.

When the uterine cavity measures more than 12 cm, the tumor is usually poorly differentiated (grade 2–3). Preoperative irradiation should begin with 5.5 weeks of external beam therapy. Using the 25-megavolt teletherapy or similar unit, 5400 rad are delivered to the pelvic midplane and lateral pelvis. External irradiation should be followed by a single application of intracavitary radium or cesium.

Using the Fletcher–Suit afterloading technique, a dose of 6000 gamma rad is given to the endometrium to a myometrial depth of 1.0 cm over a period of 48 to 72 hours. The vaginal colpostat is arranged so only 4000 rad are delivered to the vaginal surface. After external therapy, 7000 rad of intravaginal irradiation will exceed the normal tissue tolerance and may injure the bladder or rectum.

The rate and total amount of radiation applied to the bladder and rectal wall should be carefully monitored, and doses should not exceed 7000 rad to rectum. Surgery is usually delayed until 4 weeks after the cesium is removed so that the pelvic tissues can recover from the effects of combined irradiation therapy. As with the other endometrial cancer lesions, in patients in whom surgery is not contraindicated, a total abdominal hysterectomy with bilateral salpingo-oophorectomy should be performed and any suspicious pelvic or para-aortic nodes removed.

STAGE II

When histologic evidence shows that a tumor has extended to the endocervix, treatment must include the lymphatic drainage system of the lower uterine segment and the cervix. The major areas of metastasis with Stage II tumors are the pelvic nodes, including the hypogastric, the obturator, the sacral, and the common iliac nodes, and occasionally even the external iliac nodes. With undifferentiated tumors, the entire pelvic lymph system should be considered at risk for metastatic involvement.

When the cervix is involved with endometrial cancer, the incidence of pelvic lymph node metastasis is 36.5%, as shown in a review by Morrow. This rate is similar to that for a grade 3, Stage I tumor and the patient should therefore be treated with preoperative irradiation. In these more advanced cases, the treatment is similar to that for Stage Ib, grade 3 lesions. First, a midpelvic dose of 5400 rad is given over a period of 5 to 6 weeks by megavoltage external irradiation, followed by a single intracavitary application of cesium using the Fletcher–Suit afterloading method and vaginal colpostats. The dose of irradiation to the vaginal surface should be adjusted appropriately. Four weeks after irradiation therapy, a total abdominal hysterectomy and bilateral salpingo-oophorectomy is performed to remove the tumor in the uterus. Surgery should include an examination of the pelvic and para-aortic lymph nodes, and any suspicious nodes should be removed and assessed. It is now our practice to routinely sample para-aortic nodes in these cases, particularly in cases with a grade 3 lesion, removing all palpable nodes from the bifurcation of the aorta to the level of the inferior mesenteric artery, because of the high incidence of extrapelvic node metastasis. Patients who are not able to undergo surgery should be treated with full external and intracavitary irradiation.

The poor survival rate of patients with metastases to the para-aortic nodes has led to the practice of extending post-surgical irradiation to include the entire para-aortic lymph node chain. Only recently has this aggressive irradiation approach proven to be effective in controlling this metastatic disease, with 5-year actuarial survival rates approaching 60% in some studies (Komaki, 1983). More radical surgery has not improved the survival rates, and procedures such as the radical Wertheim hysterectomy and pelvic lymphadenectomy still cause excessive morbidity without significant therapeutic benefit.

STAGE III

The cure rate for endometrial adenocarcinoma that extends outside the uterus depends on control of the disease within the pelvis. Most Stage III tumors are found with an enlarged uterus, which should be removed if surgery is possible.

Treatment is similar to that for Stage II lesions. The initial approach is to deliver 5400 rad of megavoltage external radiation to the midplane of the pelvis over a period of 5 to 6 weeks. Intracavitary irradiation follows, with vaginal surface dosage limited to 4000 rad. Depending on the extent of the lesion, a second course of intracavitary brachytherapy may be required. While some clinics use a second intracavitary dose, others eliminate the intracavitary therapy completely, but increase the external beam therapy.

Four weeks following irradiation, an exploratory laparotomy should be performed if the patient is able to withstand surgery. During laparotomy any extrauterine mass should be carefully examined. Unrelated benign adnexal masses may cause errors of diagnosis and treatment. Any suspicious pelvic or para-aortic lymph nodes should be removed and evaluated, and the liver, bowel, omentum, and upper diaphragm should be examined for metastatic growths. As described for Stage II lesions, we routinely sample the para-aortic nodes in Stage III cases because of the high incidence of metastasis.

After the abdominal evaluation, a total hysterectomy with bilateral salpingo-oophorectomy should be performed if the uterus and most of the tumor can be removed without damaging the other pelvic organs. Some clinics have begun using peritoneal washings to determine whether or not implants have extended to the peritoneum, but the procedure is probably superfluous if the patient has received full pelvic irradiation.

STAGE IVa

The advanced endometrial tumor that has extended to the rectum or bladder is difficult to treat effectively. Because the tumor has extended so far, a hysterectomy is not effective, although removing the bulk of tumor in the enlarged uterus may be beneficial to irradiation therapy of the pelvis. Because Stage IVa disease usually involves metastases beyond the pelvic cavity, exenteration is not appropriate. Brunschwig used exenteration in such cases, but results were so extremely poor and the complication rate so high that the procedure was determined unsuitable even for palliative treatment.

Preoperative irradiation therapy should be structured to each patient's needs. A basic approach is to give 5400 to 6000 rad of external teletherapy to the midplane of the pelvis. For tumors in the vesicovaginal or rectovaginal septum, additional irradiation can be applied locally with interstitial radium or cesium needles, iridium wire, or vaginal cylinders.

Some patients may need a colostomy should a rectovaginal fistula result from irradiation and tumor regression. Aggressive local treatment of tumor in the bladder wall may also cause a fistula, but a urinary diversion is rarely indicated for palliative therapy.

After irradiation therapy, high doses of progestins such as 17-α-hydroxyprogesterone caproate (Delalutin), medroxyprogesterone acetate (Depo-Provera) or megestrol acetate (Megace) may be given, although the hormones provide only temporary control for about one-third of the patients. Other chemotherapeutic agents, including the combination of doxorubicin (Adriamycin) and cyclophosphamide with cis-platinum, have not been effective in giving long-term control of this tumor.

STAGE IVb

When endometrial carcinoma involves the upper abdomen or organs outside the abdomen, pelvic surgery should only be used to remove bulk cancer tissue. Although full irradiation is usually given to the abdomen and pelvis, it is not able to control the extrapelvic spread of the disease. Localized irradiation may help control pain and bleeding. An individual patient may also benefit from irradiation treatment of a lesion in the bladder or rectal wall. Progestins should be used in patients with well-differentiated tumors or high levels of progesterone receptors. Multiagent chemotherapy should be reserved for patients with less favorable prognoses.

Surgical Considerations

The technique of total abdominal hysterectomy for endometrial carcinoma differs slightly from that for benign uterine disease. In the past, surgeons began the procedure by closing the cervix with figure-of-eight sutures to prevent spread of implants to the vaginal vault. The use of preoperative or postoperative irradiation to the vaginal vault has made cervical closure an unnecessary step.

When the abdomen is opened to remove a uterus with endometrial cancer, the fallopian tubes should immediately be clamped across the cornual portion of the uterus to prevent retrograde passage of the tumor cells during the operative procedure. Since ovarian metastases occur in 5% to 10% of all cases, the ovaries and tubes should be removed, regardless of the patient's age or the stage of the tumor.

An *extrafascial* hysterectomy is performed to remove the fascia of the cervix and lower uterine segment which are rich in lymphatics. The base of the broad ligament is not clamped or cut as close to the cervix as usual, and the pubovesicocervical fascia is not separated from the uterine specimen.

A 1 to 2 cm cuff of the vaginal fornix should be removed with the cervix to ensure that the adjacent lymphatics have been removed. Excision of a wider cuff does not decrease the incidence of vaginal recurrence. The vaginal lymphatics should be studied with the rest of the surgical specimen. Preoperative or postoperative irradiation to the vaginal vault has also reduced the need for wide resection and shortening of the upper vagina.

On rare occasions, an endometrial carcinoma has been discovered during surgery for a supposedly benign disease. Although not originally planned, the ovaries and fallopian tubes must also be removed, even though the rate of metastasis to the adnexa is not high. Occasionally in a case where the uterus has been removed for benign disease and the ovaries and tubes have been left in place, histologic study discloses unsuspected endometrial carcinoma. If there is no evidence of myometrial invasion and the lesion is a well-differentiated, grade 1 tumor, the adnexa need not be removed. If the uterine disease is grade 3 or shows deep myometrial invasion, the adnexa may be treated effectively with postoperative irradiation. Alternatively, the adnexa should be removed surgically, not only to exclude a potential site of tumor metastasis but to decrease the serum estrogen level if the patient is premenopausal. In postmenopausal patients, the small risk of ovarian metastasis alone should be compared with the stage of the disease and grade of the tumor before an additional laparotomy is recommended for the specific purpose of removing the tubes and ovaries. In the presence of a poorly differentiated tumor with moderate or deep myometrial invasion, the subsequent laparotomy should include not only an adnexectomy, but a careful examination and sampling of suspicious pelvic and para-aortic nodes. Also, a thorough examination of the peritoneal surfaces, diaphragm, and abdominal viscera should be made for evidence of metastatic disease.

ALTERNATE METHOD OF TREATMENT

One other current modality of treatment of Stage I endometrial carcinoma warrants particular discussion. The debate concerns the value of preoperative irradiation followed by hysterectomy as compared to treatment primarily by hysterectomy followed by postoperative irradiation if needed. The original work of Graham in the treatment of Stage I endometrial carcinoma was reported in 1971 and is the basis of this controversy. Eighty-two patients in Graham's series received preoperative treatment with radium followed by hysterectomy. The 5-year cure rate was 76% and two patients showed vaginal

vault recurrence. Fifty-one patients were allocated for primary hysterectomy followed by vaginal treatment with radium. The 5-year cure rate was 82% and there were no cases of vaginal vault recurrence. Of interest was the fact that among the cases receiving preoperative radium, 14% died from recurrent carcinoma and 10% died from other causes. Among the group treated with primary hysterectomy and postoperative vaginal vault irradiation, only 6% died from recurrent carcinoma whereas 13% died from other causes. This clinical experiment set the stage for a raging debate that has continued until the present time.

For Stage I carcinoma of the endometrium many clinics now perform a total abdominal hysterectomy, bilateral salpingo-oophorectomy, and pelvic and para-aortic lymph node assessment as a primary procedure (Fig. 33–7). Depending on the depth of myometrial invasion and the grade of the disease, the patient either is given intravaginal cesium prior to hospital discharge or is treated with whole pelvic irradiation. A patient with a well-differentiated tumor that is confined to the endometrium or that shows minimal myometrial invasion is managed with surgery alone, since such tumors rarely metastasize to lymph nodes or to the vagina. All other patients receive vaginal cuff irradiation to reduce the incidence of vaginal vault disease. Patients with grade 2 or grade 3 tumors are evaluated in terms of the depth of myometrial invasion and the presence or absence of pelvic lymph nodes. If there is no myometrial invasion or only superficial penetration, and there is no evidence of pelvic node metastases, the patient receives vaginal vault irradiation including 7000 rad to the vaginal mucosa, which provides approximately 2500 rad to a depth of 5 mm below the surface. If pelvic lymph nodes are positive for tumor, the patient receives whole

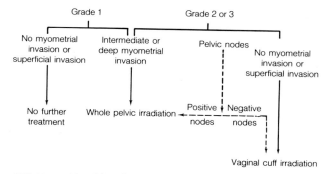

FIG. 33–7   Algorithm for treatment of endometrial carcinoma following primary treatment by total abdominal hysterectomy and bilateral salpingo-oophorectomy.

TABLE 33–8   *5-Year Survival Rates for Endometrial Carcinoma by Stage of Disease, 1973–1975*

		5-YEAR SURVIVAL	
STAGE	NUMBER TREATED	Number	Percent
I	8,550	6,340	74.2
II	1,690	970	57.4
III	822	240	29.2
IV	314	30	9.6
No stage	125	76	60.0
Total	11,501	7,656	66.6

(FIGO Annual Report, Vol 18, 1982)

pelvic irradiation regardless of the extent of the myometrial extension of the tumor. If intermediate or deep myometrial invasion is present, the patient receives, over a period of 5 to 6 weeks, 5000 rad whole pelvic irradiation that includes the upper one-half of the vagina.

To date there have been few prospective randomized studies to determine the validity of this treatment protocol, but preliminary data show no difference in the 5-year cure rates in comparison with other conventional methods of treatment, including irradiation followed by surgery. Most studies fail to show that surgery plus irradiation is superior to surgery alone, because 75% of Stage I tumors are grade 1 or grade 2 lesions. Only in the poorly differentiated, grade 3 lesion is there a significant improvement in 5-year cure rates when surgery is combined with irradiation. There appears to be little evidence to date showing that there is a therapeutic benefit to the preoperative use of whole pelvic irradiation as compared to a similar course of therapy in the postoperative period, if needed. Because of the possibility of postoperative pelvic

adhesions of the small bowel, however, postoperative irradiation carries the risk of complications such as small bowel obstruction and fistula formation.

Prognosis

Although the 5-year survival rates for Stage I endometrial carcinoma are impressive, varying from 75% to 85%, and, in some clinics, from 85% to 95%, the cure rates are not so impressive when all stages of the disease are considered. Volume 18 of the FIGO Annual Report on the Results of Treatment of Gynecological Cancer documents a 5-year survival rate of only 66.6% for 11,501 patients with all stages of endometrial carcinoma treated between 1973 and 1975 (Table 33–8). The FIGO report also shows that little improvement has occurred in the overall survival rate of 63% among patients treated between 1962 and 1968. In Table 33–9, the 5-year cure rates are correlated with the stage and grade of the disease in the FIGO report. The 5-year cure rate for patients with Stage I, grade 3 lesions (56.3%) is lower than the cure rate for those with Stage II, grade 1 (62.7%).

In a study of the literature, Morrow collected reports on 2,432 patients and found that the 5-year survival rate for all stages was similar (68%). A comparison of Morrow's data with the FIGO report shows the similarity of the survival rates for each stage of endometrial carcinoma (Fig. 33–8).

Jones reviewed the different treatment methods used between 1955 and 1974 for Stage I tumors. The review showed no statistical difference in the 5-year survival rates; patients treated with surgery had a 75% rate whereas patients treated with both surgery and irradiation had a 78% survival rate (Table 33–10). In the FIGO report, 98.6% of the 11,501

TABLE 33–9   *5-Year Survival Rates for Endometrial Carcinoma by Histologic Grade and Stage of Disease*

HISTO-LOGIC GRADE	STAGE I			STAGE II			STAGE III			STAGE IV		
	Number Treated	5-Year Survival Number	Percent	Number Treated	5-Year Survival Number	Percent	Number Treated	5-Year Survival Number	Percent	Number Treated	5-Year Survival Number	Percent
Grade 1	2783	2182	78.4	351	220	62.7	185	66	35.7	54	6	11.1
Grade 2	1536	1155	75.2	331	190	57.4	175	57	32.6	51	6	7.8
Grade 3	588	331	56.3	222	86	38.7	162	26	16.0	86	5	5.8
Not graded	843	537	63.7	110	60	54.5	79	16	20.3	40	5	12.5
TOTAL	5750	4205	73.1	1014	556	54.8	601	165	27.5	231	20	8.7

(FIGO Annual Report, Vol 18, 1982. Data based on 7596 cases reported from 69 institutions where grade of tumor was included.)

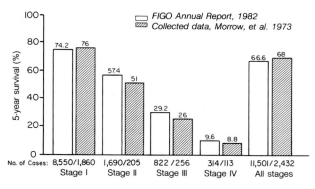

FIG. 33–8 Comparison of 5-year survival rates with endometrial carcinoma, by stage. The data, from a collected series of Morrow in 1973 and the 1982 FIGO Annual Report, show that cure rates did not improve in the 9 years between the studies.

patients were treated with surgery or irradiation or both. For a large number of patients with endometrial carcinoma, surgical treatment may not be feasible.

Irradiation Therapy

Although the cure rate of patients with advanced endometrial cancer can be improved with the adjunctive use of irradiation, patients with a well-differentiated tumor in a small uterus without myometrial invasion have an equally high survival rate without preoperative or postoperative irradiation. Some physicians continue to debate the issue, but Aalders and associates from the Norwegian Radium Hospital in Oslo have clarified this matter in a study of 540 patients with Stage I endometrial carcinoma. In a prospective randomized study that compared postoperative irradiation therapy to no irradiation therapy, there was no difference in survival among patients with grade 1 and grade 2 disease. This study recommended that external therapy was advisable primarily for patients with grade 3 lesions or those with deep myometrial invasion. This conclusion has also been supported by Piver and associates.

For patients with medical contraindications to surgery or with unresectable lesions, irradiation becomes the primary method of treatment. Despite general agreement that without surgery, survival rates are lowered by 10% to 20%, amazingly good results have been provided with sophisticated radiotherapeutic techniques.

The M. D. Anderson Hospital and other expert radiotherapeutic centers have now achieved very favorable results for the treatment of patients with serious medical complications or advanced disease, with cure rates that equal those of primary surgery and combined irradiation and surgery. As reported by Landgren and coinvestigators, a 5-year survival rate of 68% was achieved in the M. D. Anderson study, and a 10-year survival rate of 57% was achieved for patients with medical contraindications for surgery. Patients with an unresectable tumor treated with megavoltage irradiation had a 26% survival rate at both 5 and 10 years.

The M. D. Anderson series stressed the use of intrauterine and intravaginal radiation sources combined with high-voltage external irradiation, when possible, to control the central tumor and any extension to the parametrium and pelvic wall. Autopsy reports from the medically inoperable patients showed that pelvic control of the disease had been obtained in 89% of Stage Ia, 78% of Stage Ib, 82% of Stage II, and 62% of Stage III lesions.

The ideal therapeutic regimen for a patient should not be decided without considering the major factors related to the spread of endometrial carcinoma. An individualized treatment plan, as outlined in Table 33–7 and Figure 33–7, can be made with information about the histologic grade of the tumor, the size of the uterine cavity, whether myometrial invasion is predicted, and whether the tumor has extended to the cervix or outside the uterus.

Radical Surgery

Because radical hysterectomy and lymphadenectomy was used for cervical cancer, surgeons nat-

TABLE 33–10 Comparison of 5-Year Survival Rates for Stage I Endometrial Adenocarcinoma by Treatment Method, 1955–1974

TREATMENT METHOD	NUMBER OF PATIENTS	5-YEAR SURVIVAL	
		Number	Percent
Surgery alone	2392	1794	75
Irradiation and surgery	3679	2886	78

(Jones, 1975)

urally extended the use of the procedure to the treatment of endometrial carcinoma. First the disciples of Bonney from London, then the Oxford school of pelvic surgeons, including Stallworthy and Hawksworth, practiced the radical method until statistical evaluations showed clearly that a radical procedure offered no improvement in patient survival. The best 5-year survival rate reported by Lewis and colleagues and by other investigators using radical hysterectomy and lymphadenectomy to treat Stage I tumors was 71%. Better survival rates were achieved with less aggressive surgery or without irradiation.

Endometrial carcinoma spreads through the regional lymphatics and blood stream to recur at the lateral pelvic wall or outside the pelvis. It is obvious, therefore, that parametrial dissection is not useful for controlling the disease. Lymphadenectomy by the most experienced surgeon is not a complete anatomical dissection. It is no more useful than irradiation used alone for controlling spread of disease through the pelvic lymph nodes, although removing suspicious lymph nodes during a surgical procedure allows the surgeon to distinguish which patients require irradiation following surgery.

Even though Park was able to report an excellent cure rate of 91% for Stage I endometrial adenocarcinoma treated with the modified Wertheim procedure at the Walter Reed Hospital, patients had a high complication rate of 24%. Evaluation of the removed pelvic nodes showed that only 1.6% had been positive for metastatic tumor. Rutledge has also re-evaluated the role of radical hysterectomy for Stage I disease and has concluded that this procedure has a limited role, if any, in the treatment of endometrial carcinoma.

When statistics are included for Stage II disease, as Jones did in a review of 376 patients from the Walter Reed and Oxford series, the 5-year survival rate was still only 77% following simple hysterectomy with or without preoperative irradiation. An important aspect of Jones's review was that the survival rate was only 24% for the 45 patients found to have positive pelvic node involvement at surgery, even though some had been treated with irradiation after surgery. Since Onsrud has shown that removing all the nodes associated with endometrial carcinoma is not feasible, even with a radical lymphadenectomy, the adjunctive use of irradiation is obviously the better method for controlling the local spread of the disease.

Many patients with endometrial carcinoma are elderly, obese, and fraught with multiple coexisting medical problems. Radical surgical procedures in these high-risk patients are all the more traumatic and the complication rate is naturally increased.

Although some members of the Oxford group still feel that radical hysterectomy is specifically indicated for Stage Ib, grade 3 lesions with deep myometrial invasion, most investigators agree that all cases of endometrial carcinoma are treated best by a simple abdominal hysterectomy and that high-voltage irradiation is the best method for treating tumor at the pelvic wall.

Vaginal Hysterectomy

Although vaginal hysterectomy has been used occasionally for treatment of endometrial tumors, use of the procedure should be limited. When a patient is so obese that abdominal surgery would be extremely difficult, performing vaginal surgery is better than not removing the tumor. The exceedingly obese patient will tolerate vaginal surgery better, but the surgeon will have difficulty assessing the extent of the disease in the pelvis and abdomen. Examining the lateral pelvic walls and upper abdomen is impossible from the vaginal route.

Butler and colleagues from the Mayo Clinic have reported over 40 years of positive experience with the use of vaginal hysterectomy for many selective cases, mainly those with well-differentiated endometrial carcinoma and a small uterus. These patients with Stage Ia tumors had an 84% survival rate, with only one vaginal recurrence. Removing the ovaries is an important part of the treatment, and should be performed if technically feasible during a vaginal procedure.

When this procedure is required for the treatment of a patient who is not a candidate for abdominal surgery because of morbid obesity, postoperative irradiation treatment should be guided by the grade of the tumor and the extent of myometrial invasion. Only in cases with a well-differentiated lesion and either superficial or no myometrial invasion should the vaginal hysterectomy and adnexectomy alone be considered the final treatment.

Recurrent Endometrial Carcinoma

The factors that influence the recurrence of endometrial carcinoma are the extent of disease at time of initial treatment, the degree of differentiation of the tumor, the adequacy of the primary treatment, and the individual host response. More than two-thirds of all recurrent tumors develop within 2 years of initial therapy. The results are best when a recurrent tumor is well-differentiated and follows a long period of quiescence.

SITES OF TREATMENT FAILURE

The most frequent sites of recurrence of endometrial carcinoma are the upper vagina, uterus, pelvic lymph nodes, para-aortic nodes, and lungs. Dede, Plentl, and Moore reported that in 75% of their patients with recurrent endometrial carcinoma, the secondary lesion developed outside the pelvis. This is in agreement with results in a current multi-institutional study by DiSaia and colleagues in the Gynecologic Oncology Group, in which 222 patients with clinical Stage I carcinoma of the endometrium were studied. During the 36- to 72-month follow-up of this study, 79% of the recurrences occurred outside the pelvis. When definable extrauterine disease was absent at the time of the original surgery, the recurrence rate was only 7%, whereas if disease was found anywhere outside the uterus, the recurrence rate was 43%. In this study, the undifferentiated, grade 3 tumors, the tumors with deep myometrial invasion, and the tumors with either pelvic or aortic node involvement showed the highest incidence of recurrence. Curiously, of the 34 patients with recurrence among the 222 studied cases, local and distant recurrence occurred in 3% of patients treated by primary surgery with radium treatment and in 5% of those treated by primary surgery alone. Komaki and associates have demonstrated in 80 patients with Stage I, grade 3, or Stage II endometrial adenocarcinoma who were followed for periods from 3 to 18 years following completion of treatment that preoperative external whole pelvic plus intracavitary radiation treatment gave the best 5-year survival. Preoperative external irradiation to the pelvis plus intracavitary brachytherapy gave a 5-year survival of 83% in these high-risk cases, with no failures after 20 months. In comparison, survival for cases treated with intracavitary irradiation alone was only 64% at 5 years and 54% at 8 years. The 5-year survival among patients with Stage II lesions was 81% compared to 66% among patients with Stage I, grade 3 lesions. In general, residual tumor in the operative specimen at the time of surgery after preoperative irradiation was associated with a worst prognosis: patients who were found to have no residual tumor had a 5-year survival rate of 96% compared to 65% for those who were found to have residual tumor. A number of reports suggest that in cases with poor prognosis (namely, Stage I, grade 3 tumors) preoperative irradiation lowers the risk of pelvic recurrence. As shown in Table 33–11, the incidence of pelvic recurrence is higher in Stage I, grade 3 lesions when surgery alone is used than when surgery is accompanied by postoperative intravaginal irradiation. Among 171 cases in studies by Malkasian, by Salazar, and by Aalders the failure rate in the pelvis with surgery alone was 16.4%. In the abdomen or other sites, the rate was 11%. In contrast, among 198 patients treated with radiotherapy and surgery with Stage I, grade 3 tumors reported by Aalders, by Salazar, and by Komaki, the rate of failure in the pelvis was only 5.6% and in either the abdomen or distant sites the rate was 15%. This large study gives clear evidence that the more advanced tumors that require surgery and external irradiation are more likely to recur. When such recurrences are found, they are usually in distant, extrapelvic sites.

Very specific information about the original tumor and its treatment are needed to determine whether or not secondary treatment is possible. If secondary treatment is to be given, irradiation and chemotherapy are the primary methods used in an attempt to arrest recurrent growth. Additional surgery is usually only a palliative effort.

IRRADIATION FOR RECURRENT ENDOMETRIAL CARCINOMA

Irradiation therapy, whether used as a repeated procedure or for the first time, is the most common method of treating recurrent endometrial lesions. Both intravaginal and external techniques are used. Irradiation therapy is most effective for local recurrences confined to the central pelvis. The poor cure rates reported by Columbia–Presbyterian Hospital (Frick, 1973) indicate the grave prognosis for recurrent endometrial carcinoma. Even when lesions recurred in the vagina, the survival rates were only 15% to 20%. Brown and colleagues from the Mayo Clinic reported a much more favorable survival rate of 50% for 30 patients with vaginal recurrences treated with irradiation.

When preoperative intracavitary irradiation was used before the initial surgical treatment, the secondary treatment should be limited to 5000 rad of betatron or linear accelerator megavoltage delivered to the midpelvis. If no irradiation was used during the initial treatment, 5500 rad of megavoltage irradiation may be given to the whole pelvis, followed by an additional 4000 gamma rad given to the vaginal surface with vaginal ovoids. Normal tissue tolerance must be carefully observed. The total irradiation dose to the vesicovaginal wall should not exceed 8000 rad delivered to a depth of 0.5 cm. The rectovaginal wall should not be treated with doses higher than 7000 rad delivered to a depth of 0.5 cm.

TABLE 33–11 *Recurrence Rates following Stage I, Grade 3 Endometrial Carcinoma, by Treatment Type*

			FAILURE RATE		
STUDY	NUMBER OF PATIENTS	5-YEAR SURVIVAL (PERCENT)	Pelvis	Abdomen	Distant Metastases
		RADIOTHERAPY + SURGERY			
Aalders	94 (Postop ext.)	80.9	3	—	14
Salazar	59 (Preop ext.)	86	4	—	6
	12 (Preop IC)	75	1	—	1
Komaki	22 (Preop ext.)	68.2 ⎫	2	2	3
	4 (Preop ext. + IC)	75.0 ⎬ (66)*	0	1	1
	7 (Preop IC)	57.1 ⎭	1	2	0
Total	198		11(5.6%)	5(2.5%)	25(12.6%)
		INITIAL SURGERY			
Malkasian	22	58.8	4	1	5
	14 (Postop IC)	71.4			
Salazar	23	71	7	—	2
	20 (Postop IC)	70	4	—	—
Aalders	92 (Postop IC)	77.2	13	—	11
Total	171		28(16.4%)	1(0.6%)	18(10.5%)

Ext—External irradiation
IC—Intracavitary irradiation
* 5-year disease-free survival
(Komaki R, Cox JD, Hertz A, et al: Influence of preoperative irradiation on failures of endometrial carcinoma with high risk of lymph node metastasis. Am J Clin Oncol 7:661, 1984)

CHEMOTHERAPY FOR RECURRENT ENDOMETRIAL CARCINOMA

Progestins are among the main systemic agents in the treatment of advanced endometrial cancer that have produced a measurable response. Objective remission occurs in about one-third of the patients treated with progestin. Response to the hormone is best when a long, tumor-free period existed before recurrence of a well-differentiated, slow-growing tumor.

Progestins appear to work at the cellular level by slowing both DNA and RNA replication. The progestins also have a modulating affect on estrogen stimulation. Recent advances in our understanding of steroid receptor physiology have advanced our knowledge of the therapeutic action of progestational agents considerably. The intracellular effects of hormonal therapy are mediated by the interaction of the steroid and its receptor. Estrogen and progesterone cytoplasmic receptors have been shown to be markedly involved in the tumor response to hormonal therapy. Tumors that lack receptors are presumably unresponsive to a specific hormone. Therefore, in the treatment of patients with recurrent endometrial carcinoma, one might expect a good response to progesterone therapy in patients who had a high concentration of progesterone receptors in the primary tumor. Also, progestins are known to effect a reduction in available estrogen receptors, thereby decreasing the response of tumors to circulating estrogens. Progesterone also stimulates the production of 17-β estradiol dehydrogenase, which converts the active form of estradiol to a weaker estrogen, estrone. Both of these physiologic events—decreasing the number of estrogen receptors and decreasing the concentration of intracellular estradiol—have an anti-estrogenic effect on the tumor. Therefore, progesterone receptors are commonly measured at the time of initial treatment to determine the likely biologic effect of the hormone on a recurrent neoplasm. Ehrlich and associates have shown a strong correlation between the responsiveness of progestins in recurrent endometrial cancer and the presence of progesterone receptors. In their study, patients with high concentrations of progesterone receptors in the tumor responded more frequently to progesterone treatment. Many investigators have shown that levels of progesterone receptors are higher in well-differentiated than in poorly differentiated endometrial carcinoma. Limited experience to date suggests a greater than 90% correlation between receptor status and response to progestin therapy.

In 1961, Kelley and Baker reported the initial results of using 17-α-hydroxyprogesterone caproate (Delalutin) for the treatment of metastatic endometrial carcinoma. Objective remission occurred in 6 of 21 patients who had pulmonary metastases and lasted from 9 months to 4.5 years. A more recent report listed a 32% remission rate. Kistner also reported a 30% remission rate.

In a collaborative study reported by Reifenstein and colleagues, the average duration of tumor regression was 30 months. The dosage of Delalutin used was 1 g or more each week for 12 or more weeks. Patients usually showed a better response when treated for longer than 12 weeks. Of 314 women studied, 21 had complete arrest of the disease. Cure could not be considered the specific result of progestin therapy because the women in Reifenstein's study also received ancillary treatment. No correlations have been made between survival rates and the amount of drug given each week, the age of the patient, or the type of concomitant anticancer therapy provided.

Approximately 15% of all poorly differentiated tumors that were treated by Reifenstein responded to progestin therapy, indicating that a hormonal trial is warranted, even with less than favorable conditions. At one time, researchers felt that pulmonary and osseous lesions responded better than pelvic or abdominal tumors, but analysis of new data shows that pelvic metastases have a similar rate of response to progestins.

Other progestational agents have provided similar results. Deppe has made an analysis of various reports of the treatment of advanced or recurrent endometrial carcinoma with various progestational agents and found response rates varying between 30% and 49% (Table 33–12). Megestrol acetate (Megace) showed a 47% objective response rate in a combined series of studies when oral doses of 80 mg/day were given. Higher doses resulted in similar rates. Medroxyprogesterone acetate (Depo-Provera) has been tried in doses of 400 to 800 mg, three times a week for a month, then once a week for a second month, then once a month for maintenance. The results currently available show a 42% response rate, but the drug appears to give results similar to those for the other progestins used. Tamoxifen, an antiestrogen nonsteroidal agent that blocks the estrogen receptor, has also been studied by Swenerton. Unfortunately, only 30% of 10 patients showed objective response when given an oral dose of 10 mg twice daily on a continuous basis for the treatment of

TABLE 33–12 *Response to Hormonal Agents in Endometrial Carcinoma*

DRUG	NUMBER OF PATIENTS	RESPONSE (PERCENT)
Hydroxyprogesterone	384	32
Medrogestone	56	49
Medroxyprogesterone	195	41
Megestrol	125	47
Tamoxifen	10	30

(Deppe, 1982)

recurrent endometrial carcinoma. Although tamoxifen does not cause toxicity, the response is no better than that observed for progestins. However, in tumors that prove to be unresponsive to progestin, the antiestrogen tamoxifen can be used to block estrogen receptors in an effort to affect specific steroid receptor mechanisms.

Other types of chemotherapeutic agents have only been used in limited trials. In a collaborative study by the Gynecologic Oncology Group, Cohen and associates observed the response of 358 patients with advanced (Stage III and Stage IV) or recurrent endometrial cancer when treated with one of two multiagent regimens: (1) Melphalan and 5-fluorouracil daily for 4 days, repeated every 4 weeks, with Megace daily for 8 weeks; and (2) Adriamycin, 5-fluorouracil and cyclophosphamide, intravenous bolus every 21 days with Megace daily for 8 weeks. The objective response rate in patients with measurable disease was 36.8% in both groups; 36.8% of each group had stable disease and 26.4% progressed on treatment. Response was not affected by age, site of recurrence, time to first recurrence, and presence or absence of previous treatment by progestational or irradiation therapy. Grade of the tumor, however, and performance status did affect response, although 44 of 57 objective responders had undifferentiated tumors. Similar results are observed, however, with progestational agents alone. The median survival for complete responders of both groups was only 18.3 months, compared with 12.9 months for partial responders, and 8.8 months with patients with stable disease. The overall objective response rate of 36.8% for the multidrug regimens is no higher than the objective response rate for Adriamycin alone.

Based on all of these studies, progestational agents alone should be used primarily in patients with well-differentiated tumors or high levels of progesterone receptors. Cytotoxic chemotherapy should be reserved for patients with less favorable prognoses, namely those with poor tumor differentiation, absent progesterone receptors, and reduced performance status. Cis-platinum chemotherapy has been used for advanced or recurrent endometrial carcinoma by Seski and colleagues at the M. D. Anderson Hospital in 26 women, using doses at 50, 70 and 100 mg/m^2 every four weeks. An objective response was obtained in 42% of the patients but the median duration of the remission was only 5 months with a range from 2 to 11 months. Although cis-platinum was found to be definitely active against endometrial cancer, the high rate of toxicity (31%) limited the use of this agent in high doses on an outpatient basis. Currently, cis-platinum is being used more commonly with Adriamycin and cyclophosphamide along with megestrol or medroxyprogesterone. Although there are many ongoing studies that appear promising, the preferential combination of therapeutic agents has not been defined as yet. At the present time, chemical control of recurrent endometrial carcinoma is limited and temporary, but new agents, such as cis-platinum, in combination with other agents are being studied in hopes of gaining control over the recurrent disease.

Uterine Sarcoma*

The lesions categorized as uterine sarcoma comprise a diverse gross and histopathologic group of cases with varying clinical implications. The only unifying theme in this group is the origin of all of the lesions from mesoderm. There are those that arise from the myometrium, stroma, or epithelium, and from other mesodermal elements such as the pericyte. Sarcomas may be classified as follows:

Tumors of uterine muscle origin
    Primary leiomyosarcoma
    Sarcoma arising in leiomyoma
    Intravenous leiomyomatosis
Tumors primarily of stromal origin
    Stromatosis
    Stromal sarcoma
Mixed mesodermal tumors
Hemangiopericytoma
Leiomyomatosis peritonealis disseminata

The clinical staging of uterine sarcoma is imprecise since there is no official clinical staging of this disease. The most commonly applied clinical staging corresponds to the FIGO guidelines for endometrial carcinoma:

* The section on uterine sarcoma was contributed by J. Donald Woodruff, M.D.

Classification	Description
Stage I	Sarcoma confined to the endometrium
Ia	The length of the uterine cavity is 8 cm or less
Ib	The length of the uterine cavity is more than 8 cm
Stage II	Sarcoma involving the fundus and endocervix or cervix but not extending outside the uterus
Stage III	Sarcoma extending outside the uterus but confined to the pelvis
Stage IV	Sarcoma spread outside the pelvis or invading the bladder or rectum

Of the sarcomas arising from the myometrium, the most common is the sarcoma developing in the pre-existing benign leiomyoma. Sarcomatous lesions of this kind are found in approximately 0.1% to 0.2% of all removed leiomyomata. Since these lesions do arise in a pre-existing encapsulated tumor—namely, the leiomyoma—they have an excellent prognosis. The classic approach to determining malignancy in

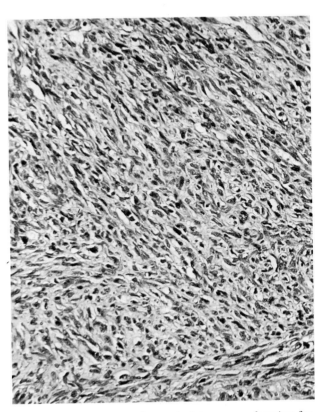

FIG. 33–9 Sarcomatous change in leiomyoma showing frequent mitoses.

a leiomyoma is to count the number of mitoses per 10 high-power fields (Fig. 33–9). Generally speaking, 10 mitoses per 10 high-power fields or more than 2 mitoses in any high-power field has been considered to be an indicator of malignancy. Even with high mitotic counts, an encapsulated lesion within the body of the uterus has an excellent prognosis. It should be appreciated that if the tumor is within the body of the uterus, adjunctive therapy, over and above hysterectomy, has not been helpful. In a series of 38 leiomyosarcomas at the Johns Hopkins Hospital, for example, there were 18 deaths, but in 14 of the 18, the tumor had extended beyond the uterine wall and invaded adjacent tissues at the time of treatment. Lesions in postmenopausal patients seem to have a worse prognosis, but this may be related to late diagnosis rather than increased malignancy.

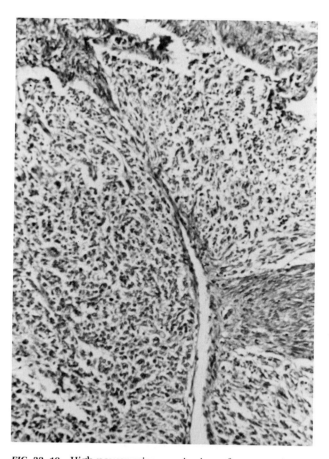

FIG. 33–10 High-power microscopic view of stromatosis uteri or endolymphatic stromal myosis. The tumor is composed of proliferating endometrial stromal cells with many mitotic figures. Although relatively benign, it infiltrates the myometrium like adenomyosis without glands.

Surgery is the treatment of choice for lesions arising in a leiomyoma. Usually, only one leiomyoma is involved in the malignant alteration, although this rule is not invariable.

Adjunctive therapy with irradiation seems to be contraindicated since there were no survivors among patients so treated in the Johns Hopkins series. However, most of these patients had extensive disease. Adriamycin has been the chemotherapeutic agent of choice. There are few survivors with extrauterine disease.

In contrast to sarcoma arising in a leiomyoma, sarcoma developing de novo in the myometrium has an extremely poor prognosis. It is approximately 5 times less common than the leiomyosarcoma in a leiomyoma. In a Johns Hopkins Hospital series of 41 cases, of 8 deaths in the entire group, 5 occurred in patients with a primary lesion in the myometrium without a pre-existing leiomyoma. De novo lesions tend to metastasize early and often to the lung, whereas the tumor developing in a leiomyoma tends to extend into the adjacent tissues.

Intravenous leiomyomatosis is a totally separate entity. These lesions involve the vascular channels and often extend from the uterus into the veins of the broad ligament. Histopathologically, they are benign. One would anticipate that the extension into the broad ligament would result in the development of thrombophlebitis and pulmonary emboli. Such has not been the case. The lesion may arise from the adjacent myometrium and extend into the vessel or may develop de novo from the muscle of the vessel wall. There seems to be no uniform agreement as to the genesis. In spite of the absence of postoperative thromboembolic phenomena, the infundibulopelvic ligaments should be clamped initially, at the time of abdominal hysterectomy, if such a lesion is expected, and the tumor should be withdrawn from the vascular channels. These tumors may be found in any age group and are generally asymptomatic, usually being discovered in the course of a hysterectomy performed for leiomyomata.

Although the lesions are histopathologically benign, in at least one documented case, sarcoma arose in this process, with extensive intravascular spread and demise of the patient.

PRIMARY STROMAL TUMORS

The most common stromal tumor is usually classified as *stromatosis*, also called *endolymphatic stromal myosis* (Figure 33–10). The typical patient is 35 to 45 years of age. Although stromatosis is generally asymptomatic, some cases produce the same complaints as adenomyosis. Stromatosis is actually

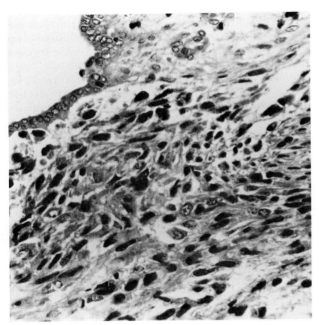

FIG. 33-11 Endometrial stromal sarcoma. High-power microscopic view, showing spindle cell pattern of stromal sarcoma cells. Bizarre nuclear changes of pleomorphism, hyperchromasia, and frequent mitoses are the features of this lesion (×250).

considered to be an adenomyosis without glandular involvement.

Since the lesions are primarily composed of proliferative stroma, mitoses occur frequently and mitotic count is not a criterion of malignant potential. Although tumors with more than 10 mitoses per 10 high-power fields are considered to be low-grade stromal sarcomas, the 10-year survival rate is almost 100% when lesions are confined to the uterus.

As with all uterine tumors, the adnexa should be evaluated during surgery. If a diagnosis of stromatosis is made by frozen section of the uterine tumor, the tubes and ovaries should be removed, regardless of the patient's age. The lesions tend to spread without gross clinical evidence of the disease. Lesions extend through the myometrium, invade the adjacent tissues, and eventually metastasize.

In a follow-up study of 33 patients reported by Thatcher and Woodruff, adjunctive progesterone treatment resulted in a high 10-year survival rate even when lesions had extended into adjacent tissue. Patients treated with irradiation had recurrences, and eventually metastases. If more than 50% of the myometrium is involved, adjunctive therapy with progestational agents (megestrol 80 mg/day) should be started. In a long-term follow-up of 9 cases so treated, no recurrence was found in 10 years.

The true stromal sarcoma is characterized by rapid mitotic activity, a loss of stromal cell differentiation, and frequent appearances of "strap cells" or rhabdomyoblasts (Fig. 33-11). The tumor is very aggressive, and the adjacent myometrium is frequently destroyed by invasion and infiltration with inflammatory cells.

The treatment for the true stromal sarcoma should be a total abdominal hysterectomy and adnexectomy. A careful histologic search should be made for epithelial elements. One area of the uterus can be invaded by stromal sarcoma, whereas mixed mesodermal tumor may exist in another area. Adjunctive chemotherapy should be used in most cases.

MIXED MESODERMAL TUMORS

Approximately 2% to 3% of all uterine malignancies are mixed mesodermal tumors, also called mixed müllerian tumors. Most of the mixed mesodermal tumors occur in postmenopausal patients between the ages of 55 and 65. The incidence of the tumor appears to be increasing. Approximately 12% to 20% of the patients have had previous pelvic irradiation, usually for cervical cancer. Patients do not have the characteristics associated with endometrial carcinoma: prolonged estrogen stimulation or obesity. The most common symptom is postmenopausal bleeding, although occasionally the polypoid tumor appears at the external os (Fig. 33-12).

Diagnosis is made by histologic sampling of the endometrium. The cellular patterns vary from one field to another. The stromal component is basically

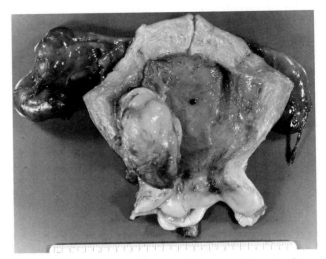

FIG. 33-12 Characteristic polypoid pattern of a mixed mesodermal tumor of the uterus in an elderly female. This tumor may appear grossly as a large endometrial polyp or an aborting submucous leiomyoma.

an endometrial sarcoma that contains rhabdomyo-blasts. The epithelial element demonstrates a wide variety of patterns from well-differentiated carcinoma to adenosquamous carcinoma. Some tumors are called heterologous, because in addition to the stromal and epithelial components, they contain tissues foreign to the endometrium, such as bone, cartilage, or adipose tissue. Heterologous tumors were originally thought to have a worse prognosis than other mixed mesodermal tumors, but all types have proven to result in similar outcomes, whether the tumor is confined within the uterus or not.

The treatment is basically hysterectomy and bilateral salpingo-oophorectomy. Evidence of extension should be evaluated as for endometrial cancer. Adjunctive irradiation has been the treatment of choice. However, the results have not been encouraging, and more recently the follow-up treatment of choice has been triple chemotherapy, mainly VAC (vincristine, actinomycin-D, and cyclophosphamide) (Table 33–13).

HEMANGIOPERICYTOMA

Hemangiopericytoma is an extremely uncommon lesion that can occur at any site, in any age group, and in either sex. In female patients, the preoperative diagnosis is usually leiomyoma, and the fundus is the most common site of origin. Although hemangiopericytomas are reported in many sizes, most are less than 10 cm in diameter. The surface of the tumor appears yellowish-brown and greasy. When analyzed histologically, the lesion is characterized by a proliferation of the cells surrounding small blood vessels. The proliferating cell is known as the pericyte of Zimmerman, although it was identified over 100 years ago by Rouget.

Although of vascular origin, the tumor is not as hemorrhagic as an angioma or an angiosarcoma.

TABLE 33–13 Chemotherapy for Uterine Sarcomas: VAC Regimen*

Vincristine: 1–1.5 mg/M² BSA†/wk. IV for 12 consecutive weeks
Actinomycin D: 0.5 mg/day IV × 5; repeat each month for 2 years
Cytoxan: 5–7 mg/kg/day IV × 5; repeat each month for 2 years

* May produce severe bone marrow depression and neutrotoxicity.
† Body surface area
(Wharton JT: Sarcomas of the Uterus. In Rutledge F, Boronow RC, Wharton JT (eds): Gynecologic Oncology. New York, John Wiley & Sons, 1976)

Because solitary tumors usually extend into the adjacent tissue, complete removal may be difficult, but surgery reported to date, including a total abdominal hysterectomy and adnexectomy, has resulted in a 5-year survival rate of almost 100% for uterine hemangiopericytomas. Tumors in other parts of the body tend to recur, to extend into adjacent tissue, and to metastasize to the lungs. No adjunctive therapy is used for treatment of a hemangiopericytoma.

LEIOMYOMATOSIS PERITONEALIS DISSEMINATA

Although the diffuse nature of this lesion may resemble that of metastatic disease, leiomyomatosis peritonealis is totally benign. Even when multifocal lesions occur, patients survive without complications. Most of the patients are diagnosed during the postpartum period or after taking oral contraceptives on a long-term basis.

The origin of leiomyomatosis is controversial. It may be a consequence of fibrosis of the peritoneal decidua, since it occurs frequently during pregnancy. The lesion is benign and needs no therapy other than histopathologic identification.

In summary, the prognosis for patients with sarcoma of the uterus is related to tumor volume, degree of encapsulation, number of mitoses, and tumor extension outside the uterus.

Bibliography

Aalders J, Abeler V, Kolstad P, et al: Postoperative external irradiation and prognostic parameters in Stage I endometrial carcinoma. Obstet Gynecol 56:419, 1980

Anderson B, Marchant DJ, Munzerider JE: Routine noninvasive hysterography in the evaluation and treatment of endometrial carcinoma. Gynecol Oncol 4:354, 1976

Antoniades J, Brady LW, Lewis GC: The management of Stage III carcinoma of the endometrium. Cancer 38:1838, 1976

Antunes CMF, Stolley PD, Rosenshein NB, et al: Endometrial cancer and estrogen use: Report of a large cancer-control study. N Engl J Med 30:9, 1979

Baggish MS, Woodruff JD: Uterine stomatosis. Clinicopathologic features and hormone dependency. Obstet Gynecol 40:487, 1972

Baggish MS, Woodruff JD: The occurrence of squamous epithelium in the endometrium. Obstet Gynecol Surv 22:69, 1967

Barber HRK, Brunschwig A: Treatment and results of recurrent cancer of the corpus uteri in patients receiving anterior and total pelvic exenteration. Cancer 22:949, 1968

Bean HA, Brant AJ, Carmichael JA, et al: Carcinoma of the endometrium in Saskatchewan, 1966–1971. Gynecol Oncol 6:503, 1978

Belgrad R, Albadawi N, Rubin A: Uterine sarcoma. Radiology 114:181, 1975

Bibbo M: Accuracy of three sampling techniques for the diagnosis of endometrial cancer and hyperplasia. J Reprod Med 27:622, 1982

Bonham DG, Bonham RJC: Cancer of the endometrium, an improved epidemiological assessment. Aust NZ J Obstet Gynecol 13:172, 1973

Bonney V: Wertheim's operation in retrospect. Lancet 1:637, 1949

Boronow RC, Morrow CP, Creasman WT, et al: Surgical staging in endometrial cancer: Clinical-pathologic findings of a prospective study. Obstet Gynecol 63:825, 1984

Boronow RC: Endometrial cancer: The emergence of therapeutic individualization. In Taymor ML, Nelson JH, Jr (Eds): Progress in Gynecology. New York, Grune and Stratton, 1983

Broders AC: Microscopic grading of cancer. In Pack GT, Livingston EM (eds): Treatment of Cancer and Allied Diseases, vol. 1. New York, Hoeber & Harper, 1941

Brown JM, Dockerty MD, Symmonds RE, et al: Vaginal recurrence of endometrial carcinoma. Am J Obstet Gynecol 100:544, 1968

Brown R: Clinical features associated with endometrial carcinoma. J Obstet Gynaecol Br Commonw 81:933, 1974

Brunschwig A: Surgical treatment of recurrent endometrial cancer. Obstet Gynecol 18:272, 1961

Butler CF, Pratt JH: Vaginal hysterectomy for carcinoma of the endometrium: Forty years' experience at the Mayo Clinic. In Gray LA (ed). Endometrial Carcinoma and Its Treatment. Springfield IL, Charles C Thomas, 1976

Cavanagh D, Praphat H, Ruffold EH: Sarcomas of the uterus. Obstet Gynecol Annu 8:413, 1979

Christopherson WM, Alberhasky RC, Connelly PJ: Carcinoma of the endometrium. II Papillary adenocarcinoma: A clinical pathological study of 46 cases. Am J Clin Pathol 77:534, 1982

Cohen CJ, Brukner HW, Deppe G, et al: Multi-drug treatment of advanced and recurrent endometrial carcinoma: A gynecological oncology group study. Obstet Gynecol 63:719, 1984

Copenhaver EH: Atypical endometrial hyperplasia. Obstet Gynecol 13:264, 1959

Cramer DW, Cutler SJ, Christine D: Trends in the incidence of endometrial cancer in the U.S. Gynecol Oncol 2:130, 1974

Creasman WT, McCarty KS Jr, Barton TK, et al: Clinical correlates in estrogen- and progesterone-binding proteins in human endometrial adenocarcinoma. Obstet Gynecol 55:363, 1980

Creasman WT, Weed JC, Jr: Carcinoma of the endometrium (FIGO stages I and II): Clinical features and management. Copelson M (ed): Gynecologic Oncology, p 569. London, Churchill Livingston, 1981

Creasman WT, Boronow RC, Morrow CP: Adenocarcinoma of the endometrium: Its metastatic lymph node potential, a preliminary report. Gynecol Oncol 4:239, 1976

Cullen TS: Cancer of the Uterus. Philadelphia, WB Saunders, 1900

Cutler BS, Forbes AP, Ingersol FM, et al: Endometrial carcinoma after stilbestrol therapy in gonadal dysgenesis. N Engl J Med 287:628, 1972

Daniel WW, Koss LG, Brunschwig A: Sarcoma botryoides of the vagina. Cancer 12:74, 1959

Dede JA, Plentl AA, Moore JG: Recurrent endometrial carcinoma. Surg Gynecol Obstet 126:553, 1968

Deppe G: Chemotherapeutic treatment of endometrial cancer. Clin Obstet Gynecol 25:93, 1982

Devore GR, Schwartz PE, Morris JM: Hysterography: A 5-year followup in patients with endometrial carcinoma. Obstet Gynecol 60:369, 1982

Dinh TV, Woodruff JD: Leiomyosarcoma of the uterus. Am J Obstet Gynecol 144:817, 1982

DiSaia PJ, Castro JR, Rutledge FN: Mixed mesodermal sarcoma of the uterus. Am J Roentgenol Rad Ther Nucl Med 117:632, 1973

Dockerty MB, Lovelady SB, Faust GT: Carcinoma of the corpus uteri in young women. Am J Obstet Gynecol 61:966, 1951

Drill VA: Relationship of estrogens and oral contraceptives to endometrial cancer in animals and women. J Reprod Med 24:5, 1980

Dunn LJ, Bradbury JT: Endocrine factors in endometrial carcinoma. Am J Obstet Gynecol 97:465, 1967

Dunn LJ, Merchant JA, Bradbury JT, et al: Glucose tolerance and endometrial carcinoma. Arch Intern Med 121:236, 1968

Edwards CL: Undifferentiated tumors. In M.D. Anderson Hospital and Tumor Institute, Houston: Cancer of the Uterus and Ovary, p 84. Chicago, Year Book Medical Publishers, 1969

Ehrlich CE, Cleary RE, Young PC: The Use of Progesterone Receptor Assay in the Management of Recurrent Endometrial Cancer, p 258. London, Baillière Tindall, 1978

Einerth Y: Vacuum curettage by the vabra method. Acta Obstet Gynecol 61:373, 1982

Ellice RM, Morse AR, Anderson WC: Aspiration cytology versus histology in the assessment of the endometrium of women attending a menopausal clinic. Br J Obstet Gynecol 88:421, 1981

Evans N: Malignant myomata and related tumors of the uterus. Surg Gynecol Obstet 30:225, 1920

Fechner RE, Kaufman RH: Endometrial carcinoma in Stein-Leventhal syndrome. Cancer 34:444, 1974

FIGO: Annual Report on the Results of Treatment in Gynecological Cancer, Vol 18. Stockholm, Radiumhemmet, 1982

Finn WF: Time, site and treatment of recurrence of endometrial carcinoma. Arch Intern Med 121:236, 1968

Fluhmann CR: Squamous epithelium in the endometrium in benign and malignant conditions. Surg Gynecol Obstet 46:309, 1928

Fox H, Sen DK: A controlled study of the constitutional stigmata of endometrial adenocarcinoma. Br J Cancer 24:30, 1970

Fremont-Smith M, Meigs JV, Graham RM, et al: Cancer of the endometrium and prolonged estrogen therapy. JAMA 131:805, 1946

Frick HC, Munnel EW, Richart RM: Carcinoma of the endometrium. Am J Obstet Gynecol 115:663, 1973

Frost JF: Gynecologic clinical cytopathology. In Novak ER, Jones GS, Jones HW (eds): Novak's Textbook of Gynecology, 9th ed, p 782. Baltimore, Williams & Wilkins, 1975

Gambrell DR Jr: Role of hormones in the etiology and prevention of endometrial and breast cancer. Acta Obstet Gynecol Scand (Suppl) 106:337, 1982

Gilbert HA, Kagan AR, Lagasse L, et al: The value of radiation therapy in uterine sarcoma. Obstet Gynecol 45:84, 1975

Goodman R, Hellman S: Postoperative irradiation in cancer of the endometrium. Gynecol Oncol 2:354, 1974

Gordan GS, Greenberg BG: Exogenous estrogens and endometrial cancer. Postgrad Med 59:66, 1976

Gordon J, Reagan JW, Finkel WD, et al: Estrogen and endometrial carcinoma. An independent pathology review supporting original risk estimate. N Engl J Med 297:570, 1977

Gore H, Hertig AT: Carcinoma in situ of endometrium. Am J Obstet Gynecol 94:134, 1966

Graham J: The value of preoperative or postoperative treatment by radium for carcinoma of the uterine body. Surg Gynecol Obstet 132:855, 1971

Gray LA Sr, Christopherson WM, Hoover RN: Estrogens and endometrial carcinoma. Obstet Gynecol 49:385, 1977

Greenwald P, Caputo TA, Wolfgang PE: Endometrial cancer after menopausal estrogens. Obstet Gynecol 50:239, 1977

Gurpide E, Tseng L, Gusberg SB: Estrogen metabolism in normal and neoplastic endometrium. Am J Obstet Gynecol 129:809, 1977

Gusberg SB: Precursors of corpus carcinoma: Estrogen in adenomatous hyperplasia. Am J Obstet Gynecol 54:905, 1947

Gusberg SB, Chen SY, Cohen CJ: Endometrial cancer: Factors influencing the choice of therapy. Gynecol Oncol 2:308, 1974

Gusberg SB, Kaplan AL: Precursors of corpus cancer: Adenomatous hyperplasia as Stage O carcinoma of the endometrium. Am J Obstet Gynecol 87:662, 1963

Hannigan EV, Freeman RS, Elder KW, et al: Treatment of advanced uterine sarcoma with vincristine, actinomycin-D and cyclophosphamide. Gynecol Oncol 15:224, 1983

Hart WR, Yoonessi M: Endometrial stromatosis of the uterus. Obstet Gynecol 49:393, 1977

Hawksworth W: The treatment of carcinoma of the body of the uterus. Proc R Soc Med 57:467, 1964

Hemsell D, Grodin JM, Brenner PF, et al: Plasma precursors of estrogen. II. Correlation of the extent of conversion of plasma androstenedione to estrone with age. J Clin Endocrinol Metab 38:476, 1974

Henderson DN: Endolymphatic stomal myosis. Am J Obstet Gynecol 52:1000, 1946

Hendricksen E: Lymphatic spread of carcinoma of the cervix and the body of the uterus. Am J Obstet Gynecol 58:924, 1949

Hendrickson MR, Kempson RL: Smooth muscle neoplasms. In Surgical Pathology of the Uterine Corpus, vol 12, p 468. Philadelphia, WB Saunders 1980

Herbst AL, Scully RE: Adenocarcinoma of the vagina in adolescence: A report of 7 cases including 6 clear cell carcinoma (so-called mesonephromas). Cancer 25:745, 1970

Herbst AL, Ulfelder H, Poskanzer EC: Adenocarcinoma: Association of maternal stilbestrol therapy with tumor appearing in young women. N Engl J Med 284:878, 1971

Herbst AL, Robboy SJ, Scully RE: Clear-cell adenocarcinoma of the vagina and cervix in girls: Analysis of 170 registry cases. Am J Obstet Gynecol 119:713, 1974

Hertig AT, Summers SC, Benglaff H: Genesis of endometrial carcinoma in situ. Cancer 2:964, 1949

Heyman K: The radiumhemmet method of treatment and results in cancer of the corpus of the uterus. J Obstet Gynaecol Br Commonw 43:655, 1936

———: Radiotherapeutic treatment of cancer corpus uteri. Br J Radiol 20:85, 1947

Hofmeister FJ: Endometrial biopsy: Another look. Am J Obstet Gynecol 118:773, 1974

Homesley HD, Boronow RC, Lewis JL: Treatment of adenocarcinoma of the endometrium at Memorial-James Ewing Hospitals, 1949–1965. Obstet Gynecol 47:100, 1984

Horowitz RI, Feinstein AR: Alternative analytic methods for case-control studies of estrogens and endometrial cancer. N Engl J Med 299:1089, 1984

———: Estrogens and endometrial cancer: Responses to arguments and current status of an epidemiologic controversy. Obstet Gynecol 65, 1985

———: New methods of sampling and analysis to remove bias in case control research: No association found for estrogens and endometrial cancer. Clin Res 25:469A, 1977

Horowitz RI, Feinstein AR, Vidone RA, et al: Histopathologic distinctions in the relationship of estrogens and endometrial carcinoma. J Am Med Assoc 246:1425, 1981

Inguilla W, Cosmi EV: Vaginal hysterectomy for the treatment of cancer of the corpus uteri. Am J Obstet Gynecol 100:541, 1968

Javert CT: Spread of benign and malignant endometrium in lymphatic system with note on coexisting vascular involvement. Am J Obstet Gynecol 64:780, 1952

Jensen EL, Ostergaard E: Clinical studies concerning the relationship of estrogens to the development of cancer of the corpus uteri. Am J Obstet Gynecol 67:1094, 1954

Jones HW III: Treatment of adenocarcinoma of the endometrium. Obstet Gynecol Surv 30:147, 1975

Kaplan SD, Cole P: Epidemiology of cancer of the endometrium. 1980

Kelley RM, Baker WH: Progestational agents in the treatment of carcinoma of the endometrium. N Engl J Med 264:216, 1961

Kempson RL, Beri W: Uterine sarcomas: Classification, diagnosis and prognosis. Hum Pathol 1:331, 1970

Kistner RW: Endometrial hyperplasia and carcinoma in situ. In Stall BA (ed): Endocrine Therapy in Malignant Disease. Philadelphia, WB Saunders, 1972

Knab DR: Estrogen and endometrial carcinoma. Obstet Gynecol Surv 32:267, 1977

Kohorn EI: Gestagens and endometrial carcinoma. Gynecol Oncol 4:398, 1976

Komaki R, Cox JD, Hartz A, et al: Influence of preoperative irradiation on failures of endometrial carcinoma with high risk of lymph node metastases. Am J Clin Oncol 7:661, 1984

Komaki R, Mattingly RF, Hoffman RG, et al: Irradiation of para-aortic lymph node metastases from carcinoma of the cervix or endometrium. Radiology 147:245, 1983

Koss LG, Schreiber K, Oberlander SG, et al: Detection of endometrial carcinoma and hyperplasia in asymptomatic women. Obstet Gynecol 64:1, 1984

Kottmeier H: Individualization of therapy in carcinoma of the corpus. In Carcinoma of the Uterus and Ovary, p 102. Chicago, Year Book Medical Publishers, 1969

Kurman RJ, Norris HJ: Mesenchymal tumors of the uterus. VI. Epithelioid smooth muscle tumors including leiomyoblastoma and clear cell leiomyoma. A clinical and pathological study. Cancer 37:1853, 1976

Lampe I: Endometrial carcinoma. Am J Roentgenol Rad Ther Med 90:1911, 1963

Landgren RC, Fletcher GH, Delclos L, et al: Irradiation of endometrial cancer in patients with medical contraindication to surgery or with unresectable lesions. Am J Roentgenol Rad Ther Nucl Med 126:148, 1976

Leis HP Jr: Endocrine prophylaxis of breast cancer with cyclic estrogen and progesterone. Int Surg 45:496, 1966

Lewis B, Cowdell R, Stallworthy JA: Adenocarcinoma of the body of the uterus. J Obstet Gynaecol Br Commonw 77:343, 1970

Lewis GC, Mortel R, Nelson HS: Endometrial cancer. Therapeutic decision and the staging process "early disease." Cancer 39:959, 1977

Lewis GC Jr, Bundy B: Surgery for endometrial cancer. Cancer 48:568, 1981

Lifshitz S, Berstein SG: Adenocarcinoma of the endometrium. In Buchsbaum HJ (ed): The menopause, p. 103. New York, Heidelberg, Springer-Verlag, 1983

Louka MH, Ross RD, Lee JH Jr, et al: Endometrial carcinoma in Turner's syndrome. Gynecol Oncol 6:294, 1978

Lyon FA: The development of adenocarcinoma of the endometrium in young women receiving long-term sequential oral contraception. Am J Obstet Gynecol 123:299, 1975

MacDonald PC, Siiteri PK: The relationship between extraglandular production of estrone in the occurrence of endometrial neoplasia. Gynecol Oncol 2:259, 1974

Mack TM, Pike MC, Henderson BE, et al: Estrogens and endometrial cancer in a retirement community. N Engl J Med 294:1262, 1976

Mahle AE: The morphological history of adenocarcinoma of the body of the uterus in relation to longevity. Surg Gynecol Obstet 36:385, 1923

Malkasian GD, Jr, Annegers JS, Fountain KS: Carcinoma of the endometrium, Stage I. Am J Obstet Gynecol 136:872, 1980

Marchese MJ, Liskow AS, Crum CP, et al: Uterine sarcomas: A clinicopathologic study, 1965–1981. Gynecol Oncol 18:299, 1984

Mazur MT, Askin FB: Endolymphatic stromal myosis: Unique presentation and ultrastructural study. Cancer 42:2661, 1978

McDonald TW, Annegers JF, O'Fallon WM, et al: Exogenous estrogen and endometrial carcinoma: Case-control and incidence study. Am J Obstet Gynecol 127:572, 1977

Montague AC-W, Swartz DP, Woodruff JD: Sarcoma arising in leiomyoma of uterus: Factors influencing prognosis. Am J Obstet Gynecol 92:421, 1965

Morrow CP, DiSaia PJ, Townsend DE: Current management of endometrial cancer. Obstet Gynecol 42:399, 1973

Nachtigall LE, Nachtigall RH, Nachtigall RD, et al: Estrogen replacement therapy II: A prospective study in the relationship to carcinoma and cardiovascular metabolic problems. Obstet Gynecol 54:74, 1979

Nolan JF, Dorough ME, Anson JH: The value of preoperative radiation therapy in Stage I carcinoma of the uterine corpus. Am J Obstet Gynecol 98:663, 1967

Norris HJ, Taylor HB: Clinical and pathological study of endometrial stroma tumors. Cancer 19:775, 1966

Novak E, Anderson DF: Sarcoma of uterus. Am J Obstet Gynecol 34:740, 1937

Novak E, Woodruff JD: Gynecologic and Obstetric Pathology, 8th ed. Philadelphia, WB Saunders 1979

Novak E, Yui E: Relation of endometrial hyperplasia to adenocarcinoma of the uterus. Am J Obstet Gynecol 32:674, 1936

Omura GA, Major FJ, Blessing JA, et al: A randomized study of Adriamycin with and without dimethyltriazenoimidazole carboxamide in advance uterine sarcomas. Cancer 52:626, 1983

Onsrud M, Kolstad P, Normal T: Postoperative external pelvic irradiation in carcinoma of the corpus. Stage I: A controlled clinical trial. Gynecol Oncol 4:222, 1976

Ostor AG, Fortune DY, Evans JH, et al: Endometrial carcinoma in gonadal dysgenesis with and without estrogen therapy. Gynecol Oncol 6:316, 1978

Park RC, Patow WE, Petty WE, et al: Treatment of adenocarcinoma of the endometrium. Gynecol Oncol 2:60, 1974

Parmley TH, Woodruff JD, Winn K, et al: Histogenesis of leiomyomatosis peritonealis, disseminata (disseminated fibrosing deciduosis). Obstet Gynecol 46:55, 1975

Perez CA, Askin F, Baglan RJ, et al: Effects of irradiation on mixed mullerian tumors of the uterus. Cancer 43:1274, 1979

Peterson EP: Endometrial carcinoma in young women: A clinical profile. Obstet Gynecol 31:702, 1968

Piver MS, Yasigi R, Blumenson L, et al: A prospective trial comparing hysterectomy plus vaginal radium and uterine radium, plus hysterectomy in Stage I endometrial carcinoma. Obstet Gynecol 54:85, 1979

Prem KA, Adcock LL, Okagaki T, et al: The evaluation of a treatment program for adenocarcinoma of the endometrium. Am J Obstet Gynecol 133:803, 1979

Price JJ, Hahn GA, Rominger CJ: Vaginal involvement in endometrial carcinoma. Am J Obstet Gynecol 91:1060, 1965

Rachmaninoff N, Climie ARW: Mixed mesodermal tumors of the uterus. Cancer 19:1705, 1966

Reagan JW, Ng ABP: The Cells of Uterine Adenocarcinoma. Baltimore, Williams & Wilkins, 1965

Reifenstein ECJ: The treatment of advance endometrial cancer with hydroxyprogesterone caproate. Gynecol Oncol 2:377, 1974

Rhoades FP: Continuous cyclic hormonal therapy. J Am Geriatr Soc 22:183, 1974

Richart RM, Ferenczy A: Endometrial morphologic response to hormonal environment. Gynecol Oncol 2:180, 1974

Rickford RBK: Involvement of pelvic lymph nodes in carcinoma of the endometrium. J Obstet Gynaecol Br Commonw 75:580, 1968

Rosenwaks Z, Wetz AC, Jones GS, et al: Endometrial pathology and estrogens. Obstet Gynecol 53:403, 1979

Rubin A: The histogenesis of carcinosarcoma (mixed mesodermal tumor) of the uterus as revealed by tissue culture studies. Am J Obstet Gynecol 77:269, 1959

Rutledge F: Role of radical hysterectomy in adenocarcinoma of the endometrium. Gynecol Oncol 2:331, 1974

Salazar OM, Bonfiglio TA, Patten SF, et al: Uterine sarcomas. Natural history, treatment and prognosis. Cancer 42:1152, 1978

Salazar OM, DePapp EW, Bonfiglio TA, et al: Adenosquamous carcinoma of the endometrium. Cancer 40:119, 1977

Schindler AE, Ebert A, Friedrich E: Conversion of androstenedione to estrone by human fat tissue. J Clin Endocrinol Metab 35:627, 1972

Schroeder R. Nordwestdeutsche Gesellschaft fur Gynakologie. Zbl Gynak 46:193, 1922

Schwartz PE, Kohorn EI, Nolton AH, et al: Routine use of hysterography in endometrial carcinoma and postmenopausal bleeding. Obstet Gynecol 45:378, 1975

Seski JC, Edwards CL, Herson J, et al: Cisplatin chemotherapy for disseminated endometrial cancer. Obstet Gynecol 59:225, 1982

Siiteri PK, Schwarz BE, MacDonald PC: Estrogen receptors and the estrone hypothesis in relation to endometrial and breast cancer. Gynecol Oncol 2:228, 1974

Silverberg E: Cancer statistics, 1984. CA 34:7, 1984

Silverberg SG, Makowski EL: Endometrial carcinoma in young women taking oral contraceptives. Obstet Gynecol 46:503, 1975

Smith DC, Prentice R, Thompson DJ, et al: Association of exogenous estrogen and endometrial carcinoma. N Engl J Med 293:1164, 1975

Spanos WJ, Wharton JT, Gomez L, et al: Malignant mixed mullerian tumors of the uterus. Cancer 53:311, 1984

Speert H: Carcinoma in the endometrium in young women. Surg Gynecol Obstet 88:332, 1949

Stallworthy JA: Surgery of endometrial cancer in the Bonney tradition. Ann R Coll Surg 48:239, 1971

Steele SJ, Scott JM, Stephens JW: Endometrial stromal sarcoma. Br J Surg 55:943, 1968

Swartz AE, Brunschwig A: Radical pan-hysterectomy and pelvic node excision for carcinoma of the corpus uteri. Surg Gynecol Obstet 105:675, 1957

Swenerton KD: Treatment of advanced endometrial adenocarcinoma with tamoxifen. Cancer Treat Rep 64:805, 1980

Tak WT, Bloedorn FG, Marchant DJ: Myometrial invasion and hysterography in endometrial carcinoma. Obstet Gynecol 50:159, 1977

Tanga R, Delgardo G: Uterine sarcoma. Int Surg 67:339, 1982

Taylor HB, Norris HJ: Mesenchymal tumors of the uterus. IV. Diagnosis and prognosis of leiomyosarcomas. Arch Pathol 82:40, 1966

Thatcher SS, Woodruff JD: Uterine stromatosis: A report of 33 cases. Obstet Gynecol 59:428, 1982

Twiggs LB, DiSaia PJ, Morrow PC, et al: Gravlee jet irrigator: Efficacy in diagnosis of endometrial neoplasia. JAMA 235:2748, 1976

Vardi JR, Tovell HMM: Leiomyosarcoma of the uterus. Obstet Gynecol 56:428, 1980

Vongtama V, Karlen JL, Piver SM, et al: Treatment results and prognostic factors in Stages I and II sarcomas of the corpus uteri. Am J Roentgenol 126:139, 1976

Vuopala A: Diagnostic accuracy and clinical applicability of cytological and histological methods for investigating endometrial carcinoma. Acta Obstet Gynecol Scand (Suppl) 22:70, 1977

Walker AM, Jick H: Declining rates of endometrial cancer. Obstet Gynecol 56:733, 1980

Weiss N, Szekely D, English D, et al: Endometrial cancer in relation to patterns of menopausal estrogen use. JAMA 242:261, 1979

Weiss WB: Progestin therapy in endometrial hyperplasia. Gynecol Oncol 2:362, 1974

Wharton JT: Sarcomas of the uterus. In Rutledge F, Boronow RC, Wharton JT (eds): Gynecologic Oncology. New York, John Wiley & Sons, 1976

Wynder EL, Escher GC, Mantel N: An epidemiological investigation of cancer of the endometrium. Cancer 19:489, 1966

Ziel HK, Finkle WD: Increased risk of endometrial carcinoma among users of conjugated estrogens. N Engl J Med 93:1167, 1975

Chapter 34

Neoplastic Ovarian Tumors

Felix N. Rutledge, M.D.

Currently, ovarian cancer is the greatest cause of death among patients with gynecologic malignancy and ranks third as a cause of death among all malignancies in women, exceeded only by carcinoma of the breast and intestine. The number of deaths resulting from ovarian cancer now exceeds that from cancer of the uterine cervix. Developments in treatment have changed the clinical course of the disease, reducing suffering and lengthening survival, yet the number of cures has increased very little. The current overall 5-year survival rate (between 15% and 30%) remains unchanged to any significant degree from previous decades. Cancer of the ovary constitutes 4.7% of all cancer in white women, affecting 1.4%, or one of every 70 women at some time during their lives. The average annual age-adjusted incidence rates are 14.2 for whites and 9.3 for blacks per 100,000 women.

The only known prevention for ovarian cancer is oophorectomy. The use of prophylactic ovarian ablation against ovarian cancer has been discussed in relation to hysterectomy for benign disease (see Chapter 11), and it is strongly advised for perimenopausal and postmenopausal patients undergoing pelvic surgery.

The quiescent nature of early developing ovarian cancer hinders its discovery while it is small. Approximately 10% of our patients with ovarian cancer were totally asymptomatic when their disease was detected by routine pelvic examination. It is estimated that only one case of ovarian carcinoma will be diagnosed for every 10,000 pelvic examinations of asymptomatic women. More than 15% of all ovarian cancers are undiagnosed until the abdomen is opened for some other reason. The differential diagnosis of ovarian enlargement is one of the most

difficult of all gynecologic diagnostic problems. Some guidelines to be applied in the diagnosis of ovarian neoplasms are:

An appreciation for the potential seriousness of a pelvic mass at any age

A sustained concern about potential cancer until the diagnosis is finally resolved

A sense of diagnostic urgency because ovarian cancers are notable for their rapid growth

A concern for preservation of fertility if prognosis is not jeopardized by less complete resection.

The physical features determined by pelvic examination are the most important distinguishing characteristics. Some ovarian tumors feel definitely benign and may be observed. For example, physiologic cysts seen in young women will usually regress spontaneously, and immediate surgery for these cysts, without clinical observation, is both unnecessary and contraindicated. Conversely, a thick-walled, semisolid cyst is more frequently neoplastic and is particularly alarming if the outer surface is irregular and the tumor cannot be displaced. Solidity and firm consistency may be deceptive signs of cancer because some very firm tumors, such as fibromas or Brenner tumors, are solid, yet benign in nature. Nodularity of the cul-de-sac of Douglas or uterosacral ligaments may be metastases, yet these, too, must be differentiated from pelvic endometriosis or organized pelvic inflammatory disease.

The patient's age is an important factor in evaluating pelvic findings because younger patients are more likely to have benign disease. During early adulthood, physiologic cysts of the ovary are quite common, whereas malignant tumors are infrequent. Patients of the older age group often have sigmoid diverticulitis, which must be distinguished from an ovarian neoplasm. Diverticular disease is more tender when palpated and often involves lower abdominal pain. In the menopausal and post-menopausal patient, an ovarian enlargement must be investigated surgically without delay. When the nature of an adnexal mass is in doubt, laparoscopy is helpful in determining the necessity for surgery. Peritoneal cavity aspiration via the cul-de-sac, as advocated by Graham and by McGowan, has limited diagnostic usefulness and some hazards. The cul-de-sac must be emptied for such a test to be safe, and the procedure may liberate into the abdominal cavity cancer cells that were previously contained within the tumor capsule or cyst wall. In the presence of clinically evident intra-abdominal fluid, a needle puncture made through the abdominal wall above the pelvic area is a safer route for study of peritoneal cytology because entry into the malignant cyst may be avoided. As with cancers in other sites, the stage of ovarian cancer dominates the prognosis and strongly influences the selection of treatment.

Classification of Ovarian Tumors

In 1964, the International Federation of Gynecology and Obstetrics (FIGO) developed a system for the clinical classification of histologic types and staging of ovarian cancer. The classification was updated in 1970. Further revisions were adopted by the General Assembly of FIGO in 1976, to be applied after July 1, 1974.

In addition, all epithelial carcinomas are graded as well differentiated (grade 1), moderately differentiated (grade 2), or poorly differentiated (grade 3).

The World Health Organization (WHO) has classified neoplastic ovarian cysts according to the cell of origin, the most frequent being the germinal epithelium tumors, followed in order of frequency by germ cell tumors, gonadal stromal tumors, and a category comprising miscellaneous tumors. Since the germinal epithelium tumors are most common they were further categorized as serous, mucinous, endometrioid, clear-cell or mesonephroid, Brenner, or undifferentiated. Each of these epithelial tumors is further defined as being benign, of low-potential malignancy, or malignant.

BENIGN EPITHELIAL TUMORS

Serous Cystadenomas

Serous cystadenomas are the most common benign epithelial tumors, accounting for 20% to 40% of be-

FIGO Clinical Classification of Carcinoma of the Ovary

Classification	Description
Stage I	Growth limited to the ovaries
Ia	Growth limited to one ovary; no ascites
	(1) No tumor on the external surface; capsule intact
	(2) Tumor present on the external surface or capsule ruptured or both
Ib	Growth limited to both ovaries; no ascites
	(1) No tumor on the external surface; capsule intact
	(2) Tumor present on the external surface or capsule ruptured or both
Ic	Tumor either stage Ia or Stage Ib, but with obvious ascites present or positive peritoneal washings
Stage II	Growth involving one or both ovaries with pelvic extension
IIa	Extension and/or metastases to the uterus and/or tubes
IIb	Extension to other pelvic tissues
IIc	Tumor either Stage IIa or Stage IIb, but with obvious ascites present or positive peritoneal washings
Stage III	Growth involving one or both ovaries with intraperitoneal metastases outside the pelvis or positive retroperitoneal nodes or both. Tumor limited to the true pelvis with histologically proven malignant extension to small bowel or omentum.
Stage IV	Growth involving one or both ovaries with distant metastases. If pleural effusion is present, there must be positive cytology to allot a case to Stage IV. Parenchymal liver metastasis equals Stage IV.
Special category	Unexplored cases that are thought to be ovarian carcinoma

nign ovarian neoplasms. They are notable for their large size, although mucinous cysts can be larger. They are named for the serous fluid they contain, which is usually straw-colored; however, if there is hemorrhage the fluid may be the color of chocolate or coffee. These cysts may be either unilocular or multilocular, and they may appear to be composed of a conglomeration of round cystic masses. They are less likely than mucinous tumors to be multilocular and more likely to be bilateral. Papillary excrescences are common, usually appearing in patches and more likely to be malignant when they cover the entire inner surface of the cyst. External excrescences occur more commonly with malignant tumors. A serous cystadenoma arises from the epithelial surface of the ovary, which is

*FIGO Histologic Classification of the Common
Primary Epithelial Tumors of the Ovary*

Classification	Description
Serous cystomas	a. Serous benign cystadenomas
	b. Serous cystadenomas with proliferating activity of the epithelial cells and nuclear abnormalities, but with no infiltrative destructive growth (low-potential malignancy)
	c. Serous cystadenocarcinomas
Mucinous cystomas	a. Mucinous benign cystadenomas
	b. Mucinous cystadenomas with proliferating activity of the epithelial cells and nuclear abnormalities, but with no infiltrative destructive growth (low-potential malignancy)
	c. Mucinous cystadenocarcinomas
Endometrioid tumors (similar to adenocarcinoma in the endometrium)	a. Endometrioid benign cysts
	b. Endometrioid tumors with proliferating activity of the epithelial cells and nuclear abnormalities, but with no infiltrative destructive growth (low-potential malignancy)
	c. Endometrioid adenocarcinomas
Clear cell tumors (Mesonephroid tumors)	a. Benign mesonephroid tumors
	b. Mesonephroid tumors with proliferating activity of the epithelial cells and nuclear abnormalities, but with no infiltrative destructive growth (low-potential malignancy)
	c. Mesonephroid cystadenocarcinomas
Undifferentiated carcinoma	Malignant tumor of epithelial structure that is too poorly differentiated to be placed in any of the other groups
Mixed epithelial tumors	Tumors composed of a mixture of two or more of the malignant groups and with no one predominant
No histology	Obvious ovarian epithelial malignant tumor by exploratory surgery, but no histology available.

mesothelial in embryonic origin. The epithelial cells are usually a single cell thickness, though often there are mixtures of columnar cells with ciliated surfaces and secretory cells as well. Cells are arranged in a complex interdigitating fashion, and few mitoses are present. Psammoma bodies may be seen in the wall of the cyst. Unilateral oophorectomy is the treatment of choice, except in the perimenopausal patient, in whom bilateral oophorectomy and hysterectomy are usually done.

Mucinous Cystadenomas

Mucinous cystadenomas are second only to serous cystadenomas in frequency of occurrence. They can attain an enormous size, and on average are much larger than serous tumors (Fig. 34–1). Their name is derived from their thick, mucinous content. Although the tumors were formerly called pseudomucinous cystadenomas because of their predominantly glycoprotein content, Fisher's histochemical studies in 1954 showed the contents to be similar to the mucin of the intestinal mucosa, namely an acid-mucopolysaccharide. As in all cystic tumors, hemorrhage may occur and change the fluid from colorless to dark brown. These tumors are notably multilocular, with walls of variable thickness and surface color that changes according to wall thickness. Thinner portions of the cyst walls are darker because the contents absorb light. The thicker areas in the wall may contain innumerable small locules that constantly increase in size; thus the tumor grows. Likewise, the cyst's contents increase by secretory action of the cells, adding to the cystic expansion. Gross papillary excrescences on the outer surface and within the cyst are characteristic of malignant change. The tumors are bilateral in 10% to 15% of cases; thus, when a unilateral tumor is encountered, the opposite ovary should be inspected carefully to make certain it does not contain a small cyst. Mucinous cysts become secondarily malignant in a small percentage of cases (Novak and Woodruff, 10%). When mucinous cystadenomas are encountered in young women, unilateral adnexal removal is indicated; in women over 40 years of age, bilateral oophorectomy is usually advisable because of the frequency of bilateral occurrence. Embryologically, these benign neoplastic cysts of the ovary are considered to be mesothelial in origin, arising from the coelomic epithelium of the ovarian surface. However, their exact origin has provoked many differing theories. Not infrequently, mucinous tumors contain mixtures of serous and endometrial elements. They are lined by a single area of tall columnar cells that resemble intestinal epithelium; often there is a variety of cells simulating the endocervical epithelium.

Although most benign serous and mucinous tumors can be diagnosed correctly by appearance, a view of the inner lining is necessary to make the diagnosis certain. The cyst should be removed intact. Because the cyst may be difficult to deliver through the abdominal opening, the surgeon is tempted to insert a trocar into these cysts to drain their contents.

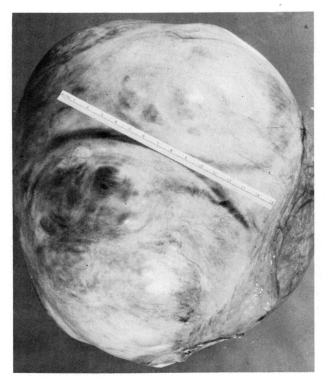

FIG. 34–1 Mucinous cystadenoma of the ovary.

Instead, the incision should be enlarged to permit the removal of the intact tumor because of the risk of seeding the peritoneum with malignant cancer cells.

Pseudomyxoma peritonei, a benign disease process involving the peritoneum, may result when a mucinous cyst ruptures and secreting cells are transplanted into the peritoneum. Sometimes pseudomyxoma peritonei is present at the time of laparotomy without evidence of cystic rupture. Although the complication is infrequent (2% to 3%), when it occurs, it can be a troublesome treatment problem and must be differentiated by frozen section study from epithelial cancer. Surgery is usually advised for removal of as much of the pseudomyxoma peritoneal implants as possible. The current technique of instilling a liter of 5% glucose and water into the peritoneal cavity as a mucolytic agent has proven quite effective. The mucopolysaccharide effusion can be removed by paracentesis an hour later and the instillation repeated as often as necessary. Laparoscopic surveillance of the peritoneal implants is an effective method of following pseudomyxoma peritonei. In most cases, adjunct chemotherapy is required to control this low-grade malignancy. This treatment avoids the necessity of a repeat laparotomy.

Brenner Tumors

Brenner tumors are rare (1% to 2% of all ovarian tumors), solid, and usually benign (99%). They are important because, like fibromas and theca cell tumors, their clinical characteristics cannot be distinguished from those of malignant tumors, and laparotomy is required for diagnosis. In addition, approximately one-third of the cases are associated with other genital cancers.

Microscopically, Brenner tumors are easily identified by characteristic islands of epithelial cells dispersed in a dense fibrous stroma. The epithelial component is transitional, with the capacity to develop squamous epithelium or mucinous epithelium (Fig. 34–2).

Brenner initially described the tumor's histology erroneously; he believed the tumor to originate from granulosa cells. The similarity of Brenner tumor cells, which have a diagonal groove across the nucleus, to Walthard's cells, which also have this distinctive grooved nucleus, led to the assumption that they had a common origin. Only recently has the origin from the surface germinal epithelium of the ovary been established for Brenner tumors. Brenner tumors, like other germinal epithelial neoplasms, arise from embryonic coelomic epithelium that has undergone metaplastic change.

The Brenner tumor develops similarly to an adenofibroma of the ovary by invaginating from the surface epithelium into the ovarian stroma. Brenner tumors are only symptomatic by large size and weight. Because their blood supply is ample, necrosis does not occur. Even during palpation there is no pain to indicate their presence. Their mobility and firm consistency resemble those of a pedunculated uterine myoma; however, since the patient is usually postmenopausal, confusion with fibroma or theca cell tumor of the ovary is more likely. All three tumors share common growth characteristics: smooth lobulated surfaces, firmness, shades of gray and yellow color, and occasionally exaggerated surface blood vessels. Roentgenograms may demonstrate foci of calcification in any of the three.

Brenner tumors are benign and oophorectomy is ample surgery; however, hysterectomy is usually advised because 10% to 15% of these patients will have endometrial hyperplasia, which is often a cause for vaginal bleeding in this older age group. Steroid hormones have been demonstrated by histochemical staining in the hyperplastic stromal cells surrounding the epithelial islands.

When metaplasia of the epithelial cells occurs, a typical mucinous epithelium may develop and, in turn, become cystic; thus, Brenner tumors are not uncommonly associated with mucinous cysts. Al-

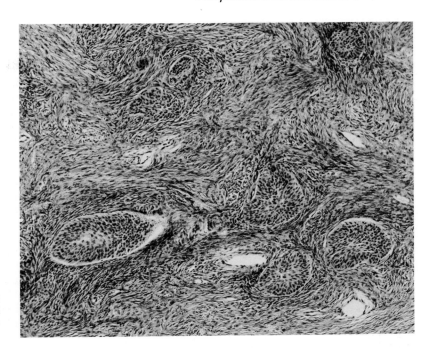

FIG. 34–2 Section of Brenner tumor. The islands of benign epithelium interspersed within the hyperplastic ovarian stroma distinguish it from the ordinary fibroma.

though this tumor is easily diagnosed histologically and easily cured by simple removal, it is a rather complex tumor that can have many histologic variations.

MALIGNANT EPITHELIAL TUMORS

The mucosa of the fallopian tube, endometrium, endocervix, and mesothelium of the peritoneal cavity that covers the ovary develop from embryonic coelomic epithelium through the intermediate development of müllerian ducts. Thus, epithelial cancers of the ovary share a common origin with other gynecologic cancers, as well as with the peritoneum. If the peritoneum holds a potential to generate these tumors, perhaps some of the peritoneal implants from serous carcinoma of the ovary are not metastases but rather separate foci of origin. This mechanism would explain how pelvic serous carcinoma could develop after both ovaries have been removed.

In the past, the reputation of mucinous tumors for being more benign than serous tumors served as a guideline for prognosis. We now understand that mucinous carcinomas are more often well-differentiated. When poorly differentiated mucinous carcinomas occur, the prognosis is not at all favorable. If the group of borderline malignancies is excluded, then Stage I serous, mucinous, and endometrioid carcinomas have similar 5-year survival: for Stage I, grade 1 and grade 2 carcinomas, the survival rate is nearly 65%. The difference in survival among epithelial types of the same stage relates mainly to the histologic grading of the tumor. Mixtures of histologic types often exist among ovarian cancers; for example, serous and endometrioid tumors often exist together. This finding is not surprising considering that both stem from the coelomic epithelium covering the ovary. Histologic categorization is only possible when there is a well to moderately differentiated pattern. A large category of undifferentiated tumors is made up primarily of serous components, and these tumors are usually quite advanced. Endometrioid carcinoma, especially, must be well differentiated before the glandular pattern can be recognized. The clinical impression of endometrioid carcinoma as a more benign tumor is probably due to the fact that it is more differentiated. This favorable impression is not true, however, for mesonephroid or clear cell carcinomas, which carry especially grave prognoses if they have extended beyond the ovary. These large clear cell tumors behave clinically as undifferentiated tumors and should be considered as grade 3 lesions.

As the study of epithelial tumors expands, more acceptance is being given to the concept that mixtures are common and that histologic grade will supersede histologic type as an indicator of clinical aggressiveness and sensitivity to treatment when surgery is incomplete. The curability of any cancer may be cast by the biologic behavior indicated by the grade of differentiation. The rapidity of division, the ability to metastasize, and resistance to drugs and ionizing irradiation are all determined by the grade of the tumor, and it appears that the tumor stage encountered at any one time is also largely determined by tumor grade.

Grading is difficult and often imprecise. Some pathologists have little confidence that grading can be done accurately because the histologic grade of cells varies significantly among different areas of a tumor mass. For clinicians, the grade of the tumor is still one of the most important prognostic factors. Tumor grade influences important decisions about the use of chemotherapy. The importance of histologic grading does not suggest that we should abandon the determination of histologic type. Histologic types of tumors, such as serous, mucinous, and endometrioid, have clinical usefulness, especially since refinements in determinations and treatment are almost certain to come.

Other observations also aid in the diagnosis and selection of the proper treatment for ovarian cancer. Awareness of the patient's age helps. For example, children and teenage girls rarely have epithelial type tumors but almost exclusively have germ cell tumors. When epithelial tumors do develop in youth, they are usually mucinous tumors. Stromal cell, Brenner, and mesenchymal tumors occur in the older age groups. Patients under 30 years of age have better differentiated tumors than older patients and a lower stage of disease at the time of diagnosis, and this is compatible with the better prognosis for patients under 40 years of age with epithelial ovarian cancer. Epithelial tumors generally do not cause stimulation of the endometrium, nor do they influence menstruation. In a general sense, they are nonfunctional; yet, they may produce some sex steroids. They also have hormone receptors and may be retarded by hormone treatment. However, there is no evidence that estrogen replacement therapy is harmful if youthful patients with ovarian cancer are given hormone supplements when bilateral oophorectomy is necessary. Dembo and Bush have shown that tumor grade and postsurgical residual tumor volume are the most important prognostic variables, followed by stage, age, and cell type of origin.

Mucinous Carcinoma

Mucinous carcinoma has been assigned a mesothelial origin, although these tumors relate less to other epithelial tumors than do the serous types. Benign mucinous cysts of the pelvic peritoneum are not found, but serous cysts of the peritoneum do occur. The columnar epithelium resembles the mucosal lining of the intestine. Some intestinal enzymes are produced by mucinous tumors. These tumors show notably elevated CEA (carcinoembryonic antigen) serum levels. Mucinous carcinoma constitutes approximately 10% of ovarian malignancies.

Serous Carcinoma

Like mucinous lesions, serous tumors may be as large as 15 cm in diameter. Often, the major portion of the mass is cystic and, when the tumors are well-differentiated, psammoma bodies are present. Grade 3 lesions are more solid and less papillary, and there is a greater likelihood for areas of necrosis in the middle of the tumor. The epithelium of the more differentiated tumors shows a variety of cells identifiable as tubal epithelium. This epithelium may include ciliated cells and mucin-producing cells. Serous carcinoma constitutes approximately 45% of ovarian malignancies.

Endometrioid Carcinoma

The origin of ovarian endometrioid carcinoma continues to be debated, and little progress toward resolution has been made over the past 20 years. There is strong evidence that these tumors develop from a müllerian origin through a process of coelomic metaplasia. The potential for the coelomic epithelium to develop structure, such as endometrium, is now accepted, and metaplasia of the coelomic epithelium covering the ovary can thus account for an endometrioma of the ovary as well as for endometrioid carcinoma of the ovary. Both occurrences have been observed in the same patient.

There seems to be a clear relationship between the existence of endometriosis and the development of endometrioid carcinoma of the ovary. Ovarian endometriosis is associated with about 10% to 15% of the cases, and pelvic endometriosis occurs in approximately 28%. The incidence does not warrant prophylactic resection of endometriosis to prevent endometrioid carcinoma of the ovary. However, surgery may be necessary to establish a diagnosis when there is an adnexal mass. Very rarely can a pathologist demonstrate a transformation between benign endometriosis and adenocarcinoma of the ovary, a requirement that was mandated originally by Sampson.

Endometrioid carcinoma of the ovary is associated with endometrial carcinoma in 15% to 26% of patients. This association necessitates determining whether the ovarian carcinoma has metastasized to the endometrium or the reverse, or whether a primary endometrial carcinoma and a primary endometrioid carcinoma of the ovary developed independently.

Endometrioid carcinoma is usually made up predominantly of glandular tissue. However, a patient will occasionally show an overshadowing of the stromal components. An endometrioid carcinoma must be at least moderately well-differentiated, otherwise it is not recognized histologically. The epithelium shows intracellular mucin, and occasionally there are subnucleic vacuoles like those noted in the endometrium under progestational stimulation. Some show clear histologic patterns, and not infrequently the tumors are mixed with small amounts of serous and mucinous epithelium.

Clear Cell Carcinoma

Perhaps one of the most controversial of the epithelial carcinomas is the clear cell (mesonephroid) variety. Unlike the serous or mucinous types, it does not present an intermediate gradation between the well-differentiated and the undifferentiated type. Most often it is undifferentiated. It has not been convincingly demonstrated that this cancer is distinct from endometrioid carcinoma of the ovary; however, it is associated more often with endometriosis than is endometrioid carcinoma of the ovary. Clear cell carcinoma seems to originate from endometriosis in approximately 25% of the reported cases. The histology is rendered very distinctive by a clear cell vacuolated cytoplasm that contains an abundance of glycogen. Occasionally, short papillae are seen, and the epithelium covering the papillae is of the hobnail variety.

It is not difficult to understand why this tumor was originally believed to arise from remnants of primitive mesonephric tubules since these large clear cells are reminiscent of hypernephroma. The tumor is solid and rarely bilateral. Of special interest is the association with hypercalcemia in approximately 30% of the patients. The calcium-mobilizing action of the tumor may complicate treatment. The median survival time is shorter than for other histologic types of ovarian epithelial carcinoma. The prognosis has generally been very poor and control by all three treatment methods has been disappointing.

GERM CELL TUMORS

The pathology of germ cell tumors is complex. Not only do the individual tumors contain multiple patterns, but also there are often mixtures containing elements of other types. A diagnosis often requires special technical processing of the tissue, and consultation among pathologists may be required for diagnostic confirmation.

Although gynecologists are urged to develop skills in the gross pathology and histopathology of ovarian tumors, this is not practical or necessary for germ cell tumors. It is important for the pathologist to be diligent in fixing and sampling these large tumors and to search comprehensively for the correct diagnosis. Treatment must be individualized for each tumor type. In obtaining a basic knowledge of germ cell tumors, clinicians should be aware of the following factors:

Ovarian tumors in children and young adults are usually of the germ cell type.

When epithelial cancer appears in youth, it is usually a well-differentiated mucinous variety.

With a well-differentiated epithelial tumor, there may be no need to remove the normal-appearing contralateral ovary or uterus, since only a small proportion of patients have involvement of both ovaries.

An accurate diagnosis of dysgerminoma is of major clinical importance, for an error can lead to inappropriate treatment.

A clear cell tumor in children may be either embryonal or endodermal sinus type, but the distinction is of minimal clinical importance.

Testing for tumor products aids diagnosis and helps in monitoring the success of treatment.

Interpretation of histopathology has been immensely aided by the development of immunopathology. Some tumors produce specific substances to which an antibody can be produced, and fluorescent staining and radioactive tagging of specific cells is now possible through immunologic techniques. Specific cells with secretory functions or receptor capacity can be identified, and many diagnostic tests can be performed on preserved specimens, as with a paraffin preparation. To date, these techniques are used mostly in research. However, those methods found practical will soon be introduced to laboratories. In time, with development of monoclonal antibody technology, we hope to have a new therapy involving the use of tumor products of germ cell tumors.

In spite of the many advances in diagnostic methods, germ cell tumors as a group remain complex. Though they share some clinical and pathologic features, each has distinctive properties that merit restating.

Mature Teratomas

Mature teratomas are cystic and benign. The term *dermoid* was formerly applied to them because their contents resembled cysts of the dermis that also contained squamous epithelium and elements of skin appendages (Figs. 34–3 and 34–4). The products of these tissues become the cyst's contents. Typically, these contents consist of oily sebaceous material that is liquid at body temperature. Thus,

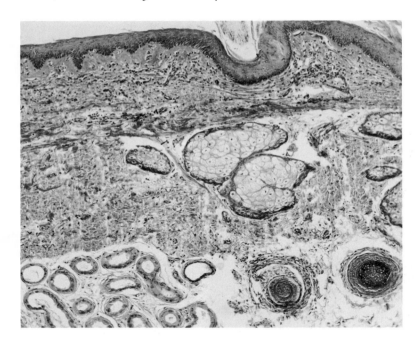

FIG. 34–3 Wall of a dermoid cyst, showing stratified squamous epithelial surface, sebaceous glands, sweat glands, and hair follicle.

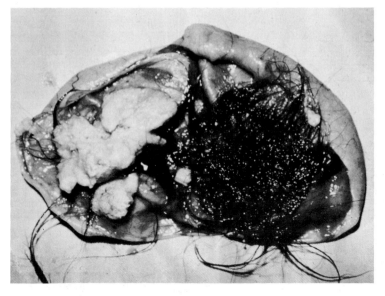

FIG. 34–4 Dermoid cyst of ovary. Cyst has been opened and sebaceous contents and a ball of hair are pouring forth.

the dermoid is soft when palpated *in situ*. When allowed to cool, the content becomes firm and no longer feels cystic.

Mature teratomas account for 27% of all primary ovarian neoplasms and 38% of those that are benign. They do not appear before menarche but may occur at any later age. They are usually discovered in the late teenage years during pelvic examination. They range from small, microscopic lesions to very large tumors, but they are usually no larger than 10 cm. Large-sized mature teratomas may be present and

asymptomatic for a long time before discovery, and recovery is usually complete on removal. The small risk of infarction or rupture, along with the small chance of malignancy (1% to 2%), give sufficient reason for prompt removal.

Mature teratomas occasionally cause pain when they twist their vascular pedicle. The vascular pedicle is ample and usually permits the tumor to seek a comfortable space, usually posterior to the uterus. Because of the tumor's weight, it often settles in the lowest part of the pelvic cavity; however, mature teratomas are notable for positioning anterior to the respective broad ligament, where they are easily palpated and are occasionally obvious to the patient. This rather distinctive trait is clinically useful and often permits preoperative diagnosis.

Mature teratomas may be diagnosed by roentgenography of the abdomen, which can show the presence of bone or rudimentary teeth lying free within the cyst or incorporated within the cyst wall. The roentgenographic shadow of the cyst often creates a "halo" effect along the surface of the tumor. This shadow is produced by the sebaceous material rather than by the hair that is often found as part of the cyst's content. Although epidermal elements predominate, there are endodermal and mesodermal elements. The epithelium is most frequently skin, gastrointestinal, respiratory, salivary gland, and neuroepithelium tissue. Occasionally, only one epidermal element is present, and this often forms tumors of a highly differentiated tissue type, such as struma ovarii (thyroid) or carcinoid.

Approximately 5% to 10% of mature teratomas are bilateral, and sometimes the contralateral dermoid will be subclinical in size. Routinely incising the contralateral ovary during laparotomy when it appears normal is no longer a recommended procedure. We have learned that such practice is conducive to formation of cysts and adhesions about the ovary and may be a source of pain or infertility.

Surgery for mature teratomas can be conservative because only the tumor needs excision. The clear limits of the tumor allow separation by blunt dissection from the uninvolved ovarian tissue along an avascular plane (Fig. 34–5). Although the ovary may be distorted by the tumor, its function remains normal. Since mature teratomas present at the age when fertility is crucial, every effort should be made to shell out the tumor and to conserve the ovary. Typically, the residual ovarian tissue is flattened on the surface of the cyst. Often the first impression appears unfavorable for preservation; yet, generally speaking, the boundaries of the uninvolved part of the ovary can be identified and separation can be accomplished.

Small amounts of thyroid are frequently found in ovarian teratomas. Rarely, the thyroid tissue appears to overgrow all other elements, and such tumors may be properly called struma ovarii. The potential for struma ovarii to produce hyperthyroidism has fascinated clinicians for years, but in fact it rarely does so. Of the more than 400 reported cases of struma ovarii, only about 40 (10%) have been found to be metabolically active and to have produced hyperthyroidism. The products of these tumors occasionally become clinically important, and although the possibility is remote, errors in management have occurred. It is a disservice to the patient to ablate the normal thyroid with radioactive

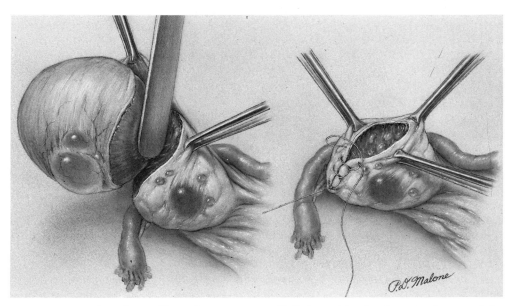

FIG. 34–5 Resection of a small cyst from an ovary. (*Left*) An incision has been made around the ovary near the junction of the cyst wall and normal ovarian tissue. The knife handle is a convenient instrument for shelling out the cyst. (*Right*) The defect in the ovary is closed with a continuous lock stitch of No. 3-0 or smaller delayed-absorbable suture on an atraumatic needle. A subcapsular suture may be placed along the undersurface of the tunica to prevent ovarian and tubal adhesions.

iodine when an ovarian struma is at fault. Not only is the histologic picture of the thyroid tissue unmistakable, but its true nature can be demonstrated by determination of its iodine content. Radioactive iodine uptake has been demonstrated in the thyroid tissue in the ovary, although the ovarian struma is usually not overactive. Fewer than 20 cases (5%) have been reported in which struma ovarii have metastasized to the liver, bone, brain, mediastinum, and other extra-ovarian sites.

Immature Teratomas

Immature and mature teratomas must be closely related, since they share the unusual ability to produce tumor from ectoderm, endoderm, and mesoderm. The immature ovarian teratoma grows rapidly and appears in children or young girls. The mature (benign) variety usually appears 10 or more years later.

Although the composition of a malignant teratoma is very mixed and the extradermal elements are always prominent, some are monodermal. In the immature teratoma group, there is a range of malignancies classified by the proportion of well-differentiated components. Evaluation of the maturity of the neuroepithelium, a common component, has been helpful to clinicians in establishing the prognosis of individual tumors. Some patients with seemingly serious tumor spread have been observed to tolerate peritoneal metastasis without treatment if the metastases are composed of mature glial tissue. In the past some patients with these conditions were treated excessively. Studies by Norris, Zirkin, and Benson, and by Robboy and Scully, have added a new dimension to clinical management by providing the following guidelines.

An immature teratoma shares characteristics common to other germ cell tumors, such as large size, rapid growth, central necrosis, and hemorrhage. Symptoms caused by pressure of the tumor on adjacent pelvic organs are also frequent. In comparison with the mature teratoma, the immature tumor is highly malignant and presents very different problems in treatment. Surgical excision, which is adequate for the mature teratoma, rarely cures the immature type; therefore, postoperative chemotherapy has become an important type of adjunctive therapy.

Germ cell tumors are rarely bilateral. Therefore, a normal-appearing contralateral ovary should be preserved.

The immature teratoma is radioresistant, and therefore postoperative roentgen therapy has little effect on unresected masses or on the prevention of recurrence. The most successful adjunctive therapy has been multiagent chemotherapy. Experience at the M. D. Anderson Hospital first demonstrated that combinations of vincristine, actinomycin-D, and cyclophosphamide (VAC) were effective, both in the prevention of recurrences and in obtaining regression where there is unresectable tumor present. The VAC combination may be modified by substitution of adriamycin for actinomycin-D. A more recent combination of vinblastine, bleomycin, and cis-platinum (VBP) has also shown activity with this disease and may ultimately become the preferred treatment when the histology is grade 3.

The VBP combination is more toxic than VAC; thus, considering the small improvement of VBP over VAC, the latter is preferred when prognostic factors are better. Gallion and colleagues noted in their review that 2-year to 7-year survival with single-agent adjunctive chemotherapy was 64% in comparison to a 77% response with combination chemotherapy. This suggests that less toxic single-agent treatment may be adequate for some patients.

The first patients treated successively with VAC at M. D. Anderson Hospital had treatment continuing for 24 months whenever it could be tolerated. When the toxic effects of vincristine appeared, the chemotherapy was continued with cyclophosphamide alone. The current protocol terminates chemotherapy after 12 months if the second-look operation proves negative, or if any residual disease is composed entirely of mature glial tissue. Some physicians are now advising much shorter periods of adjunctive chemotherapy and earlier second-look procedures. More experience is needed to determine the optimum number of courses of chemotherapy and to determine which patients are suited for surgery alone and which for surgery accompanied by VAC, VBP, or single-agent chemotherapy. There is little support for postoperative irradiation as a treatment method. One cannot judge the therapeutic results for an immature teratoma without relating survivals to the histologic grade. Norris, Zirkin, and Benson note survival as 81% for grade 1; 60% for grade 2; and 30% for grade 3. Gallion and colleagues' review of patients with a pure immature teratoma recorded the influence of stage alone:

Stage	Number of Patients	2-year Survival
Ia	65	65%
Ic	3	33%
II	15	40%
III	19	32%
IV	2	50%

It is expected that these survivals will be improved by adjunctive chemotherapy as applied in recent years.

Dysgerminoma

Dysgerminoma, the most common germ cell tumor, is unique because of its sensitivity to irradiation and its greater tendency for bilateral occurrence (11%) as compared to other germ cell tumors. This tumor comprises 1% to 2% of all ovarian neoplasms. The tumor is also notorious for lymphatic metastasis. Along with other germ cell tumors, the dysgerminoma grows rapidly, becomes large, and is prone to necrosis, hemorrhage, and rupture. It occurs during youth, although the average patient age is one or two decades older than that of patients with other germ cell tumors. The dysgerminoma often contains elements of embryonal carcinoma or choriocarcinoma and may develop from a benign gonadoblastoma. It is this risk of progression of a gonadoblastoma to a dysgerminoma that is the basis for gonadectomy in females with gonadal dysgenesis and a Y-containing genotype. The majority of dysgerminomas develop in normal ovaries.

Dysgerminomas are hormonally inactive, although they may produce small amounts of α-fetoprotein or human chorionic gonadotropin (hCG) when they are of a mixed variety. These tumor products from a dysgerminoma indicate components of endodermal sinus cancer and trophoblastic cells. The products of a dysgerminoma do not interfere with fertility and, thus, are not uncommonly discovered during pregnancy (15%).

The symptoms are not distinctive. Pain signals the tumor's presence in 50% of the patients. The histopathologic diagnosis is not difficult. The cells resemble primordial germ cells and have a potential for differentiation into either embryonic or extraembryonic tissue. The cells are of uniform size and the intervening stroma is interspersed with clusters of lymphocytes, which aid in the diagnosis of this tumor.

The curability of this tumor is nearly 100%, and even when recurrences develop, 70% of patients are cured. Seventy-five percent of all recurrences occur within 1 year of the original diagnosis. Failure to cure happens most often when there is a mixture with radioresistant components from other germ cell tumor types. When such foreign elements are present, they survive irradiation and regrow as pure forms with their own characteristic histologic patterns. A thorough search by multiple sampling of the tumor for these other germ cell components is vitally important for determining the appropriate treatment. For example, a dysgerminoma with embryonal or choriocarcinoma components should be treated with multiagent chemotherapy rather than roentgen therapy, which would otherwise be the ideal adjunct treatment for dysgerminoma. The high frequency of lymph node metastasis dictates that a para-aortic lymphadenectomy should be done for a more accurate staging of the disease. Conservative therapy consisting of unilateral salpingo-oophorectomy may be performed in the absence of intra-abdominal or para-aortic node metastases. If para-aortic node or intra-abdominal metastases are detected, total abdominal hysterectomy and bilateral salpingo-oophorectomy followed by whole-abdomen irradiation is the treatment of choice. An irradiation boost is given to the para-aortic, mediastinal, and supraclavicular lymph node regions if the para-aortic nodes are involved with tumor. Chemotherapy, similar to that for immature teratoma, is indicated when the extent of disease precludes the use of curative irradiation therapy.

Endodermal Sinus Tumors

Among germ cell tumors, endodermal sinus tumors are second to dysgerminoma in frequency of occurrence. They are aggressive, highly malignant cancers afflicting girls and young women. Until the development of chemotherapy, the usual survival ranged between 12 and 18 months. Clinically, these tumors grow rapidly to reach a diameter as large as 30 cm and spread extensively throughout the peritoneal cavity. Metastases to the liver add to the problems of therapy. The duration of illness is short, the tumor is large, and there is pain. Hemorrhage and necrosis produce signs and symptoms of an acute abdominal catastrophe. As with dysgerminoma, spread to the lymph nodes is an important aspect of the metastatic pattern.

Much clinical experience from earlier years has been lost because the pathogenesis and histology were uncertain and patients were diagnosed erroneously. The endodermal sinus tumor was confused with renal carcinoma, clear cell carcinoma of the ovary, and embryonal carcinoma. Currently, the endodermal sinus tumor is believed to arise from germ cells that differentiated from extraembryonic tissue. They arise from the yolk-sac remnants and migrate with the germ cells to the ovarian analog. Endodermal sinus tumors differ from embryonal tumors by retaining some yolk-sac and vitelline structures in their architecture and by producing specific tumor products, such as α-fetoprotein. The endometrial sinus tumor can be distinguished microscopically by a loose network of microcysts, among which appears a pseudopapillary pattern produced by epithelial cells arranged endwise about a capillary. This unique microscopic structure is named the *Shiller–Duval body*. The presence of α-fetoprotein tumor products is strongly indicative of this type of tumor, for while other types of germ cell tumors produce this product, the quantity is much larger in the endodermal sinus tumor. It can be measured in the serum and can also be demonstrated by immunoperoxidase stains in the cells of the endodermal sinus tumor. Alpha-fetoprotein concentrations tend to correlate with the stage and extent of the disease. Treatment consists of surgical removal of all visible tumor, followed by combination chemotherapy. Preservation of the contralateral ovary is indicated when it appears normal, since the disease rarely occurs bilaterally.

In 1976, Kurman and Norris extended Teilum's 1976 observations, directing subsequent research toward correct histogenic classification. These reports, as well as those by Jimerson and Woodruff, who studied 41 patients in 1977, emphasized the lethal character of this disease. Survivals were rare, although the majority of endodermal sinus tumors are Stage Ia. In 1975, Smith and Rutledge showed improved survival with multiagent chemotherapy, and in 1983 Gershenson and colleagues extended this report with a current analysis of the experience at the M. D. Anderson Hospital with 41 patients. Notable features in this series were:

Stage	Patients (Percent)
I	21 (51%)
IIb	5 (12%)
III	15 (37%)

Symptoms (median duration)	4 weeks
Palpable mass	76%
Fever	32%
Median diameter	17 cm

Results of Chemotherapy

Drugs	Number of Patients	2-Year Survival
ActFuCy	5	40%
VAC	22	72%
Velban-bleomycin	2	100%

These results show responsiveness of this tumor to chemotherapy. Since there are few recurrences after 2 years, the projected 5-year survival should exceed 65%. It is hoped that more extended median survivals will be observed as observation time lengthens. In the use of multiagent chemotherapy there is a significant improvement of survival in Stages I and II, but this is yet to be demonstrated in Stage III. There is no effective second-line chemotherapy following the use of one of the above multiagent regimens. There is an occasional cure by oophorectomy alone, but most patients require adjunctive treatment. Multiagent chemotherapy is recommended adjunctively after complete or incomplete removal of the tumor by surgery and after recurrence when surgery fails.

Embryonal Carcinoma

Embryonal carcinoma is the least differentiated of the germ cell tumors and may be considered a stem tumor from which a teratoma, endodermal sinus tumor, or choriocarcinoma may develop. It is closely related to the endodermal sinus tumor by the production of α-fetoprotein and to choriocarcinoma by the production of hCG. Embryonal carcinoma may develop in any of three cellular directions or combinations: (1) embryonal, teratomatous structures, (2) extraembryonal (yolk sac or vitelline [endodermal sinus]), or (3) choriocarcinoma.

The embryonal tumor resembles other germ cell tumors in gross appearance and symptomatology. It is soft, friable, and prone to necrosis and hemorrhage. The size ranges from 5 cm to 25 cm in diameter, and the surface capsule is penetrated in about one-third of the cases. Histologically, the tumor contains a variety of cellular patterns and is notable for variations in histologic appearance. Histologically, the tumor contains high mitotic activity and bizarre-appearing nuclei. Often the cells are arranged in syncytial patterns. The cells may be large, with extensive vacuolization; the stroma is notably scanty; there are multinucleated giant cells; and syncytiotrophoblastic cells can be identified by immunoperoxidase stain for hCG.

Although these tumors are usually hormonally inactive, when trophoblastic cells are present there may be sufficient hCG production to excite precocious puberty, to result in a positive pregnancy test, and to produce vaginal bleeding in a young child. Since the capsule is often penetrated by the tumor cells, hemorrhagic ascites is frequent. Pain is frequent and severe and is often dealt with on an emergency basis.

The treatment is the same as for endodermal sinus tumors: complete surgical resection of the cancer followed with vincristine, adriamycin, and cyclophosphamide chemotherapy. If unresectable residual tumor is present, the surgery is followed with vinblastine, bleomycin, and cis-platinum chemotherapy. For Stage Ia disease, unilateral oophorectomy is ample surgery, since this tumor rarely develops in both ovaries. However, para-aortic lymph node sampling and assessment is mandatory for all malignant germ-cell tumors to determine the presence or absence of occult lymphatic spread. Irradiation treatment has not been proven to be effective. Beta hCG and alpha fetoprotein levels should be followed during and after therapy for both embryonal carcinoma and endodermal sinus tumors.

STROMAL TUMORS

Stromal tumors comprise granulosa cell, theca cell, Sertoli–Leydig cell, gynandroblastoma and unclassified sex cord tumors (listed in declining frequency). Stromal tumors represent 3% to 5% of malignant ovarian tumors. They have received much attention in the literature because of their hormonal production, which may be estrogenic or androgenic. Theca cell tumors are consistently estrogenic, but granulosa cell tumors may produce testosterone and progesterone, as well as estradiol; thus, some granulosa cell tumors are virilizing. When this occurs, the androgen secretion usually stems from stromal cell hyperplasia within the ovary. Gynandroblastomas are rare stromal tumors that include both theca cell tumor and arrhenoblastoma elements and may produce both estrogen and androgen.

The effects of the hormonal secretions of ovarian stromal tumors (80% are active) may be the most notable symptoms. Inappropriate menstruation at the wrong age should alert the clinician to the possibility of granulosa cell or theca cell tumors. When androgens are produced, oligomenorrhea or amenorrhea, hirsutism, breast atrophy, alopecia, vocal cord changes, and skeletal muscle hypertrophy occur. A small increase in the incidence of adenocarcinoma of the endometrium can be expected among these patients because of the excess estrogen secretion. Such adenocarcinomas have a favorable prognosis because of their low grade and superficial myometrial invasion.

Granulosa Cell Tumors

A granulosa cell tumor may develop at any time from premenarche to late menopause. The size varies from nonpalpable to 10 cm to 15 cm in diameter. Since this tumor often grows slowly there is a longer time span within which to discover the less symptomatic, smaller neoplasm. The slower growth also allows the vascular supply to keep pace with the tumor so that rupture occurs less frequently than with germ cell tumors. Mixtures of granulosa and theca cell elements are common in a tumor that is called a granulosa cell tumor. In the firm, compact tumor there is a large theca cell component, but if the composition of the tumor is pure granulosa cells, it is softer. Cysts may partially surface, thereby causing the tumor to grossly resemble a teratoma.

Although some granulosa cell tumors have a benign, slow growth, others are more malignant, with rapid growth and recurrence following soon after

excision. Women below age 40 have the more benign tumor. This observation is reliable enough to support unilateral oophorectomy for a Stage Ia lesion when fertility is desired or when the diagnosis becomes known postoperatively and the contralateral ovary has not been removed. In women past the childbearing age, bilateral oophorectomy and hysterectomy are warranted. Postoperative irradiation to the pelvic region or the entire abdomen may be considered; however, there is no consensus regarding the need or benefit of postoperative irradiation. When there is a large theca cell component, the granulosa cell tumor is more benign. Unfortunately, when the histology is wholly granulosa cells, assessing the degree of anaplasia is not very helpful in predicting clinical behavior. Since the true malignancy of this tumor cannot be determined until the patient has been followed for 10 to 20 years, it is preferable to consider all granulosa cell tumors as malignant. Kottmeier had 5-year cure rates of 68% for granulosa and theca cell tumors grouped together, but 10% recurred 5 or more years later. Patients who exhibited late recurrences had slow-growing tumors. For these patients another operation for resection might succeed for a long interval.

A granulosa cell tumor may be confused histologically with a small-cell, undifferentiated serous carcinoma of the ovary or with a fallopian tube cancer. Carcinoid tumors are occasionally mistaken for granulosa cell tumors, but the resemblance is only superficial since the granulosa cell tumor has few mitoses. Some granulosa cells arrange in small circles and resemble ova with a homogenous, pink center containing proteinaceous material. This complex is termed a Call–Exner body and is characteristically present in 50% of these tumors. In addition, nuclear grooving is typical for sex cord tumors, and if observed may help distinguish the granulosa tumor from other tumors with similar size cells, compactness, and architectural arrangement.

If surgery is incomplete or recurrence develops, or if irradiation treatment is not appropriate, chemotherapy should be used. Chemotherapeutic drugs are less effective for stromal tumors of the ovary than for epithelial types. Most of the reports in the literature deal with single-agent therapy, but the frequency of tumor response is low. The new trend is to use multiagent therapy, but there is little experience available by which to judge results. Among the few patients at M. D. Anderson who received actinomycin-D, 5-fluorouracil, and cyclophosphamide (ActFuCy), two had long-term, complete regression of tumor.

Theca Cell Tumors

A pure theca cell tumor is benign and is often called a thecoma. Cases reported in the literature as "malignant thecoma" are probably fibrosarcomas of the ovary. Theca cell tumors are notable for causing postmenopausal uterine bleeding because of their estrogenic production. Endometrial hyperplasia and adenocarcinoma should be looked for when a firm ovarian tumor is discovered in a postmenopausal woman. Hysterectomy with bilateral salpingo-oophorectomy cures almost 100% of these tumors.

Sertoli–Leydig Cells (Arrhenoblastoma)

This rare ovarian neoplasm has more notoriety in the scientific literature than its clinical importance merits. Hormonal function and masculinization of patients (80%) make case-reporting interesting. Breast atrophy, reduced subcutaneous fat, amenorrhea, changes in body contour, hypertrophy of the clitoris, excess body hair, acne, and deepening of the voice are all symptoms that point to elevated plasma androgens. These findings plus an ovarian mass indicate a need for pelvic laparotomy, but prior to surgery a serum level of DHEA-sulfate for adrenal hyperplasia is helpful in the differential diagnosis. The test makes use of the presence of high serum levels of dehydroepiandrosterone sulfate and cortisone suppression of the adrenals.

Histologically, the tumor consists of a combination of tubules and interstitial cells of Leydig. Some tumors contain a hyperplasia of the Sertoli cells that line the glandular component (tubules) of the neoplasm and may produce an elevation in the serum estrogen level.

Some Sertoli–Leydig cell tumors are malignant, even when the histologic pattern appears innocuous. Regional recurrences and distant metastases may ultimately cause death. Few data are available about radiosensitivity and chemotherapy responsiveness because of the rarity of this tumor. Although the same Sertoli–Leydig cell tumor may imply a mixture of the relatively distinctive types of cells, some tumors are pure. Excessive testosterone production and virilization cause the most spectacular clinical changes, while there is estrogen production in 20% of the cases. These tumors have an *in vitro* capacity to synthesize androstenedione and testosterone from progesterone and pregnanolone. They may occur in youth and are unilateral in 90% to 95% of cases. Conservative surgery is advised in younger patients, since the risk of malignancy is low and removing the contralateral ovary is not important for cure. Malignancy is unusual, and there is little prophylaxis because it is impossible to identify malignant varieties by histology. As with granulosa cell tumors, the prognosis correlates poorly with the histologic pattern.

Surgical Treatment of Ovarian Cancer

In the earliest stages and with the most favorable histologic types, ovarian cancers are frequently cured by surgery alone. Customarily, the treatment employs three therapeutic modalities: resection, irradiation, and chemotherapy.

Surgery is the most curative treatment. Multiple operations are often required during the management of advanced disease.

The surgeon treating ovarian cancer assumes a serious responsibility. Skill in pelvic surgery alone is not enough; the disease itself must be well understood. The surgeon should be technically able to resect large, advanced pelvic tumors as well as the metastases that frequently involve upper abdominal organs. The surgeon must be able to correct problems of the intestinal tract that are a consequence of cancer therapy and be able to search out metastases that may be subclinical. The extent of surgery required varies with the stage, cell type, and grade of the cancer. The overall cure rate based on stage of disease is shown in Table 34–1 (see p. 899). There has been little improvement in the past 30 years because 70% or more of the tumors are at advanced stages (III or IV) when diagnosed. In discussing the recommended treatment, the classification of ovarian cancer by cell type will be used as an organizational structure.

EPITHELIAL CANCER

There is no significant difference in the treatment of the various histologic types of epithelial ovarian tumors. In general, excision is considered the first line of treatment because more patients are cured by excision than by irradiation or chemotherapy without excision. The role of surgery, therefore, is of the utmost importance. Still, surgery alone is limited to the most favorable conditions, as in grade 1 and Stage Ia lesions. For the remainder of cases, postoperative adjunctive irradiation or chemotherapy, or both, should be employed, even though the resection may appear complete. Additionally, laparotomy is needed for accurate staging, which is essential in designing a comprehensive treatment plan.

Conventional surgical treatment for epithelial ovarian cancer is bilateral salpingo-oophorectomy and hysterectomy, although there are a few exceptions to this castrating treatment. An exception, for example, occurs when the contralateral ovary appears normal as in cases of Stage Ia, grade 1 disease. With willingness to accept the small risk that the contralateral ovary may be harboring subclinical metastases or even originate another cancer, the contralateral ovary may be saved. This deviation from standard treatment would be for the preservation of fertility; conservation of an ovary solely for hormone production would not be justified, since hormonal replacement therapy is highly effective.

Treatment by unilateral oophorectomy does not meet with universal acceptance. Taylor of Columbia University, Decker and, later, Williams and Dockerty from the Mayo Clinic support such treatment with an experience involving a small series of patients. Taylor and associates stipulated that the lesion must be a well-differentiated mucinous type. The Mayo Clinic studies allow for grade 1, Stage Ia mucinous or serous types. Kottmeier of Stockholm had the largest experience and thus spoke with the greatest authority in supporting selective conservatism for these special conditions. The dictum for all other patients however, remains the removal of both ovaries whenever possible, along with all resectable extra-ovarian disease.

Bilateral Salpingo-Oophorectomy and Hysterectomy

There are several factors that call for the removal of both ovaries and the uterus, even though one ovary may appear normal and the uterus may be asymptomatic. The contralateral ovary may contain a subclinical cancer and the corpus may harbor subclinical metastasis or even another primary tumor. A contralateral ovary proved normal at the time of surgery has a strong potential for developing a new lesion in the future. Removal of the ovaries without concomitant removal of the uterus could lead to difficulties should estrogen replacement therapy be elected: the endometrium could be stimulated to hyperplasia, thus causing excessive uterine bleeding. Because there is small risk of exogenous estrogen producing an endometrial carcinoma, replacement therapy is generally advised in younger patients.

There are advantages and disadvantages to removing the uterus. For some surgeons, hysterectomy is considered bad practice because the ovarian cancer, which may be incompletely removed, may then invade the top of the vagina and create vaginal bleeding and offensive vaginal discharge. When there is unresectable metastasis within the cul-de-sac of Douglas, hysterectomy may be difficult and hazardous. Kottmeier recommended conserving the uterus and using it as a receptacle for intracavitary radium. He used this method to increase the dose of irradiation to the pelvic cavity, thus accomplish-

ing a more effective dose of irradiation by external therapy with a low complication incidence. Irradiation from within the corpus has never been a popular practice in the United States, but its theoretical value is sound. For the majority of patients with epithelial carcinoma, the minimum standard resection is bilateral salpingo-oophorectomy and hysterectomy.

Omentectomy

The omentum is a frequent site of the earliest intra-abdominal metastases. Often omental metastases cannot be felt, and omentectomy therefore has value for correct staging. Opinions vary about the value of routine omentectomy for a normal-appearing omentum. Advocates favor removal as prophylaxis against recurrence in this organ, whereas others believe that removal is not effective. Whether or not the surgeon advocates omentectomy routinely, it is important that adequate sampling of the normal-looking omentum be routine procedure at the time of primary surgery and during any subsequent second-look laparotomy. Removal of the omentum containing metastases reduces tumor bulk and will be discussed in the section on tumor reduction.

Lymphadenectomy

For many years clinicians have been impressed by the intraperitoneal spread of epithelial cancer of the ovary, even to the point of ignoring the lymphatic pathway. With the development of lymphangiography and computerized tomography, lymph-node metastasis is discovered more easily. The frequency of positive nodes is high, and while we still expect little therapeutic value from lymphadenectomy, sampling of this node group has become a basic part of staging and valuable in the determination of completeness of treatment during second-look operations. The para-aortic nodes and pelvic lymphatics are important pathways of spread and sites of residual cancer when the intraperitoneal metastases are cured.

Biopsy and Staging

The importance of correct staging during initial laparotomy has not been fully appreciated by many surgeons. The failures have included incomplete exploration of the upper abdomen and failure to obtain specimens from sites notable for subclinical metastasis. In early stages these biopsies may yield evidence of metastases not clinically obvious. When biopsies provide the only pathologic specimens, it is important that the specimen is a viable tissue. As tissue necrosis is common, a satisfactory tissue sample is more certain if the samples are large and from several sites. Samples may be distorted by mishandling or poor fixation; thus, large pieces of cancerous tissue will be more likely to have areas of suitable viability. When the cancer of the ovary is very extensive, biopsy may be the only accomplishment of the primary laparotomy.

Cancer cells free within the peritoneal cavity have been recognized by the FIGO Committee as an indicator of unfavorable prognosis. Collection of peritoneal fluid for cytologic search for malignant cells is a routine staging procedure and a vital diagnostic tool.

In recent years we have learned that subclinical metastasis of the Stage I and II disease often exists. When surgery alone is employed, the incidence of failure for treatment of Stage I disease is 25% and for Stage II disease is 50%. The poor results of surgery alone, even when all tumor has seemingly been removed, can be explained on the basis of inadequate staging, which is usually a result of inadequate sampling in the areas where subclinical metastases are present.

THE SECOND-LOOK OPERATION

With the increased use of chemotherapy in the management of ovarian cancer, exploratory laparotomy to assess the effectiveness of chemotherapy has been utilized more frequently. The primary purpose of the second-look operation is to determine whether chemotherapy has eradicated ovarian cancer and whether the drugs can be discontinued.

The M. D. Anderson Hospital has had a large experience with this procedure. The findings and the subsequent course of the disease have been reviewed and updated on several occasions. A recent review of 10 years' experience (1971–1981) by Wharton and Edwards examined 246 second-look operations for patients who had Stage III and IV epithelial cancer of the ovary. There were 113 patients with residual cancer visible at laparotomy but not palpable prior to surgery. Of the 246 patients, 50 had microscopic residual cancer detectable only after histology study of tissue samples. In 83 patients, studies were negative both clinically and microscopically. Of the 83 patients, 16 had been treated previously with chemotherapy after metastases were resected or with unresected metastasis no greater than 2 cm in diameter. With these ideal conditions and with a negative second-look operation, 1 of the 16 patients (6%) had disease recurrence. Of the remaining 67 negative patients, 29% had recurrences. The median recurrence interval was 18.5 months. By Berkson Gage statistical methods the projected estimates for 2-year survival rate was 99%

and for 5-year survival was 85%. None of the patients younger than 40 years of age who had negative second-look operations developed recurrence, and none of the patients of any age with grade 1 cancers developed recurrence. Patients with grade 2 cancers had a recurrence incidence of 20%, while those with grade 3 tumors had a recurrence incidence of 27%. No cancer was present after 1 year mean duration of chemotherapy in grade 3 tumors.

Some of the patients who have been observed beyond 5 years have developed recurrence indicating that at least one-quarter of patients who have negative second-look laparotomy will eventually develop recurrent ovarian cancer.

When clinical trials are conducted to evaluate the cancericidal action of a specific drug, an assessment by laparotomy is more accurate than assessment by clinical evaluation, even when the clinical evaluation is supported by computerized tomography, sonography, and other techniques. The surgically determined response to chemotherapy provides the most accurate assessment and the best current information about how nearly the drug therapy has approached a complete cancer kill.

Whereas a negative second-look procedure is unreliable assurance of a cure, a second-look laparotomy that demonstrates residual cancer not evident before surgery can indicate a need for continued treatment. There are exceptions, however, such as cases where metastases are composed mainly of mature glial cells, as mentioned in the discussion of immature teratomata, and in grade 1 epithelial cancers. The information gained by second-look laparotomy is contributing greatly to a store of knowledge that will ultimately permit accurate predictions about the clinical course of a patient's disease without the need for laparotomy. The role of second-look laparotomy is changing as knowledge about the interaction of chemotherapy and the cancers is revealed by the procedure itself. The ultimate goal is to eliminate this surgery whenever possible, and the prospects for accomplishing this goal are good.

A complete search of all potential sites for metastases within the abdominal cavity is obviously impossible, since this disease spreads by both peritoneal implantation and the lymphatic system. The number of potential sites is large, and some areas are inaccessible. For these reasons, no patient can be said with certainty to be cured. Nevertheless, a reasonable clinical approach is to assume that if the most frequent sites for metastases available to investigation at laparotomy are found to be negative, then the less common sites for metastases are negative also. To give this assumption credibility, tissue sampling must be extensive, and the second-look laparotomy must be more than a simple exploratory laparotomy. In addition to excision of the ovaries, if they are still present, a major portion of the omentum must be removed. Samples of the pelvic wall lymph nodes and para-aortic nodes must be collected, and multiple biopsies of the peritoneum, the paracolic gutters, and the diaphragmatic peritoneum are also recommended. The search should always include a sample of peritoneal fluid collected for cytologic examination upon entering the abdomen, at the time of staging and tumor resection, as well as at the second-look operation.

There are basic surgical techniques that can ensure greater safety and completeness for second-look operations. The incision should give easy access to all parts of the abdominal cavity. Since the diaphragm is most difficult to expose, the incision must extend as near the rib margin as possible. Loops of intestine can be expected to be adherent to the anterior abdominal wall, especially to an old incisional scar. Patients who have had episodes of partial intestinal obstruction should have a bowel preparation in case intestinal resection is necessary. Long-term chemotherapy may damage heart, liver, lungs, kidneys, and bone marrow. The adequacy of these organ functions should therefore be confirmed preoperatively. For some patients with early-stage disease and favorable prognostic factors, a second-look operation is unnecessary.

When prophylactic chemotherapy has failed, the second-line form of therapy may have such a low success rate that continued efforts at treatment are not worthwhile. On failure of initial treatment, several options may be considered:

To discontinue all treatment if the disease is indolent. Such a decision may be acceptable with well-differentiated histologic types.
To employ external radiation therapy or intraperitoneal isotope radiation.
To change cytotoxic drugs.
To change to hormone therapy.

Patients with clinically evident residual cancer may be candidates for tumor-reductive surgery, but they may not qualify for second-look laparotomy, which, by strict definition, serves to determine completeness of treatment.

Patients who have received high-dose radiation to the entire abdomen and pelvis are at a greater risk from surgery and the related complications of the second-look procedure. The procedure therefore may not be justified for these especially high-risk patients.

Patients who have had multiple abdominal operations and those who have extensive intra-abdominal adhesions cannot be satisfactorily explored. They, too, are at a greater risk of serious surgical complications.

Peritoneoscopy (Laparoscopy)

Peritoneoscopy (laparoscopy) has had some trials as a substitute for laparotomy but has proved inadequate for searching out metastases and reaching all areas of the peritoneal cavity. Peritoneoscopy is useful in screening out patients who have readily apparent metastases. Even when peritoneoscopy proves useful, the information provided is less than that gained from laparotomy. The amount and size of the tumor burden is not revealed, and there is no opportunity for tumor-reductive resection. While opinion is divided on this subject, these disadvantages outweigh any benefits peritoneoscopy may offer as a substitute for laparotomy.

CYTOREDUCTIVE SURGERY FOR ADVANCED OVARIAN CANCER

Within the past 20 years, the prevalent philosophy regarding the role of resection for advanced cancer has reversed. Formerly, partial resection of a cancerous mass was held to be worthless in the control of cancer. Some considered such surgery potentially harmful because it might facilitate cancer spread, and because even short-term pain relief accomplished by reducing pressure was not worth the discomfort caused by the operation. Therefore, many patients simply had biopsy at laparotomy with no effort being made to resect if the dissection would prove lengthy and hemorrhage could be expected. This attitude still prevails among some surgeons, but it is no longer an acceptable stance.

Today's surgeon must be mentally and technically prepared to aggressively resect large pelvic masses and to move into the upper abdomen to remove metastases that may require intestinal resection, colostomy, or splenectomy (either alone or in combination). Resection need not be complete so long as a significant reduction of tumor mass and the total tumor cell burden is accomplished.

The potential benefit to the patient of radical surgery with incomplete resection is dependent on the adjunctive treatment used to deal with the unresectable residual tumor. Without chemotherapy or irradiation therapy to follow through with a continuous attack on the cancer, rapid regrowth will erase the initial accomplishment of surgery. One can reasonably question the value of such partial resection if chemotherapy is capable of reducing large masses (when the cancer is sensitive to the treatment). If the cancer is insensitive, then chemotherapy cannot be an adjunctive therapy and the value of tumor-reductive surgery again comes under question. However, tumor-reductive surgery has several benefits. Most cures are accomplished by removal of the cancer, and the resection can include those tissues with higher risk of containing subclinical metastases. When total resection is impossible, as is generally the case, the anticancer effectiveness of either irradiation therapy or chemotherapy is improved when employed postoperatively in close sequence after removal of a major portion of the tumor.

In the late stages of cancer of the ovary, intestinal function is often significantly disturbed. The relief of intestinal obstruction by tumor resection improves nutrition and therefore helps the patient to tolerate the toxicity of irradiation therapy or chemotherapy. Removal of cancer invading the bowel lessens sepsis. Sepsis is especially dangerous should chemotherapy cause severe leukopenia. Removal of large tumor masses lessens pain; thus, there is an immediate benefit from such operations. The bladder and rectal functions may be further improved by surgically removing the compression created by large pelvic cancer masses.

Too often, patients with advanced cancer of the ovary are declared inoperable before resectability has been amply tested. Tenacious effort is necessary and a reluctant surgeon may fail to complete the needed resection if cancer was not suspected in the preoperative diagnosis. If the physical evidence indicated less serious disease, such as myomata, endometriosis, or functional cyst of the ovary, the surgical team will not be prepared for the diagnosis. Should the intestinal tract not be prepared for resection, and the patient's permission for colostomy was not obtained, cytoreductive surgery may be deferred. The surgeon may not be accustomed to operating on the upper abdominal organs and may not have made provision for consultation or assistance. If the incision was too restrictive, tumor in the upper abdomen cannot be resected adequately.

A repeat attempt at tumor resection after proper preparation may still be warranted. If a repeat laparotomy is being contemplated, several considerations will aid in reaching a decision.

Initially, a review of the findings observed at the initial laparotomy should be made. If metastases are multiple, if small peritoneal excrescences are widely distributed over the abdominal wall and viscera, or if there is a smooth coating of cancer over the abdominal viscera, surgery will not be effective. The presence of large para-aortic nodes or parenchymal metastases to the liver also indicates that resection is not possible. When the metastases infiltrate deeply into vital organs in multiple sites, the dissection needed for removal would be too destructive.

If a large volume of tumor can be removed by resection of an intestinal segment, this should be done. In preparation, the bacterial flora of the bowel should be lowered by adequate antibiotic preparation, and the patient must consent to the operation.

Repeated surgery can be avoided by thorough groundwork prior to the initial procedure. Preparation begins with the surgeon, who is most effective when knowledgeable of the growth pattern of cancer of the ovary. The surgeon should have confidence in performing dissection of any part of the abdominal cavity. Preparation may include corrective treatment for a vital organ function prior to operation. Since aggressive tumor-reductive surgery is stressful for the patient and prone to complications, the physical strength and general medical health of the patient, including cardiopulmonary and renal reserve, must be assessed carefully. Patients with advanced ovarian cancer can be too ill for an extensive operation. For such an operation to be beneficial, postoperative complications must not be excessive nor the recovery period prolonged. Otherwise, the accomplishments of the resection are lost to cancer regrowth. Patients with a large pleural effusion and large abdominal ascites usually have impairment of oxygenation. Others may be physically weak or essentially bedridden, and unless these problems can be corrected, an operation should be cancelled because of the risk of excessive postoperative respiratory complications and high mortality. Patients who have lost large portions of body mass through depleted nutrition and serum protein depletion are not suited for immediate surgery. Hyperalimentation, however, may correct this deficiency.

An alternative treatment plan for such gravely ill patients could be to proceed directly with chemotherapy in an effort to reduce the tumor volume while improving nutrition and restoring function to the organs vital for postoperative recovery. This treatment plan assumes that a diagnosis of malignancy can be established without laparotomy or has been established by previous laparotomy and tumor biopsy without resection.

In summary, patients selected for surgery should have ample physical strength, body chemistry deficiencies replaced, associated diseases treated, and surgical preparations completed. The first avenue of approach to patients who are to be treated surgically is through exploration of the abdomen, for only by this approach can the surgeon determine whether conditions are suitable for successful tumor reduction therapy. Laparoscopy is of little value in determining resectability, and it is both technically difficult and hazardous when the cancer is extensive.

Large metastatic masses of cancer located within reach of the surgeon are usually attached to organs that are not vital. The omentum with metastatic cancer usually detaches if adherent to a neighboring structure; however, it may be necessary to remove a segment of transverse colon along with the omentum (Fig. 34-6). If the splenic flexure of the colon is involved, the spleen or gastrohepatic ligament may also be incorporated, or the gall bladder may be included in the mass. Resection of the omentum involved with metastatic cancer may require only omentectomy; however, the surgeon must be prepared for complex resection.

The ileocecal region is another area where the intestine is often involved with advanced ovarian cancer. Resection of the right colon along with the necessary portion of small bowel can significantly relieve a large tumor burden. The proximity of the sigmoid colon to the ovaries causes this section of the bowel to become involved as primary growth in the ovary expands. The sigmoid colon can often be freed from the cancer, but even when this is impossible, resection is practical and beneficial if significant tumor reduction is accomplished. More than one bowel segment resection may be necessary; good surgical judgement will control the duration of the operation, the blood loss, and the amount of intestinal tract sacrifice.

It is important for the surgeon to be aware of the abdominal cavity compartments, for these provide access to metastases and an approach to resection. When the normal anatomy of the abdominal cavity is distorted by large pelvic masses, these anatomical spaces become important to the surgeon because they are the most avascular pathways for circumscribing the tumor for removal.

Certain techniques can make the abdominal approach to advanced ovarian cancer more efficient and safer. The vertical incision, preferably midline, can be extended the entire length of the abdomen if necessary. Entering the abdominal cavity above the umbilicus is suggested because intestines are less prone to become adherent to the anterior abdominal wall at this level, especially if the patient has had an incision below the umbilicus for previous surgery. Even without prior surgery, the anterior abdominal wall above the umbilicus is safer for entry because the omentum may intervene between the abdominal wall and the underlying intestines.

Multiple metastases are generally encountered in advanced ovarian cancer; thus, the surgeon must

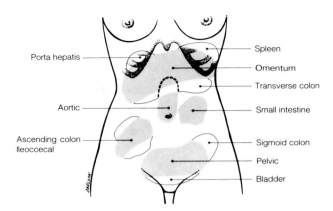

FIG. 34-6 Sites within the abdomen commonly involved in metastases from ovarian cancer. Some of these metastases require resection of a part of the organ harboring the cancer.

decide in what order they must be resected. The ovarian masses themselves have a high priority because they provide the most representative tissue for the pathologists to use in determining whether the cancer had its origin in the ovary. Effective chemotherapy depends on accurate histologic diagnosis, and cancers originating from other organs would be less responsive to drugs chosen for cancer assumed to have developed from the ovary. The best tissue samples for making the exact distinction, therefore, come from the ovary.

Masses producing intestinal obstruction need resection because functioning intestines are vital to postoperative recovery. Masses producing such obstruction should have a high priority on the resection list; however, since removal of intestinal obstructions is likely to involve contamination of the abdomen by bowel contents, it is advisable to perform this part of the procedure last. Omental masses usually contain a large volume of cancer that can be resected without sacrifice of any significant vital function. This resection can be performed at any time, but it is not uncommon for the transverse colon to be involved; thus, segmental resection of this structure may be necessary.

When multiple masses at different sites must be resected, the largest and most troublesome cancer will usually be in the pelvic cavity. On initial assessment of a pelvic mass it may appear that removal is impossible; yet, persistent dissection will often accomplish effective removal. There are techniques that will facilitate this dissection. Since ovarian masses commonly involve the peritoneum of the pelvic wall, the bladder, and the sigmoid colon, there are advantages to approaching the resection through the retroperitoneal spaces. Although the cancer may be adherent to the peritoneum, it rarely

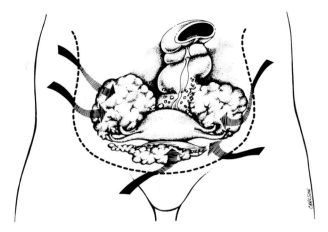

FIG. 34-7 Arrows indicate the direction for the dissection to surround the cancerous masses within the pelvis. The retroperitoneal path is easier and safer.

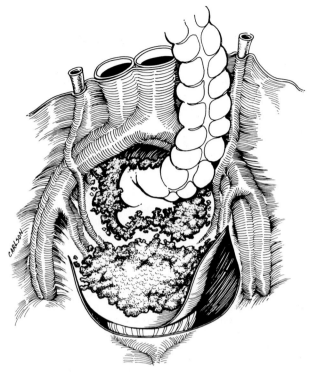

FIG. 34-9 For some patients the peritoneal covering of the bladder is involved with implants of cancer and must be removed.

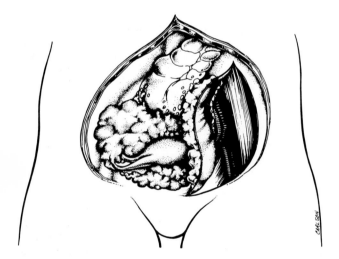

FIG. 34-8 The retroperitoneal space is best entered along the pelvic brim where the ovarian blood vessels can be ligated and the course of the ureter identified.

penetrates, and the best method for detaching the cancer is from outside the peritoneum. The blood supply to the cancer originates behind the peritoneum, and here blood vessels can be ligated for better control of hemorrhage. By using the retroperitoneal approach (Fig. 34-7) the pelvic peritoneum is removed, which, since normal-appearing peritoneum often contains microscopic metastases, is more curative. By using this technique the ureters are exposed early and kept in view during the entire dissection of the pelvic cancer, so that the risk of ureteral injury is lessened.

The retroperitoneal dissection for removal of pel-

vic masses can begin at the pelvic brim near the ovarian vessels where the ureter crosses the brim (Fig. 34-8). The course of the ureter is established and the ovarian blood vessels are ligated. The ureter is kept in view while the dissection progresses along the pelvic wall to the depths of the pelvic cavity. The peritoneum, with the attached cancer, is rolled medially as these tissues are freed. The round ligament is then divided, the uterine and superior vesical vessels are ligated, and the peritoneal covering of the bladder is removed if there is cancer implantation (Fig. 34-9).

The cul-de-sac is often filled with cancer, and the conventional methods for separating the bladder from the uterus, and the vagina from the rectum cannot be used. An alternative resection may be possible if the vagina can be divided anteriorly, allowing the posterior cul-de-sac cancer to be separated from the rectosigmoid (Fig. 34-10). When the cancer cannot be separated from the rectosigmoid, segmental intestinal resection should be considered. Segmental resection with reanastomosis would be preferred. If necessary, however, sigmoid colostomy and closure of the distal end (Hartmann's pouch) may be performed.

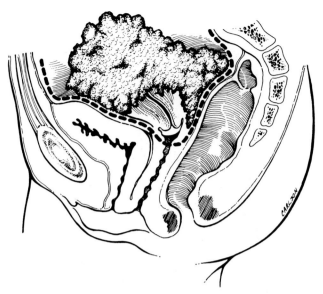

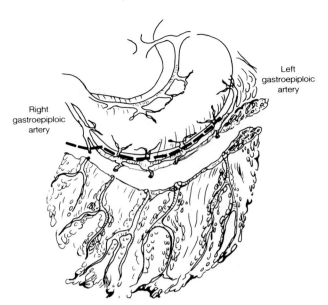

FIG. 34-10 When ovarian cancer incorporates the uterus and a hysterectomy is needed, usually the tumor is freed from the sigmoid and lifted from the cul-de-sac before the upper vagina is transected to complete the hysterectomy. When this order of resection cannot be accomplished because of the cancerous mass, the reverse sequence may be attempted; access may be easier through the anterior cul-de-sac. The vagina can be divided, and the tumor in the posterior cul-de-sac can be freed by retrograde dissection.

FIG. 34-11 Site of excision of gastrocolic component of omentum in a total omentectomy. Partial omentectomy at the level of the transverse colon is safer and usually as effective as the higher level indicated by the broken line; however, a large part of the omentum between stomach, spleen, and splenic flexure of the colon will remain.

Omentectomy for Tumor Reduction

A partial omentectomy is a simple operation, but the complete procedure is much more difficult. For a total omentectomy, the gastroepiploic blood vessels and the short gastric vessels can be exposed and a direct approach can be employed for removal (Fig. 34–11). The short gastric vessels should be ligated by suturing and not by free-hand tying, which may allow them to slip free and bleed. The stomach often distends after omentectomy during the postoperative period, and the expanded stomach may dislodge ligatures not sutured into the serosa of the stomach wall. The partial omentectomy leaves the gastrocolic ligament and a portion below the spleen; however, this is a safer operation and usually ample. An indirect approach may be necessary.

The omentum thickened by cancer distorts and conceals the location of the blood vessels in the area. A safer approach may be to begin dissection beneath the omental mass by separating the ascending colon. This dissection gains entry into the lesser omental sac, and the position of the blood supply to the area may become clearer. Exposure of the retrogastric space is helpful should splenectomy be needed; also,

this maneuver is protective of the middle colic artery.

Para-aortic Lymphadenectomy

The retroperitoneal nodes are important in the spread pattern of ovarian cancer. Total dissection of these nodes to reduce the cancer burden is not feasible; however, sampling of nodes in this area to search for metastases is essential for staging. We employ one or more of three approaches to the para-aortic nodes. One approach is directly beneath the mesentery of the small intestine. In this region, caution is needed to avoid dissecting too high and encountering the blood supply to the ileum or injuring the second portion of the duodenum. The right ureter should be identified and protected when this pathway to the aortic nodes is used. The thin vena cava is very vulnerable to damage and may be the greatest potential source of danger in dissecting this area. The surgeon should also be alert to the location of the superior mesenteric artery, since this is one of the more important structures that needs to be protected. The inferior mesenteric is also nearby, but it is much less important and can be sacrificed if necessary.

Another approach to the aortic nodes is to free

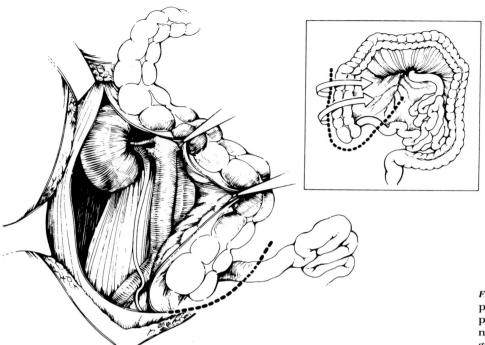

FIG. 34-12 The precaval and para-aortic area can be exposed by dividing the peritoneum of the right paracolic gutter and rolling the ascending colon medially.

the right colon by dividing the peritoneum of the right colic gutter and rotating the bowel toward the midline (Fig. 34–12). The proximal colon and terminal ileum can be rotated upward in a manner that is the reverse of its embryological development. Again, the right ureter will be exposed and should be separated from its attachment to the colon mesentery. The ureter can be deflected from the area of dissection. Essentially the same technique can be used on the left side with similar precautions. The inferior mesenteric artery is more vulnerable (Fig. 34–13) from the left paracolic gutter approach. A third method is to approach the para-aortic lymph nodes by opening the peritoneum at the bifurcation of the aorta and continuing the dissection cephalad to the region of the renal vessels.

After the intra-abdominal operation has been completed and abdominal closure is approached, special consideration should be given to the fact that the patient has advanced cancer and reduced ability to heal in the abdominal wall. In general, we use nonabsorbable sutures employing a stitch of Smead-Jones design. The Smead-Jones suture is essentially a pulley-type stitch of substantial unabsorbable material that penetrates the abdominal fascia, muscle, and peritoneum about 2.5 cm from the edge of the incision and then continues over and picks up the edge of the fascia on both sides

and then passes through the opposite fascia, muscle, and peritoneum. If the peritoneum retracts, it should be grasped and pulled flush with the incision edge before the suture is passed through the abdominal wall. If the abdominal cavity has been grossly contaminated by intestinal contents or if an area of infection has been released, the peritoneum, muscle, and fascia are sutured but the remaining abdominal wall is not approximated immediately. In the skin, subcutaneous sutures are placed but are not tied for 3 or 4 days until it is evident that infection is not going to occur.

SUMMARY

Hysterectomy with bilateral salpingo-oophorectomy, with or without omentectomy, and para-aortic lymph node sampling, is adequate surgery for early or moderately advanced cancer of the ovary. When the cancer is confined and easily removed, patients are managed well by this more conservative resection. However, patients with advanced disease deserve a maximum surgical effort. These surgical principals reflect a change in our philosophy of management over recent years.

The concept of treating ovarian cancer by aggressive surgery and sometimes radical resection, which may or may not be complete, is new and

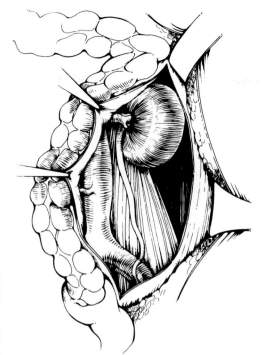
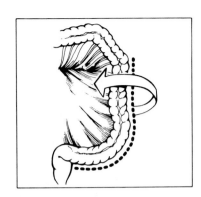

FIG. 34–13 The descending colon can be retracted to expose the left para-aortic area. Since the inferior mesenteric vessel restricts exposure of this side when directed from the right, this left side approach is useful for the dissection of aortic nodes.

still being tested. This approach has been made feasible by the development of more effective irradiation therapy machines and active cancericidal drugs for postoperative treatment. The concept is not applicable to many cancers of other sites in the body, because the remaining cancer is not as sensitive to chemotherapy. The tumor-reductive therapy sets the stage for more effective chemotherapy. Long-term remissions and cures are now possible for advanced cancers even when surgery is incomplete.

Still, cytoreductive surgery for advanced metastases is in the clinical trial and research stage. Evidence is clear that small metastases have a better prognosis than large metastatic lesions. However, it has not been established whether a small tumor volume achieved by resection has the same prognosis as an unresected small tumor.

Adjunctive Treatment for Ovarian Cancer

In recent years we have come to recognize that almost all patients with epithelial cancer of the ovary require more than maximum surgical resection. In earlier years, no additional treatment was advised after surgery for early-stage cancers of the ovary. The inadequacy of surgery alone for Stages I and II disease was slowly recognized. The survival rate for Stage I cancer treated by surgery alone was

noted to be only 65% to 75% at 5 years. Also, it was evident that irradiation of the pelvic region did not prevent recurrences in early-stage disease. Finally, when biopsies of the diaphragm and paracolic lymph gutters became routine procedure for Stage I and II lesions, it became known that subclinical metastases had often occurred. This more thorough search discovered small metastases that had been missed by the usual procedure of blindly palpating in the upper abdominal cavity. It is now recognized that not only is direct visual inspection important, but so is routine sampling of the peritoneum, para-

TABLE 34–1   *5-Year Survival Rates for Ovarian Epithelial Cancer by Stage of Disease*

STAGE	NUMBER OF CASES	5-YEAR SURVIVAL (PERCENT)
Ia	940	69.0
Ib	227	63.9
Ic	157	50.2
IIa	251	51.7
IIb and IIc	672	42.4
III	2,074	13.3
IV	933	4.1
Total	5,254	30.6

(Data from FIGO Annual Report, Vol 18, 1982)

aortic lymph nodes, and the omentum in order to discover subclinical metastases. A study of peritoneal cytology does not always indicate these metastases.

EXTERNAL IRRADIATION THERAPY

External therapy to the abdomen is the oldest of the currently used adjunctive therapies. At first, postoperative treatment was prescribed because surgery had not removed all of the cancer; later, however, the treatment was also prescribed for patients who had all visible tumor removed but needed additional treatment to avoid recurrences. The earlier techniques often directed irradiation only to the area of known residual disease, usually within the pelvis. Even when irradiation was employed adjunctively as prophylaxis after what seemed to be complete resection, only the pelvic region was treated. It is now recognized that irradiation of inoperable ovarian cancer is not successful if the residual tumor mass is large, that is, greater than 2 cm in diameter. Clinical experience has also shown that irradiation of the lower abdomen alone to prevent recurrence is unsuccessful because recurrence often occurs in the upper abdomen. The technical requirements for safe, successful pelvic and abdominal irradiation therapy are well known, but many patients do not qualify when the necessary guidelines are applied.

Technically, there is no obstacle to delivering the required dosage. Megavoltage machines in current use have sufficient energy to deliver a greater dose than can be tolerated. These new machines have removed the limitations imposed for a long time by intolerance of the skin. Intense irradiation reaction in the skin from lower-energy machines was a great impediment to irradiation therapy for many years. The depth dose can now be delivered and distribution can be controlled by a variety of techniques, such as open-field, large-portal, whole-abdomen irradiation; multiportal large-field irradiation; or moving-strip techniques to the entire abdomen. Often the dosage to the pelvis is intensified by additional treatment, the pelvic boost.

Each technique has some advantage; no single technique has been proved superior. Additional refinements, such as rotational therapy, are used for special problems, but still lacking is the ability to broaden the difference between the biological damage we call cancericidal action and normal-tissue damage we call toxicity or complications. This differential is so narrow for bowel tissue that unavoidable serious bowel injury is expected in approximately 5% of the patients who have whole-abdomen irradiation and pelvic boost. This injury

incidence would be greater if the dosage needed to eradicate gross cancer were administered.

The liver and kidneys also impose limitations on irradiation of the abdomen. If the cancer has spread to the parenchyma of the liver and kidney, external irradiation is unwarranted because these organs will tolerate only 2000 to 2500 rads at the rate of approximately 200 rads per day, which is well below the effective irradiation dose for tumor control. Thus, cancer in close proximity to the kidney and liver precludes a full dose. Although parenchymal metastases to the liver from epithelial cancer of the ovary are unusual, metastases to the surface of the liver, diaphragm, and pericolic gutters are common.

Clinical guidelines for using external irradiation therapy are as follows.

Tumor masses must be small. The maximum size has not been established, but approximately 2 cm has been generally accepted as a guideline. The location within the abdomen is important because:
1. a large dose is more tolerable within the pelvis than in the mid or upper abdomen;
2. metastases in the vicinity of the liver and kidney are in relative sanctuary areas because these organs require special protection.

Patients who have large and recurrent ascites or morbid obesity present additional problems in external irradiation dosimetry. The variations in dosage and depth and the instability of the portals reduce precision in placement and targeting of the therapy.

Irradiation treatment of tumors in growing children should be avoided if possible because their growth may be stunted by epiphyseal irradiation. Irradiation therapy should not be withheld in children or young women with metastases from a dysgerminoma, since this tumor is very sensitive to this therapy.

One of the acute effects of irradiation is depression of blood cell formation. Neutropenia, thrombocytopenia, and anemia are regular consequences. This happens with whole-abdomen therapy because bone marrow is damaged in the vertebral bodies and iliac bones. Patients who have previously received protracted chemotherapy may already have profound and persistent bone marrow depression to the degree that planned full-dosage irradiation must be abandoned. Incomplete irradiation is inadequate for cancer kill but can cause chronic intolerance to future chemotherapy.

Simultaneous administration of full-intensity chemotherapy and full-dosage irradiation is not tolerable unless the irradiation is confined.

It has not been proved that irradiation and chemotherapy are wholly incompatible, and there remains some optimism that each may augment the other if the dosage, sequence, and duration can be adjusted. Preirradiation chemotherapy of shorter duration may both reduce the size of inoperable masses to a point where they are suitable for irradiation and leave sufficient bone marrow reserve to support both treatments. There is some prospect that persistent but small-sized residual cancer after protracted chemotherapy may be vulnerable to external irradiation therapy, which can accomplish a final kill. Intraperitoneal radiophosphorus is also being tested for this role, but it currently offers no improvement over whole-abdomen megavoltage therapy.

Grade 1 epithelial tumors have a special clinical course. The second-look laparotomy may find minimal cancer, although continued chemotherapy fails to destroy the disease. With alkylating agent chemotherapy, the patient is exposed to a 5% to 9% risk of leukemia or other bone marrow disease that could be more lethal than the cancer itself. Irradiation treatments may be valuable under these conditions.

CHEMOTHERAPY

During the 1950s and 1960s alkylating agents were used effectively in chemotherapy. Thiotepa, chorambucil, cyclophosphamide, and melphalan were the most popular drugs, and these were given singularly, with similar results in most cases. A combination of drugs to be administered simultaneously was proposed as a treatment method in 1960 for patients who failed single-agent treatment or who required more aggressive treatment because of advanced cancer.

In 1972, Smith and coworkers reported a 47% response from 494 patients treated with melphalan. Complete regression among these patients was 20%. In addition, multiagent therapy had been tested and compared with single-agent melphalan by randomized clinical trial. The combination of actinomycin-D, 5-fluorouracil, and cyclophosphamide (ActFuCy) reflected no superiority for combination chemotherapy but did exhibit a greater toxicity. Failure of this combination to increase the response percentage was disappointing, although the failure of this initial effort at multiagent therapy was perhaps due to drug choice. The selection was based on combining an antimetabolite with an antibiotic and an alkylating agent, intending to include the simultaneous effect of drugs with different actions.

Realizing the potential for combination chemotherapy to ultimately prove superior, we approached the selection of drugs for combination in a different manner. With counseling from the National Cancer Institute a series of randomized clinical trials were started to test the cancericidal action of single agents available for such combination prior to applying them together. The plan was to establish drug activity when used alone and then to use the drugs in combination in the future. During these clinical trials, two new drugs were tested and accepted: hexamethylmelamine and cis-platinum. The advantage of combination chemotherapy was clearly established in 1978 by studies at the National Cancer Institute employing hexamethylmelamine, cyclophosphamide, methotrexate, and 5-fluorouracil (HexaCAF). In these studies, 80 previously untreated patients were selected randomly to receive only melphalan or HexaCAF. The response rate was assessed using the criteria listed in Table 34–2. The rate of complete remission was 33% for HexaCAF versus 16% for melphalan. Median survival times were 29 months and 17 months, respectively. Thus, the HexaCAF was clearly superior. These results were so convincing that a movement toward combination chemotherapy has almost replaced single-

TABLE 34–2   *Criteria of Response to Chemotherapy used at M.D. Anderson Hospital*

CLINICAL	SURGICAL
COMPLETE	
No clinically detectable disease persisting 3 months or longer.	No visible disease at time of second-look laparotomy. A complete surgical response is further defined, based on review biopsies, as being microscopic positive or microscopic negative.
PARTIAL	
Reduction of 50% or more in palpable tumor masses, calculated by the sum of two perpendicular diameters, which persisted 3 months or longer.	50% or greater reduction in the sum of tumor masses measured at time of second-look operation.
NO RESPONSE	
No tumor regression detectable after two or more courses of chemotherapy or appearance of new lesions or effusions.	

TABLE 34-3 Chemotherapeutic Agents

GENERIC NAME	TRADE NAME + SYNONYMS	DOSAGE RANGE*
Alkylating agents		
Cyclophosphamide	Cytoxan	6–8 mg/kg/day I.V. or orally for 5 days every 21–28 days, *or*
		100–150 mg/day orally, as tolerated, *or*
		500–1000 mg/M² I.V. every 28 days
Melphalan	Alkeran	0.2 mg/kg/day orally for 5 days every 28 days
Chlorambucil	Leukeran	0.2 mg/kg/day orally until toxicity
Antimetabolites		
Methotrexate	Mexate	40–50 mg/M²/day I.V. or I.M. every 2–3 weeks
5-Fluorouracil (5-FU)	Fluorouracil	400–500 mg/M² I.V. every 7–14 days
	Adrucil	
Antibiotics		
Doxorubicin HCL	Adriamycin	40–60 mg/M² I.V. every 28 days
	Adria	(Maximum accumulated dose 450–550 mg/M²)
Dactinomycin	Cosmegen	0.5 mg/day I.V. for 5 days every 28 days
	Actinomycin-D	
Bleomycin		10 units/M² I.V. or I.M. weekly (maximum accumulated dose 200 units/M²)
Vinca alkaloids		
Vincristine sulfate	Oncovin	1.5–2.0 mg/M² I.V. weekly (adult maximum dose 2 mg) until neurotoxicity
Vinblastine sulfate	Velban	4–10 mg/M² I.V. every 1–2 weeks
Hormones		
Medroxyprogesterone	Depo-Provera	250 mg I.M. weekly
Megestrol acetate	Megace	160–320 mg/day orally in divided doses
Heavy metals		
Cis-diamminedichloro-platinum	Cis-platinum, cisplatin, Platinol	20 mg/M²/day I.V. for 3–5 days, *or*
		50–100 mg/M² I.V. day 1 every 28 days
Other		
Hexamethylmelamine		8 mg/kg/day orally as tolerated
VP-16 (Etoposide)	Vepesid	50–60 mg/M²/day I.V. for 5 days every 2–4 weeks

MULTIAGENT (COMBINATION) CHEMOTHERAPY

PAC
Cis-platinum		50 mg/M² I.V. day 1
Adriamycin		50 mg/M² I.V. day 1
Cytoxan		500–750 mg/M² I.V. day 1
		every 28 days
		(reduce doses for prior irradiation)

HEXA-CAF
5-FU		600 mg/M² I.V. days 1 and 2
Methotrexate		40 mg/M² I.V. days 1 and 8
Cytoxan		150 mg orally days 1 to 14
Hexamethylmelamine		150 mg/M² orally days 1 to 14
		every 28 days

Cytoxan and Cis-platinum
Cytoxan		1000 mg/M² I.V. day 1
Cis-platinum		50 mg/M² I.V. day 1
		every 28 days

TABLE 34-3   *Chemotherapeutic Agents (Continued)*

GENERIC NAME	DOSAGE RANGE*
CHAD	
Cis-platinum	50 mg/M² I.V. day 1
Adriamycin	25 mg/M² I.V. day 1
Cytoxan	600 mg/M² I.V. day 1
Hexamethylmelamine	150 mg/M² orally days 8 to 21
	every 28 days
CHAP	
Cis-platinum	50 mg/M² I.V. day 1
Adriamycin	30 mg/M² I.V. day 1
Cytoxan	150 mg/M² orally days 2 to 8
Hexamethylmelamine	150 mg/M² orally days 2 to 8
	every 28 days
HAC	
Hexamethylmelamine	4 mg/kg orally days 1 to 14
Adriamycin	40 mg/M² I.V. day 1
Cytoxan	200 mg/M² orally days 1 to 5
	every 28 days
VAC	
Vincristine	1.5–2 mg/M² I.V. (maximum adult dose 2 mg) weekly
	for 8–12 weeks or until neurotoxicity
Actinomycin-D	0.5 mg/day I.V. days 1 to 5
Cytoxan	8–10 mg/kg/day I.V. days 1 to 5
	every 28 days
VBP	
Vinblastine	0.3 mg/kg I.V. in 2–4 divided doses day 1
Bleomycin	15 units/day continuous I.V. infusion for 5 days
Cis-platinum	100 mg/M² I.V. day 1
	every 21–28 days
VBP	
Vinblastine	0.3 mg/kg I.V. day 1, every 21 days
Bleomycin	15–30 units I.V. weekly, for 12 weeks
Cis-platinum	20 mg/M²/day I.V. for 5 days, every 21 days
VP-16 Regimen	
VP-16	100 mg/M²/day for 3 to 5 days, every 21–28 days
Cis-platinum	20 mg/M²/day for 5 days, every 28 days
Bleomycin	30 units I.V. weekly for 12 weeks

* Dosages are frequently different when the agent is given in combination with other agents. In addition, dosages often must be modified because of differences in patient tolerance or clinical condition.

agent treatment. A number of combination chemotherapy protocols have recently been initiated, although they differ in dosage, interval between treatments, route of administration, and the criteria for measuring anticancer action. The treatment is not complex. All the combinations employing cis-platinum produce very similar results.

Progress in chemotherapy has slowed because no new superior drugs have become available. Oncologists are now left to try to improve treatment by using different schemes of drug combinations, and treatment intervals (Table 34–3). The specific agents and dose ranges of the available chemotherapeutic agents are listed. The cytotoxic effect of these agents is produced by disrupting the orderly metabolic pathway of DNA biosynthesis and replication as outlined (Fig. 34–14).

Combination drug therapy has demonstrated a greater percentage rate of responses and longer duration of remission for advanced disease, but with greater toxicity. However, the superiority over single-agent chemotherapy administered postoperatively for Stage I and II disease (which has been totally excised) is still debatable. Since the toxicity

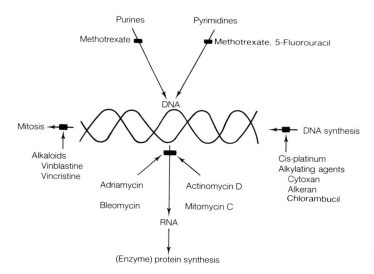

FIG. 34–14 Sites of interruption of cell metabolism and replication by various chemotherapeutic agents.

for single-agent therapy is considerably less than for the combinations, it is adequate treatment as prophylaxis against recurrence from subclinical metastases. However, combination chemotherapy after failure with a single agent has had meager results.

Melphalan, cyclophosphamide, Adriamycin, hexamethylmelamine, and cis-platinum, are the most frequently employed drugs for epithelial carcinoma of the ovary. Melphalan causes only mild nausea and vomiting, but thrombocytopenia restricts its protracted use, and when it is combined with other drugs, the schedule for administration may be disrupted by thrombocytopenia. Used alone, there is minimal alopecia. It is an excellent single-agent therapy with regard to safety, provided the bone marrow is monitored, and has a good response percentage and survival time.

The cancericidal action of cyclophosphamide equals that of melphalan, but it is more useful as the alkylating agent in combination multiagent treatment. Nausea and vomiting are more severe than with melphalan, and bone marrow depression is more notable for leukopenia. The patient's acceptance of cyclophosphamide is limited due to the alopecia associated with its use. Like melphalan, cyclophosphamide is a good drug to choose when single-agent adjunctive treatment is indicated.

The cardiac toxicity of Adriamycin, which becomes very dangerous beyond an accumulated dose of 450 to 550 mg/M², restricts the duration of its use. It is contraindicated for some older patients, including those with a history of heart failure or previous mediastinal irradiation. Skill acquired after many years of use has added some variability to the maximum accumulated dosage, especially for younger patients. While Adriamycin is a popular component of multiagent drug treatment, it is not an outstanding single-agent therapy for epithelial ovarian cancers. There is some doubt that the added toxicity it contributes when used in combination is worth its limited, additional antitumor action in ovarian cancer chemotherapy.

Hexamethylmelamine was proven in clinical trials to equal melphalan for inducing tumor regression; however, this drug is given orally for 2 weeks each month, and many patients stay in a constant state of nausea from the drug. Also, neurotoxicity develops as the total dose of the drug accumulates. Nevertheless, hexamethylmelamine remains a useful addition to ovarian cancer chemotherapy treatment.

Cis-platinum remains the superior drug for this disease, whether used alone or in combination. Response percentages are greater and remissions are longer than those associated with any other single drug. When combined with alkylating agents, the cancericidal action is augmented. Nausea and vomiting associated with its administration are severe and often interfere with patient compliance. Repeated courses of cis-platinum lead to neuro- and renal toxicity, and, like Adriamycin, it is restricted by total accumulated dose.

Alkylating agents have been used longer, and the results are more extensively recorded. Most of the results recorded are experiences with Stage III and Stage IV ovarian cancers. The response percentages range from 35% to 65%, and the median survival from 10 months to 14 months.

Chemotherapy requires close monitoring of toxicity by the physician prescribing the drugs. Often, the gynecologist must be responsible, or share in the responsibility, even if a chemotherapist manages the treatment. This situation exists because patients continue to rely on gynecologists for guidance and because often the patient does not understand which symptoms are caused by drugs and which are due to cancer. Gynecologists must be knowledgeable of chemotherapeutic toxicity in order to serve their patients' needs.

The common side effects of chemotherapy are well documented and usually predictable. Patients react individually with a wide range of tolerance. Different drugs often have some toxicity in common, yet they usually have some distinctive actions as well. Some symptoms are frequent and some uncommon.

The most frequent and consistent drug toxicity develops in tissues proliferating rapidly. Bone marrow and upper intestinal mucosa are examples of organs that metabolize quickly. Other toxicities, such as neurotoxicity, deafness, paresthesia, and motor weakness, are peculiar to certain drugs. Neurotoxicity is produced by cis-platinum, vincristine, vinblastine, and hexamethylmelamine. Renal toxicity from cis-platinum is serious and requires periodic monitoring with creatinine clearance testing and routine evaluation of serum BUN and creatinine before each treatment. Hepatotoxicity for methotrexate and Adriamycin can be serious and is increased when excretion is impaired. The adequacy of liver and renal function becomes especially important for methotrexate, Adriamycin, and cis-platinum tolerance. Severe impairment may preclude the use of some drugs or at least require dosage reduction when damage to the liver and kidney is less serious.

Cis-platinum appears to produce the best cancericidal action, and its power is enhanced when other drugs are administered concomitantly. When first-line chemotherapy fails, other drugs should be tried although their prospects for success are meager even if cis-platinum was a part of the first chemotherapy regimen.

There are certain basic factors to be considered in the chemotherapeutic management of ovarian cancer, including prognostic factors and toxicity. Prognostic factors have been identified and they guide management. They help to decide how radical the treatment must be and how closely the therapy may approach serious toxicity for maximum cancer control. The most important indicators are the stage and grade of the lesion and the residual volume. Significant but less influential factors are age and some special histologic types.

The benefits of chemotherapy are best measured by tumor regression, duration of remission, and survival time. The best results in these categories usually occur in patients with early-stage disease or well-differentiated tumors and in patients below age 40. When the stage is advanced, the best results are with well-differentiated carcinomas in patients below age 40 and with metastases less than 2 cm in diameter. Recurrences and regrowth are the rule in chemotherapy.

Bibliography

Afridi MA, Vongtama V, Tsukada Y, et al: Dysgerminoma of the ovary, radiation therapy for recurrence and metastases. Am J Obstet Gynecol 126:190, 1976

Alderman SJ, et al: Postoperative use of radioactive phosphorus in Stage I ovarian cancer. Obstet Gynecol 49:659, 1977

Aure JC, Hoeg K, Kolstad P: Clinical and histologic studies of ovarian carcinoma, a long term follow-up of 990 cases. Obstet Gynecol 37:1, 1971

Barber HRK, Graber EA: The PMPO syndrome (postmenopausal palpable ovary syndrome). Obstet Gynecol 38:921, 1971

Barber HRK, Kwon TH: Current status of the treatment of gynecologic cancer by site: Ovary. Cancer 38:610, 1976

Barlow JJ, Piver MS: Single agent versus combination chemotherapy in the treatment of ovarian cancer. Obstet Gynecol 49:609, 1977

Bateman JC: Chemotherapy of solid tumors with triethylene thiophosphoramide. N Engl J Med 252:21, 879, 1955

Bateman JC, Winship T: Palliation of ovarian carcinoma with phosphamide drugs. Surg Gynecol Obstet 102:347, 1956

Berkson J, Gage RP: Calculation of survival rates for cancer. Proc Staff Meetings Mayo Clinic 25:270, 1950

Boiman RE, Holzaepfel JH, Barnes AC: Intra-arterial nitrogen mustard in advanced pelvic malignancies. Am J Obstet Gynecol 72:1319, 1956

Brenner F: Das Oophoroma follicurare. Frankfurt Z Pathol 1:150, 1907

Bush TS, et al: Treatment of epithelial carcinoma of the ovary: Operation, irradiation, and chemotherapy. Am J Obstet Gynecol 127:692, 1977

Cangir A, Smith J, Van Eys J: Improved prognosis in children with ovarian cancers following modified VAC (vincristine sulfate, dactinomycin, and cyclophosphamide) chemotherapy. Cancer 42:1234, 1978

Clark DGC, Hilaris BS, Ochoa M: Treatment of cancer of the ovary. Clin Obstet Gynecol 3:159, 1976

Copeland LJ: Malignant gynecologic tumors. In Sutow WW, Fernbach DJ, Vietti TJ (eds): Clinical Pediatric Oncology, 3rd ed. St. Louis, CV Mosby, 1983

Copeland LJ, Wharton JT, Rutledge FN, et al: Role of "third-look" laparotomy in the guidance of ovarian cancer treatment. Gynecol Oncol 15:145, 1983

Creasman WT, Rutledge FN: The prognostic value of peritoneal cytology in gynecologic malignant disease. Am J Obstet Gynecol 10:773, 1971

Curling DM, Hudson CN: Endometrial tumors of the ovary. Br J Obstet Gynaecol 82:405, 1975

Curry SL, Smith JP, Gallagher HW: Malignant teratoma of the ovary: Prognostic factors and treatment. Am J Obstet Gynecol 131:845, 1978

Decker DG, Mussey E, Williams TJ, et al: Rating of gynecologic malignancy, epithelial ovarian cancer. In the 7th National Cancer Proceedings. Philadelphia, JB Lippincott, 1973 deLima OL: Disgerminoma do ovário. Contribuição para o seu estudo anatomoclinico. Docenta-Livre na Regencia da Cadeira de Clinica Ginecológica da Escola Paulista de Medicina. São Paulo, 1966

Dembo AJ, Bush RF: Choice of postoperative therapy based on prognostic factors. Int J Oncol Biol Phys 8:893, 1982

Edwards CL, Herson J, Gershenson DM, et al: A prospective randomized clinical trial of melphalan and cis-platinum versus hexamethylmelamine, Adriamycin, and cyclophosphamide in advanced ovarian cancer. Gynecol Oncol 15:261, 1983

Ehrlich CE, Einhorn L, William SS, et al: Chemotherapy for stage III–IV epithelial ovarian cancer with cis-diaminochichlorplatinum II, Adriamycin, and cyclophosphamide: A preliminary report. Cancer Treat Rep 63:281, 1979

Ehrlich CE, et al: Response "second-look" status and survival in stage III–IV epithelial ovarian cancer trialed with cis-dichlorodiamine platinum (3) (cis-platinum) Adriamycin (ADR) and cyclophosphamide (CXT). ASCO, C:416, 1980

Fazekas JT, Maier JG: Irradiation of ovarian carcinoma: A prospective comparison of the open field and moving-strip techniques. Am J Roentgenol 120:118, 1974

Feldman GB, Knapp RC: Lymphatic drainage of the peritoneal cavity and its significance in ovarian cancer. Am J Obstet Gynecol 119:991, 1971

Felmus LB, Pedowitz P: Clinical malignancy of endocrine tumors of ovary and dysgerminoma. Obstet Gynecol 29:344, 1967

FIGO: Annual Report on the Results of Treatment in Gynecological Cancer, vol 18, Stockholm, 1982

Fisher ER: "Pseudomucinous" cystadenomas: A misnomer. Obstet Gynecol 4:616, 1954

Forney JP, DiSaia PJ, Morrow CP: Endodermal sinus tumor. A report of two sustained remissions treated postoperatively with a combination of actinomycin-D, 5-flurourouracil and cyclophosphamide. Obstet Gynecol 45:186, 1975

Fox H, Agrawal K, Langley FA: A clinicopathological study of 92 cases of granulosa cell tumor of the ovary with special reference to the factors influencing prognosis. Cancer 35:231, 1975

Fox H, Langley FA: Tumors of the Ovary. Chicago, Year Book Medical Pub, 1976

Gallion H, van Nagell JR, Jr, Donaldson ES, et al: Immature teratoma of the ovary. Am J Obstet Gynecol 146:361, 1983

Gershenson DM, Del Junco G, Copeland LJ, et al: Mixed germ cell tumors of the ovary: Obstet Gynecol 64:200, 1984

Gershenson DM, Del Junco G, Herson J, et al: Endodermal sinus tumor of the ovary: The M. D. Anderson experience. Obstet Gynecol 61:194, 1983

Gershenson DM, Wharton JT, Herson J, et al: Single agent cis-platinum therapy for advanced ovarian cancer. Obstet Gynecol 61:194, 1983

Gottschalk S: Ein neuer Typus einer klein cystischen bösartigen Eierstockgeschwulst. Arch Gynakol 59:676, 1899

Graham J, Burstein P, Graham R: Prognostic significance of pleural effusion in ovarian cancer. Am J Obstet Gynecol 106:312, 1970

Green TH, Jr: Hemisulfur mustard in the palliation of patients with metastatic ovarian carcinoma. Obstet Gynecol 13:383, 1959

Green W, Gancedo H, Smith R, et al: Pseudomyxoma peritonei: Nonoperative management and biochemical findings. Cancer 36:1834, 1975

Greenwald EF: Ovarian tumors. Clin Obstet Gynecol 18:61, 1975

Griffiths CT, Grogan RH, Hall TC: Advanced ovarian cancer, primary treatment with surgery, radiotherapy and chemotherapy. Cancer 29:1, 1972

Hallgrimsson J, Scully RE: Borderline and malignant Brenner tumors of the ovary: A report of 15 cases. Acta Pathol Microbiol Immunol Scand (Sect A-80, Suppl)223:56, 1972

Hirabayashi K, Graham J: Genesis of ascites in ovarian cancer. Am J Obstet Gynecol 106:492, 1970

Hreshchyshyn MM: Single-drug therapy in ovarian cancer: Factors influencing response. Gynecol Oncol 1:220, 1973

Hull MGR, Campbell GR: The malignant Brenner tumor. Obstet Gynecol 42:527, 1973

International Federation of Gynecology and Obstetrics: Classification and staging of malignant tumours in the female pelvis. Acta Obstet Gynecol Scand 50:1, 1971

Ireland K, Woodruff JD: Review: Masculinising ovarian tumors. Obstet Gynecol 31:2, 83, 1976

Jimerson GK, Woodruff JD: Ovarian intraembryonal teratoma: I. Endodermal sinus tumor. Am J Obstet Gynecol 127:73, 1977

Jones LA, Edwards CL, Freedman RS, et al: Estrogen and progesterone receptor titers in primary epithelial ovarian carcinomas. Int J Cancer 33:567, 1983

Julian CG, Woodruff JD: The biologic behavior of low-grade papillary serous carcinoma of the ovary. Obstet Gynecol 40:860, 1972

Knapp RC, Friedman EA: Aortic lymph node metastases in early ovarian cancer. Am J Obstet Gynecol 119:1013, 1974

Kottmeier HL: Carcinoma of the female genitalia. Abraham Flexner Lecture Series, no 11. Baltimore, Williams & Wilkins, 1953

Krepart G, Smith JP, Rutledge F, et al: The treatment for dysgerminoma of the ovary. Cancer 41:987, 1978

Kurman RJ, Norris HJ: Embryonal carcinoma of the ovary: A clinicopathologic entity distinct from endodermal sinus tumor resembling embryonal carcinoma of the adult testes. Cancer 38:2420, 1976

Lewis GC, Jr: Chemotherapy of ovarian tumor. In Pitkin RM (ed): Year Book of Obstetrics and Gynecology. Chicago, Year Book Medical Publishers, 1976

Masterson JT, Calome RJ, Nelson J: A clinical study on the use of chlorambucil in treatment of cancer of the ovary. Am J Obstet Gynecol 79:1002, 1960

Masterson JG, Nelson JH, Jr: The role of chemotherapy in the treatment of gynecologic malignancy. Am J Obstet Gynecol 93:1102, 1965

McCormack TP, Riddick DH: Hormonal function of a granulosa cell tumor. Obstet Gynecol 48(Suppl)1:18S, 1976

McGowan L, Bunnag B: A morphologic classification of a peritoneal fluid cytology in women. Int J Gynecol Obstet 11:173, 1973

Meyer R: Der tumor Ovarii Brenner. Zentralbl Gynakol 65:770, 1932

Moore JG, Brandkamp W, Burns WL: Evaluation of chemotherapy in ovarian and cervical cancer by tissue culture methods. Am J Obstet Gynecol 77:780, 1959

Norris HJ: Functioning tumors of the ovary. Excerpta Medica 364:219, 1975

Norris HJ, Zirkin HJ, Benson WL: Immature (malignant) teratoma of the ovary: A clinical and pathologic study of 48 cases. Cancer 37:2359, 1976

Novak ER: Granulosa cell ovarian tumors as cause of precocious puberty, with report of 3 cases. Am J Obstet Gynecol 26:505, 1933

Novak ER, Woodruff JD: Gynecologic and Obstetric Pathology. 8th ed. Philadelphia, WB Saunders, 1979

Pedowitz P: Dysgerminoma. Am J Obstet Gynecol 86:693, 1963

Peterson WF: Malignant degeneration of benign cystic teratomas of ovary: A collective review of the literature. Obstet Gynecol Surv 12:793, 1957

Piver MS: Radioactive colloids in the treatment of Stage Ia ovarian cancer. Obstet Gynecol 40:42, 1972

Piver MS, Barlow JJ, Yazigi R, et al: Melphalan chemotherapy in advanced ovarian carcinoma. Obstet Gynecol 51:352, 1978

Piver MS, Lele SB, Barlow JJ: Cyclophosphamide, hexamethylmelamine, doxorubicin, and cis-platin (CHAD) as a second-line chemotherapy for ovarian adenocarcinoma. Cancer Treat Rep 65:85, 1981

Piver MS, Lele SB, Barlow JJ, et al: Second-look laparoscopy prior to proposed second-look laparotomy. Obstet Gynecol 55:571, 1980

Piver MS, Shashikant L, Barlow JJ: Preoperative and intraoperative evaluation in ovarian malignancy. Obstet Gynecol 48:312, 1976

Robboy SJ, Scully RE: Ovarian teratoma with glial implants on the peritoneum: An analysis of 12 cases. Hum Path 1:643, 1970

Schellhas HF: Malignant potential of the dysgenic gonad: No. 1. Obstet Gynecol 44:298, 1974

Schiller W: Zur Histogenese der Brennerschen Ovariatumoren. Arch Gynäkol 157:65, 1934

Schwartz PE, Smith JP: Treatment of ovarian stromal tumors. Am J Obstet Gynecol 125:402, 1976

Scully RE: Gonadoblastoma: A gonadal tumor related to the dysgerminoma (seminoma) and capable of sex hormone production. Cancer 25:1340, 1970

Serov SF, Scully RE, Sobin LH: International histological typing of ovarian tumors. No. 9. Geneva, World Health Organization. Symposium on Ovarian Carcinoma. Monograph 42 by the National Cancer Institute

Smith JP, Delgado G, Rutledge FN: Second-look operation in ovarian carcinoma postchemotherapy. Cancer 38:1438, 1976

Smith JP, Rutledge F: Advances in chemotherapy for gynecologic cancer. Cancer 36:669, 1975

Smith JP, Rutledge F, Wharton JT: Chemotherapy of ovarian cancer: New approaches to treatment. Cancer 30:1565, 1972

Smith WG, Day TG, Smith JP: The use of laparoscopy to determine the results of chemotherapy of ovarian cancer. J Reprod Med 18:257, 1977

Stanhope C, Smith JP, Rutledge FN: Second trial drugs in ovarian cancer. Gynecol Oncol 5:52, 1977

Stenwig JT, Hazenkamp J, Beecham JB: Granulosa cell tumors of the ovary: A clinicopathological study of 118 cases with long term follow-up. Gynecol Oncol 7:136, 1979

Surveillance Epidemiology and End Results: Incidence and Mortality Data 1973 to 1977. Young JL, Jr, Percy CL, Asire A (eds). Bethesda, Maryland, National Cancer Institute, 1981

Tait L: On the occurrence of pleural effusion in association with disease of the abdomen. Med Chir Soc Trans 75:109, 1891

Talerman A: Gonadoblastoma associated with embryonal carcinoma. Obstet Gynecol 43:138, 1974

Taylor HC, Long ME: Problems of cellular and tissue differentiation in papillary adenocarcinoma of the ovary. Am J Obstet Gynecol 70:753, 1955

Te Linde RW: Granulosa cell tumors of the ovary and their relation to postmenopausal bleeding. Am J Obstet Gynecol 20:552, 1930

Teilum G: Special tumors of the ovary and testes and related extragonadal lesions. Comparative pathology and histological identification. Philadelphia, JB Lippincott, 1976

Thigpen T, Shingleton H, Homestey H, et al: Cis-dichlorodiamineplatinum (II) in the treatment of gynecologic malignancies. Phase II trials by the Gynecologic Oncology Group. Cancer Treat Rep 63:1549, 1979

Tobias JS, Griffiths CT: Management of ovarian cancer: Current concepts and future prospects. N Engl J Med 294:16, 1976

Vogl SE, et al: Cyclophosphamide (C), hexamethylmelamine (H), Adriamycin (A), and diaminedichloroplatinum (D) "CHAD" versus melphalan (M) for advanced ovarian cancer (OvCa)—a randomized prospective trial of the Eastern Cooperative Group. C-548, ASCO, 1981

Vogl SE, Bernzweig M, Kaplan B, et al: CHAD and HAD regimens in advanced ovarian cancer: Combination chemotherapy including cyclophosphamide, hexamethylmelamine, Adriamycin, and cisdichlorodiaminoplatinum II. Cancer Treat Rep 63:311, 1979

Wangensteen OH, Lewis FJ, Tougen LA: The "second-look" in cancer surgery. Lancet 71:303, 1951

Webb MJ, Malkasian GD, Jr, Jorgensen EO: Factors influencing ovarian cancer survival after chemotherapy. Obstet Gynecol 44:564, 1974

Wharton JT, Edwards CL: Cytoreductive surgery for common epithelial tumors of the ovary. Clinics in Obstet Gynecol 10(2), 1983

Wharton JT, Herson J, Seski JC, et al: Prognostic factors, toxicity analysis, and activity of second-line agents in patients with Stage III and IV carcinoma of the ovary treated with melphalan (L-PAM). (in press)

Wharton JT, Herson J, Edwards CL, et al: Single agent Adriamycin followed by combination hexamethylmelamine-cyclophosphamide for advanced ovarian carcinoma. Gynecol Oncol 14:262, 1982

Wharton JT, Rutledge FN, Smith JP, et al: Hexamethylmelamine: An evaluation of its role in the treatment of ovarian cancer. J Obstet Gynecol 7:83, 1979

Wilkinson EJ, Friedrich EG, Holty TA: Alpha-fetoprotein and endodermal sinus tumor of the ovary. Am J Obstet Gynecol 116:711, 1973

Williams TJ, Dockerty MB: Status of the contralateral ovary in encapsulated low-grade tumors of the ovary. Surg Gynecol Obstet 143:763, 1976

Woodruff JD, Markley RL: Struma ovarii. Obstet Gynecol 9:707, 1957

Young RC, Chabner B, Hubbard SP, et al: Advanced ovarian adenocarcinoma: A prospective clinical trial of melphalan (L-PAM) versus combination chemotherapy. N Engl J Med 299:1261, 1978

Young RC, Deker DG, Wharton JT, et al: Staging laparotomy in early ovarian cancer. JAMA

Young RC, DeVita VT, Chabner BA: Chemotherapy of advanced ovarian carcinoma: A prospective comparison of phenylalanine mustard and high dose cyclophosphamide. Gynecol Oncol 2:489, 1974

Index

An *f* following a page number indicates a figure; a *t* indicates tabular material.